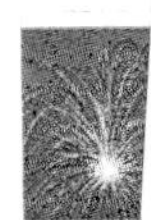

Manual of Oncologic Therapeutics

Third Edition

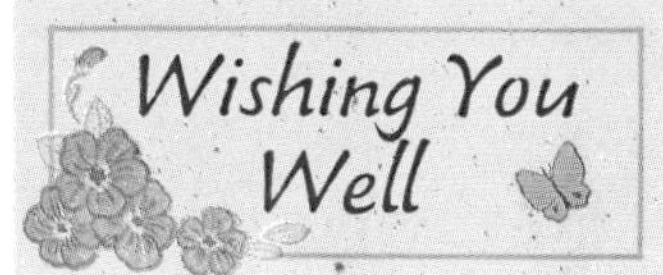

MANUAL OF ONCOLOGIC THERAPEUTICS

Third Edition

John S. Macdonald, M.D.
Professor of Medicine
Chief, Division of Medical Oncology
Medical Director
Temple University Cancer Center
Philadelphia, Pennsylvania

Daniel G. Haller, M.D.
Professor of Medicine
Associate Chief for Clinical Affairs
Hematology/Oncology Division
Department of Medicine
University of Pennsylvania Medical Center
University of Pennsylvania School of Medicine

Robert J. Mayer, M.D.
Professor of Medicine
Harvard Medical School
Clinical Director
Department of Medicine
Dana-Farber Cancer Institute

With 107 Contributors

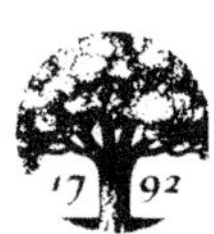

J. B. Lippincott Company
Philadelphia

Dedicated to our wives, Suzanne, Eileen, and Jane

ASSISTANT EDITOR: Eileen Wolfberg
PRODUCTION EDITOR: Virginia Barishek
COVER DESIGNER: Larry Pezzato
PRODUCTION AND EDITING SERVICES: Caslon, Inc.
COMPOSITOR: Digitype
PRINTER/BINDER: R. R. Donnelley & Sons Company/Crawfordsville

Third Edition

 Printed in the United States of America. For information write J. B. Lippincott Company, 227 East Washington Square, Philadelphia, Pennsylvania 19106.

6 5 4 3 2 1

Library of Congress Catalog Card Number 89-647334

ISSN 1046-638X
ISBN 0-397-51394-1

∞This Paper Meets the Requirements of ANSI/NISO Z39.48-1992 (Permanence of Paper).

The authors and publisher have exerted every effort to ensure that drug selection and dosage set forth in this text are in accord with current recommendations and practice at the time of publication. However, in view of ongoing research, changes in government regulations, and the constant flow of information relating to drug therapy and drug reactions, the reader is urged to check the package insert for each drug for any change in indications and dosage and for added warnings and precautions. This is particularly important when the recommended agent is a new or infrequently employed drug.

CONTRIBUTORS LIST

Dennis J. Ahnen, M.D.
Associate Professor of Medicine
University of Colorado School of Medicine
Clinical Investigator
Department of Veterans Affairs Medical Center
Associate Director for Cancer Prevention and Control
University of Colorado Cancer Center
Denver, Colorado

Carmen J. Allegra, M.D.
Chief, NCI-Navy Medical Oncology Branch
Naval Hospital Bethesda
National Cancer Institute
Bethesda, Maryland

Carol L. Alter, M.D.
Assistant Professor
Director, Psychosocial Services
Temple University Cancer Center
Philadelphia, Pennsylvania

Kenneth C. Anderson, M.D.
Massachusetts General Hospital
Dana-Farber Cancer Institute
Harvard Medical School
Boston, Massachusetts

Karen Antman, M.D.
Division of Medical Oncology
Columbia-Presbyterian Medical Center
Columbia University
New York, New York

Frederick R. Appelbaum, M.D.
Director, Division of Clinical Research
Member, Fred Hutchinson Cancer Research Center
Professor of Medicine
University of Washington
Seattle, Washington

James O. Armitage, M.D.
Department of Internal Medicine
Section of Oncology/Hematology
University of Nebraska Medical Center
Omaha, Nebraska

Deborah M. Axelrod, M.D.
Assistant Clinical Professor
Albert Einstein College of Medicine
Director, Louis Venet, M.D. Comprehensive Breast Service
Department of Surgery
Beth Israel Medical Center
New York, New York

Rita Axelrod, M.D.
Temple University Cancer Center
Philadelphia, Pennsylvania

Richard R. Barakat, M.D.
Gynecology Service
Department of Surgery
Memorial Sloan-Kettering Cancer Center
New York, New York

Philip J. Bierman, M.D.
Department of Internal Medicine
Section of Oncology/Hematology
University of Nebraska Medical Center
Omaha, Nebraska

Ronald Bleday, M.D.
Assistant Professor of Surgery
Harvard Medical School
Chief, Section of Colorectal Surgery
New England Deaconess Hospital
Boston, Massachusetts

George J. Bosl, M.D.
Head, Division of Solid Tumor Oncology
Memorial Sloan-Kettering Cancer Center
New York, New York

Linda S. Callans, M.D.
Assistant Professor of Surgery
Department of Surgery
Hospital of the University of Pennsylvania
Philadelphia, Pennsylvania

George P. Canellos, M.D.
William Rosenberg Professor of Medicine
Harvard Medical School
Chief, Division of Medical Oncology
Dana-Farber Cancer Institute
Boston, Massachusetts

Bruce D. Cheson, M.D.
Head, Medicine Section
Clinical Investigations Branch
Cancer Therapy Evaluation Program
Division of Cancer Treatment
National Cancer Institute
Bethesda, Maryland

George Chin, M.D.
Rocky Mountain Health Center
Denver, Colorado

Raphael S. Chung, M.D.
Chairman and Program Director
Department of Surgery
Meridia Huron Hospital
Cleveland, Ohio

Marta A. Dabezies, M.D.
Associate Professor of Medicine
Temple University School of Medicine
Philadelphia, Pennsylvania

John M. Daly, M.D.
Lewis Atterbury Stimson Professor
Chairman, Department of Surgery
Cornell University Medical College
Surgeon in Chief
The New York Hospital
New York, New York

Maria de Carvalho, R.N., M.S.N., O.C.N.
Clinical Nurse Educator
Cancer Nursing Service
Warren Grant Magnuson Clinical Center
National Institutes of Health
Bethesda, Maryland

Malcolm M. DeCamp, Jr., M.D.
Assistant Professor of Surgery
Harvard Medical School
Associate Surgeon
Division of Thoracic Surgery
Brigham and Women's Hospital
Boston, Massachusetts

Thomas F. DeLaney, M.D.
Associate Professor of Radiology
Boston University School of Medicine
Chief, Department of Radiation Oncology
Boston University Medical Center
Boston, Massachusetts

George D. Demetri, M.D.
Assistant Professor of Medicine
Harvard Medical School
Dana-Farber Cancer Institute
Boston, Massachusetts

ZoAnn E. Dreyer, M.D.
Baylor College of Medicine
Texas Children's Hospital
Houston, Texas

Daniel B. Dubin, M.D.
Department of Dermatology
Harvard Medical School
Boston, Massachusetts

Anthony D. Elias, M.D.
Department of Medicine
Dana-Farber Cancer Institute
Harvard Medical School
Boston, Massachusetts

Gerald A. Ferretti, D.D.S., M.S.
Department of Pediatric Dentistry
University of Kentucky
Lexington, Kentucky

Robert W. Finberg, M.D.
Laboratory of Infectious Diseases
Dana-Farber Cancer Institute
Boston, Massachusetts

Howard A. Fine, M.D.
Division of Cancer Pharmacology
Dana-Farber Cancer Institute
Boston, Massachusetts

Richard I. Fisher, M.D.
Dorothy W. and J. D. Stetson Coleman Professor of Oncology
Director, Division of Hematology/Oncology
Director, Oncology Institute
Loyola University Stritch School of Medicine
Maywood, Illinois

R. Armour Forse, M.D. Ph.D.
Associate Professor of Surgery
Harvard Medical School
Chief, Division of General Surgery
New England Deaconess Hospital
Boston, Massachusetts

Kevin R. Fox, M.D.
Assistant Professor of Medicine
University of Pennsylvania School of Medicine
Philadelphia, Pennsylvania

Michael A. Friedman, M.D.
Associate Director
Cancer Therapy Evaluation Program
Division of Cancer Treatment
National Cancer Institute
Bethesda, Maryland

Jose P. Garcia, M.D.
Department of Surgical Oncology
Brigham and Women's Hospital
Boston, Massachusetts

Glenn E. Gerber, M.D.
Assistant Professor of Medicine
University of Chicago
Chicago, Illinois

Lynn H. Gerber, M.D.
Chief, Department of Rehabilitation Medicine
National Institutes of Health
Bethesda, Maryland

Jon Glass, M.D.
Temple University Hospital
Philadelphia, Pennsylvania

Donna Glover, M.D.
Director, Hematology/Oncology
Presbyterian Hospital
Philadelphia, Pennsylvania

Richard J. Gralla, M.D.
Director
Ochsner Cancer Institute
New Orleans, Louisiana

Jean L. Grem, M.D.
NCI-Navy Medical Oncology Branch
Naval Hospital Bethesda
National Cancer Institute
Bethesda, Maryland

Dupont Guerry, IV, M.D.
Professor of Medicine
University of Pennsylvania School of Medicine
Hematology-Oncology Division
Department of Medicine
University of Pennsylvania Medical Center
Philadelphia, Pennsylvania

Lee Helman, M.D.
Senior Investigator
Molecular Genetics Section
Pediatric Branch
National Cancer Institute
Bethesda, Maryland

Marc E. Horowitz, M.D.
Baylor College of Medicine
Texas Children's Hospital
Houston, Texas

Susan Molloy Hubbard, R.N., M.S., O.C.N.
Director, International Cancer Information Center
Associate Director
National Cancer Institute
Bethesda, Maryland

Daniel C. Ihde, M.D.
Professor of Medicine
Chief, Division of Medical Oncology
Department of Internal Medicine
Washington University School of Medicine
St. Louis, Missouri

Charlotte D. Jacobs, M.D.
Associate Professor of Medicine
Stanford University School of Medicine
Stanford University Medical Center
Stanford, California

Richard Allen Johnson, M.D.
Instructor
Harvard Medical School
Division of Dermatology
New England Deaconess Hospital
Boston, Massachusetts

Philip W. Kantoff, M.D.
Director of Genitourinary Oncology
Assistant Professor of Medicine
Harvard Medical School
Dana-Farber Cancer Institute
Boston, Massachusetts

Ira Kelberman, M.D.
Assistant Professor of Medicine
Gastroenterology Section
Department of Medicine
Temple University School of Medicine
Philadelphia, Pennsylvania

David Kelsen, M.D.
Gastrointestinal Oncology Service
Division of Solid Tumor Oncology
Department of Medicine
Memorial Sloan-Kettering Cancer Center
New York, New York

M. Margaret Kemeny, M.D.
Chief, Division of Surgical Oncology
North Shore University Hospital—Cornell University Medical College
Manhasset, New York

Timothy J. Kinsella, M.D.
Professor and Chair
Department of Human Oncology
University of Wisconsin–Madison Medical School
Madison, Wisconsin

Michael L. Kochman, M.D.
Assistant Professor of Medicine
Division of Gastroenterology
University of Pennsylvania School of Medicine
Philadelphia, Pennsylvania

Benjamin Krevsky, M.D., M.P.H.
Associate Professor of Medicine
Gastroenterology Section
Department of Medicine
Temple University School of Medicine
Philadelphia, Pennsylvania

Edward J. Lee, M.D.
Associate Professor
University of Maryland Cancer Center
University of Maryland School of Medicine
Associate Professor of Medicine and Oncology
University of Maryland Medical Systems
Baltimore, Maryland

Michael M. Lieber, M.D.
Professor of Urology
Mayo Medical School
Consultant in Urology
Mayo Clinic
Rochester, Minnesota

Charles J. Lightdale, M.D.
Professor of Clinical Medicine
Columbia University College of Physicians and Surgeons
Director, Clinical Gastroenterology
Columbia-Presbyterian Medical Center
New York, New York

David R. Macdonald, M.D., F.R.C.P.C.
Associate Professor
Departments of Clinical Neurological Sciences and Oncology
University of Western Ontario
Attending Neurologist
London Regional Cancer Centre
London, Ontario, Canada

John S. Macdonald, M.D.
Professor of Medicine
Chief, Division of Medical Oncology
Medical Director
Temple University Cancer Center
Philadelphia, Pennsylvania

Ian T. Magrath, MB, BS, FRCP, FRCPath
Head, Lymphoma Biology Section
Pediatric Branch
National Cancer Institute
Bethesda, Maryland

Donald H. Mahoney, Jr., M.D.
Baylor College of Medicine
Texas Children's Hospital
Houston, Texas

Maurie Markman, M.D.
The Cleveland Clinic Cancer Center
Department of Hematology/Medical Oncology
The Cleveland Clinic Foundation
Cleveland, Ohio

Robert Mashal, M.D.
Instructor, Department of Medicine
Dana-Farber Cancer Institute
Harvard Medical School
Boston, Massachusetts

Charles L. McGarvey, III, M.S., P.T.
Chief, Physical Therapy Section
Department of Rehabilitation Medicine
Warren G. Magnuson Clinical Center
National Institutes of Health
Bethesda, Maryland

Joan E. Mollman, M.D.
Department of Neurology
University of Pennsylvania Medical Center
University of Pennsylvania School of Medicine
Hospital of the University of Pennsylvania
Philadelphia, Pennsylvania

Craig Nichols, M.D.
Associate Professor of Medicine
Indiana University School of Medicine
Indianapolis, Indiana

Angela Ogden, M.D.
Baylor College of Medicine
Texas Children's Hospital
Houston, Texas

C. Kent Osborne, M.D.
Division of Medical Oncology
University of Texas Health Science Center
San Antonio, Texas

Michael P. Osborne, M.D.
Professor of Surgery
Cornell University Medical College
Chief, Breast Service
Department of Surgery
The New York Hospital
Cornell Medical Center
New York, New York

Robert T. Osteen, M.D.
Department of Surgical Oncology
Brigham and Women's Hospital
Boston, Massachusetts

Harlan Pinto, M.D.
Oncology Section
Veterans Administration Medical Center
Palo Alto, California
Assistant Professor of Medicine
Stanford University School of Medicine
Stanford, California

Philip A. Pizzo, M.D.
Chief of Pediatrics
Head, Infectious Diseases
National Cancer Institute
Uniformed Services University for the Health Sciences
Bethesda, Maryland

David G. Poplack, M.D.
Elise C. Young Professor of Pediatric Oncology
Department of Pediatrics
Baylor College of Medicine
Director, Texas Children's Cancer Center
Children's Hospital
Houston, Texas

Beth Popp, M.D.
Pain Service
Department of Neurology
Memorial Sloan-Kettering Cancer Center
New York, New York

Russell K. Portenoy, M.D.
Associate Professor of Neurology and Neuroscience
Cornell University Medical College
Director, Analgesic Studies and Associate Attending Physician
Pain Service
Department of Neurology
Memorial Sloan-Kettering Cancer Center
New York, New York

John H. Raaf, M.D., D.Phil.
Professor of Surgery
Case Western Reserve University
Chief of Surgery
Cleveland Veterans Administration Medical Center
Cleveland, Ohio

Martin N. Raber, M.D.
Professor and Chairman
Department of Clinical Investigation
M.D. Anderson Cancer Center
Houston, Texas

Peter M. Ravdin, M.D., Ph.D.
Division of Medical Oncology
University of Texas Health Science Center
San Antonio, Texas

Ted P. Raybould, D.M.D.
Department of Pediatric Dentistry
University of Kentucky
Lexington, Kentucky

Michael F. Reed, M.D.
Clinical/Research Fellow in Surgical Oncology
Harvard Medical School
Boston, Massachusetts

Jerome P. Richie, M.D.
Professor and Chief
Division of Urology
Brigham and Women's Hospital
Boston, Massachusetts

Kevin E. Salhany, M.D.
Division of Anatomic Pathology
Department of Pathology and Laboratory Medicine
University of Pennsylvania School of Medicine
Philadelphia, Pennsylvania

Leonard Saltz, M.D.
Gastrointestinal Oncology Service
Division of Solid Tumor Oncology
Department of Medicine
Memorial Sloan-Kettering Cancer Center
New York, New York

Scott Saxman, M.D.
Assistant Professor of Medicine
Indiana University School of Medicine
Indianapolis, Indiana

Charles A. Schiffer, M.D.
Professor of Medicine and Oncology
Head, Division of Hematology
Head, Division of Hematologic Malignancies
University of Maryland Cancer Center
University of Maryland School of Medicine
Baltimore, Maryland

Sandra Schnall, M.D.
Associate Professor of Medicine
Temple University Cancer Center
Philadelphia, Pennsylvania

Lynn M. Schuchter, M.D.
Assistant Professor of Medicine
University of Pennsylvania School of Medicine
Hematology-Oncology Division
Department of Medicine
University of Pennsylvania Medical Center
Philadelphia, Pennsylvania

Michael V. Seiden, M.D.
Massachusetts General Hospital
Dana-Farber Cancer Institute
Harvard Medical School
Boston, Massachusetts

Claudia A. Seipp, R.N., O.C.N.
Oncology Nurse Clinician
Surgery Branch
National Cancer Institute
Bethesda, Maryland

Brenda Shank, M.D., Ph.D.
Radiation Oncology Department
Mount Sinai Medical Center
New York, New York

Charles L. Shapiro, M.D.
Dana-Farber Cancer Institute
Boston, Massachusetts

Jeffrey Sklar, M.D., Ph.D.
Professor, Department of Pathology
Director, Division of Diagnostic Molecular Biology and Molecular Oncology
Department of Pathology
Brigham and Women's Hospital
Harvard Medical School
Boston, Massachusetts

Malcolm Smith, M.D.
Head, Pediatric Section
Clinical Investigations Branch
Cancer Therapy Evaluation Program
National Cancer Institute
Bethesda, Maryland

Arthur J. Sober, M.D.
Associate Professor of Dermatology
Harvard Medical School
Associate Chief of Dermatology
Massachusetts General Hospital
Boston, Massachusetts

C. Philip Steuber, M.D.
Baylor College of Medicine
Texas Children's Hospital
Houston, Texas

Paul C. Stomper, M.D.
Director, Mammography Center at Roswell Park
Director of Diagnostic Radiology
Roswell Park Cancer Institute
Associate Professor of Radiology
School of Medicine and Biomedical Sciences
State University of New York at Buffalo
Buffalo, New York

David J. Sugarbaker, M.D.
Associate Professor of Surgery
Harvard Medical School
Chief, Division of Thoracic Surgery
Brigham and Women's Hospital
Boston, Massachusetts

Tate Thigpen, M.D.
Professor of Medicine
Director of the Division of Oncology
Department of Medicine
University of Mississippi School of Medicine
Jackson, Mississippi

Anne Lewis Thurn, Ph.D.
Scientific Review Administrator
PDQ Editorial Boards
International Cancer Information Center
National Cancer Institute
Bethesda, Maryland

Peter G. Traber, M.D.
Chief, Division of Gastroenterology
T. Grier Miller Associate Professor of Medicine
University of Pennsylvania School of Medicine
Philadelphia, Pennsylvania

Richard S. Ungerleider, M.D.
Chief, Clinical Investigations Branch
Cancer Therapy Evaluation Program
National Cancer Institute
Bethesda, Maryland

Nicholas J. Vogelzang, M.D.
Professor of Medicine
University of Chicago
Chicago, Illinois

Robert L. Vogelzang, M.D.
Professor of Radiology
Director of Vascular and Interventional Radiology
Northwestern University
Chicago, Illinois

Robert E. Wittes, M.D.
Chief, Medicine Branch
National Cancer Institute
National Institutes of Health
Bethesda, Maryland

Norman Wolmark, M.D.
Director, Division of Surgical Oncology
Department of Surgery
Allegheny General Hospital
Pittsburgh, Pennsylvania

Alan Yagoda, M.D.
Professor of Clinical Medicine
Division of Medical Oncology
Columbia-Presbyterian Medical Center
New York, New York

PREFACE

This is the third edition of *The Manual of Oncologic Therapeutics*. The first two editions were edited by Robert Wittes, M.D., of the National Cancer Institute. The third edition passes on to new editorship. It was felt appropriate to produce the third edition of *The Manual of Oncologic Therapeutics* with multiple editors. Three editors, all experienced clinical oncologists and investigators, will bring to the work a variety of perspectives and experiences that will hopefully enrich the usefulness of *The Manual of Oncologic Therapeutics*.

It is important to understand the concept upon which we base this book. Clearly, there are a number of excellent textbooks of oncology. These range from comprehensive textbooks attempting to encompass all the most important aspects of the basic and clinical science of oncology to discipline-oriented works and disease-oriented volumes, which by necessity have a smaller scope. The operative word in our minds in producing *The Manual of Oncologic Therapeutics* was "manual." In medicine "manual" implies a useful reference that may be repetitively accessed to help clinicians with specific problems. It is important to understand that we have not attempted to build a comprehensive oncologic textbook. Our goal is to update and expand the previous editions of *The Manual of Oncologic Therapeutics* so that the third edition will be a useful tool for the next several years to clinicians and clinical investigators caring for cancer patients. We do not envision a cover to cover reading of this work. Rather, we see this as valuable, sound information, which will be in the clinic, in the office, and on the hospital oncology and general medical units where medical students, residents, fellows, and attending physicians may quickly find information relevant to particular clinical problems.

Because of the design and the purpose of *The Manual of Oncologic Therapeutics*, the editing of this work was somewhat different from the editing of other oncologic textbooks. For example, we did not assiduously attempt to prevent duplication of information. Thus, if similar information on molecular biology or epidemiology was important to the context of a number of chapters, we permitted it to be repeated in these chapters. A more specific example involves endoscopy. Although we have chapters on endoscopy describing the principles and approaches to endoscopic management of patients, we certainly did not eliminate practical reference to endoscopy in the various chapters discussing gastrointestinal and lung tumors. We are aiming to be able to have a reader pick up *The Manual of Oncologic Therapeutics*, turn to a chapter, and find a concise but relatively complete review of a subject. We do not want a reader to find it necessary to search through an index or table of contents to learn important pieces of information bearing upon the clinical problem in question.

The third edition's major divisions grew out of a review of the usefulness of the organization of the first two editions of the work. Section I reviews important procedures that are relevant to the staging, diagnosis, and management of patients with neoplastic disease. We have substantially updated chapters where appropriate and have included an additional chapter that discusses the burgeoning use of endoscopic ultrasound in oncology.

Section II is a new section that attempts to put the techniques of immunodiagnosis and molecular genetic analysis of malignant tissue into context for the clinician. We hope that the discussions of tumor markers, PCR techniques, and flow cytometry will give clinicians a cogent and concise reference to the ways these techniques are being applied in malignant disease in the 1990s.

Section III reviews the common therapeutic approaches used in the management of cancer patients and has been updated with new authors and an expansion of the chemotherapy chapter.

Section IV discusses the most common tumors and the therapeutic approach to patients with these diseases. There have been extensive changes in the authorship of this section from the previous edition. Each chapter is required to stand alone as a concise and clear guide to the managing clinician of not only the appropriate management of a particular disease in the mid-1990s, but also, as a description of the important disease-related research questions that require the participation of patients in clinical trials.

Section V discusses regional therapy, which has become a progressively more important area of oncology with the availability at many institutions of well-trained interventional radiologists highly capable of catheterizing vessels of an increasing variety of organs.

Section VI discusses oncologic emergencies. Each chapter is organized to provide the clinician with a rapid review of diagnosis and therapy.

Section VII addresses the important area of supportive care and has been updated to emphasize the importance of pain control. A new chapter has been added on the use of growth factors and cytokines in the supportive care of the cancer patient.

Section VIII has been expanded because of the increasing use of transplantation techniques in both hematologic malignancies and solid tumors. To accomplish this, the section now consists of two chapters, one on allogeneic transplant and the other on autologous transplant. The autologous transplant chapter addresses the evolving data on the use of peripheral blood stem cells in the support of high-dose chemotherapy for hematologic malignancies and solid tumors.

Finally, Section IX updates the important area of paraneoplastic syndromes.

The appendices are aimed at providing useful practical information to clinicians on the objective evaluation of toxicity and therapeutic efficacy of treatments. This section has also been updated and expanded to give physicians information on how to access computerized databases on cancer care and research.

In the preface of *The Manual of Oncologic Therapeutics*, 2nd edition, Dr. Robert Wittes appropriately pointed out that one must be very cautious about publications that purport to present state-of-the-art therapy. His point was that it is rare in oncology for us to have anywhere near acceptable, much less perfect, therapy for malignant disease. The treatments and approaches to particular diseases discussed in the various editions of *The Manual of Oncologic Therapeutics* represent working drafts that provide clinicians with descriptions of the best care available but fall far short of being definitive elucidations of the approach to patients with malignant disease.

We concur with Dr. Wittes. We wish to emphasize with the third edition of *The Manual of Oncologic Therapeutics* that clinicians managing cancer patients must understand that the best therapy for malignant disease is almost always a well-designed research clinical trial. There is no doubt that oncology has made major strides over the last 20 years and that those strides have been reflected in patients living longer with better quality of life. We have cured diseases today that we could not cure 20 years ago. However, we wish to reiterate that in using *The Manual of Oncologic Therapeutics* readers should realize that it serves as a guide to help with current management. However, it is also critical that in managing a patient the clinician know that one of the first bits of information that should be ascertained is the availability of an appropriate clinical trial in which the patient may be enrolled. Only through this constant evaluation and testing of new approaches to treatment will progress continue to be made in therapy of neoplastic disease.

We hope *The Manual of Oncologic Therapeutics* will be a useful milepost on the way to improved understanding of the management of malignant disease. We have reached an exciting point in oncology in 1994. We have experienced a burgeoning of information on the molecular biology and the molecular genetics of cancer. This knowledge has led to an understanding of the molecular differences between normal and neoplastic cells. The beauty of this information is that it allows research oncologists to develop therapy targeted specifically at the cancer cell, taking advantage of carefully defined molecular differences between cancer and normal cells. With this knowledge base, it is a short step to designing specific clinical trials to test important treatments based upon molecular concepts. To the patient and the clinician, these types of treatments with their specificity and decreased toxicity will represent a true renaissance in oncology.

John S. Macdonald, M.D.
Daniel G. Haller, M.D.
Robert J. Mayer, M.D.

ACKNOWLEDGMENTS

The Editors wish to thank Stuart Freeman and Eileen Wolfberg at J.B. Lippincott Company, whose constant encouragement and support facilitated the realization of this volume. The Editors also wish to acknowledge our enormous gratitude to Ms. Deborah Ann Skrocki, without whose superb organizational skills, technical expertise, and unending patience this volume would not have been possible.

CONTENTS

I. PROCEDURES FOR BIOPSY AND ENDOSCOPY

I. PROCEDURES FOR BIOPSY AND ENDOSCOPY

1. SKIN BIOPSY IN THE DIAGNOSIS AND MANAGEMENT OF MALIGNANCY

Arthur J. Sober

The skin biopsy is a simple procedure that is an invaluable diagnostic aid in the evaluation of potential skin cancers. Several techniques may be employed for cutaneous biopsy, including punch (trephine), incisional, and excisional biopsies. Table 1–1 lists the indications for each type of biopsy.

Biopsy punches are available in diameters ranging from 2 mm to 8 mm. For suspected basal cell carcinoma, a 2- to 3-mm punch is usually sufficient (Table 1–2). For Bowen's disease (squamous cell carcinoma in situ), a punch that is at least 3 mm in diameter is suggested. For squamous cell carcinoma or malignant melanoma, a punch that is at least 4 mm in diameter allows the pathologist to obtain a specimen of sufficient size for diagnosis. Punch biopsies are of limited value in the evaluation of processes involving deeper structures of skin (subcutis), because the fat often is left behind when the plug of skin is removed. In addition, punch biopsies are less than optimal when broad specimens are needed, such as in the differentiation of keratoacanthoma from squamous cell carcinoma where the border, deep margin, as well as a central portion of the lesion should be included for accurate assessment. In this instance, incisional biopsy is preferred.

In general, total excisional biopsy with close margin is the best choice for melanoma because the pathologist has the entire specimen to evaluate and, if the lesion is benign, definitive treatment has been achieved. Serial sections of the specimen allow determination of maximum tumor thickness, which can then be used to plan the extent of surgical therapy and to predict prognosis. At times, lesser procedures (punch or incisional biopsy) may be necessary for the evaluation of melanoma, and available data do not show that the prognosis worsens when these types of biopsy are performed.[1] When incisional or punch biopsy is performed, the final determination of prognosis must be deferred until the complete tumor specimen is examined following definitive therapy. Excisional biopsy with wide margins is not necessary to establish the diagnosis of melanoma and does not result in improved prognosis compared to less aggressive biopsy procedures.[2] Table 1–2 indicates the best area for biopsy of a suspected melanoma if incisional or punch biopsy is to be performed.

TECHNIQUES FOR PERFORMING SKIN BIOPSIES

1. Prepare the area with an alcohol wipe.
2. With a 30-gauge needle inject sufficient local anesthetic with epinephrine (usually 0.2 to 1 ml of solution) to produce blanching in the area of the biopsy (avoid epinephrine when biopsying a digit).
3. Clean the area with either soap, alcohol, iodine, or an iodophore-containing cleanser.
4. Select the appropriate biopsy technique.

TABLE 1–1. INDICATIONS FOR VARIOUS TYPES OF SKIN BIOPSY

TYPE OF BIOPSY	INDICATIONS
Punch (trephine)	Basal cell carcinoma Bowen's disease (squamous cell carcinoma in situ) Melanoma (occasional) Squamous cell carcinoma (occasional) Internal malignancies metastatic to skin
Incisional	Keratoacanthoma Squamous cell carcinoma Melanoma (occasional) Internal malignancies metastatic to skin
Shave	Any elevated lesion on a contoured surface such as pinna of ear or nose
Excisional (narrow margins)	Melanoma (procedure of choice) Any of the other types of cutaneous malignancy

A. Punch Biopsy
   (1) Before injecting anesthetic, mark the border of the lesion. (The lesion may disappear after the injection of anesthetic.)
   (2) Stretch the skin between the thumb and index or middle finger (Fig. 1–1).
   (3) Place the punch at right angles to the skin surface (Fig. 1–1).
   (4) Rotate and advance the punch with firm downward pressure until the subcutis is reached.
   (5) Remove the punch.
   (6) Gently elevate the core of tissue with forceps or the point of a needle, and sever the base with a pair of scissors or a scalpel (Fig. 1–2).
   (7) The site can be left unsutured, if small, or it can be closed with one or two sutures.
   (8) Remove the sutures in 5 to 7 days for a facial lesion, or 7 to 14 days for lesions of the trunk or extremities.

B. Incisional or Wedge Biopsy
   (1) Before injecting anesthetic, outline the area to be sampled with an ellipse (Fig. 1–3).
   (2) Prepare the site as for punch biopsy.
   (3) Incise the area outlined by the ellipse with a scalpel blade.
   (4) Lift the specimen and sever the base with either scissors or the scalpel blade.
   (5) Suture as needed for closure.
   (6) Remove the sutures as for punch biopsy.

C. Excisional Biopsy
   This biopsy is performed in the same manner as for an incisional biopsy, with the exception that the entire lesion is within the ellipse.

D. Shave Biopsy
   (1) Prepare the site as described above.
   (2) Place a small amount of local anesthetic beneath the lesion; this will elevate the lesion above the plane of the surface.
   (3) With a No. 15 scalpel blade held parallel to the skin surface, slide the blade across the base of the lesion in one smooth stroke, if possible.
   (4) Hemostasis is achieved with very light electrodesiccation, topical solutions such as Monsel's (ferric subsulfate), Gelfoam, or by direct pressure.

POSTBIOPSY WOUND CARE

For most biopsy sites no special care is required other than washing with soap and water once daily. For biopsies in which two or more sutures have been placed, cleaning the area twice a day (beginning 48 hours after the procedure) with hydrogen peroxide, then drying it, and covering it with an antibacterial ointment (bacitracin, povidone-iodine, or Bactroban) should prevent bacterial infection.

TABLE 1–2. SITES OF BIOPSY FOR INCISIONAL OR PUNCH BIOPSY

TUMOR	SUGGESTED LOCATION FOR BIOPSY
Basal cell carcinoma	Rolled border
Keratoacanthoma	Pie-shaped section from edge to center
Squamous cell carcimoma	Pie-shaped section from edge to center
Melanoma	
If flat	Darkest area
If raised	Most raised portion

HANDLING OF SPECIMENS

1. Place each biopsy into a separate container that is properly labeled with the patient's name, date, and some method of identifying the original location maintained in the patient's record and on the biopsy laboratory slip.
2. If multiple biopsies are being performed, label all containers before beginning so that the chance of confusing the tissue samples is reduced.
3. If indicated in your office practice or institution, a consent form for the biopsy procedure should be signed prior to beginning the procedure.

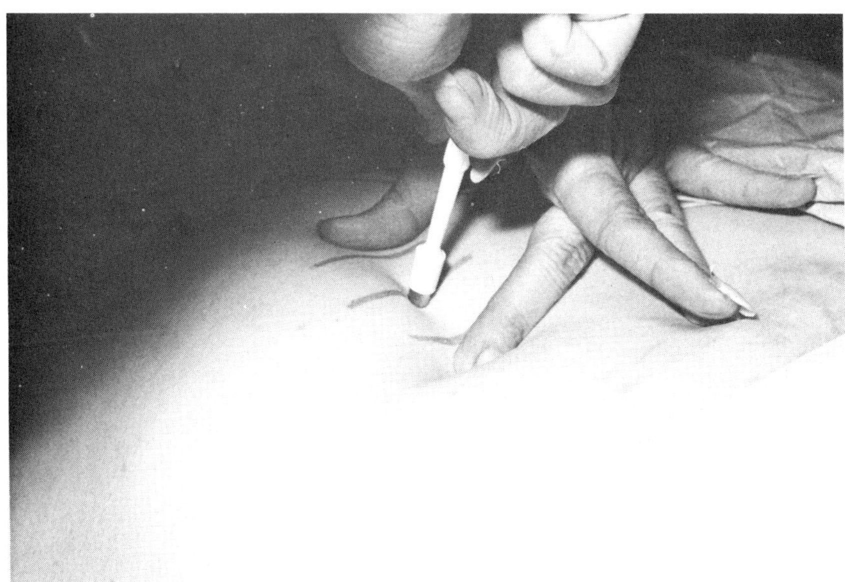

Figure 1–1. In punch biopsy the skin is stretched between the thumb and index or middle finger, and the punch is positioned at right angles to the skin surface.

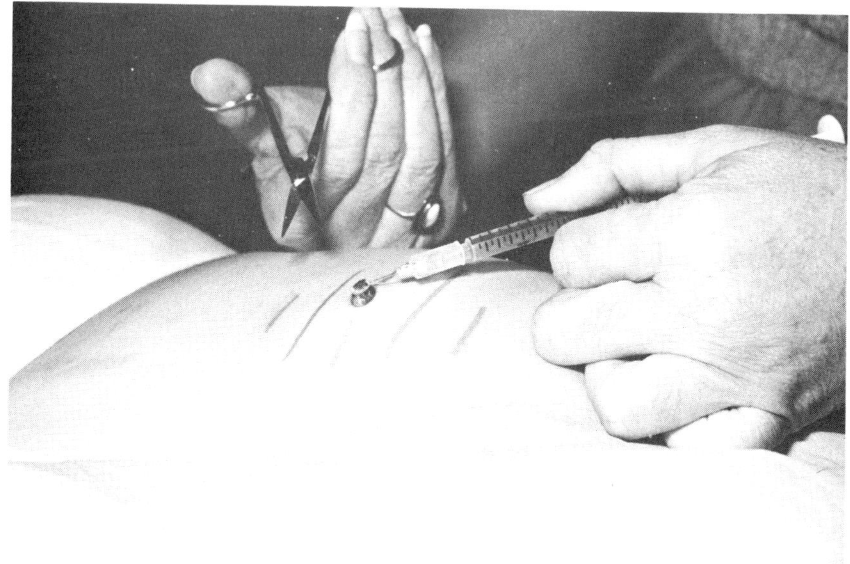

Figure 1–2. To obtain the specimen in punch biopsy, the core of tissue is elevated with forceps or the point of a needle and the base is severed with a pair of scissors.

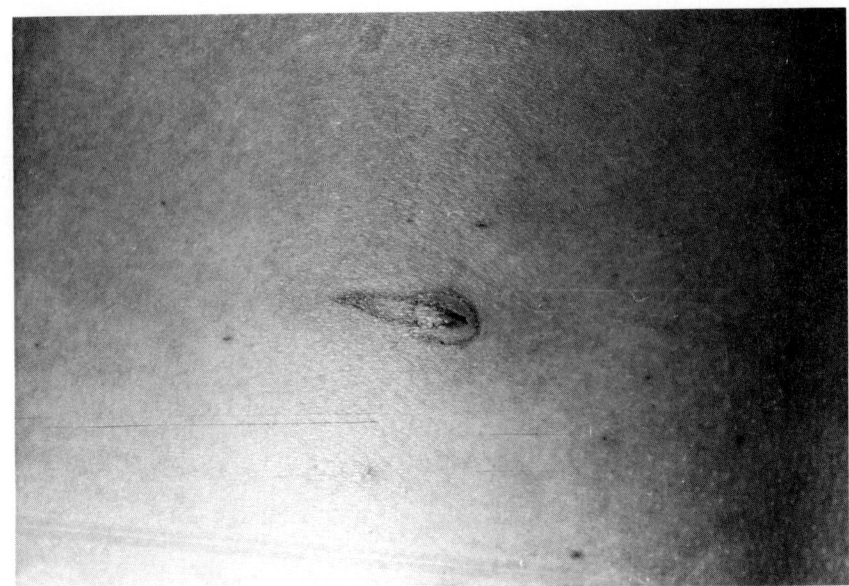

Figure 1–3. In incisional biopsy the area to be sampled is outlined with an ellipse prior to injecting anesthetic.

REFERENCES

1. Lederman JS, Sober AJ. Does biopsy type influence survival in clinical Stage I cutaneous melanoma? J Am Acad Dermatol 13:983–987, 1985
2. Lederman JS, Sober AJ. Wide excision as the initial diagnostic procedure in the management of cutaneous melanoma. J Dermatol Surg Oncol 12:697–699, 1986

John S. Macdonald, Daniel G. Haller, Robert J. Mayer, Eds. *Manual of Oncologic Therapeutics*, Third Edition.

2. BIOPSY AS A PRELUDE TO DEFINITIVE OPERATIVE THERAPY FOR BREAST CANCER

Norman Wolmark
John S. Macdonald

The increasing acceptance of breast-preserving operations has elevated the importance of the initial breast biopsy and calls for a technique involving careful planning and meticulous attention to operative detail. The breast biopsy should be carried out by experienced breast clinicians — ideally the same physicians who will perform the definitive operation, should the lesion prove to be malignant.

Although the presence of a palpable persistent mass or dominant nodule remains the most common indication for breast biopsy, the biopsy of nonpalpable, mammographically diagnosed abnormalities is being performed with increasing frequency. Each of these situations is discussed separately because each has unique ramifications. This chapter does not address those special circumstances in which breast biopsy is performed for skin or nipple changes or persistent nipple discharge.

BIOPSY OF A PALPABLE DOMINANT MASS

The clinician must formulate a strategy that not only will establish a diagnosis but also will take into account the subsequent management of the patient, most notably the likelihood of a breast-preserving operation. The first step in establishing a diagnosis of a palpable lesion should be fine-needle aspiration cytology. If malignant cells are detected, this procedure circumvents an open biopsy and enables the surgeon to proceed directly with definitive therapy (breast-preserving operation or mastectomy). It must be emphasized that fine-needle aspiration may accurately diagnose cytologic malignancy, but it cannot differentiate between invasive and intraductal carcinomas. Fine-needle aspiration can also establish the presence of a benign fluid-filled gross cyst and thus obviate the need for further intervention. If the needle aspiration cytology is not definitive — that is, tumor cells are not present and the lesion is not a gross cyst — definitive diagnosis must be established using an open biopsy. It is absolutely critical that both the surgeon and the patient be in agreement on the definitive operative therapy to be undertaken should the lesion prove to be malignant. This agreement must be established before, not following, the breast biopsy, because the selection of a breast-preserving cancer operation will influence the approach to the biopsy, and conversely, an injudiciously performed breast biopsy can eliminate the possibility of a subsequent breast-preserving operation.

Before any operative procedure on the breast, bilateral mammography is essential for assessing the nature of the dominant lesion, the surrounding breast parenchyma, and the contralateral breast. In patients who are being considered for breast-preserving operations, it is necessary to rule out the presence of diffuse microcalcifications that are beyond the scope of the contemplated resection.

TECHNIQUE OF OPEN BREAST BIOPSY

If there is even a remote possibility that the lesion is malignant, the open biopsy should be performed under the assumption that the lesion is, in fact, malignant and in such a manner as to ensure that the patient may have a breast-preserving operation, should that option be appropriate. Accordingly, the open biopsy should consist of a definitive lumpectomy or segmental mastectomy. Thus, the procedure should both establish a diagnosis and serve as the mammary component of the breast-preserving operation. The breast incision should be curvilinear and positioned directly over the palpable mass (Fig. 2–1). The popular technique of using a circumareolar incision for a lesion located a good distance from the incision is to be condemned (Fig. 2–2). Although the circumareolar incision achieves a superior cosmetic result, the process of burrowing through a major expanse of breast tissue to reach a remote lesion significantly compromises the ability to perform a segmental mastectomy at either the initial or subsequent operation. Furthermore, the use of radial rather than curvilinear incisions achieves suboptimal cosmetic results and thus has been abandoned. The lesion must be removed with a rim of normal tissue throughout the entire circumference (Fig. 2–3). This does not mean that a fixed amount of normal tissue be resected (*e.g.*, 2 cm in all directions), but rather that only the amount of tissue necessary to achieve histologically tumor-free margins be removed. The underlying pectoralis fascia need not be disturbed, and an ellipse of skin may or may not be included. The specimen must be oriented by the surgeon at the time of operation so the pathologist can adequately assess the margins. Margins of resection are tinted with ink before the specimen is sectioned and diagnosis is established by frozen section. If the lesion proves to be malignant and the

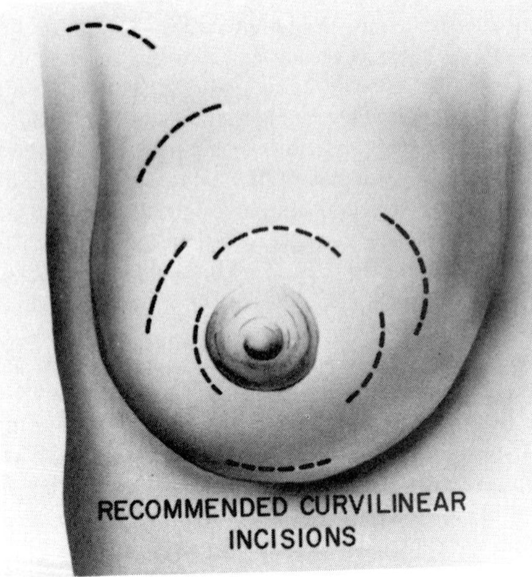

Figure 2–1. In open breast biopsy, the breast incision should be curvilinear and should be positioned directly over the mass.

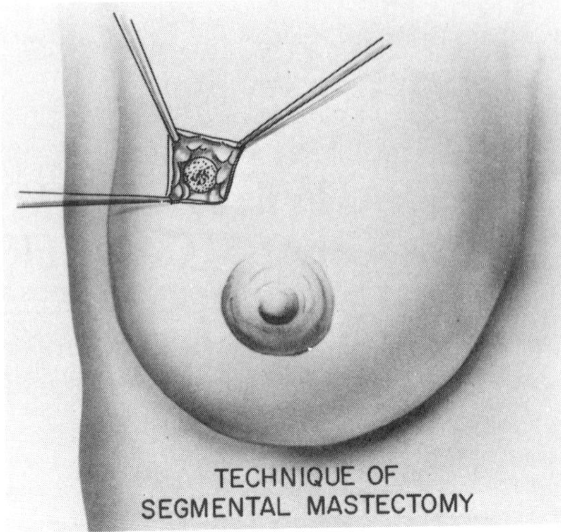

Figure 2–3. The lesion must be removed with a rim of normal tissue throughout the entire circumference in order to achieve margins that are histologically tumor-free.

margins have been shown to be free of tumor, the surgeon need not further disturb the breast and may proceed directly with an axillary dissection (if a breast-preserving operation is considered appropriate). If tumor involves one of the margins, the surgeon can return to the resection site and remove more breast tissue in the appropriate area in order to establish a tumor-free perimeter. If the excised lesion proves to be benign, the surgeon has performed a slightly wider operation than might otherwise have been contemplated, but this consequence is far preferable to having inadequately resected a malignant lesion. The procedure is completed by cosmetic reapproximation of the skin, without oblitera-

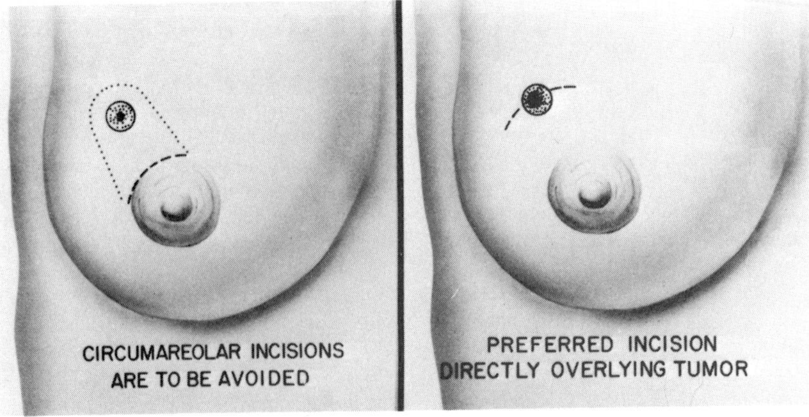

Figure 2–2. A circumareolar incision for a lesion located remote from the areola should be avoided; incisions should be made directly over the tumor.

tion of the underlying dead space, with sutures or drainage devices.

Because assessment of hormone receptor status and, possibly, oncogene status and DNA content may provide valuable prognostic information and guide treatment, it is the surgeon's responsibility to provide tissue for these studies. Typically, tissue immediately placed in liquid nitrogen will suffice, although receptors may be determined by immunohistochemical techniques using fixed tissue. The optimum approach to a breast-preserving operation in the management of malignant lesions is to perform the biopsy and definitive segmental resection at the same time. The surgeon confronted with the prospect of performing a breast-preserving operation after a biopsy has been carried out previously (by the same or another surgeon) is faced with the major dilemma of not knowing the confines of the tumor or, for that matter, its precise location. The not infrequent presence of a hematoma from a previous biopsy is a further confounding influence. On the other hand, if the patient and surgeon have agreed that a mastectomy is to be performed as the definitive operation, the prerequisites described previously for biopsy are largely irrelevant; the only stipulation is that the biopsy incision be placed in such a manner that it will be encompassed by the elliptical incision fashioned for the subsequent mastectomy.

BIOPSY OF A NONPALPABLE, MAMMOGRAPHICALLY DETECTED LESION

In the case of a nonpalpable, mammographically detected lesion, the surgeon strives to meet the same prerequisites outlined for the management of a palpable dominant nodule. This is made more difficult by the fact that the location of the lesion must be established by radiographic methods. Most commonly, the area of microcalcifications or other sinister mammographic finding is identified with the use of a radiopaque marker inserted under mammographic control. Once the needle or wire has been positioned, the surgeon has a reasonable estimate of the location of the suspicious mammographic findings. The same principles as for a palpable nodule are now applied. A curvilinear incision is made over the putative lesion, and the excision is effected so as to achieve histologically free margins. Before the lesion is oriented for the pathologist, it is subjected to specimen mammography to ensure that all the mammographic abnormalities have been included in the resected specimen. The same procedure that has been outlined for palpable masses is now followed.

ONE-STEP VERSUS TWO-STEP OPERATIVE APPROACH

The increasing popularity of breast-preserving operations has also had a significant influence on the interval between biopsy and the definitive operative procedure for breast malignancy. When breast-preserving operations were first offered as an "alternative" unencumbered by the availability of reliable data, the two-step operative approach seemed desirable. Employing this method resulted in the postponement of the definitive operation following the biopsy so that the patient could avail herself of consultation and alternatives to mastectomy. The two-step approach was also advocated as a procedure that resulted in less psychological trauma than the standard practice in which a patient was anesthetized without knowing whether the mass was malignant and whether she will awake with or without a breast. With the establishment of the breast-preserving operation as a standard method of breast cancer therapy, the two-step procedure has become an anachronism.

The optimum time to perform a lumpectomy or segmental mastectomy for cancer is at the time of the initial biopsy. It becomes even more critical, therefore, for the decision relative to subsequent therapy to be discussed and agreed on before the biopsy. For this reason, the use of needle aspiration represents a significant advance. Armed with the diagnosis, one can intelligently discuss the options available to the patient before to any open operative procedure. The one-step operation will undoubtedly gain in popularity for patients who are candidates for breast-preserving operations.

BIBLIOGRAPHY

Fisher B. Reappraisal of breast biopsy prompted by the use of lumpectomy. JAMA 253:3588, 1985

Fisher B, Bauer M, Margolese RG et al. Five-year results from the NSABP trial comparing total mastectomy to segmental mastectomy with and without radiation in the treatment of breast cancer. N Engl J Med 312:665–673, 1985

Fisher B, Wolmark N, Fisher ER, Deutsch M. Lumpectomy and axillary dissection for breast cancer: Surgical, pathological and radiation considerations. World J Surg 9:692–698, 1985

Harris JR, Morrow M, Bonadonna X. Cancer of the breast. In DeVita VT, Hellman S, Rosenberg SA (eds). Cancer: Principles and Practice of Oncology. Philadelphia, JB Lippincott, 1993:1264–1332

Veronesi U, Saccozzi R, Del Vecchio M et al. Comparing radical mastectomy with quadrantectomy, axillary dissection and radiotherapy in patients with small cancers of the breast. N Engl J Med 305:6–11, 1981

John S. Macdonald, Daniel G. Haller, Robert J. Mayer, Eds. *Manual of Oncologic Therapeutics*, Third Edition.

3. LYMPH NODE BIOPSY

Kevin E. Salhany

Lymph node biopsies generally include biopsies for primary diagnosis, staging, and lymph node dissections for carcinoma or melanoma. Indications for diagnostic lymph node biopsies include suspected lymphoma or metastatic tumor, persistent lymphadenopathy, lymphadenopathy associated with unexplained fever or weight loss, and persistent or recurrent adenopathy following therapy in patients known to have had lymphoma.[1] Lymph node biopsies in treated lymphoma patients should be performed to confirm recurrence of lymphoma, to evaluate for histologic transformation or progression to higher grade lymphoma, and to rule out a new lymphoma or second malignancy. The differential diagnosis for unexplained lymphadenopathy includes metastatic tumor, lymphoma, infectious lymphadenitis, and reactive lymphadenopathy.

Communication among the oncologist, surgeon, and pathologist before diagnostic lymph node biopsies is essential to ensure that the biopsy is appropriately handled and worked up. Accurate diagnosis depends on biopsy of an appropriate lymph node with adequate tissue for ancillary studies, careful biopsy technique, rapid transport to the pathology department, and proper lymph node work-up. Diagnostic lymph node biopsies should be performed by experienced surgeons, and should be removed intact with as little trauma as possible to prevent crush artifact and distortion of nodal architecture. In general, the largest accessible lymph node should be biopsied even though this may require deeper exploration. Lymph nodes 2 cm or larger are preferred, but they should be at least 1 cm. Smaller lymph nodes are less likely to be diagnostic and often provide insufficient tissue for a complete work-up. Cervical lymph nodes usually provide better biopsies than inguinal lymph nodes because of the high frequency of chronic lymphadenitis and scarring in inguinal nodes.[1]

Once removed, the fresh lymph node should be placed in a container of sterile normal saline to prevent tissue desiccation and sent immediately to the pathology department to determine the nature of the process and to confirm whether adequate diagnostic tissue is available. If an infectious etiology is suspected, intraoperative cultures of one of the ends of the lymph node should be taken; otherwise, the lymph node should be sent intact. Clear instructions should be given to the pathologist indicating the purpose of the lymph node biopsy to prevent mishandling of the specimen. The pathologist should immediately examine touch imprints of the fresh lymph node to determine the basic nature of the process. Frozen sections of lymphomas or reactive lymph nodes generally are not indicated unless the touch prep is inadequate to determine if lesional tissue is present,[1,2] but may be performed if adequate tissue is available to complete the lymphoma work-up. If frozen sections must be performed, only part of the specimen should be frozen, and the surgeon should be prepared to obtain more fresh tissue to complete the diagnostic work-up if necessary. The diagnostic work-up for lymphoma includes preparation of air-dried touch imprints, representative B5- or formalin-fixed sections for routine histology, a representative section snap-frozen (−70°C) for frozen section immunohistochemistry and possible molecular diagnostic studies, a small portion fixed in glutaraldehyde for possible ultrastructural studies, and at least 1 cc of fresh tissue to make cell suspensions for immunophenotyping by flow cytometry, flow cytometric DNA analysis, cytogenetics, and molecular genetics.[1,2]

If the initial lymph node examination suggests an infectious process, tissue should be send for culture. Hormone-receptor analysis and DNA analysis can be performed in the case of metastatic breast carcinoma if the lymph node is received fresh. Tissue should be fixed in glutaraldehyde for poorly differentiated malignant neoplasms in case electron microscopy is needed.

Lymph node biopsies for staging and lymph node dissections in patients with documented carcinoma or melanoma do not require the same precautions and detailed work-up required for initial lymphoma diagnoses. However, these lymph nodes should be sent to the pathology department fresh, whenever possible, so that hormone receptor studies or other special studies may be performed on grossly positive nodes, if indicated. Frozen sections of lymph nodes for intraoperative staging of prostatic, endometrial, and lung carcinoma are commonly performed during radical resections, but should be limited to cases in which the results will influence surgical management. It is sometimes useful to obtain a quick gross estimate of the number of lymph

Supported in part by Grant #IRG-135L from the American Cancer Society nodes from the pathologist during surgery to determine if the lymph node dissection is adequate. In staging laparotomies for Hodgkin's disease, the spleen and lymph node biopsies should be sent fresh to the pathology department immediately so they may be quickly examined and fixed to ensure optimal histologic preservation. Frozen sections are not indicated in staging laparotomies for Hodgkin's disease.

REFERENCES

1. Stansfeld AG. Indications, technique and applications for lymph node biopsy. In Stansfeld AG, d'Ardenne AJ (eds). Lymph Node Biopsy Interpretation. 2nd ed. Edinburgh, Churchill Livingstone, 1992:29.
2. Collins RD. Lymph node examination: What is an adequate workup? Arch Pathol Lab Med 109:796, 1985.

John S. Macdonald, Daniel G. Haller, Robert J. Mayer, Eds. *Manual of Oncologic Therapeutics*, Third Edition.

4. DIAGNOSTIC PROCEDURES RELATED TO THE THORAX

Michael F. Reed
Malcolm M. DeCamp, Jr.
David J. Sugarbaker

BRONCHOSCOPY

Bronchoscopy is the most commonly employed procedure for the diagnosis of pulmonary disease. Rigid bronchoscopy was introduced in the late nineteenth century and remains the indicated method of diagnosis and therapy in certain select circumstances. In most cases, the flexible fiberoptic bronchoscope is now the instrument of choice. Flexible bronchoscopy, developed by Ikeda in 1970, provides accurate visualization of the tracheobronchial tree, and its widespread use has revolutionized the management of intrathoracic disease.

Rigid Bronchoscopy

Adult open-tube rigid bronchoscopes are available with internal diameters of up to 9 mm. Assisted ventilation can be provided by a side-arm channel. A closed system exists with the lens in place. The larger diameter of rigid bronchoscopes, compared with flexible bronchoscopes, facilitates passage of instruments for biopsy and suctioning and allows easier and more rapid removal of foreign bodies. The rigid bronchoscope also provides control of the patient's airway, which is essential in evaluating or treating obstructing lesions of the trachea. The rigid instrument is effective for dilating strictures and is ideal for performing laser therapy. The indications for rigid bronchoscopy thus include evaluation and control of massive hemoptysis, foreign body removal, examination and treatment of tracheal and main-stem bronchial lesions, and laser bronchoscopy.

The procedure is limited to these few indications because it also has a number of drawbacks. Rigid bronchoscopy usually requires general anesthesia. Visualization is limited to the oropharynx, larynx, trachea, and the main-stem and lobar bronchi. Although angled telescopes may improve visualization of the segmental level, instrumentation, including biopsy, is feasible only for structures under direct vision. This technique provides a low yield for tissue diagnosis of peripheral lesions because smaller airways are not accessible by rigid bronchoscopy.

TECHNIQUE

Rigid bronchoscopy is typically performed in an operating room. Once general anesthesia is achieved, the patient is placed in the supine position with the neck flexed and the chin extended. The examiner elevates the epiglottis with the tip of the lubricated bronchoscope and visualizes the vocal cords. The scope is then inserted into the trachea. The anesthesiologist maintains ventilation by using the side-arm channel or a Venturi jet ventilating adaptor. The trachea, carina, main-stem and lobar bronchi, and all segmental orifices are systematically examined. All lesions are biopsied and brushed under direct visualization. Large, obstructive lesions may be "cored out" with the scope and extracted. This is often useful when lobar or whole-lung collapse limits therapy. Bleeding is controlled by using electrocautery.

Flexible Bronchoscopy

Although rigid bronchoscopy continues to play a vital role in select situations, most practitioners employ flexible fiberoptic bronchoscopy as an initial diagnostic modality. Flexible fiberoptic bronchoscopes range from 1.8 to 6 mm in external diameter. The smallest bronchoscopes have no channel, whereas the larger instruments have channels of up to 2.6 mm in internal diameter. The most common indication for fiberoptic bronchoscopy is the evaluation of suspected carcinoma of the lung. Other clinical settings that warrant the procedure include hemoptysis, diffuse lung disease, lung abscess, aspiration, pneumonia in immunocompromised individuals, and oxygenation or ventilation problems in intubated patients. When a patient is evaluated for lung cancer, fiberoptic bronchoscopy facilitates tissue diagnosis, contributes to staging, and assists in the determination of resectability.

The flexible fiberoptic bronchoscope possesses certain distinct advantages over rigid bronchoscopes. The smaller diameter and flexibility permit evaluation of peripheral bronchi and also allow placement of the bronchoscope through an endotracheal tube. Technologic advances in illumination and fiberoptics provide superior visualization and allow photography or video monitoring. Multiple channels permit insertion of small brushes, forceps, needles, and laser fibers. Flexible fiberoptic bronchoscopy may be performed in an outpatient setting because it requires only topical anesthesia and mild sedation for satisfactory patient comfort, thereby obviating the need for an operating room, general anesthesia, and anesthesiologist.

Flexible fiberoptic bronchoscopy is still frequently used

in the operating room during difficult placement of an endotracheal tube, before thoracotomy to verify resectability of a lung mass, and after lung resection in order to evaluate the bronchial stump and to suction secretions before extubation. However, it may also be employed in an endoscopy suite, in an intensive or intermediate care unit, or in the emergency department. The disadvantages of flexible fiberoptic bronchoscopy are primarily related to its smaller diameter. Biopsy specimens are smaller and suctioning is much less efficient.

The flexible fiberoptic bronchoscope may be inserted transnasally, transorally, through an endotracheal tube, or through a rigid bronchoscope. The main advantage of the nasal route is the ability to perform the procedure in an outpatient setting by using topical anesthesia. Drawbacks include patient discomfort and the inability to withdraw the bronchoscope freely during the procedure, thereby limiting biopsy size to samples that fit through the operating channel. The transoral route has the benefit of superior patient comfort. The bronchoscope may be more easily removed multiple times. Brushes and forceps need not be pulled through the bronchoscope, and better samples are obtained. Disadvantages include excessive gagging and the occasional need for endotracheal intubation in high-risk patients.

TECHNIQUE

When flexible bronchoscopy is performed on an awake patient, sedation is appropriate. Premedication with atropine prevents bradycardia, limits bronchial secretions, and diminishes reflex bronchoconstriction. Supplemental oxygen is administered during the procedure. Monitoring should include pulse oximetry, noninvasive blood pressure readings, and electrocardiography. Initial topical anesthesia is provided by a nebulizer. Subsequently the vocal cords, trachea, and carina are anesthesized by injecting topical anesthesia through the bronchoscope or by cricothyroid membrane puncture with a 25-gauge needle.

As the bronchoscope is advanced, all anatomical structures are examined, starting with the pharynx and vocal cords and proceeding to the trachea, followed by a systematic survey of the tracheobronchial tree. Manifestations of tumor involvement, which are frequently subtle, including widening and fixation of the carina, increased or purulent secretions, mucosal friability, increased submucosal vascularity, irregular bronchial folds, mucosal thickening, indistinct cartilage rings, loss of sharpness of the spurs between separate bronchi, and obvious masses.

All suspicious areas require biopsy. Specimens are obtained by brushings, forceps biopsy, and bronchial washings. The techniques are complementary and the diagnostic yield increases when all three methods are used. Brushings are performed by vigorously passing the bronchial brush across the lesion, then withdrawing the instrument from the bronchoscope and wiping the bristles across a glass slide that is immediately fixed with alcohol. The region is then biopsied by using the forceps to grasp and avulse small tissue fragments. Multiple specimens are obtained from different locations on the lesion because certain sites might contain only necrotic tumor. Fluoroscopic guidance in targeting a peripheral lung lesion increases the diagnostic yield and lessens the chance of pneumothorax. An increased number of specimens results in a higher sensitivity; at least four biopsy specimens per lesion is the recommended number. Washings are obtained by performing bronchoalveolar lavage. The tip of the bronchoscope is wedged in the subsegmental bronchus of interest, and 20 ml saline solution is injected then suctioned into a trap. This is repeated until 100 ml is collected.

If an intrathoracic lesion, whether a primary tumor or an enlarged lymph node, is not visible endobronchially, transbronchial needle aspiration is an alternative method of obtaining tissue. It should be performed before brushing or forceps biopsy to avoid false-positive aspirations. The technique is useful for the evaluation of lesions not invading a bronchus, such as suspicious paratracheal and subcarinal lymph nodes, submucosal bronchial masses, and peripheral lesions. When transbronchial needle biopsy of mediastinal masses is anticipated, a computed tomographic (CT) scan of the chest is mandatory before bronchoscopy to accurately locate the lesion. Fluoroscopic guidance is indicated when transbronchial needle aspiration of a peripheral lesion is performed. Complications such as bleeding, infection, and pneumothorax are rare. However, needle biopsy should be limited to one hemithorax to avoid bilateral pneumothoraces. When transbronchial needle aspiration is considered, precise understanding of parabronchial vascular anatomy is essential.

LASER BRONCHOSCOPY

Palliative therapy for patients with obstructing lesions of the trachea and main-stem bronchi has traditionally relied on rigid bronchoscopy. More recent technologic advances have added flexible fiberoptic bronchoscopy with laser therapy to the armamentarium. A procedure that uses the benefits of all three techniques has proved effective in providing palliation to patients with certain endotracheal and endobronchial masses. The rigid bronchoscope provides airway control and facilitates debulking of large tumors, whereas the flexible fiberoptic bronchoscope, passed through the rigid instrument, allows the use of flexible fiber-directed laser therapy with improved visualization and accurate targeting of the laser. neodymium:yttrium aluminum garnet (Nd:YAG) and potassium titanyl phosphate (KTP) are two frequently used lasers.

Patient selection is critical when endobronchial laser resection is being considered. Ideal candidates are individuals with obstructions of the trachea or main-stem bronchi that arise from upper-lobe tumors or mediastinal masses. Middle-

or lower-lobe tumors frequently result in masses that are not amenable to this therapy because the restoration of aeration requires creation of a channel to a normal bronchus distally. Thorough outpatient evaluation before laser therapy aids in patient selection, namely the identification of those with patent distal bronchi who would benefit from the procedure. Clinical indications include inspiratory wheezing and a recent chest radiograph that verifies aeration of the lung. Flexible bronchoscopy should be employed to locate the lesion and to verify airway patency. In fact, suctioning during fiberoptic bronchoscopy may temporarily improve pulmonary function and thus make the patient a better candidate for general anesthesia.

Laser resection is indicated only for endobronchial masses. Bronchial obstruction secondary to extrinsic compression is not an indication for laser therapy. Normal vascular and bronchial anatomy may be distorted by external compression. Where an external mass compresses a vascular structure, laser vaporization carries an increased risk of significant, potentially fatal, hemorrhage. In this clinical setting, the placement of an endobronchial stent and/or urgent radiation therapy or brachytherapy provide safer methods of achieving bronchial patency.

TECHNIQUE

Laser resection must be performed in an operating room, and the procedure carries unique requirements for both anesthetic and surgical techniques. To prevent airway fires during laser use, the fraction of inspired oxygen (FiO_2) must be maintained at or below 0.4%. Vigilant monitoring by pulse oximetry is therefore mandatory. If desaturation occurs, requiring an increased FiO_2, laser vaporization must be temporarily halted until an FiO_2 of no more than 40% is resumed. Although some anesthesiologists prefer Venturi ("jet") ventilation during rigid bronchoscopy, we have found that this method often results in the passage of tissue and tumor fragments into the distal bronchi during laser resection. We therefore advocate traditional ventilation by the side-arm channel of the ventilating rigid bronchoscope.

As with routine rigid bronchoscopy, suitable general anesthesia is achieved first, and then the patient is positioned supine with the neck flexed and chin extended. The rigid bronchoscope is passed through the mouth. The flexible bronchoscope is then introduced, and, if a tissue diagnosis has not yet been obtained, biopsies are taken and sent for frozen section. The laser fiber is then passed through the bronchoscope and well past the tip of the bronchoscope to avoid damaging the instrument with the activated laser.

The "ready beam" is used to target the laser accurately; vaporization begins at the free margin of the mass and proceeds toward its base in the bronchial wall. Intermittent removal of the fiberoptic instruments may allow introduction of larger forceps to debulk large pieces of the tumor. Reintroduction of the flexible scope and use of the unfocused laser provide hemostasis. Refocusing the laser permits pinpoint resection of the tumor, especially near the bronchial wall. Before the laser is removed, the tip should be allowed to cool to avoid damaging the channel of the flexible bronchoscope.

After the procedure, patients are given dexamethasone for 48 hours to minimize edema. An overnight hospital stay permits pulse oximetry for the first 12 postoperative hours in a monitored setting. Clinical improvement in pulmonary function occurs during the subsequent week as edema recedes.

In addition to the potential complications associated with rigid and flexible bronchoscopy, endobronchial laser resection carries certain risks. Intraoperative fires may occur, especially when the laser is activated in the presence of high oxygen partial pressures. Laser damage to surrounding structures may result in hemorrhage or airway perforation, especially if the operator does not sufficiently account for the extent of tissue destruction that always occurs below the surface during vaporization. This last risk may be diminished, and longer palliation achieved, if the resection is repeated in 1 month. By performing two procedures, the surgeon may elect a strategy in which the first resection results in a conservative debulking. During the second procedure, visualization is improved and accurate targeting of the laser makes resection of residual tumor near the bronchial wall, or nearby vascular structures, much safer.

THORACENTESIS

Thoracentesis may be useful for obtaining a diagnosis, staging, or, in selected cases, providing therapeutic benefit for patients with malignancy. Examination of pleural fluid allows the clinician to discriminate a transudate from an exudate, a malignant effusion from a benign effusion, and a sterile process from an empyema. Although large effusions may be clinically discerned with percussion, prudence dictates careful localization of smaller fluid collections by using plain radiographs, ultrasonography, or CT. When a diagnostic procedure is planned, fluid may be obtained with a relatively small needle (20- to 22-gauge). Similarly, a short intravenous catheter may be used to avoid leaving a needle within the chest.

A therapeutic tap should be entertained only for symptomatic patients. This approach should be selected when a chest tube or more definitive operative drainage is ill-advised, such as for the relief of dyspnea in a terminal patient or in the setting of coagulopathy. Therapeutic drainage of an effusion will benefit only a patient with a significant volume of pleural fluid. The procedure requires a longer, soft catheter, which can be positioned dependently within the chest and connected either to a three-way stop or to a vacuum bottle to facilitate complete evacuation of unloculated pleural fluid. The technique of thoracentesis is similar to that described elsewhere in this book for closed-tube thoracostomy.

CLOSED PLEURAL BIOPSY

The technique of closed pleural biopsy is of value in the evaluation of pleural-based masses or thickening with little or no associated pleural effusion. In the setting of a concomitant pleural effusion, the diagnostic yield is usually better with analysis of the fluid itself. When a percutaneous pleural biopsy is desired, a backward-biting needle, such as that described by Abrams or Cope, is the preferred instrument. Multiple passes of this device are necessary to yield a sample sufficient for histologic examination. Because it is a blind percutaneous procedure, the need for adequate radiographic localization is paramount.

Although the diagnostic accuracy of a pleural biopsy may be inferior to that of thoracoscopy, it can be safely performed in the outpatient setting. When a definitive diagnosis is achieved, the risk of a general anesthetic may be avoided. A common clinical dilemma is the differentiation of metastatic adenocarcinoma from an epithelial-type mesothelioma. A simple closed biopsy is unlikely to yield sufficient tissue for the battery of histologic, immunohistochemical, and ultrastructural studies necessary to make the appropriate pathologic discrimination. In patients who have a high suspicion for pleural mesothelioma and who otherwise display reasonably good general health, operative thoracoscopy for more generous pleural biopsies under direct vision is recommended.

PERCUTANEOUS LUNG OR MEDIASTINAL BIOPSY

With universal access to interventional CT, the practice of percutaneous fine-needle aspiration biopsy of solid organs has been extended to the lungs and mediastinum. This technique commonly employs a long (22-gauge or finer) needle that yields only cytologic information. The procedure is helpful for peripheral or pleural-based lesions, especially if extensive disease is suspected and surgery is to be avoided. Pneumothorax complicates fine-needle aspirations within the thorax in 10% to 50% of cases.

When malignancy is high in the differential diagnosis and a benign fine-needle aspirate is obtained, sampling bias should be suspected and more aggressive means of biopsy should be employed. Similarly, in certain cases of positive cytology from a fine-needle aspirate, clinical skepticism is warranted. One example of this would be a fine-needle biopsy diagnosis of small cell carcinoma. At times, this may be indistinguishable by cytologic examination from benign carcinoid or neuroendocrine non–small cell carcinoma. These ambiguities make treatment decisions difficult and sway many clinicians to prefer mediastinoscopy or video-assisted thoracoscopy to obtain more definitive tissue samples.

MEDIASTINOSCOPY

Planning appropriate therapeutic strategies for patients with non–small cell carcinoma of the lung requires accurate surgical-pathologic staging. Current treatment options consist of one or more modalities, notably surgical resection, both thoracoscopically and by traditional thoracotomy, radiation therapy, and chemotherapy, including preoperative (neoadjuvant) protocols. Surgical resection remains the mainstay of treatment for Stage I and II disease. Recent trials suggest that certain select Stage IIIA lung cancers, which have T3 primary tumors or involvement of ipsilateral mediastinal lymph nodes (N2), may be treated with neoadjuvant chemotherapy followed by surgical resection, resulting in pathologic downstaging and improved survival. Cancers of Stages IIIB and IV are unresectable, and radiation therapy and/or chemotherapy remain the modalities of choice.

Accurate staging, for which mediastinoscopy is an important tool, separates patients who are candidates for surgery from those who have unresectable disease. Dwight Harken observed that metastatic spread to the mediastinal lymph nodes removed during pneumonectomy correlated with much worse survival. Daniels (1949) and Harken (1954) pioneered methods of biopsying cervical and mediastinal lymph nodes. In 1959, Carlens described an improved technique in which he introduced a mediastinoscope through a small midline suprasternal incision to provide access to bilateral paratracheal nodes as well as hilar and carinal lymph node groups. This technique allowed preresectional identification of patients for whom thoracotomy would prove futile.

The level of lymph node involvement correlates with prognosis. Naruke noted this relationship and, in 1978, introduced a thoracic lymph node map that illustrates the various lymph node groups and assigns them to specific nodal levels (N0, N1, N2, or N3). A modified version of Naruke's map is depicted in Figure 4–1. When Mountain and colleagues proposed the new international staging system for non–small cell lung cancer in 1986, the level of lymph node involvement served as the principal prognostic determinant (Table 4–1). Assessment of mediastinal lymph node spread is essential for two reasons. First, accurate staging is mandatory in appropriately treating any patient with lung cancer. Second, new therapeutic modalities can be evaluated only by clinical trials in which homogeneity of staged groups is verified.

The principal noninvasive method for evaluating mediastinal lymph node spread is by CT. On pathologic examination of patients with lung cancer, enlarged mediastinal nodes frequently prove to be inflammatory and show no evidence of metastatic involvement. A number of studies have verified that one third of patients with lung cancer who have mediastinal nodal enlargement on CT prove to have no evidence of metastasis after biopsy or resection. For this reason,

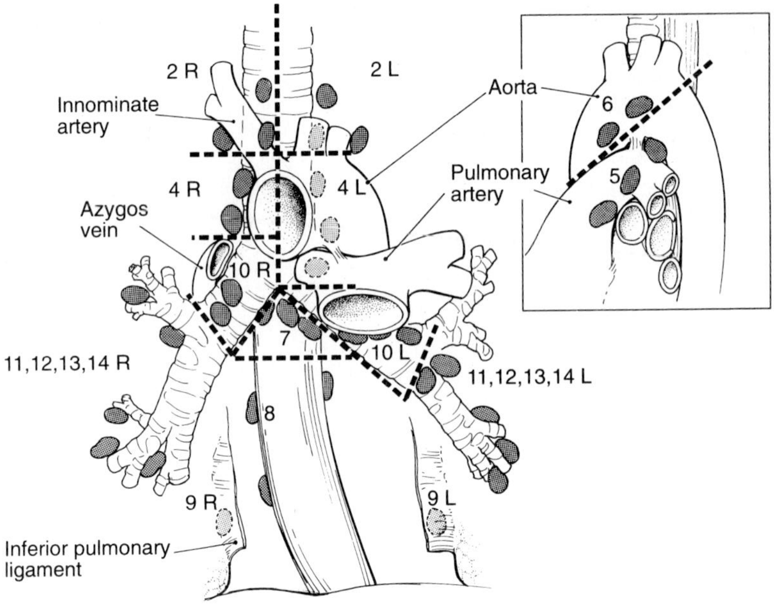

Figure 4–1. Illustration of lymph node locations. *Key*: (2) upper paratracheal nodes, (4) lower paratracheal nodes, (5) aortopulmonary nodes, (6) anterior mediastinal nodes, (7) subcarinal nodes, (8) paraesophageal (below carina) nodes, (9) pulmonary ligament nodes, (10) tracheobronchial angle nodes, (11–14) intrapulmonary nodes. (nodal stations 1 and 3 are not shown.) Adapted from Naruke T, Suemasu K, Ishikawa S. Lymph node mapping and curability at various levels of metastasis in resected lung cancer. J Thorac Cardiovasc Surg 76:832–839, 1978

TABLE 4–1. NODAL STATIONS FOR STAGING LUNG CANCER

Superior mediastinal nodes		
	2 (R or L)	Upper paratracheal*
	4 (R or L)	Lower paratracheal*
	10 (R or L)	Tracheobronchial angle*
Aortic nodes		
	5	Aortopulmonary*
	6	Anterior mediastinal*
Inferior mediastinal nodes		
	7	Subcarinal (ipsilateral to both sides)*
	8 (R or L)	Paraesophageal
	9 (R or L)	Pulmonary ligament
Intrapulmonary nodes		
	11 (R or L)	Interlobar
	12 (R or L)	Lobar
	13 (R or L)	Segmental
	14 (R or L)	Subsegmental
N0	No regional lymph node spread	
N1	Metastasis to ipsilateral intrapulmonary nodes (11, 12, 13, 14)	
N2	Metastasis to ipsilateral superior mediastinal (2, 4, 10), ipsilateral aortic (5, 6), or ipsilateral inferior mediastinal nodes (7, 8, 9)	
N3	Metastasis to contralateral lymph nodes, ipsilateral or contralateral scalene nodes, or supraclavicular nodes	

*Indicates nodal stations evaluable by mediastinoscopy.

demonstration of mediastinal nodal enlargement by CT is an absolute indication for mediastinoscopy.

We believe that there are additional relative indications for mediastinoscopy. Although patients with N2 disease were treated nonoperatively in the past, recent studies show that neoadjuvant chemotherapy improves resectability, results in pathologic downstaging, and may lead to improved survival, thus transforming the goal of mediastinoscopy from merely determining feasibility of resection to also identifying patients with Stage IIIA disease who might benefit from preresectional chemotherapy. Although the rate of false-positive CT scans leads to the absolute need for mediastinoscopy in the setting of CT-demonstrated nodal enlargement, the chance of a false-negative CT result also affects the decision to perform mediastinoscopy. Because surgical resection of N2 disease results in poor survival and neoadjuvant therapy might be especially useful among patients with microscopic N2 disease, identification of the patients with false-negative CT scans should improve therapeutic outcome. Therefore, the presence of predicters of increased risk of mediastinal spread serves as a relative indication for mediastinoscopy.

Increased risk of mediastinal spread, regardless of CT findings, is noted with large (>3-cm) tumors and centrally located tumors. CT detection of mediastinal spread has an accuracy of 79% for central tumors vs. 90% for peripheral tumors, whereas the frequency of mediastinal spread for central and peripheral lesions is 37% and 15%, respectively. The histologic subtype of the primary tumor is also a predictor of the risk of mediastinal spread, with N2 metastasis occurring in only 19% of those with squamous histology, compared with 35% of patients with adenocarcinoma, 46% with large cell carcinoma, and 65% with small cell carcinoma.

Mediastinoscopy also plays a vital role when a needle biopsy of a peripheral nodule reveals small cell cytology. Because cells of neuroendocrine phenotypes may appear cytologically similar but are treated quite differently, mediastinoscopy provides tissue for accurate pathologic diagnosis, thereby avoiding treating a well-differentiated neuroendocrine tumor with modalities appropriate for small cell lung cancer.

In the clinical setting of more than one primary tumor, the highest-stage lesion determines prognosis. Thus, accurate staging in this circumstance requires determination of mediastinal nodal involvement.

Hoarseness resulting from vocal cord paralysis may be secondary to left recurrent laryngeal nerve compression by aortic nodal enlargement. This also represents a relative indication for mediastinoscopy.

In addition to the presence of a predictor of increased risk of mediastinal lymph node metastasis, a final relative indication for mediastinoscopy is the intent to enroll a patient in a clinical trial comparing treatments for Stage IIIA and/or Stage IIIB disease. Inaccurate staging, and the resulting mix of patients with N2 and N3 disease would lead to a loss of homogeneity among staged groups and might alter the results or mask improved therapeutic outcomes for a specific stage.

In summary, we advocate mediastinoscopy for the following relative indications:

1. Anticipated use of neoadjuvant regimen.
2. Large primary lesion (>3 cm, *i.e.*, T2 or T3).
3. Primary lesion located in the central one third of the thorax.
4. Biopsy-proven adenocarcinoma or large cell carcinoma.
5. Stage I lesion with small cell cytology.
6. Multiple primary lung masses.
7. Left vocal cord paralysis.

TECHNIQUE

Mediastinoscopy is typically performed in the operating room while the patient is under general anesthesia. For most lesions, cervical mediastinoscopy is the procedure of choice. However, if a left upper-lobe mass is present, anterior mediastinoscopy, as described by McNeill and Chamberlain, is the initial procedure because the subaortic and aortopulmonary (Levels 5 and 6) nodes are not accessible *via* the suprasternal incision. Some thoracic surgeons advocate the use of video-assisted thoracoscopic surgery for biopsy of these nodes draining the left upper lobe. If the Level 5 or 6 nodes exhibit metastatic involvement, resection is deferred and cervical mediastinoscopy is performed to evaluate the N3 nodes.

For cervical mediastinoscopy, the patient is placed supine with the neck extended. A 3-cm horizontal incision is made superior to the suprasternal notch. Dissection is carried down through the pretracheal fascia. The surgeon's finger is inserted, and digital dissection anterior to the trachea results in minimal hemorrhage and allows access into the mediastinum for palpation.

The cervical mediastinoscope is then inserted. The sucker tip is the only instrument used for dissection within the mediastinum because of the risk of injuring vascular structures with sharp objects. The appropriate nodes are then biopsied with forceps. After biopsy of the paratracheal (Levels 2 and 4) and tracheobronchial angle (Level 10) nodes, the subcarinal nodes (Level 7, which are considered ipsilateral to both sides) are biopsied. Nodes need not be removed in their entirety. In fact, removing an intact node makes disruption of its vascular pedicle more likely, and more bleeding will occur. Small biopsy samples are sufficient for both frozen and permanent sections. In the rare case that significant hemorrhage is encountered, the scope is left in place to facilitate tamponade of the bleeding vessels. If packing and hemostatic materials do not result in hemostasis, or if hemorrhage is significant, thoracotomy should be performed on the side ipsilateral to the lesion to allow subsequent resection. Fortunately, the complication rate of cervical mediastinoscopy is low. A retrospective review of 1000 mediastinoscopies at Toronto General Hospital demonstrated a morbidity of 2.3% and no mortality.

THORACOSCOPY

Thoracoscopy has been performed by thoracic surgeons for over 50 years, usually for the diagnosis of pleural disease and for treatment of effusions and empyemas. Recent advances in fiberoptic, video, and instrument technology have significantly increased the number of applications of the technique. Thoracoscopy allows visualization of the complete visceral and parietal pleural surface, provides access for biopsy of lung parenchyma, and facilitates biopsy of mediastinal masses. Three or four small incisions suffice where, in the past, a large thoracotomy was necessary. If therapeutic resection is performed, a limited thoracotomy is sufficient. The small incisions are much less painful and result in shorter hospital stays and minimal loss of pulmonary function.

TECHNIQUE

Thoracoscopy should be performed in the operating room, while the patient is under general anesthesia, by a thoracic surgeon because rapid conversion to thoracotomy may be required. A double-lumen endotracheal tube is inserted, and single-lung ventilation of the contralateral lung is maintained while atelectasis of the ipsilateral lung is achieved when pneuomothorax is induced. Insufflation is rarely necessary. Trocars are introduced through small, 2- to 3-cm incisions. Location of ports anteriorly, laterally, and posteriorly permit different angles of access and facilitate "triangulation," allowing efficient manipulation of anatomical structures. Endoscopic instruments, including the camera, electrocautery, grasping forceps, scissors, clip applicators, and staplers, may be shifted between trocars to provide different views and appropriate angles for instrument use. Video monitoring with the camera provides excellent visualization for the surgeon and assistants. Once the procedure is completed, a chest tube is left in place through one trocar site and is typically removed the following day. The use of thoracoscopic surgery reduces the length of hospital stay as well as duration of recovery.

Common indications for thoracoscopy include lung, mediastinal, pleural, and pericardial disease when tissue diagnosis is required. Bullous disease, pericoronal and pleural effusions, and peripheral lung nodules may be treated by using thoracoscopic techniques. Video-assisted thoracoscopic surgery, using a limited thoracotomy, allows for pulmonary resection. It also has been used to assist in esophageal procedures, including esophagectomy, vagotomy, staging of esophageal cancers, and in the treatment of severe gastroesophageal reflux disease or achalasia. As the techniques improve, other indications for thoracoscopic surgery will certainly evolve.

REFERENCES

1. Carlens E. Mediastinoscopy: A method for inspection and tissue biopsy in the superior mediastinum. Dis Chest 36:343–352, 1959
2. Daniels AC. A method of biopsy useful in diagnosing certain intrathoracic diseases, Dis Chest 16:360–367, 1949
3. Faber LP, Warren WH. Endoscopic examinations. In Shields TW (ed). General Thoracic Surgery. 3rd ed. Philadelphia, Lea & Febiger, 1989:245–264
4. Harken DE, Black H, Clauss R, Farrand RE. A simple cervicomediastinal exploration for tissue diagnosis of intrathoracic disease. With comments on the recognition of inoperable carcinoma of the lung. N Engl J Med 251:1041–1044, 1954
5. Luke WP, Pearson FG, Todd TRJ et al. Prospective evaluation of mediastinoscopy for assessment of carcinoma of the lung. J Thorac Cardiovasc Surg 91:53–56, 1986
6. McNeill TM, Chamberlain JM. Diagnostic anterior mediastinotomy. Ann Thorac Surg 2:532–539, 1966
7. Mentzer SJ, Sugarbaker DJ. Thoracoscopy and video-assisted thoracic surgery. In Brooks DC (ed). Current Techniques in Laparoscopy. Philadelphia, Current Medicine, 1994: 20.1–20.12
8. Mountain CF. A new international staging system for lung cancer. Chest 89(suppl):225S–233S, 1986
9. Naruke T, Suemasu K, Ishikawa S. Lymph node mapping and curability at various levels of metastasis in resected lung cancer. J Thorac Cardiovasc Surg 76:832–839, 1978
10. Sugarbaker DJ, Mentzer SJ, Strauss G et al. Laser resection of endobronchial lesions: Use of the rigid and flexible bronchoscopes. Oper Tech Otolaryngol Head Neck Surg 3:93–97, 1992

John S. Macdonald, Daniel G. Haller, Robert J. Mayer, Eds. *Manual of Oncologic Therapeutics*, Third Edition.

5. LOWER GASTROINTESTINAL ENDOSCOPY

Ira Kelberman
Benjamin Krevsky

Endoscopic evaluation of the lower gastrointestinal tract generally refers to flexible sigmoidoscopy or colonoscopy (Figure 5–1). These procedures are performed with flexible fiberoptic or electronic video endoscopes. The two procedures differ in the extent of examination and requirements for patient preparation and care.

Flexible sigmoidoscopy has replaced rigid proctosigmoidoscopy for most diagnostic examinations. The flexible sigmoidoscope is more comfortable for patients and affords a more comprehensive visual examination of the rectum and sigmoid colon. The flexible sigmoidoscope is useful for diagnostic examinations and therapeutic procedures in the distal colon. This procedure is rapid and requires minimal patient preparation.

Colonoscopy refers to the endoscopic examination of the entire large intestine, allowing for diagnoses and therapeutics from cecum to anal canal. In addition, the terminal ileum may often be evaluated via intubation of the ileocecal valve. Unlike sigmoidoscopy, colonoscopy requires a complete bowel preparation, conscious sedation, and cardiorespiratory monitoring. The procedure usually takes from 30 minutes to 1 hour to complete.

INDICATIONS

The indications for lower gastrointestinal endoscopy may be classified as diagnostic, therapeutic, or cancer screening.

For diagnostic purposes, flexible sigmoidoscopy is useful for evaluation of disease processes limited to the distal colon. Examples include assessment of anal discomfort, minor rectal bleeding (in adults under 35 years of age), evaluation of diarrhea, and examination of distal colonic anastomoses.

Diagnostic colonoscopy is used to investigate gastrointestinal bleeding clinically manifest by gross blood, melena, or occult bleeding. Because the gastrointestinal tract is the most common site of blood loss, colonoscopy is used to evaluate unexplained iron deficiency anemia. Colonoscopy is useful in evaluating inflammatory bowel disease, when information regarding severity or biopsy verification of diagnosis is needed for treatment decisions, or for cancer surveillance. Chronic diarrhea of uncertain etiology should be evaluated by colonoscopy. Abnormalities found on lower gastrointestinal barium studies should be investigated by colonoscopy to verify the abnormality and to establish a tissue diagnosis.

The timing and best method for colon cancer screening and surveillance remain controversial. However, flexible sigmoidoscopy and colonoscopy remain the cornerstones for identifying and treating patients with colonic neoplasia. The American Cancer Society recommends flexible sigmoidoscopy in asymptomatic patients without significant risk factors for colon cancer starting at age 50, with follow-up examinations every 3 to 5 years. Patients with a history of colonic neoplasia, ulcerative colitis, or Crohn's colitis, or a strong family history of colon cancer, require periodic complete colonoscopy for adequate surveillance of colon cancer and polyps. Although some authorities have recommended screening colonoscopy in asymptomatic adults, this concept has not been generally accepted.

Therapeutic interventions via lower gastrointestinal endoscopy are performed with a colonoscope. The flexible sigmoidoscope is used only where treatment will be limited to the sigmoid colon or rectum or in patients who have undergone significant colonic resections. Colonoscopy is used for removal of colonic polyps by snare electrocautery or "hot" biopsy forceps. Various modalities for cautery of bleeding colonic lesions may be implemented with a colonoscope. These include monopolar and bipolar electrocautery, the heater probe, laser, or local injection therapy with agents such as epinephrine. Palliation of obstructing colonic tumors can be performed through the colonoscope using laser energy. Other therapeutic interventions afforded by the colonoscopy include decompression of severe colonic dilatation, removal of foreign bodies, and reduction of colonic volvulus.

CONTRAINDICATIONS

General contraindications to flexible sigmoidoscopy or colonoscopy include an uncooperative patient or medical instability in which the risk of the procedure outweighs the benefit of endoscopic intervention. Lower intestinal endoscopy is generally contraindicated in patients with a perforated viscus, severe acute diverticulitis, or fulminant colitis.

RISKS AND COMPLICATIONS

The risks of colonoscopy include cardiopulmonary as well as gastrointestinal complications. Hypotension and hypoventilation may be precipitated by the agents used for intravenous sedation. Hypotension and bradycardia may result from vagal stimulation during colonoscopic manipulation. Abdominal

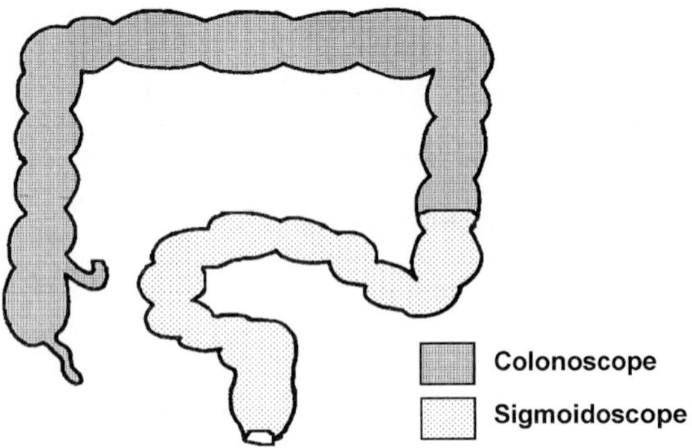

Figure 5–1. Anatomy of the colon and extent of examinations. The flexible sigmoidoscope permits visualization of the distal lower intestine, as indicated by the light shading. The colonoscope permits examination of the entire colon, as indicated by the dark shading, in addition to the area observed on sigmoidoscopy.

discomfort from colonic distention or endoscope movement is not uncommon, but it is usually transient. Significant bleeding occurs in only about 1% of polypectomies and may present up to 14 days after the procedure. Perforation may be caused by pressure at the endoscope tip, at the apex of a "loop" formed by the shaft of the colonoscope, at cautery sites following polypectomy, or by gaseous overdistention. The overall complication rate for diagnostic colonoscopy is less than 1%, with complication rates of about 1% for procedures involving polypectomy.

THE PROCEDURE

For flexible sigmoidoscopy, an overnight fast and two phosphate enemas given within 2 hours of the examination are adequate preparation. Colonoscopy, however, requires a complete bowel cleansing. One of two bowel preps is commonly used: either a polyethylene glycol-electrolyte solution for gut lavage (*e.g.*, Golytely or Colyte) or an oral sodium phosphate bowel prep (*e.g.*, Fleet Phospho-soda). The former is safer for patients who cannot tolerate sodium or phosphate loads or fluid/volume shifts, but it requires a larger volume ingestion.

Pre-procedure laboratory tests include a complete blood count and coagulation parameters (PT/PTT). Other laboratory tests are obtained as dictated by the patient's medical history. Informed consent is obtained by careful explanation of the procedure, the indications, and the risk of complications to the patient.

Because of the risks of sedation and the procedure itself, heart rate, blood pressure, and pulse oxymetry monitoring in addition to nurse and physician observation are recommended during colonoscopy. Vital sign monitoring is not necessary during flexible sigmoidoscopy. For colonoscopy intravenous access is also essential, allowing for administration of sedation and maintenance of access for emergency administration of drugs, fluids, or blood products.

Antibiotic prophylaxis is used during colonoscopy in patients with known valvular heart disease, implanted prosthetic devices, or immune compromise. Oral antibiotics (*e.g.*, amoxicillin) or intravenous regimens (*e.g.*, ampicillin and gentamycin) may be used depending on patient circumstance. Vancomycin is substituted for ampicillin in penicillin-allergic patients.

Sedation is rarely required for flexible sigmoidoscopy. Conscious sedation is used during colonoscopy. Combinations of narcotic analgesic (*e.g.*, meperidine or fentanyl) and a benzodiazepine (*e.g.*, midazolam or diazepam) are used. The level of sedation is titrated to the individual patient.

Colonoscopy and flexible sigmoidoscopy are begun with the patient in the left lateral decubitus position. Following a careful digital rectal examination to assess for the presence of stool or masses, the endoscope tip is inserted. Advancement of the endoscope is achieved by multiple manipulations. Because the anatomy of the colon includes flexures and angulations, various techniques of advancement (torque, "jiggling," application of external abdominal pressure, changing patient position) are used to thread the instrument proximally.

During advancement and careful withdrawal of the colonoscope, direct visualization of the mucosa is achieved. This permits the identification of any abnormalities. Pathologic examination may also be provided because the suction/instrument channel of the endoscope allows the passage of biopsy forceps. Therapeutic interventions are performed by the introduction of forceps, snares, coagulation probes, injection catheters, or laser fibers through the colonoscope channel. In addition, new imaging techniques are being developed for use during colonoscopy. Endoscopic ultrasonography or spectral analyses (for processing reflected light) may be used for better characterization of mass and vascular lesions.

Patients undergoing flexible sigmoidoscopy rarely require postprocedure care and are free to resume their normal activities and diet immediately after the procedure. After colonoscopy, patients are observed for signs of altered blood pressure, hypoventilation, perforation, and bleeding. During recovery from sedation, the patient is progressively advanced from stretcher, to semirecumbent position, to ambulation before discharge. Reversal agents such as naloxone or flumazenil may be used in more deeply sedated individuals. The patient is advised not to drive a motor vehicle or operate machinery on the same day. Diet and activity are advanced as rapidly as tolerated. Patients are instructed to contact their physician should signs of a complication evolve, and appropriate medical follow-up is arranged.

BIBLIOGRAPHY

American Society for Gastrointestinal Endoscopy. Appropriate use of gastrointestinal endoscopy. Manchester, MA, August, 1992, pp. 1–11

Blackstone MO. Endoscopic Interpretation. New York, Raven Press, 401–421, 1984

Cotton PB, Williams CB. Practical Gastrointestinal Endoscopy. 3rd edition. Oxford, Blackwell Scientific Publications, 1990

Drossman DA. Manual of Gastroenterologic Procedures. 3rd ed. New York, Raven Press, 1993

Keefe EB, Schrock TR. Complications of Gastrointestinal Endoscopy. In Sleisenger MH, Fordtran JS (eds). Gastrointestinal Disease. 5th ed. Philadelphia, WB Saunders, 301–308, 1993

John S. Macdonald, Daniel G. Haller, Robert J. Mayer, Eds. *Manual of Oncologic Therapeutics*, Third Edition.

6. UPPER GASTROINTESTINAL ENDOSCOPY

Benjamin Krevsky

The field of gastrointestinal endoscopy (from the Greek *skopeo*, to examine, and *endon*, within) has made astounding advances in the past decade. Only 10 years ago, all endoscopes contained fiberoptic bundles for imaging and were rather thick. While at the time these were excellent diagnostic tools, their therapeutic capabilities were quite limited. Instruments of the day permitted examination of the esophagus, stomach, and duodenum but left most of the small intestine unexamined.

Current instruments are highly sophisticated and extremely useful in the diagnosis and management of cancer involving the upper gastrointestinal tract. Contemporary gastroscopes either use fiberoptic imaging systems or state-of-the-art miniature video cameras. The cameras, located at the leading edge of the instrument, permit a high-resolution digital image to be obtained. This image can be displayed on a video monitor for several people or an entire auditorium to watch at once. The procedure is easily videotaped for later review, for example, for a surgeon to review preoperatively. High-quality photographic images can be obtained immediately for documentation, as a basis for later comparison, and for patient education. The instruments are much thinner today. While standard instruments in the early 1980s were 11 mm (35 Fr) in diameter, they are now 9 mm (28 Fr) in diameter. Gastroscopes as thin as 7 mm (23 Fr) are occasionally used. Therapeutic endoscopy — for hemostasis, tumor ablation, occlusion of tracheoesophageal fistulas, dilation, and other procedures — is now commonly performed. Finally, instruments have been developed, such as enteroscopes, which can extend the range of the endoscope beyond the ligament of Treitz, all the way to the terminal ileum.

INDICATIONS

The general indications for upper gastrointestinal endoscopy (esophagogastroduodenoscopy) are too numerous to list in their entirety. The major indications can be broken down into two classes: diagnostic and therapeutic.

Endoscopy is a simple, relatively safe, and effective means for obtaining diagnostic information and tissue samples in patients with upper gastrointestinal malignancies. The ability to obtain biopsy specimens under direct visual control for histopathological examination and brush cytology specimens has permitted a 95% diagnostic yield. The occasional examinations in which specimens show negative results are usually in submucosal lesions. Fortunately, repeat attempts are often successful. Also, endoscopists have recently started using needle biopsy techniques for deep lesions, similar to those already in use for bronchoscopy. While some practitioners obtain barium studies prior to endoscopy, most are going straight to endoscopy to start the diagnostic, staging, and tumor grading process.

Esophagogastroduodenoscopy is commonly used to make a definitive diagnosis when an abnormal upper gastrointestinal series has been obtained from a symptomatic patient. In addition to the ability to obtain tissue specimens, the endoscopist can determine the anatomical position of a tumor, its length, and the degree of luminal compromise. Although endoscopy is often used as a first-line study in the investigation of upper gastrointestinal complaints such as dyspepsia, early satiety, anorexia, and epigastric pain, most authorities still recommend a barium esophagram as the first diagnostic test in dysphagia.

There are numerous other diagnostic uses for esophagogastroduodenoscopy. One is the evaluation of iron deficiency anemia, especially if the lower gastrointestinal tract is normal. Acute gastrointestinal hemorrhage is occasionally from a tumor, although chronic hemorrhage with iron deficiency is the more common presentation. Endoscopy is useful in the evaluation of a patient with known cancer but a new symptom, to search for metastases or new tumors. Esophagogastroduodenoscopy is performed both at the time of diagnosis of a gastric ulcer to rule out cancer and again at healing. The inflammation surrounding an ulcerated cancer sometimes leads to negative biopsy results; however, after 4 to 6 weeks of therapy, a repeat biopsy may be positive for cancer. Endoscopy is useful to assess the efficacy of treatment, whether surgery, radiation, or chemotherapy and also to evaluate for the complications of therapy (*e.g.*, mucositis, stricture, and so forth).

Surveillance is an important use of endoscopy. The classic example is Barrett's epithelium. While the precise surveillance schedule remains controversial, it is clear that Barrett's epithelium is a premalignant lesion. Regular endoscopy with multiple biopsies can often detect the high-grade dysplasia that is premonitory to, or even coincident with, adenocarcinoma. Other indications for surveillance include achalasia or a prior history of adenomatous polyps of the upper gastrointestinal tract.

Therapeutic endoscopy has become a major adjunct to surgery, chemotherapy, and radiation therapy in the care of cancer patients. Energy can be applied through an endoscope in many forms. Electrocautery energy, similar to the surgical Bovie can be applied through the instrument channel. This energy can be used to cut, as in a polypectomy; to cauterize, as in hemorrhage; or to ablate, as in intraluminal reduction of tumor size. The heater probe, a small nonstick capsule with a heating element inside, is useful for the control of bleeding. The laser — in particular the Neodymium: Yttrium Aluminum Garnet (Nd:YAG) laser — is a form of high-energy infrared light, which can be applied under direct vision with high precision. At low energy levels, it coagulates tissue. At higher energy levels, it vaporizes tissue almost instantly.

Control of bleeding has become an important use of endoscopy. Gastric adenocarcinomas, esophageal cancers, and leiomyosarcomas are all known to bleed. This bleeding can be controlled in a matter of minutes with electrocautery, the heater probe, or a laser.

Management of stenoses is often a problem in upper gastrointestinal tract cancer. These can arise at the site of surgical anastomoses, from radiation, from infiltration of tumor (*e.g.*, from a pulmonary primary tumor), or from the primary tumor itself. Dilation can be performed successfully with mercury-filled bougies, or tapered wire-guided plastic dilators (Savary type). When the stenosis is too tortuous or narrow, through-the-scope balloon dilators can be used under direct vision. While dilation is highly successful for radiation strictures, its effectiveness is often short-lived in cancerous stenoses. In such cases, the laser has proven a valuable tool for opening the lumen quickly, safely, and effectively. Prolongation of survival has been demonstrated in esophageal cancer through the use of laser tumor ablation. Electrocautery can also be used for this purpose, but experience with this technique is much more limited than with the laser.

When the laser is not available, or a tracheoesophageal fistula is present, stents can be inserted into the esophagus. These are plastic tubes inserted after dilatation, so that the swallowed food and medications bypass the tumor or fistula, permitting the resumption of oral intake. Unfortunately, the insertion of stents is a high-risk procedure, and they tend to migrate. Also, because of their limited size (11 mm or less internal diameter), the patient usually can only eat a puréed diet. Anything more solid is apt to get stuck.

The percutaneous endoscopic gastrostomy (PEG) is an important adjunct in the nutritional management of cancer patients. It is inserted endoscopically and can be used for nutritional support in about 24 hours. The presence of a PEG permits many patients to switch from parenteral to enteral nutrition. It also ensures that nutritional support can be maintained during periods of anorexia or when the esophagus is blocked. When no longer needed, removal is usually a simple, nonendoscopic procedure.

Foreign bodies are a common problem in patients with esophageal cancers, resulting in a complete obstruction. In most cases, the foreign body is an inadequately chewed piece of meat. These objects can be removed from the area of narrowing with an endoscopic snare, forceps, or basket, and an overtube to protect the airway. The use of a Foley catheter to pull out an impaction is not recommended, since the object can easily fall into the trachea, thus converting an esophageal occlusion into an airway occlusion.

CONTRAINDICATIONS

The contraindications to esophagogastroduodenoscopy are few and, on the whole, broad. In general, the procedure is contraindicated when the risk to the patient's life or health outweighs the potential benefits of the procedure. More specific contraindications include lack of cooperation and a perforation that is highly suspected or known to have occurred.

RISKS AND COMPLICATIONS

Esophagogastroduodenoscopy is well tolerated even in elderly and debilitated patients. The use of conscious sedation, extracorporeal monitoring, and the availability of reversal agents permit the performance of endoscopy with a high degree of comfort and safety. Although complications do occur, the risk of a major complication such as perforation is about 1 in 1000. Complications can be secondary to the medications used, aspiration, cardiac events, infections, and therapeutic misadventures. Specifically, complications may include perforation, hemorrhage, distention, pacemaker dysfunction, endocarditis, aspiration pneumonia, hypoxemia, hypotension, and myocardial infarction (among others).

THE PROCEDURE

Patient preparation for the procedure is individualized and helps ensure a safe and effective outcome. Knowing the indication for the procedure, in light of the underlying illness(es), allows the endoscopist to be prepared for all eventualities. Meeting with the patient beforehand also permits a rapport to develop, which is highly beneficial for allaying anxiety and reducing the amount of sedative required.

Before the procedure, a coagulation profile is obtained, with particular attention to the patient's history. Depending on the circumstances, tests ranging from only a complete blood count (CBC) to a whole profile including manual platelet count, prothrombin time (PT), partial thromboplastin time (PTT), and bleeding time may be appropriate. Nonsteroidal anti-inflammatory drugs (NSAIDs) and aspirin are discontinued for a week if possible. Endocarditis prophylaxis is administered in the presence of immunosuppression, prosthetic valves, prior endocarditis, and prior rheumatic fever. The route (oral vs. intravenous) and type of antibiotics depend on the individual patient's circumstances.

After a fast of at least 8 hours (longer if obstructed), the patient is brought to the endoscopy suite where informed consent is obtained. Intravenous sedation is administered by the endoscopist with monitoring. Rarely is general anesthesia used. Albeit sedated, the patient is usually able to answer questions during the procedure. A spray to numb the oropharyngeal mucosa is administered. The patient is positioned in the left lateral decubitus position, and the tip of the endoscope is inserted into the mouth through a "bite block." Under direct observation, the instrument is advanced through the esophagus, stomach, and pylorus, to the duodenum. The gut is then examined again on withdrawal of the instrument, and any biopsies or therapeutic maneuvers are performed. A typical diagnostic examination takes about 10 minutes.

POSTPROCEDURE CARE

After the examination or treatment, the patient is brought to a recovery area and is monitored while the sedation wears off. Reversal agents are sometimes administered, most commonly naloxone for meperidine and flumazenil for diazepam or midazolam. The patient does not have anything to eat or drink for about 2 hours because of the risk of aspiration. Since the effects of sedation may last several hours despite a sense of well-being, a friend or relative is asked to help the patient get home. Operation of motor vehicles or dangerous equipment is proscribed for 12 to 24 hours.

ENTEROSCOPY

Enteroscopy is a new application of upper gastrointestinal endoscopy which can lengthen the extent of examination all the way to the terminal ileum. Three major types of enteroscopy have evolved: sonde, "push," and intraoperative.

Intraoperative enteroscopy has been performed for years, using colonoscopes. After a laparotomy is performed, the instrument is introduced through the mouth or an incision in the duodenum. The surgeon then passes the instrument manually while the endoscopist observes intraluminally. The development of effective sonde and push enteroscopes should make the use of intraoperative enteroscopy less commonplace.

Sonde enteroscopy utilizes a long thin endoscope that is passed nasally and allowed to pass by peristaltic action to the distal ileum. Preparation and performance of the procedure are much like that for routine upper gastrointestinal endoscopy. However, unlike the 10-minute esophagogastroduodenoscopy, sonde enteroscopy may take 4 to 6 hours.

Push enteroscopy uses a specially modified gastroscope that is approximately 2500 cm in length. This instrument permits an excellent examination of the upper gastrointestinal tract to a distance of about 100 cm past the ligament of Treitz. Biopsy, electrocautery, and laser therapy are all possible with this instrument. While much faster than the sonde examination (only 30 to 45 minutes), it is also less comprehensive.

BIBLIOGRAPHY

American Society for Gastrointestinal Endoscopy. Appropriate use of gastrointestinal endoscopy. Manchester, MA, August, 1992:1–11

Cotton PB, Williams CB. Practical Gastrointestinal Endoscopy. 3rd ed. Oxford, Blackwell Scientific Publications, 1990

Gilbert DA, Buelow RG, Chung RSK et al. Status evaluation: enteroscopy. Gastrointest Endosc 37:673–677, 1991

Keefe EB, Schrock TR. Complications of gastrointestinal endoscopy. In Sleisenger MH, Fordtran JS (eds.). Gastrointestinal Disease: Pathophysiology, Diagnosis, Management. 5th ed. Philadelphia, W.B. Saunders, 1993: 301–308

Krevsky B. Enteroscopy: exploring the final frontier. Gastroenterology 100:838–844, 1991

Krevsky B. Palliation of advanced esophageal cancer: a (laser) light at the end of the tunnel. Gastroenterology 101: 1748–1750, 1991

Sivak MV Jr, ed: Gastroenterologic Endoscopy. Philadelphia, WB Saunders, 1987

John S. Macdonald, Daniel G. Haller, Robert J. Mayer, Eds. *Manual of Oncologic Therapeutics*, Third Edition.

7. ENDOSCOPIC RETROGRADE CHOLANGIO-PANCREATOGRAPHY

Marta A. Dabezies
Benjamin Krevsky

Endoscopic retrograde cholangiopancreatography (ERCP) is a specialized adaptation of gastrointestinal endoscopy. It is performed with a side-viewing instrument, thus allowing a direct view of the papilla of Vater which is located on the medial wall of the second portion of the duodenum. Once identified, the papilla can be cannulated using a catheter inserted through the biopsy channel of the endoscope, and radiopaque contrast can be instilled into the pancreatic and biliary ductal systems. A variety of diagnostic and therapeutic instruments can be introduced into either ductal system in a similar manner.

INDICATIONS

ERCP provides detailed diagnostic information about the duodenum, biliary system, and pancreas, and also provides access to the ductal systems for nonoperative therapy, especially for patients with obstructive jaundice. ERCP is frequently used to further delineate abnormalities noted on computed tomography or ultrasonography, such as dilated biliary ducts or pancreatic enlargement. It is the study of choice in patients with suspected ampullary carcinoma because it provides direct visualization of the papilla and the means to obtain biopsy specimens.

ERCP is frequently performed for the evaluation of the jaundiced patient. Not only can ERCP establish the presence or absence of obstruction, it can also define the site of obstruction. Biliary obstruction has many causes, including intrinsic tumor, stone disease, extrinsic compression from pancreatic carcinoma or chronic pancreatitis, inflammatory conditions such as sclerosing cholangitis, metastatic disease to the porta hepatis, ampullary lesions, and ductal injury from previous surgery or hepatic artery chemotherapy infusion. These entities can usually be differentiated by ERCP. When ERCP suggests the presence of malignant biliary obstruction, tissue samples can be obtained for biopsy and cytology.

ERCP is also useful in the evaluation of pancreatic disease. It is used to demonstrate ductal anatomy before surgery. It may also help to differentiate pancreatic cancer (which has an abrupt cut-off of the duct) from chronic pancreatitis (in which there is usually irregular ductal enlargement). Occasionally the pancreatogram in patients with acute or recurrent pancreatitis demonstrates congenital pancreatic anomalies such as pancreas divisum (incomplete fusion of the major and minor ductal systems).

The therapeutic applications of ERCP are as important as the diagnostic applications. This is particularly true for patients with obstructive jaundice, in whom successful palliation can be achieved in approximately 85% of cases. Patients with malignant strictures of the bile duct or occlusion secondary to adenopathy can be palliated by endoscopic stent placement. Conventional endoscopic stents range from 7 fr to 11.5 fr. These tend to become occluded by a combination of bacterial biofilm and biliary sludge, but can be expected to remain patent for 3 to 6 months. Expandable metal stents with a diameter of 1 cm have recently been introduced. Unfortunately these may also occlude due to a combination of mucosal hyperplasia and biliary sludge. Expandable metal stents probably maintain luminal patency in the biliary tree somewhat longer than conventional plastic stents. Whether this justifies their increased cost remains to be seen. Balloon dilation of biliary strictures can also be performed but is somewhat more successful for benign than malignant strictures. When temporary drainage is required, a nasobiliary catheter can be inserted endoscopically. This allows bile flow to be measured and provides access to the bile duct for repeated cholangiograms.

CONTRAINDICATIONS

Because ERCP is an extension of upper gastrointestinal endoscopy, the only contraindications are those applying to esophagogastroduodenoscopy. These include recent myocardial infarction or cerebrovascular accident, in which setting ERCP may have an appreciable risk of a life-threatening cardiovascular complication, and obstruction of the pharynx or upper gastrointestinal tract rendering the procedure impossible. Small bowel obstruction, suspected perforation, and lack of patient cooperation are strong relative contraindications. A history of anaphylaxis to radiographic contrast agents is a relative contraindication, but patients with a history of milder allergic reactions can undergo ERCP safely using non-ionic contrast agents after pretreatment with corticosteroids and diphenhydramine.

RISKS AND COMPLICATIONS

The most common complication of ERCP is the development of postprocedure pancreatitis. Although elevated amylase can be seen in 67% of patients, presumably secondary to contrast-induced chemical irritation of the pancreas, clinically significant pancreatitis occurs in less than 3% to 5% of patients. Other complications include cholangitis, intestinal perforation, and cardiorespiratory complications similar to those seen in upper gastrointestinal endoscopy. When biliary obstruction is present, antibiotics are usually given before the procedure to diminish the risk of cholangitis. Sphincterotomy carries a slightly increased risk, including a 1% to 2% risk of hemorrhage or perforation.

THE PROCEDURE

ERCP can be divided into its endoscopic and radiologic portions. It may be performed in either the gastrointestinal endoscopy suite or in radiology, depending on the availability of high quality fluoroscopy and x-ray equipment within an institution. After an overnight fast, patients are sedated with a combination of intravenous narcotics and benzodiazepines in a manner similar to upper gastrointestinal endoscopy. The side-viewing endoscope is inserted blindly into the stomach and under direct vision into the duodenum. Once the papilla is identified, a 5 Fr catheter is inserted via the biopsy channel of the endoscope and radiopaque contrast is instilled under fluoroscopic guidance. Only enough contrast as is needed to demonstrate the ductal systems is used, as overfilling can lead to pain and complications.

If an abnormality that requires further intervention is detected, a sphincterotomy is usually performed by replacing the injection catheter with one that has an electrocautery wire near its tip. It is usually possible to make an incision up to 1 cm in length. This is ample to allow passage of cytology brushes and biopsy forceps, and to insert stents or remove stones. Most ERCP equipment can be inserted over a guide wire placed into the bile duct or pancreatic duct at the time of the initial cannulation.

POSTPROCEDURE CARE

Postprocedure care is identical to that given following upper gastrointestinal endoscopy, except that heavier doses of sedation may be required for ERCP and patients may require longer or more intensive monitoring. Patients may have significant abdominal distention from air insufflation and should be encouraged to pass gas. Any patient undergoing sphincterotomy or other invasive therapy should be monitored overnight in a hospital because of the risk of delayed complications such as hemorrhage.

BIBLIOGRAPHY

Bilbao MK, Dotter CT, Lee TG, Katon RM. Complications of endoscopic retrograde cholangiopancreatography (ERCP). A study of 10,000 cases. Gastroenterology 70:314, 1976

Cotton PB. Critical appraisal of therapeutic endoscopy in biliary tract diseases. Annual Review of Medicine 41:211, 1990

Cotton PB, Williams CB. Practical Gastrointestinal Endoscopy. 3rd ed. Oxford, Blackwell Scientific Publications, 1990

Domschke W, Foerster E. Endoscopic implantation of large-bore self-expanding biliary mesh stent. Gastrointest Endosc 36:55, 1990

John S. Macdonald, Daniel G. Haller, Robert J. Mayer, Eds. *Manual of Oncologic Therapeutics*, Third Edition.

8. ENDOSCOPIC ULTRASOUND

Benjamin Krevsky

There are times when contrast roentgenography, computed tomographic (CT) scanning, magnetic resonance imaging, transcutaneous ultrasound, and flexible endoscopy do not provide adequate information to clinically stage a lesion. Endoscopic ultrasound (EUS) — the marriage of the flexible endoscope with an ultrasound imaging system — was developed to fill that gap.

At present there are three type of endoscopic ultrasound imaging systems. The most prevalent system (Olympus America, Inc.) incorporates a rotating transducer into the most distal tip of an endoscope's insertion tube. After endoscopic visual control is used to place the transducer next to the area to be imaged, the transducer rotates, giving a 360° view of the region. The depth of image penetration depends on the frequency of ultrasound. Typically 7.5 or 12 MHz frequencies are used. Image detail is excellent to a depth of several centimeters. Usually, the various muscle layers of the gastrointestinal (GI) tract can be identified, and accurate staging comparable to histologic or surgical staging can be performed. Another system incorporates a static transducer at the endoscope tip (Pentax Precision Instrument Corporation). This system reduces motion artifact and permits Doppler blood flow measurement to be performed. Unfortunately, the 100° imaging sector makes it difficult to precisely identify the region being imaged. Miniaturized, thin probes (Fuginon and Microvasive, among others) can be inserted through the working channel of an endoscope to image a specific location with great precision. Because these probes can be manufactured to use higher frequencies they can obtain more detailed information. They also are advantageous because they are used with conventional endoscopes.

INDICATIONS

The primary use of endoscopic ultrasound is for staging at the time of diagnosis. Tumors of the esophagus, stomach, pancreas, small intestine, and colon can all be imaged with this technology. The intestinal wall is usually seen as a five-layered structure, representing the mucosa, muscularis mucosa, submucosa, lamina propria, and adventitia. Invasion through each layer can be identified (Figure 8–1). The concordance of EUS with surgery is 90% for tumor invasion and 84% for node detection. It is more accurate than CT scanning for the determination of invasion and nodes (CT scanning is less than 60% accurate compared to 84% for EUS).

Other uses for EUS are to evaluate for postoperative recurrence, guidance of biopsies, evaluation of subepithelial lesions (*e.g.*, lipomas), and evaluation of small pancreatic lesions.

Endoscopic ultrasound has few limitations, but these are clinically relevant. Assessment of the depth of invasion may be inaccurate in the presence of inflammation. Small nodes or microscopic metastases may not be detected. Large inflammatory nodes can be mistaken for cancerous nodes. The large scope size prevents full evaluation of lesions that are tightly stenotic. Limited penetration makes it difficult to see distant metastases. Finally, there is a long learning curve for the endoscopists who do the examination. Therefore, examinations are best performed in active centers that do a lot of these examinations.

CONTRAINDICATIONS

The contraindications for endoscopic ultrasound are the same as for routine diagnostic endoscopy. EUS is often done at the same time as the diagnostic procedure.

COMPLICATIONS AND RISKS

Worldwide experience with endoscopic ultrasound is small, but in general it appears to be as safe as routine diagnostic endoscopy. There have been several reported cases of perforation during passage through a tight stenosis. Also, the instillation of water to improve imaging can lead to electrolyte imbalance or aspiration.

THE PROCEDURE

Both the procedure itself and postprocedure care are similar to that for routine upper GI endoscopy or colonoscopy, according to the region being examined. No special preparation or medications are required. EUS adds about 10 to 15 minutes to the total examination time.

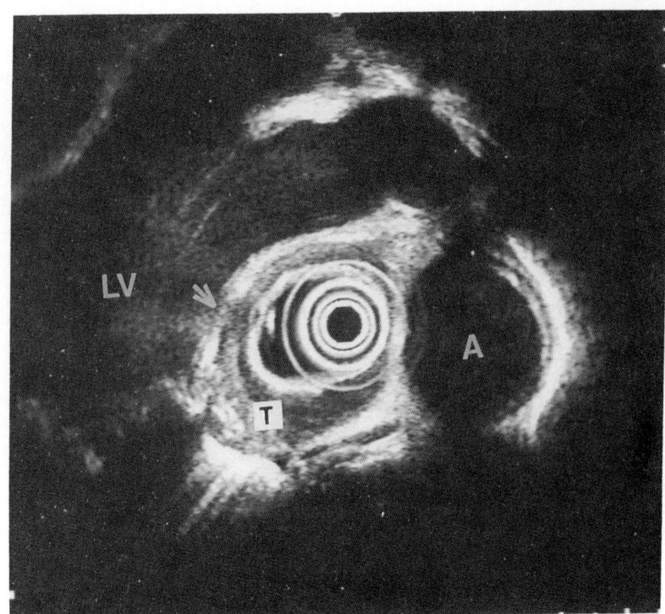

Figure 8–1. Endoscopic ultrasound image (12 MHz) from a patient with adenocarcinoma of the esophagus. The concentric white circles in the center of the field are artifacts of the transducer. *A*, aorta; *LV*, left ventricle; *T*, tumor. The arrow indicates invasion of the pericardium near the left ventricle by tumor.

BIBLIOGRAPHY

Botet JF, Lightdale C. Endoscopic sonography of the upper gastrointestinal tract. AJR 156:63–68, 1991

Botet JB, Lightdale DJ, Zauber AG et al. Preoperative staging of esophageal cancer: Comparison of endoscopic US and dynamic CT. Radiology 181:419–425, 1991

Gilbert DA, Marino AJ Jr, Jensen DM et al. Status evaluation: Endoscopic ultrasonography. Gastrointest Endosc 38:747–749, 1992

Lightdale CJ, Botet JF. Esophageal carcinoma: Pre-operative staging and evaluation of anastomotic recurrence. Gastrointest Endosc 36:S11–S16, 1990

Rösch T, Lorenz R, Classen M. Endoscopic ultrasonography in the evaluation of colon and rectal disease. Gastrointest Endosc 36:533–539, 1990

9. GENITOURINARY TRACT: PROCEDURES FOR DIAGNOSIS, BIOPSY, AND ENDOSCOPY

Jerome P. Richie

The accessibility of the lower urinary tract without requirement for an open surgical incision has differentiated urology from other surgical fields. Intervention may be for the purpose of diagnosis or for therapeutic intervention. Procedures may be performed under local anesthesia or may require regional or general anesthesia, depending on the complexity of the procedure. Availability of flexible fiberoptic endoscopes has facilitated bedside or office-based endoscopic procedures for the purpose of diagnosis.

Because manipulation of the urinary tract may result in significant injury, thorough knowledge of anatomy and careful attention to detail is essential. Prophylactic antibiotics may decrease the risk of sepsis, especially when the urinary tract is infected. Generous use of a water-soluble lubricant and low-pressure irrigation will minimize the likelihood of morbidity.

Direct visualization of both the anterior and posterior urethra as well as the bladder neck and bladder can be accomplished by cystourethroscopy. This procedure is used for the diagnosis of lower urinary tract disease and is an essential part of the evaluation for hematuria. Access to the upper urinary tract also can be accomplished cystoscopically. The most common indication for cystourethroscopy is for evaluation of microscopic or gross hematuria. The combination of endoscopic direct visualization with radiographic visualization allows one to determine the etiology of urinary tract bleeding in a substantial number of patients. Cystoscopic access to the upper tract can allow for a collection of specimens for cytology, access for brush biopsy, direct visualization by ureteroscopy, or injection of dilute contrast material through small catheters to visualize the ureter, renal pelvis, and calyces. With the addition of fluoroscopy, diagnostic and therapeutic procedures of the lower and upper urinary tract can be performed reliably.

URETHROSCOPY

Urethroscopy and cystoscopy can be performed using either rigid or flexible endoscopes. Advantages of rigid endoscopy include impressive optics secondary to the use of a rod lens system with solid rods to conduct light with minimal loss, ease of manipulation and orientation, a larger working channel for therapeutic intervention, and a larger intraluminal opening for better water flow with improved visualization. Especially in the patient with active bleeding, the ability to empty the bladder periodically as well as higher flow rates allows more effective visualization.

Flexible endoscopy has the advantages of greater comfort for the patient, ease of passage of the instrument, especially in patients with enlarged prostate or elevation of the bladder neck, and ability to visualize the anterior bladder and bladder neck by deflection of the tip of the instrument.

Especially in the male patient, inspection of the urethra with a straight-ahead or zero-degree telescopic lens can be helpful. Strictures or narrowing of the urinary tract can be identified, and short circumferential strictures may be incised under direct vision using a cold-knife urethrotome. An incision is generally made at 12 o'clock to minimize the risks of hemorrhage.

CYSTOSCOPY

The use of fiberoptic telescopes of varying size has allowed complete examination of the interior of the bladder. Urethroscopy as described above is performed using a straight-ahead or oblique (30°) lens, and inspection of the bladder is carried out with 30°, 70°, and 120° lenses to visualize the entire intravesical surface. The 30° lens allows one to inspect the base and anterolateral aspect of the bladder, whereas a 70° to 90° lens is used to view the bladder dome and part of the posterior wall. The anterior bladder neck and the posterior bladder neck in a patient with a median lobe or very enlarged prostate are visualized with a 120° lens. Suprapubic pressure will facilitate identification of abnormalities in the dome of the bladder.

At the beginning of endoscopy, urine can be obtained for cytological Papanicolaou (Pap) smear. Visualization of the entire intravesical mucosa is then performed to identify papillary or solid tumors. Increased vascularity may indicate carcinoma in situ. Flexible endoscopes may be used to diminish patient discomfort, but they lack a working sheath for biopsy capability. Inspection of the bladder should also include visualization of the ureteral orifices to evaluate the color of efflux of urine from each kidney as well as to evaluate the possibility of papillary tumors emerging from the ureteral orifice.

PERCUTANEOUS ENDOUROLOGY

Percutaneous access to the kidney was first described in 1955. With improvement in techniques and instrumentation, the percutaneous approach, in contrast to retrograde instrumentation, can give access for diagnosis and treatment of selected lesions. First and foremost, a percutaneous puncture route should be chosen for straight-forward access. The percutaneous placement, using either ultrasound, fluoroscopy, or occasionally computed tomographic (CT) scanning, allows access to the upper tract. Dilation by serial fascial dilators or balloon dilators will then allow placement of a larger rigid tube to allow for therapeutic interventions. In addition to treatment of benign disorders, percutaneous approaches have been described for resection of low-grade renal pelvic tumors in selected patients. Electroresection and electrocoagulation can be used, but more commonly, Neodymium:YAG laser coagulation is used for treatment of urothelial tumors in the renal pelvis. Recurrence rates have not yet been determined, but will certainly be higher in high grade lesions; therefore, this approach should be considered only in selected patients with low-grade tumors.

TRANSURETHRAL BIOPSY

Resectoscopes with a 26 to 28 Fr. sheath (8 to 9 mm in diameter) can be used for transurethral surgery to eradicate a transitional cell tumor of the bladder. A cold cup can be used to obtain specimens of mucosa for random biopsies to evaluate for dysplasia or carcinoma in situ. A wire cutting loop with electrocautery can be used to resect and fulgurate the tumors throughout the bladder. Resection of a bladder tumor should begin with a cold cup biopsy of the top of the tumor for histology without cautery artifact. Then the deeper portion of the tumor, along with some of the underlying bladder musculature, is resected and sent separately for pathologic review. In addition to resecting the tumor, a deep biopsy is obtained at the base to evaluate for the presence or absence of muscular invasion. Adequate hemostasis is essential.

With low-grade papillary tumors, simple fulguration of smaller lesions may suffice once histology has been obtained from some of the bladder tumors. Occasionally, laser therapy can be used for destruction of some of these bladder tumors, as discussed in the next section of this chapter. In patients with extensive broad-based and sessile-appearing tumors, complete resection may be difficult or impossible. Attempts at complete resection may lead to perforation, with potential spillage of tumor cells outside the bladder, converting the patient to a stage T3B or C tumor. In such cases, adequate resection into the muscle wall to document the presence of muscle invasion is sufficient. A tumor overlying the ureteral orifice should be resected without regard to the orifice. Fulguration should be limited, however, because of the possibility of scarring with subsequent obstruction. The ureteral stent may be left indwelling for several days or weeks after resection to allow healing.

Tumors that arise in a bladder diverticulum should be biopsied rather than resected completely. Because a diverticulum is an out-pouching of the bladder mucosa, muscle backing is minimal. Transurethral resection should not be attempted because of the high risk of bladder perforation.

LASER

Lasers can be used through flexible or rigid endoscopes. Many types of lasers have been used for the treatment of bladder tumors. Because laser energy may be selectively absorbed by tumors and vascular tissues, the argon laser has been used, but only for small tumors. The Neodymium:YAG laser has a penetration depth of up to 1.5 cm, and, therefore, can be used on larger tumors. This laser has adequate coagulation, but it does have more risk of injury because of its higher penetration. Neodymium:YAG laser has been used with reasonable tumor control. The disadvantage of the laser is the lack of adequate tissue for pathologic diagnosis.

PROSTATE

Carcinoma of the prostate is the most common malignancy in men, with an estimated 200,000 new cases and 38,000 deaths predicted for 1994. Although traditionally thought to be a disease of older men, with increased awareness prostate cancer has been diagnosed in men beginning in their late 30s. The incidence increases progressively until it reaches a peak in the eighth decade of life. A wide range of therapeutic options is available to individual patients.

The availability of prostate specific antigen, a protein serease bound to alpha-one antichymotripsin and circulating in the blood stream, has allowed earlier detection of prostate cancer. This blood test, coupled with the ease of biopsy under ultrasound guidance, has resulted in an increased ease of diagnosis of prostate cancer.

Transrectal ultrasonography is an efficient modality for evaluating the prostate and facilitating prostatic biopsy. The diagnosis of cancer on transrectal ultrasound is based on the hypoechoic appearance of prostatic nodules when viewed by ultrasound. The highly cellular compact nature of the malignancy minimizes the interface between cells, and, therefore, minimizes internal echoes. Not all prostate cancers, however, are hypoechoic; it is estimated that approximately 33% of prostate cancers may be isoechoic.

Ultrasonography can be used to visualize the prostate in both transaxial and sagittal planes. Separate or combined probes can be introduced into the rectum to allow visualization of the entire prostate, especially the peripheral zone in which most cancers arise. Biopsy can be performed using a spring-loaded device that allows an inner trocar to be advanced under ultrasound guidance. The rapidity of the procedure results in minimal patient discomfort, and, therefore, no need for anesthesia. High-quality samples can be obtained with a relatively low complication rate. The predominant complications are bleeding or infection. If a hypoechoic area is identified on ultrasound, this area can be biopsied directly under ultrasound guidance. In patients with elevated prostate-specific antigen but no palpable or visual abnormalities, biopsies can be taken from the base, middle, and apex of each side of the prostate, giving six sector biopsies to evaluate for the presence or absence of prostate cancer. In patients who have had negative biopsies in the past, the anterior or transition zone should be biopsied because of the remote possibility of prostatic cancer arising in this area.

The technique of ultrasonography has enhanced the ability to visualize the majority of the prostate, especially the peripheral zone. Ultrasonography, along with the spring-loaded biopsy gun, has increased the urologist's ability to accurately diagnose prostate cancer, generally in an earlier stage in which the disease is potentially more curable.

John S. Macdonald, Daniel G. Haller, Robert J. Mayer, Eds. *Manual of Oncologic Therapeutics*, Third Edition.

10. LIVER BIOPSY

Charles J. Lightdale

The method chosen to obtain a specimen of liver tissue for histologic diagnosis depends on the clinical setting and the results of liver imaging. In patients with liver disease, the history and physical examination suggest the correct diagnosis more than 90% of the time. In addition, commonly available blood tests help indicate the probability of biliary obstruction, cholestasis, infiltration, or hepatocellular disease. Ultrasound and computed tomography (CT) have revolutionized the approach to the jaundiced patient, because they often permit one to distinguish between intrahepatic and extrahepatic cholestasis. These imaging modalities have also proved more successful than radionuclide scans in differentiating focal from diffuse liver disease. For focal lesions, biopsies are performed more accurately using CT or ultrasound for guidance, or they can be done under direct vision via peritoneoscopy. Percutaneous liver biopsy performed without such guidance has been called "blind" and is best suited to diffuse liver disease.

Studies have shown an overall yield of 40% to 50% for diagnosis of malignant liver disease by a single percutaneous biopsy. These figures are somewhat misleading, because the yield of an unguided biopsy depends a great deal on the amount of liver consumed by tumor and the location of the malignant tissue. In advanced liver malignancy, the likelihood of positive findings with unguided biopsy is approximately 70%, whereas in early disease, the probability of the needle striking cancerous tissue is 30% or less. Two biopsies combined with aspiration cytology adds 10% to 20% to the yield of blind technique. Biopsies are routinely performed using a transthoracic approach to the right lobe. The results of unguided biopsies are more likely to be positive if scans indicate malignant liver tissue in the lateral right lobe.

Aiming a needle at a scan-indicated defect in the liver greatly increases the diagnostic yield of percutaneous biopsy for malignant liver disease. Radionuclide scans are unsatisfactory as guides, particularly with a subcostal approach, because of the risk of puncturing major blood vessels, bile ducts, the gallbladder, or adjacent viscera. Cysts, possibly echinococcal, cannot be differentiated from other types of lesions by scan defects. Such risks can be avoided by using ultrasound or CT to guide biopsy needles, or by using peritoneoscopy for direct-vision biopsy. The accuracy of these methods is 80% to 90%, and they are the procedures of choice for diagnosing malignant liver disease.

Needle biopsy of the liver has proved highly effective in diagnosing diffuse liver diseases, such as hepatitis and fatty metamorphosis. A typical percutaneous aspiration biopsy specimen measures only about 1.2 mm × 20 mm and weighs at most about 15 mg, equal to about 0.001% of the total liver mass. The more focal the disease, the less accurate such biopsies become. The false-negative sampling error in cirrhosis for a single blind percutaneous aspiration biopsy is in the range of 20% to 25%.

TECHNIQUE

Most percutaneous biopsies are performed using an aspiration needle method described by Menghini. The technique appears simple but requires dexterity and attention to detail for maximum safety. It is best learned under the supervision of an experienced teacher. The key elements of the Menghini method are a very brief intrahepatic phase, lasting a fraction of a second, and the use of a small-bore needle, usually 1.2 mm in caliber. The method has been divided into the following stages:

1. After local anesthesia, a skin incision of approximately 2 mm is made using a pointed scalpel.
2. The biopsy needle with attached syringe is pushed into the subcutaneous tissue.
3. Approximately 1 ml of saline solution is injected to expel any tissue fragments from the needle.
4. While aspiration on the syringe is maintained and the patient holds his breath in expiration, the needle is quickly inserted into the liver and then withdrawn from the patient.
5. Saline solution is injected from the syringe through the needle to expel the liver tissue into a specimen container.

Biopsies are classically done with a transthoracic approach through an intercostal space. This avoids the risk of puncturing other viscera. The pleural space is punctured, but if proper technique is maintained, this is of no consequence. Using percussion, the point of maximum liver dullness is established in an intercostal space. The biopsy site should be in this space, between the anterior and midaxillary lines.

A variety of aspiration needles for liver biopsy are available, including disposable needle-and-syringe combinations. Cutting needles, such as the Vim-Silverman and Tru-Cut needles, and a subcostal approach may be used by some experts, but such methods are considered to increase the risk of blind liver biopsy. New, thin, spring-loaded cutting needles (the so-called "gun" biopsy method) have recently been marketed as easy to use and more reliable, but their expense has not yet been justified in sufficiently large studies.

RISKS AND CONTRAINDICATIONS

Blood clotting abnormalities are the most frequently encountered contraindications. Prothrombin time and platelet count should be routinely measured before biopsy. Liver bleeding time is not directly correlated with these parameters, but experience has shown that excessive bleeding is more likely if the prothrombin time is more than 2 seconds over control and if the platelet count is below 100,000. There is a gray zone of risk, and some clinicians perform biopsies in patients with slightly longer prothrombin times and with lower platelet counts. A partial thromboplastin time is usually included in the prebiopsy evaluation as an additional screen for clotting factor abnormalities or circulating anticoagulants. Any abnormalities detected or any suggestion of a bleeding diathesis in the medical history merits a thorough coagulation work-up before biopsy.

When a liver biopsy is essential, it can still be done safely if the clotting abnormalities can be at least temporarily corrected. This is usually accomplished by transfusion of fresh frozen plasma or platelets. The use of a thin biopsy needle appears to decrease the risk of postbiopsy bleeding. Transjugular needle biopsy of the liver is a specialized radiologic technique available in some centers, where biopsy through a hepatic vein is accomplished with a catheter-guided technique. This method appears to add safety in patients with a bleeding diathesis.

Patients must be cooperative during percutaneous liver biopsy. Belligerent, hysterical, stuporous, delirious, psychotic, or comatose patients should not undergo biopsy unless movement and breathing can be controlled to avoid lacerating the liver. Other contraindications are skin infections at the biopsy site; right-sided pneumonia, empyema, or subphrenic abscess; peritonitis; obstructive jaundice; cholangitis; and suspicion of hydatid disease. Ascites will make percutaneous liver biopsy more risky and difficult, as will a small and cirrhotic liver. Ultrasonography, CT, or peritoneoscopy-guided biopsy is preferable in this setting.

Pain is common after liver biopsy; it is often referred to the right shoulder or right hypochondrium. The pain is usually mild and transient, disappearing after 1 to 2 hours. This type of pain is probably caused by a small amount of bleeding into the subcapsular or subdiaphragmatic space. A transient friction rub of no significance may develop over the biopsy site.

Peritonitis from bile leakage is rare except in obstructive jaundice. Penetration of abdominal viscera is rare if the transthoracic approach is used, with the right kidney being most commonly injured. Injury to pleural or intercostal blood vessels may occur. Bacteremia is uncommon.

The most frequent and serious complication is prolonged bleeding from the liver biopsy site. This occurs in 0.1% to 0.2% of biopsies and may require transfusion and emergency surgery. Postbiopsy hemobilia has been described, as have hepatic arteriovenous fistula and arterial aneurysm.

The mortality rate for Menghini-type biopsy has been reported as approximately 0.015%. Series reporting the use of cutting needles have had higher mortality rates, ranging from 0.04% to 0.17%.

PATIENT PREPARATION

Patients should fast for 6 to 8 hours before liver biopsy; however, a light diet for patient comfort and to promote emptying of the gallbladder may be allowed. Aspirin and nonsteroidal anti-inflammatory agents should be avoided for a week before biopsy. A recent prothrombin time, partial thromboplastin time, and platelet count should be obtained, and significant abnormalities corrected, as discussed previously. Blood type should be determined. Some clinicians routinely cross-match blood for possible transfusion, but most do this only in a high-risk setting.

The most common local anesthetic used is lidocaine, and patients should be questioned about possible allergic reactions. Because patients should be cooperative for the procedure, adequate time should be allowed to establish a calm atmosphere. Highly anxious patients who cannot be calmed with a "vocal local" may sometimes require a mild preprocedure sedative or tranquilizer. Some clinicians routinely give all patients intravenous conscious sedation for liver biopsy, most commonly using an agent such as midazolam at levels comparable to those for gastrointestinal endoscopy.

POSTPROCEDURE CARE

The patient should be examined closely for signs of blood loss. Pulse and blood pressure should be measured frequently, usually at half-hourly intervals for the first 2 to 4 hours after biopsy, then hourly for another 4 hours. Abdominal swelling and pain lasting more than 1 to 2 hours after the biopsy suggest intra-abdominal bleeding. Many clinicians routinely measure hematocrit and hemoglobin 4 to 8 hours after biopsy. Others measure these parameters only if bleeding is suspected clinically. Blood transfusions should be used as needed, and surgical consultation should be obtained promptly if serious bleeding occurs.

After Menghini-type liver biopsy, some physicians position the patient on the right side for 1 to 3 hours, and some add a towel roll under the biopsy site to help tamponade postbiopsy bleeding. These maneuvers are of unproven benefit. Patients are routinely maintained at strict bed rest for 24 hours. It has become evident, however, that the great majority of postbiopsy complications appear in the first few hours after biopsy. If the patient is without symptoms and stable after 6 to 8 hours, many physicians allow ambulation to a nearby bathroom and chair. In a stable patient, a light meal may be given 3 to 4 hours after biopsy.

At some centers, outpatient percutaneous aspiration liver biopsy has become routine. After 6 to 8 hours of observation in the hospital after the biopsy, stable patients are discharged to rest at home. No increase in morbidity and mortality from liver biopsy has been documented using this approach.

BIBLIOGRAPHY

Conn HO, Yesner R. Re-evaluation of needle biopsy in the diagnosis of metastatic cancer of the liver. Ann Intern Med 59:53–58, 1963

Ferrucci JT. Liver tumor imaging. Cancer 67 (4 suppl):1189–1195, 1991

Janes CH, Lindor KD. Outcome of patients hospitalized for complications after outpatient liver biopsy. Ann Intern Med 118:96–98, 1993

Menghini G. One-second biopsy of the liver—Problems of its clinical application. N Engl J Med 283:582–585, 1970

Nord HJ. Biopsy diagnosis of cirrhosis: Blind percutaneous versus guided direct vision techniques—A review. Gastrointest Endosc 28:102–104, 1982

John S. Macdonald, Daniel G. Haller, Robert J. Mayer, Eds. *Manual of Oncologic Therapeutics*, Third Edition.

11. LUMBAR PUNCTURE

Jon Glass

Neurologic dysfunction in the cancer patient may be caused by direct or indirect effects of cancer, or by infection. Although this causes serious morbidity, rapid diagnosis and therapy may often improve outcome. Lumbar puncture (LP) provides valuable diagnostic information, and is an important adjunct in the therapy of neoplastic diseases.

INDICATIONS

In the cancer patient, LP is indicated in the evaluation of suspicion of neoplastic meningitis as well as central nervous system (CNS) infections, especially opportunistic infections and meningitis. It is also useful in newly diagnosed or known disease, in the therapy of neoplastic or infectious meningitis, and in assessing the response of known disease to therapy.

CONTRAINDICATIONS

Infection over the LP site is the only absolute contraindication, because meningitis may result. Sepsis is a relative contraindication, as blood-borne organisms may be introduced into the cerebrospinal fluid (CSF). Increased intracranial pressure and bleeding diatheses are relative contraindications. Intracranial pressure (ICP) may be elevated due to a focal mass lesion, such as an intra- or extraparenchymal neoplasm, abscess, or hemorrhage. In such cases, the neurologic examination usually reveals lateralizing focal signs. Nonlocalized processes, such as multiple metastases, hydrocephalus, infectious and neoplastic meningitis, and certain metabolic encephalopathies, may not produce focal neurologic signs, rather causing mental status changes, headache, and, in some instances, papilledema. If any of these is present, a head CT or MRI should be performed before LP. In all cases, the fundi should be examined for papilledema. If LP is absolutely necessary in the setting of increased ICP, neurosurgical consultation should be obtained, and the patient pretreated with corticosteroids and mannitol. Neurologic difficulties due to spinal block may worsen following an LP, and a partial block may be made complete.

Bleeding diatheses are also relative contraindications, and such patients requiring LP should be pretreated with fresh-frozen plasma and/or platelet transfusion as indicated.

TECHNIQUE

Blood glucose should be measured within 15 minutes of the start of the examination. Proper positioning is essential. The patient is placed in the lateral decubitus position, with the back parallel to the bed, and the knees and neck maximally flexed. The L3–L4 or L4–L5 interspace is located; the L4 vertebra is at the level of the top of the superior iliac crests. In young children, the L4–L5 or L5–S1 interspaces are used. The area around the interspace is washed three times with povidone-iodine solution and again three times with alcohol, removing all iodine, and draped sterilely. The skin and subcutaneous tissues may be locally anesthetized. A 20- or 22-gauge spinal needle is inserted, perpendicular to the back and angled toward the umbilicus, with the bevel facing up (this allows splaying of the fibers of the dura, which are positioned longitudinally). The needle is advanced slowly, and the stylet may be removed frequently to assess for return of CSF. When the dura is pierced and the subarachnoid space entered, a characteristic "pop" is felt. Care should be taken not to advance the needle too far, as trauma to the epidural venous plexus may produce a bloody tap. When CSF flow is obtained, its pressure is measured with a manometer. This requires full patient relaxation, which may be facilitated by lessening knee and neck flexion. Once CSF flow has been established, it should be allowed to flow freely into the tubes for collection. Slow CSF flow can usually be corrected by turning the needle or slightly advancing it or withdrawing it. CSF should never be suctioned with a syringe. After the fluid is collected, the stylet is replaced and the needle withdrawn slowly. The patient is advised to remain lying, preferably in the prone position, for 2 to 12 hours.

On occasion, difficulties in obtaining CSF in the lateral decubitus position necessitate use of the sitting position. The spine should be completely straight, and the patient should lean forward onto a table. The bevel should be parallel to the long axis of the body. Should measurement of opening pressure be required, the patient can be carefully placed in the lateral decubitus position following CSF return. Under fluoroscopic control, CSF can be obtained from the lumbar region. In cases of spinal block, CSF can be sampled from the cisterna magna. These procedures should be performed only by qualified personnel. In rare instances, a ventricular tap may be needed for collection of CSF; this procedure should be performed by a neurosurgeon. In cases where prolonged administration of antineoplastic or antimicrobial therapy is required, placement of an intraventricular reservoir provides rapid access to the CSF and improved drug distribution.

CSF COLLECTION AND EXAMINATION

In all cases, red and white blood cell counts and white blood cell differential should be obtained on the first and last tubes, and protein and glucose concentrations should be performed. Traumatic taps can be distinguished from subarachnoid hemorrhage by clearing of the red blood cells by the last tube and by the lack of a yellowish tinge in the supernatant after centrifugation (xanthochromia). In cases of a traumatic tap, protein and WBC levels may be artificially elevated; actual levels may be estimated by deducting 1 mg/dl of protein and 1 WBC for every 1000 RBC; however, this value varies widely between patients. In cases of subarachnoid hemorrhage, rapid RBC lysis may artificially increase the WBC count. The remainder of the examination is based on clinical suspicion. Suspected neoplastic meningitis warrants the removal of at least 8 ml of CSF for cytologic examination. Although fresh CSF is preferred, an equal volume of 50% alcohol may be added when a delay in processing is anticipated. In addition, when indicated, CSF should also be evaluated for opportunistic infections such as mycobacteria and fungi. The cellular reaction in the immunocompromised patient may be meager or absent; when infectious meningitis is suspected, CSF should be immediately brought to the lab for culture, and light microscopy examinations for bacterial, fungi, and mycobacteria should be performed. Other tests, including antibody titers, evaluations of bacterial and fungal antigens, viral cultures, protein electrophoresis, and biochemical markers for neoplastic meningitis (such as LDH, α-fetoprotein, and β-hCG) should be performed as indicated.

COMPLICATIONS

The most common complication of LP is positional headache, appearing when the patient sits or stands and resolving when he or she returns to a horizontal position. Although usually seen in the first 1 to 3 days and lasting no more than 7 to 10 days, it may persist for weeks. This can be treated with bed rest, fluid, and analgesics. As its development is usually due to a persistent CSF leak at the puncture site, risk can be minimized by using the smallest possible gauge needle. Less often, localized back pain or radicular pain (from injury to a nerve root) may occur. Other complications include meningitis, arachnoiditis, transient sixth nerve palsy, spinal subdural hematoma, and herniation in the setting of increased ICP. When an unexpectedly large opening pressure is noted, minimal CSF should be collected, prompt neurosurgical consultation obtained, and the patient treated with corticosteroids, mannitol, and (if necessary) hyperventilation.

John S. Macdonald, Daniel G. Haller, Robert J. Mayer, Eds. *Manual of Oncologic Therapeutics*, Third Edition.

12. BONE MARROW ASPIRATION AND BIOPSY

Edward J. Lee
Charles A. Schiffer

Bone marrow aspiration and biopsy are cytologic and histologic methods, respectively, of assessing the bone marrow. The indications may vary from an abnormality in blood cell production to the need to stage a patient with a nonhematologic malignancy before or during therapy. This procedure is fundamental to the diagnosis and appropriate therapy of all patients with acute leukemia, myelodysplastic syndromes (MDS), and non-Hodgkin's lymphomas (NHL) and of some patients with nonhematologic malignancies that frequently involve the bone marrow, such as small cell undifferentiated lung cancer and adenocarcinoma of the breast.

Bone marrow aspiration and biopsy complement each other, and each has its limitations. Aspiration produces a monolayer of cells that may be stained with a variety of techniques to allow specific diagnosis to be made. Bone marrow aspiration is the procedure of choice when a hematologic malignancy or disorder is suspected because individual cells may be examined with accuracy. Romanovsky (including Wright and Giemsa) stains are the standard initial approach and are sufficient to identify acute leukemia, MDS, or the presence of some nonleukemic malignant processes such as NHL and solid tumors. Cytochemical stains such as myeloperoxidase, Sudan black, periodic acid-Schiff, and others can distinguish between acute lymphocytic and myeloid leukemia in most patients, a distinction that is critical to appropriate therapy.

In contrast, biopsy results in thicker sections and reduces the ability to characterize single cells. This can be critical in the differential diagnosis. For example, distinguishing between 20% and 50% myeloblasts on biopsy may be difficult and thus cloud the distinction between MDS and acute leukemia. In addition to standard hematoxylin and eosin staining, biopsies may be stained for reticulin and for a variety of enzymes, proteins, or markers. Bone marrow biopsy is the definitive procedure for assessing marrow cellularity, the presence and extent of fibrosis or granulomata, and the presence and nature of any nonhematologic malignancy. When aspiration is unsuccessful, biopsy represents the only means of obtaining diagnostic material. Properly prepared aspirates and biopsies can also be studied with monoclonal antibodies allowing immunophenotyping of hematopoietic and nonhematopoietic cells.

There are few contraindications to a carefully planned and performed bone marrow aspiration and biopsy. If severe thrombocytopenia (<20,000/μl) is present and platelet transfusion is planned, one should perform the procedure after transfusion rather than before. However, the procedure may be done safely even with extremely low platelet counts. A sternal site is probably preferred for an aspirate in the presence of hemostatic abnormalities; less soft tissue overlies the sternum than the iliac crest, allowing pressure to be applied more directly at the site of the puncture. Patient comfort is also improved because hematomas are smaller and do not interfere with sitting or ambulation. Biopsies from the sternum are contraindicated, however, and should be taken from the iliac crest. Therefore, the site of the procedure may depend on the information required. In obese patients, correction of coagulation abnormalities before a biopsy is preferred.

Sternal marrow aspiration should not be performed in patients with thoracic aortic aneurysms, because accompanying erosion of the posterior table of the sternum can result in puncture. Patients with lytic bone disease of ribs or sternum should not have sternal aspirates because of the possibility of fracture. Aspirates should be done with extreme caution in patients with multiple myelomas or osteoporosis. In patients receiving anticoagulation therapy, heparin should be discontinued temporarily before the procedure and should not be restarted until hemostasis is ensured. Warfarin therapy is not a contraindication to sternal aspiration, but a biopsy procedure preferably should be done with normal coagulation studies.

STERNAL ASPIRATION

The patient should be supine, without elevation of head or trunk. The important landmarks to be identified are the sternal angle of Louis and the lateral borders of the sternum in the second intercostal space (ICS). The skin is cleaned and a fenestrated drape placed so that the procedure may be carried out in a sterile fashion. The skin, subcutaneous tissues, and periosteum are infiltrated with a local anesthetic such as 1% lidocaine. Local anesthetics produce a burning sensation, and infiltration of skin and periosteum may cause pain. As with all procedures, it is wise to warn the patient of each sensation to avoid unexpected movements and contamination of the field. The infiltration should be accomplished with a 25-gauge needle, and the surface of the bone should be "sounded" during periosteal infiltration. All sternal aspiration needles should have a guard that prevents inadvertent penetration of the posterior table of the sternum. This guard is adjusted according to the distance from skin to periosteum identified during infiltration. Following the infiltration and preparation of the aspiration needle, a 2-mm superficial skin incision should be made with a surgical blade. The incision should be placed in the midsternum, within the area previously anesthetized, and should run laterally at the level of the second ICS. The aspiration needle with guard is then introduced into this incision and is advanced carefully to contact the periosteum. A corkscrew motion is often helpful when advancing the needle. If adequate anesthesia has been obtained, the patient will report only "pressure" and not sharp pain — the distinction is important. If sharp pain is noted, local anesthesia may not be adequate. The needle is then advanced, again with rotation, until fixed in the bone. The newer disposable needles are extremely sharp, and the sense of "give" often felt after the tip of the needle has passed from cortex into the marrow may not be appreciated. Therefore, since the sternum may be only 1 cm thick, we recommend not advancing the needle once it is felt to be fixed in bone. Bone marrow is obtained by removing the obturator, affixing a 10- to 12-ml syringe, and aspirating briskly. One milliliter is sufficient material because any excess will be diluted by peripheral blood. This aspiration is usually accompanied by a few seconds of pain, which can be quite significant and cannot be prevented. Again, it is best to make patients aware of when the pain will occur to allow them to prepare. Spicules of bone marrow are quite friable and easily obtained in this manner unless significant fibrosis is present or the bone marrow is tightly packed with leukemia or other malignancy. For patients in whom multiple aspirates are needed, such as for cytogenetic or immunophenotyping analyses, it is advisable to rotate and slightly advance the needle to be assured of obtaining representative bone marrow rather than peripheral blood.

If no material is obtained and no pain is felt, it is possible that the marrow space has not yet been entered. The obturator can be replaced, and the needle carefully advanced 2 mm to 3 mm. The same procedure for aspiration is repeated. If unsuccessful, the needle should be withdrawn, the landmarks reviewed, and the needle reintroduced within the anesthetized area. If blood without marrow is obtained after aspiration, then the needle should be completely withdrawn and either flushed to remove clot, or replaced with a new needle.

Once marrow has been obtained, smears are prepared. Many techniques produce adequate results. One method is to expel the aspirated marrow promptly onto a glass slide placed at an angle in a small Petri dish such that the blood runs into the dish. The spicules, which represent only a small amount of the aspirated material, usually adhere to the slide. Smears can then be prepared by using a glass coverslip to pick up spicules. The coverslip with the spicules is placed so that capillary action allows spreading of cells between slide and coverslip or coverslip and coverslip, and the initial coverslip is then pulled gently in a direction parallel to the flat surface to produce the smear. Much practice is necessary before good smears are reliably produced.

POSTERIOR ILIAC CREST ASPIRATION AND BIOPSY

A number of needles permit adequate sampling. We will discuss only the use of the Jamshidi needle — one that permits both aspiration and biopsy.

The patient is positioned prone, although many physicians prefer that the patient be placed in a lateral decubitus position. The site usually used is the posterior superior iliac spine. This may be identified and defined in all but the most obese patients. In some patients who have had radiation therapy to the pelvis, the anterior iliac crest may provide a better sample. The area to be sampled is prepared and anesthetized in a manner similar to that described for the sternal aspirate. The aspiration needle is again fixed in bone and aspiration attempted. Since the cortex is thicker, it may be necessary to advance the needle or reposition it to be sure of reaching the marrow cavity. Once the aspiration has been accomplished, the biopsy is done by advancing the capped needle without the obturator with a twisting motion. Discomfort often occurs during this procedure, but only rarely is it necessary to premedicate patients with meperidine or midazolam (Versed) in low doses. Indeed, the use of conscious intravenous sedation should be carried out only if the patient will be monitored and parameters such as respiratory, pulse, blood pressure, and oxygen saturation are measured frequently, as respiratory depression may occur, particularly after a procedure has been completed. Once the needle has been advanced to the desired length of the biopsy (1.5 cm to 2 cm is recommended), the needle is rotated briskly first in one direction, then the opposite. The needle is then "rocked" gently by exerting pressure perpendicular to the shaft of the needle in all four directions. The purpose of these last two maneuvers is to separate the biopsy from the bone. The needle is then removed slowly while rotating gently, and the biopsy is removed by pushing it up the needle to the hub with a stylet provided specifically for this purpose. If the aspiration attempts have been unsuccessful and either acute leukemia or tumor involvement of marrow is suspected, it is often appropriate to touch the biopsy specimen to slide before placing it in fixative, saline, or culture medium. These touch preparations can then be processed with cytologic rather than histologic methods and can add substantially to the diagnostic information.

AFTERCARE

In all patients with any hemostatic abnormality, the puncture site should be directly compressed for 5 to 10 minutes. Direct manual pressure is clearly the method of choice. In addition, in any patient who has had a posterior iliac spine procedure, the site should be compressed to minimize hematoma formation. A pressure bandage should then be applied and should remain in place for 18 to 24 hours. The major complications of the procedure are bleeding and infection. Both can be minimized by careful technique during and after the procedure.

John S. Macdonald, Daniel G. Haller, Robert J. Mayer, Eds. *Manual of Oncologic Therapeutics*, Third Edition.

13. LAPAROSCOPY

Ronald Bleday
R. Armour Forse

Laparoscopy is becoming more widely applied to general surgical procedures. This phenomenon is mostly attributable to improved technology, particularly better video cameras. Biliary surgery, in which the standard of care for the removal of a noninflamed gallbladder is now laparoscopic cholecystectomy, has led the way in laparoscopic surgery. As surgeons have gained more experience with the instruments and the techniques of laparoscopy they are increasingly applying these skills to both the diagnosis and treatment of intraabdominal malignancies.

DIAGNOSTIC LAPAROSCOPY

The initial use of diagnostic laparoscopy was in gynecologic oncology. In three separate reviews on the use of laparoscopy in diagnosing ovarian malignancies in patients with cysts that appeared benign on imaging studies, between 2% and 4% of the cysts were found to be malignant.[1,2] In women over the age of 50, 32% of cysts were found to be malignant and associated with advanced disease.[3] The advantage of the laparoscope over other radiologic studies is that it can provide a tissue sample as well as a diagnostic exploration. Laparoscopy is also being applied to both the diagnosis and treatment of endometrial carcinoma; however, the protocols are still developing.

For nongynecologic tumors within the abdomen, the application of the laparoscope for staging is just beginning to evolve. In patients with primary and metastatic hepatic malignancies, laparoscopy is now being used before resection to decrease the negative laparotomy rate and increase the rate of resectability. In a recent study from the New England Deaconess Hospital, 29 patients underwent staging laparoscopy prior to a planned laparotomy for resection of a hepatic malignancy that had been judged to be resectable by both preoperative computed tomography (CT) scan and ultrasonography. In this study, 12 patients had primary hepatic malignancies and 17 had metastatic malignancies. In 14 of the 29 patients (48%), laparoscopy demonstrated evidence of unresectability. Four patients with primary disease had unsuspected cirrhosis, while 10 of 17 patients with metastatic lesions had small peritoneal metastases or other metastases outside the liver seen on laparoscopy and, therefore, were deemed unresectable for cure. In 15 of the 29 patients in whom no metastatic disease outside the liver or cirrhosis was seen, laparotomy was performed. Four of these patients were found to have unresectable disease not identified laparoscopically. All four of these patients had previous surgery with significant adhesions in the right upper quadrant that had precluded adequate visualization of the area. Overall there were no significant complications from the laparoscopy in this study. Also, when those patients who had been ruled out for resection by laparoscopy were compared to matched historical patient controls who underwent a laparotomy without resection, there was a significant difference in the length of stay. Laparoscopically staged patients had an average of stay of 1.2 days (±0.5), whereas laparotomy staged patients stayed 6.6 days (±1.6).[4] The conclusion of this study was that if resectable disease can be ruled out with laparoscopy, patient morbidity and length of stay will be decreased. We now perform a diagnostic laparoscopy before any laparotomy for resection of either a primary or metastatic hepatic malignancy.

New technology is also progressing to increase the usefulness of the laparoscope in obtaining a more precise view of the liver parenchyma before a laparotomy. An ultrasound probe is now being developed to go through a 10/11-mm laparoscopic trocar to perform intraoperative ultrasound of the liver. Not only will this technology increase our ability to stage a patient, but there is the potential for combining laparoscopic intraoperative ultrasound with laparoscopically applied hepatic cryosurgery so as to be able to perform curative surgery on tumors of the liver without a major abdominal incision.

Pancreatic carcinoma is often unresectable, and laparoscopy may provide a very cost-effective and minimally invasive method by which to differentiate between resectable and nonresectable patients. The initial work on the use of laparoscopy for pancreatic carcinoma was done by Warshaw.[5] In his study, laparoscopy, combined with either CT or MRI, was able to determine unresectability in more than 90% of the unresectable patients. When all three tests were negative, 78% of pancreatic tumors were found to be resectable. Other authors have had similar results.[6,7] In these studies, the main advantage of laparoscopy appears to be its ability to see peritoneal and omental deposits that are not visible on preoperative radiologic investigations. Cytology on peritoneal washings is also being evaluated to see if laparoscopy plus washings of the peritoneal cavity are predictive of outcome. One of the main reasons to rule out unresectable patients with pancreatic cancer is that they can now be palliated with a biliary stent using endoscopic retrograde cholangiopancreatography (ERCP). Because few patients truly need a duodenal bypass for pancreatic cancer, preoperative staging along with laparoscopy can keep patients out of the hospital, allowing palliation using minimally invasive techniques.

Laparoscopy may be very useful in staging patients for either palliative treatments or curative treatments in gastric carcinoma. In particular, diagnostic laparoscopy may allow for more accurate preoperative staging so that neoadjuvant multimodality therapy could possibly be carried out to allow for a greater cure rate with this otherwise very aggressive disease. One study found that laparotomy can be avoided in up to 40% of patients in whom diagnostic laparoscopy showed evidence of either metastasis or unresectable advanced disease.[8] In another series, diagnostic laparoscopy was found to be more sensitive and overall more accurate than preoperative CT scan and ultrasound in determining the resectability of patients with gastric carcinoma.[9] Again, laparoscopy appeared to be best at seeing extranodal intraperitoneal disease.

Finally, laparoscopy is starting to be used in the staging of Hodgkin's disease. Dissection of the periaortic lymph nodes, a liver biopsy, and even laparoscopically-assisted splenectomy is now being done to help stage patients with Hodgkin's lymphoma in the same manner as an open laparotomy. If protocols using a laparoscope and comparing it to the accuracy of open laparotomy can be developed, this laparoscopic staging technique can help determine the type of therapy used (*i.e.*, radiotherapy vs. chemotherapy) and in determining certain radiotherapy ports. Work in this field is still in its infancy and more data will be needed before recommendations can be made on its use.

LAPAROSCOPIC-ASSISTED INTESTINAL RESECTIONS FOR CANCER

The laparoscope has been useful in laparoscopic colectomy for colorectal cancer. The technique for laparoscopic-assisted colon resection has been previously described.[10] The technique is actually a laparoscopic-assisted operation in which part of the procedure is done using the laparoscope, then a small incision is made and the procedure is completed in the traditional manner. In particular, exploration and mobilization of the colon can be done with the laparoscope and laparoscopic instruments. Ligation of the vascular pedicle is also becoming more easily performed with laparoscopic clips and vascular stapling devices; however, resection of the bowel and anastomosis often is still done in an extracorporeal fashion.

The main question with laparoscopic-assisted colectomy for colorectal cancer is whether it provides the same specimen as traditional open techniques and whether there is any unique biologic alteration with the laparoscopic procedure that leads to any change in survival or in recurrence. There have been several reports of wound recurrences at trocar sites in patients undergoing laparoscopic-assisted colectomy.[11] In our experience, however, we have not had any unique problems with the laparoscope and, in an analysis of our first 12 laparoscopic-assisted colectomies versus data from our tumor registry in the 2 years before the use of a laparoscope, we found no statistically significantly difference in the proximal margin, distal margin, specimen size, tumor size, lymph node count in the lymphovascular pedicle, or operative time (Table 13–1). There were significant differences in the time to enteral feeding and in the length of stay, both favoring the laparoscopic-assisted approach (see Table 13–1). We also analyzed the data of patients who had their operation started with a laparoscopic-assisted approach but who were then soon converted to the traditional technique due to adhesions or other factors. These patients tended to have a length of stay and a time to enteral feeding similar to patients undergoing traditional open colectomy (see Table 13–1).

TABLE 13–1. LAPAROSCOPIC VERSUS NONLAPAROSCOPIC SURGERY FOR COLON CANCER

PARAMETER	LAPAROSCOPIC-ASSISTED COLECTOMY (n = 12)	LAPAROSCOPIC-ASSISTED COLECTOMY CONVERTED TO OPEN PROCEDURE (n = 6)	OPEN COLECTOMY (n = 29)
Proximal margin (cm)	9.4 ± 1.3	11.5 ± 1.3	11.9 ± 2.3
Distal margin (cm)	5.3 ± 1.4	12.0 ± 6.9	6.8 ± 0.9
Specimen size (cm)	17.4 ± 2.0	28.7 ± 5.6	20.5 ± 2.0
Tumor size (cm)	3.7 ± 0.6	4.5 ± 0.9	4.2 ± 0.5
Number of lymph nodes	10.6 ± 2.1	14.2 ± 3.6	10.6 ± 1.2
Operative time (min)	232 ± 21	270 ± 30	284 ± 23
Enteral feeds (days)	3.3 ± 0.4	6.5 ± 1.7*	5.1 ± 0.2*
Length of stay (days)	6.1 ± 0.5	12.0 ± 1.9*	12.3 ± 1.8*

Data are expressed as mean ± SE.
* = $p \leq 0.05$ by Analysis of Variance (ANOVA) and Games-Howell test vs. LAC.

A national randomized intergroup trial is being organized to directly assess the results of the laparoscopic-assisted colectomy for the resection of colorectal cancer versus traditional surgery. This type of study will be the only way to determine the length of stay and survival benefits of the two procedures.

LAPAROSCOPIC-ASSISTED RESECTIONS OF OTHER INTRAPERITONEAL ORGANS FOR CANCER

Surgeons are beginning to explore the application of laparoscopic-assisted techniques for other oncologic problems. Laparoscopic-assisted splenectomy is being performed for Hodgkin's disease, and all other aspects of the staging process for Hodgkin's disease are being perfected. Experimental work is also being performed on laparoscopic adrenalectomy, nephrectomy, and retroperitoneal node biopsy. The laparoscope can now be used for laparoscopic appendectomy and may be useful in patients with small carcinoids of the appendix. Clearly, the advantages in terms of decreased morbidity that have been seen with laparoscopic-assisted techniques need to be evaluated for each disease where it can be applied. Only with prospective trials can the surgical community honestly and fully assess the laparoscope's role in the diagnosis and treatment of intraabdominal malignancy.

REFERENCES

1. Mage G, Wattiez A, Canis M et al. Contribution of celioscopy in the early diagnosis of ovarian cancers. Ann Chiru 45:525–528, 1991
2. Martin DC. Laparoscopic treatment of ovarian endometriomas. Clin Obstet Gynecol 34:452–459, 1991
3. Pint C, Felgeres A, Colau JC. Ovarian cysts in women over 50 years of age. A retrospective study from 1979 to 1989 at Foch Medicosurgical Center. J Chirurg 127:528–532, 1990
4. Babineau TJ, Lewis WD, Jenkins RL et al. The role of staging laparoscopy in the treatment of hepatic malignancy. Am J Surg 167:151–155, 1994
5. Warshaw AL, Gu ZY, Wittenberg J, Waltman AC. Preoperative staging and assessment of resectability of pancreatic cancer. Arch Surg 125:230–233, 1990
6. Ivanov S, Keranov S. Laparoscopic assessment of the operability of pancreatic cancer. Khirurgiia-Sofia 42:12–14, 1989
7. Cuschieri A. Laparoscopy for pancreatic cancer: Does it benefit the patient? Eur J Surg Oncol 14(1):41–44, 1988
8. Krisplani AK, Kapur BM. Laparoscopy for pre-operative staging and assessment of operability in gastric carcinoma. Gastrointest Endosc 37:441–443, 1991
9. Watt I, Stewart I, Anderson D et al. Laparoscopy, ultrasound and computed tomography in cancer of the oesophagus and gastric cardia: a prospective comparison for detecting intra-abdominal metastases. Br J Surg 76:1036–1039, 1989
10. Bleday R, Babineau TJ, Forse RA. Laparoscopic surgery for colon and rectal cancer. Seminars in Surgical Oncology 9:59–64, 1993
11. Fusco MA, Paluzzi MW. Abdominal wall recurrence after laparoscopic-assisted colectomy for adenocarcinoma of the colon. Dis Colon Rectum 36:858–861, 199

John S. Macdonald, Daniel G. Haller, Robert J. Mayer, Eds. *Manual of Oncologic Therapeutics*, Third Edition.

14. GYNECOLOGY: PELVIC EXAMINATION AND BIOPSY TECHNIQUES

Richard R. Barakat

GYNECOLOGIC EXAMINATION

The gynecologic examination is an essential part of the evaluation of any female patient with cancer, and it is an essential screening procedure for all women. The examination should be performed annually beginning with the onset of sexual activity (or ages 18 to 21 years in women who are not sexually active) and should continue the rest of the woman's life. A gynecologic examination should consist of a careful gynecologic history and examination of the supraclavicular, axillary, and inguinal lymph nodes; the breasts; the abdomen; the external and internal genital organs; and the rectum.

GYNECOLOGIC DIAGNOSTIC PROCEDURES

Papanicolaou Smear

After inserting a water-moistened speculum and visualizing the cervix, a Pap smear is performed. The Pap smear consists of two separate specimens: the endocervical sample and the ectocervical sample. The endocervical specimen can be obtained by using a rubber bulb and glass cannula to aspirate the endocervical mucus, or one can moisten a small cotton swab and sample the endocervix. The ectocervix is then scraped circumferentially with a wooden or plastic spatula and the sample smeared on a glass slide. The Pap smear slides are immediately fixed by immersion in 95% ethyl alcohol or by spraying with a commercial fixative.

Colposcopy

Colposcopy of the cervix and vagina is indicated as part of the evaluation of any patient with an abnormal Pap smear. A large vaginal speculum is used, and the cervix and upper vagina are washed liberally with 3% or 4% acetic acid. After examining the vaginal fornices, the cervix is examined. Abnormal cervical patterns consist of white epithelium, mosaic patterns, punctation, and abnormal vasculature. Examples of these abnormalities can be found in most basic colposcopy textbooks.

Special Stains

TOLUIDINE BLUE STAIN

Toluidine blue is a vital stain that stains areas of the vulvar epithelium that have nuclei in the keratin layer (parakeratosis). The vulva is painted with a 1% aqueous solution of toluidine blue dye and, after drying, is washed with a 1% solution of acetic acid. The toluidine blue dye that persists indicates areas to be biopsied. The test is usually reserved for patients with known dysplasia or for patients being followed because of previous dysplastic lesions.

LUGOL'S STAIN

When painted with a 90% Lugol's solution, the normal vagina and cervix stain dark brown. Dysplastic epithelium does not stain. Such areas are called "Lugol's positive" and should be biopsied. Immature metaplasia and epithelial abrasions do not stain and account for false-positive areas. Lugol's staining is an adjunct to colposcopic examination for localizing potentially abnormal areas.

Biopsy Procedures

VULVAR BIOPSY

Any suspicious vulvar lesion should be biopsied. After infiltration of the area to be biopsied with 1% lidocaine, a Keye's dermal biopsy instrument is used to remove a 2-, 4-, or 6-mm tissue sample, including a normal skin margin. The small plug of tissue is excised with fine scissors. Application of a silver nitrate stick to the base of the biopsy site usually controls bleeding, and sutures are rarely necessary. The patient should be told to expect a slight amount of bleeding from the site; the application of an antibiotic gel to the site two times daily for 2 to 3 days will decrease the chance of local infection. The location of the biopsy should be labeled for the pathologist and a drawing made in the patient's chart indicating the location of the biopsies.

VAGINAL BIOPSY

Vaginal biopsies can be performed with cervical biopsy instruments, although a skin hook to tent up the tissue to be biopsied is helpful. Most patients have some sensation of pain with a vaginal biopsy, and local anesthesia is required, particularly when more than one biopsy is to be performed. Lidocaine 1% may be used with a 24- or 25-gauge spinal needle. Biopsy specimens should be submitted in separate containers that are carefully labeled with the location of the biopsy.

CERVICAL BIOPSY

Numerous instruments are suitable for cervical biopsy, and no particular instrument is best for all situations. It is best to have a small selection of several types of instruments available, and the physician should become familiar with one or two instruments that he or she finds most suitable. Cervical biopsy can usually be performed without anesthesia; bleeding is quite easily controlled by applying a silver nitrate stick or Monsel's solution (ferric subsulfated) to the biopsy site. All biopsy specimens should be submitted in separate containers that are accurately labeled with the site of the biopsy. There may be some spotting following a cervical biopsy, but significant bleeding is extremely unusual. In order to minimize bleeding, the patient should be instructed to refrain from coitus for 48 to 72 hours following biopsy.

ENDOCERVICAL CURETTAGE

Endocervical curettage is indicated for the evaluation of the endocervix above the area that can be visualized by the colposcope, and it is an essential part of the evaluation of the patient with an abnormal Pap smear. This procedure is performed with a Kevorkian curette, a small, sharp curette designed specifically for endocervical curettage. It is important that the curettage be performed thoroughly, beginning at the 12 o'clock position and proceeding clockwise or counterclockwise until the entire endocervical canal has been scraped. One helpful technique for obtaining the specimen from the endocervical curettage is to use a glass rod attached to a suction bulb to aspirate the mucus, blood, and fragments of tissue from the endocervical curettage. Although endocervical curettage does not require any form of anesthesia, it can be uncomfortable and the patient should be cautioned to expect menstrual-like cramps during the procedure.

CONE BIOPSY

Cone biopsy of the cervix is indicated as a diagnostic procedure for patients who have unsatisfactory colposcopy and in patients in whom invasive cancer cannot be excluded on the basis of biopsy. It is also used in patients who have such widespread cervical dysplasia that accurate sampling of the entire area by biopsy is not feasible. Cone biopsy can be used as a therapeutic procedure to remove all areas of premalignant tissue, preserving the uterus for childbearing. This procedure requires overnight hospitalization or observation in a day surgical unit.

More recently, biopsy and treatment of cervival dysplasia has been accomplished with the use of the loop electrosurgical excision procedure (LEEP). Electrosurgical excision of cervical dysplasia has the advantage of being performed under local anesthesia on an outpatient basis. The procedure is tolerated very well by patients and provides a tissue specimen for histopathologic evaluation.

ENDOMETRIAL BIOPSY

Endometrial biopsy is the best method for the evaluation of patients with abnormal uterine bleeding. Various instruments have been designed for this procedure; all consist of some type of curette or cannula that is inserted through the cervix into the uterine cavity. Endometrial tissue is scraped from the uterine wall and aspirated mechanically into a syringe or reservoir. An alternate method of obtaining endometrial samples is with the Pipelle endometrial suction curette. Histopathologic results obtained in this manner appear to correlate very well with endometrial curettings. The procedure is usually performed without an anesthetic but does cause menstrual-like cramping that can occasionally be relatively severe. Possible complications of the procedure are perforation of the uterine cavity and a vasovagal response to cervical instrumentation that occasionally causes a significant drop in blood pressure and may require treatment with atropine. The patient may experience spotting for 3 to 4 days following the procedure. The major limitation of the procedure is the inability to pass the curette through the cervical canal in some patients. Unfortunately, this occurs more frequently in postmenopausal patients, who are most likely to require endometrial biopsy. If the endometrial sample is inadequate or if the procedure cannot be performed because the instrument cannot pass through the cervix, the patient must be scheduled for dilatation and curettage.

The indications for dilatation and curettage include the evaluation of abnormal uterine bleeding and, in some cases, treatment of abnormal bleeding. The advantages of the procedure as compared with endometrial biopsy are that patients with cervical stenosis can be sampled and a more complete sampling of the endometrium can be obtained. The disadvantage is the requirement of a general or regional anesthetic.

Evaluation of the Adnexal Mass

The presence of an adnexal mass in a premenarchal girl or postmenopausal woman requires evaluation by exploratory surgery. In the reproductive age group a large percentage of adnexal masses are functional ovarian cysts that will resolve spontaneously. Such masses are almost always cystic, smooth, unilateral, freely mobile, and less than 8 cm in size. If the above conditions are not present or if the mass becomes larger or fails to resolve after observation for two menstrual cycles, exploratory laparotomy is indicated.

Ultrasonography or computed tomographic (CT) scan are occasionally used in the evaluation of patients with a possible adnexal mass and can be helpful in certain limited circumstances. If a pelvic mass is palpated on pelvic examination, ultrasound and CT scan will not add a significant amount of information. These procedures can be helpful, however, in the evaluation of patients in whom the pelvic examination is less than satisfactory. Patients who are obese or who have a high risk of ovarian neoplasms (such as patients with familial ovarian cancer) may well benefit from routine screening by ultrasonography. When combined with color flow Doppler, transvaginal ultrasound may help differentiate benign from malignant ovarian masses preoperatively on the basis of increased tumor vascularity.

Fine-Needle Aspiration

Fine-needle aspiration is performed by placing a small-bore needle (usually 25- or 26-gauge) into a mass and aspirating cells that are then smeared on a slide and stained in the Papanicolaou manner. Special needle guides are available to assist in the performance of these procedures per vagina or per rectum, and various syringe holders allow one-handed aspiration and make the procedure more convenient, but this technique is easily performed with instruments readily available to any physician. The materials needed to perform the procedure consist of 25- or 26-gauge spinal needles with stylets and 20-gauge syringes and materials for performing Pap smears. If abnormal areas can be palpated (such as superficial lymph nodes or abdominal or pelvic masses), the procedure can be performed by the physician at the bedside or in the office. For lesions that cannot be palpated, such as lung lesions, retroperitoneal nodules, or enlarged nodes, the procedure is performed using CT scan, ultrasound, or fluoroscopic guidance. Fine-needle aspiration is particularly helpful in the evaluation of patients with palpable masses on pelvic or rectal examination. One should *not*, however, perform fine-needle aspiration in the patient with an undiagnosed pelvic mass where the potential of ovarian carcinoma exists, because perforating an otherwise unruptured carcinoma may precipitate spread of the disease through the peritoneal cavity.

BIBLIOGRAPHY

Coppleson M. Gynecologic Oncology. Fundamental Principles and Clinical Practice. London, Churchill Livingstone, 1981

Friedrich EG. Vulvar Disease. Major Problems in Obstetrics and Gynecology. Vol 9. Philadelphia, WB Saunders, 1976

Greenhill JP. Office Gynecology. 8th ed. Chicago, Year Book Medical Publishers, 1965

Sevin B, Greening SE, Nagi M et al. Fine needle aspiration cytology in gynecologic oncology. I. Clinical aspects. Acta Cytol 23:277, 1976

John S. Macdonald, Daniel G. Haller, Robert J. Mayer, Eds. *Manual of Oncologic Therapeutics*, Third Edition.

15. MAMMOGRAPHY-DIRECTED BIOPSIES

Paul C. Stomper

INDICATIONS FOR MAMMOGRAPHY

Mammography screening has resulted in a reduction of approximately 20% to 30% in breast cancer mortality in women aged 50 and older in most large prospective randomized trials. These trials included limited compliance among the group of women assigned to undergo routine mammography screening as well as crossover from the control group assigned to routine follow-up according to their physicians' directions. Case-controlled studies in which populations of women who had 100% compliance for screening mammography were compared with populations of women who had not undergone mammography show a reduction in mortality of 50% or more.

The mortality reduction benefit for women under age 50 has not yet been conclusively shown due to the lack of statistical power, short-term follow-up, and problems with randomization and quality control in modern trials. The International Union Against Cancer (UICC) consensus in 1993 was that the available data can support a range of guidelines including recommendations to begin screening at age 40 or to begin at age 50 (Geneva, Switzerland meeting, 1993). Most screening guidelines assume a mortality reduction benefit in younger women and recommend screening at 1- to 2-year intervals for women between the ages of 40 and 50 and annually thereafter. Earlier mammographic screening should be considered for women at high risk including those with a family history of breast cancer, previous breast biopsy showing atypical hyperplasia, or prior breast cancer.

Aside from screening of asymptomatic women, mammography should also be performed for presence of any symptom or finding on physical exam that raises the suspicion of breast cancer and before any form of breast surgery.

MAMMOGRAPHY TECHNIQUE

High-quality mammography requires dedicated mammography equipment, experienced mammography technologists, skilled interpretation by radiologists, and proper management of equivocal or suspicious findings. The most widely preferred technique, film-screen mammography, requires compression of the breast between a parallel plastic compression plate and an underlying film-screen cassette holder during the x-ray exposure. This causes no or mild discomfort for most women. Screening mammography consists of craniocaudad and medial-lateral oblique images of each breast. If a suspicious or equivocal finding is observed, additional specialized projections of an area of the breast are often obtained. Breast ultrasound is used predominantly only as an adjunct to mammography to distinguish solid masses from cysts.

MAMMOGRAPHY INTERPRETIVE CRITERIA

Breast cancer has a wide range of mammographic appearances. The two general categories are poorly circumscribed soft tissue masses and clustered microcalcifications — variable-sized and variable-shaped calcium particles measuring 40 μm to 1 mm in diameter and numbering greater than 4 to 5 per cm^3. Although mammography is very sensitive for the detection of clinically occult early-stage breast cancers, there is a significant overlap in the mammographic appearance between these cancers and many benign entities. This is related to the fact that there is little difference in gross morphology, especially among those mammographic appearances of lesser predictive value for malignancy (the more well-circumscribed masses and the nonlinear, granular-type calcifications with more well-defined edges and greater homogeneity of size and shape).

The minimum threshold for recommending biopsy of lesions of lower predictive value is controversial. Short-interval (6-month) mammographic follow-up is an acceptable alternative to biopsy for mammographic lesions of very low predictive value (*i.e.*, less than 1%). Several studies have shown that the small percentage of very low suspicion lesions that were followed carefully and later shown to be cancer were still detected at an early, curable stage. As high-resolution mammographic images and the use of accessory views become more uniform practice, it appears possible to develop more reproducible criteria upon which to base biopsy recommendations.

The most specific mammographic feature of malignancy is the spiculated mass, a three-dimensional density with radiating spicules that histologically consists of infiltrating or, less commonly, intraductal cancer surrounded by reactive fibrosis. Although some benign lesions may mimic this appearance, a spiculated mass is associated with a greater than 90% chance of being breast cancer.

Approximately 40% of clinically occult, mammographically detected cancers are noncalcified soft tissue densities. Only one third of these appear as spiculated masses. Approximately 25% appear as irregularly outlined masses. Another 25% present as less specific, round, oval, or lobulated masses with indistinct borders. Less than 10% of clinically occult, noncalcified cancers presented as areas of architectural distortion of dense parenchymal tissue. Less than 5% present as well-defined, round, oval, or lobulated masses with completely well-defined borders. Small, well-defined masses or nodules have a very low predictive value for malignancy, ranging from 0 to 2% in several studies, and are not biopsied by most mammographers unless they exhibit interval growth on serial mammograms or are larger than 10 to 15 mm. Short interval (6-month) follow-up mammography is often recommended for small, well-defined nodules seen on the first or baseline mammogram and adequately imaged to document the well-defined margins.

Mammographic microcalcifications are seen in approximately 60% of clinically occult cancers. Histologically, these usually represent intraductal calcifications in areas of necrotic tumor, usually comedocarcinoma or calcifications in mucin-secreting tumors such as the cribriform or micropapillary subtypes of intraductal cancer. Although the classic linear and branching type of microcalcifications usually associated with comedocarcinoma are of higher predictive value for malignancy (approximately 70%), this type of calcification comprises only half of the malignant microcalcification clusters. A significant proportion of biopsy-proven malignant microcalcification clusters are of the granular type — nonlinear-irregular calcifications of varying size and shape. Although granular-type microcalcifications have a lesser predictive value for malignancy (approximately 20%) due to the higher prevalence of benign lesions with this type of calcifications, most of these microcalcification clusters should also be viewed with suspicion and biopsied.

PREDICTIVE VALUE OF MAMMOGRAPHY

Large series of needle localization procedures for clinically occult lesions performed in the United States showed that mammography had a predictive value of between 20% and 30%. (Predictive value is defined as the number of cancers detected divided by the total number of biopsies performed for clinically occult lesions deemed suspicious by the mammographer. Lobular carcinoma in situ is considered to be benign.) The overall percentage of biopsies based on mammographic recommendations that show cancer can vary between mammography centers and is increased by the following factors:

1. The increasing age of the women being screened
2. The presence of previous mammograms of the same women for comparison (incident in contrast to prevalent or baseline screening)
3. The level of expertise of the mammographer(s).

Other factors that should be considered when comparing the predictive value of mammography between mammography clinics include:

1. Whether the lesions biopsied were truly clinically occult and detected by mammography only
2. The percentage of cancers detected by mammography only that were ductal carcinoma in situ (DCIS)
3. The percentage of cancers detected that were minimal invasive cancers (smaller than 1 cm)
4. The percentage of invasive cancers detected that were axillary node negative.

As more women undergo screening mammography and have serial mammograms available for comparison to permit the interpretation of suspicious interval change, the overall predictive values for mammography-prompted biopsies should increase.

MAMMOGRAPHY-GUIDED BIOPSY TECHNIQUES

Accurate guidance for the biopsy and accurate histologic diagnosis of nonpalpable abnormalities detected by mammography are essential. The optimal selection and implementation of biopsy methods described below require close collaboration among the diagnostic radiologist, surgeon, and pathologist.

NEEDLE LOCALIZATION AND OPEN SURGICAL BIOPSY

Mammographically-guided hookwire localization followed by open surgical excisional biopsy is the most commonly used method for biopsy of nonpalpable abnormalities. The hookwire localization technique uses a standard mammography unit with a specialized plastic compression plate that contains an aperture surrounded by grid-coordinate markings so that the needle containing the hookwire can be placed through the aperture within 5 to 10 mm of the mammographic lesion. After the needle depth relative to the lesion is determined with a perpendicular mammographic projection obtained with the needle in place, the needle is removed over the hookwire, leaving the hookwire in place to guide open surgical excision. The surgical excision can be performed in an outpatient setting under local anesthesia. Precise preoperative hookwire localization allows accurate removal of the nonpalpable lesion with minimal, if any, resulting cosmetic deformity. Patients are sent home shortly after the biopsy and usually return to routine activity within 24 hours.

SPECIMEN RADIOGRAPHY AND MAMMOGRAPHIC-PATHOLOGIC CORRELATION

Specimen radiography and mammographic-pathologic correlation of the biopsy specimen are essential to confirm that all or an adequate sample of the mammographic lesion has been excised and to guide the pathologist to the precise location of the suspicious mammographic finding. Specimen radiography should be performed on clinical mammography systems or dedicated specimen radiography units. Specimen radiography has been shown to be an accurate means of confirmation of excision for both calcified and noncalcified soft tissue mammographic lesions. Specimen radiography is not an accurate predictor of histologic margin status of malignant lesions. For small microcalcification clusters (less than 10 to 15 mm), gross sectioning of the operative specimen into 1- to 2-cm sections and re-radiographing the sections is recommended to precisely guide the pathologist to the location of the abnormalities. Because histologic calcifications are often seen in tissue without mammographic microcalcification, the presence of histologic calcifications cannot be assumed to represent the suspicious mammographic calcifications without strict mammographic-pathologic correlation.

FINE-NEEDLE ASPIRATION

Fine-needle aspiration of clinically occult mammographic abnormalities can acquire samples for cytologic analysis. The optimization of results for this method requires accurate placement and multiple passes of 20- to 22-gauge needles into the mammographic abnormality under grid-coordinate or stereotactic mammographic guidance or under breast ultrasound guidance. Disadvantages of fine-needle aspiration cytology include sampling errors and the need for an experienced cytopathologist. Insufficient sampling rates occur in approximately 10% of cases.

As with fine-needle aspiration cytology of clinically palpable masses, there is some limitation in the sensitivity for detection of malignancy. Reported sensitivities of fine-needle aspiration of nonpalpable lesions range from 77% to 97%. Cytologic analysis will not differentiate invasive from noninvasive breast carcinomas. Depending on management philosophy, a positive fine-needle aspiration cytology may expedite therapy and allow a surgeon to perform a wide excision or lumpectomy during the first surgical procedure. A negative fine-needle aspiration cytology associated with a suspicious mammographic finding requires histologic evaluation. Whereas fine-needle aspiration of clinically palpable lumps may provide a rapid and convenient diagnosis of breast carcinoma during the initial clinical visit, image-guided fine-needle aspiration often requires a second visit to the mammography clinic and may ultimately add nonbeneficial time and expense if it does not provide a sufficient rate of definitive diagnoses.

Fine-needle aspiration of the fluid contents of masses that by ultrasound are indeterminate for the presence of simple, benign cysts is a highly effective procedure that prevents unnecessary excisional biopsies for cysts. Lesions that completely or nearly completely resolve or collapse and yield benign-appearing fluid or cytologically benign fluid upon aspiration are considered benign and do not warrant further intervention.

CORE BIOPSY

Large-needle core biopsy has several advantages over fine-needle aspiration cytology as a cost-effective alternative to needle localization and excisional biopsy. Decreased insufficient sampling rates and the ability to perform histologic examination increase the ability of core biopsy to make definitive diagnoses, especially of mammographically indeterminate lesions.

Needle core biopsies consist of three to five or more samples from various regions of a mammographic lesion obtained with 14- to 16-gauge needles and a spring-triggered biopsy gun under local anesthesia. These are performed under ultrasound guidance or stereotactic radiographic guidance using add-on stereotactic devices for upright clinical mammographic units or specialized tables with stereotactic equipment.

The optimal clinical application of core biopsy has yet to be determined. Although some physicians feel that core biopsies of very-low-suspicion lesions (less than 1% chance of malignancy) would decrease patient anxiety during follow-up, most physicians feel that 6-month follow-up is the appropriate management of low-suspicion lesions and that core biopsies would only add significant costs to mammography screening programs. For indeterminate lesions, the initial reported accuracy of core biopsy in small series is encouraging. Parker and coworkers showed 96% agreement between core biopsy and surgical biopsy in 102 patients. Multicenter studies of larger numbers of patients are underway to determine the overall accuracy of core biopsy as compared to surgical biopsy and the types of mammographic lesions most suitable for core biopsy diagnosis. A definitive diagnosis of malignancy by core biopsy may allow a therapist to discuss treatment alternatives with the patient and eliminate one of the surgical procedures. However, some therapists prefer more extensive pathologic knowledge of the tumor (*e.g.*, the presence or absence of an extensive intraductal component or minimal invasion) before deciding on breast-conserving therapy versus mastectomy as well as on the need for axillary dissection.

MOLECULAR MARKER ASSAYS

Mammography-directed biopsy methods can provide fresh-tissue, lesion-specific samples of clinically occult lesions for molecular marker assays including estrogen and progesterone receptors, DNA analysis, and oncogenes. Earlier clinical studies of these markers used gross tissue samples of palpable masses only or paraffin-fixed histologic blocks. Small nonpalpable lesions that occupied less than 10% to 15% of the histologic block sections were often excluded from these studies to avoid excessive contamination from adjacent benign tissue in methods that processed the entire tissue sample (in contrast to immunohistochemical methods). Lesion-specific material can be provided by the *in vivo* needle aspirate or core biopsy itself or even the needle washings after the biopsy sample is extracted for diagnosis. *In vitro* specimen radiography-guided aspiration of the operative specimens of clinically occult lesions as small as 2 mm also has been shown to provide adequate fresh-tissue, lesion-specific samples for flow cytometric DNA analysis as well as other markers.

BIBLIOGRAPHY

Jackson VP. The status of mammographically-guided fine-needle aspiration biopsy of nonpalpable breast lesions. Radiol Clin of North Am 30:155–166, 1992

Kopans DB, Lindfors KK, McCarthy KA et al. Spring hookwire breast lesion localizer: Use with rigid-compression mammographic systems. Radiology 157:537–538, 1985

Kopans DB, Feig SA. The Canadian National Breast Screening Study: A critical review. AJR 161:755–760, 1993

Miller AB, Baines CJ, To T, Wall C. Canadian National Breast Screening Study. Breast cancer detection and death rates among women aged 40-49. Can Med Assoc J 147:1459–1476, 1992

Parker SH, Lovin JD, Jobe WE et al. Nonpalpable breast lesions: Stereotactic automated large-core biopsies. Radiology 180:403–407, 1991

Sickles EA. Periodic mammographic follow-up of probably benign lesions: Results in 3,184 consecutive cases. Radiology 179:463–468, 1991

Stomper PC, Gelman RS. Mammography in symptomatic and asymptomatic patients. Hematology/Oncology Clinics of North America 3:611–640, 1989

Stomper PC, Stewart CC, Penetrante RB et al. Flow cytometric DNA analysis of clinically occult breast lesions using specimen mammography-guided fresh tissue needle aspirates: Eighty case experience. Radiology 185:415–422, 1992

John S. Macdonald, Daniel G. Haller, Robert J. Mayer, Eds. *Manual of Oncologic Therapeutics*, Third Edition.

II. BIOLOGIC MARKERS OF MALIGNANCIES

16. CIRCULATING TUMOR MARKERS

George J. Bosl

Circulating tumor markers are biologic substances that are either produced by a tumor or released by the host. They are quantitated by an assay of serum or plasma. The concentration of the marker in the blood represents a balance between production and clearance. Some tumors are efficient producers of a marker and others are not. For a few histologically proven malignancies, the presence of a tumor marker can determine therapy, and in others the marker can aid in following the patient and evaluating the efficacy of treatment. Four points about tumor markers deserve emphasis:

1. Markers *cannot* be used to make a diagnosis of cancer. Although an increased level may raise the suspicion of cancer, a diagnosis of cancer is not possible without histologic proof. Conversely, normal marker values do not imply the absence of cancer, but rather that the cancer may not be producing the marker.
2. With very few exceptions, which are discussed later in the chapter, markers are not valuable as screening tools.
3. The primary role of a tumor marker is to monitor the course of the disease. Therefore, tumor markers must be assayed serially — before, during, and after the completion of therapy.
4. Although there is a general relationship between higher tumor marker values and a greater extent of disease, elevated concentrations of a tumor marker in the absence of other clinical or radiographic evidence of disease may in special circumstances be an indication to initiate treatment.

This chapter discusses the clinically relevant markers that aid in detection and treatment of malignancies.

HUMAN CHORIONIC GONADOTROPIN

Human chorionic gonadotropin (HCG) is composed of an alpha and a beta subunit. The alpha subunits of luteinizing hormone (LH), follicle-stimulating hormone, and thyroid-stimulating hormone are structurally identical. The beta subunits are immunologically distinct. The radioimmunoassay for the beta subunit of HCG detects nanogram quantities of protein. Results are usually recorded in "milli-international units per milliliter (mIU/ml)"; for each standard a linear relationship exists between nanograms and milli-international units. The use of "mIU/ml" does not permit an accurate comparison of values determined by different laboratories.

An increased concentration of HCG is most frequently found in patients with germ cell tumors of gonadal and extragonadal origin and gestational trophoblastic disease. Classically, choriocarcinoma produces HCG. Because both cytotrophoblasts and syncytiotrophoblasts are required to make the histologic diagnosis of choriocarcinoma, and because only syncytiotrophoblasts secrete HCG, the presence of an elevated serum level of HCG does not necessarily mean that histologically verifiable choriocarcinoma *is* present. Other epithelial malignancies such as breast, gastrointestinal, bladder, and small and non-small cell lung cancers can rarely produce HCG; this sometimes occurs in association with histologically documented choriocarcinomatous differentiation/metaplasia. In patients with choriocarcinoma,

HCG levels are invariably increased. Between 20% and 60% of men with germ cell tumors will have increased HCG levels, depending on the stage of disease, and these elevations are often associated with gynecomastia. Embryonal carcinoma and mixed tumors with syncytiotrophoblasts often produce HCG. An elevated serum level of HCG may occasionally be found in patients with seminoma (about 15% of advanced cases) because of the occasional presence of syncytiotrophoblasts. However, this does not change the prognosis of seminoma, stage for stage. Therefore, an elevated HCG level in a patient with a seminoma does *not* imply that a nonseminomatous component is present, and management decisions should be guided by the histologic diagnosis. Many reports suggest that in patients with advanced metastatic disease, the absolute value of HCG is inversely related to prognosis.

Serial monitoring of HCG levels is an important part of the management of patients with germ cell tumors and gestational trophoblastic disease. Both HCG and alphafetoprotein (AFP) (see following section) should be measured in all patients with germ cell tumors, because recurrence may be heralded by one or both markers and the markers elevated at relapse may be discordant with those seen at the initial diagnosis. Frequent assays may detect a rise in HCG level around the fifth day of chemotherapy, presumably due to release of the protein into the patient's circulation. Treatment should be continued until the levels have returned to normal.

The half-life of clearance of HCG from the blood is approximately 30 hours, a fact that is often used in patient management. Effective treatment, whether it be surgery, radiation therapy, or chemotherapy should cause prompt cessation of marker production. Repeated blood sampling will demonstrate either normal or slow clearance; slow clearance implies incomplete treatment. Conversely, values that are decreasing and still above the normal may be within the expected half-life clearance and not reflect active disease. Rising or persistently elevated values even in the absence of clinically or radiographically detectable disease imply active disease, but a normal HCG value does not exclude active tumor. Thus, treatment can be started on the basis of repeatedly abnormal values and at a time of minimal tumor volume. There is one exception: in a patient who is hypogonadal after chemotherapy or bilateral orchiectomy, low but "elevated" levels of HCG may be measured. This may be due to cross-reactivity with LH or pituitary secretion of HCG; the beta subunit of LH is very similar to that of HCG. Thus, in a male patient with a slightly elevated (but not rising) HCG, testosterone should be administered in order to suppress pituitary gonadotropin secretion. The HCG should then return to normal. Frequent use of marijuana has also been reported to be associated with high HCG levels that are unrelated to cancer.

Immunohistochemical stains for HCG have been used in the assessment of anaplastic tumors of unknown primary site and histogenesis. Midline tumors or pulmonary nodules with a histologic diagnosis of anaplastic carcinoma occasionally show a positive immunohistochemical stain for HCG. However, this is not specific for a germ cell tumor. Recent studies have shown that an isochromosome of the short arm of chromosome 12 is a specific cytogenetic marker of germ cell tumors and can be detected in fresh tumor tissue using conventional and molecular cytogenetic techniques.

ALPHA-FETOPROTEIN

Alpha-fetoprotein (AFP) is produced by the fetal liver, yolk sac, and gastrointestinal tract and is rapidly cleared from the blood shortly after birth. It is present in the serum of pregnant women in the second and third trimester, and in nearly all patients with ataxia telangiectasia. As a tumor marker, it is useful primarily in the management of patients with hepatoma and germ cell tumors of testicular, extragonadal, and ovarian origin. As with HCG, a highly specific and sensitive radioimmunoassay exists that can detect nanogram quantities. The standard unit is ng/ml.

In patients with germ cell tumors, the presence of an elevated serum level of AFP is absolute evidence of the presence of a nonseminomatous cell type. Elevated levels are typically detectable in the serum of patients with endodermal sinus tumor (yolk sac tumor), but AFP is also frequently seen in patients with embryonal carcinoma. Tumors producing both AFP and HCG have separate cellular populations that produce the two markers. A patient with "seminoma" and an increased AFP should be managed as if a nonseminomatous cell type were present. In both hepatoma and germ cell tumors, higher values generally correlate with greater tumor border, and the frequency of increased AFP levels increases with stage of disease. However, many patients with both hepatomas and germ cell tumors will have normal values. Therefore, normal values do not exclude either diagnosis. In patients with germ cell tumors, about 80% of patients with advanced disease will have increased levels of either AFP or HCG or both. In populations at high risk for hepatoma, including those of Asian and Eskimo extraction chronically infected with the hepatitis B or C viruses, AFP screening can result in early detection of hepatoma and resection when a single tumor is present.

As with HCG, serial measurements of AFP before, during, and after treatment are essential. A rise in the serum level of AFP may be detected shortly after the start of chemotherapy in germ cell tumor patients, and rising or persistently elevated levels imply active disease.

After effective treatment, the serum half-life of AFP is about 5 days. A significant deviation from the expected half-life (greater than 7 days) is nearly always the result of active tumor. Falsely elevated levels of AFP are rare. However, massive hepatic regeneration can result in transiently elevated AFP levels. Therefore, in a patient with an elevated AFP following treatment for a germ cell tumor or hepatoma but no clinical or radiographic evidence of disease, repeat assays should be performed. Because germ cell tumors are curable even in the most advanced stages, a persistently elevated or rising AFP level is evidence of recurrent disease, and treatment can be initiated on the basis of the marker value alone.

Immunohistochemical stains for AFP can be used in a fashion similar to those for HCG. The same group of patients with anaplastic carcinomas of midline origin, without an obvious primary site, may be found to have a positive immunohistochemical tumor stain for AFP, suggesting a germ cell tumor. However, since AFP can be rarely detected serologically or immunohistochemically in other tumors, positive staining in a tumor of uncertain histogenesis is not specific for a particular disease.

CARCINOEMBRYONIC ANTIGEN

Carcinoembryonic antigen (CEA) is an oncofetal glycoprotein, and was originally described in patients with colon cancer. Subsequent studies have demonstrated that an elevated serum level of CEA is commonly found in patients with lung cancer, colon cancer, gastric cancer, breast cancer, pancreas cancer, and other similar cancers of epithelial origin. As with other tumor markers, a general direct relationship exists between the magnitude of the elevated value of CEA and the extent of disease and prognosis. CEA is not specific for malignancy, and low levels can be found in benign conditions such as inflammatory bowel disease, pulmonary tuberculosis, and cirrhosis, and in smokers. However, these "false-positives" are usually less than 10 ng/ml.

CEA should be followed before, during, and after treatment. Unlike AFP and HCG, rising levels of CEA are not usually used to initiate systemic chemotherapy. The diseases for which CEA is a useful marker tend to be resistant to chemotherapy, and the major value of a rising level of CEA is to motivate a search for a removal of a localized recurrence in the asymptomatic patient who has no other evidence of disease. For example, in colon cancer an increasing level of CEA may justify an exploratory laparotomy in an attempt to resect a solitary recurrence. Some of these highly selected patients will have prolonged survival. However, such exceptions are unusual and decisions should be made with care. The role of regular CEA monitoring in curatively resected patients is controversial, with recent data suggesting that although elevation of postoperative CEA values may correlate with recurrence of cancer, very few patients attain prolonged survival as a result of resection of disease detected by elevation of CEA.

LACTATE DEHYDROGENASE

Increased levels of lactate dehydrogenase (LDH) occur in patients with virtually all malignancies. It is a ubiquitous enzyme consisting of many isoenzymes and is located in essentially all normal body tissues. Although increased levels of LDH may represent hepatic metastases, LDH is strongly correlated with tumor bulk and has been reported to be an important prognostic variable in patients with germ cell tumors, malignant lymphomas, and several other tumors. Isoenzyme assays have been reported to be useful, but they provide little additional information as to the value of LDH itself and are not routinely ordered. Because of the widespread expression of LDH in normal body tissues, particularly the liver and the heart, elevated serum levels of LDH do not necessarily imply recurrent or progressive disease. Other causes of increased levels of LDH must be considered (*e.g.*, myocardial infarction and hepatitis). Therefore, treatment for a malignancy should not be based solely on the presence of a rising or persistently elevated LDH level.

PROSTATE SPECIFIC ANTIGEN

Prostate specific antigen (PSA) has become a useful marker in the management of patients with prostate cancer. It is highly specific for disorders of the prostate and is one of three immunohistochemical stains that are tissue/disease-specific (the others are thyroglobulin for thyroid cancer and HMB-45 for malignant melanoma). Neither cystoscopy nor digital rectal examination causes increased PSA levels. However, any disorder of the prostate, including benign hypertrophy, biopsy, and prostatitis can result in elevated PSA levels. PSA should be measured in all patients suspected of having prostate cancer. Elevated levels are found in patients with both locoregional disease and metastatic disease. Tumor grade and serum PSA level may be independent prognostic factors for survival after therapy in patients with organ-confined disease. Serum levels should return to normal after successful therapy. Persistently elevated values indicate residual active disease. Recent studies suggest that measurement of PSA levels is useful as a screening tool. PSA combined with digital rectal examination can detect prostate cancer at an earlier stage than digital rectal examination alone. An increasing number of patients are being diagnosed with organ-confined disease. Although this may result in better survival, there is no prospective recognized trial that supports this hypothesis because prostate cancer has a variable natural history and no curative systemic treatment exists for micrometastases (unlike breast cancer, for which adjuvant chemotherapy clearly increases survival). Therefore, the exact value of screening for prostate cancer with serum PSA levels remains unclear.

PSA has also been shown to be a useful surrogate for response to treatment. A decline or increase of PSA by 50% or more over three consecutive samples has been used to screen new drugs for activity against the hormone-refractory prostate cancer. Thus, the usefulness of serial PSA determinations continues to evolve.

ACID PHOSPHATASE

Acid phosphatase (AP) is a nonspecific intracellular enzyme normally found in the prostate gland, erythrocytes, and platelets. It is useful primarily in following patients with prostate cancer but is a less specific measure of prostate cancer than PSA. A prostate-specific AP will be present in the serum of up to 70% of patients with metastatic disease. The only other disease that may have an increased level of AP is Gaucher's disease. Thus, AP levels are rarely indicated in women. Although AP levels are not useful for screening men for prostate cancer, the serum AP level usually follows the course of metastatic disease. An elevated AP level in a patient with organ-confined disease is sometimes a criterion for a decision against radical prostatectomy. Rectal examination may lead to transiently increased AP levels. Therefore, blood should be drawn before a rectal examination is performed.

CA-125 AND CA 15-3

CA-125 is a useful tumor marker for ovarian cancer. It is present during embryonic development of the coelomic epithelium and is present on adult structures derived from it but not in the normal adult ovary. Elevations of CA-125 can be observed occasionally in benign conditions, and it has been reported to cycle with the mentrual cycle. It has been found in about 80% of ovarian cancers and is useful for monitoring epithelial ovarian tumors. Measured preoperatively in women with a pelvic mass, elevated values predict the diagnosis of ovarian cancer. Its presence may precede clinical evidence of disease by months. It is not useful as a screening tool in the general population of women although it may be useful in screening women with a high familial risk of ovarian cancer. The combined use of CA-125 and transvaginal ultrasound are under study, but there is no current role for these two tests in screening for ovarian cancer in the general population. CA-125 should be measured in all patients with suspected or known ovarian cancer and at regular intervals during and after therapy as a monitor of response and recurrence. Like other markers, persistently elevated or rising levels of CA-125 imply active disease and may be used to prompt an exploratory laparotomy. Like AFP and HCG, a decline of CA-125 at half-life (4 to 7 days) is associated with a better prognosis than when the decline is prolonged. CA-125 levels may occasionally be elevated in a wide variety of epithelial malignancies.

CA 15-3 is a high-molecular-weight plycoprotein antigen that has been found circulating at high levels in the serum of breast cancer patients. It has been reported to be useful in the management of patients with metastatic disease and for follow-up after breast cancer surgery. Elevated levels generally correlate with the burden of metastatic disease, but CA 15-3 is infrequently elevated in patients with stage I or stage II disease. It is more sensitive than CEA in the management of breast cancer patients. Elevated values have been reported in patients with benign breast, lung, and liver disease. It has no value as a screening test.

IMMUNOGLOBULINS

Probably the oldest tumor marker is the circulating monoclonal immunoglobulin (Ig) found most commonly in patients with multiple myeloma, Waldenstrom's macroglobulinemia, or, less commonly, the non-Hodgkin's lymphomas. Patients with multiple myeloma may have increased IgG, IgA, IgE, or IgD levels. The first two are far more common than the latter two. IgM is found in patients with Waldenstrom's macroglobulinemia. Electrophoretic techniques are routinely used to distinguish between the Ig types in patients with multiple myeloma, and the quantity of Ig produced is linked to the staging system and in general correlates (as do nearly all tumor markers) with the extent of disease. These values should be followed serially and will provide a reflection of the disease's activity.

Many causes of increased Ig levels are not related to the presence of a plasma cell dyscrasia or malignant lymphoma. Benign monoclonal Ig spikes that do not reflect occult multiple myeloma can be detected in the protein electrophoreses of elderly patients.

CALCITONIN

Calcitonin is produced normally by the C cells of the thyroid gland. It is ectopically produced by medullary carcinoma of the thyroid and less commonly by small cell lung cancer. It is primarily used to follow patients with medullary thyroid cancer and to screen families suspected of having multiple endocrine neoplasms. In families with the multiple endocrine neoplasia syndrome, medullary carcinoma of the thyroid, pituitary adenomas, parathyroid adenomas, and pheochromocytomas may be transmitted in an autosomal dominant pattern. In such families, calcitonin levels should be obtained after calcium and pentagastrin stimulation to detect medullary thyroid cancer in the earliest possible stage and thereby prolong survival in those patients who are found to have the disease in its occult form. Thyroidectomy is required in such patients. This is a major exception to the rule that tumor markers are not useful for screening purposes.

SEROTONIN

Serotonin is produced ectopically by carcinoid tumors. Serotonin itself is not readily measurable, but it is degraded to 5-hydroxyindoleacetic acid (5-HIAA), which is easily measured in urine. Not all carcinoid tumors, however, produce

5-HIAA. Those of foregut (lung, stomach) and hindgut (rectum) origin do not make serotonin, whereas those of ileal origin usually do. In general, increased 5-HIAA levels indicate hepatic metastases. A 24-hour urine sample should be tested to quantitate the amount of 5-HIAA excreted. Values above 150 mg/24 hours generally imply a poor prognosis. Patients with values less than this are often followed (in the absence of tumor-related symptoms) without therapy. 5-HIAA can be used diagnostically as well. In a patient with a tumor of unknown origin, but for which there exists the suspicion of a carcinoid, an increased 5-HIAA can be considered diagnostic.

CATECHOLAMINES

Abnormally high levels of catecholamines may be found in patients with neuroblastomas and pheochromocytomas. Levels of epinephrine and norepinephrine as well as their catabolic products (metanephrines and vanillylmandelic acid) are accurate tumor markers for these rare malignancies.

STEROID HORMONES

The normal endocrine hormone products of adrenal, ovarian, and testicular function may be used as tumor markers for malignancies of these organs. About two thirds of patients with malignancies of the adrenal gland may produce measurable quantities of cortisol, androgens, and estrogens. The rare malignant testicular Leydig cell tumor may produce the same hormones. Granulosa-theca tumors of the ovary produce estrogens and precocious puberty in girls and endometrial hyperplasia and carcinoma or cystic breast hyperplasia in women. Rarely, ovarian tumors may be masculinizing (arrhenoblastomas). Plasma assays for cortisol, estradiol, and testosterone, and urine assays for 17-hydroxysteroids and 17-ketosteroids will be useful both in diagnosis and in following the course of these diseases.

Glucocorticoids may be produced in response to adrenocorticotropic hormone-producing tumors. These patients will present with Cushingoid features, which prompts the physician to order these hormone assays.

OTHERS

Rarely, other tumor products may be used as specific tumor markers.

Glucagon is a marker for glucagon-producing pancreatic islet cell tumors. A specific syndrome of abnormal glucose tolerance, dermatitis (necrolytic migratory erythema), anemia, weight loss, and stomatitis (Mallinson's syndrome) accompanies this disease. Insulin is a marker for insulin-producing pancreatic islet cell tumors; gastrin-producing pancreatic islet cell tumors (Zollinger-Ellison syndrome) are marked by gastrin; and thyroglobulin marks carcinoma of the thyroid.

BIBLIOGRAPHY

Bajorin DF, Bosl GJ. The use of serum tumor markers in the prognosis and treatment of germ cell tumors. PPO Update 6:1–11, 1992

Bates SE, Longo DL. Use of serum tumor markers in cancer diagnosis and management. Semin Oncol 14:102–138, 1987

Bosl GJ, Geller NL, Bajorin D. Serum tumor markers and patient allocation to good-risk and poor-risk clinical trials in patients with germ cell tumors. Cancer 67:1299–1304, 1991

Catalona WJ, Smith DS, Ratliff TL et al. Measurement of prostate-specific antigen as a screening test for prostate cancer. N Engl J Med 324:1156–1161, 1991

Colmer R, Ruibai A, Salvador L. Circulating tumor marker levels in advanced breast carcinoma correlated with the extent of metastatic disease. Cancer 64:1674–1681, 1989

Daly L, Ferguson J, Cram GP et al. Comparison of a novel assay for breast cancer mucin to CA15-3 and carcinoembryonic antigen. J Clin Oncol 10:1057–1065, 1992

Gerber GS. Prostate specific antigen. PPO Update 7:1–8, 1993

Hayes DF, Zurawski VR Jr, Kufe DW. Comparison of circulating CA15-3 and carcinoembryonic antigen levels in patients with breast cancer. J Clin Oncol 4:1542–1550, 1986

Kane RA, Littrup PJ, Babaian R et al. Prostate-specific antigen levels in 1695 men without evidence of prostate cancer. Findings of the American Cancer Society National Prostate Cancer Detection Project. Cancer 69:1201–1207, 1992

Kelly WK, Scher HI, Mazumdar M et al. Prostate-specific antigen as a measure of disease outcome in metastatic hormone-refractory prostate cancer. J Clin Oncol 11:607–615, 1993

Lange PH. Prostatic specific antigen in diagnosis and management of prostate cancer. Urology 36:25–29, 1990

Malakasian GD, Knapp RC, Lavin RT et al. Preoperative evaluation of serum CA-125 levels in premenopausal and postmenopausal women patients with pelvic masses: Discrimination of benign from malignant disease. Am J Obstet 159:341–346, 1988

Moertel CG, Fleming TR, Macdonald JS et al. An evaluation of the carcinoembryonic antigen (CEA) test for monitoring patients with resected colon cancer. JAMA 270:943–947, 1993

Muto MA, Cramer DW, Brown DL et al. Screening for ovarian cancer: The preliminary experience of a familial ovarian cancer center. Gynecol Oncol 51:12–20, 1993

Oesterling JE. Prostate specific antigen. A critical assessment of the most useful tumor marker for adenocarcinoma of the prostate. J Urol 145:907–923, 1991

Oesterling JE. Prostate-specific antigen. Improving its ability to diagnose early prostate cancer. JAMA 267:2236–2238, 1992

O'Shaughnessy A, Check JH, Nownuozi K, Lurie D. CA-125 levels measured in different phases of the menstrual cycle in screening for endometriosis. Obstet Gynecol 81:99–103, 1993

Pons-Anicet DM, Krebs BP, Mira R, Namer M. Value of CA15-3 in the followup of breast cancer patients. Br J Cancer 55:567–569, 1987

Rustin G, Gennings J, Nelstrop A et al. for the North Thames Cooperative Group. Use of CA-125 to predict survival of patients with ovarian carcinoma. J Clin Oncol 7:1667–1671, 1989

Sevelda P, Vavra N, Schemper M, Salzer H. CA-125 as an independent prognostic factor for survival in patients with epithelial ovarian cancer. Am J Obstet Gynecol 161:1213–1216, 1989

Silver HK, Archibald BL, Ragaz J, Colman AJ. Relative operating characteristic analysis and group modeling for tumor markers: Comparison of CA15-3, carcinomembryonic antigen, and mucin-like carcinoma-associated antigen in breast carcinoma. Cancer Res 51:1904–1909, 1991

Tondini C, Hayes DF, Gleman R et al. Comparison of CA15-3 and carcinoembryonic antigen in monitoring the clinical course of patients with metastatic breast cancer. Cancer Res 48:4107–4112, 1988

Toner GC, Geller NL, Tan C et al. Serum tumor marker half-life during chemotherapy allows early prediction of complete response and survival in nonseminomatous germ cell tumors. Cancer Res 50:5904–5910, 1990

John S. Macdonald, Daniel G. Haller, Robert J. Mayer, Eds. *Manual of Oncologic Therapeutics*, Third Edition.

17. POLYMERASE CHAIN REACTION IN THE DIAGNOSIS AND MONITORING OF CANCER

Robert Mashal
Jeffrey Sklar

Since 1980 there have been important advances in the understanding of the molecular genetic events that underlie the development of malignancy. A powerful new technique, the polymerase chain reaction (PCR), has greatly simplified the analysis of the genetic changes that are the consequences of these events and has facilitated the development of tests that use these changes as markers for the diagnosis and monitoring of cancer. Although the field of molecular cancer testing is still in its infancy, it is likely to play an increasingly important role in the routine management of patients with cancer as the clinical significance of the many new discoveries in the molecular genetics of cancer becomes better understood. In this chapter, we briefly review the principles of PCR, outline the types of applications and markers for which the technique is best suited, and present several examples of the use of the technique in the laboratory evaluation of patients with cancer.

ELEMENTS OF THE TECHNIQUE

PCR permits the efficient *in vitro* amplification of relatively short segments of DNA from complex mixtures of DNA when there exists some *a priori* knowledge of the nucleotide sequences immediately surrounding the region of DNA to be amplified. In general, PCR has two major applications. First, it provides a method for rapidly purifying a particular region of DNA, such that this region can be more easily characterized. Second, large quantities of the DNA product can be amplified from even a single copy of template DNA, making possible the highly sensitive detection of very small amounts of target sequence.

The principle behind PCR is outlined in Figure 17–1. The key ingredients in the technique are a DNA template (usually total genomic DNA extracted from a tissue specimen), DNA polymerase, two oligonucleotide primers, and deoxynucleoside triphosphates. During the reaction, DNA polymerase polymerizes deoxynucleoside triphosphates into strands of DNA according to the nucleotide sequence specified by the two separate strands of the template. DNA polymerase cannot, however, initiate DNA synthesis *de novo* from any point on the DNA; rather, it can only add nucleotides to the 3′ end of a pre-existing piece of nucleic acid already annealed to single-stranded template. In the PCR reaction, these 3′ ends are provided by two short, single-stranded oligonucleotides known as primers, which vary from about 15 to 40 nucleotides in length. The primers are designed to be complementary to the specific sequences on the two strands of the template flanking the segment to be amplified, with one primer complementary to each strand. Automated machines have been devised for the synthesis of these oligonucleotides according to any sequence the operator dictates.

PCR proceeds through a series of cycles of DNA synthesis. Each cycle involves three steps: denaturation, primer annealing, and extension. During the denaturation step, the double-stranded DNA template is rendered single-stranded by heating the reaction mixture. The mixture is then cooled to permit annealing of the primers to their complementary sequences in the single strands. The primers included in the reaction are present at such a large molar excess relative to the template that after the double-stranded template is denatured into single strands, the sequences complementary to the primers are rapidly bound by primers, one on each strand, with their 3′ ends directed toward the region to be amplified. After annealing, the DNA polymerase adds nucleotides to the primers as directed by the sequence of the template. The product of this first cycle is two new strands of DNA, each having indeterminate length, and beginning with one of the two primers at its 5′ end. In the next cycle of denaturation, annealing, and primer extension these strands serve as a template for DNA synthesis, which this time produces complementary strands of a precise size, with each strand having a primer embedded at one end and a sequence complementary to the other primer at the opposite end. In theory, each subsequent cycle doubles the amount of product fragments, all of which are of the same size, determined by the relative positions of the sequences in the original template DNA complementary to the oligonucleotide primers.

Assuming doubling of the PCR product occurs during each cycle of primer extension, 2^n copies of the product are generated after n cycles of PCR for each copy of template added at the start of the reaction. In other words, about 10^6 fragments result after 20 cycles of amplification from a single template. PCR is now performed in automated incubators called thermal cyclers, which rapidly heat and cool the reaction mixture to the proper temperatures required for denaturation, annealing, and primer extension. Because the three steps of each cycle last for about 5 to 10 minutes, standard amplifications of 20 to 30 cycles can be completed con-

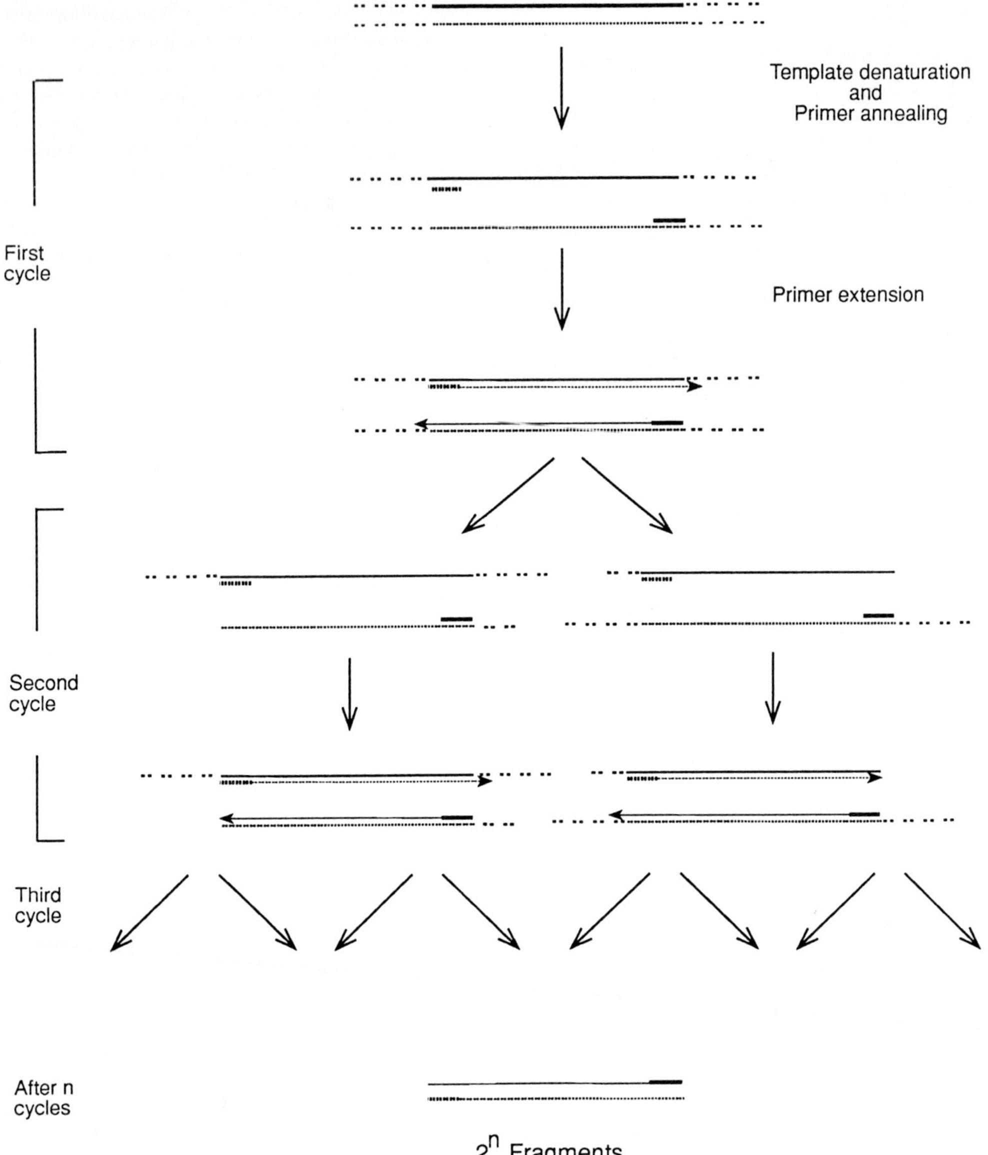

Figure 17–1. Schematic representation of the polymerase chain reaction. Double-stranded DNA, which serves as a template, is first heat-denatured and then cooled to allow annealing with the single-stranded oligonucleotide primers. After annealing, DNA polymerase extends the primer with dexoyribonucleotides in a sequence complementary to that of the template DNA. After a second cycle of heat denaturation, the primers now anneal to both the original template DNA and the additional strands created in the cycle of DNA synthesis. The doubling of DNA continues in subsequent cycles, such that in theory, after n cycles, 2^n copies of PCR product accumulate for each copy of template DNA at the start of the reaction. The overwhelming majority of these PCR products are fragments of a size precisely determined by the relative positions of the primer-complementary sequences in the template DNA.

veniently in 2 or 3 hours. A third development that has been critical to making PCR practical (after DNA synthesizers and thermal cyclers) has been the purification of heat-resistant DNA polymerases isolated from bacteria found in thermal hot springs and deep sea geothermal vents. These polymerases can withstand the high temperatures of denaturation and annealing, so that no fresh ingredients need to be added after the start of the reaction.

Analysis of the PCR product may involve a number of procedures. For example, the reaction mixture may be applied to a nylon membrane, followed by hybridization with a radiolabeled oligonucleotide complementary to the sequences expected to be amplified. The products may also be subjected to nucleotide sequence analysis, with or without prior cloning in bacteriophage vectors. However, post-amplification analysis of the product most often includes some type of gel electrophoresis, usually in agarose or polyacrylamide gels to assess the size of the product fragment or to gain partial information about the sequence of the fragment. Two electrophoretic methods widely used for identifying sequence differences in PCR products without having to engage in detailed nucleotide sequence analysis are single-strand conformational polymorphism electrophoresis (SSCP) and denaturing gradient gel electrophoresis (DGGE).

The basic PCR technique has been modified for a variety of purposes. One very useful modification with particular relevance for the clinical testing for cancer involves the amplification of nucleotide sequences from RNA. In this procedure, termed RT-PCR, using the retroviral enzyme reverse transcriptase, a cDNA copy of the RNA is first synthesized from the RNA extracted from cells. The cDNA is then subjected to PCR, with the strand of DNA complementary to the cDNA being produced during the first cycle of primer extension. Thereafter, the amplification continues through the standard process of exponential fragment amplification.

ADVANTAGES AND DISADVANTAGES

The principal advantages of PCR lie in its sensitivity, speed, and simplicity. Sufficient DNA for analysis can be obtained from extremely small quantities of cells, as might be found in a needle biopsy specimen or in a body fluid such as urine, sputum, or cerebrospinal fluid. If a specific marker sequence can be used to identify a particular cell, one such cell can be detected in as many as 10^5 total cells—a threshold determined only by the maximal amount of genomic DNA that can be conveniently assayed in a single reaction tube (about 2 μg, or the equivalent of about 2×10^5 cells).

Another advantage of PCR is that, in contrast to the Southern blot procedure, for instance, PCR can be used to analyze partially degraded DNA, such as the highly fragmented DNA that is obtained on extraction of nucleic acids from formalin-fixed and paraffin-embedded tissue sections. This feature of PCR greatly expands the number of retrospective studies that can be carried out, since paraffin-embedding of tissues is the routine procedure for the preparation of histologic tissue sections and pathology departments store blocks of embedded tissues for long periods of time.

As useful as PCR is, it also has several significant disadvantages, some of which are intrinsic to the method and cannot be entirely overcome. For example, under most circumstances PCR is performed only when the DNA sequence on either side of the region of interest is known. Therefore, if DNA sequence is known only on one side of a region, amplification is not ordinarily attempted, although partial solutions to this problem have been developed for amplifications of restiction fragments. These involve the ligation of a short piece of defined DNA sequence to the end of a fragment opposite the site of known sequence within the fragment (this version of PCR is referred to as anchored PCR). Also, circularization of DNA fragments and amplification around the circle using two back-to-back primers has been successful in some situations (this version is referred to as inverse PCR). Specificity of amplification can sometimes be a problem in PCR. Given the complexity of eukaryotic nuclear DNA (about 3×10^9 base pairs per haploid genome), it is remarkable in many respects that primers 20 nucleotides long can distinguish between the many sequences in the genome related to them to the extent that they do. Many sequences probably undergo some level of amplification, but it is only the products with sequences best matching the primers that compete effectively for primer extension. Nevertheless, nonspecific products occasionally are generated during PCR. To avoid these undesired amplification products, computer programs have been written to help select primers having optimal sequences within the regions surrounding the target DNA for a specific PCR amplification. Additionally, the cycling temperatures, principally that of annealing, and the concentration of magnesium in the reaction mixture can be varied to reduce the relative amounts of nonspecific by-products. Also, radiolabeled oligonucleotides can be used as hybridization probes to demonstrate specific amplification or identify the proper fragment within a gel. Finally, a common practice to suppress nonspecific amplification is to perform a second round of PCR using a set of primers (referred to as nested primers) complementary to sequences contained within the region targeted for amplification, inside the positions of two original primers used in the first round of cycles.

The nonquantitative nature of PCR represents another drawback. As products accumulate during successive cycles of PCR, the molar ratio of primer to template fragment decreases. As a result, in the later cycles some strands of the fragment anneal to each other rather than to primer; these fragments are not copied during the extension step. Furthermore, at least some polymerase probably becomes inactivated after repeated exposure to high temperature. These and other factors contribute to a plateau effect achieved after about 30 to 40 PCR cycles. Therefore, determination of the amount of starting template in the reaction is not straightforward. Various strategies have been proposed in response to this problem, including the co-amplification of another template added to the reaction mixture present in known amounts. However, this strategy is fraught with potential error, and probably the safest approach is to simply dilute the template until no specific product can be obtained, similar to the procedure of limiting dilution employed to quantitate antigen with antibody.

As mentioned earlier, PCR is ordinarily restricted to the amplification of products less than a few kilobases long. Large sequences are usually amplified in pieces rather than as one big fragment. Recently, modifications in the PCR technique have been suggested to permit amplification of DNA sequences as long as 35 kilobases in length. However, at the same time, the size limitation of conventional PCR has certain advantages. For example, by positioning primers to complement cDNA sequences on either side of an exon junction, amplification from cDNA can be distinguished from that derived from genomic DNA because, if the intron in the genomic DNA is large enough, PCR will not occur across it.

Perhaps the most important disadvantage associated with PCR relates to the extreme sensitivity of the technique. Since only a single copy of template can generate large amounts of product, contamination of a reaction by exogenous template, usually in the form of previously amplified product from a similar reaction, can give rise to false positive results. There are, however, several procedures by which this problem can be minimized. Most molecular diagnostic laboratories now have ultraclean set-up rooms containing laminar flow hoods into which no PCR products are introduced. Reagents are added to reaction mixtures with pipette tips containing aerosol barriers to prevent the inadvertent passage of products from pipetting apparatuses. Reaction mixtures are often treated with ultraviolet irradiation to inactivate any DNA prior to the addition of template and polymerase. Furthermore, control reactions which contain no template are routinely run in parallel with test reactions to check for possible contamination of reagents.

TYPES OF MARKERS

PCR amplification is useful in the molecular analysis of cancer when the DNA or RNA of the tumor differs from that of the normal DNA or RNA of the surrounding tissue. Tumor DNA and RNA can differ from that of normal tissue in many different ways.

Point Mutations

Point mutations are an important difference separating cancerous from normal cells. Ideally, to detect point mutations, the amplification would be specific for the mutated sequences. Sometimes this may be possible, particularly when the specific mutation is known, either because the mutation has previously been identified or because mutations at a certain site are often found in a type of cancer (for example, mutations in codons 12, 13, and 61 in the *RAS* family of oncogenes). In such situations, competitive PCR can be performed using a primer that matches the mutant nucleotide at its 3′ end and is radiolabelled with ^{32}P at its 5′ end. This primer is mixed with a competing unlabeled primer that matches the normal sequence at its 3′ end, and amplification is performed with a third nonspecific primer that generates product with either of the other two primers. Alternatively, a primer can be constructed with its 3′ end just short of the mutant base and a mismatch within its sequence near the 3′ end so that successful amplification of the mutant sequence creates a restriction site. Amplification of the mutant sequence can be checked for by digestion of the PCR product with the appropriate restriction endonuclease.

These approaches to the detection of point mutations do not work well, however, when there are relatively large amounts of normal cells present in the specimen. Furthermore, most point mutations occur at multiple sites within oncogenes or tumor suppressor genes in different cancers. Therefore, if detection is to be attempted using point mutations as markers, PCR is usually combined with some other technique for the detection of point mutations. These techniques include detailed nucleotide sequence analysis; hybridization with radiolabeled, mutation-specific oligonucleotides under stringent conditions; SSCP electrophoresis; and DGGE.

Chromosomal Translocations

As a group, chromosomal translocations are among the best markers for detection of cancer cells by PCR. Different chromosomal translocations are associated with specific subtypes of cancer, and detection of a chromosomal translocation within a biopsy specimen can therefore yield important diagnostic and prognostic information. From a technical point of view, detection by PCR is in principle straightforward. Primers complementary to DNA on either side of the breakpoint will yield a product only from cells containing the translocation, since these complementary sequences lie on separate chromosomes in cells lacking the translocation. Without any competition from products derived from normal DNA, amplification of DNA across the breakpoints of chromosomal translocations achieves the theoretical maximum in sensitivity (one cell in a total of 10^5). Thus, chromosomal translocations are excellent markers for detection of minimal disease.

This situation pertains to those translocations, such as the t(14;18)(q32;q31) of follicular small cleaved lymphoma, in which the breaks are relatively tightly clustered within the DNA of the two participating chromosomes and products can be amplified directly from genomic DNA. However, in most translocations, the chromosomal breaks are much more heterogeneous, as in the Philadelphia chromosome of chronic myelogenous and acute lymphoblastic leukemias. Often the breaks are spread over considerable distances within large introns of genes spanning the site of breakage, and recombination between the chromosomes gives rise to chimeric genes across the translocation breakpoint. As a result, although the breaks in the DNA are heterogeneous, the structure of the chimeric gene transcript is conserved among cases containing the same type of translocation. This fact has been used to detect the presence of translocations by RT-PCR of the RNA transcribed from the chimeric gene using primers complementary to exonic sequence in each of the two fused genes. The method is at least as sensitive as direct PCR of DNA across translocation breakpoints. The presence of the relatively long intron sequences between the two exons blocks amplification from any genomic DNA which invariably contaminates the RNA preparation.

Antigen Receptor Gene Rearrangements

Rearrangements of immunoglobulin and T-cell receptor genes represent highly useful markers for the diagnosis of lymphocytic cancers. These markers are not specific for cancer, because normal lymphocytes contain rearrangements of these genes. However, detection of uniform rearrangements within a specimen can be used to screen for monoclonality of lymphocytes, an important criterion of cancer.

There are seven antigen receptor genes, three coding for immunoglobulins and four coding for T cell receptors. In the germline, each of these genes contains several multimembered sets of discontinuous gene segments known as V and J segments, and sometimes a third set of D segments. During early lymphocyte differentiation, one member of each of these families is brought together through DNA recombination, leading to a continuous V(D)J sequence. Just before joining of these segments, novel sequences are created at the junctions between segments by the combined effects of variably sized, short deletions of DNA from the ends of the segments together with insertions of varying numbers of random nucleotides between the deleted ends. These novel sequences are specific for individual lymphocytes and any clonal progeny of that lymphocyte, including a malignant clone that might arise from the transformation of a normal lymphocyte. In normal immune responses, the lymphocytes tend to represent many different clones, while in cancers, only one clone is present.

In some of the antigen receptor genes (primarily the immunoglobulin heavy chain gene and the gamma and delta T cell receptor genes), it has been possible to amplify sequences across the V(D)J junction using primers designed to be complementary to conserved regions in the V and J segments. As these conserved sequences are many kilobasepairs apart in the germline, non-rearranged genes will not amplify during PCR. The uniformity of the PCR products is then evaluated based on the size of the product on a polyacrylamide gel or by some method to assess the sequence at the junction (for example, DGGE). Additionally, if the junctional sequence is determined, this marker can be used to monitor residual disease during therapy.

Tumor-Specific RNA

Aside from the chimeric gene transcripts produced from chromosomal translocations, sensitive detection of metastatic tumor cells may be accomplished through RT-PCR of normal messenger RNA molecules. These RNAs are ordinarily found in tissues at the site of the primary tumor, but their presence would not be expected at another site unless metastasis to that location had occurred. RT-PCR is potentially a highly sensitive way to accurately stage a cancer to the level of one in 10^5 total cells. The major impediment facing this approach is that many tissues express low levels of many different genes, even those usually considered to be tissue-specific (a phenomenon referred to as illegitimate transcription). So far only a few genes with the degree of tissue specificity necessary for this type of RT-PCR assay have been found.

APPLICATIONS TO CANCER DETECTION

PCR has been applied for virtually every diagnostic purpose for which conventional histopathologic and other methods have been used, including primary diagnosis, staging, determination of prognosis, monitoring therapy, and detecting residual disease. One additional diagnostic purpose that is related to cancer but is not readily accomplished by any other method concerns the identification of asymptomatic individuals who have a familial predisposition to cancer. Several different forms of cancer predisposition have been identified, some involving single types of cancer and some involving multiple cancers. Of those forms for which the causative genetic lesions have been characterized so far (for example, the Li-Fraumeni syndrome, familial colon cancer, neurofibromatosis, and multiple endocrine neoplasia type II), the bulk of the mutations seem to be base substitutions. PCR is likely to play a central role in the detection of these mutations and in deciding which patients need careful monitoring and possibly prophylactic therapy.

As discussed previously, the great sensitivity of PCR for detecting nucleic acid markers of cancer make this technique especially well suited for functions that involve finding very small amounts of disease. Examples of such applications include the examination of bone marrow for cancer in patients under evaluation for autologous transplantation and screening of bone marrow for micrometastases in patients being considered for localized therapeutic modalities. However, in these contexts it should be noted that detection of cancer cells by PCR does not provide information about the clonogenic potential or even the viability of cells. RT-PCR may be more informative in this regard than is direct

PCR of genomic DNA because of the lesser stability of RNA relative to DNA, but the significance of PCR results in predicting relapse ultimately can be decided only through studies of long-term clinical outcomes and correlations with test results.

A brief description of the application of PCR in cancer diagnosis from the perspective of specific diseases follows.

Myeloid Leukemias

Perhaps the single most commonly employed application of PCR to cancer diagnosis at present is the detection of the Philadelphia chromosome, the t(9;22)(q34;q11), in chronic myeloid leukemia (CML) and a subset of cases with acute lymphoid leukemia (ALL). This translocation fuses the 5′ portion of the *BCR* gene on chromosome 9 to the 3′ portion of the *ABL* oncogene on chromosome 22, and results in the production of a chimeric transcript in leukemic cells. The positions of the break in *BCR* tend to be more toward the 5′ end of the gene in the majority of ALL cases, and this distinction is useful in separating *de novo* ALL from CML in lymphoid blast crisis. Both types of translocations are detected by RT-PCR using exonic primers complementary to sequences on each side of the breakpoint. Molecular detection of this translocation has proven to be more sensitive than conventional cytogenetics because of either submicroscopic chromosomal rearrangements or cryptic rearrangements obscured by complex, abnormal karyotypes. RT-PCR has also been employed for the detection of minimal residual disease following bone marrow transplantation in CML. The clinical significance of this finding is still under investigation, but persistent detection of the fusion transcript appears likely to be an early marker of recurrent disease.

DNA fragments surrounding the breakpoints of several additional chromosomal translocations commonly found in acute myelogenous leukemia have recently been cloned and sequenced. The best studied is the t(15;17)(q22-24;q11-q21) of acute promyelocytic leukemia (APL). This translocation joins the retinoic acid receptor alpha gene on chromosome 17 to the *PML* gene on chromosome 15. Detection of the fusion transcript by RT-PCR has therapeutic implications because of the high rate of remission achieved by therapy with all transretinoic acid in this particular subtype of AML. As in CML, detection of the fusion transcript appears to be useful in the monitoring of minimal residual disease in patients with APL.

Lymphocytic Cancers

The most general marker for lymphocytic cancer is clonal antigen receptor gene rearrangement. Analysis of clonal antigen receptor gene rearrangements for diagnostic purposes usually is performed by Southern blot hybridization. This analysis detects virtually all rearrangements but suffers from disadvantages routinely associated with Southern blot hybridization, including the long interval to produce results, the need for radioactive hybridization probes, and the requirement for DNA from at least 100,000 to 1,000,000 cells. Especially because of the latter issue, PCR has particular diagnostic value when only small numbers of tumor cells are available for analysis; for example, in lymphocytoses in cerebrospinal fluid associated with lymphomas of the central nervous system and skin biopsy specimens containing possible early T-cell lymphoma. Also, as has already been discussed, PCR has been used to amplify sequences at the V(D)J junction as markers for minimal residual disease in ALL.

The t(14:18)(q32;q31) found in about 90% of follicular small cleaved lymphoma, the most common type of non-Hodgkin's lymphoma in the United States, joins the immunoglobulin heavy chain gene on chromosome 14 with the anti-apoptosis gene *BCL-2* on chromosome 18. In most cases DNA across the translocation breakpoint can be amplified using one of two sets of primers and genomic DNA. The major complication with the application of PCR to detect this marker is that it is often possible to amplify products from normal hyperplastic lymph nodes. Dilution analysis shows that the translocation is present in these tissues in very low numbers, close to the limit of detection by PCR. This problem does not arise when analyzing blood or bone marrow, and it has been demonstrated that patients receiving purged marrow autografts (14;18)(q32;q31) translocations detectable by PCR have a significantly worse prognosis.

Solid Tumors

Although molecular diagnosis has not been explored as systematically for solid tumors as it has in hematopoietic cancers, a number of model studies have indicted the potential of PCR in the diagnosis of solid tumors. All of the different types of markers discussed previously are relevant to these tumors, except for antigen receptor gene rearrangements. Several outstanding examples follow.

Several solid tumors carry specific chromosomal translocations. The best studied to date is the t(11;22) translocation of Ewing's sarcoma, which fuses the genes *EWS* on chromosome 22 with the *FLI* gene on chromosome 11. Detection of the fusion transcript by RT-PCR has diagnostic relevance and has also been used as a marker for minimal residual disease. It is likely that this type of analysis will be extended to other solid tumor types with characteristic chromosomal translocations as more of these specific breakpoints are described at the molecular level.

Among point mutations in cancer, those found in the *RAS* family of oncogenes offer the best markers for primary diagnosis since these mutations seem to be restricted to only a few codons, as mentioned earlier. For example, PCR amplification of *RAS* mutations from cells collected in the pancreatic juice by retrograde cholepancreatic endoscopy has been demonstrated as a feasible method for early diagnosis of pancreatic cancer.

Mutations in the *TP53* tumor suppressor gene represent the single most common genetic alteration in cancer but are problematic markers for primary diagnosis because the mutations occur at many different positions within the gene. Consequently, *TP53* mutations have been investigated as markers for monitoring of early relapse rather than for primary diagnosis, involving repetitive testing over time for the same mutation. For example, to screen patients for recurrent bladder cancer, the *TP53* gene is amplified from the original tumor and the mutation within the gene determined (about 50% of bladder carcinomas contain such mutations). Once the mutation within the gene is known, cells in urinary sediments can be screened for the mutation by amplification of the appropriate region of *TP53* gene and application of one of the several methods for identifying sequence changes within the amplified DNA.

Tissue-specific RNA as a marker for micrometastasis has the advantage that no preliminary work-up is necessary before applying PCR to detect small numbers of metastatic cells. For example, prostate specific antigen (PSA) is produced by normal prostate tissue and many prostate tumors but not by normal peripheral blood cells. Detection of PSA mRNA in the peripheral blood by RT-PCR has been demonstrated as a method for detecting circulating tumor cells in peripheral blood. The clinical significance of this finding is under study. Likewise, RT-PCR detection of mRNA transcripts for keratin 19 has been used to detect micrometastatic breast cancer in bone marrow.

BIBLIOGRAPHY

Bishop JM. Molecular themes in oncogenesis. Cell 64:235–248, 1991

Kruzrock R, Gutterman JU, Talpaz M. The molecular genetics of Philadelphia chromosome-positive leukemias. N Engl J Med 319:990–998, 1988

Lee M-S, Chang K-S, Cabanillas F et al. Detection of minimal residual cell carrying the t(14;18) by DNA sequence amplification. Science 237:175–178, 1987

Moreno JG, Croce CM, Fischer R et al. Detection of hematogenous micrometastasis in patients with prostate cancer. Cancer Res 52:6110–6112, 1992

Rowley JD, Aster JC, Sklar J. The clinical applications of new DNA diagnostic technology on the management of cancer patients. JAMA 270:2331–2337, 1993

Sidransky D, von Eschenbach A, Tsai YC et al. Identification of p53 gene mutations in bladder cancers and urine samples. Science 252:706–709, 1991

Sklar J. Principles of molecular cell biology of cancer: Molecular approaches to cancer diagnosis. In DeVita VT, Hellman S, Rosenberg SA (eds). Cancer: Principles and Practice of Oncology. Philadelphia, JB Lippincott, 1993:92–113

Yamada M, Wasserman R, Lange B et al. Minimal residual disease in childhood B-lineage lymphoblastic leukemia. Persistence of leukemic cells during the first months of treatment. N Engl J Med 323:448–455, 1990

John S. Macdonald, Daniel G. Haller, Robert J. Mayer, Eds. *Manual of Oncologic Therapeutics*, Third Edition.

18. FLOW CYTOMETRY

Dennis J. Ahnen
George Chin

Flow cytometry is a technically sophisticated but conceptually simple method for quantitatively measuring one or multiple parameters of a suspension of isolated cells. Flow cytometry has long been used for a wide variety of analyses in the research laboratory. Flow cytometric analysis of cellular antigens and/or DNA content is becoming increasingly useful in clinical oncology.

METHODOLOGY

The flow cytometer is able to rapidly measure and record the intensity of fluorescence of individual cells or nuclei. For most clinical applications, the technique involves preparation of isolated cells (or nuclei) from a tissue of interest, tagging the cells with a fluorescent label that binds quantitatively to one or more specific cellular constituents. The flow cytometer disperses the fluorescent-labeled cells into single droplets of saline and passes the droplets in single file through a laser light source that excites the fluorescent label, and a fluorescence detector records the intensity of fluorescence of each individual cell. The fluorescence data is usually displayed in a histogram that plots the number of cells as a function of the intensity of fluorescence. Some flow cytometers have the capacity to separate (sort) cells on the basis of the intensity of fluorescence. The sorting capacity is used in the research laboratory primarily to isolate a population of cells or nuclei that has a cellular parameter of interest.

The strengths of flow cytometric analysis are that the technique can rapidly and reproducibly quantitate one or more cellular parameters on a large number of suspended cells (5000–10,000 cells per second). The disadvantages of the technique are that the cells must be dispensed into a single-cell suspension to obtain reliable results (this is obviously easier with leukemias than solid tumors) and that the analysis is done on all the cells in the suspension (tumor cells and stromal cells) so that the histologic and spatial relationships of the measured parameters within the tissue are lost.

CLINICAL USE

The two most common clinical uses of flow cytometry are in the phenotypic characterization of leukemias and lymphomas and the analysis of DNA content to determine ploidy status and/or proliferative rate.

Leukemia and Lymphoma Phenotyping

Flow cytometry is widely used to augment histologic evaluation in the diagnosis and classification of leukemias and lymphomas. The expression of many cellular antigens is regulated during differentiation of B and T lymphocytes. Monoclonal antibodies have been made to many such antigens, and the antibodies have been classified into "cluster of differentiation" (CD) groups so that antibodies with comparable specificity are given the same CD number. The expression of CD antigens can be measured flow-cytometrically by incubating aliquots of the isolated cells (leukocytes from blood, bone marrow cells, lymph nodes, tumor mass) with a panel of fluorescently-labeled antibodies directed against CD antigens and measuring the intensity of fluorescence of the cell populations. The pattern of expression of CD antigens is used to determine the cell lineage phenotype of the cells.

Flow cytometric phenotyping can be useful in establishing the diagnosis of leukemia. For example, chronic lymphocytic leukemia (CLL) can be differentiated from a benign lymphocytosis because CLL cells have a common phenotype (B cell differentiation markers CD19, CD20 and CD22, with paradoxical expression of the T cell marker CD5 and weak expression of either kappa or lambda light chains). Similarly, flow cytometric phenotyping can help differentiate myeloid from lymphoid leukemias or T-cell from B-cell lymphomas, and phenotyping allows a subclassification of the lymphomas and leukemias into more homogenous groups.

Figures 18–1 and 18–2 illustrate the typical expression of CD antigens during normal B and T cell differentiation and in malignancies of B and T cell origin. Flow cytometry cannot replace histologic evaluation of the tissue; for example, the distinction between nodular and diffuse lymphomas cannot be made by phenotyping the tumors.

DNA Analysis

Flow cytometric analysis of DNA content is performed by incubating isolated nuclei with a dye such as propidium iodide that binds quantitatively to DNA. In normal cell populations (Fig. 18–3), most cells have two copies of each chromosome (2N DNA); these cells appear as the main peak of the DNA histogram of normal tissue. A small fraction of the cells of any tissue are in the process of DNA synthesis and cell division. Cells in G2 and M phases of the cell cycle have four copies of each chromosome (4N DNA) and appear as a peak

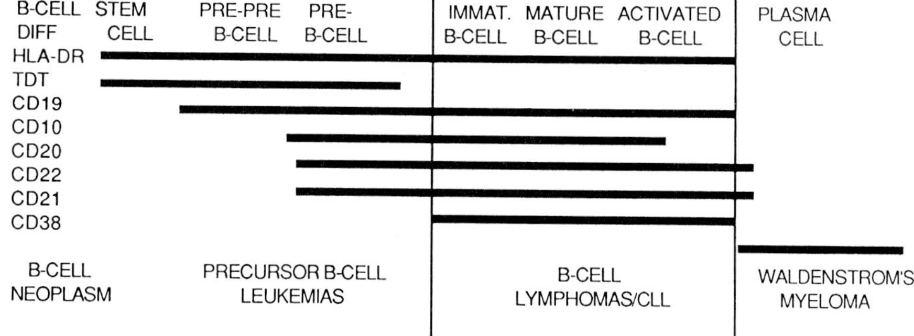

Figure 18–1. Immunophenotype of B cells during normal differentiation and of B-cell neoplasms. *CLL,* chronic lymphocytic leukemia; *TDT,* terminal deoxynucleotidyl transferase. (Modified from Cassman J, Chused T, Fischer R et al. Diversity of immunophenotypes of lymphoblastic lymphoma. Cancer Res 43:4486, 1983.

of cells with fluorescence twice as intense as the 2N peak (Fig. 18–3). Cells that are synthesizing DNA in preparation for cell division (S phase of the cell cycle) have fluorescent intensities intermediate between the 2N and 4N peaks. The percentage of the cells in each region of the histogram (2N, 4N peaks or the S phase region) can be quantitated by the flow cytometer. The percentage of cells in the S and G2/M phases of the cell cycle is a measure of the proliferative rate of the tissue.

The ploidy status of a cell population can also be determined by flow cytometric analysis of DNA content. Diploid cells by definition have 2N DNA content. Aneuploid cell populations appear on the DNA histogram as a peak of cells with a DNA content that is distinctly different from the 2N peak (Fig. 18–4). Most aneuploid cell populations have DNA contents somewhere between the 2N and 4N peaks. Tetraploid cell populations (aneuploid populations with near-4N DNA) can be distinguished from the normal G2/M cell population by expanding the vertical scale of the histogram. If there is a tetraploid cell population, a G2/M peak

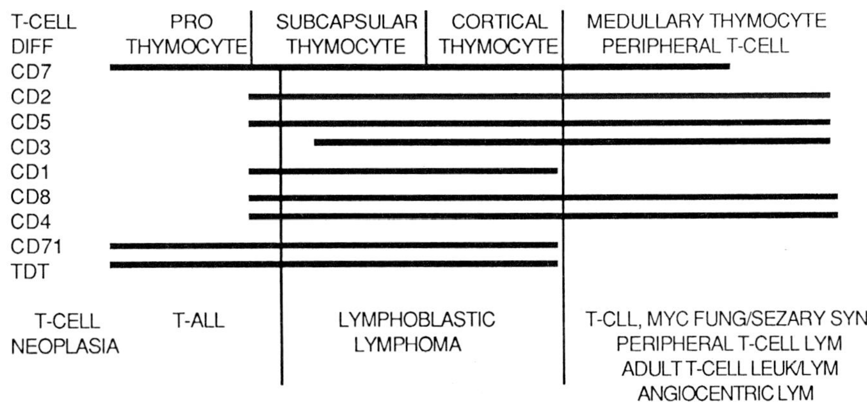

Figure 18–2. Immunophenotype of normal T-cell differentiation and T-cell malignancies. *T-ALL,* T-cell acute lymphocytic leukemia; *T-CLL,* T-cell chronic lymphocytic leukemia; *TDT,* terminal deoxynucleotidyl transferase. (Modified from Longo DL, DeVita VT Jr, Jaffe ES et al. Lymphocytic lymphomas. In DeVita VT Jr, Hellman S, Rosenberg SA (eds). Cancer: Principles and Practice of Oncology. 4th ed. Philadelphia, JB Lippincott 1993; 1868.)

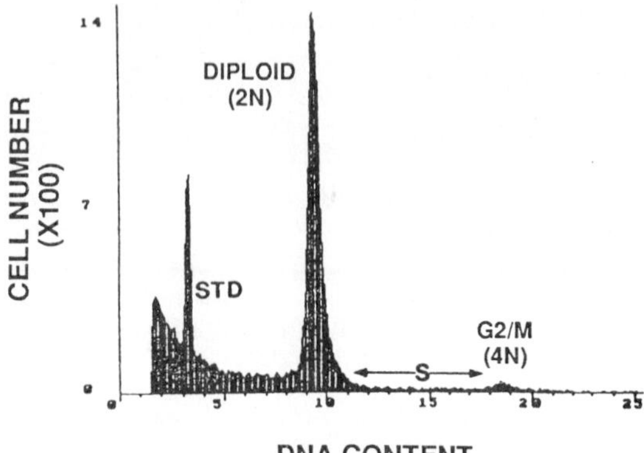

Figure 18–3. Flow cytometric analysis of DNA content. Normal tissues contain predominantly cells that contain two copies of each chromosome (diploid or 2N). Cells in G2 and M phases of the cell cycle have completed DNA synthesis but have not yet divided and thus have 4N DNA. Cells in S phase of the cell cycle are synthesizing DNA and have DNA contents between the 2N and 4N peaks. An internal standard (STD) of known DNA content (chicken or fish RBCs) is included in each sample to allow direct quantitation of the amount of DNA in each of the other peaks.

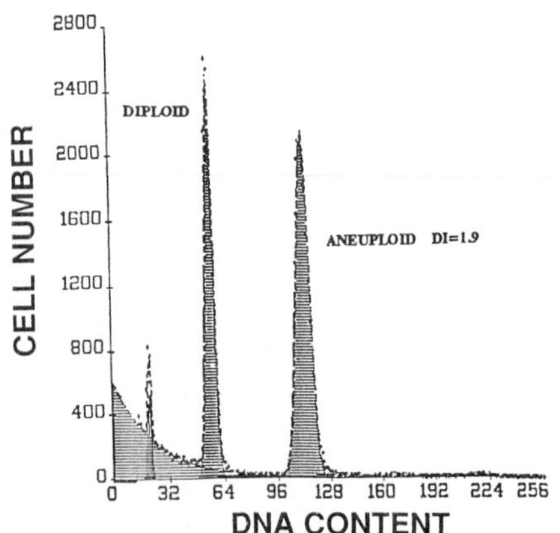

Figure 18–4. DNA histogram of tissue containing an aneuploid cell population. In addition to the diploid peak, a large peak of cells with 1.9 times as much DNA as the diploid peak (DNA index or DI = 1.9) is present in this colon cancer. The flow cytometer can calculate the DI of the aneuploid peak and the percentage of cells in the aneuploid population as well as the proliferative rate (% S or % S + G2 + M) of both the diploid and the aneuploid cell population.

for the tetraploid population should be detectable in the 8N DNA region of the histogram.

Flow cytometric analysis of proliferation and ploidy status is of clinical value in selected cases to supplement histology in the differentiation between benign and malignant tumors. Some ovarian tumors, for example, can be difficult to classify histologically because they have a higher mitotic activity than the usual benign ovarian tumor, but do not show invasion into the stroma. These tumors have been called ovarian tumors of low malignant potential. The majority (50% to 90%) of these tumors are diploid, but patients with aneuploid tumors have a much worse outcome. Similarly, ploidy status can occasionally be helpful to distinguish between osteoblastomas and osteosarcomas and between benign fibrous tumors and fibrosarcomas. Analysis of ploidy status is occasionally of value to confirm the cytologic diagnosis obtained by fine-needle aspiration of a mass or in the evaluation of cells in pleural effusions or ascites.

The more common clinical use of flow cytometric analysis of DNA content is as a prognostic tool. Ploidy status has been shown to influence prognosis in several cancer types (ovarian, early stage breast, colorectal, and bladder). A high proliferative rate has been shown to have prognostic importance in breast cancer and tends to correlate with aneuploidy in many tumor types.

BREAST

Between 50% and 90% of breast cancers are aneuploid. Aneuploidy tends to occur more frequently in tumors that are poorly differentiated, have a high proliferative activity, and/or are estrogen and progesterone receptor negative. In general, patients with aneuploid breast cancers have a poorer survival than those with diploid tumors. In patients with node-positive breast cancer, it is not clear that ploidy status provides independent prognostic information, but in early node-negative breast cancer both ploidy status and proliferative activity have prognostic significance. In this group, diploid tumors are associated with the best survival, aneuploid and tetraploid tumors with DNA content between 2 and 4N have intermediate survival, and the small group of hypodiploid and hypertetraploid tumors (5% to 10%) appear to be associated with the poorest survival.

An association has been seen between a high proliferative rate (S or S + G2/M phase fraction) and prognosis with both node-negative and node-positive invasive breast cancer. However, the subset of patients with diploid tumors that have a high proliferative rate (% S by flow cytometry) have a prognosis as poor as the group with aneuploid tumors.

COLORECTAL

About 60% of all colorectal cancers are aneuploid; interestingly, right-sided colon cancers (cecum, ascending and transverse colon) are less frequently aneuploid than left-sided colon and rectal cancers. Most studies demonstrate a pattern of increasing frequency of aneuploidy with advancing Dukes stage. Numerous studies have confirmed that patients with diploid colorectal tumors have a long-term survival about 10% to 20% greater than those with aneuploid tumors. Some, but not all, of the studies have shown that the prognostic significance of ploidy status is independent of the other prognostic factors (stage and differentiation), but clearly stage is of greater prognostic importance than ploidy status. Proliferative rate has been reported to be of greater prognostic value than ploidy status in a few studies, but this has not been extensively evaluated.

Aneuploidy is not strictly a feature of malignant colonic mucosa. About 20% of benign adenomatous polyps contain aneuploid cell populations. In the setting of chronic ulcerative colitis, patches of aneuploid mucosa can be detected in histologically normal-appearing mucosa. In this setting, ploidy status is being evaluated as a predictive factor for subsequent cancer risk.

BLADDER

In superficial transitional cell carcinoma of the bladder, ploidy status has been shown to provide useful prognostic information. In general, aneuploidy is seen more frequently in tumors with a higher histologic grade, but even within grades the presence of aneuploid stem lines correlates with poorer survival. DNA flow cytometry of urine or bladder irrigation specimens does not appear to be useful for routine screening or in the evaluation of hematuria, but is useful in patients with bladder cancer, in the follow-up of patients with a previous history of bladder cancer, or for screening when there is a high level of suspicion of the disease. In established tumors, ploidy status is most useful in stratifying grade 2 superficial (Ta, T1, T1) tumors. In this group, ploidy status is predictive for stage progression to muscle invasion and metastasis. Tumors with multiple aneuploid populations appear to have a worse prognosis that those with a single tetraploid or aneuploid population and diploid tumors are associated with the best prognosis.

In patients with superficial bladder cancer treated by transurethral resection, the presence of nontetraploid aneuploidy in a bladder irrigation indicates recurrent tumor (a diploid histogram does not exclude recurrence, however). After intravesical therapy of superficial bladder cancers, detection of a nontetraploid aneuploid population is an indicator of treatment failure.

OVARY

About 60% of ovarian cancers are aneuploid. Numerous studies have demonstrated a correlation between ploidy status and survival in patients with ovarian cancer; patients with diploid tumors have more prolonged survival than those with aneuploid tumors. In some studies, the S phase fraction has also been found to correlate with survival.

QUALITY CONTROL

As with any other technique, flow cytometric analysis must be performed in a standardized manner. Quality control issues include methods of tissue procurement, sample processing, instrument standardization, and data interpretation. Higher quality flow cytometry generally can be performed on fresh tissue than on fixed-paraffin-embedded material. Genetic heterogeneity within cancers is not uncommon so that multiple (minimum of 3) sites of the tumor should be evaluated. Variations in the mathematical models to determine % S and % G2/M phase as well as differences in tissue processing will produce different proliferative values. For this reason, no standard range of normal proliferative rate should be used; the normal range should be determined in each laboratory relative to internal laboratory controls. Performed properly, flow cytometry will become an increasingly useful tool in the clinical care of patients with cancer.

BIBLIOGRAPHY

Ahnen DJ. Abnormal DNA content as a biomarker of large bowel cancer risk and prognosis. J Cell Biochem 16G:143–150, 1992

Bauer KD. Quality control issues in DNA content flow cytometry. Ann NY Acad Sci 677:59–77, 1993

Braylan RC. Flow cytometric DNA analysis in the diagnosis and prognosis of lymphoma. Am J Clin Pathol 99:374–380, 1993

Clark GM. Applicability of flow cytometry in breast cancer. Ann NY Acad Sci 677:379–383, 1993

Dressler LG, Seamer MT, Owens MA et al. DNA flow cytometry and prognostic factors in 1331 frozen breast cancer specimens. Cancer 61:420–427, 1988

Duque RE. Flow cytometric analysis of lymphomas and acute leukemias. Ann NY Acad Sci 677:309–325, 1993

Frierson HF Jr. Flow cytometric analysis of ploidy in solid neoplasms: Comparison of fresh tissues with formalin-fixed paraffin-embedded specimens. Hum Pathol 19:290–294, 1988

Givan AL. Flow Cytometry — First Principles. New York, Wiley-Liss 1992:135–149

Hood DL, Petras RE, Edinger M et al. DNA ploidy and cell cycle analysis of colorectal carcinoma by flow cytometry: A prospective study of 137 cases using fresh whole cell suspensions. Am J Clin Pathol 93:615–620, 1990

Jaffe ES, Cossman J. Immunodiagnosis of lymphoid and mononuclear phagocytic neoplasms. In Rose NR, Friedman H, Fahey JL (eds). Manual of Clinical Laboratory Immunology. 3rd ed. Washington, DC: American Society of Microbiology, 1986:779

Kallioniemi OP, Blanco G, Alarackko M et al. Improving the prognostic value of DNA flow cytometry in breast cancer by combining DNA index and S-phase fraction: A proposed classification of DNA histograms in breast cancer. Cancer 62:2183–2190, 1988

Merke DE, McGuire WL. Ploidy, proliferative activity and prognosis: DNA flow cytometry of solid tumors. Cancer 65:1194–1206, 1990

Reinherz EL, Haynes BF, Nadler LM et al. Leukocyte typing II. Human T lymphocytes. Vol. 1. New York, Springer-Verlag, 1987

Riley RS. The flow cytometer: Historical developments and present applications. In Riley RS, Mahin EJ, Ross W (eds). Clinical Applications of Flow Cytometry. New York, Igaku-Sholin 1993:3–13

Wersto RP, Liblit RL, Koss LG. Flow cytometric DNA analysis of human solid tumors: A review of the interpretation of DNA histograms. Hum Pathol 22:1085–1098, 1991

Williams DM, O'Connor S, Grant JW et al. Rapid diagnosis of malignancy using flow cytometry. Arch Dis Child 68:393–398, 1993

John S. Macdonald, Daniel G. Haller, Robert J. Mayer, Eds. *Manual of Oncologic Therapeutics*, Third Edition.

III. COMMON THERAPEUTIC PROCEDURES

19. VASCULAR ACCESS FOR CANCER THERAPY

Jose P. Garcia
Robert T. Osteen

Safe and effective access to the circulation is crucial to the implementation of cancer therapy. Access must be tailored to the specific condition and needs of each patient. Health professionals should possess a basic understanding of the different access devices available and the risks and benefits of each.

INDICATIONS

Not all patients undergoing treatment for cancer will require long-term central venous access. Patients receiving short-term intravenous bolus injections of chemotherapeutic agents usually do well with peripheral access. Central venous access is indicated in the following situations: inadequate peripheral veins, need for frequent access for administration of chemotherapy, total parenteral nutrition (TPN), frequent administration of blood products, need for blood sampling, home infusion of intravenous fluids or antibiotics, acute leukemia, high grade lymphoma, or patients who are undergoing bone marrow transplantation.

LIMITATIONS

The patient being treated for cancer is susceptible to bleeding disorders, infections, and venous sclerosis or thrombosis. Cytotoxic drugs are chemical irritants that can cause sclerosis of small peripheral veins with low flow. As repeated cannulation diminishes the number of usable veins, the risk of extravasation increases. Chemotherapeutic agents can cause severe damage when extravasation into subcutaneous tissue occurs.

Most cytotoxic drugs suppress the bone marrow, which leads to thrombocytopenia and granulocytopenia. Thrombocytopenia can play a major role in determining the site of cannulation. Percutaneous placement of central venous catheters should not be attempted in patients with platelet counts less than 30,000. Subclavian vessels are not accessible for manual compression if bleeding occurs from needle puncture. If an open venotomy is to be performed, however, platelet counts in the 10,000 to 15,000 range are acceptable. Patients with a prothrombin time greater than 15 seconds should receive fresh frozen plasma before percutaneous line placement. Patients should be off heparin for 4 hours before percutaneous central vein cannulation. Leukemic patients with abnormal bleeding indices or disseminated intravascular coagulopathy may need to be treated with chemotherapy before central line placement. Hypercoagulable patients are susceptible to line thrombosis.

Fever and bacteremia are common problems associated with chemotherapy-induced granulocytopenia. Every effort should be made to identify and treat any fever source before placement of indwelling catheters.

Patients with a mastectomy, lymphoma involving chest subcutaneous tissue, steroid acne, previous radiation treatment, and superior vena cava syndrome may have limited access to central veins. The patient's pulmonary and mental status also affects catheter placement. Some patients are unable to lie flat because of dyspnea secondary to malignant effusions. An implantable device that cannot be removed accidentally may be preferable for the patient with a confused mental status.

COMPLICATIONS

Central venous catheters should be optimally positioned with the tip 3 cm above the superior vena cava–right atrium junction. Bleeding should not be a major problem if bleeding indices have been corrected. Injury to the carotid or subclavian arteries is uncommon. Rare bleeding complications include lacerations of the subclavian vein, hemothorax and cardiac tamponade. Most postoperative bleeding is from the subcutaneous tunnel, not the venotomy site. A pressure dressing is usually sufficient for hemostasis.

The incidence of pneumothorax following central vein cannulation has been reported to range from less than 1% to 6% and is directly related to the site of cannulation and the experience of the surgeon. Pneumothorax from an open venotomy of the cephalic or external jugular veins should not occur.

Central venous catheters should be placed with the patient supine or in the Trendelenburg position to decrease the risk of air embolism. Inspiration can pull air into the vein, and amounts of 70–100 cc of air in the venous system can be lethal. Patients should be instructed to clamp the line before disconnecting the Luer-Lok cap prior to flushing. Air embolism has been reported with breaks in the line, usually where the Luer-Lok adapter fits into the tubing.

Other rare complications associated with placement of central venous catheters include chylothorax, injury to the sympathetic chain, and catheter embolization. Extravasation is usually seen in peripheral catheters, although tunneled central lines can break between the skin surface and the venotomy site. Implantable systems need to be accessed carefully so as to not extravasate at the reservoir site.

Infection is the most common complication of indwelling catheters. There are three types of infections: at the skin–catheter interface external to the Dacron cuff; tunnel infections between the cuff and the venotomy site; and septicemia. The risk of infection can be reduced if strict sterile technique is observed. Peripheral catheters should be replaced every 72 hours to decrease the risk of infection. Designated TPN ports should not be violated for other uses. Some studies have suggested an increased rate of infection with multiple lumen lines.

Infection at the exit site has been reported to be as high as 50%. These infections are within 2 cm of the catheter exit site. Peripheral catheters should be removed immediately. Central venous catheters with exit site infections can usually be treated with oral antibiotics for 10 days and local care. Catheter removal is rarely required. In the nondiabetic, dicloxacillin 250 mg four times daily is sufficient. Neutropenic patients should be treated with intravenous antibiotics. Vancomycin is usually the antibiotic of choice. The rate of exit site infections may be reduced by the application of povidone-iodine ointment at the skin–catheter interface.

Tunnel infections between the Dacron cuff and the venotomy site track subcutaneously along the catheter. These infections are characterized by the presence of erythema, induration, and tenderness more than 2 cm from the tract. Approximately 60% to 80% of tunnel infections will require catheter removal even if treated with appropriate intravenous antibiotics.

Local infections can lead to the more serious complication of septic thrombophlebitis, which most commonly occurs in patients receiving TPN. Septic thrombophlebitis is marked by infection of the catheter lumen and any associated clot. This type of infection is usually refractory to IV antibiotics and requires at the least removal of the catheter and sometimes removal of the involved vein.

Patients with indwelling catheters who exhibit clinical features consistent with sepsis need a thorough fever search. Blood cultures to confirm sepsis should be drawn from all ports and a peripheral site. Gram-positive organisms account for 60% to 70% of infections, gram negatives for 20% to 30%, and fungal infections 5% to 10%. Polyurethane central venous catheters should be removed and empiric antibiotics, usually vancomycin and an aminoglycoside, started. If the line is changed over a wire, the catheter tip should be cultured and a new site used if the culture is positive. More than 80% of coagulase negative staphylococcal sepsis involving external catheters or implantable devices can be cleared with a 10-day course of IV vancomycin. If cultures from any port are positive after 48 to 72 hours, the catheter must be moved. Patients with persistently positive blood cultures following line sepsis should have an echocardiogram to rule out endocarditis.

The incidence of catheter-related sepsis for polyurethane catheters has been reported at 0.6 cases per 100 catheter days. Hickman, Broviac, and Groshong catheters are four times less likely to be associated with sepsis than polyurethane catheters. In the largest reported study of silicone catheters, the incidence of sepsis was only 0.14 infections per 100 catheter days. This study also showed that double-lumen catheters do not have a higher rate of infection than single-lumen catheters. The rate of infection was increased ten-fold in patients with catheter thrombosis. Implantable devices have the lowest incidence of sepsis, which has been reported at 0.001 cases per 100 catheter days.

Catheter thrombosis is the second most common complication of indwelling catheters. Catheter thrombogenicity and pliancy are directly related — only polyurethane and silicone elastomers less than 16×10^6 N · m^2 are sufficiently pliant to assure a very low incidence of thrombotic complications. Thrombosis may be caused by catheter malposition or small-diameter tubing. The overall incidence of major vein thrombosis is unknown. A 29.5% incidence of thrombosis has been reported using small Broviac catheters, whereas the larger Hickman catheters have rates in the 4% to 10% range. Catheter thrombosis may also be caused by compression of the catheter between the clavicle and the first rib if percutaneous puncture of the subclavian vein is too medial.

AVAILABLE DEVICES

Central venous catheters can be divided into three categories: short-term polyurethane catheters; silicone catheters (Hickman, Broviac, Groshong); and implantable devices (Port-A-Cath, Passport). The Broviac catheter was developed for TPN administration, and later modifications gave way to Hickman catheters, which are ideal for chemotherapy. Implantable devices have gained widespread use because of the low complication and infection rates.

Polyurethane catheters are available with up to three lumens. These catheters routinely are placed in the subclavian or internal jugular vein and the position documented by chest radiograph. The Hickman, Broviac, and Groshong catheters are barium-impregnated silicone catheters with low thrombogenicity and have little tendency to form fibrin sleeves. The Hickman catheter has a larger bore and thicker wall than the Broviac and is most commonly used in adults. These catheters can be either single- or double-lumen, and the largest bore available is 1.6 mm. The Groshong catheter has a valve at the tip that opens only during aspiration or infusion, thereby avoiding the need for heparin flushes, which makes it ideal for patients who are allergic to heparin. The Groshong catheter may have a higher incidence of malfunction than the Hickman catheter.

Several implantable devices are now available that consist of a barium-impregnated silicone catheter and an injection port containing a self-sealing silicone septum for percutaneous puncture. A straight or right-angled Huber needle must be used to access the port. The technique for placement is similar to that of the Hickman catheter except for the creation of a subcutaneous pocket on the anterior chest wall for the reservoir. Port-A-Cath devices are either single- or double-lumen; Passport catheters are single-lumen only. Central venous catheters of all types are best placed under fluoroscopy to insure proper positioning. They can usually be placed with local anesthesia and light intravenous sedation.

Success with implantable venous access devices led to the development of long-term access for the peritoneum, the epidural space, and the arterial system. The most commonly used arterial access is for hepatic arterial chemotherapy in patients with metastatic colorectal cancer. Regional chemotherapy has the advantage of causing minimal systemic toxicity while exposing the tumor to a high dose of the drug. Early experience was frustrated by stiff radiographic catheters and external pumps, but a totally implantable arterial infusion device is now available. Catheter placement in the gastroduodenal artery requires a laparotomy. Reported complications include catheter occlusion, rupture, dislocation, and arterial bleeding. Gastrointestinal ulceration and pancreatitis can occur if cytotoxic agents are misdirected into the stomach and duodenal arterial system. The overall complication rate for internal pumps have been reported at 0.07 cases per 100 catheter days.

SELECTION OF DEVICE

If central access is needed for only a few days, percutaneous placement of a polyurethane catheter may be the best choice. Patients who require intermittent bolus of nonvesicant chemotherapy, long-term outpatient chemotherapy, infrequent blood work or transfusions, or who have very active lifestyles would be better served with implantable devices. Patients who require frequent blood sampling, TPN, continuous infusion of chemotherapy, and simultaneous administration of multiple medications are candidates for Hickman or Groshong catheters. Patients with acute leukemia or undergoing bone marrow transplantation should have external catheters placed. Implantable devices require less care and do not need daily flushings like the external catheters. The advantage of the Passport is that it can be placed via a peripheral vein. Flow through implantable devices is limited by the 19-gauge Huber needle, and they are more expensive than external catheters. Percutaneous catheters are easier to remove than implantable devices.

INSERTION TECHNIQUE

Any accessible vein of the neck or upper trunk may be used. For a cut-down, a visible external jugular vein is a reasonable first choice. An alternative is the cephalic vein lying in the deltopectoral groove, which can be successfully cannulated approximately 75% of the time. If these attempts are unsuccessful, percutaneous puncture of the internal jugular or subclavian vein can be performed. The saphenous vein is associated with an increased incidence of vein thrombosis and is used only as a last resort.

A wide area of the neck and chest should be prepared to allow access to the cephalic, subclavian, external, and internal jugular veins. Permanent catheters must be appropriately positioned with the aid of fluoroscopy or chest radiograph. A catheter positioned in an innominate vein may be acceptable if it cannot be negotiated into the superior vena cava.

For percutaneous insertion, the vein is punctured and a J-wire is inserted and passed into the right atrium. If difficulty is encountered in passing the wire, repositioning the neck or shoulder might help. The needle may be bent slightly to slip it under the clavicle for puncture of the subclavian vein. It is important to enter the subclavian vein without angulation between the skin and the venopuncture site. The introducer sheath is larger and more flexible than the needle and any angulation of the track may crimp the sheath and prevent the catheter from being fed through the bore. The catheter should be placed lateral enough to allow for a gentle angulation. The vein is cannulated with a vessel dilator and a 12 Fr Teflon peel-away sheath is passed over the J-wire. The exit site for the cannula must be chosen low enough on the chest (about nipple level) to allow the patient to see and change the dressing. The catheter should exit the skin medial to the breast and lateral to the sternum. Friction between the catheter and the skin overlying a large breast can cause irritation if the catheter site is too lateral. Shorter tunnels are less painful and decrease the risk of bleeding in patients with bleeding disorders. The Dacron cuff should be positioned approximately 3 cm from the exit site. Long tracts between the skin and cuff increase the risk of local infection and make removal of the catheter more difficult.

The catheter of an implantable system is placed similar to that for the external catheter except that insertion of the catheter in the cephalic vein may be attempted first to make it possible to use one incision for catheter insertion and reservoir implantation. The reservoir is placed in a subcutaneous pocket in a convenient location on the anterior chest wall and sutured to the pectoralis muscle fascia. The skin incision should not lie over the septum. The skin surface should be parallel to the diaphragm of the reservoir. The subcutaneous tissue should be thinned out to allow easy puncture of the septum. Passport catheters are placed via peripheral veins.

INDICATIONS FOR REMOVAL

The most common reason for catheter removal is infection. Catheter-related infections not responsive to appropriate antibiotic therapy (24 hours in neutropenic, 72 hours in non-neutropenic) should be removed. Other reasons for removal include relapse of infection after an appropriate antibiotic course, catheter tip culture positive (for polyurethane catheters), and isolation of Candida or bacillus species. Some external catheters may be repaired after rupture, but sterility is compromised, the risk of infection is increased, and the diameter of the lumen is decreased.

MAINTENANCE

Manipulation of external central venous catheters should be by strict aseptic technique. The catheter must be clamped before accessing the port. Four cc. of blood should be discarded, prior to drawing blood or starting an infusion to remove heparin from the line. Hickman and Broviac catheters should be flushed twice daily with 2.5 ml of 25U/ml or 5 ml of 10U/ml heparin. Groshong catheters require only a saline flush weekly. The exit site should be cleaned twice daily with hydrogen peroxide and povidone-iodine should be applied. Opsite dressings tend to macerate the skin less than other dressings.

To access implantable systems after the skin has been prepared with betadine solution and wiped with alcohol, the hub of the diaphragm is grasped between the thumb and the index finger and the Huber needle is inserted perpendicular to the port septum. The needle position should be verified by aspiration of blood. The system is flushed with 20 ml of sterile saline followed by 5 ml of 25U/ml heparin after use or every 4 weeks, whichever is more frequent.

Catheter thrombosis, a common problem with indwelling catheters, usually results from a clot at the catheter tip or obstruction of the catheter by the vein wall. If blood cannot be withdrawn, the catheter should be flushed with 3 ml (percutaneous) or 6 ml (implantable) of 1 : 1000 heparin solution. Excessive pressure can rupture silicone tubing. Polyurethane catheters will withstand much higher pressures. Tuberculin syringes are ideal for flushing. If flushing fails, 3 ml of 5000 IU urokinase may be instilled (6 ml for an implantable device). This step can be repeated at 5 and 30 minutes if unsuccessful at first. Attempts to free the clot by reaming a silicone catheter with a stiff wire are never successful. A recent prospective trial found a significant reduction in the incidence of catheter thrombosis (from 38% to 10% over 90 days) with the administration of 1 mg of Coumadin daily beginning 3 days after insertion. Patients exhibiting clinical symptoms of vein thrombosis should have a venogram. Confirmed thrombosis can be treated with streptokinase infusion and catheter removal. If patency is re-established, heparin or Coumadin may be considered.

Central vein catheters are crucial to the care of the cancer patient but can lead to significant complications. The clinician must fully evaluate the needs of each patient and weigh the risks and benefits of these devices.

BIBLIOGRAPHY

Marx AB, Landmann J, Harder FH. Surgery for vascular access. Current Problems in Surgery 27:7–15, 1990

O'Donnell JF, Coughlin CT, Lemarbre PJ. Selected procedures in medical oncology. Oncology for the House Officer 14:200–209, 1992

Pasquale MD, Campbell JM, Magnant CM. Groshong versus Hickman catheters. Surg Gynecol Obstet 174:408–410, 1992

Pessa ME, Howard RJ. Complications of Hickman-Broviac catheters. Surg Gynecol Obstet 161:257–260, 1985

Tilney NL, Kirkman RL, Whittemore AD, Osteen RT. Vascular access for dialysis and cancer chemotherapy. Adv Surg 19:248–270, 1986

Wilmore DW, Brennan MF, Harken AH et al. Infection associated with intravascular devices. American College of Surgeons Care of the Surgical Patient, Vol 2, 9:4:5–8. New York, Scientific American, 1993

John S. Macdonald, Daniel G. Haller, Robert J. Mayer, Eds. *Manual of Oncologic Therapeutics*, Third Edition.

20. CLOSED-TUBE THORACOSTOMY

Michael F. Reed
Malcolm M. DeCamp, Jr.

INDICATIONS

Closed tube thoracostomy is frequently used in the management of effusive pleural disease and pneumothorax.

Among cancer patients, malignant pleural effusion is the most common indication for tube thoracostomy. Although any malignancy may cause pleural effusion, nearly two thirds of malignant pleural effusions are a result of breast cancer, lung cancer, and lymphoma. Collectively, an additional 15% are secondary to reproductive, genitourinary, and gastrointestinal neoplasms. Malignant pleural mesothelioma causes pleural effusion in 80% to 90% of patients, but diagnosis of these effusions may prove difficult and require more invasive techniques.

Pleural effusions in a cancer patient may occur secondary to a benign condition or as a result of therapy. For this reason, achieving an accurate diagnosis of the effusion is imperative.

Malignant effusions are exudative with a high protein content (>3 g/100 ml), lactic dehydrogenase (LDH) level (pleural LDH–to–serum LDH ratio > 0.6), and specific gravity (>1.015). Most malignant pleural effusions have a volume of greater than 500 ml at presentation. Typical presenting complaints include cough, dyspnea, and chest pain. Tachypnea, labored breathing, dullness to percussion, and tracheal deviation are characteristic findings on physical examination. Fever should raise the suspicion of coexistent infection. Empyema may be excluded by assessing fluid pH (<7.2 suggests likely progression to empyema) and by culture.

The diagnosis of pleural effusion is primarily made by using radiologic studies. Upright posteroanterior (PA) and lateral chest radiographs demonstrate blunting of the costophrenic angles with small effusions. Larger volumes will appear as partial or complete opacification of a hemithorax. For smaller effusions, or to demonstrate mobility of the fluid, lateral decubitus films may be employed. Ultrasonographic evaluation is useful in the evaluation of a loculated effusion. Computed tomography (CT) may occasionally be indicated in the evaluation of very small, complex, or loculated effusions.

Pneumothorax is another setting in which tube thoracostomy may be required. In the cancer patient, pneumothorax may be seen after central venous line insertion, especially with subclavian placement, after intercostal nerve blocks, and with fine-needle aspiration of an intrathoracic mass. The risk of pneumothorax is estimated at 20% during fine-needle aspiration of the lung. If the pneumothorax is small and asymptomatic, the air may be withdrawn with a small catheter. If, however, the pneumothorax is large, if it recurs after catheter drainage, or if the patient is symptomatic, tube thoracostomy is indicated.

TECHNIQUE OF INSERTION

When a thoracostomy tube is being placed, the patient is ideally positioned upright, sitting comfortably. For a patient who is unable to sit up, the preferred technique is to place the patient in the lateral decubitus position with the uninvolved hemithorax down. The affected chest is prepared in a sterile fashion with an iodine-based solution, and towels are draped to establish a sterile field.

In the case of effusions, the tube placement site is in the sixth or seventh intercostal space at the midaxillary line for free-flowing effusions. For pneumothorax, the tube should be placed superiorly, ideally in the fifth intercostal space at the midaxillary line. When a loculated effusion is present, tube placement depends on the location of the collection. Ultrasonographic guidance may be particularly useful in locating a loculated effusion, choosing an insertion site, and verifying appropriate placement. Right-angle chest tubes are preferred when the loculated effusion is located in the costophrenic sulcus.

Patient discomfort can be minimized through the use of premedication with meperidine, morphine, or fentanyl, as well as a benzodiazepine. The skin is locally anesthetized with lidocaine by first raising a skin wheal with a 25-gauge needle, then infiltrating the deeper layers, down to the pleura, with a 20-gauge needle. A 2- to 3-cm incision, large enough to admit the index finger, is made through the skin and into the subcutaneous tissue. Before proceeding further with dissection, the anchoring sutures should be placed. Ideally, they are placed before insertion of the thoracostomy tube for the following reasons: suturing is technically simpler without the tube in the way; placement of a suture in the center of the wound allows a tighter seal when the tube is removed and diminishes the chance of drainage or pneumothorax; and suturing before tube placement avoids damage to the tube. Two sutures are inserted, one vertical mattress stitch at the middle of the incision and one simple suture at the anterior end. They are left untied until after the tube is inserted.

Once the anchoring sutures are in place, the subcutaneous tissue is dissected by using a blunt clamp. The dissection is carried over the superior edge of a rib to avoid damaging the intercostal vessels that run under the inferior edge of the ribs. The pleura is punctured with the clamp. Trocars for the placement of thoracostomy tubes should be avoided because of the potential damage to the underlying structures during trocar insertion.

After the pleura has been opened, a finger is inserted to verify the absence of adhesions. A 28- to 32-French chest tube is then inserted by using a clamp at the tip for guidance. The open end of the tube is also clamped to prevent fluid spillage and open pneumothorax. The tube is directed cephalad for free-flowing effusions. A basilar collection is better drained with a right-angled tube directed posteriorly toward the diaphragm into the costovertebral sulcus.

Once inserted the appropriate distance, the tube is fixed in place with the sutures. The simple suture at the end of the incision is tied to the tube. The mattress stitch is left untied and is wrapped around the tube and securely taped to it. An airtght dressing, petroleum gauze covered with dry gauze, for example, is applied. The thoracostomy tube is connected to a three-chamber drainage system set at 20-cm water suction. A chest radiograph is immediately obtained to verify tube placement. Daily films are useful to monitor tube position and function, as well as efficacy of drainage and lung re-expansion.

Complications of tube thoracostomy include air leak, bleeding, and injury to viscera. An air leak, caused by damage to the lung, is managed by continued suction. More serious complications, such as hemorrhage resulting from injury to the intercostal vessels or intrathoracic vessels or injury to viscera, may require prompt laparotomy or thoracotomy to repair the damage. Complications are minimized by the careful placement of the skin incision and meticulous technique during tube insertion. Digital confirmation of a free pleural space is paramount.

A thoracostomy tube should be removed when drainage is less than 50 ml/24 hours. An airtight dressing, such as petroleum gauze covered with dry gauze, is prepared. The anchoring suture at the anterior end of the incision is cut. The mattress suture is untaped and unwrapped from the tube. With the patient exhaling or performing a Valsalva maneuver, the tube is rapidly pulled out in a single motion. The dressing is simultaneously applied to prevent air leakage and subsequent pneumothorax. The mattress stitch is tied down to seal the wound, and the dressing is tightly fixed in place with elastic tape. A chest radiograph is obtained to document the absence of pneumothorax. A follow-up film obtained 24 hours later is indicated to document the absence of fluid reaccumulation.

SCLEROSIS

When tube thoracostomy has been performed for a malignant pleural effusion, sclerotherapy should be considered to prevent recurrence of the effusion. Sclerotherapy is futile until adequate evacuation of the effusion has been documented by film because it is effective only when the visceral and parietal pleurae are in contact. The efficacy of visceral-parietal pleural symphysis is enhanced when drainage is less than 100 ml in 24 hours. Sclerotherapy is also contraindicated for suspected or proven pleural infections (empyema).

The more commonly utilized sclerosing agents include talc, bleomycin, tetracycline (not currently available in the United States in the intravenous formulation), and doxycycline. The patient should be premedicated with a narcotic and, if feasible, an anxiolytic. The sclerosing agent is mixed with 100 ml lidocaine and is instilled through the thoracostomy tube, which is then clamped. The patient's position is changed every 15 minutes for 4 hours to distribute the sclerosing agent over the entire pleural surface. Full right and left lateral decubitus positioning, as well as steep Trendelenburg and reverse Trendelenburg positioning, is optimal. The chest tube is then unclamped and returned to suction. Daily chest films verify lung expansion and absence of recurrent effusion. The tube may be removed the day after the procedure.

BIBLIOGRAPHY

Hausheer FH, Yarbro JW. Diagnosis and treatment of malignant pleural effusion. Semin Oncol 12:54, 1985

McFadden PM, Jones JW. Tube thoracostomy: Anatomical considerations, overview of complications, and a proposed technique to avoid complications. Mil Med 150:681, 1985

Miller KS, Sahn SA. Chest tubes. Indications, technique, management and complications. Chest 91:258, 1987

Robinson LA, Fleming WH, Galbraith TA. Intrapleural doxycycline control of malignant pleural effusions. Ann Thorac Surg 55:1115, 1993

Ruckdeschel JC. Management of malignant pleural effusion: An overview. Semin Oncol 15:24, 1988

Webb WR, Ozmen V, Moulder PV et al. Iodized talc pleurodesis for the treatment of pleural effusions. J Thorac Cardiovasc Surg 103:881, 1992

John S. Macdonald, Daniel G. Haller, Robert J. Mayer, Eds. *Manual of Oncologic Therapeutics*, Third Edition.

21. RADIOTHERAPY: IMPLICATIONS FOR GENERAL PATIENT CARE

Brenda Shank

It has been estimated that 50% of cancer patients will require radiation therapy (RT) at some point in the course of their illness. For some, RT will be curative, either alone or in conjunction with surgery or chemotherapy. In others, it will be palliative. In nearly all patients who receive RT, however, there will be some side effects. The term **recall phenomenon** refers to a process in which a reaction in a previously irradiated area is enhanced or repeated when a chemotherapeutic agent that acts as a radiation sensitizer, such as dactinomycin or doxorubicin, is given weeks or months after completion of irradiation. Surgical intervention may also increase the probability of morbidity; for example, performance of multiple abdominal surgical procedures increases the incidence of small bowel obstruction after pelvic irradiation.

This chapter focuses on the acute and chronic side effects of RT for each organ system commonly affected and considers general management of these problems. Acute effects are those defined as occurring within days or weeks of treatment and are primarily related to edema, parenchymal cell death and loss, and inflammation. Chronic changes occur months to years later and generally are related to stromal changes such as fibrosis.

It is the radiation oncologist's responsibility to minimize morbidity of treatment by targeting the tumor area as accurately as possible, avoiding normal critical structures or minimizing the dose to these areas. Computed tomography (CT) and magnetic resonance imaging (MRI) have proved extremely valuable in delineating the target volume, normal structures, and patient contour at multiple levels within the patient's body. Thus, treatment plans may be optimized by using multiple fields and blocking of normal tissues. Three-dimensional (3D) treatment planning, using sophisticated computer techniques and state-of-the-art imaging, allow one to better target the tumor with minimal radiation to normal critical structures. However, even with these techniques, some normal tissue always will be treated, and side effects are possible, especially when radical RT is used, treating to high curative doses.

SYSTEMIC EFFECTS

With the exception of total body irradiation (TBI), RT is local therapy and side effects are confined to the region of treatment. However, many patients do experience some generalized symptoms of malaise, fatigue, loss of appetite, and depression. The etiology of these symptoms is unclear, and it is impossible to separate the radiation effects from the psychological and emotional effects of coping with cancer and body changes due to treatment. Frequently, emotional support and reassurance that these are normal responses to treatment are all that are necessary.

SKIN

Although skin reactions are less common in this era of high-energy photon-beam treatment and sophisticated treatment planning, they are still encountered in high-dose therapy for tumors at or near the skin surface, such as chest wall recurrences after mastectomy for breast cancer, soft-tissue sarcomas of extremities, or pelvic sites that include the perineum such as vulvar or anal cancer. If retreatment of an area has been done, or if careful planning has not been done and overlapping fields have been used, reactions may be severe and persistent. Concomitant chemotherapy may also enhance such reactions.

Acute reactions appearing after 3500 to 4000 cGy may consist of erythema, dry desquamation with pruritus, and moist desquamation. This generally responds best to keeping the area clean and as dry as possible; if symptomatic, the reaction may be treated with local measures, such as topical vitamin A & D ointment or baby oil for dry desquamation, or a light dusting of cornstarch in moist intertriginous areas, such as under the breast or in the groin. Severe pruritus or moist desquamation may benefit from cleansing the area with a 1:1 solution of hydrogen peroxide and normal saline and may require treatment with a topical corticosteroid (1% hydrocortisone). Another helpful regimen has been an integrated treatment combining cleansing with a moisturizer/wetting agent combination (*e.g.*, Cara-Klenz) with subsequent application of an aloe vera gel extract (*e.g.*, Carrington Dermal Wound Gel). In all cases, patients should wear loose, soft clothing over the affected area and should try to keep the area open to air when at home. They may also use Telfa pads (without tape on affected skin) to protect moist areas from clothing. Rarely, a patient may develop a pruritic rash that originates in the area of treatment but spreads extensively ouside the treatment fields. This allergic phenomenon may require a systemic antihistamine (such as diphenhydramine) and topical corticosteroid, as well as discontinuation of any suspect drugs.

At no time during treatment or the recovery period should patients use any perfumes, soaps, powders, lotions, or deodorants containing scents, heavy metals, or irritating chemicals on irradiated areas. Shaving in irradiated areas should be avoided, or performed only with an electric shaver. Patients should protect irradiated areas from the sun by means of sunscreens, protective clothing, or shades. They should avoid heat to the irradiated areas (sunlamps, heating pads, or hot water bottles) and avoid swimming in either chlorinated or salt water. Tepid baths and showers are usually permissible, but soaps should not be used in the irradiated area.

Epilation occurs to some degree with doses of 1500 cGy or greater but is usually transient with doses ≤4000 cGy. A wig, scarf, or turban may provide great psychological benefit if hair loss occurs on the head, and patients should be warned in advance so that preparations may be made. Anhydrosis, which may be temporary or permanent depending on the dose, requires no treatment other than reassurance.

Other possible late skin changes, which progress with time, are usually seen after doses exceeding 4500 cGy. These include hyperpigmentation or hypopigmentation, telangiectasia, ulceration, and fibrosis, which, if extensive, can be quite painful. For severe, debilitating late skin changes, reconstruction with well-vascularized tissue from outside the irradiated area may be done.

ORAL CAVITY AND PHARYNX

Because high doses of radiation are used for curative treatment in head and neck cancer (≥6000 cGy), toxicity of treatment is frequent, as the cumulative dose exceeds 4500 cGy and often is severe, with oral mucositis, pain, and anorexia most common in the acute phase, and xerostomia and dental caries in the chronic phase. The patient population with head and neck cancer has many other factors that contribute to morbidity, such as the abuse of alcohol and tobacco, and poor dental and oral hygiene. Therefore, prevention is the first consideration before initiating therapy. All patients being treated in the head and neck area (including mantle treatment for Hodgkin's disease or TBI) should see a dentist who is skilled in working with cancer patients. If extractions are necessary, they should be performed at least 14 days before irradiation of that region. Extractions *after* irradiation of the mandible should be avoided, because this is a frequent cause of osteoradionecrosis of the mandible. Dental care should include not only dental repair and treatment of other mouth problems, but also instruction in daily fluoride prophylaxis to be used for the duration of life for prevention of dental caries. During treatment, patients should gargle as frequently as 10 to 15 times a day with a solution of salt and baking soda (1 teaspoon of each in 1 quart of water), and also irrigate the mouth with the same solution by means of a gravity-feed irrigation bag. For painful swallowing, patients sometimes find it helpful to gargle, swish, and swallow 15 ml of 2% lidocaine (Xylocaine Viscous) solution. Patients should be instructed to discontinue use of alcohol and tobacco and to avoid mouthwashes that contain alcohol. They should also avoid very hot or cold foods, spicy foods, and acidic foods such as tomatoes or citrus fruits and juices. Social service intervention for referral to appropriate support groups may help.

The mucositis experienced by these patients, along with the loss of taste and altered taste sensations, contributes to weight loss. Nutritional counseling can be extremely helpful, with recommendations with regard to foods that overcome the loss of taste, nutritional supplements, and written material designed specifically for head and neck cancer patients. In a minority of patients, a nasogastric feeding tube or a percutaneous gastrostomy may be indicated for nutritional support. Increasing the amount of liquids with meals helps to overcome the xerostomia brought on by salivary irradiation. Artificial saliva preparations such as a mixture of sorbitol with sodium carboxymethylcellulose and methylparaben (*e.g.*, Salivart), or a preparation containing a mucoprotective factor from the yerba santa plant (Mouth Kote), may increase comfort between meals. Sialogogues, such as pilocarpine, can increase salivary flow and minimize symptoms, with only minor side effects, predominantly sweating. The optimum dose schedule from several studies is 5 mg orally three times daily. (See Chap. 58 for a detailed discussion of nutritional support).

In marrow transplant patients who are at high risk for reactivating herpes simplex infection, prophylactic oral or intravenous acyclovir is highly effective in preventing this complication. Oral candidiasis is usually treated successfully with oral nystatin (nystatin USP dissolved in water) or clotrimazole (Mycelex in troche form). Newer techniques of decreasing the severity of oral mucositis include the use of G-CSF (granulocyte-colony stimulating factor).

GASTROINTESTINAL TRACT

Esophagus

With moderate doses of irradiation (≥4000 cGy), patients may develop an esophagitis manifested primarily by pain, especially on swallowing. Antacids, a soft bland diet, and, occasionally, swallowing a preparation of 2% lidocaine such as Xylocaine Viscous before meals may help. Esophagitis usually subsides 7 to 10 days after completion of irradiation. One should be alert to possible superimposed *Candida* infection, especially if the patient is immunocompromised. Treatment consists of either oral nystatin (Mycostatin) or ketoconazole (Nizoral), or clotrimazole (Mycelex) troches.

Stomach

Radiation gastritis may occur with moderate doses (≥4500 cGy) but is usually readily treatable with antacids and a bland diet. Nausea and vomiting may be controlled by prochlorperazine maleate (Compazine), ondansetron (Zofran), or simply by lowering the dose per fraction of daily radiation treatments.

Small Intestine

Upper abdominal or even pelvic irradiation may include a significant portion of small bowel, and because doses around 4500 cGy may frequently be employed for curative intent, radiation enteritis is fairly common. This is manifested by nausea and vomiting, diarrhea, crampy abdominal pain, anorexia, and occasionally gastrointestinal bleeding. These may be managed conservatively by antiemetics (Compazine, Tigan, Zofran) and antidiarrheal agents (Lomotil, Imodium, Kaopectate). Phenothiazines should be avoided, however, in patients receiving TBI in the standing position because orthostatic hypotension is a frequent side effect of these drugs. Diet should generally be bland and have low fat, low residue, and low gluten content. Milk products and flatulence-producing foods such as onions, peas, and beans should generally be avoided. Antiflatulence medications such as simethicone (*e.g.*, Mylicon or Phazyme) may also help. Dietary supplements may be necessary to control weight loss (*e.g.*, Sustacal, Ensure, Meritene, Isocal, or Carnation Instant Breakfast). Electrolyte balance and fluid intake should be maintained. In one clinical study, patients with diarrhea responded to aspirin (presumably by anti-prostaglandin action) after failing to respond to other conventional treatments.

Late effects occasionally include malabsorption, small bowel obstruction with adhesions, and perforation or fistula when doses ≥5000 cGy are given. Malabsorption may be managed by dietary alterations or by hyperalimentation, but the other sequelae may have to be managed by surgical intervention.

Colon and Rectum

Proctosigmoiditis is the most common large bowel injury potentially occurring after doses exceeding 5500 cGy. It is manifested by bleeding, tenesmus, and pain. A low-residue bland diet and the use of a stool softener (*e.g.*, Colace) may give relief. Although steroid enemas have been advocated, they have not been shown to be useful. Occasionally, surgical intervention such as diversion may be necessary for severe intractable symptoms.

Anus and Perianal Area

The anal mucous membrane and perianal skin are very sensitive to radiation when doses >5000 cGy are given, probably because of moisture, trauma, and bacterial contamination. The external area should be kept as clean and dry as possible during treatment, and a thin layer of cornstarch may be applied. Sitz baths with mild soap and tepid water may also help. For pain and discomfort, a combination corticosteroid-anesthetic cream (*e.g.*, Corticaine) may be applied.

Liver

When all or most of the liver is irradiated to 3000 cGy, or even less when combined with chemotherapeutic agents, an acute radiation hepatitis may be seen, generally consisting of malaise, nausea, fever, and increased abdominal girth and weight gain associated with ascites. Liver function tests will be abnormal, and a liver scan done at this time will demonstrate decreased uptake in the area of the radiation port. Veno-occlusive disease (VOD) of the liver has been seen frequently in patients who undergo bone marrow transplantation. VOD is less when fractionated TBI regimens are used compared with single dose TBI regimens. The treatment approach is to control the symptoms of nausea and correct any fluid and electrolyte imbalance.

ENDOCRINE SYSTEM

Pituitary

Irradiation of the pituitary for an adenoma, or incidentally as a result of irradiation of brain or nasopharynx, may result in a variety of endocrine abnormalities with doses as low as 3500 cGy, including decreased growth hormone resulting in decreased growth velocity in children, which parallels the biochemical abnormality. In adults, increased prolactin or thyroid-stimulating hormone (TSH) or even decreased cortisol may be seen. RT that includes the pituitary in a child or an adult with a reasonable long-term prognosis requires a consultation with an endocrinologist for baseline hormonal studies and continued follow-up with hormonal replacement if needed.

Thyroid

Many patients who have been treated in the neck area with doses ≥2400 cGy will later develop hypothyroidism, which may be only chemical or may be clinically evident. Patients who have undergone marrow transplantation are more likely to have abnormal T4 levels and elevated TSH with single dose TBI than with fractionated TBI. Even asymptomatic hypothyroidism should be treated with thyroid hormone replacement to avoid chronically elevated TSH levels, which have been implicated in the long-term development of thyroid cancer after radiation therapy to the neck area.

LUNG

Clinically significant radiation pneumonitis, consisting of cough, fever, dyspnea, and chest pain, may be encountered 2 to 3 months after completion of RT to a significant volume of lung (≥2000 cGy to both lungs or ≥4000 cGy to one third of one lung). In marrow transplant patients, interstitial pneumonitis has been a significant problem (incidence of about 20% whether or not TBI is used for cytoreduction). Fractionated TBI regimens result in a significantly lower incidence of pneumonitis than do single-dose TBI regimens. Rales may be present and there may be an elevated white count, but sputum cultures are negative unless there is a superimposed infection. The radiologic picture initially may be one of a "ground glass" appearance in the area that was irradiated, but this may extend outside the irradiation fields as well.

Symptoms may subside without treatment, but if treatment is needed, prednisone, 15 mg four times daily, may be given. When treatment is stopped, it is important to slowly taper the steroid to prevent the precipitous return of symptoms. Patients should avoid environmental irritants such as smoke, exhaust fumes, and perfumes. Using a humidifier and sleeping with several pillows may make it easier to breathe. Occasionally, oxygen may be required in a severe case, but care should be taken to use the minimum effective concentration so as not to further damage the alveolar interface.

Chronic changes include shortness of breath and cyanosis. The chest radiograph then shows an area of fibrosis, frequently mimicking almost exactly the radiation fields. There may also be a loss of lung volume with an elevated diaphragm and shifted mediastinum. Again, steroids may be helpful. Antibiotics may be required if superimposed infections occur.

CARDIOVASCULAR SYSTEM

Heart

Pericarditis may result from moderate doses of radiation (≥4000 cGy) to most of the heart. Pericarditis usually presents with dyspnea or precordial pain, any time from during the course of irradiation (rarely), or, more commonly, from 6 months to a few years after irradiation is completed. Steroids or nonsteroidal anti-inflammatory drugs such as ibuprofen (*e.g.*, Motrin, Advil) in a dosage of 400 mg three times a day may be used. Pericardial effusions may also occur, sometimes without any symptoms. They tend to resolve without surgical intervention, although occasionally a pericardial window may be required. More serious, however, are constrictive pericarditis and tamponade, which rarely are seen now because of careful treatment planning to avoid delivery of a high dose of radiation to the entire heart. Pericardiectomy is usually necessary in such cases.

Vascular System

Some of the consequences described above have been attributed to small vessel disease in the myocardium as well as to fibrosis of the myocardium and pericardium. In addition, there have been instances of myocardial infarction in young people who have been irradiated to the heart. This has been considered to be due to accelerated coronary atherosclerosis. Other blood vessels have generally been considered quite resistant to radiation. However, there have been many reports of radiation damage of arteries, manifested as accelerated atherosclerosis, especially at high-dose junctions of fields (≥4500 cGy). Vascular surgery may be done without excess morbidity in such situations when necessary.

GENITOURINARY SYSTEM

Bladder

During pelvic irradiation for tumors of the rectum, prostate, cervix, or bladder, an acute cystitis may occur after ≥3000 cGy, with dysuria, frequency, nocturia, urgency, and sometimes hematuria. Urinalysis and cultures should be performed, and any infection should be treated with appropriate antibiotics. With negative cultures, the irritative symptoms may be treated with phenazopyridine (Pyridium), 100 mg to 200 mg three times daily, which acts as an analgesic; patients should be warned that their urine will become orange or red. Foods and beverages that are bladder irritants, such as alcohol and caffeinated beverages, should be avoided. Patients should be instructed to force fluids and to acidify their urine — for example, by drinking cranberry juice. After high-dose radiation (≥6000 cGy), chronic symptoms of frequency, urgency, and nocturia may occur if the bladder has become fibrosed and contracted. The diagnosis may be established by cystoscopy and/or a cystogram. Treatment is an ileal loop diversion if symptoms are uncontrolled by conservative measures such as limiting fluid intake before bedtime.

Kidneys

Kidney damage rarely occurs with modern radiotherapeutic techniques, because great care is usually taken not to exceed 2000 cGy to the kidneys and to spare one kidney entirely. Symptoms include headache, dyspnea, nausea, and vomiting, and the patient may become hypertensive and anemic. Laboratory findings may be only proteinuria in early or mild cases, but may also include elevated serum blood urea nitrogen and creatinine. Treatment consists of bed rest, low-protein and low-salt diet, and, potentially, blood transfusions, hypotensive medications, and/or dialysis. With significant nephritis of one kidney, when the other has been spared, nephrectomy may be required.

Ovaries and Testes

Patients may become infertile after even low doses to the gonads (150–300 cGy to the testes or ovaries); women may become amenorrheic and experience menopausal symptoms.

However, this is not invariable even after a total dose of 2000 cGy, and patients should be advised to use birth control if they do not want children. With higher doses to the testes and ovaries (≥3000 cGy), infertility is nearly certain.

Vagina

Patients with irradiation doses to the vagina exceeding 5000 cGy may experience dyspareunia due to mucosal alterations (loss of secretions) and to constriction of the vagina. Using lubricants as well as vaginal dilators for several months after completion of radiation therapy, especially prior to late fibrotic changes, may be of benefit. One effective vaginal moisturizer (Replens vaginal gel) is a mixture of lubricants intended to duplicate the normal vaginal condition; the use of a pre-filled applicator three times a week is recommended.

CENTRAL NERVOUS SYSTEM

Brain

During cranial irradiation, patients may experience headache, nausea, and vomiting, and papilledema may be observed, all suggesting increased intracranial pressure. Dexamethasone, 4 mg four times daily, usually prevents these symptoms and signs. Several weeks to a few months after cranial irradiation (≥1800 cGy) combined with intrathecal chemotherapy, a somnolence syndrome has been described, primarily in children, in which patients sleep for excessive periods of time. It is transient, lasting 3 to 14 days, and occurs about 6 weeks after a course of irradiation. It has been suggested, but not proven, that children exhibiting this syndrome preferentially develop late learning disabilities and seizure disorders. Prednisone coverage (15 mg/m^2/day) during cranial irradiation can lower the incidence of this syndrome in children. Some patients also experience transient ear pain and/or hearing loss during cranial irradiation. If infection is ruled out, no intervention is necessary.

The most serious chronic effect of RT is brain necrosis, which is a significant risk only with doses greater than 5000 cGy and can completely mimic tumor recurrence in symptoms, signs, and radiographic appearance, although there is the possibility of distinguishing the two by means of positron emission tomography. The only treatment is excision of the necrotic area, if possible. Other late symptoms, such as short-term memory loss and visual memory disturbances, have been described at doses as low as 3000 cGy (300 cGy fractions) when radiation has been combined with aggressive chemotherapy. CT scan abnormalities, such as white matter changes, calcifications, and ventricular dilatation, have also been seen with combined regimens. The relative contribution of radiation and chemotherapy to these changes has yet to be determined but treatments using lower doses/fraction (≤2000 cGy) appear to be less morbid. Supportive care is the only treatment known.

Spinal Cord

Generally, there are no symptoms during radiation treatment, but a few months after irradiation of the cervical or thoracic spinal cord to doses of ≥4000 cGy, approximately 10% of patients may experience electric shock-like sensations shooting into one or more extremities on neck flexion (Lhermitte's sign). These sensations are transient, lasting 1 to 6 months, apparently related to a temporary demyelination, and do not presage any late morbidity. Radiation myelopathy, which occurs months to years after irradiation, usually occurs only after doses ≥5000 cGy. This devastating complication may result in progressive paresthesias, loss of motor function, and/or loss of bowel and bladder function. It may be difficult to differentiate from tumor recurrence. There is no known effective therapy.

EYE

The lens of the eye is sensitive to relatively low doses of irradiation; total doses of about 1000 cGy can produce cataracts, especially if given in a single dose. Patients treated near the eye who report blurred or deteriorating vision should be evaluated ophthalmologically. In some, lens replacement surgery may be indicated if vision is sufficiently impaired. Acutely, conjunctivitis or keratitis may occur. Infection, if proven, should be treated with appropriate antibiotics. If infection is absent, steroid eyedrops may help.

BLOOD

Large-field irradiation, such as is used in treatment of Hodgkin's disease or in large pelvic fields, may result in significant bone marrow suppression, especially if chemotherapy has also been employed. If leukopenia or thrombocytopenia is significant, treatment may have to be interrupted. Anemia, if it occurs, is usually seen later, after completion of treatment, unless aggressive chemotherapy was given before treatment. Transfusion should be considered if the hemoglobin falls to levels of 9 g/100 ml or less. Patients with thrombocytopenia should avoid any aspirin-containing medications and should report any signs of bleeding. Other precautions include avoiding anything that might traumatize the skin or mucous membranes, such as douches, suppositories, or hard toothbrushes. Patients should use only an electric razor for shaving.

BONE

Impairment of bone growth may be seen in children who have received more than 2000 cGy to bone, leading to malformation or shortening, and decreased height if several vertebral bodies are irradiated. The younger the child, the greater the effect. Impairment of bone growth due to bone irradiation should be differentiated from growth effects due to pituitary irradiation, which is potentially treatable by growth hormone replacement.

A more serious complication of bone irradiation is osteonecrosis, which may occur with doses greater than 6000 cGy to bone and at even lower doses, especially in combination with chemotherapy. The most common location is the mandible, which is treated to high doses in most head and neck cancers and which is subject to trauma from dental extractions or infections. Prevention by means of careful treatment planning and dental care is most important. Any dental extractions after radiation therapy to the area should be done with antibiotic coverage and careful closure of the mucosa. If necrosis does occur, treatment usually includes antibiotics and careful debridement. Occasionally, resection of the involved bone may be required. Necrosis of the heads of the long bones, fortunately an uncommon occurrence, may require joint replacement or bone grafting.

CARCINOGENESIS

A major concern in cancer treatment with radiation and/or chemotherapeutic agents is carcinogenesis. With radiation, prerequisites for presumptive diagnosis of a radiation-induced cancer are that the tumor must be within the field of irradiation and of a histology different from the original cancer. There is usually a latent period of at least 4 years for solid tumors and at least 2 years for leukemia induction. The most common cancers related to radiation treatment are leukemias, thyroid carcinoma, and soft-tissue and bone sarcomas. Physicians should be alert to the potential for such malignancies in follow-up. Patients who have been treated in the area of the thyroid should have a careful physical examination every 2 years with surgical intervention if a palpable nodule develops. Most thyroid carcinomas have occurred in patients who have received relatively low doses of irradiation for benign disease ($\leq$1500 cGy), whereas higher therapeutic doses used for treatment of malignancies more commonly result in hypothyroidism. It has been difficult to assess the probability that a given malignancy in an irradiated patient has been the result of that irradiation. A report in 1985 from the National Institutes of Health has provided tables that are useful in assessing such probabilities, based on the type of cancer, age of the patient at exposure, and latent period from exposure to development of the cancer.

Multiple malignancies are quite common in cancer patients even without radiation therapy, especially in head and neck and lung cancer patients, whose predisposing factors increase their general risk for other malignancies in these areas. Some patients belong to "cancer families," in which a variety of cancers are common, such as endometrium, breast, and colon carcinoma. The bottom line is that any patient with a previous cancer should always be considered at a higher risk for a second malignancy, and good interim histories and physical examinations must be done on a regular basis.

BRACHYTHERAPY: SPECIAL CONSIDERATIONS

Most of the preceding discussion applies to brachytherapy as well as to external beam treatments, but there are a few special considerations. **Brachytherapy** is the use of radioactive sources close to or within the tumor as opposed to a beam directed from some distance (teletherapy or external beam treatment). A high dose of radiation can be given to a small volume of tumor or tissue at risk for residual tumor while sparing most surrounding normal tissue from the effects of radiation. The radioactive material may be encapsulated (*e.g.*, seeds), in the form of wires, or in solution such as colloidal chromic phosphate P-32 solution. Two primary methods of delivery are by means of intracavitary or interstitial implants. In an intracavitary implant, the radioactive sources are placed temporarily into a body cavity and radiation is delivered into the area adjacent to this cavity. In an interstitial implant, the radioactive material is inserted directly into the tissue where the radiation is to be delivered and may be temporary or permanent. Temporary implants are either low-dose rate, in which the radioactive sources are removed after hours to days, or high-dose rate, in which the sources are removed after several minutes. Permanent implants remain in place, with their radioactivity gradually decaying and the dose being delivered over a period of months. Most modern brachytherapy is carried out with radionuclides such as ^{192}iridium, ^{137}cesium, and ^{125}iodine. These radionuclides have replaced radium, previously the most commonly used isotope, due to the hazards associated with the decay product of radium, radon gas.

Brachytherapy procedures are performed under local or general anesthesia, with patients being hospitalized for a few days. Temporary implants are removed before the patient leaves the hospital, and special radiation precautions are taken during the hospital stay to reduce radiation exposure to personnel or visitors. Because total radiation exposure to others depends on the duration of exposure and proximity to the sources, personnel are usually instructed to perform their duties expeditiously, and visitors are instructed to stay near the door of the room and to visit for only a limited period of time, until the implant is removed and radioactive warning signs are taken down. Once the implant is removed, there is no residual radioactivity. Frequently, the patient and the family need to be reassured of this fact.

For permanent implants, an isotope with relatively low activity and energy is usually used, such as ^{125}I, and few precautions need to be taken on discharge from the hospital. The patient may be given instructions concerning the length of time and how close he or she may spend in proximity to children or someone of child-bearing age, and told when no further precautions of any sort are necessary. At some institutions, the patient is given a form containing this information before discharge. It should be made clear to the patient and family that at no time can another person become contaminated with radiation by touching the patient.

BIBLIOGRAPHY

Anseline PF, Lavey IC, Fazio VW, et al. Radiation injury of the rectum: Evaluation of surgical treatment. Ann Surg 194:716, 1981

Ch'ien LT, Aur RJA, Stagner S et al. Long-term neurological implications of somnolence syndrome in children with acute lymphocytic leukemia. Ann Neurol 8:273, 1980

Daly TE. Dental care in the irradiated patient. In Fletcher GH. Textbook of Radiotherapy. 3rd ed. Philadelphia, Lea and Febiger, 1980:229

Duffner PK, Cohen ME, Voorhess ML et al. Long-term effects of cranial irradiation on endocrine function in children with brain tumors: A prospective study. Cancer 56:2189, 1985

Ewer MS, Benjamin RS. Cardiac complications. In Holland JF, Frei E, Bast RC, et al (eds). Cancer Medicine. 3rd ed. Philadelphia, Lea and Febiger, 1993:2345

Glatstein E, Carter SK. The chronic toxicity of cancer treatment. In Carter SK, Glatstein E, Livingston RB (eds). Principles of Cancer Treatment. New York, McGraw-Hill, 1982:221

Jao S-W, Beart RW Jr, Gunderson LL. Surgical treatment of radiation injuries of the colon and rectum. Am J Surg 151:272, 1986

Johnson JT, Ferretti GA, Nethery WJ et al. Oral pilocarpine for post-irradiation xerostomia in patients with head and neck cancer. N Engl J Med 329:390, 1993

Larson DL. Management of complications of radiotherapy of the head and neck. Surg Clin North Am 66:169, 1986

Lawson JA. Surgical treatment of radiation-induced atherosclerotic disease of the iliac and femoral arteries. J Cardiovasc Surg 26:151, 1985

Mandell LR, Walker RW, Steinherz P, Fuks Z. Reduced incidence of the somnolence syndrome in leukemic children with steroid coverage during prophylactic cranial radiation therapy: results of a pilot study. Cancer 63:1975, 1989

Marks G, Mohiudden M. The surgical management of the radiation-injured intestine. Surg Clin North Am 63:81, 1983

Meadows AT, Silber J. Delayed consequence of therapy for childhood cancer. CA—A Cancer J for Clin 35:271, 1985

Mould JJ, Adam NM. The problem of avascular necrosis of bone in patients treated for Hodgkin's disease. Clin Radiol 34:231, 1983

Oberfield SE, Allen JC, Pollack J et al. Long-term endocrine sequelae after treatment of medulloblastoma: Prospective study of growth and thyroid function. J Pediatr 108:219, 1986

Report of the National Institutes of Health Ad Hoc Working Group to Develop Radioepidemiological Tables. Washington, D.C., National Institutes of Health, 1985. Publication No. 85-2748.

Scanlon EF, Berk RS, Khandekar JD. Postirradiation neoplasia: A symposium. Curr Probl Cancer 3:4, 1978

Shank B. Radiation therapy: Side effects and their management. Prim Care & Cancer 6:49, 1986

Vikram B, Strong EW, Shah JP, Spiro R. Second malignant neoplasms in patients successfully treated with multimodality treatment for advanced head and neck cancer. Head Neck Surg 6:734, 1984

Wright WE, Haller JM, Harlow SA, Pizzo PA. An oral disease prevention program for patients receiving radiation and chemotherapyl. J Am Dent Assoc 110:43, 1985

John S. Macdonald, Daniel G. Haller, Robert J. Mayer, Eds. *Manual of Oncologic Therapeutics*, Third Edition.

22. CHEMOTHERAPY: THE PROPERTIES AND USES OF SINGLE AGENTS

Jean L. Grem
Maria de Carvalho
Robert E. Wittes
Carmen J. Allegra

In this chapter we describe some of the clinically relevant properties of the single agents that constitute the principal building blocks for effective contemporary systemic therapy. We have included the most commonly used agents as well as some investigational drugs that show particular promise and may become commercially available in the near future. This chapter of the manual is not intended as a substitute for personal familiarity with the clinical properties of these drugs or a grasp of the relevant literature. These agents should be administered only by medical personnel who have had adequate hands-on training in their use or who are being closely supervised by others with such training.

For most of the agents described in this chapter, information is provided in six categories: (1) pharmacology, (2) therapeutic uses, (3) details of administration, (4) precautions and dose modifications, (5) drug interactions, and (6) toxicity. The descriptions of therapeutic uses are not meant to be restrictive; many agents are under investigation in areas for which efficacy has not yet been established and thus may be employed in ways not mentioned here or in the disease chapters of the manual.

Under "Details of Administration" we have tried to include clinically relevant information that will permit delivery of drug according to best current practice. Much of the data on recommended dose and schedule of single agents may have only borderline relevance to common contemporary practice, which relies heavily on drug combinations. Nevertheless, this information may be relevant to the care of individual patients. None of this information should be regarded as an endorsement of therapeutic strategies that are obviously inadequate (*e.g.*, the use of asparaginase or procarbazine alone for the treatment of acute lymphoblastic leukemia or Hodgkin's disease, respectively).

Because drug stability may depend on the temperature and duration of storage in solution as well as the solvent or vehicle used, particular care should be given to these details. Also, as with all drugs, one should not assume that two or more agents can be dissolved together and administered from the same bottle or into the same tubing, unless compatibility under these specific conditions has been previously established.

A good description of how to modify the dose of anticancer agents in various clinical circumstances is a particularly difficult problem. The pharmacology and clinical effects of most anticancer agents have not been subjected to systematic study under conditions of abnormal major organ function; the careful studies of carboplatin in the setting of abnormal renal function stand in contrast to the general trend. The interested reader should consult the article by Sulkes and Collins for a fuller discussion of these issues and their implications for optimal use of cytotoxic agents. For agents about which information is lacking, therefore, the best practice is to use a careful empirical approach that considers what is known about the pharmacology and disposition of the agent under conditions of normal organ function, together with the clinical status of the patient. These modifications should be undertaken only by the experienced clinician.

We also must point out that while fear of inducing intolerable toxicity is appropriate, so should be the fear of underdosing patients whose chance of long-term palliation or cure depends on the delivery of full drug doses. Uncritical readiness to reduce doses in anticipation of toxicity or in reaction to mild and reversible side effects is as much to be condemned as heedless disregard of patient safety in an attempt to be as aggressive as possible. Walking this fine line represents the art of medical oncology. The descriptions of drug toxicity presented in this chapter concentrate on those that are clinically most important and are not meant to be an exhaustive list of every side effect that has ever been imputed to the particular agent.

Anticancer agents are highly reactive molecules, and interactions with other antineoplastic drugs, as well as with agents from many other therapeutic classes, are an ever-present possibility. Information about drug–drug interactions are available from the literature only on a sporadic basis, mostly as case reports rather than from systematic pharmacologic study. Moreover, the common use of anticancer agents in combination confounds the interpretation of many case reports that allege interactions between specific cancer drugs and noncancer drugs. The information included under the heading Drug Interactions should, therefore, be regarded as incomplete and tentative. For cancer patients on active treatment with chemotherapy or biologic response modifiers, physicians should monitor plasma levels of those drugs whose levels determine therapeutic effect and toxicity (*e.g.*, digitalis derivatives, antiarrhythmics, anticonvulsants, anticoagulants), unless specific data are available that rule out the likelihood of such interactions.

Three of the investigational cytotoxic agents described in

this chapter have been placed in a special treatment investigational new drug (IND) category (Group C) that permits the National Cancer Institute (NCI) to provide these drugs for the treatment of patients in certain disease categories outside the usual clinical trials context (Table 22-1). The criteria for placing a drug into Group C include evidence of reproducible clinical benefit to patients at an acceptable toxic cost; a Group C application must be approved by the Food and Drug Administration (FDA) before a drug can be made available under this mechanism. For some of these drugs, the NCI requires the reporting only of adverse drug reactions; for others, certain baseline patient information and outcome data are required. For information about obtaining any of the three cytotoxic agents listed in Table 22-1 for the treatment of particular patients outside of a clinical trial, call the NCI Drug Management and Authorization Section of the Investigational Drug Branch at (301) 496-5725.

ALKYLATING AGENTS

Alkylating agents react strongly with various nucleophilic substances to form covalent linkages. A variety of chemical groups (sulfhydryl, carboxyl, imidazole, phosphate, and amino) may serve as targets in biologic systems. The cellular effects of alkylating agents are probably related chiefly to the alkylation of components of DNA; the N7 position of guanine is particularly susceptible, although a number of other sites may be alkylated as well. Reaction of alkylating agents with susceptible sites may lead to depurination, strand breaks, the formation of DNA inter- or intrastrand crosslinks, or the formation of links between a DNA strand and protein. These reactions may have profound effects on DNA replication and transcription and are thought to be responsible for the principal clinical effects of these agents: cytotoxicity, mutagenesis, and carcinogenesis.

Although alkylation takes place in both proliferating and nonproliferating cells, the proliferating compartment is preferentially sensitive to the killing effects of these drugs. Cells in any phase of the cell cycle are susceptible, although late G1 and S are more vulnerable phases than G2, M, or early G1. Agents that result in glutathione depletion, such as buthioninessulfoximine (BSO), may enhance the cytotoxicity of the alkylating agents.

TABLE 22–1. NCI DRUGS AVAILABLE UNDER GROUP C DISTRIBUTION

DRUG	GROUP C INDICATION
Amsarcrine	Refractory acute nonlymphoblastic leukemia
Erwinia asparaginase*	Acute lymphoblastic leukemia patients allergic to the *Escherichia coli* preparation
Azacitidine	Refractory acute nonlymphoblastic leukemia

Acquired resistance to the killing effects of alkylating agents is a clinical problem. Mechanisms of resistance are diverse and may include decreased accumulation of drug by resistant cells, an increase in inactivation of active alkylating metabolites, increased repair of alkylating agent–induced damage (*e.g.*, guanine 0^6-alkyl transferase), and an increase in the intracellular content of chemical groups, such as free thiols (*e.g.*, glutathione), that can compete with other targets and neutralize drug intracellularly. The extent of clinical cross-resistance between the various alkylating agents is unclear. Although some types of acquired resistance *in vitro* to one alkylator may be associated with increased resistance to others, this is not always the case, and patients who have failed treatment containing one member of this class may still respond to other alkylators.

The alkylating agents in clinical use fall into five chemical classes:

1. The nitrogen mustards (mechlorethamine, cyclophosphamide, ifosfamide, chlorambucil, and melphalan)
2. The ethylenimines (thiotepa, hexamethylmelamine)
3. The alkyl sulfonates (busulfan)
4. The nitrosoureas (carmustine, lomustine, semustine, streptozocin)
5. The triazines (dacarbazine).

Although they share common mechanisms of action, these agents differ markedly in chemical reactivity and stability, pharmacology, and clinical uses. For example, the nitrogen mustards are quite variable in their chemical stability and reactivity. The enhanced lipophilicity of the nitrosoureas allows them to pass across the blood–brain barrier; this property may account in part for their utility in treating tumors of the central nervous system (CNS). Like the nitrogen mustards, they are extensively biotransformed *in vivo*. Nitrosoureas produce a variety of chemical effects on biologic molecules, including alkylation, carbamoylation, and inhibition of DNA repair. In any particular clinical circumstance, the choice of an alkylating agent depends on the known activity of the agent for the tumor in question, the spectrum of toxicities, the preferred route of administration, the status of major organ function, desired onset of action, and the experience of the individual physician.

Although differing in degree and time course, alkylating agents have many common biologic effects, including myelosuppression and immunosuppression. Prolonged use commonly results in amenorrhea in women and oligospermia or azoospermia in men. Although individual patients treated with chemotherapy have fathered or borne children successfully, the extent of reversibility of chemotherapy-induced amenorrhea or azoospermia requires further study. Reversibility is by no means guaranteed and appears to depend in part on the age of the patient (for women experiencing treatment-induced amenorrhea, the younger the patient, the more likely the resumption of menses), the cumulative dose of drug, and the length of time off therapy. Younger women tolerate higher doses of drug before cessation of menses than older women.

Alkylating agents are teratogenic in experimental animals; clinical experience suggests that exposure in the first trimester is associated with an increased incidence of fetal malformations, although administration during the second or third trimester appears not to be.

All alkylating agents should be regarded as carcinogenic. Most reported cases of second malignancies following exposure to alkylators are acute leukemias, although an increased incidence of bladder cancer following cyclophosphamide therapy is also well documented. The risk of secondary acute leukemia appears to depend on total dose of drug and duration of follow-up. For patients with ovarian cancer surviving for 10 years after alkylator treatment, the risk may be as high as 5% to 10%. Available data from recent breast adjuvant chemotherapy trials and from studies of combination chemotherapy in Hodgkin's disease suggest somewhat lower risks. Aside from the increased incidence of bladder cancer following cyclophosphamide administration, there is no firm evidence that the incidence of any specific solid tumor is increased as a result of exposure to alkylating agents.

A number of alkylating agents in common use can produce pulmonary injury; these include busulfan, cyclophosphamide, chlorambucil, and several nitrosoureas. The toxicity usually presents with the characteristic radiographic and functional manifestations of interstitial pneumonitis, alveolitis, and fibrosis. The clinical course is variable but is often relentlessly downhill. The syndrome may sometimes appear insidiously months or years after the last dose of alkylator. The probability of developing pulmonary toxicity appears roughly dose-related for several alkylators, although no clear dose–response relationship appears to exist for busulfan. Glucocorticoids have been used as treatment; however, their efficacy is uncertain. The principal clinical problem is distinguishing drug-induced lung damage from infection or progressive cancer, and an aggressive diagnostic approach including lung biopsy may be required.

Mechlorethamine

PHARMACOLOGY

Mechlorethamine (nitrogen mustard) is the prototype of the polyfunctional alkylating agent; it was, in fact, the first nonhormonal antineoplastic agent to enter clinical trials. An analogue of mustard gas, it is very soluble in water and alcohol. One chlorethyl moiety of the molecule undergoes intramolecular cyclization with release of a chloride ion and formation of a highly reactive intermediate that may attack nucleophilic groups. The second chlorethyl moiety may then react via an identical mechanism to produce a species crosslinked between two alkylated nucleophils.

The parent drug is highly reactive with a chemical and biologic half-life of a few minutes. The drug binds rapidly to tissues. The principal route of degradation is by spontaneous hydrolysis, although some enzymatic demethylation also occurs. Whereas less than 0.01% is excreted in the urine as unmetabolized drug, up to half of the inactive metabolites are cleared renally.

THERAPEUTIC USES

Currently, the major systemic indication for mechlorethamine is in combination with vincristine, procarbazine, and prednisone (MOPP) for the treatment of Hodgkin's disease and other lymphomatous states. It is also used occasionally as a sclerosing agent intrapleurally for malignant effusions and may be applied topically as a dilute solution or ointment for mycosis fungoides.

DETAILS OF ADMINISTRATION

Mechlorethamine is supplied in vials of 10 mg mechlorethamine hydrochloride and 100 mg sodium chloride and is reconstituted with 10 ml sterile water, resulting in a 1 mg/ml solution; this should be prepared immediately prior to administration. Mechlorethamine is a powerful vesicant and should be prepared and administered with care. Proper handling procedures include the use of gloves and a biologic safety cabinet. Inhalation of the powder or vapors or their contact with skin or mucous membranes must be avoided. The drug should be injected over a few minutes through the tubing of a freely running intravenous infusion. As a single agent, the dose is 0.4 mg/kg (10–12 mg/M^2) every 4 to 6 weeks, given as a single dose; dividing the dose over 2 to 4 days increases the duration of nausea and vomiting, and there is no evidence that this schedule is more effective. The intracavitary dose is 12 mg/M^2, which produces systemic toxicity approximately equivalent to that of intravenously administered drug. For topical application, use 10 mg of drug dissolved in 60 ml of tap water or as a 0.01% ointment preparation.

If the drug comes in contact with skin, the area should be flushed with copious amounts of water. Following the flush with water, the area should be bathed with a 2% sodium thiosulfate solution. If the drug is extravasated into surrounding tissue during administration, any excess should be aspirated; the area may then be infiltrated with a 4% sodium thiosulfate solution in an attempt to neutralize residual mechlorethamine. This should be followed with ice packs applied to the area for 6 to 12 hours to minimize local reaction (see Practical Guidelines for Chemotherapy Administration at the end of this chapter). The affected tissues will initially become indurated and, for large enough infiltrations, may eventually slough.

DOSE MODIFICATIONS

The dose-limiting toxicity of mechlorethamine is myelosuppression; therefore, patients who have received extensive prior chemotherapy or radiotherapy may tolerate only reduced doses of the drug. Furthermore, because intracavitary dosing causes systemic toxicity, appropriate dose reduction is also required by this route in hematologically compromised patients.

DRUG INTERACTIONS

Agents which deplete cellular glutathione levels may enhance the cytotoxic effects of mechlorethamine.

TOXICITY

Hematologic suppression is dose limiting. Depression of lymphocytes occurs within 24 hours of injection; granulocytes and platelets decline within 6–8 days and recover by 2–3 weeks. Nausea and vomiting are often severe, occurring within the first 1–3 hours and persist for up to 24 hours. Alopecia is less marked than with cyclophosphamide. The drug is sclerosing and must not be allowed to extravasate paravenously (see Practical Guidelines for Chemotherapy Administration at the end of this chapter). Maculopapular skin eruptions do not appear to be allergic in origin and do not contraindicate continuation of therapy. Hyperpigmentation often follows topical administration.

Cyclophosphamide

PHARMACOLOGY

Cyclophosphamide is a cyclic phosphamide ester of mechlorethamine; the monohydrate is lipid soluble. The parent compound is inactive; hepatic microsomal oxidation leads to the generation of the active alkylating metabolite phosphoramide mustard. Acrolein, a secondary product, is responsible for the cystitis associated with cyclophosphamide exposure. Some degree of selective cytotoxicity may be conferred by phosphamidases and phosphatases in neoplastic cells.

Cyclophosphamide is principally cleared by hepatic metabolism to inactive metabolites that are eliminated primarily by the kidneys; renal failure thus results in prolonged blood levels of active and inactive metabolites of cyclophosphamide, but apparently not in increased toxicity. After doses of 6 mg to 80 mg/kg, the plasma half-life is 4 to 10 hours. Recent studies have documented at least 90% bioavailability of the oral preparation.

THERAPEUTIC USES

Cyclophosphamide, the most versatile alkylating agent, has a very broad spectrum of activity and is an integral part of contemporary regimens for the treatment of non-Hodgkin's lymphomas, chronic lymphocytic leukemia, multiple myeloma, small cell lung cancer, carcinomas of the breast and ovary, and a number of pediatric tumors, including bone and soft tissue sarcomas and neuroblastoma. In very high doses, cyclophosphamide, in combination with total-body irradiation and bone marrow transplantation, may be curative in patients with acute leukemia and chronic myelogenous leukemia. Because of its immunosuppressive properties, it has been used in various nonneoplastic settings, including severe rheumatoid arthritis, Wegener's granulomatosis, nephrotic syndrome in children, and allograft rejection.

DETAILS OF ADMINISTRATION

Cyclophosphamide is supplied as 25- and 50-mg tablets and as a powder for parenteral administration in 100-mg, 200-mg, 500-mg, 1-g, and 2-g vials. It is dissolved by adding 5 ml of sterile water for every 100 mg of drug. The agent may be difficult to dissolve, and vigorous shaking in a mechanical shaker may be necessary. The solution should be inspected for complete reconstitution before it is administered. The tablets and unreconstituted powder are stable at room temperature; reconstituted drug is chemically and physically stable for 24 hours at room temperature and for 6 days at 4°C.

If reconstituted in preservative-free sterile water, the drug should be used promptly. The drug may be infused as reconstituted or may be diluted further in a convenient volume of 5% dextrose in water or 0.9% sodium chloride solution and given by rapid or slow intravenous infusion. The oral preparation of cyclophosphamide may be better tolerated when taken with or immediately following meals.

The parenteral form has been administered intravenously, intramuscularly, intrapleurally, and intraperitoneally, although only intravenous administration is commonly used now. A large number of dose schedules have been explored for both initial and subsequent therapy; however, since cyclophosphamide is most commonly given in combination with other chemotherapeutic drugs, the dose and schedule depend on the specific regimen used.

When used as a single agent, an appropriate intravenous regimen is 1000 mg to 1500 mg/m^2, repeated about every 3 weeks for patients with normal bone marrow function. More conservative dosing may be indicated for elderly or heavily pretreated patients. If oral administration is desired, a suitable schedule is 2 mg to 3 mg/kg (50–100 mg/m^2) daily. By either route, doses may be modified upward or downward depending on patient tolerance to therapy, particularly the extent of leukopenia.

DOSE MODIFICATIONS

Patients who have had a history of cytotoxic chemotherapy or who have had radiation therapy to a large proportion of marrow-bearing areas are likely to develop greater degrees of myelosuppression from a given dose of cyclophosphamide than those without these pretreatment characteristics; such patients may require some decrease in the dose of drug used initially. Patients whose bone marrow is infiltrated with tumor may also be more sensitive to the myelosuppressive effects of cyclophosphamide. Because the aim of treatment is to kill the neoplastic cells, however, dose reduction may be counterproductive. Therefore, the use of lower doses of drug in anticipation of toxicity is a matter for expert clinical judgment. Since the drug's active metabolites are excreted by the kidneys and since the drug is activated by the liver, one might anticipate that abnormalities in the function of these organs would have a significant effect on the choice of dose. While systematic data on this point are few, available information suggests doses need not be modified in the setting of either renal or hepatic insufficiency. However, the drug should be administered with great caution to patients in severe renal failure.

DRUG INTERACTIONS

Allopurinol prolongs the half-life of cyclophosphamide metabolites and may increase myelosuppression. An increased leukopenic effect is possible in patients receiving chronic barbiturate therapy; similar effects should be watched for in the presence of other drugs that induce hepatic microsomal enzyme activity, such as phenytoin and chloral hydrate. The clinical impact of any of these interactions has been inconsistent. Glucocorticoids decrease the activity of this enzyme system and may decrease the extent of activation of a dose of cyclophosphamide. The clinical importance of this effect is uncertain, but should be considered in the presence of fluctuating doses of glucocorticoids. Cyclophosphamide has also been reported to increase the effect of succinylcholine, presumably by its inhibitory effect on pseudocholinesterase. Cyclophosphamide has also been associated with an increased anticoagulant effect when used with these agents. It also may increase the cardiotoxic potential of doxorubicin and presumably other anthracyclines.

TOXICITY

The myelosuppression induced by cyclophosphamide is manifested mainly as leukopenia, although thrombocytopenia can also occur, particularly at higher doses or in patients with reduced marrow reserve. Alopecia is common, and nausea and vomiting can be severe at high doses, although the drug is usually fairly well tolerated at conventional doses. A unique effect of cyclophosphamide and its analogue ifosfamide is acute sterile hemorrhagic cystitis; this may occur in up to 10% of patients treated with cyclophosphamide. This varies in severity from asymptomatic hematuria to fulminant hemorrhage that may require urologic intervention (see Chap. 56). The cystitis is produced by active metabolites of cyclophosphamide. It can be largely prevented by adequate hydration before and after intravenous treatment with frequent voiding and by ensuring that patients receiving oral treatment are chronically well hydrated. With very high dose administration, consideration should be given to the simultaneous use of N-acetylcysteine or sodium mercaptoethanesulfonate (mesna) (see section on Ifosfamide for a description of mesna administration). Late sequelae include bladder contracture and fibrosis, and cases of bladder cancer have been reported. Other side effects include stomatitis, skin and nail hyperpigmentation, interstitial pulmonary fibrosis, gonadal dysfunction, syndrome of inappropriate antidiuretic hormone secretion, and, at very high doses, cardiac toxicity.

Ifosfamide

PHARMACOLOGY

Ifosfamide is an oxazaphosphorine nitrogen mustard differing from cyclophosphamide in the placement of the chloroethyl groups. Whereas in cyclophosphamide both chloroethyl groups are attached to the exocyclic nitrogen, in ifosfamide one of the chloroethyl groups is attached to the endocyclic ring nitrogen. Ifosfamide is activated at a slower rate than cyclophosphamide by the hepatic mixed-function oxidase system because of a lower affinity of parent compound for the activating enzymes. Because this 4-hydroxylation reaction is slower than with cyclophosphamide, dechloroethylation results in a higher proportion of inactive metabolites, thus accounting for the higher doses of ifosfamide required clinically.

At lower individual doses of ifosfamide (1.6–2.4 g/m^2), such as are commonly given when the total dose is divided over 3 to 5 days, plasma decay appears monoexponential, with a half-life of about 7 hours. In all, about 55% to 60% of an administered dose is recovered in the urine; roughly 15% is recovered in the urine as unchanged drug. By contrast, with single doses of 3.8 g to 5 g/m^2, elimination is biexponential, with a terminal half-life of 15 hours. Total urinary recovery may account for 80% of an administered dose, and about 50% to 55% may be recovered as unchanged drug. These comparisons suggest that a given total dose may be more active biologically if it is fractionated over several days.

THERAPEUTIC USES

Ifosfamide has important clinical activity in a number of malignancies. In some testicular cancer patients failing two or more previous attempts at remission induction with combination chemotherapy, ifosfamide-containing combinations (usually with cisplatin and etoposide or vinblastine) appear to induce durable complete remissions. Combinations containing this drug have significant activity as second-line treatment in resistant non-Hodgkin's lymphomas. The drug has significant activity in soft tissue sarcomas of both children and adults. In children, combinations of ifosfamide and etoposide are the focus of several current trials; in adults, studies are attempting to define the extent to which ifosfamide can increase the activity of standard therapy (doxorubicin alone or with dacarbazine). It is not yet clear whether ifosfamide offers unique therapeutic advantages over cyclophosphamide when equivalently myelosuppressive doses of the two drugs are employed.

DETAILS OF ADMINISTRATION

Ifosfamide is supplied in 1- and 3-g vials and is reconstituted by adding sterile water for injection USP (20 ml/g). The currently recommended single-agent schedule of ifosfamide is

1.2 g/m^2 per day of drug for 5 consecutive days to deliver a total of 6 g of drug. This schedule is generally repeated at 3- to 4-week intervals.

At these doses, it is necessary to administer mesna (sodium mercaptoethane sulfonate) concomitantly with ifosfamide. Mesna is a thiol compound that limits the urothelial toxicity associated with the administration of ifosfamide and cyclophosphamide. It functions solely as a uroprotector, has no cytotoxic activity, and even at high doses does not interfere with the cytotoxic activity of the oxazaphosphorines. The recommended administration schedule is to administer an initial dose of mesna at 20% of the ifosfamide dose (on a g/m^2 basis) at the same time as the ifosfamide dose, with additional doses of mesna, each at 20% of the ifosfamide dose, 4 and 8 hours after every ifosfamide dose. Alternatively, mesna can be given by continuous intravenous infusion for the duration of the ifosfamide course (*e.g.*, over 5 days for a 5-day course); each day the infused dose of mesna (in g/m^2) should equal that day's dose of ifosfamide. On the last day of treatment, the infusion should end 12 to 16 hours after the last dose of ifosfamide. Currently the manufacturer recommends that an ifosfamide dose of 1.2 g/m^2 be accompanied by mesna 240 mg/m^2 intravenous bolus at hours 0, 4, and 8 following start of ifosfamide, on each day that ifosfamide is administered. The mesna dose should be modified in proportion with ifosfamide dose adjustments.

DOSE MODIFICATIONS

Dose modifications have not been firmly established. However, the general guidelines given for cyclophosphamide are probably appropriate.

DRUG INTERACTIONS

Because ifosfamide undergoes hepatic activation by microsomal enzymes, interaction is potentially possible with drugs such as barbiturates, phenytoin, and chloral hydrate. The same interactions reported for cyclophosphamide might also be anticipated for ifosfamide; however, they remain to be demonstrated. See comments in later sections on CNS-active agents.

TOXICITY

As the dose of ifosfamide alone is escalated in the absence of uroprotection, hemorrhagic cystitis is dose limiting. In the presence of uroprotection (adequate hydration, bladder irrigation, fractionated schedule, mesna administration), myelosuppression, particularly leukopenia, becomes dose limiting. CNS toxicities, manifested as confusion, lethargy, and occasionally seizures, are usually transient and resolve with discontinuation of the drug. Minimizing the use of narcotics, antiemetics, and other CNS-active agents, whenever possible, may lessen the incidence of these side effects. Nausea and vomiting, alopecia, and hyponatremia are also seen. The drug's potential for producing clinical nephrotoxicity is largely abrogated by mesna, although evidence of subclinical renal damage of varying degrees has been documented, and there are case reports of overt severe renal failure with high-dose ifosfamide therapy despite mesna administration.

Melphalan

PHARMACOLOGY

Melphalan is a rationally designed synthetic product formed from nitrogen mustard and the amino acid phenylalanine. Synthesis was originally motivated by the hope that the phenylalanine moiety would impart some selective cytotoxicity against melanoma, which takes up phenylalanine for the synthesis of tyrosine and ultimately melanin; this promise was never fulfilled. Melphalan appears to have a rather broad spectrum of activity. It is practically insoluble in water and only slightly soluble in alcohol. Melphalan enters cells by the L-amino acid carrier system that also transports the amino acids phenylalanine, leucine, and glutamine. Thus, the drug's uptake from plasma or ascitic fluid may be influenced by the ambient amino acid concentration.

After oral administration, bioavailability is quite variable; between 20% and 50% of an administered dose is excreted unchanged in the stool. The drug has biphasic elimination from plasma, with an alpha half-life of about 70 minutes and a beta half-life of about 160 minutes. Melphalan is principally eliminated by chemical hydrolysis to inactive products. Urinary recovery amounts to approximately 50% of a dose within the first 24 hours of administration; however, only 10% to 15% of an administered dose is excreted as parent compound in the urine. The drug is about 60% protein bound; serum from jaundiced patients may bind the drug less completely.

THERAPEUTIC USES

Only the oral form of melphalan is commercially available. Melphalan has significant activity in multiple myeloma and in carcinomas of the breast and ovary. For all of these indications, it is used most commonly in combination with other agents. Although the parenteral formulation is still investigational, it has been extensively used by the intra-arterial route in certain centers for the isolation-perfusion treatment of metastatic melanoma limited to the extremity. High doses of parenteral melphalan, alone or in combination, have also been studied recently with autologous bone marrow rescue in a variety of tumor types, including neuroblastoma, colorectal cancer, myeloma, melanoma, and leukemia.

DETAILS OF ADMINISTRATION

The oral dosage form of melphalan is commercially available as 2-mg tablets. A parenteral formulation, which is still investigational, is available for clinical trials from Burroughs-Wellcome Company or from the Investigational Drug Branch, Division of Cancer Treatment, NCI. The following comments all pertain to oral administration. Melphalan has been given in a variety of dose schedules. For the treatment of multiple myeloma, the drug has been given at 0.25 mg/kg daily for 4 to 7 days every 4 to 6 weeks. For ovarian cancer, a variety of dose schedules are recommended; one of these aims to deliver a total of 1 mg/kg divided over 5 days, repeated every 4 to 5 weeks. The NSABP adjuvant trials in breast cancer used a schedule of 0.15 mg/kg/day for 5 days, repeated at 6-week intervals. Alternatives that do not adjust dose by body surface area or weight (*e.g.*, 6 mg daily for 2 to 3 weeks, then off for 2 to 4 weeks, then 2 to 4 mg daily as tolerated by counts) are not recommended. Fasting patients absorb the drug more rapidly and cimetidine may decrease the bioavailability of melphalan.

DOSE MODIFICATIONS

Because the predominant toxicity is hematologic, the dose may need to be reduced in patients with compromised marrow function. Similarly, lower doses should be considered in patients with either compromised renal or liver function because of excretion and protein-binding considerations, respectively.

DRUG INTERACTIONS

Administration of melphalan with cyclosporine increases the risk of nephrotoxicity. In cell culture tamoxifen can inhibit uptake of melphalan.

TOXICITY

The dose-limiting toxicity of melphalan is leukopenia and thrombocytopenia, generally occurring 2 to 3 weeks following a course of treatment and returning to normal by 4 weeks. Some patients, particularly those who are elderly or heavily pretreated, may require up to 6 weeks for full count recovery. Nausea and vomiting are usually mild but may be substantial with high intermittent dose schedules. Alopecia is much less severe than with cyclophosphamide. Diarrhea and stomatitis are very uncommon with the oral preparation but are the principal dose-limiting toxicities when the drug is given parenterally at very high (*i.e.*, transplant) doses. Dermatitis and pulmonary fibrosis have been reported, usually in patients receiving the drug over prolonged periods. The drug is probably more leukemogenic than some other alkylators (*e.g.*, cyclophosphamide).

Chlorambucil

PHARMACOLOGY

An aromatic derivative of mechlorethamine, chlorambucil has the same mechanism of action as the other derivatives of nitrogen mustard.

The drug is rapidly and almost completely absorbed following oral administration. It is metabolized to phenylacetic acid mustard (PAAM), which also has bifunctional alkylating activity. Peak plasma concentration of the alkylating metabolite occurs within 2 to 4 hours; in fasting patients, the area under the concentration-time curve of PAAM is about 45% greater than that of chlorambucil. The drug and its metabolites appear to be extensively bound to plasma and tissue proteins. It is not known whether chlorambucil crosses the blood–brain barrier. Terminal plasma half-lives of chlorambucil and PAAM are 1.5 and 2.5 hours, respectively. The drug is extensively metabolized in the liver to PAAM. Both chlorambucil and PAAM are principally cleared by chemical hydrolysis to inactive metabolites that are then excreted predominantly by the kidneys. Less than 1% of administered drug is excreted in the urine as chlorambucil and PAAM.

THERAPEUTIC USES

Chlorambucil has the slowest onset of action of any of the bifunctional alkylating agents. Its major clinical uses at present are in the treatment of chronic lymphocytic leukemia, macroglobulinemia, and the indolent non-Hodgkin's lymphomas. It is also occasionally employed in the treatment of ovarian and breast cancer and has useful activity in patients with multiple myeloma. As with cyclophosphamide, its lympholytic effects have motivated its use in various nonmalignant conditions in which immunosuppression is desired.

DETAILS OF ADMINISTRATION

Chlorambucil is available in 2-mg tablets. The usual initial dose is 0.1 mg to 0.2 mg/kg given as a single daily dose for 3 to 6 weeks, at which point bone marrow suppression may necessitate some lowering of the dose. The drug can usually be continued at 2–4 mg orally daily. Chlorambucil may also be administered by an intermittent schedule initially at a dose of 0.4 mg/kg and repeated every 4 weeks. Absorption is most rapid if the drug is taken on an empty stomach, although the AUC of the drug and its phenylacetic acid metabolite is unchanged.

DOSE MODIFICATIONS

As with other myelosuppressive agents, those patients with significant decreased marrow reserve for any reasons may not tolerate full-dose therapy.

DRUG INTERACTIONS

No drug interactions have been reported.

TOXICITY

Chlorambucil is among the best tolerated of antineoplastic agents. Myelosuppression is dose limiting but is generally slow in onset and is easily reversible when the drug is discontinued. Nausea is usually mild or nonexistent. The drug is occasionally responsible for alopecia, skin rashes, and rare hepatotoxicity. Pulmonary fibrosis with chlorambucil use has also been reported. As with other agents of this class, azospermia, amenorrhea, and secondary leukemia are risks of treatment. Isolated cases of allergic skin reaction, drug fever, and immune hemolysis have been reported.

Thiotepa

PHARMACOLOGY

Thiotepa, an ethylenimine derivative, is a polyfunctional alkylating agent bearing three aziridine groups. The drug functions through transformation into active quaternary ethylenimonium ions, which attack DNA in the same manner as the mechlorethamine derivatives. It may also release aziridine intracellularly.

Following intravenous administration, plasma concentrations of drug decline in a biexponential fashion (alpha half-life, ~10 min; beta half-life, ~2 hours). Tepa, the major metabolite, which itself has antiproliferative activity, is detectable almost immediately; by 2 hours after injection, the plasma concentration of tepa is equal to or greater than that of thiotepa and persists longer in plasma. Very little thiotepa or tepa appears in the urine, but total urinary excretion of alkylating agent activity in the first 24 hours accounts for about 30% of the administered dose. It is not known whether thiotepa or its metabolites are distributed into milk. Absorption from the gastrointestinal (GI) tract or from body cavities is incomplete, ranging from 10% to 100%, and appears to be enhanced by extensive tumor infiltration or mucosal inflammation, as following radiotherapy or after surgery. Systemic administration produces cerebrospinal fluid (CSF) concentrations of drug equivalent to that of plasma.

THERAPEUTIC USES

For systemic therapy thiotepa has been largely superseded by other alkylating agents, although it is still used occasionally for the treatment of metastatic breast cancer, ovarian cancer, and the lymphomas; in these settings it is employed in combination with other agents. Thiotepa's principal use at present is for the intravesical treatment of superficial bladder cancer (carcinoma in situ, early-stage transitional cell carcinoma), where significant response can be attained in upwards of two thirds of patients. Thiotepa is also employed for the intracavitary treatment of malignant effusions in the pleural or pericardial spaces; it is very well tolerated by this route because it is not a local vesicant and because of the low incidence of significant GI side-effects. Intraperitoneal administration does not, however, carry much of a regional advantage compared to the systemic route. The drug is also under investigation for the treatment of meningeal carcinomatosis by the intrathecal route, although pharmacologic data suggest no significant regional advantage for intraventricular or intrathecal over systemic administration. High-dose intravenous administration, followed by bone marrow transplantation, is also a focus of study, since the maximum tolerated dose in the transplant setting appears to exceed the conventional maximum tolerated dose by more than 50-fold.

DETAILS OF ADMINISTRATION

Thiotepa is commercially available in vials containing 15 mg, with 80 mg of sodium chloride and 50 mg of sodium bicarbonate. It is reconstituted by adding 1.5 ml of sterile water to yield an isotonic solution of 10 mg/ml. This solution is chemically stable for 5 days when stored in the refrigerator. However, the final solution contains no preservative and should therefore be discarded within 24 hours. This solution should be protected from light.

Because the drug is not sclerosing, it has been given by a great variety of routes (intravenous, intramuscular, subcutaneous, intracavitary); the intravenous route is usually preferred for systemic therapy. The usual dose for single-agent treatment is 0.3 mg to 0.4 mg/kg by rapid intravenous injection every 1 to 4 weeks. An alternative schedule is 0.2 mg/kg intravenously daily for 4 days every 2 to 4 weeks. For intrapleural space installation, thiotepa may be given at a dose of 0.8 mg/kg after the intrapleural space has been drained of fluid; this treatment may be repeated weekly, although failure to control pleural fluid accumulation with the initial treatment of a chest tube and intrapleural chemotherapy generally does not bode well for future control. For intravesical administration, doses range from 30 mg to 60 mg, given in 30 ml to 60 ml of sterile water by catheter into the bladder cavity at weekly intervals for 4 weeks.

DOSE MODIFICATIONS

The same general guidelines apply as for other alkylating agents.

DRUG INTERACTIONS

Thiotepa may inhibit pseudocholinesterase activity; therefore, succinyl choline should be administered cautiously if used in close temporal proximity to thiotepa.

TOXICITY

Myelosuppression is dose related and cumulative; the predominant effect is leukopenia, with a nadir at 10 to 14 days. Intracavitary administration may result in significant systemic absorption of drug with resultant myelosuppression. This drug causes much less nausea and vomiting at conventional doses than does mechlorethamine. Pain at the injection site, anorexia, dizziness, headache, hives, and bronchoconstriction are very uncommon. As with all alkylating agents, interference with fertility should be anticipated. Intravesical administration can result in lower abdominal discomfort, bladder irritability, and rarely hemorrhagic cystitis.

Hexamethylmelamine

PHARMACOLOGY

Hexamethylmelamine (HMM) consists of a triazene ring with dimethylamino groups at each of the three carbons. Although the drug bears structural similarities to intermediates in the metabolism of nitrogen mustard and to other known alkylating agents such as triethylenemelamine (TEM), it is not certain that it functions as an alkylating agent *in vivo*. HMM itself is inactive, and metabolic activation by hepatic microsomal P-450 mono-oxygenases appears necessary for cytotoxicity. The drug does not appear to be cross-resistant with bifunctional alkylators of the nitrogen mustard type. Because HMM bears some structural similarities to agents such as azacitidine, and because the drug inhibits incorporation of thymidine and uridine into DNA and RNA, respectively, some investigators have proposed antimetabolite mechanisms of action, for which there is no direct evidence.

The bioavailability of the oral preparation is highly variable. HMM is rapidly but variably N-demethylated in the liver; urinary excretion is largely in the form of the various methylmelamine metabolites along with melamine itself. About 60% to 70% of an administered dose is excreted as metabolites within the first 24 hours. The identity of the active antitumor agent(s) is unknown. The terminal plasma half-life ranges from 5 to 10 hours; 62% of the metabolites are recovered in the urine during the first 24 hours after administration. A recently developed parenteral formulation in Intralipid 10% appears to provide more consistent plasma drug concentrations.

THERAPEUTIC USES

HMM has demonstrated activity against a number of solid tumors, including ovarian cancer, small cell lung cancer, lymphoma, and endometrial and cervical cancer. It has been used extensively in combination chemotherapy programs in ovarian cancer.

DETAILS OF ADMINISTRATION

The drug is supplied as a 50-mg capsule containing lactose and calcium stearates. Capsules should be stored in a tightly sealed bottle at room temperature (15° to 30°C). Dosage ranges from 4 mg to 12 mg/kg per day have been investigated. The usual duration of therapy has been 21 to 90 days, depending on the dose of other concurrent cytotoxic agents and the severity of GI toxicity. The total daily dose should be given in four divided increments (after meals and at bedtime). The recommended dose/schedule is an intermittent schedule of 260 mg/m^2 by mouth, four times daily in four divided doses for 14–21 days in a 28-day cycle. This appears well tolerated and active as second-line therapy for ovary cancer. In combination with other cytotoxics, doses in the 150–200 mg/m^2 range for 14 days appear to be well tolerated.

DOSE MODIFICATIONS

The same general guidelines apply as for other alkylating agents.

DRUG INTERACTIONS

Administration of HMM to patients taking antidepressants (tricyclics or MAO inhibitors) has been associated with the appearance of severe orthostatic hypotension. In murine models phenobarbitol increases the metabolism and decreased the antitumor effects of HMM. Cimetidine can prolong the half-life of HMM through inhibition of hepatic metabolism.

TOXICITY

Nausea and vomiting may be severe and dose limiting; this effect seems related to the cumulative dose of drug. Myelosuppression appears also to be related to cumulative dose and/or time on treatment. Neurotoxicity may be a prominent feature of drug effect after extended periods of therapy. Both central (somnolence, lethargy, mood changes) and peripheral (loss of deep tendon reflexes, paresthesias, ataxia) effects may be evident. The etiology of the neurotoxicity is unknown, but the side effects usually abate when the drug is discontinued.

Busulfan

PHARMACOLOGY

Busulfan is an alkyl sulfonate not chemically related to mechlorethamine. The drug is highly toxic to bone marrow precursors but exhibits little toxicity to lymphocytes and the GI tract.

Busulfan is well absorbed after oral administration; elimination half-life is approximately 2.5 hours. The drug undergoes extensive biotransformation; 12 metabolites have been isolated thus far, but most have not been chemically identified. Metabolites are slowly eliminated via urinary excretion. Less than 1% of the parent compound is found in urine, and most of the drug is excreted as metabolites, principally, methane sulfonic acid (10%–50% of the dose within 24 hours). After oral administration of high doses, CSF concentrations of drug rapidly increase and are similar to plasma levels.

THERAPEUTIC USES

The principal clinical use of busulfan is in chronic myelocytic leukemia (CML); although not curative, the drug can induce good control of blood counts in about 90% of patients with previously untreated disease. Several weeks of continuous therapy may be required to reduce the leukocyte count to desired levels. Busulfan is less effective in CML patients who lack the Philadelphia chromosome, and the drug is ineffective in patients with CML in blast crisis. Busulfan is also sometimes used in patients with polycythemia vera and essential thrombocythemia whose disease cannot be controlled by other means. Because of its rather high degree of selectivity for bone marrow–derived cells, busulfan is currently being explored in relatively high doses, in combination with cyclophosphamide and bone marrow transplantation, in patients with acute leukemia.

DETAILS OF ADMINISTRATION

Busulfan is commercially available as 2-mg tablets. Therapy is generally initiated with doses of 4 mg to 8 mg, depending on the initial white blood cell (WBC) count. Starting at the high dose produces a more rapid effect but also increases the chance of overshoot and prolonged aplasia; accordingly many physicians begin therapy at a fixed dose of 4 mg. Counts should be monitored weekly and drug discontinued when the WBC count has fallen to 10,000 to 20,000/μl. The patient is then monitored off drug until the WBC count rises again, at which point therapy is reinstituted as outlined above. Some physicians prefer to employ maintenance therapy (1 to 3 mg daily), but there is no evidence that this is better than intermittent courses as required by the level of WBC. (See Chapter 41 for further discussion.)

DRUG INTERACTIONS

In murine models, phenytoin and phenobarbital decrease the lethality of high-dose busulfan, possibly by inducing drug-metabolizing enzymes. This interaction, if it exists in humans, is of potential concern in the treatment or prophylaxis of busulfan-related seizures in the transplant setting.

TOXICITY

Myelosuppression is dose limiting; the WBC count begins to fall after about 10 days of therapy and continues to fall for about 2 weeks after discontinuation. Thrombocytopenia and anemia are also seen. Full recovery from drug-induced myelosuppression may take weeks after discontinuation. Occasional skin hyperpigmentation, amenorrhea, and gynecomastia may be associated with busulfan administration. With long term use, the drug has rarely produced a mixed alveolar and interstitial pneumonitis characterized by cough, progressive dyspnea, pulmonary fibrosis, and ultimately respiratory insufficiency. Gastrointestinal side effects are generally mild or nonexistent. High doses of busulfan in the transplant range are associated with generalized seizures in some patients. In the transplant setting, hepatotoxicity is dose limiting; the probability of developing veno-occlusive disease appears related to the extent of drug exposure (AUC). At standard doses, hepatotoxicity has been reported (reversible cholestasis with focal necrosis) but appears to be extremely rare.

Carmustine

PHARMACOLOGY

Spontaneous decomposition of carmustine (BCNU) yields a chloroethyldiazonium hydroxide that can alkylate proteins and nucleotides in DNA leading to the formation of interstrand or intrastrand DNA crosslinks and DNA-protein crosslinks. Decomposition also produces an isocyanate molecule that may result in the carbamoylation of proteins, including enzymes. Carbamoylation may inhibit DNA polymerase, DNA repair, and the synthesis and processing of RNA. It is currently suspected that the alkylating activity of the nitrosoureas is responsible for the therapeutic activity of these compounds, while the carbamoylating activity contributes largely to toxicity.

Intravenously administered carmustine is rapidly degraded; plasma concentration curves reflect a distribution half-life of about 6 minutes and a beta-phase half-life of about 70 minutes. In studies using radiolabeled drug, prolonged levels of plasma radioactivity were detected, probably reflecting intrahepatic circulation of metabolites and/or protein binding. Carmustine is rapidly metabolized with approximately 30% of metabolites eliminated in the urine within the first 24 hours and up to 70% within 96 hours. Some of these metabolites are active cytotoxic agents. The drug and/or its metabolites readily cross the blood–brain barrier; cerebrospinal fluid concentrations of radioactivity range from 15% to 70% of simultaneous plasma levels after intravenous administration.

THERAPEUTIC USES

In the course of its development, carmustine has been incorporated into a large number of combinations in a wide variety of tumor types. Presently, however, its use in conventional doses is largely restricted to the therapy of malignant brain tumors, Hodgkin's disease, and multiple myeloma. For brain tumors, it is an effective adjuvant to local therapy (surgery and radiotherapy). For the lymphomas and myeloma, it is most commonly used in combination with other agents. Recent investigations have explored very high doses with autologous bone marrow rescue, either as a single agent or in combination against brain tumors, malignant melanoma, and other solid tumors, with variable results; its use in the transplant setting remains investigational.

DETAILS OF ADMINISTRATION

Carmustine is commercially available in a 100-mg vial as a white lyophilized powder, highly soluble in alcohol and poorly soluble in water. Carmustine is reconstituted with 3 ml of absolute alcohol followed by 27 ml of sterile water. Reconstituted solution may be further diluted with sodium chloride or 5% dextrose in water. Accidental contact of the skin with reconstituted solution has produced transient hyperpigmentation of the exposed area.

The usual single-agent dose is 200 mg/m^2 given intravenously over 1 to 2 hours every 6 weeks. This may be divided into two equal doses given over 2 successive days to lessen the acute side effects, but this is generally not necessary. In the treatment of mycosis fungoides, carmustine has been applied topically as a hydroalcoholic solution or ointment in concentrations of 0.05% to 0.4% one to two times daily. The usual topical dosage is 10 mg daily for 6 to 8 weeks. If response is inadequate, after a rest interval of 6 weeks, a second course of topical therapy with 20 mg daily (up to 30 days) may be tried.

DOSE MODIFICATIONS

There are no standardized guidelines for dose modifications in the presence of hematologic toxicity. (See the section on

Dose Modification under Lomustine for reasonable guidelines.)

DRUG INTERACTIONS

Cimetidine has been reported to increase myelosuppression, and amphotericin B may enhance cellular uptake of carmustine. *In vitro* the nitrosoureas have been reported to decrease the antifungal effect of amphotericin B.

TOXICITY

Myelosuppression is the usual dose-limiting toxicity. The white count nadir generally occurs 4 to 6 weeks after administration whereas thrombocytopenia tends to appear a little earlier (3 to 4 weeks). Myelosuppression tends to increase with successive cycles of therapy. Nausea and vomiting may be severe and occur within 2–3 hours after drug administration. Hepatotoxicity, generally mild and reversible, has been reported in up to about 25% of patients. Rare but serious adverse effects include interstitial pneumonitis and fibrosis and progressive renal damage. The probability of drug-induced interstitial pneumonitis appears to be dose related; patients receiving cumulative doses in excess of 1400 mg/m^2 are at particular risk. Optical neuritis and atrophy as well as hemorrhagic glaucoma may result from regional administration into the carotid artery below the level of the ophthalmic artery. Although the drug is not a vesicant, too rapid intravenous infusion may produce a burning pain at the infusion site.

Lomustine

PHARMACOLOGY

Lomustine (CCNU) is a nitrosourea derivative that has both chlorethyl and cyclohexyl side chains. The mechanism of action is the same as that of carmustine.

Lomustine is rapidly absorbed from the GI tract and is rapidly and completely metabolized. Intact drug cannot be detected in plasma or urine; peak plasma levels of metabolites occur in about 3 hours following administration of an oral dose, and the plasma half-life of metabolites is 16 to 48 hours. Approximately 50% of radioactive drug is excreted as metabolites in the urine during the first 12 hours after administration. Radiolabeled drug and/or metabolites cross the blood–brain barrier rapidly; cerebrospinal levels of radioactivity are about 50% of simultaneous plasma concentrations. Intact drug cannot be detected in the cerebrospinal fluid.

THERAPEUTIC USES

Lomustine has clinically useful activity in the lymphomas and brain tumors, with lower levels of activity in a variety of other solid tumors. Single-agent data suggest greater activity against Hodgkin's disease than carmustine has.

DETAILS OF ADMINISTRATION

The drug is available commercially as 10-mg, 40-mg, and 100-mg capsules. The usual single-agent dose is 130 mg/m^2 given every 6 to 8 weeks. Patients who have compromised bone marrow function should probably receive reduced doses of 100 mg/m^2 with subsequent dosage adjustment as needed to maintain adequate bone marrow function.

TABLE 22–2. GUIDELINES FOR DOSE MODIFICATIONS FOR MYELOSUPPRESSION CAUSED BY PREVIOUS LOMUSTINE ADMINISTRATION

NADIR AFTER PRIOR DOSE (CELL/mm^3)		
LEUKOCYTES	PLATELETS	PERCENTAGE OF PRIOR DOSE TO BE GIVEN
≥4000	≥100,000	100
3000–3999	75,000–99,999	100
2000–2999	25,000–74,999	70
<2000	<25,000	50

DOSE MODIFICATIONS

Reasonable guidelines for dose modifications in the presence of myelosuppression from previous lomustine courses are outlined in Table 22-2.

DRUG INTERACTIONS

Like carmustine, lomustine may interact with cimetidine, amphotericin B, and phenytoin.

TOXICITY

The spectrum of toxicities is similar to carmustine; myelosuppression is delayed, and nausea and vomiting may be severe. Although vomiting generally does not occur for 2 to 6 hours following a dose, it may occur sooner on repeated dosing or when lomustine is given in combination with other agents. If vomiting occurs soon after ingestion, the vomitus should be inspected for intact capsules; if these are identified with certainty, the drug should be readministered. Stomatitis, alopecia, and transient hepatotoxicity are infrequent and generally are mild.

Semustine

PHARMACOLOGY

Semustine (methy-CCNU) is the 4-methyl derivative of lomustine. The mechanism of action is the same as that of carmustine.

The drug is rapidly absorbed after oral administration and is not detectable in either plasma or urine because of rapid metabolism. The chloroethyl moiety has a half-life of about 36 hours. As with carmustine and lomustine, the drug penetrates the blood–brain barrier well.

THERAPEUTIC USES

Semustine has single-agent activity against the lymphomas, brain tumors, melanoma, and adenocarcinomas of the stomach, colon, and rectum. Semustine is no longer in active clinical development.

DETAILS OF ADMINISTRATION

Semustine is not commercially available. NCI's investigational formulation is as 10-mg, 50-mg, and 100-mg capsules for oral administration. The usual single-agent dose is 200 mg/m^2 orally. Because of the delayed and cumulative myelosuppressive effects, the drug is administered at intervals of at least 6 weeks.

DOSE MODIFICATIONS

No standardized guidelines exist. (See section on Dose Modifications under Lomustine for reasonable guidelines.)

DRUG INTERACTIONS

No drug interactions have been reported. The possibility of interactions similar to those for carmustine must be considered.

TOXICITY

The toxicity of semustine is similar to that of carmustine and lomustine. Nephrotoxicity manifested as renal failure has been noted, especially at cumulative doses greater than 1500 mg/m^2. The histologic picture is similar to radiation nephritis. Proteinuria and urinary sediment abnormalities are inconstant findings; the kidneys may appear abnormally small radiographically. The drug is leukemogenic in humans; risk is probably proportional to total cumulative dose and to time at risk (*i.e.*, length of follow-up).

Streptozocin

PHARMACOLOGY

Streptozocin, a naturally occurring antibiotic isolated from streptomyces, is a glucosamine-1-methyl-nitrosourea that differs from other clinically active nitrosoureas in the absence of a chloroethyl side chain and in the presence of a D-glucopyranose moiety, which renders the drug water soluble. In addition to its inhibitory effects on DNA synthesis, it has potent inhibitory effects on pyridine nucleotide metabolism and on some key enzymes involved in gluconeogenesis. The drug undergoes spontaneous decomposition *in vivo* to produce methylcarbonium ions that cause DNA interstrand crosslinking; the alkylating activity of streptozocin is relatively weak compared with that of the other nitrosoureas. Streptozocin also carbamoylates amino acids and proteins via the formation of organic isocyanates. The drug also inhibits the alkyltransferase that may participate in alkylator-induced DNA damage; accordingly streptozocin is being explored in combination with other alkylators.

Intravenous administration is associated with rapid and extensive metabolism; no intact drug remains in the plasma after 3 hours. Elimination is triphasic, with a terminal half-life of 40 hours. Approximately 10% to 20% of an intravenous dose is excreted into the urine within 24 hours, principally as metabolites. The metabolites distribute into the cerebrospinal fluid, and levels are detectable for at least 24 hours. There is considerable variation among patients in streptozocin distribution to the cerebrospinal fluid.

THERAPEUTIC USES

The principal use of streptozocin is for islet cell tumors of the pancreas. It is the most active single agent for this disease; current evidence suggests that the combination of streptozocin and 5-fluorouracil is superior to streptozocin alone (see Chap. 36). Adriamycin plus streptozocin represents a reasonable choice for therapy of islet cell cancers. The drug also has some activity against metastatic carcinoid tumors. It is also active in advanced Hodgkin's disease and has been used in combination with other agents for this disease, as well as for adenocarcinomas of pancreatic and colorectal origin.

DETAILS OF ADMINISTRATION

Streptozocin is available commercially in 1-g vials. The drug is reconstituted with 9.5 ml of either dextrose injection USP or 0.9% sodium chloride injection (USP) to form 100 mg/ml. As a single agent, the usual regimen is 1 g/m^2 given intravenously weekly for 4 weeks; an alternative is 500 mg/m^2 intravenously daily for 5 days, repeated every 6 weeks. Slow infusions prevent local discomfort at the infusion site.

DOSE MODIFICATIONS

In patients in whom creatinine clearance is below 25 mg/min, the dose should be reduced by 50% to 75%.

DRUG INTERACTIONS

Streptozocin is toxic to pancreatic beta cells; administration may be followed acutely by significant hypoglycemia and more chronically by glucose intolerance. Potentially significant interactions may, therefore, exist with any agent affecting glucose tolerance. Because of the drug's nephrotoxicity, other potentially nephrotoxic drugs should be given with streptozocin only when absolutely required and then with great care.

TOXICITY

The dose-limiting toxicity may either be gastrointestinal or renal. Severe nausea and vomiting are not very responsive to conventional antiemetics such as pitenothiazines. Streptozocin may either aggravate or cause duodenal ulcers. Renal toxicity is manifested by proteinurea and azotemia. Permanent tubular damage may occur. Myelosuppression is usually mild, but streptozocin may potentiate the marrow toxicity of some other drugs. Mild hepatic toxicity is usually transient. The drug may cause burning when injected into the vein.

Dacarbazine

PHARMACOLOGY

Dacarbazine was synthesized as a chemical analogue of the purine precursor 5-amino-imidazole-4-carboxamide, in the hope that it would function as an antimetabolite. It turned out, however, that dacarbazine undergoes metabolic activation by the NADPH-dependent mixed function oxidase system to yield the methyldiazonium ion, an active species that can methylate sensitive sites on nucleic acids. In addition, dacarbazine is light sensitive and yields photodecomposition products that might be responsible for some of this compound's cytotoxicity in tissue culture. Dacarbazine inhibits synthesis of DNA and, to a lesser extent, RNA.

Extensive metabolism follows intravenous administration; the terminal plasma half-life is about 40 minutes, with about 20% binding to plasma proteins. Approximately 40% of parent drug is found in the urine within the first 24 hours. There is some renal tubular secretion. Dacarbazine has a limited ability to cross the blood–brain barrier.

THERAPEUTIC USES

Dacarbazine is probably the most active single agent for the treatment of metastatic melanoma. Responses occur in about 25% of patients; visceral disease responds much less frequently than metastases that are limited to skin and lymph nodes. Dacarbazine is active against Hodgkin's disease and is a component of the doxorubicin, bleomycin, and vinblastine (ABVD) regimen. It has a response rate of about 15% against the soft-tissue sarcomas of adulthood and is commonly combined with doxorubicin.

DETAILS OF ADMINISTRATION

Dacarbazine is commercially available in 100-mg and 200-mg vials, which must be protected from light and stored at 2° to 8°C. Discoloration of dacarbazine powder to pink indicates some decomposition. The 100-mg vial is reconstituted with 9.9 ml of sterile water and the 200-mg vial with 19.7 ml of sterile water for injection (USP), resulting in concentrations of 10 mg/ml. The solutions are stable for 8 hours at 20°C or for 72 hours at 4°C. The reconstituted solution may be further diluted in up to 500 ml of 5% dextrose in water or 0.9% sodium chloride solution and remains stable for at least 24 hours when stored at 4°C or for 8 hours at room temperature. Dacarbazine forms a precipitate with hydrocortisone sodium succinate. Reconstituted solution may be administered by intravenous push over a 1-minute period or, preferably, infused over a 15- to 30-minute period.

The regimen frequently used for adult patients with malignant melanoma is 250 mg/m^2 daily for 5 days. Treatment cycles are repeated every 3 to 4 weeks.

DOSE MODIFICATIONS

As usual, the drug should be used with caution in patients with bone marrow compromise or abnormal liver or renal function, although no validated guidelines exist for dose modification under these circumstances.

DRUG INTERACTIONS

Dacarbazine activation may be increased by phenytoin or phenobarbital. Experimental evidence indicates that xanthine oxidase may be inhibited, although it is not clear that this is significant clinically; effects additive to those of allopurinol and potential enhancement of toxicity if given along with azathioprine or mercaptopurine might be anticipated from such an interaction.

TOXICITY

Dacarbazine is one of the most emetogenic of chemotherapeutic agents; onset is usually within 1 to 3 hours of drug administration. In the absence of effective antiemetic therapy, the nausea and vomiting may be so severe as to constitute the dose-limiting toxicity. This may be accompanied by generalized malaise, low-grade fever, and myalgia. If the nausea and vomiting can be abrogated, myelosuppression is dose limiting, although at the doses specified above, myelosuppression is generally mild. Depression of the white blood cell count usually predominates over thrombocytopenia and resolves by 3 weeks in most patients.

Diarrhea occurs in some patients. Too rapid infusion of undiluted reconstituted drug causes pain along the injection site. Patients should be warned against direct sun exposure for a day or so after receiving a dose; direct sunlight produces facial flushing, facial paresthesias, and lightheadedness.

Acute hepatic vascular toxicity resulting in death has been reported in at least 15 patients (~0.01%) treated with dacarbazine as a single agent; this appears to result from occlusion of small and medium-sized veins and differs pathologically from veno-occlusive disease of other causes.

PLANT DERIVATIVES

The common periwinkle plant (*Vinca rosea Linn*) was believed for many generations to have beneficial medicinal properties. Extracts that caused bone marrow suppression in rats led to the isolation of two active alkaloid anticancer agents. The vinca alkaloids are large and complex molecules; vincristine and vinblastine differ only in methyl (vinblastine) or formyl (vincristine) side chains on the parent molecule. Both drugs bind to tubulin with high affinity and prevent the assembly of microtubules.

The mandrake plant, a source of Native American folk remedies, is also the source of podophyllotoxin, of which etoposide and teniposide are semisynthetic derivatives. They are structurally unrelated to the vinca alkaloids and do not share a common mechanism of action. They may, however, exhibit cross-resistance with the vinca alkaloids and other natural products via the phenomenon of multidrug resistance.

Paclitaxel is found in the bark of the Western yew tree; other closely related compounds such as taxotere may be isolated from material derived from other members of the Taxus family.

Vincristine

PHARMACOLOGY

Vincristine sulfate is the salt of an asymmetric dimeric alkaloid. Vincristine causes reversible mitotic arrest through binding to cytoplasmic precursors of the spindle. The drug is

M-phase-specific, blocking proliferating cells as they enter metaphase. It may also inhibit RNA synthesis through effects on DNA-dependent RNA polymerase. The neurotoxicity of vincristine may be related to its relative polarity; indeed, vincristine has the greatest polarity of this series of compounds, and vinblastine the least.

Vincristine is extensively bound to tissue components. Peak plasma levels are about 0.4 μm with a terminal half-life of about 24 hours. The primary route of elimination of the drug and its metabolites is by the liver into the bile and feces; 70% is excreted in the feces and 5% to 16% in the urine. Therefore, patients with obstructive liver disease may be more susceptible to vincristine neurotoxicity. There is minimal entry into the central nervous system (CNS). The drug is unpredictably absorbed from the GI tract.

THERAPEUTIC USES

Vincristine has a broad spectrum of clinical activity. The drug is an important component of curative drug combinations in acute lymphoblastic leukemia, Hodgkin's disease, the intermediate and aggressive non-Hodgkin's lymphomas, Wilms' tumor, Ewing's sarcoma, and childhood rhabdomyosarcoma. Combinations of vincristine and cyclophosphamide produce high remission rates in the treatment of neuroblastoma. The drug is also used with cyclophosphamide and dactinomycin as an adjunct to surgery and/or radiation therapy in the treatment of rhabdomyosarcoma. Finally, vincristine is also commonly used in combinations against small cell lung carcinoma, breast carcinoma, and multiple myeloma.

DETAILS OF ADMINISTRATION

Vincristine is available in 1-mg, 2-mg, and 5-mg vials. Each ml contains 1 mg of vincristine sulfate, 100 mg of mannitol, 1.3 mg of methylparaben, and 0.2 mg of propylparaben. The drug is light sensitive and should be stored at 2° to 8°C. Vincristine should be administered into the tubing of a freely running intravenous infusion of normal saline or dextrose solution.

The normal dose in children is 2 mg/m^2; in adults it is 1.4 mg/m^2 weekly. The practice of capping the adult dose at a maximum of 2 mg should be discouraged. The injection may be completed in 1 minute, or the dose may be diluted in a large volume and administered slowly over several hours or longer by continuous infusion.

Vincristine is very irritating and must be given only intravenously. Care should be taken to ensure that the needle is properly positioned in the vein to avoid extravasation. If leakage occurs into paravenous tissue, it may cause considerable irritation. If irritation occurs, the injection should be stopped immediately (see Practical Guidelines for Chemotherapy Administration at the end of this chapter).

DOSE MODIFICATIONS

It is common practice to reduce the administered dose in the presence of significant hepatic dysfunction. Reasonable guidelines would stipulate a 50% reduction for bilirubin greater than 3. Although many clinicians reduce the dose of vincristine in the presence of a mild peripheral neuropathy, this practice should be discouraged, particularly if the drug is being used in combinations with curative intent. In the presence of significant neuropathy, such as painful paresthesias, peripheral motor weakness, cranial nerve palsies, or ileus, the drug may have to be held until reversal of the toxicity. When the drug is employed in a clearly palliative setting, a somewhat more liberal attitude about dose reduction or lengthening of intervals between doses in the presence of moderate toxicity may be justifiable. These decisions require expert medical judgment.

DRUG INTERACTIONS

Vincristine increases the accumulation of methotrexate in tumor cells; methotrexate reaches higher steady-state levels in humans with acute myeloblastic and lymphoblastic leukemia cells in the presence of vincristine at concentrations greater than 0.1 μm. The clinical significance of this interaction needs further study. Asparaginase may decrease hepatic clearance of vincristine. Vincristine may decrease oral bioavailability of digoxin.

TOXICITY

The dose-limiting side effect of vincristine is neurotoxicity. Mild neuropathy presenting with sensory impairment, loss of deep tendon reflexes, and paresthesias is common. Less often one may see severe painful paresthesias, ataxia, foot drop, and cranial nerve palsies. Autonomic effects include severe constipation, abdominal pain, and ileus. Clinically significant hematologic toxicity is unusual. Dermatologic effects and alopecia occur in 20–70% of patients. Other rare side effects include CNS depression and syndrome of inappropriate secretion of antidiuretic hormone (SIADH).

Vinblastine

PHARMACOLOGY

Vinblastine sulfate is the salt of a dimeric alkaloid containing both indole and dihydroindole moieties. The drug crystallizes critical microtubular proteins of the mitotic spindle. In high concentrations, vinblastine exerts complex effects on nucleic acid and protein synthesis. It may also cause a rearrangement of binding sites in the protein of microtubular units, permitting polymerization of the tubule proteins to protofibrils.

Like vincristine, vinblastine is rapidly distributed into body tissues. About 75% is bound to plasma proteins. The drug has a triphasic plasma clearance; the terminal half-life approximates 20 hours. Oral absorption is unpredictable. The drug is partially metabolized to deacetyl vinblastine, but most of the drug is ultimately excreted intact in the bile with some enterohepatic circulation; approximately 20% is excreted in the urine. Obstructive liver disease may therefore increase the toxicity of this drug. Very little of the drug penetrates the CNS.

THERAPEUTIC USES

Vinblastine is a component of curative treatment regimens for advanced Hodgkin's disease and testicular cancer. For the former, it is most often used in combination with doxorubicin, bleomycin, and dacarbazine (ABVD). Vinblastine, cisplatin, and bleomycin in combination (VPB) is an established treatment regimen for advanced nonseminomatous germ cell tumors. Vinblastine is also useful in the palliative treatment of breast carcinoma, mycosis fungoides, Kaposi's sarcoma, and choriocarcinoma. Slow intravenous infusions have reportedly been effective in some cases of refractory idiopathic thrombocytopenic purpura.

DETAILS OF ADMINISTRATION

Vinblastine is supplied in 10-mg vials at a concentration of 1 mg/ml without excipients. The lyophilized drug should be diluted with normal saline solution containing phenol or benzyl alcohol as preservative; other solutions are not recommended by the manufacturer. This solution may be stored in the refrigerator for 30 days without significant loss of potency. Vinblastine should be administered through the side arm of a freely running intravenous infusion. The injection may be completed in 1 minute. The needle should be positioned properly in the vein to ensure that no extravasation or spillage occurs. Alternatively, the dosage may be diluted in a large volume (100 ml) intravenous infusion and administered over a longer period of time (30 minutes). If leakage accidentally occurs in the surrounding tissue, it may cause considerable damage. The injection should be discontinued immediately (see Practical Guidelines for Chemotherapy Administration).

When vinblastine is used as single-agent therapy, most adults with relatively normal marrow function tolerate 5 to 12 mg/m^2 weekly without difficulty. The manufacturer recommends a starting dose of 3.7 mg/m^2 intravenously for adults and 2.5 mg/m^2 intravenously for children. Treatment is repeated weekly with gradual escalation (in increments of about 1.8 mg/m^2 per week for adults and 1.25 mg/m^2 per week for children) until dose-limiting leukopenia is encountered. The manufacturer recommends a maximum dose of 18.5 mg/m^2 weekly for adults or 12.5 mg/m^2 for children; these doses are substantially in excess of those that the vast majority of patients are likely to tolerate.

DOSE MODIFICATIONS

A reasonable dose modification for hepatic dysfunction is as outlined for vincristine.

DRUG INTERACTIONS

Vinblastine may decrease the pharmacologic effects of phenytoin and increase methotrexate accumulation by tumor cells. The clinical significance of the latter interaction requires further study. Acute bronchospasm has been noted with vinblastine in patients with a recent exposure to mitomycin-C.

TOXICITY

Leukopenia is the usual dose-limiting toxicity. The nadir occurs within 5 to 10 days of administration. Thrombocytopenia and anemia are uncommon. The drug is generally well tolerated; nausea, if it occurs at all, is mild and controlled by antiemetic agents. Stomatitis and constipation are seen more frequently at higher doses or with continuous infusions. Neurologic and dermatologic complications are much less common than with vincristine and usually occur in patients on prolonged therapy. Other side effects include mild reversible alopecia, rashes, and photosensitivity reactions. The drug is a local vesicant if extravasation occurs. High doses may lead to general myalgias and sometimes pain referred to the tumor itself. Finally, continuous infusion regimens may lead to transient hepatitis.

Etoposide

PHARMACOLOGY

Etoposide is a semisynthetic derivative of podophyllotoxin. The presence of a hydroxyl group at the C4′ position of the C-ring is associated with the drug's ability to induce DNA strand breaks, an effect that appears to be mediated by interaction with topoisomerase II. This interaction may be responsible, at least in part, for the drug's cytolytic activity. The drug is cell-cycle dependent, inducing G2 phase arrest.

Etoposide undergoes rapid distribution and metabolism with a large apparent volume of distribution. The drug is approximately 94% bound to serum proteins; neither etoposide nor its metabolites readily penetrate the CNS, although high doses produce measurable levels of drug and metabolites in both CNS tumor tissue and the CSF. The terminal half-life ranges from 6 to 8 hours in adults with normal organ function. About 40% of the dose is excreted in the urine as unchanged drug and metabolites within 48 hours. The drug is metabolized predominantly at the D-ring to produce a pharmacologically active hydroxyacid. Absorption following oral administration is variable, and a two-fold increase in dose by the oral route is necessary to achieve the same effect as with systemic administration.

THERAPEUTIC USES

Etoposide is a key component of curative combination chemotherapy for disseminated nonseminomatous testicular carcinoma; the combination of etoposide and cisplatin, with bleomycin, is an established regimen for the treatment of nonseminomatous testicular carcinoma. Etoposide is also extremely active in non-Hodgkin's lymphoma and has been incorporated into several aggressive regimens for intermediate grade non-Hodgkin's lymphoma. It is probably the most active single drug against small cell lung carcinoma and has therefore been incorporated into various combinations, including CAV (with cyclophosphamide and doxorubicin), ECHO (with cyclophosphamide, doxorubicin, and vincristine), and with cisplatin. The combination of ifosfamide and etoposide has good activity against pediatric sarcomas, particularly Ewing's sarcoma. The drug has also been used in the treatment of refractory acute myelogenous leukemia, non–small cell lung carcinoma, and Kaposi's sarcoma.

DETAILS OF ADMINISTRATION

The drug is supplied for parenteral use in 100-mg vials. Each ml contains 20 mg of etoposide, 2 mg of citric acid, 30 mg of benzyl alcohol, 80 mg of polysorbate 80, 650 mg of polyethylene glycol 300, and 30.5% alcohol. Etoposide should be administered in a 5% dextrose solution or a 0.9% sodium chloride solution, in concentrations of 0.2 or 0.4 mg/ml. Etoposide concentrate for injection must be diluted before administration, in either glass or plastic polyvinyl chloride containers. Etoposide solutions containing 0.1 mg to 0.4 mg/ml in 0.9% sodium chloride or 5% dextrose solutions have been passed through several commercially available filters, such as a .22-micron Millex-GS filter, without decomposition. Because hypotension following rapid intravenous administration has been reported, it is recommended that etoposide solutions be administered over 30- to 60-minute periods. To avoid possible skin reactions, the use of gloves is recommended. In the event that exposure does occur, wash affected areas of skin immediately with soap and water.

The usual dose for etoposide is 50 mg to 100 mg/m^2/daily on days 1 to 5, or 100 mg/m^2/daily on days 1, 3, and 5 every 3 to 4 weeks in combination with other drugs. Recent work has shown that this dose is substantially less than the true maximum tolerated dose, with or without bone marrow transplant. Except in the treatment of Kaposi's sarcoma associated with acquired immunodeficiency syndrome (AIDS), etoposide is rarely used as a single agent.

For oral use a 50-mg capsule is available. Bioavailability is roughly 50%; therefore, the recommended oral dose is 2 times the intravenous dose.

DOSE MODIFICATIONS

In renal failure the dose should probably be reduced in rough proportion to the reduction in creatinine clearance.

DRUG INTERACTIONS

No drug interactions have been reported.

TOXICITIES

The dose-limiting side-effect of etoposide is leukopenia with a nadir in approximately 7–15 days; thrombocytopenia is seen less frequently. Nausea and vomiting are seen in about 35% of patients but are seen more frequently with the oral preparations. Anorexia and diarrhea occur in less than 15% of patients. Rapid intravenous administration may be associated with transient hypotension. Anaphylactoid reactions have been reported in up to 2% of patients and may be severe. The associated bronchospasm may be responsive to antihistamine therapy. Reversible alopecia and peripheral neuropathy are also occasionally seen. Administration of high doses to patients with glioma has produced acute reversible neurological deterioration in several cases 9–10 days following therapy. Treatment with dexamethazone resulted in rapid reversal of the abnormalities.

Teniposide

PHARMACOLOGY

Teniposide is a semisynthetic podophyllotoxin. The drug is insoluble in water and is dissolved in a mixture of organic solvents for clinical use. The drug probably works by a similar mechanism of action as described for etoposide, *i.e.*, inhibition of topoisomerase II.

Like etoposide, teniposide is extensively bound to serum proteins (>99%) and shows minimal entry into the CNS. The pharmacokinetics differ somewhat from etoposide. The pharmacokinetic profile is biphasic, with a terminal half-life of 5 hours. About 40% of the administered dose is excreted in the urine. Metabolites account for 80% of drug excreted in the urine.

THERAPEUTIC USES

Teniposide has been shown to be highly active in combination in certain pediatric hematologic malignancies. Teniposide plus cytarabine appears to be highly effective salvage therapy for initial induction failures in childhood acute lymphocytic leukemia (ALL); the drug has also been incorporated into the consolidation phase of several experimental programs. Teniposide plus doxorubicin plus bleomycin has been shown to be active salvage therapy for both Hodgkin's and non-Hodgkin's lymphoma. Teniposide has also shown activity against Kaposi's sarcoma, multiple myeloma, and small cell and non–small cell lung cancer. Investigational protocols continue to define the role of this drug in all of these diseases.

DETAILS OF ADMINISTRATION

Teniposide is supplied as a 50-mg ampule containing benzyl alcohol, 150 mg; N,N-dimethyl-acetamide, 300 mg; polyoxyethylated castor oil, purified, 2.5 g; and maleic acid (sufficient quantity to adjust to pH 5.1; in absolute alcohol). Solutions of teniposide should be diluted to a final concentration of no more than 1 mg/ml in non-DEHP containers such as glass or polyolefin, since the solvents can leach plasticizers from, for example, PVC containers. Teniposide solutions at concentrations less than 0.4 mg/ml are stable for 24 hours at room temperature. However, solutions of 1 mg/ml should be administered within 4 hours to avoid precipitation. To avoid precipitation during preparation and administration, agitation of the dissolved drug should be minimized, and the drug should be given as soon after preparation as possible. Refrigeration is not recommended. Teniposide should be infused over 45 to 60 minutes to prevent hypotension during administration. Extravasation should be avoided, and a 5- to 10-ml flush of normal saline before administering the drug should be given to check the vein for patency.

Teniposide is generally used at doses of 150 mg to 170 mg/m^2 twice weekly for 4 weeks in combination therapy for childhood or adult ALL. For solid tumors, weekly doses of 60 mg to 80 mg/m^2 intravenously are used, but more aggressive protocols have used up to 60 mg/m^2 daily for five days.

DOSE MODIFICATIONS

Hepatic metabolism and excretion may play an important role in teniposide's disposition, but the relationship between hepatic dysfunction and drug clearance has not been worked out.

DRUG INTERACTIONS

No drug interactions have been reported.

TOXICITIES

Leukopenia is dose limiting, with the nadir occurring at approximately day 7; thrombocytopenia may occur as well. Rapid intravenous administration leads to transient hypotension. Nausea, vomiting, and diarrhea are seen in about 30% of patients, and transient alopecia may also occur, especially on the higher dose 5-day schedules. Mucositis has been reported in up to three fourths of patients. Allergic reactions are seen in about 5% of patients and may be severe; most symptoms can be alleviated by stopping the infusion and administering diphenhydramine. Liver function test abnormalities, nephrotoxicity, and neurotoxicity occur uncommonly.

Paclitaxel

PHARMACOLOGY

Paclitaxel is a novel diterpene derivative originally isolated from the bark of the Western yew (*Taxus brevifolia*). The molecule consists of a complex oxetan ring structure with ester side chains at the 2, 4, 10, and 13 positions of the central ring. Both total synthesis and a semisynthesis using taxane precursors derived from Taxus sources appear feasible and may also be commercially viable. The drug is poorly soluble in water; several research groups are seeking water-soluble derivatives by side-chain modification. The drug acts by binding to a specific site on tubulin, promoting its polymerization, and stabilizing the resulting microtubules. The drug also binds directly to tubulin oligomers and preformed polymerized tubulin. Resistance may be on the basis of mdr-1 gene expression or more likely by the evolution of tubulin mutants that no longer bind drug.

Paclitaxel has a triphasic disappearance from the plasma following intravenous injection. The alpha, beta, and gamma half-lives are approximately 11 minutes, 2 hours, and 21 hours, respectively. The drug is highly bound to serum proteins (>97%). Only about 5% of injected drug appears to be excreted by the renal route. Extent of metabolism *in vivo* is unknown although at least 11 metabolites have been found in man.

THERAPEUTIC USES

Development of paclitaxel was hindered for years by the great difficulty in obtaining adequate quantities from natural sources. The drug has important activity in resistant or relapsed ovarian cancer; about 30% of patients who have failed initial combination chemotherapy containing cisplatin or carboplatin respond, the majority with partial rather than complete responses. Studies of paclitaxel in breast cancer have demonstrated activity comparable to doxorubicin. In preliminary studies, paclitaxel showed some activity in several additional tumor types not notably sensitive to standard agents (melanoma, non–small cell lung cancer); follow-up studies are in progress.

DETAILS OF ADMINISTRATION

Paclitaxel is supplied as a concentrated solution of 300 mg per ampule (5 ml). Each ml contains 6 mg paclitaxel, 527 mg of Cremaphor EL (polyoxyethylated castor oil), and 49.7% (V/V) alcohol. This concentrate must be diluted 1:15 to 1:20 in saline or 5% dextrose before intravenous administration. These solutions are stable for up to 27 hours at room temperature. Paclitaxel should be administered through an in-line filter (0.22 μm). Because paclitaxel contains Cremaphor EL, which is capable of leaching plasticizer from polyvinyl chloride containers, the drug should be mixed in glass or non–DHEP-containing vessels. Bolus administration in phase I studies was attended by an unacceptably high rate of anaphylactoid reactions, probably due to the formulation; lengthening the infusion time to at least 3 to 6 hours and premedication with antihistamines and corticosteroids have largely obviated this problem. The drug is currently recommended to be given at a dose of 135 mg/m^2 as a 24-hour continuous infusion every 3 weeks. The drug is also being tested with shorter (3-hour) and longer (96-hour) infusions in an attempt to find the optimal clinical schedule. Combination studies with other active agents and studies of high-dose administration with hematopoietic growth factors are in progress.

DOSE MODIFICATIONS

Insufficient information exists at present. Patients with prior therapy may require dose reductions, as may patients with hepatic dysfunction, although no specific guidelines are available. More detailed pharmacologic study is needed.

DRUG INTERACTION

Ketoconazole may inhibit paclitaxel metabolism.

TOXICITY

Aside from anaphylactoid reactions, which occur sporadically despite the precautions listed above, the major side effects seen in trials to date appear to be bone marrow suppression (principally neutropenia, resolved in most patients by the second to third week), nausea and vomiting, alopecia, and a sensory peripheral neuropathy. Sinus bradycardia of no hemodynamic significance is seen in about one third of patients treated at active dose levels. Significant cardiac arrhythmias, including ventricular tachyarrhythmias and varying degrees of A-V block, have also occurred in a small percentage of treated patients; risk factors for occurrence of cardiac complications have not yet been defined but prior history of cardiac dysfunction should prompt caution in the use of paclitaxel.

Taxotere

PHARMACOLOGY

Taxotere is a semisynthetic analogue of Paclitaxel whose starting material is extracted from the needles of *Taxus brevifolia*. Like Paclitaxel, taxotere's mechanism of action also appears to be through the formation and stabilization of intracellular microtubule bundles.

Taxotere has a biexponential disappearance from the plasma with a terminal half-life of approximately 3 hours. Urinary excretion of the drug is minimal.

THERAPEUTIC USES

Based on preliminary clinical trials, taxotere appears to have activity in the treatment of patients with breast, ovarian, and non–small cell lung cancer.

DETAILS OF ADMINISTRATION

Taxotere is supplied as an investigational agent being developed by Rhone-Poulenc-Rorer Pharmaceuticals, Inc. (Collegeville, Pennsylvania). The drug is supplied as a concentrated solution containing 15 mg of taxotere per ml in a 1 : 1 solution of polysorbate 80/Tween 80 and alcohol. The concentrate should be diluted in 5% dextrose to a final concentration not exceeding 0.3 mg/ml. Diluted solutions of taxotere are stable for at least 8 hours at room temperature. The optimal schedule for the administration of taxotere has not been defined. Recommended dose for taxotere given as a 1-hour infusion daily for 5 days every 21 days is 12 mg/m^2/day. A 6- or 24-hour infusion of the drug given every 3 weeks was found to be well tolerated at a dose of 90–100 mg/m^2.

DOSE MODIFICATIONS

Insufficient information exists at present and no specific guidelines are currently available.

DRUG INTERACTION

There are no known drug interactions.

TOXICITY

The dose-limiting toxicity of taxotere has been found to be neutropenia. Anaphylactoid reactions have been seen on occasion, and patients have been successfully retreated with the addition of steroids and histamine antagonists. Other toxicities that have been noted include rash, alopecia, and thrombocytopenia. Notably, neurologic and cardiac toxicities have not been reported. A capillary leak syndrome consisting of pleural effusions and peripheral edema of uncertain etiology has been described. Current investigations are attempting to define the mechanism of this toxicity and preventive measures.

ANTITUMOR ANTIBIOTICS

The antitumor antibiotics in common clinical use are natural products isolated from the culture broth of various species of streptomyces. They produce tumoricidal and antimicrobial effects by direct inhibition of DNA and/or RNA synthesis. The cytotoxic potency of these drugs prevents their clinical use as antibacterial agents. They exhibit a variety of effects on different phases of the cell cycle; kinetically they behave as phase-nonspecific agents. Many of the side effects of this group of drugs are similar to the alkylating agents, while others, such as the cardiotoxicity of the anthracyclines or the pulmonary and skin reactions of the bleomycins, are characteristic of individual agents or chemical classes.

The extent to which the antibiotics are carcinogenic or leukemogenic in humans is unknown; there is no direct evidence implicating any of them, as there is for the alkylators. Doxorubicin and mitomycin are positive in the Ames test, induce sister chromatid exchanges, and are carcinogenic in animals. Actinomycin D is carcinogenic in animals but negative in the Ames test. Bleomycin appears negative in both but can cause sister chromatid exchanges. Because all of these agents are employed most commonly in complex combinations, it seems unlikely that definitive human data will be forthcoming, and it is probably safest to regard these compounds as potential human carcinogens or leukemogens.

Daunorubicin

PHARMACOLOGY

Daunorubicin, an anthracycline glycoside antibiotic, has a tetracycline-ring structure to which the sugar daunosamine is linked. Compounds of this class all have quinone and hydroquinone moieties on adjacent rings that permit electron transfer reactions. The drug inhibits DNA synthesis and DNA-dependent RNA synthesis by intercalating between base pairs of the DNA helix and inducing its uncoiling. Daunorubicin also inhibits the activity of topoisomerase II, thus leading to the further induction of DNA strand breaks. The compound also appears to produce cellular damage through free-radical formation. The drug is maximally cytotoxic in the S or G2 phases at intermediate doses but behaves kinetically as phase nonspecific at higher doses.

Daunorubicin is rapidly metabolized in the liver and distributed in tissues as unchanged drug and metabolites. Plasma elimination is triphasic, with a terminal half-life of about 18 hours. The principal metabolic product formed by aldo-keto reductase is daunorubicinol, which has antineoplastic activity. Cleavage of the glycosidic bond yields metabolites that are devoid of antitumor activity but that may be involved in cardiac and other toxicity. An estimated 40% of the drug is eliminated by biliary excretion; the cumulative excretion in the urine is 25% of combined drug and metabolites. Because the drug is extremely irritating to tissues and has poor bioavailability, it must be administered intravenously.

THERAPEUTIC USES

Daunorubicin is used mainly in combination regimens for remission induction in acute myelogenous leukemia. As a single agent it produces complete remissions in 30% to 50% of patients. In combination with cytarabine, with or without thioguanine, it produces complete remissions in 60% to 80% of patients. It is not effective in the prophylaxis of meningeal leukemia. Daunorubicin is also used in combination with vincristine and prednisone for remission induction in acute lymphocytic leukemia. The drug appears also to have activity in a number of pediatric and adult solid tumors, but possible wider use outside the setting of leukemia has been preempted by doxorubicin.

DETAILS OF ADMINISTRATION

Daunorubicin is supplied for injection in 20-mg vials with 100 mg of mannitol. When reconstituted with 4 ml of sterile water for injection, each ml contains 5 mg of daunorubicin hydrochloride. The reconstituted solution is stable for 24 hours at room temperature or 48 hours when refrigerated and should be protected from sunlight. Daunorubicin should only be administered intravenously. The desired dose should be injected into the tubing of a freely flowing intravenous infusion of 5% dextrose in water or 0.9% sodium chloride. It should not be mixed or administered in the same tubing with other drugs or heparin.

Dosage is 30 mg to 60 mg/m^2 intravenously daily for 3–5 days, repeated every 3 to 4 weeks. Within this range, the dose of 60 mg/m^2 is usually reserved for single-agent use, with 45 mg/m^2 being the dose commonly used in combination therapy. Severe tissue necrosis will occur if extravasation occurs during administration. In case of extravasation, as much infiltrated drug as possible should be aspirated. Although no specific treatments are of proven value for tissue damage, the local reaction may be partially abrogated by infiltrating the area with an injection of 50 mg to 100 mg of hydrocortisone sodium succinate and/or 5 ml of 8.4% sodium bicarbonate and by applying cold compresses. If the infiltration is severe, the patient may subsequently require excision of the area with skin grafting and plastic surgery (see Practical Guidelines for Chemotherapy Administration).

DOSE MODIFICATIONS

Daunorubicin must be used with particular caution in patients with a history of heart disease. Hepatic or renal impairment may enhance the toxicity of usual doses of daunorubicin (see Doxorubicin).

DRUG INTERACTIONS

Daunorubicin is physically incompatible with heparin sodium and with dexamethasone phosphate.

TOXICITY

The dose-limiting toxicity is hematologic, predominantly leukopenia, with the mean nadir at 10 days. Severe bone marrow hypoplasia is the aim of treatment in acute myeloblastic leukemia. Both acute and chronic cardiac toxicity may occur. Acutely with drug administration, the electrocardiogram may show nonspecific abnormalities, sinus tachycardia, heart block, and ventricular irritability. Cumulative dose-dependent cardiomyopathy, ultimately manifested by congestive heart failure, occurs in approximately 1% to 2% of patients at a total dosage of 550 mg/m^2 and in about 12% at a total dose of 1000 mg/m^2. Children appear to be more sensitive than adults. Cardiac failure may occur at total lower doses in patients who have received radiation therapy to a port including the heart (see Doxorubicin).

Nausea and vomiting are usually mild, lasting 24 to 48 hours; prophylactic antiemetics may help. Stomatitis is infrequent, occurring as early as 5 to 7 days. Other effects include reversible alopecia and red urine (not hematuria). Extravasation of daunorubicin produces severe local irritation and can lead to tissue necrosis.

Idarubicin

PHARMACOLOGY

Idarubicin (4-demethoxydaunorubicin) is an analogue of daunorubicin, lacking the methoxyl group of the C-4 position of the aglycone. It has a higher therapeutic index than either doxorubicin or daunorubicin in a variety of murine leukemias and tumors, including MS-2 sarcoma, and both solid and ascitic sarcoma 180. The drug was eight times more potent than daunorubicin when administered to mice with L-1210 and PP8 leukemia. The drug binds to DNA with a marked inhibitory effect on nucleic acid polymerases and is more active than daunorubicin in inhibiting RNA synthesis and mouse fibroblast proliferation. It is also a potent inhibitor of topoisomerase II and this along with its ability to form free radicals certainly contributes to cytotoxicity.

Following rapid intravenous injection, the plasma disappearance of idarubicin is triphasic and similar to that seen for doxorubicin, with a terminal half-life of approximately 22 hours. Following either intravenous or oral administration, there is an accumulation and prolonged retention of the active metabolite 13-idarubicinol, with elevated plasma levels persisting for more than 8 days after administration of the drug. This metabolite may contribute to the drug's overall cytotoxicity.

By both intravenous and oral routes, idarubicin appears to be concentrated and retained in tissues to a proportionately greater extent than daunorubicin.

THERAPEUTIC USES

Idarubicin is active against Hodgkin's and indolent non-Hodgkin's lymphomas, carcinoma of the breast, and in acute lymphoblastic and nonlymphoblastic leukemia. Activity against ANLL has been shown both as a single agent and in combination with other chemotherapeutic agents, where idarubicin appears at least as effective, and probably more effective than daunorubicin both in CR rates and survival. Oral idarubicin has demonstrated activity in approximately 25% of untreated patients with advanced breast cancer and cross-resistance with other anthracyclines may not be complete. The relative merit of oral versus intravenous idarubicin has yet to be established. In breast cancer, idarubicin appears to be less active than doxorubicin at equivalently myelosuppressive doses.

DETAILS OF ADMINISTRATION

The drug is supplied in sterile glass vials containing 5 and 10 mg of idarubicin. The vial is reconstituted with 5 and 10 ml of sterile water or normal saline to a concentration of 1 mg/ml and can be used up to 72 hours thereafter when stored at room temperature and 7 days with refrigeration. The desired dose is withdrawn into a syringe containing 10 ml to 15 ml of normal saline and is administered by intravenous injection over a 10- to 15-minute period through the side arm of a freely running infusion. In combination with AraC in the induction therapy of ANLL, a dose of 12 mg/m^2 daily for 3 consecutive days has been used most frequently. By mouth, as a single agent, doses of 45 mg/m^2 per course, divided over 3 days, are effective and well tolerated in the treatment of solid tumors.

DOSE MODIFICATIONS

Idarubicin is not significantly eliminated through the kidneys, so dose modification for renal dysfunction is not indicated unless renal impairment is severe. Since the drug is significantly metabolized by the liver, dose modifications should be considered for abnormal liver function. There are no pharmacologically validated recommendations at present, but the same recommendations as those for epirubicin are a reasonable guide. These are as follows: reduce the dose by 50% when the bilirubin is elevated 1.3 to 2 times normal and/or enzymes are increased 1.1 to 2 times normal. If the bilirubin is elevated between 2.1 and 5 times normal and/or enzymes are increased 2.1 to 5 times normal, the dose is reduced by 75%. The drug is discontinued if the bilirubin or enzymes exceed 5 times normal. (See comments under Doxorubicin.) Further study is required.

DRUG INTERACTIONS

There are no known *in vivo* drug interactions to date; based on doxorubicin data, mixing with heparin sodium is not advised.

TOXICITY

Idarubicin by injection at equally myelosuppressive doses causes less severe nausea, vomiting, alopecia, and mucositis than doxorubicin or daunorubicin. In patients with solid tumors, leukopenia is more often observed than thrombocytopenia; 10 mg to 12.5 mg/m^2 of idarubicin by injection produces about the same degree of myelosuppression as 60 mg/m^2 of doxorubicin and 40 mg to 45 mg/m^2 of oral idarubicin.

Doxorubicin

PHARMACOLOGY

Doxorubicin is an anthracycline glycoside antibiotic differing structurally from daunorubicin at the 8 position, where a hydroxyacetyl group replaces an acetyl group. Like daunorubicin, doxorubicin forms a complex with DNA by intercalation between base pairs, leads to the formation of free radicals, and inhibits topoisomerase II, all of which contribute to inhibition of DNA synthesis and DNA-dependent RNA synthesis. Doxorubicin is active throughout the cell cycle.

Doxorubicin is widely distributed in plasma and tissues, with a triphasic plasma clearance. The terminal half-life of drug and metabolites is approximately 30 hours. The drug is rapidly metabolized by the liver to yield an active metabolite (doxorubicinol) and a number of metabolites (aglycones) that have no antitumor effect but may be associated with cardiac and other toxicities. Approximately 50% of the dose is excreted in the bile within 7 days. Less than 5% of the drug is excreted in the urine; penetration of the cerebrospinal fluid is poor. The drug is not stable in gastric acid and is not absorbed from the GI tract.

THERAPEUTIC USES

This drug has an exceptionally broad spectrum, with significant antitumor activity in the hematologic malignancies, sarcomas of soft tissues and bone, and carcinomas of breast, lung, stomach, prostate, bladder, testis, thyroid, ovary, and uterus, as well as some epidermoid carcinomas. It is part of some curative combination and/or multimodality regimens in the leukemias (although the balance of opinion favors daunorubicin or idarubicin as the anthracycline of choice in acute leukemia), the diffuse lymphomas, sarcomas, breast cancer, and small cell lung cancer. It is employed widely in other tumor types, alone and in combination, for palliation of advanced disease. The drug does not have useful activity in renal cell carcinoma, colorectal cancer, or malignant melanoma.

DETAILS OF ADMINISTRATION

Doxorubicin hydrochloride is supplied in 10-mg, 20-mg, 50-mg and 100-mg vials, with 50 mg, 100 mg, 250 mg, and 500 mg of lactose, respectively. The 10-mg, 20-mg, 50-mg, and 100-mg vials are reconstituted with 5 ml, 10 ml, 25 ml, and 50 ml respectively, of 0.9% sodium chloride injection or sterile water for injection, giving a final concentration of 2 mg/ml of doxorubicin. Bacteriostatic diluents are not recommended. The reconstituted solution is stable for 24 hours at room temperature and for 48 hours under refrigeration and should be protected from sunlight. The dose should be injected into the tubing of a freely running intravenous infusion of 0.9% sodium chloride or 5% dextrose solution and administered slowly over a period of not less than 3 minutes; the rate of injection should depend on the size of the vein and the dose.

Local erythematous streaking along the vein and/or facial flushing may indicate too rapid administration. A stinging or burning sensation may be a symptom of extravasation, but extravasation may occur without these symptoms. If extravasation occurs, the administration of the drug should be stopped immediately. Although no particular intervention has been demonstrated to be effective, irrigation of the site with copious amounts of saline, local infiltration with corticosteroids, and application of cold compresses may possibly alleviate the local reaction (see Practical Guidelines for Chemotherapy Administration). Should the skin reaction progress or be exceptionally large, plastic surgery may subsequently be required.

The usual single-agent dose is 60 mg to 75 mg/m^2 given intravenously every 21 days; less may be appropriate for patients with inadequate bone marrow reserve from age or prior therapy. Alternative doses and schedules have also been explored (*e.g.*, 20 mg/m^2 intravenously once weekly by bolus, or 60 mg/m^2 by continuous infusion over 48 to 96 hours every 3 weeks). Current data suggest that low-dose weekly regimens or continuous infusion schedules decrease the cumulative risk of cardiac toxicity without significant compromise in antitumor effect. Administration of the iron chelator ICRF-187 with doxorubicin appears to decrease doxorubicin's cardiotoxicity significantly without an important decrease in antitumor effect. The drug appears to have a steep dose–response curve; some investigators have employed bolus doses in the 90 mg to 120 mg/m^2 range with impressive response rates but also a substantial incidence of cardiac toxicity. Doses in this range should not be administered outside clinical trials. (See section on Toxicity for comments on cardiac monitoring).

DOSE MODIFICATIONS

Particular caution is necessary for patients with preexisting heart disease. Most physicians regard the presence of congestive heart failure, compensated or uncompensated, as a contraindication to doxorubicin administration. Some, however, recommend the use of continuous-infusion regimens even in the presence of compensated organic heart disease or in patients with risk factors for the development of doxorubicin cardiomyopathy (*e.g.*, hypertension, prior radiation therapy to the heart).

Doses should be reduced in the presence of severely impaired hepatic function, but validated guidelines for dose attenuation under these circumstances are not available. Conventional guidelines (*e.g.*, 50% of full dose for bilirubin between 2 and 3; 25% of full dose for bilirubin between 3 and 5; hold drug for bilirubin greater than 5) probably result in significant underdosing of patients with mild or moderate hepatic dysfunction. Further study is required.

DRUG INTERACTIONS

Doxorubicin precipitates in the presence of heparin and of 5-fluorouracil. Amphotericin B may increase tumor cell uptake of doxorubicin and thus may partially reverse doxorubicin resistance in tumor cells; it is not clear whether this effect is exploitable clinically. Cyclophosphamide or mitomycin administration may increase the risk of cardiac toxicity and mercaptopurine, the risk of hepatotoxicity. Doxorubicin may decrease the oral bioavailability of digoxin. Barbiturates may enhance doxorubicin's clearance.

TOXICITY

The toxicity of doxorubicin is similar to that of daunorubicin. The major acute dose-limiting toxicity is hematologic; leukopenia has a median nadir at 10 to 15 days. Anemia and thrombocytopenia are much less common and generally less severe.

Stomatitis occurs uncommonly with single-dose administration but more frequently on multiple-day schedules. Nausea and vomiting are usually mild to moderate on the day of administration. Alopecia is virtually universal, beginning between the third and fourth week from the initial dose. The drug may cause hyperpigmentation of the skin, especially the nail beds. As noted above, the agent is locally necrotizing if injected subcutaneously. Doxorubicin may cause reactivation of tissue reactions in areas of previous irradiation ("recall" phenomenon).

Both acute and chronic cardiac toxicity may occur. Acute effects include nonspecific ST-segment and T-wave changes and occasionally a pericarditis–myocarditis syndrome. Chronic cardiotoxicity usually presents as congestive heart failure and has a 5% incidence rate as the total doxorubicin dose approaches 550 mg/m^2 (by bolus administration); above this cumulative dose the incidence of congestive heart failure increases significantly. Prior mediastinal irradiation, significant hypertension, or coadministration of cyclophosphamide or mitomycin increases the risk of toxicity. Treatment of drug-induced cardiomyopathy is the same as for congestive heart failure of any cause.

Monitoring the cardiac status of patients receiving significant total doses of doxorubicin is an important feature of treatment; unfortunately, a simple, inexpensive, sensitive, and widely applicable technique does not exist. The endomyocardial biopsy appears to reflect drug-related myocardial damage in a manner that is linear with dose; this test has good predictive value and little morbidity in experienced hands but is not widely available. Of the many possible noninvasive approaches, the most widely employed is serial determination of the left-ventricular ejection fraction (LVEF) by radionuclide cardiography. Determination of LVEF at rest and, if possible, with exercise at various total doses of doxorubicin (*e.g.*, 0, 150, 300, 450 mg/m^2, and more frequently as the total dose approaches and exceeds 550 mg/m^2) is a reasonable approach; significant decrease in the LVEF from baseline or decrease to below normal levels indicates myocardial functional impairment and should prompt cessation of further doxorubicin administration.

Epirubicin

PHARMACOLOGY

Epirubicin (4′ epidoxorubicin) is an anthracycline antibiotic differing from doxorubicin in the epimerization of the hydroxyl group in position 4′ of the amino sugar moiety. In preclinical screening, the antitumor activity is similar to that of doxorubicin, but the drug has greater activity in Lewis lung carcinoma, MS-2 sarcoma, and xenografts of human melanoma. In chronic toxicity studies, epirubicin was quantitatively less toxic than doxorubicin.

The serum decay curve of epirubicin is triphasic, with a beta half-life of 1.3 to 2.6 hours and a gamma half-life of 30 to 38 hours. The volume of distribution (1430 liters/m^2) indicates significant tissue distribution. Eleven percent of the dose is eliminated in the urine over the first 48 hours. As with doxorubicin, plasma clearance is significantly reduced in patients with abnormal liver function tests.

THERAPEUTIC USES

Epirubicin is active in a variety of tumors including breast carcinoma, ovarian cancer, soft tissue sarcoma, lung cancer, non-Hodgkin's lymphoma, leukemias, and gastric cancer. It seems apparent that epirubicin has a spectrum of activity and toxicity similar to that of doxorubicin but is less potent by a factor of about 1.3. Early comparative trials in breast cancer indicated that epirubicin produced response and survival rates equivalent to doxorubicin with less cardiotoxicity and less acute toxicity, particularly myelosuppression.

The major interest in epirubicin is now in exploring higher doses and alternative schedules, so as to exploit the improved safety profile of this drug. In particular, at very high doses such as 180 mg/m^2, there appears to be considerably less mucositis than with comparable myelosuppressive doses of doxorubicin.

DETAILS OF ADMINISTRATION

This drug is not yet commercially available in the United States. Epirubicin is supplied as a red-orange lyophilized powder in vials containing 10 mg of epirubicin with 50 mg of lactose, and in vials containing 50 mg of epirubicin with 250 mg of lactose. It is prepared for intravenous injection by reconstitution with 5 ml (for 10 mg) and 25 ml (for 50 mg) sodium chloride injection (0.9%). The drug should be administered by injection into the side arm of a freely flowing solution of saline or 5% dextrose, with care to avoid extravasation. Reconstituted epirubicin is stable for 24 hours at room temperature.

DOSE MODIFICATIONS

Because only 11% of the drug is excreted in the urine in the first 48 hours, dose modification for renal dysfunction is not indicated unless renal impairment is severe.

Since the drug is significantly metabolized by the liver, dose modification is required for abnormal liver function. The current recommendations are 50% reduction when the bilirubin is elevated 1.3 to 2 times normal and/or enzymes are increased 1.1 to 2 times normal. If the bilirubin is elevated between 2.1 and 5 times normal and/or enzymes are increased 2.1 to 5 times normal, the dose is reduced by 75%. The drug is discontinued if the bilirubin or enzymes exceed 5 times normal (see Doxorubicin).

DRUG INTERACTIONS

There are no known drug interactions to date. However, based on doxorubicin data, mixing with heparin sodium is not advised.

TOXICITY

Epirubicin at dose levels identical to doxorubicin appears to have lower acute toxicity than its parent compound with particular reference to myelosuppression, stomatitis, vomiting, alopecia, and acute cardiac changes. Myelosuppression is dose related with nadir at approximately 10 days after therapy, returning to normal by day 21. Partial alopecia is universal; nausea and vomiting occur frequently. No renal or hepatic toxicity has been seen to date.

While uncommon, chronic cardiac toxicity has been reported in patients receiving epirubicin. For the few patients in whom cardiac toxicity has been noted, the median dose received has been approximately 1100 mg/m^2.

Dactinomycin

PHARMACOLOGY

Dactinomycin (actinomycin D), a phenoxazine pentapeptide antibiotic, is the major component of a mixture of actinomycins produced by *Streptomyces parvullus*. The drug intercalates between guanine-cytosine base pairs in DNA and inhibits DNA-dependent ribosomal and messenger RNA synthesis. Actively proliferating cells are more sensitive than quiescent cells to the cytotoxic effects; the drug is primarily cell-cycle nonspecific.

Dactinomycin is poorly absorbed orally. Following intravenous administration of [3H]dactinomycin, the isotope is rapidly distributed into tissues and has a prolonged biologic and tissue half-life; the terminal plasma half-life is approximately 36 hours. The drug does not penetrate into the central nervous system. Approximately 30% of the drug is recovered in the urine and feces after one week, and it has significant retention in nucleated cells including granulocytes and lymphocytes. A more specific radioimmunoassay indicates a much shorter half-life of dactinomycin in humans compared to the radiolabeled studies ($\alpha = 0.8$ minutes, $\beta = 3.5$ hours).

THERAPEUTIC USES

Dactinomycin is used as a component of combination regimens together with surgery and/or radiation therapy for nephroblastoma, rhabdomyosarcoma, and Ewing's sarcoma. In nephroblastoma (Wilms' tumor), dactinomycin is generally combined with vincristine, surgery, and, in Groups II and III, radiation therapy; these regimens produce 2-year relapse-free survival rates of 80% to 90%. The drug is used with cyclophosphamide vincristine and doxorubicin in the treatment of rhabdomyosarcoma. It has also been used for regional perfusion, alone or more commonly with other agents, as an adjunct to radiation therapy for the local control of Ewing's sarcoma and rhabdomyosarcoma, although most current regimens emphasize systemic rather than regional administration.

Dactinomycin has been incorporated into combinations for advanced nonseminomatous testicular cancer, although equivalently effective regimens without dactinomycin are also available. As a single agent, it is as effective as methotrexate in the initial treatment of patients with nonmetastatic gestational choriocarcinoma; 90% or more of patients are cured with either agent.

DETAILS OF ADMINISTRATION

Dactinomycin (Cosmegen) is commercially available in 0.5 mg vials with 20 mg of mannitol. It is reconstituted by adding 1.1 ml of sterile water for injection *without preservatives*. The resulting solution (at a concentration of approximately 0.5 mg/ml) should be clear and gold in color and is stable at room temperature for at least 2 months after reconstitution. Since no preservatives are in the solution, however, any unused portions should be discarded after 24 hours to minimize possible bacterial growth. The drug should be administered only intravenously because of irritation to tissue. The desired dose of the reconstituted solution should be injected over a few minutes into the tubing of a freely flowing intravenous infusion to reduce the risk of local reaction due to extravasation of the drug. An in-line cellulose ester membrane filter should not be used during administration of dactinomycin solutions, since the drug binds to the filter.

Dactinomycin is extremely damaging to soft tissues and causes a severe reaction if extravasation occurs. If extravasation does occur, as much infiltrated drug as possible should be aspirated. Although no specific treatments are of proven value in preventing or reducing tissue damage, cold compresses should be applied. Some advocate prompt infiltration with 50 mg to 100 mg of hydrocortisone sodium succinate and/or isotonic sodium thiosulfate injection (4.14% of the pentahydrate salt) (see Complications of Parenteral Therapy, p. 132).

Various dosage schedules are employed. For adults, some suggest 500 µg intravenously daily for 5 days (but should not exceed 15 µg/kg daily or 400 to 600 µg/m^2 daily). For children, either 15 µg/kg intravenously daily for 5 days may be given or a total dose of 2.5 mg/m^2 intravenously divided over a 1-week period; a second course may be given after 3 weeks provided all signs of toxicity have disappeared.

The usual perfusion doses of dactinomycin are 50 µg/kg for the pelvis or a lower extremity and 35 µg/kg for an upper extremity, and the drug is usually diluted in 150–500 ml of physiologic solutions.

PRECAUTIONS AND DOSE MODIFICATIONS

Dactinomycin is immunosuppressive, and should not be given before live virus vaccinations or during an active viral infection because of the risk of developing a severe generalized disease. Dactinomycin appears to potentiate the effects of radiotherapy, and can cause radiation recall. The dose of dactinomycin may need to be reduced in patients who have received prior radiotherapy. Dosage should be based on ideal body weight or body surface area in obese or edematous patients.

DRUG INTERACTIONS

Unexpected hepatic toxicity was described in children with Wilms' tumor; although dose and schedule were important factors, the administration of other hepatotoxic agents, especially halogenated inhalation anesthetics such as enflurane and halothane, was associated with these severe toxic reactions.

TOXICITIES

The major dose-limiting toxicity is hematologic; the onset of thrombocytopenia and leukopenia occurs within 7 days after treatment, and leukocyte and platelet nadirs are usually seen at 14 and 21 days. Nausea and vomiting usually occur within a few hours, may be severe, and may represent the acute dose-limiting toxicity. Vomiting may persist for 4 to 20 hours; antiemetics may be helpful. Stomatitis, proctitis, and diarrhea are possible manifestations of the drug's effect on the gastrointestinal mucosa. Hepatic toxicity includes ascites, hepatomegaly, transaminitis, hyperbilirubinemia and veno-occlusive disease. Skin erythema, desquamation, and hyperpigmentation occur, especially in previously irradiated areas. The drug also may induce an acneiform eruption, which is reversible after therapy is discontinued. Alopecia usually begins 7 to 10 days after administration of the drug and is also reversible. Other toxicities include malaise, fatigue, lethargy, fever, myalgia and hypocalcemia.

Plicamycin

PHARMACOLOGY

Plicamycin (mithramycin) is an antibiotic produced by *Streptomyces plicatus*, and has a complex crystalline structure consisting of a polycyclic chromophobic group with attached sugars. In the presence of divalent cations, especially magnesium, the drug forms complexes with DNA; it selectively inhibits transcription of guanine-cytosine containing DNA, thereby inhibiting DNA-directed synthesis of RNA. In addition, plicamycin lowers serum calcium by a direct effect on osteoclasts: the drug appears to block the ability of osteoclasts to respond to parathyroid hormone. The calcium-lowering effects are independent of the tumoricidal activity, and are achieved with lower doses than required for antineoplastic activity. Plicamycin has recently been shown to cause differentiation of chronic myelogenous leukemia blasts, and can inhibit transcriptional activity of a transfected human *c-myc* gene.

The pharmacology of plicamycin is not well characterized. In animal studies, plicamycin distributes to the Kupffer cells of the liver, renal tubular cells, along formed bone surfaces, and in areas of active bone resorption. Twenty-five percent of radiolabeled drug is excreted in the urine within 2 hours and 40% within 15 hours. Cerebrospinal fluid levels equivalent to blood levels are achieved 4 to 6 hours after dosing. The drug is much less potent when administered orally.

THERAPEUTIC USES

Because of its severe toxicity, plicamycin has not been systematically evaluated. Its use as an antitumor agent has been essentially restricted to patients with disseminated germ cell tumors of the testis, especially embryonal carcinoma, that are refractory to standard combination chemotherapy. Currently, with effective second- and even third-line combination regimens available (see Chap. 33), the use of plicamycin is even more limited.

Plicamycin is mainly used to treat patients with severe hypercalcemia unresponsive to other methods of treatment (see Chap. 33). The dose needed to treat hypercalcemia is much lower than the antitumor dose, and toxicity is generally not severe. The drug has caused symptomatic benefit in hypercalcemia associated with Paget's disease.

DETAILS OF ADMINISTRATION

Plicamycin (Mithracin) is available as a lypophilized mixture of plicamycin, mannitol, and disodium phosphate for intravenous administration. Each vial contains 2500 μg of plicamycin and 100 mg of mannitol. Intact vials should be stored in the refrigerator at 2° to 8°C. Each vial is reconstituted with 4.9 ml of sterile water for injection using only gentle shaking, to give a slightly yellow but clear solution with a final concentration of 500 μg/ml. Fresh solution should be prepared on each day of therapy. The calculated dose should be added to 1 liter of 5% dextrose and 0.9% sodium chloride injection and infused over a period of 4 to 6 hours.

The antitumor dose is individualized according to clinical and hematologic response. If the patient has abnormal fluid retention, the patient's ideal weight is used to calculate the dosage. In the treatment of testicular tumors, the dosage recommended by the manufacturer is 25 μg to 30 μg/kg once daily for 8 to 10 days or until toxicity requires discontinuance of the drug. Daily dosage should not exceed 30 μg/kg, and more than a 10-day course of therapy is not recommended. Tumors responsive to plicamycin generally show a response within 3 to 4 weeks after initial therapy. Additional courses are given at monthly intervals.

For the treatment of the hypercalcemia of malignancy, one approach is to give 25 μg/kg daily for 3 to 4 days. Additional courses at intervals of 1 week or more may be given if the initial course is successful. This dose usually reduces the elevated calcium concentrations to within normal range within 24 to 48 hours. If response is not observed or remains inadequate 48 hours after the initial dose, an additional course may be given. An approach that may be safer (and is equally effective) is to give an initial dose of 25 μg/kg and observe the response of the serum calcium; most patients will show a significant drop within 48 to 72 hours. A second dose (25 μg/kg) can then be given 3 to 4 days after the first. Control of the serum calcium level often can then be maintained with single weekly doses. Ordinarily plicamycin is used only after failure of saline infusions and induction of saline diuresis.

PRECAUTIONS AND DOSE MODIFICATIONS

Plicamycin should not be administered to patients with preexisting thrombocytopenia, coagulation disorder, or bleeding diathesis. The drug should be used with extreme caution in patients with impaired bone marrow function, and in patients with preexisting renal or hepatic impairment.

The dose should be reduced in patients with abnormal hepatic and kidney function. However, validated guidelines for dose reduction under these circumstances are not available.

DRUG INTERACTIONS

No drug interactions have been reported.

TOXICITY

In antitumor doses, plicamycin causes major toxicities to the bone marrow, liver, and kidneys. Severe coagulation defects may occur due to the combination of thrombocytopenia and depression of soluble clotting factors. Leukopenia and anemia may also be seen. Hepatic toxicity is characterized by significant elevations of serum glutamic-oxaloacetic transaminase and lactate dehydrogenase; prothrombin times are also significantly elevated in one fourth of patients. Renal toxicity is manifested by increased serum creatinine and proteinuria.

Decreases in serum phosphate concentration and urinary excretion of calcium may accompany the lowering of serum calcium concentrations. After discontinuation, transient rebound hypercalcemia may occur. The drug also causes nausea, vomiting, diarrhea, and stomatitis; there is marked variation among patients and tolerance to these side effects. Neurologic manifestations include severe headache and irritability. Dermatologic toxicity is manifested by a progressive blushing in the face with thickening and coarsening of the skin folds in about one third of patients. If extravasation occurs, local irritation and cellulitis may occur at the injection site.

Mitomycin

PHARMACOLOGY

Mitomycin (mitomycin-C), an antibiotic produced by *Streptomyces caespitosus*, undergoes activation intracellularly: bioreduction of the quinone moiety yields an opened aziridine ring and exposure of an alkylating site at C1; enzymatic modification of the carbamate side chain exposes the second (crosslinking) site at C10 for alkylation. Activated mitomycin causes crosslinking of DNA chains by binding at the N2 and O6 positions of adjacent guanine residues in the minor groove, thereby interfering with DNA synthesis. Oxygen free radicals have been suggested to contribute to cytotoxicity from mitomycin. Cytotoxic effects are greatest when cells are treated in late G1 and early S phase. Resistance to mitomycin has been attributed to an increase in specific cytosolic proteins (possibly a glutathione transferase), as well as "multidrug" resistance mediated by overexpression of P-glycoprotein.

The drug is poorly absorbed orally. Following intravenous administration of 10 mg/m^2, peak concentrations of about 1 μg/ml are typically achieved; mitomycin is rapidly cleared from plasma, with α and β half-lives of 8 and 48 minutes, respectively. Mitomycin is widely distributed in tissues; metabolism by the liver and other tissues is the primary means of inactivation. Pharmacokinetics are not altered in patients with impaired hepatic function. Mitomycin distributes into bile and ascites; maximum biliary levels of 0.5 μg/ml were achieved after 2 hours, and were 5-fold higher than simultaneous plasma levels during the elimination phase. Less than 10% of an intravenous dose is excreted in the urine as active drug.

THERAPEUTIC USES

Mitomycin has shown antitumor activity against a number of solid tumors, including carcinomas of the stomach, pancreas, colon, breast, head and neck, lung, and cervix. The combination of mitomycin, fluorouracil, and doxorubicin (FAM) has been widely used against advanced stomach cancer. Certain mitomycin-containing combinations are useful as second- or third-line therapy in metastatic breast cancer. The use of mitomycin and 5-FU together with radiation therapy induces a high incidence of durable complete remissions in patients with anal cancer. In patients with squamous cancer of the head and neck, preliminary data suggest that mitomycin may be an effective radiosensitizer.

Intravesical treatment has been used in patients with carcinoma of the bladder. Topical installations of 1 mg/ml aqueous solutions, 20 mg total per instillation, may be used, with retention of the solution for 3 hours. The procedure is repeated three times weekly for up to 20 installations per course. Other regimens involve a single instillation of 40 mg in 40 ml of water following transurethral resection of the tumor, with four additional instillations during the year following tumor resection.

DETAILS OF ADMINISTRATION

Mitomycin (Mutamycin) is available in 5-, 20-, and 40-mg vials containing twice the amount of mannitol by weight. The vials should be reconstituted by adding 10, 40, or 80 ml of sterile water to 5-, 20-, and 40-mg vials, respectively, to yield a clear purple solution containing approximately 0.5 mg/ml mitomycin and 1 mg/ml mannitol. The vial should be shaken to enhance dissolution. If the product does not dissolve promptly, the vial should be allowed to stand at room temperature until clear. The reconstituted solution should be protected from light if not used within 24 hours, and is stable for 14 days when refrigerated or for 7 days at room temperature. This reconstituted solution may be further diluted with a 5% dextrose in water injection, 0.9% sodium chloride injection, or lactated Ringer's solution to a concentration of 20–40 μg/ml; these solutions are stable for 3 hours, 12 hours, and 24 hours, respectively.

The usual initial dosage of single agent mitomycin is 20 mg/m^2 intravenously every 6 to 8 weeks. Thereafter, subsequent doses should be adjusted according to the hematologic toxicity. Because of cumulative myelosuppression, patients should be carefully reevaluated after each course of therapy before administering additional therapy.

PRECAUTIONS AND DOSE MODIFICATIONS

Because of the risk of severe bone marrow suppression and renal toxicity, mitomycin should be avoided in patients with preexisting thrombocytopenia and leukopenia, impaired renal function, substantial prolongation of the prothrombin or bleeding time, coagulation disorders, or bleeding diatheses. A history of hypersensitivity to the drug is also a contraindication.

Because of the cumulative myelosuppression produced by this drug, particular caution is advised in patients with bone marrow compromise and in all patients as the number of treatment cycles increases. Abnormalities of liver or kidney function do not appear to alter the drug's pharmacokinetic behavior.

DRUG INTERACTIONS

No drug interactions have been established. Coadministration with or following doxorubicin appears to increase the risk of cardiotoxicity.

TOXICITY

The most frequent toxic effect of mitomycin is cumulative myelosuppression manifested by thrombocytopenia and leukopenia. The myelosuppression occurs relatively late (3 to 8 weeks) and becomes progressively more marked with subsequent dosing. Nausea and vomiting may occur within 1 to 2 hours following administration. Vomiting is usually mild, but nausea and anorexia may persist for 2 to 3 days. Alopecia, mucocutaneous toxicity, and renal toxicity may be seen. Severe soft tissue ulcers may occur if the drug extravasates. Renal toxicity with elevated serum creatinine levels and glomerular dysfunction may occur. Microangiopathic hemolytic anemia (the hemolytic-uremic syndrome) is a feared complication of mitomycin therapy, and may be delayed in onset. Afflicted patients exhibit thrombocytopenia, circulating schistocytes, and acute renal insufficiency, and may also have cardiopulmonary decompensation. This toxicity may be progressive and fatal even if treatment is discontinued; recently, serial blood perfusion over protein A columns has successfully treated some patients with mitomycin-associated microangiopathic hemoytic anemia. Interstitial pneumonitis may also appear in treated patients; discontinuance of drug and corticosteroid administration may slow the progression and or resolve the process in many cases. Veno-occlusive disease of the liver has been reported after high-dose mitomycin therapy with autologous marrow support.

Bleomycin

PHARMACOLOGY

The bleomycins are a family of sulfur-containing glycopeptides that are fermentation products of *Streptomyces verticillus*. The bleomycin A2 and B2 fractions represent 55–79% and 25–32% of the total weight, respectively, of the commercially available drug. The active conformation juxtaposes six nitrogens in a "ring" which can bind metals; the bleomycin–iron complex is thought to be the active form. Bleomycin binds to DNA; DNA strand damage is thought to result from oxygen free radicals that are generated by the bleomycin–iron–oxygen complex, and results in both single-stranded and double-stranded breaks in DNA; the net result is inhibition of DNA synthesis. Bleomycin is cell cycle phase specific, and is most active in the G2 and M phases; cell progression out of G2 phase is blocked. The cytosolic enzyme bleomycin hydrolase, a cysteine protease, is responsible for its inactivation. Variations in tissue distribution of this enzyme account for the toxicity profile of bleomycin and its relative bone marrow-sparing effects. *In vitro*, agents containing sulfhydryl groups, hydrogen peroxide and ascorbic acid inactivate bleomycin.

After intravenous administration, bleomycin is rapidly distributed to body tissues with an initial plasma half-life of about 20 minutes, followed by a slower elimination phase of 2 to 3 hours. About half of a dose can be recovered in the urine at 24 hours, but only 20–40% is the active drug. Tissue inactivation occurs rapidly, especially in the liver and kidney. In animals, bleomycin is mainly distributed to skin, lungs, kidney, peritoneum, and lymph nodes. In patients with renal failure, the half-life is significantly prolonged; bleomycin clearance correlates fairly well with creatinine clearance. Prior use of nephrotoxic drugs such as cisplatin can reduce bleomycin clearance. The drug is not active by the oral route. The drug is well absorbed following intramuscular and subcutaneous injection.

THERAPEUTIC USES

Bleomycin has significant activity in a number of tumors, and its relative lack of myelosuppressive toxicity makes it attractive for combination with other drugs. It is a component of curative combination regimens in testicular cancer, the diffuse lymphomas, and Hodgkin's disease, although the extent of its contribution to the therapeutic activity of these regimens has generally not been delineated. It is also extensively employed, alone or in combination, for the treatment of squamous cell cancers of many sites, notably head and neck, cervix, penis, vulva, and skin. It is also reasonably effective as intrapleural treatment of malignant pleural effusions.

DETAILS OF ADMINISTRATION

Bleomycin is commercially available in vials containing 15 units. The powder is stable under refrigeration. For intramuscular or subcutaneous injection, the contents of the vial may be dissolved with 1–5 ml sterile water, sodium chloride, 5% dextrose, or bacteriostatic water for injection. For intravenous administration, the vial should be reconstituted with at least 5 ml of physiologic saline or glucose, and administered slowly over 10 minutes. A reconstituted solution of bleomycin in 5% dextrose, sodium chloride, or 5% dextrose containing heparin (at 100 U/ml or 1000 U/ml) is stable for 24 hours at room temperature.

The usual dosage for squamous cell and testicular carcinomas is 10 to 20 U/m^2 given either subcutaneously, intramuscularly, or intravenously once or twice weekly. Continuous infusion regimens at doses of 5 to 15 U/m^2 daily for 4 to 7 days are also well tolerated and may have greater activity than intermittent bolus schedules, although this has not been definitively shown. For lymphomas, any of several schedules may be employed in combination therapy. Lymphoma patients seem to be prone to a low incidence of anaphylactoid reactions to bleomycin. Accordingly, it has been the practice in many clinics to administer a test dose of 1 to 2 units; if no reaction occurs, full-dose treatment commences. If administration of cumulative doses greater than 300 units is undertaken, pulmonary function must be monitored with particular care. Even at lower total doses than this, monitoring of pulmonary function at appropriate intervals is strongly recommended. Vital capacity and the carbon monoxide diffusing capacity are probably the most meaningful parameters to follow. Decreases in either one by 25% or more should prompt cessation of bleomycin.

When used as a sclerosing agent to control malignant pleural effusions, 50–60 units (not to exceed 40 U/m^2) has been diluted with 50–100 ml 0.9% sodium chloride or 5% dextrose injection and instilled into the chest through a thoracostomy tube. The tube is then clamped for up to 24 hours, and the drug is distributed by periodic rotation of the patient. The fluid is then removed. About half the dose is absorbed systemically.

PRECAUTIONS AND DOSE MODIFICATIONS

Bleomycin should be avoided or used only with extreme caution in patients with substantial renal impairment. Although no validated guidelines are available for relating the dose reduction to quantitative measures of renal function, it seems reasonable to decrease the dose in a manner that is roughly proportional to the decrease in creatinine clearance below normal. Patients with known allergy or idiosyncratic reaction to the drug should not be rechallenged. The drug should be administered with extreme caution to any patient with substantial pulmonary function impairment. Although it is not clear if these patients are more susceptible to bleomycin-associated lung damage, any preexisting decrease in pulmonary reserve means that a patient will not tolerate a given degree of bleomycin-induced lung damage as well as a patient with normal pulmonary function. Anaphylactoid reactions may occur in patients with lymphoma; test doses are recommended, as noted previously. Because of the increased risk of serious pulmonary toxicity with high total doses, it is prudent to restrict the cumulative dose of bleomycin to less than 300 units.

DRUG INTERACTIONS

Bleomycin given in close temporal proximity to irradiation produces a greater-than-additive effect, possibly because of free-radical effects on DNA. Synergistic pulmonary toxicity has been reported in patients receiving bleomycin following previous irradiation. To minimize the risk of pulmonary toxicity in patients undergoing surgery who have received bleomycin, the inspired oxygen concentration should be maintained at approximately that of room air during surgery and the postoperative period. Combination therapy including bleomycin may decrease the serum concentration of digoxin and phenytoin.

TOXICITY

The most serious toxicity is pulmonary; interstitial pneumonitis occurs in approximately 10% of treated patients. The risk of this toxicity is related to both age and cumulative dose, although there is wide variation among patients in the cumulative dose required to produce clinically significant pulmonary damage. Radiologic studies and pulmonary function tests do not distinguish between bleomycin injury and the numerous other possible causes of reticulonodular, infiltrative, or consolidative patterns on chest x-ray. Nor are there reliable predictive tests to indicate which patients are destined to develop pulmonary damage. Treatment consists of cessation of bleomycin and avoidance of other agents or maneuvers likely to damage the lungs. The value of corticosteroids is uncertain.

The most frequent adverse effect of bleomycin is mucocutaneous toxicity, which occurs in over half of treated patients, and is the most frequent dose-limiting side effect when the drug is used aggressively. Desquamation of the skin of hands, feet, and pressure areas may be seen, together with hardening and tenderness of the fingertips, ridging of the nails, hyperpigmentation, and/or pruritic erythema. These are usually evident within 1 to 3 weeks and are largely reversible, although the hyperpigmentation may be very long-lasting. Mucositis is ordinarily the acute dose-limiting toxicity and may be very severe if drug is not stopped when the first signs of mucositis appear. Alopecia is common. Raynaud's phenomenon has been reported after bleomycin therapy.

Allergic reactions include fever and chills following injection, and more rarely, hypotension and cardiorespiratory collapse. Gastrointestinal effects are less common. Bleomycin does not produce significant bone marrow toxicity.

Mitoxantrone

PHARMACOLOGY

Mitoxantrone is a synthetic antracenedione that has a symmetrical structure consisting of a tricyclic planar chromophore and two basic side chains. Mitoxantrone intercalates into DNA; positively charged nitrogens on the two alkyl side chains interact electrostatically with the negatively charged ribose phosphates on DNA, thus stabilizing the intercalation process. Mitoxantrone also inhibits the activity of topoisomerase II. As a consequence, the drug causes DNA interstrand and intrastrand crosslinking and DNA-protein crosslinks, and inhibits both DNA and RNA synthesis. The drug also binds to cytokeratin 8, a cytoskeletal protein, which may interfere with cell division. Mitoxantrone is cytotoxic against both cycling and nonproliferating cells, although rapidly proliferating tissues are more sensitive. Mitoxantrone can induce cell cycle arrest in G_2 phase.

Mitoxantrone pharmacokinetics show that the drug has rapid initial half-life (ranging from 2.4–15 minutes) due to distribution of drug into erythrocytes, leukocytes, and platelets. The β phase ranges from 17 minutes to 3 hours, and is believed to result from redistribution of drug from blood cells and into various tissues. The drug is approximately 78% bound to plasma proteins. The terminal half-life is long, and has been reported to vary from 3 to 12 days. The mean plasma clearance is 210 to 600 ml/min, but renal clearance is ≤20 ml/min. The highest tissue concentrations are found in the liver, pancreas, thyroid, spleen, heart, and bone marrow, and prolonged retention can occur. Hepatobiliary elimination of the drug is important, and about 25% of the dose is recovered in the feces within 5 days of dosing. Patients with severe hepatic dysfunction (bilirubin >3.4 mg/dl) may have a lower total body clearance and higher area under the plasma-concentration time curve than patients with normal or mild to moderate hepatic impairment.

THERAPEUTIC USES

Mitoxantrone is approved for use in combination with cytosine arabinoside in remission induction for acute nonlymphoblastic leukemia. It also has activity in breast carcinoma and ovarian carcinoma. Randomized trials in breast cancer suggest that mitoxantrone therapy has a slightly lower response rate than doxorubicin, but is better tolerated and is associated with less cumulative cardiac toxicity. Combinations including mitoxantrone are active in relapsed or refractory nonlymphoblastic leukemia and poor-prognosis lymphoma.

DETAILS OF ADMINISTRATION

Mitoxantrone is commercially available as a sterile blue aqueous solution in vials containing 20 mg, 25 mg, and 30 mg at a concentration of 2 mg/ml mitoxantrone base. The drug is stable for 2 years from manufacture. Before use, the concentrated solution must be diluted to at least 50 ml with sodium chloride or 5% dextrose for injection. The drug is then administered slowly into the tubing of a freely running intravenous infusion over a period of at least 3 minutes; infusion over 15 to 30 minutes is recommended. Drug administration should be followed by an intravenous flush with the appropriate diluent. Local erythema or streaking along the vein of infusion may mean that the drug is being administered too rapidly. A burning or stinging sensation may indicate extravasation or infiltration, in which case the infusion should be terminated immediately and restarted in another vein.

For leukemia, in combination with cytosine arabinoside, the usual dose is 12 mg/m^2 daily for 3 consecutive days. Mitoxantrone has also been given as a continuous infusion for 5 days in relapsed acute leukemia. For solid tumors, single-agent doses are either 10 mg to 14 mg/m^2 intravenously every 3 weeks, or 3–4 mg/m^2 daily for 3 to 5 days every 4 weeks.

PRECAUTIONS AND DOSE MODIFICATIONS

In heavily pretreated patients with solid tumors and poor marrow reserve, the initial dose may need to be reduced. Severe liver impairment may decrease clearance.

DRUG INTERACTIONS

No drug interactions have been reported.

TOXICITY

The principal toxicity of mitoxantrone is myelosuppression; granulocytes are primarily affected with a median nadir at day 12. Thrombocytopenia is relatively mild. Other toxicities include nausea and vomiting (mild to moderate in 30% of patients), alopecia in 10% to 15% of patients, occasional mucositis, and, more rarely, elevations in liver function tests. Patients should be warned that urine may be blue in color after drug administration.

One of the major, long-term toxicities is cardiac toxicity, which can vary from transient electrocardiographic changes to decreases in ventricular ejection fraction, or even severe congestive heart failure. Particular caution should therefore be used when the drug is given to patients with preexisting heart disease or a history of anthracycline administration. It appears that the cardiotoxicity of mitoxantrone is less than that of the anthracyclines. In patients who have not received prior anthracyclines or mediastinal radiation, the incidence of cardiac toxicity increases with cumulative doses ≥160 mg/m^2; in patients previously treated with anthracyclines, the cumulative dose should not exceed 120 mg/m^2. Diagnostic indications for discontinuing mitoxantrone therapy include endomyocardial biopsy evidence of cariomyopathy, and/or a ≥20% drop in cardiac ejection fraction.

ANTIMETABOLITES

Antimetabolites are compounds that bear a structural similarity to a naturally occurring substance such as a vitamin, nucleoside, or amino acid. An antimetabolite interacts with cellular enzymes in one of three ways:

1. By substituting for a metabolite that is normally incorporated into a key molecule, such as DNA or RNA, and thus disrupting cellular function
2. By competing with a normal metabolite for occupation of the catalytic site of a key enzyme
3. By competing with a normal metabolite that acts at an important enzyme regulatory site or other important receptor

Most antimetabolites are cell cycle phase specific with greatest activity during S phase. Their successful use is often highly schedule dependent in animal systems and probably also in humans, although the relation of their clinical effects and schedule of administration has generally been incompletely defined.

As a class, the antimetabolites are often considered to present minimal risk of carcinogenesis and/or leukemogenesis. This seems a reasonable inference from the available evidence, with the proviso that the evidence itself is rather sketchy. Moreover, at least one member of this class (mercaptopurine) is carcinogenic in *in vivo* test systems. It seems unlikely that direct human evidence will be forthcoming for most of these compounds, because only one (fluorouracil) has been given as a single agent to large numbers of patients who are available for long-term follow-up.

Methotrexate

PHARMACOLOGY

Methotrexate (originally known as amethopterin) is a folic acid analogue with substitution of an amino group for a hydroxyl group on the fourth position of the pteridine ring, and a methyl group on the amino nitrogen between the pteridine ring and the benzoyl group. Methotrexate enters cells by an active membrane transport system; a low affinity entry mechanism has been described at high extracellular concentrations. Methotrexate is a substrate for folylpolyglutamate synthetase; methotrexate polyglutamates have a more prolonged intracellular half-life than the monoglutamate form. Methotrexate inhibits dihydrofolate reductase (DHFR), the enzyme which converts dihydrofolate to tetrahydrofolate, thus leading to partial depletion of tetrahydrofolate and accumulation of dihydrofolate and 10-formyldihydrofolate. Decreased availability of 5,10-methylenetetrahydrofolate and 10-formyltetrahydrofolate interferes with the *de novo* synthesis of thymidylate (a precursor of thymidine triphosphate, which is needed for DNA synthesis) and purines, respectively. Further, methotrexate- and dihydrofolate-polyglutamates directly inhibit glycinamide ribonucleotide- and aminoimidazole carboxamide ribonucleotide-transformylases, enzymes involved in *de novo* purine synthesis, as well as thymidylate synthase. The cytotoxicity of methotrexate can, in part, be circumvented by leucovorin (5-formyltetrahydrofolate), thymidine, and hypoxanthine (a purine precursor). Glutamate residues are removed intracellularly enzymatically by a hydrolase, and efflux from the cell occurs through several mechanisms. Mechanisms of resistance to methotrexate include impaired membrane transport, defective polyglutamation, increased DHFR content through gene amplification, and reduced affinity of DHFR for methotrexate.

Following oral administration of low doses (7.5 to 45 mg/m^2), methotrexate is rapidly absorbed, but absorption is incomplete and variable with a range of 23% to 95%. Further, with doses $\geq$30 mg/m^2, methotrexate absorption is saturable, and the fraction absorbed declines as systemic drug exposure plateaus. Therefore, increasing the dose of methotrexate may not improve poor bioavailability. The water soluble salt, methotrexate sodium, is used for parenteral administration. Methotrexate is approximately 50% bound to plasma proteins. Following intravenous administration of conventional doses, the initial and terminal half-lives are 2–3 hours and 8–10 hours, respectively, and methotrexate is excreted primarily as the intact drug in the urine. Methotrexate is actively secreted in the proximal renal tubule. With high-dose regimens ($\geq$1 g/m^2), however, methotrexate can be metabolized by 7-hydroxylation in the liver. At conventional doses, the drug does not reach therapeutic concentrations in the cerebrospinal fluid, since levels are roughly 5–10% of plasma levels. Cerebrospinal fluid levels within the cytotoxic range may be obtained, however, after administration of high doses. The aqueous solubility of both methotrexate and 7-hydroxymethotrexate are markedly influenced by pH, and both are poorly soluble in acidic urine. Significant third-space fluid accumulations, such as pleural or abdominal effusions, may act as a reservoir for methotrexate after high-dose administration, and slow release from third spaces may increase drug toxicity. Methotrexate undergoes enterohepatic circulation, and about 10% is excreted in the feces. Intestinal bacteria can deactivate methotrexate by removing glutamate residues. Peritoneal dialysis and hemodialysis are not effective in clearing methotrexate.

THERAPEUTIC USES

As one of the oldest drugs in the oncologist's armamentarium, methotrexate has been explored in many clinical settings and over a huge range of dose and schedule variations; leucovorin rescue has permitted administration of methotrexate over more than a four-log dose range. The drug is part of contemporary curative strategies in several tumor types, including childhood acute lymphoblastic leukemia, osteogenic sarcoma, non-Hodgkin's lymphoma, and gestational choriocarcinoma. In combination with other agents, the drug is commonly used in the treatment of breast cancer in both the advanced and adjuvant settings and for metastatic bladder cancer. It has long been regarded as the single-agent standard for squamous head and neck cancers, although it induces remissions in only a minority of these patients; further, response durations are usually very short.

Certain high-dose regimens have shown activity against brain tumors. Intrathecal administration is effective treatment for involvement of the cerebrospinal fluid and meninges with lymphoblastic leukemia; it is also the most widely used chemotherapeutic drug for meningeal carcinomatosis. Methotrexate is used in cases of extensive psoriasis resistant to other forms of therapy and in many other noncancer settings (such as rheumatoid arthritis) as an immunosuppressant.

DETAILS OF ADMINISTRATION

Methotrexate is available from various manufacturers in multiple dosage forms and strengths (Methotrexate Sodium Injection, Folex:

1. As a preservative-free parenteral preparation in vials containing either 20, 25, 50, 100, 200, or 250 mg; a 1-g vial has become available recently.
2. As a low-sodium sterile preparation in 100-mg vials

3. In a vial containing preservatives (benzyl alcohol 0.9%, and sodium chloride 0.63%) in 2.5 mg/ml and 25 mg/ml
4. As 2.5-mg tablets for oral use.

Methotrexate sodium injections in powder should be protected from light and stored at 15° to 30°C. For dose preparations requiring reconstitution, concentrations should be no greater than 25 mg/ml with an appropriate sterile, preservative-free medium such as sodium chloride or 5% dextrose.

If intrathecal injections are required, solutions containing 1 mg/ml methotrexate should be prepared using preservative-free 0.9% sodium chloride injections or Elliot's B solution as a diluent. *Methotrexate solutions containing preservatives should never be administered intrathecally.* Intrathecal dosing is currently recommended on the basis of age: a maximum dose of 12 mg for patients greater than 3 years old; 6 mg for infants $\leq$1 year old; 8 mg for patients 1 to 2 years old, and 10 mg for patients 2 to 3 years old. Regardless of the method used to determine intrathecal methotrexate dosage, the dose should be carefully checked prior to administration to minimize the risk of inadvertent intrathecal overdose. For treatment of meningeal leukemia or carcinomatosis, doses are repeated twice weekly until the cerebrospinal fluid clears, then at weekly intervals for one or more additional doses. For CNS prophylaxis, the interval of administration is less frequent.

Systemic methotrexate may be administered orally, intravenously, or intramuscularly. Individual administered doses have varied from 2.5 mg to 30 g/m^2. When used as a single agent for adult patients with normal renal function, conventional-dose regimens without leucovorin most commonly consist of 30–50 mg/m^2 once a week; doses may be cautiously escalated each week until dose-limiting toxicities (stomatitis, myelosuppression) are encountered. For solid tumors, there is no evidence that more frequent dose administration is superior to weekly administration.

High-dose methotrexate with leucovorin rescue is an integral part of current standard therapy for osteosarcoma and is used extensively in experimental programs for other tumors, including acute lymphoblastic leukemia, intermediate and aggressive non-Hodgkin's lymphomas, and head and neck cancer. In general, rigorous evidence from controlled trials showing that high doses are actually superior to conventional doses in these settings is lacking. Nevertheless, the putative pharmacologic advantages over lower doses ensure that clinical investigations with high-dose methotrexate will continue.

With attention to several crucial factors, high doses of methotrexate can be administered safely. Lack of attention to these factors, however, can result in devastating toxicity. These factors include (1) patient selection — patients should have normal renal function and must be able to understand and follow instructions; (2) adequate hydration; (3) adequate urinary alkalinization; (4) monitoring of serum methotrexate levels and creatinine levels before and after therapy; and (5) proper leucovorin administration.

Various schedules of methotrexate/leucovorin have been explored. The dose of methotrexate in these "high-dose" regimens has ranged from 100 mg/m^2 to 30 g/m^2 given every 1 to 3 weeks; most regimens involving a dose $\geq$1 g/m^2 employ an intravenous infusion over 6 to 36 hours, sometimes with part of the dose administered as a loading dose. Shorter infusion times of 1 to 2 hours have also been used, since the associated higher peak methotrexate levels are theoretically desirable. Leucovorin is used in doses sufficient to compete with methotrexate cellular influx, promote efflux, and reestablish intracellular pools of reduced folates. Leucovorin administration generally follows methotrexate after a delay of 2 to 24 hours to allow peak methotrexate activity while providing protection for normal cells during most of the interval during which serum methotrexate concentrations exceed 1×10^{-8} M. The general rule is that the longer the delay in leucovorin rescue, or the higher the serum level, the greater the dose of leucovorin required. Following 6-hour infusions, methotrexate plasma concentrations above 5×10^{-6} M at 24 hours or 5×10^{-7} M at 48 hours predict for toxicity; with 24 to 36 hour methotrexate infusions, concentrations above 5×10^{-7} M at 48 hours predict for toxicity.

Adequate hydration and urinary alkalinization are essential to prevent the precipitation of methotrexate in the renal tubules and urinary tract, an event that may cause obstructive renal failure, with retention of methotrexate and devastating toxicity. Sufficient bicarbonate should be administered to ensure a urinary pH of 7 or higher at the time of methotrexate administration and for 48 hours thereafter.

The following regimens have been recommended.

1. Prehydration: For 12 hours prior to treatment, ensure adequate urine flow and pH with 1.5 l/m^2 (5% dextrose in water, 0.45%–0.9% saline) with 100 mEq sodium bicarbonate and 20 mEq of potassium chloride per liter. (In highly cooperative patients, equivalent hydration and alkalinization can be achieved by the oral route on an outpatient basis with careful nursing instruction.) Urine pH must be 7 or higher at time of drug administration, and urine flow should exceed 100 ml/hr.
2. Drug administration
   a. Jaffe regimen: 50 to 250 mg/kg of methotrexate is given intravenously over 6 hours. Continue hydration as above with 3 l/m^2 for 24 hours. Begin leucovorin 2 hours after end of infusion at 15 mg/m^2 intramuscularly every 6 hours for 7 doses. Then monitor as described below.
   b. NCI regimen: bolus administration of 50 mg/m^2 methotrexate given intravenously, followed by a 36-hour infusion of methotrexate at a dose of 1.5 gm/^{2}. At 36 hours begin an intravenous infusion of 200 mg/m^2 leucovorin over 12 hours. At 48 hours, give leucovorin, 25 mg/m^2, intramuscularly or intravenously every 6 hours for 6 doses.
3. Monitoring methotrexate levels: At 48 hours determine

TABLE 22–3. ADMINISTRATION OF LEUCOVORIN FOR METHOTREXATE LEVELS OVER 5×10^{-7}M

DRUG LEVEL	DOSE OF LEUCOVORIN (q 6 hours × 8 doses)
5×10^{-7}M	15 mg/m²
1×10^{-6}M	100 mg/m²
2×10^{-6}M	200 mg/m²

the serum methotrexate level; give further leucovorin for levels above 5×10^{-7} M as outlined in Table 22-3.

Methotrexate levels are determined every 48 hours with leucovorin doses adjusted as outlined in Table 22-3 until drug concentration is less than 5×10^{-8} M.

The administration of high-dose methotrexate should be performed only by physicians and nurses experienced in its use and familiar with the appropriate techniques of hydration, alkalinization, and the monitoring of serum methotrexate levels to minimize the risk of severe toxicity. In addition, physicians administering high-dose methotrexate should follow meticulously the particular protocol on which the treatment being planned is based; ad hoc variations in the dose, schedule, and timing of the methotrexate or the leucovorin may have unpredictable consequences for the therapeutic index.

PRECAUTIONS AND DOSE MODIFICATIONS

The administration of methotrexate to patients with abnormal renal function results in increased systemic drug exposure and the potential for overwhelming toxicity. Accordingly, methotrexate should not ordinarily be used to treat patients with abnormal renal function. If no other therapeutic options exist and methotrexate is deemed essential to the patient, the dose should be attenuated in rough proportion to the reduction in creatinine clearance, and the treating physician should be prepared to monitor serum methotrexate levels serially and administer leucovorin as necessary until serum methotrexate levels have fallen below 5×10^{-8} M. Methotrexate should be administered cautiously to patients with ascites or pleural effusions.

DRUG INTERACTIONS

Potentially important interactions can occur with other protein-bound drugs such as salicylates, sulfonamides, phenytoin, and para-amino benzoic acid; these drugs displace methotrexate from its protein-binding sites in the blood, causing an increase in the serum levels of free drug. Certain nonabsorbable oral antibiotics used in gut sterilization may decrease the intraluminal metabolism of methotrexate and thereby increase the plasma concentration. Nonsteroidal antiinflammatory agents, salicylates, and probenecid may decrease the renal clearance of methotrexate. The action of oral anticoagulants, such as warfarin, may be potentially increased by methotrexate. Amphotericin B may alter cell membrane structure and permeability and increase cellular uptake of methotrexate. In the setting of renal failure, oral activated charcoal and cholestyramine may increase intestinal binding of methotrexate and increase its fecal excretion. Ceftriaxone and sulfamethoxazole increase the renal clearance of methotrexate. Bacterial carboxypeptidase G_1 can deactivate methotrexate by removing its terminal glutamate residue. The toxicity of high-dose methotrexate in the setting of renal failure may be partially rescued with pharmacologic doses (8 g/m² per day by continuous infusion) of thymidine; an investigational formulation is available from the Division of Cancer Treatment of the National Cancer Institute under the special exception mechanism.

Methotrexate may have significant interactions with other antineoplastic agents. Sequential administration of methotrexate followed 24 hours later by fluorouracil increases the formation of fluorouridine monophosphate and thus increases fluorouridine triphosphate incorporation into RNA. Pretreatment with inhibitors of thymidylate synthase antagonizes methotrexate toxicity. L-asparaginase blocks the toxicity and antitumor activity of methotrexate. Methotrexate pretreatment may increase cytosine arabinoside nucleotide formation.

TOXICITY

The usual dose-limiting toxicities are myelosuppression and mucositis. Leukopenia and thrombocytopenia occur 4 to 14 days after drug administration. A second phase of leukopenia may occur rarely 12 to 21 days after drug administration. Stomatitis and diarrhea are common and are indications for interruption of therapy until resolution. Nausea and vomiting are generally mild but may be more severe after high doses of drug. Acute hepatic dysfunction (elevation of hepatic enzymes) is usually reversible, subclinical, and seen more frequently in patients receiving high-dose therapy. Chronic hepatic fibrosis may result from long-term low-dose treatment, as is given to patients with psoriasis or with acute lymphoblastic leukemia in remission; the incidence of this complication may approach 25% of patients treated for more than 5 years. Nephrotoxicity is uncommon with low doses of methotrexate, although dehydrated, malnourished patients are at significant risk. Renal tubular obstruction and injury may occur with high-dose therapy. The drug may produce skin rashes, usually of maculopapular type.

Methotrexate pneumonitis is a self-limited process characterized by fever, cough, and an interstitial infiltrate. Biopsies have revealed inconstant findings, and there is no consensus about the etiology of this condition; the relationship of the interstitial infiltrates to methotrexate administration is unclear in many cases. Therapy involves withholding methotrexate and ruling out infectious or neoplastic causes of the clinical picture.

Neurotoxicity has been reported with intrathecal methotrexate and/or high-dose systemic methotrexate with or without craniospinal radiation. Acute chemical arachnoiditis, with signs of meningeal irritation, may occur after intrathecal injection, and is ameliorated by dose reduction or omission. A transient encephalopathy has been reported in 15% of leukemia/lymphoma patients following high-dose systemic methotrexate. Subacute onset or chronic demyelinating leukoencephalopathy is characterized by personality changes, intellectual decline, seizures, paresis, cranial nerve palsies, dysarthria, seizures and coma. Unfortunately, no treatment is available.

Fluorouracil

PHARMACOLOGY

Fluorouracil (5-FU) is a uracil analogue with the substitution of a fluorine atom in place of hydrogen on the C5 position of the pyrimidine ring. 5-FU readily enters cells and undergoes complex metabolism to its active nucleotide forms. Incorporation of fluorouridine triphosphate (FUTP) into RNA interferes with RNA processing and function, and 5-FU-tRNA inhibits enzymes involved in post-transcriptional modification of incorporated uracil bases. Inhibition of thymidylate synthase by fluorodeoxyuridine monophosphate (FdUMP) leads to depletion of thymidine triphosphate (dTTP) and accumulation of deoxyuridine monophosphate (dUMP). dTTP depletion interferes with DNA synthesis and repair. Incorporation of fluorodeoxyuridine triphosphate and deoxyuridine triphosphate into DNA may affect DNA stability. Mechanisms of resistance include deletion of enzymes involved in 5-FU anabolism, increased thymidylate synthase content, qualitative changes in thymidylate synthase, inadequate levels of 5,10-methylenetetrahydrofolate to promote and maintain stability of the thymidylate synthase ternary complex (enzyme-FdUMP-reduced folate cofactor), and increased activity of catabolic pathways.

Following intravenous administration, the plasma half-life of 5-FU is 8 to 12 minutes. As the dose increases, 5-FU displays non-linear pharmacokinetics, with saturable clearance. Clearance is several-fold faster with infusions than with bolus administration, and circadian variation in 5-FU pharmacokinetics has been described. About 90% of 5-FU is eliminated by metabolism (50% catabolism, 40% anabolism), and less than 10% is renally excreted as unchanged drug. Dihydropyrimidine dehydrogenase, which is widely distributed in tissues including liver and gastrointestinal mucosa, reduces 5-FU to the inactive metabolite dihydrofluorouracil. Subsequent catabolic steps occur in the liver: dihydrofluorouracil is enzymatically converted to α-fluoroureidopropionic acid, then to fluoro-β-alanine and urea. 5-FU and its catabolites undergo biliary excretion and enterohepatic circulation. The drug has extremely variable absorption from the gastrointestinal tract after oral administration.

THERAPEUTIC USES

The drug is used widely in the treatment of carcinomas of diverse histologies and sites of origin, including adenocarcinomas of breast, colon, rectum, stomach, and pancreas, squamous carcinomas of head and neck, esophagus, skin, and anal carcinoma. Curiously, the drug appears to have no role against the tumors that are most sensitive to chemotherapy: the leukemias, lymphomas, testicular cancer, and most pediatric cancers. Data on the activity of 5-FU in these tumors are either lacking or suggest inactivity.

In breast carcinoma it is usually used in combination therapy with cyclophosphamide, vincristine, and methotrexate or doxorubicin. For gastrointestinal malignancies, it may be used either alone or in combination with other agents, including doxorubicin, mitomycin, or semustine. The combination of 5-FU and leucovorin is now commonly employed. 5-FU in conjunction with levamisole, an immunomodulator, is considered standard adjuvant therapy for patients with node-positive colon carcinoma. Current trials in head and neck and esophageal cancer are exploring cisplatin and 5-FU in combination with surgery and/or radiation therapy.

DETAILS OF ADMINISTRATION

The drug is commercially available (Fluorouracil Injection, Adrucil) for injection as a 50 mg/ml solution in 10-ml vials or ampules, and as 20-, 50-, and 100-ml vials. These should be stored at room temperature and protected from light. The solution may discolor slightly during storage, but potency and safety are not adversely affected. If a precipitate occurs from exposure to low temperatures, the drug should be redissolved by heating to 60°C (140°F) with vigorous shaking. 5-FU is administered by intravenous injection; further dilution is not required. The drug is an irritant; although not a true vesicant, extravasation should be avoided. 5-FU should not be mixed physically with diazepam, doxorubicin, cytarabine, or methotrexate. The drug is very alkaline and should not be mixed with acidic products.

5-FU has been administered as a single agent in a variety of ways:

1. "Loading schedules," such as 12–15 mg/kg (500–600 mg/m^2) given by intravenous bolus daily for 5 consecutive days; on resolution of toxicity (generally by day 28), 10–15 mg/kg (350–600 mg/m^2) is then given by intravenous bolus each week. Alternately, repeated cycles of the daily for 5 consecutive days schedule are repeated at 3- to 4-week intervals as tolerated.
2. Weekly intravenous bolus schedules using 12 mg to 15 mg/kg (500–600 mg/m^2) as tolerated.
3. Continuous intravenous infusion regimens. In general, as the duration of infusion increases, the highest tolerated daily dose decreases. Some commonly employed schedules include
   a. 1000 mg/m^2 daily for 4–5 consecutive days, repeated every 3 to 4 weeks

b. A protracted infusion 200–300 mg/m^2 daily for several weeks until the appearance of side effects; the infusion is restarted after complete resolution of toxicity
c. 2600 mg/m^2 as a 24-hour infusion weekly.

Oral administration is not recommended because of erratic absorption. Topical 5-FU in either a solution or cream is used in the treatment of actinic keratoses (see Chap. 37).

In order to maximize the effectiveness of 5-FU and circumvent mechanisms of drug resistance, investigators have attempted to modulate the activity of 5-FU by the addition of other agents. The combination of 5-FU and leucovorin is one such combination, because the maintenance of high concentrations of reduced folates intracellularly will lead to greater and more prolonged inhibition of thymidylate synthase. A recent meta-analysis of randomized trials in patients with advanced, measurable colon cancer has shown increased activity of 5-FU in combination with leucovorin (response rate about 25%) over 5-FU alone (response rate about 12%), without an impact on survival. Similar investigations are ongoing for stomach and breast cancers. A recently published National Surgical Breast and Bowel Project (NSABP) adjuvant trial in Stage B and C colon cancer showed superiority of 5-FU plus leucovorin given on a weekly schedule compared to a combination of semustine, vincristine and 5-FU in terms of disease-free and overall survival. Other current investigational strategies include modulation of 5-FU with interferon α, N(phosphonacetyl)-L-aspartic acid, sequential methotrexate followed by 5-FU, and delayed uridine rescue.

PRECAUTIONS AND DOSE MODIFICATIONS

Like most antineoplastic agents, 5-FU has a narrow therapeutic index. In a particular patient the dose required to produce mild stomatitis is often only slightly below the dose that will produce life-threatening gastrointestinal ulceration. The presence of any stomatitis or diarrhea on a day 5-FU is scheduled to be administered should mandate deferral of treatment until resolution of the toxicity. Patients with deficiency of dihydropyrimidine dehydrogenase (an autosomal recessive disorder) may have life-threatening or fatal toxicity if treated with 5-FU or floxuridine. The activity of this enzyme can be measured in peripheral blood mononuclear cells in specialized laboratories for research purposes.

DRUG INTERACTIONS

Sequential methotrexate followed by 5-FU increases 5-FU cytotoxicity; the basis for this effect is methotrexate-associated accumulation of phosphoribosylpyrophosphate, which favors the direct conversion of 5-FU to fluorouridine monophosphate, and consequently increased FUTP incorporation into RNA. A 24-hour interval appears to be superior to a 1-hour interval in some preclinical and clinical studies. Leucovorin increases the intracellular pools of 5,10-methylenetetrahydrofolate mono- and polyglutamate, which in turn may increase the extent and duration of FdUMP-mediated thymidylate synthase inhibition. In preclinical studies, pharmacologic doses of thymidine circumvent the FdUMP-mediated blockade of thymidylate synthase and favor formation of the ribonucleotide metabolites of 5-FU, thus enhancing FUTP incorporation into RNA. In clinical studies, however, thymidine blocked the catabolism of 5-FU to dihydrofluorouracil; the half-life of 5-FU was thus markedly prolonged, resulting in severe toxicity without an apparent improvement in anticancer activity. Chronic cimetidine therapy inhibited 5-FU catabolism to dihydrofluorouracil in subhuman primates, resulting in an increased systemic to 5-FU, while ranitidine did not affect 5-FU clearance. N-(Phosphonacetyl)-L-aspartate (PALA), an inhibitor of aspartate carbamoyltransferase, an enzyme in the *de novo* pyrimidine synthetic pathway, has been shown in preclinical systems to enhance FUTP formation and RNA incorporation, and can modulate both the RNA- and DNA-directed cytotoxic effects of 5-FU. Delayed administration of pharmacologic concentrations of uridine in some preclinical models selectively increases the rate of recovery of normal tissues from 5-FU-associated inhibition of RNA and DNA synthesis. In contrast, concurrent administration of uridine antagonizes 5-FU cytotoxicity by interfering with its anabolism to FUTP and its subsequent incorporation into RNA. Allopurinol, after conversion to oxypurinol ribonucleotide, interferes with the enzyme orotidylate decarboxylase, thus causing a buildup in orotic acid; the latter blocks 5-FU activation to FUMP by the enzyme orotate phosphoribosyltransferase. Tissues including normal host tissues which primarily use the *de novo* pathway for 5-FU anabolism to FUMP would theoretically be protected from 5-FU cytotoxicity, whereas tumors capable of anabolizing 5-FU through salvage pathways would not be protected. However, clinical studies using systemic allpurinol with 5-FU suggested the combination did not appear to result in an improved therapeutic index. Interferons α, β, and γ enhance the toxicity of 5-FU in some preclinical models. The type of interferon which optimally potentiates 5-FU toxicity varies depending on the tumor cell type. The underlying mechanism(s) are undoubtedly complex and may differ in various tumors; however, interferon α has been shown to increase FdUMP metabolism and to enhance 5-FU-associated DNA damage. Interferon γ has been shown to block the acute 5-FU–mediated increase in thymidylate synthase protein content, thus maintaining inhibition of thymidylate synthase. Interferon α pretreatment decreased the leukopenia resulting from weekly bolus 5-FU administration in mice, presumably due to an interferon-mediated induction of proliferative arrest in interferon-sensitive bone marrow progenitor cells. In some clinical studies, interferon α administered on a consecutive daily schedule decreased 5-FU clearance in individual patients, thus resulting in a higher systemic exposure. Interferon α decreased [^{3}H]5-FU catabolism in peripheral blood mononuclear cells isolated from patients receiving the combination of interferon α, 5-FU and leucovorin, suggesting a possible basis for the decreased 5-FU clearance.

TOXICITY

The dose-limiting toxicity of 5-FU depends largely on the schedule of administration. Continuous infusion regimens or consecutive daily bolus schedules are generally limited by gastrointestinal toxicity, manifested primarily as mucositis or diarrhea, while intermittent bolus schedules tend to produce bone marrow suppression. Severe and life-threatening mucositis and diarrhea can occur; therefore, maintaining adequate hydration is imperative, and early intervention and aggressive supportive care are required. Anorexia, nausea, and vomiting may accompany therapy by any schedule, but these are usually mild and transient. Hair loss frequently occurs. Cutaneous toxicity includes reversible maculopapular rash, skin hyperpigmentation, and enhanced reactions with ultraviolet light and photosensitivity. Ocular toxicity (conjunctivitis, blepharitis, epiphora) also occurs frequently, and excessive lacrimation is the most common symptom. Long-term continuous infusion may produce palmar plantar erythrodysesthesia (the "hand-foot syndrome"), which consists of painful paresthesias and hyperpigmentation of the skin on the palmar surfaces of the hands and feet; these symptoms resolve slowly on discontinuation of drug. Neurologic toxicity comprised of somnolence, cerebellar ataxia, and upper motor neuron signs may occur. Neurologic toxicity has generally occurred with high-dose 5-FU or intensive daily schedules, and has also been prominent in some studies in which 5-FU was combined with modulators such as thymidine, interferon α, PALA and allopurinol. Patients treated with 5-FU infrequently may develop anterior chest pain, arrythmias, and myocardial ischemia, with or without infarction during drug administration. Patients with preexisting heart disease appear to be at increased risk of this complication, which may be due to transient coronary vasospasm. Cardiac toxicity appears to occur more often with infusional schedules.

Floxuridine

PHARMACOLOGY

Floxuridine (fluorodeoxyuridine, FUDR) is the deoxyribonucleoside derivative of 5-FU. Floxuridine enters cells by the facilitated nucleoside transport mechanism. When administered clinically, floxuridine can be converted to 5-FU by thymidine phosphorylase (which can then be subsequently metabolized by the usual anabolic and catabolic pathways), or be directly converted intracellularly to FdUMP by thymidine kinase. Inhibition of thymidylate synthase results in DNA-directed toxicity. With continuous infusion schedules, the drug appears to be preferentially anabolized to FdUMP, whereas conversion to 5-FU is prominent following single intravenous bolus doses. Floxuridine is a cell cycle phase-specific agent with marked cytotoxicity in S phase.

THERAPEUTIC USES

By intravenous bolus, floxuridine has been administered according to schedules similar to those for 5-FU at approximately twice the daily dose: *e.g.*, 30 mg/kg (1100 mg/m^2) for 5 consecutive days. A 14-day continuous intravenous infusion at 0.15 mg/kg/day (5–6 mg/m^2 per day) has been used as the "systemic" therapy arm in randomized comparisons with hepatic arterial infusions (HAI) of floxuridine. When given systemically as a single agent, however, floxuridine appears to offer no particular advantages over 5-FU. There is emerging interest, however, in combining leucovorin with systemic floxuridine. Floxuridine is currently approved for administration by HAI for the palliative management of patients with metastatic adenocarcinoma confined to the liver. When given by HAI, floxuridine has pharmacologic advantages over 5-FU, including a much higher first-pass hepatic extraction rate (up to 90% of floxuridine is removed from the circulation on one pass through the liver), and peripheral venous levels are consequently relatively low. The most frequently used regimen is a 14-day continuous HAI regimen: although higher doses have been given, 0.2 mg/kg per day is the currently recommended dose. Randomized trials with carefully selected patients with apparent metastatic disease confined to the liver have shown that the response rate to HAI floxuridine is higher than that achieved with single-agent systemic 5-FU or floxuridine, and the time to hepatic disease progression is longer. In general, however, the overall time to disease progression and overall survival are not improved. In these trials, about one fourth of patients progressing on the systemic arm have subsequently responded to HAI of floxuridine. HAI of floxuridine is limited by hepatic toxicity and catheter-related complications.

DETAILS OF ADMINISTRATION

Floxuridine is available as a powder in 500-mg vials, which are reconstituted with 5 ml of sterile water for injection, resulting in a concentration of 100 mg/ml. A preservative-free solution consisting of 5 ml of 100 mg/ml is also commercially available. The reconstituted solution should be stored at 2° to 8°C and used within 2 weeks. This reconstituted solution may be further diluted in 5% dextrose in water or in 0.9% sodium chloride for injection. An infusion pump is used to overcome pressure in the hepatic artery and to ensure a uniform infusion rate. Heparin (100 to 200 U/ml) may be added to the floxuridine infusate.

PRECAUTIONS AND DOSE MODIFICATIONS

The manufacturer recommends that the drug should be used with particular caution in patients with bone marrow compromise or impaired liver or kidney function. No established guidelines are available for dose modification under these circumstances.

DRUG INTERACTIONS

See the corresponding section under 5-FU, since many of the same interactions might be anticipated.

TOXICITY

When the drug is employed in regional infusions, potential adverse effects due to catheter placement and position include arterial ischemia, thrombosis bleeding at the insertion site, blockage of the catheter, embolism, and infection. Accidental slippage of the catheter into the arterial supply of the stomach or duodenum can lead to ulceration within the infused area. Careful surgical technique by an experienced surgeon can minimize these complications. Division and ligation of the hepatic arteries distal to the point of cannulation that supply the superior border of the distal stomach and proximal duodenum can reduce these toxic effects. Hepatic toxicity is manifested by liver function abnormalities (elevation of transaminases and alkaline phosphatase), cholestatic jaundice, and occasionally biliary sclerosis. Liver enzymes must be monitored carefully, and therapy should be interrupted if elevations of alkaline phosphatase and/or SGOT occur. Although floxuridine may be reinstituted at a lower dose once the liver enzymes normalize, most patients become progressively intolerant. The clinical picture may not improve in some cases after therapy is discontinued.

Side effects of systemic administration include bone marrow suppression, nausea, vomiting, diarrhea, and stomatitis; these are quite uncommon with regional administration into the hepatic artery.

Fludarabine Phosphate

PHARMACOLOGY

Fludarabine phosphate (2-fluoro-arabinosyl-adenosine monophosphate, 2-F-ara-AMP) was originally synthesized in an effort to make analogues of vidarabine (9-β-D-arabinofuranosyladenine, ara-A) which would be resistant to adenosine deaminase. Fludarabine (2-F-ara-A) has poor solubility, whereas the monophosphate salt has good aqueous solubility. *In vivo,* the drug is rapidly converted in plasma to 2-F-ara-A, which enters cells by the facilitated nucleoside transport mechanism. 2-F-ara-A is then phosphorylated to the 5′-monophosphate derivative, F-ara-AMP, by deoxycytidine kinase, and then is converted to the di- and triphosphate level by pyrimidine mono- and diphosphate kinases, respectively. F-ara-ATP inhibits several enzymes important for DNA synthesis and repair, including ribonucleotide reductase, DNA polymerase α, DNA primase, and DNA ligase I. F-ara-ATP can be incorporated into nascent DNA chains as a false nucleotide, and appears to interfere with chain elongation. Induction of apoptosis occurs in some cancer cell lines. Potential mechanisms of resistance include deletion of deoxycytidine kinase, decreased capacity for nucleoside transport, and qualitative and quantitative changes in target enzymes.

Initial pharmacokinetic studies described a very short initial half-life of 0.6 hours, followed by a subsequent distribution phase with a half-life of 10 hours. More sensitive assays have revealed a terminal half-life of 30 hours. The total body clearance correlates with creatinine clearance. In leukemic cells, the intracellular half-life of F-ara-ATP is about 15 hours. In patients receiving conventional doses of F-ara-AMP (20–25 mg/m^2 daily for 5 days), about 24% of an injected dose is excreted into the urine as F-ara-A; renal elimination is much greater (40–60%), however, with high doses ≥80 mg/m^2. Fludarabine phosphate has good bioavailability after oral dosing (about 75%).

THERAPEUTIC USES

Striking degrees of antitumor activity have been observed in several types of lymphoproliferative disorders, including chronic lymphocytic leukemia (CLL), Hodgkin's disease, the more indolent non-Hodgkin's lymphomas, and mycosis fungoides. Activity in CLL patients who have failed alkylators (about 50% major responses) and in the indolent non-Hodgkin's lymphomas appear particularly promising. The drug appears to lack significant activity in the major classes of adult epithelial cancers.

DETAILS OF ADMINISTRATION

Fludarabine phosphate (Fludara) is commercially available as a white, lyophilized solid cake. Each vial contains 50 mg of fludarabine phosphate, 50 mg of mannitol, and sodium hydroxide to adjust pH to 7.7. The vials should be stored under refrigeration between 2° and 8°C. The drug should be prepared for parenteral use by aseptically adding 2 ml sterile water for injection; the white cake should dissolve within 15 seconds, and will contain fludarabine phosphate at 25 mg/ml. The product may be diluted in 100–125 ml of 5% dextrose of 0.9% sodium chloride. The reconstituted product has no antimicrobial preservatives and thus should be used within 8 hours of preparation. An investigational oral formulation has recently entered clinical trials. The most common dose schedule is 25 mg/m^2 by intravenous infusion over approximately 30 minutes daily for 5 consecutive days, with treatment recycled every 4 weeks as tolerated.

PRECAUTIONS AND DOSE MODIFICATIONS

Elderly patients may have increased risk of neurologic toxicity. Patients with renal insufficiency should be treated with extreme caution. Patients with bone marrow impairment should be closely monitored for excessive toxicity. Fludarabine phosphate may cause tumor lysis syndrome in patients with advanced bulky lymphoma or CLL.

DRUG INTERACTIONS

The combination of fludarabine phosphate and pentostatin (deoxycoformycin) was associated with an unacceptably high (22%) incidence of fatal pulmonary toxicity in an investigational study in patients with refractory CLL. Therefore, the use of fludarabine phosphate in combination with pentostatin is not recommended by the manufacturer.

TOXICITY

Myelosuppression (granulocytopenia, thrombocytopenia and anemia) is the most common dose-limiting toxicity. Although resolution of hematologic toxicity generally permits retreatment at 28-day intervals, myelosuppression may be severe and cumulative. Immunosuppression may occur, and viral, bacterial and other opportunistic infections, particularly pneumonia, may be problematic. Other common toxicities include fever, chills, nausea and vomiting, malaise, fatigue, anorexia, and weakness. Diarrhea and mucositis may occur. Elevation of serum transaminases and serum creatinine may occur. High doses of fludarabine ($\geq$95 mg/m^2 per day for 5 days) during the initial Phase I testing was associated with catastrophic CNS toxicity, characterized by delayed onset, progressive encephalopathy, visual disturbances, and death. The pathological correlate appears to be demyelination. The incidence of devastating neurotoxicity is clearly dose-related. At the currently recommended doses, weakness, somnolence and fatigue may occur; however, some patients have experienced agitation, confusion, paresthesias, visual disturbance and coma, although these toxicities are uncommon. Tumor lysis syndrome, which has occurred only rarely with the current doses, may include hyperuricemia, hyperphosphatemia, hypocalcemia, metabolic acidosis, hematuria, urate crystalluria, and renal failure. Pneumonitis in the absence of a definite infectious cause may occur and is characterized by dyspnea, cough and interstitial infiltrate. Skin rash and edema may occur.

Mercaptopurine

PHARMACOLOGY

Mercaptopurine (6-MP) is a purine antimetabolite that is converted intracellularly by the enzyme hypoxanthine-guanine phosphoribosyltransferase to the ribonucleotide derivative, thioinosinic acid (TIMP). TIMP interferes with several *de novo* purine synthetic reactions, including the initial step in the purine biosynthetic pathway, and the formation of adenosine monophosphate (AMP) and xanthine monophosphate (the precursor of guanosine monophosphate, GMP) from inosinic acid (IMP). In addition, mercaptopurine can be methylated to form 6-methylthioinosinic acid (MTIMP, also referred to as 6-methylmercaptopurine ribonucleotide), which is also a potent inhibitor of *de novo* purine synthesis. Mercaptopurine can be converted to 6-thioguanine (deoxy)ribonucleotides, which upon further phosphorylation to the triphosphate level, can be incorporated into RNA and DNA. The drug is a powerful immunosuppressant; humoral immunity is affected more strongly than cellular immunity. Attempts to modify the molecule led to the discovery of azathioprine and allopurinol.

Mercaptopurine is inactivated by xanthine oxidase to thiouric acid. Oxidation of the sulfhydryl group of MTIMP also inactivates the drug; dethiolation also occurs. The bioavailability of oral mercaptopurine is limited because of extensive first-pass metabolism in the liver and gastrointestinal mucosa by xanthine oxidase. Less than 20% of the administered dose is absorbed, and only one third of children studied achieve cytotoxic plasma concentrations with conventional doses. There is considerable inter- and intrapatient variation in bioavailability. Concomitant food administration decreases mercaptopurine absorption, and time of day may also affect efficacy: in one study, administration in the evening appeared to be superior to morning dosing. Following a standard dose of 75 mg/m^2, peak plasma levels of about 70 ng/ml (1 μM) are obtained 1–2 hours after oral dosing; however, the area under the plasma concentration versus time curve (AUC) varied about five-fold. The elimination half-life was 1–1.5 hours. Following intravenous administration of 75 mg/m^2, in contrast, peak plasma levels were 70-fold higher. At conventional doses, clearance is primarily hepatic; renal excretion may account for 20–40% of the administered dose with higher doses. Approximately 30% of the dose is protein bound. With continuous infusions, mean steady-state levels in the 1 to 10 μM range can be maintained.

THERAPEUTIC USES

Current use of mercaptopurine is almost entirely restricted to its incorporation into maintenance regimens for acute leukemia. Although it is also clearly capable of inducing remissions in some patients, its relatively slow effect and the existence of more active regimens have relegated its use to the maintenance setting. It also has some activity in patients with chronic myelocytic leukemia who are no longer responding to busulfan or hydroxyurea. Mercaptopurine has also been used in the transplant setting with corticosteroids to prevent graft rejection.

DETAILS OF ADMINISTRATION

Mercaptopurine is supplied in 50-mg tablets (Purinethiol). The usual maintenance dosage is 1.5–2.5 mg/kg daily. When used for induction, the usual dosage is 2.5 mg/kg daily (70 mg/m^2 for children or 80–100 mg/m^2 for adults); if no clinical improvement or toxicity occurs after 4 weeks, the dose may be increased to 5 mg/kg daily. If an abnormally large or rapid fall in leukocyte or platelet count occurs, mercaptopurine should be discontinued.

PRECAUTIONS AND DOSE MODIFICATIONS

The drug should be used with special caution in patients with abnormal liver function. The risk of hepatotoxicity increases in this setting; hepatic fibrosis leading to death has occurred. The appearance of liver function abnormalities should usually prompt discontinuation of mercaptopurine until the abnormalities clear. Patients receiving allopurinol should receive a dose reduction of the oral mercaptopurine dose by 50% to 75%. The drug should be used cautiously with other hepatotoxic drugs. See the section on thioguanine for a discussion of variations in thiopurine methyltransferase activity as a determinant of thiopurine toxicity.

DRUG INTERACTIONS

Allopurinol blocks the enzymatic oxidation of mercaptopurine to thiouric acid. Pharmacokinetic studies of the effect of allopurinol pretreatment on the disposition of oral and intravenous mercaptopurine indicated a five-fold increase in the plasma AUC of oral mercaptopurine; in contrast, the AUC of intravenous mercaptopurine was not affected. No therapeutic advantage has been gained with the combination of allopurinol and oral mercaptopurine, however, because the toxicity of mercaptopurine is increased. In addition, allopurinol may antagonize the antileukemic activity of mercaptopurine by increasing hypoxanthine levels. Mercaptopurine decreases the hypoprothrombinemic effect of warfarin.

TOXICITY

The major dose-limiting effect is myelosuppression, which may not occur for several weeks; recovery after cessation of drug is usually fairly prompt. The drug causes nausea, vomiting, and anorexia in approximately 25% of patients. Stomatitis and diarrhea are seen more commonly with large doses. Other side effects include drug fever, eosinophilia, rash, and occasional cases of pancreatitis. Hepatotoxicity with frank jaundice has been associated with mercaptopurine administration in 10% to 40% of adult patients in various reported series. Intrahepatic cholestasis and hepatic parenchymal necrosis may both be present in varying proportions, but the mechanism of this effect is not clear. Periodic monitoring of liver function tests during treatment is desirable in order to detect early signs of hepatic dysfunction, at which point the drug should be discontinued until recovery. Patients receiving mercaptopurine should be assumed to be immunosuppressed.

Thioguanine

PHARMACOLOGY

Thioguanine (6-TG) is a structural analogue of guanine in which a sulfhydryl group replaces a hydroxyl group in the C6 position. Thioguanine is metabolized by hypoxanthine-guanine phosphoribosyltransferase to the ribonucleotide derivative, 6-thioguanylic acid (TGMP). TGMP interferes with several *de novo* purine synthetic reactions, including the initial step in the purine biosynthetic pathway, and the formation of AMP and xanthine monophosphate (the precursor of GMP) from IMP. TGMP and its deoxyribonucleotide derivative can be further anabolized to the triphosphate level, and then be incorporated into RNA and DNA. The extent of incorporation into DNA appears to correlate with the production of strand breaks and cellular cytotoxicity; DNA-protein crosslinks have also been described. The drug appears to be S phase specific. Thioguanine can also interfere with cell surface glycoprotein synthesis. Thiopurine methyltransferase is the enzyme responsible for mediating the methylation of both mercaptopurine and thioguanine; S-adenosylmethionine is the methyl donor. Subsequent conversion of the methylated purine sulfonic acid derivative to oxypurines liberates inorganic sulfate, thus deactivating the drug. A pharmacogenetic determinant of susceptibility to thiopurine toxicity is low levels of thiopurine methyltransferase; patients with relative deficiency of this enzyme may have higher intracellular levels of thioguanine nucleotides and a higher risk for severe myelosuppression.

Thioguanine, like mercaptopurine, has variable and incomplete bioavailability following oral administration. Peak concentrations in blood occur 2 to 4 hours after oral dosing; 10-fold variation in plasma levels have been noted after a common dose. Food intake seems to decrease thioguanine absorption. After intravenous administration, the plasma half-life has ranged from 25 to 240 min (median, 90 minutes). The drug does not enter the CNS. Clearance is predominantly by hepatic metabolism. Only trace quantities of parent drug are excreted in the urine. Unlike mercaptopurine, deamination is minimal, and allopurinol does not affect its bioavailability.

THERAPEUTIC USES

Thioguanine has been used primarily in the treatment of acute nonlymphoblastic leukemia in combination with cytarabine, with or without daunorubicin. It is most commonly used as part of induction regimens, but has sometimes been incorporated into consolidation or maintenance programs. Thioguanine has activity in chronic myelogenous leukemia, and has been used as part of combination chemotherapy regimens in the blastic phase of the disease when single agents are no longer effective. It is not known to be clinically useful for other neoplasms, although an investigational intravenous formulation is currently being evaluated in Phase II studies sponsored by the Division of Cancer Treatment of the National Cancer Institute.

DETAILS OF ADMINISTRATION

Thioguanine is available as 40-mg tablets (Thiopurine Tabloid), which should be stored at room temperatures between 15° and 30°C. Oral suspensions of thioguanine containing 40 mg/ml may be prepared from the commercially available tablets; to do this, the tablets should be crushed and mixed with a suspending agent (*e.g.*, cologel) equal to one third of the final volume, then brought to final volume with a 2:1 mixture of a simple syrup (*e.g.*, wild cherry syrup). The resulting suspension is stable for at least 84 days when stored in an amber glass bottle at room temperature. The drug is best administered on an empty stomach, because food appears to slow absorption and reduce peak plasma levels.

The single-agent dose of thioguanine is approximately 2 mg/kg daily. The total daily dose calculated to the nearest multiple of 20 mg may be given at one time. In the absence of response or dose-limiting toxicity, the dose should be escalated. As noted previously, however, the drug is almost never given singly. The usual dose of thioguanine in combination therapy for induction of remission in patients with acute leukemia is generally 75–200 mg/m^2 daily in one or two divided doses for 5 to 7 days. Maintenance dosages and schedules vary with the regimen.

PRECAUTIONS AND DOSE MODIFICATIONS

The drug should be given cautiously to patients with renal or hepatic dysfunction; pharmacologically validated rules for dose modification are not available.

DRUG INTERACTIONS

There is no apparent interaction with allopurinol, in contrast to mercaptopurine and azothioprine. The drug should be used cautiously with other hepatotoxic drugs.

TOXICITY

The major dose-limiting toxicity is hematologic, which is dose-related and manifested by granulocytopenia, thrombocytopenia and anemia. Myelosuppression usually occurs gradually over 2–4 weeks, but may produce marrow hypoplasia. Intravenously administered drug is 2.5-fold more potent in inducing myelosuppression than the same dose orally. Nausea, vomiting, and anorexia may occur but are generally of only mild severity. Stomatitis and diarrhea may occur, and can necessitate dosage reduction. Hepatic dysfunction is less common than with mercaptopurine; however, elevations of liver enzymes and even jaundice have been described.

Cytarabine

PHARMACOLOGY

Cytarabine (9-β-D-arabinofuranosyl cytosine, cytosine arabinoside, ara-C) is a deoxycytidine antagonist that differs from deoxycytidine by virtue of a stereotypic inversion of the 2′-hydroxyl group of the sugar moiety. The drug enters cells by the facilitated nucleoside transport mechanism, and the rate-limiting step in intracellular anabolism is the phosphorylation by deoxycytidine kinase to the 5′-monophosphate derivative, ara-AMP. Ara-AMP is subsequently phosphorylated to the di- and triphosphate derivatives by pyrimidine mono- and diphosphate kinases, respectively. Ara-CTP inhibits DNA polymerase α. Ara-CTP is also incorporated into DNA, and can interfere with DNA chain elongation during both semiconservative DNA replication and DNA repair, thus resulting in DNA fragility. Ara-C treatment can induce apoptosis in some cancer cell lines. There are also possible effects on phospholipid synthesis and the structure and function of the cell membrane. The drug is S-phase specific. Ara-C and Ara-CMP are inactivated by cytidine deaminase and deoxycytidylate deaminase, respectively. Resistance mechanisms include deletion of deoxycytidine kinase, expansion of dCTP pools (increased CTP synthase activity), increased cytidine deaminase activity, decreased capacity for nucleoside transport, and decreased intracellular retention of Ara-CTP following drug removal.

Both cytidine deamininase and deoxycytidylate deaminase are widely distributed in the body. Oral administration is not effective because of extensive and rapid deamination within the gut, with less than 20% systemic availability. After intravenous bolus administration, cytarabine is rapidly cleared with biphasic elimination: the initial half-life is 7–20 minutes, while the terminal half-life has been estimated to range from 0.5–2.5 hours. The deamination product, ara-U, has a half-life of 3–6 hours, and is excreted predominantly in the urine, with some biliary excretion. During continuous intravenous administration, steady-state plasma levels of Ara-C increase linearly up to about 5 μM (the range achieved with 100 mg/m^2/hour); thereafter, deamination is saturated and plasma levels can increase unpredictably. Cerebrospinal fluid levels are approximately 50% of the plasma levels during infusions. There is little cytidine deaminase activity in cerebrospinal fluid; intrathecal administration of 50 mg/m^2 cytarabine yields peak concentrations of 1 mM; Ara-C levels fall slowly with a half-life of 2 hours, and cytotoxic concentrations (≥0.4 μM) are maintained for 24 hours.

THERAPEUTIC USES

"Conventional doses" of cytarabine, 100 mg/m^2 daily for 7 days as a continuous intravenous infusion, are primarily used in induction therapy of acute nonlymphoblastic leukemia (ANLL), nearly always in combination with an anthracycline ±6-thioguanine; 200 mg/m^2 daily is used when cytarabine is given as a single agent. It is also a component of consolidation, maintenance, and intensification regimens after remission is attained. Combinations including cytarabine are also employed for the blastic phase of chronic myelogenous leukemia, with much less effectiveness than for *de novo* ANLL. The use of high doses of cytarabine (*e.g.*, 3 g/m^2 over 2 hours every 12 hours for 6 to 12 doses, or 100 mg/m^2/hour for 24 hours) is currently being examined in several randomized trials in both front-line and maintenance settings. Low doses of cytarabine (continuous infusion of 5–10 mg/m^2 daily) have been employed in elderly patients in an attempt to induce differentiation of leukemic cells and provide effective therapy with less toxicity. This approach can induce remissions in some patients but is not devoid of toxicity, and it is not clear to what extent cytotoxicity rather than differentiation is responsible for the clinical effect. Intrathecal cytarabine is used to treat meningeal leukemia and other meningeal neoplasms; the most frequent regimen is 30 mg/m^2 (in 5–10 ml of an isotonic, preservative-free solution) twice weekly until the CSF clears, followed by one additional dose.

Cytarabine has no clearly useful activity in solid tumors, although it has been incorporated into certain active combinations for the non-Hodgkin's lymphomas. Evidence of *in vitro* synergism with cisplatin has motivated some trials of this two-drug combination in both systemic and intracavitary approaches. The studies of systemic administration have not yielded promising results, and definitive intracavitary trials are pending.

DETAILS OF ADMINISTRATION

Cytarabine is available as a sterile, lyophilized powder in 100- and 500-mg glass vials; 1- and 2-g vials are also available. These vials should be stored at 15°–30°C. A diluent is supplied: bacteriostatic water for injection with 0.945% benzyl alcohol. For reconstitution, 5 ml of diluent is added to the 100 mg vial; 10 ml is added to 500 mg- and 1-g vials, while 20 ml is added to the 2-g vials; the resultant solutions contain 20, 50, 100 and 100 mg/ml, respectively. The resulting solution may be stored at room temperature and is stable for 48 hours; the manufacturers recommend, however, that the solutions be used as soon as possible after reconstitution. The reconstituted solution can be further diluted with 5% dextrose or 0.9% sodium chloride injection for intravenous infusion. *Because of the potential toxicity of large amounts of benzyl alcohol, the manufacturers recommend that the diluent containing this preservative should* not *be used for intrathecal administration, in neonates, or if high-dose regimens are employed.* Preservative-free 0.9% sodium chloride injection, Elliot's B solution (for intrathecal injection), or other isotonic buffered diluents can be used to reconstitute cytarabine under these circumstances.

PRECAUTIONS AND DOSE MODIFICATIONS

Elderly patients have a high incidence of neurotoxicity with high-dose cytarabine regimens. Neurotoxicity with high-dose cytarabine may occur much more frequently in patients with impaired renal function (evidenced by an elevated serum creatinine).

DRUG INTERACTIONS

High concentrations of ara-U (such as that produced during high-dose cytarabine regimens) can decrease deamination of cytarabine through feedback inhibition of cytidine deaminase. Deamination is blocked by tetrahydrouridine (which should be added to blood collection tubes for accurate determination of cytarabine plasma levels). Interference with the DNA incorporation of cytarabine (*e.g.*, by pretreatment with thymidylate synthase inhibitors) may antagonize its cytotoxicity. Cytarabine-mediated interference of DNA repair potentiates the cytotoxicity of alkylating agents and platinum analogs. Inhibitors of ribonucleotide reductase (such as fludarabine, hydroxyurea) decrease competing pools of dCTP, thereby enhancing cytarabine anabolism and DNA incorporation.

TOXICITY

Myelosuppression is the dose-limiting toxicity, especially leukopenia and thrombocytopenia. Megaloblastosis of the bone marrow is quite common, although clinically significant anemia is not. Myelosuppression is dose-dependent. Anorexia, nausea, and vomiting occur commonly. Gastrointestinal epithelial ulceration may occur, manifested by mucositis, diarrhea, ileus and abdominal pain. An acute cytarabine syndrome characterized by fever, myalgia, bone pain, maculopapular rash, conjunctivitis, malaise and occasional chest pain has been described, and occurs 6 to 12 hours after dosing; corticosteroids may alleviate the symptoms. The drug may occasionally produce transient hepatic dysfunction manifested by elevated liver enzymes at conventional doses; features typical of intrahepatic cholestasis and pancreatitis may be seen with high-dose regimens. Neurotoxicity, chiefly presenting as cerebellar dysfunction with or without a cerebral component, is also a disturbing feature of very high-dose administration; this is usually reversible but may take months to resolve and occasionally is permanent. Significant neurotoxicity appears uncommon at cumulative doses of ≤ 36 g/m^2. Neurotoxicity may also be reduced by longer intravenous administration over ≥ 3 hours. Conjunctivitis, responsive to topical steroids, and hydradenitis are seen with high doses of drug. Pulmonary toxicity, cardiomyopathy, and a syndrome of sudden respiratory distress are possible, but rare, complications of high-dose regimens.

Azacitidine

PHARMACOLOGY

Azacitidine (azacytidine) is an analogue of cytidine which differs by a substitution of nitrogen for the C_5 in the pyrimidine ring. This substitution renders the triazine ring chemically unstable in aqueous solutions. Azacitidine is transported into the cell by the facilitated nucleoside transport mechanism, and is metabolized to its 5′-monophosphate derivative by uridine/cytidine kinase. Upon further phosphorylation to the triphosphate level, it can be incorporated into RNA, disrupting the synthesis and processing of both nuclear and cytoplasmic species; consequently, protein synthesis is inhibited. It is also incorporated, although to a lesser extent, into DNA, leading to inhibition of DNA synthesis. An important consequence of its DNA incorporation is inhibition of DNA methylation, which allows enhanced expression of a wide variety of genes. It is a cell cycle phase specific agent, with greatest cytotoxic effects exerted in S phase.

Pharmacokinetic data are limited and are based on studies of [^{14}C]-labeled drug. The plasma half-life of total radioactivity (parent drug plus metabolites) after intravenous bolus administration is about 3.5 hours, but after 30 minutes, less than 2% of [^{14}C] counts reflect intact parent drug. Azacitidine is deaminated by cytidine deaminase, which is found in high concentrations in liver, granulocytes, and intestinal epithelium, and in lower concentrations in plasma. The drug undergoes extensive metabolism and chemical decomposition, and a variety of metabolic products have been identified in the urine of beagle dogs. The disposition and metabolism in humans is incompletely characterized. Subcutaneous drug administration yields rapid and fairly efficient absorption. The drug does not penetrate the cerebrospinal fluid well. Negligible amounts of the drug appear to be excreted in the feces.

THERAPEUTIC USES

The main use of azacitidine is in both adult and pediatric acute nonlymphoblastic leukemia, with some activity seen in acute lymphocytic leukemia. The drug is generally used in the maintenance phases of initial therapy or in relapse; combinations with other agents, including vincristine, prednisone, daunorubicin, cytarabine, etoposide, and amsacrine, are the rule. The drug has little clinical activity in human solid tumors.

DETAILS OF ADMINISTRATION

Azacitidine is not commercially available. It is available for investigational purposes from the Division of Cancer Treatment of the NCI and also, under NCI's Group C program, for the treatment of patients with relapsed acute leukemia who are unlikely to respond to existing standard therapies and are unable to enter clinical trials. It is supplied in a 100-mg vial with mannitol (100 mg). The drug may be reconstituted with 19.9 ml of sterile water for injection, with each ml containing 5 mg of azacitidine and 5 mg of mannitol. The reconstituted solution hydrolyzes at room temperature and should be used within 30 minutes to ensure maximum potency. Azacitidine can be further diluted for continuous infusion at concentrations of 2 mg/ml. Lactated Ringer's solution may be the best diluent because it not only provides a pH of around 6.5, but 90% potency is maintained for up to 15 hours at room temperature. Concentrations of less than 2 mg/ml should be avoided, since the drug is more unstable in dilute solution. For continuous infusion, a new solution should be prepared every 8 to 12 hours.

Various intravenous schedules are employed in acute nonlymphoblastic leukemia: (1) 100 mg to 250 mg/m^2 biweekly, or (2) 150–400 mg/m^2 daily for 5 days either by bolus or continuous infusion. The latter schedule is often employed in combination therapy. Continuous infusion is preferable, and is associated with much less gastrointestinal toxicity than with bolus dosing. Daily subcutaneous administration of 30 to 85 mg/m^2 can be tolerated for up to 10 days.

PRECAUTIONS AND DOSE MODIFICATIONS

To minimize the risk of severe and potentially fulminant hepatic toxicity, some authors recommend that the drug be avoided in patients with extensive liver metastases, liver dysfunction, and/or hypoalbuminemia.

DRUG INTERACTIONS

Tetrahydrouridine, an inhibitor of cytidine deaminase, can increase the cytotoxicity of azacitidine.

TOXICITY

The dose-limiting side effect is hematologic, with a leukopenic nadir occurring between 2 and 4 weeks. Thrombocytopenia is seen less frequently; both the leukopenia and thrombocytopenia are dose-dependent. Severe anemia is unusual. Gastrointestinal toxicity, including nausea, vomiting, and diarrhea, can be profound. After bolus administration, these side effects occur within 1 to 2 hours and last for 4 to 5 hours. Antiemetic prophylaxis shows some benefit, and continuous infusion appears to reduce these gastrointestinal effects substantially. Hepatotoxicity is a rare but potentially serious complication. Neuromuscular side effects (weakness, lethargy, and muscle pain) have occurred rarely. A transient fever may be seen during and up to 24 hours after drug administration.

Cladribine

PHARMACOLOGY

Cladribine (2-chloro-2′-deoxy-β-D-adenosine, 2-CdA) is a synthetic purine deoxyribonucleoside antimetabolite that is resistant to adenosine deaminase. 2-CdA is metabolized intracellularly to its 5′-triphosphate form (2-CdATP); deoxycytidine kinase catalyzes the initial, rate-limiting phosphorylation step to 2-CAMP. 2-CdATP can be incorporated into DNA, and is associated with enhanced DNA fragility and strand breaks. 2-CdA inhibits the enzymes DNA polymerase, DNA ligase, and ribonucleotide reductase, which leads to inhibition of both DNA and RNA synthesis. Depletion of nicotine adenine dinucleotide (NAD) and ATP occurs in lymphocytes treated with 2-CdA, presumably a consequence of increased activity of the DNA repair enzyme poly (ADP-ribose) polymerase; these biochemical effects may represent an important component of cytotoxicity. Apoptosis may reflect the final common pathway for cytotoxicity. 2-CdA is toxic to both actively dividing and quiescent lymphocytes and monocytes; treatment is accompanied by an accumulation of cells in the G_1/S phase junction.

Pharmacokinetic data from a trial in which 2-CdA was given as a 7-day continuous intravenous infusion (0.09 mg/kg per day) revealed a steady-state plasma level of 6 ng/ml (0.02 μM). When given as a 2-hour infusion (0.12 mg/kg), the mean end-of-infusion plasma level was 48 ng/ml (0.17 μM), and the terminal half-life was 5.4 hours. Bioavailability is 97% and 50% after subcutaneous and oral administration, respectively. The drug is approximately 20% protein bound.

THERAPEUTIC USES
2-CdA has recently been approved as first- or second-line therapy for patients with hairy cell leukemia. 2-CdA also has some activity in previously treated low-grade non-Hodgkin's lymphomas, cutaneous T-cell lymphomas and mycosis fungoides, and acute and chronic nonlymphocytic leukemias. Acute and chronic lymphocytic leukemias are less responsive.

DETAILS OF ADMINISTRATION
The drug is commercially available (Leustatin) as a clear, colorless, sterile, preservative-free, isotonic solution. Each vial contains 10 mg (1 mg/ml), and should be stored at 2° to 8°C, protected from light. To prepare a single daily dose, the calculated dose (0.09 mg/kg) should be added to an infusion bag containing 500 ml 0.9% sodium chloride injection, and infused by vein over 24 hour. Once diluted, the solution should be used promptly or stored in the refrigerator for no more than 8 hours. 5% Dextrose should not be used as the diluent because of increased degradation of 2-CdA. To prepare a 7-day infusion, bacteriostatic 0.9% sodium chloride injection (containing 0.9% benzyl alcohol) should be used. The appropriate amount of 2-CdA for the 7 days should be passed through a sterile 0.22-μm hydrophilic syringe filter as the solution is added to the infusion reservoir. Then, the diluent should also be passed through the filter to bring the total volume to 100 ml. Admixtures for the 7-day infusion have demonstrated acceptable stability for at least 7 days.

PRECAUTIONS AND DOSE MODIFICATIONS
The effect of renal and hepatic dysfunction on 2-CdA clearance and the safety of 2-CdA administration in such patients has not been established.

DRUG INTERACTIONS
There are no known clinical drug interactions. The drug should be used cautiously with other myelosuppressive agents.

TOXICITY
Severe granulocytopenia occurs in the majority of hairy cell patients, while severe anemia and thrombocytopenia occur in about 37% and 12%, respectively. Prolonged depression of CD4-lymphocytes is noted. Myelosuppression is dose-related and usually reversible. Fever occurs in two thirds of patients, and infection can be documented in about 30%. Other common toxicities include fatigue, nausea, rash, headache, and injection site reactions. High doses of 2-CdA (4–9 times higher than the recommended dose) used in conjunction with high-dose cyclophosphamide and total body irradiation as preparation for marrow transplant was associated with severe, irreversible, neurologic toxicity (paraparesis/quadriparesis) and/or acute renal failure in 45% of patients treated for 7–14 days.

Pentostatin

PHARMACOLOGY
Pentostatin (2′deoxycoformycin) is an adenosine analogue produced by *Streptomyces antibioticus*. It is a potent transition-state inhibitor of adenosine deaminase (ADA), which deaminates adenosine to inosine and deoxyadenosine to deoxyinosine. Although ADA is detectable in virtually all mammalian tissues, its activity is greatest in lymphoid tissue. Children with congenital ADA deficiency have severe combined B- and T-cell immunodeficiency, lymphopenia, hypogammaglobulinemia, and numerous systemic infections. Therefore, it was postulated that an inhibitor of ADA might be useful in the treatment of lymphoproliferative disorders. *In vitro*, pentostatin induces cytotoxicity associated with increased cellular levels of dATP. Other effects include depletion of NAD and ATP, inhibition of ribonucleotide reductase, inhibition of DNA and RNA synthesis, and DNA damage. The drug is toxic to nonreplicating as well as to dividing cells, and the precise basis for its toxicity in lymphoid neoplasms and hairy cell leukemia is not fully understood.

Following rapid intravenous infusion of 2–10 mg/m^2 per day, its plasma clearance in humans is biphasic, with a terminal half-life of about 5 hours; peak plasma levels are in the 1–5 μM range. By 24 hours, about 90% of an administered dose is recovered in the urine. Total body clearance of drug correlates with creatinine clearance. Hence, renal function is a critical determinant of pentostatin's pharmacologic behavior and is an important variable in assessing which patients should be treated with the drug. Pharmacodynamic studies indicate that ADA in lymphocytes is maximally inhibited by doses of 4 mg/m^2. The drug is a very tight binding inhibitor, and prolonged inhibition of the enzyme occurs after drug administration; this observation provides the rationale for an intermittent dosing schedule.

THERAPEUTIC USES
Pentostatin is very active in previously untreated hairy cell leukemia (overall response rate ≥ 90%; CR > 50%), and is also effective in patients who have failed interferon α therapy (overall response rate 86%; CR = 58%). Two major Phase III trials comparing pentostatin with interferon α have been conducted: one in hairy cell leukemia patients who have relapsed after splenectomy, the other in patients who have never been treated. The drug also has activity in cutaneous T-cell lymphoma/mycosis fungoides and chronic lymphocytic leukemia; some patients with HTLV-1–associated adult T-cell leukemia/lymphoma have responded to pentostatin.

DETAILS OF ADMINISTRATION
Initial clinical trials in acute leukemia with high-dose pentostatin were complicated by severe toxicity. With proper selec-

tion of patients having normal renal function and adequate performance status, it is possible to administer the currently recommended doses of pentostatin safely. Pentostatin is commercially available as a sterile, lyophilized powder in 10-mg vials (Nipent). Intact vials should be stored in a refrigerator (2° to 8°C). Good performance status and normal renal function are essential for the safe administration of pentostatin. The recommended dose is 4 mg/m^2 given intravenously every other week. The drug should be reconstituted in 5 ml sterile water for injection and mixed thoroughly to obtain complete dissolution of a solution yielding 2 mg/ml. Pentostatin may be administered over 5 minutes, or further diluted in 25–50 ml 5% dextrose or 0.9% saline and given over 20–30 minutes. Patients should receive hydration with 500–1000 ml of 5% dextrose in 0.5% normal saline or equivalent before drug administration, and an additional 500 ml should be given after the drug.

PRECAUTIONS AND DOSE MODIFICATIONS

Patients with mild to moderate impairment of renal function (elevated serum creatinine or blood urea nitrogen) or a poor performance status of 3 should receive reduced doses; the dose reduction can be in proportion to renal impairment. The drug should not be given to patients with a performance status of 4 or to patients with severely impaired renal function. In the presence of infection and neutropenia, therapy should be withheld until the infection has been treated.

DRUG INTERACTIONS

Administration of pentostatin with vidarabine (ara-A) results in striking inhibition of ara-A deamination. An unacceptably high incidence of pulmonary toxicity occurred in patients with CLL treated with a combination of pentostatin and fludarabine phosphate. There is anecdotal evidence that allopurinol may increase the toxicity (particularly cutaneous toxicity) of pentostatin.

TOXICITY

Toxicity is dose- and schedule-dependent; pretreatment renal function and performance status clearly affect the nature and severity of toxicities. Previous studies demonstrated that higher doses were capable of producing serious renal toxicity, neurologic toxicity (including seizures and coma), and cardiopulmonary toxicity. With currently recommended doses, pentostatin causes myelosuppression (granulocytopenia and lymphocytopenia, thrombocytopenia and anemia), immunosuppression, nausea and vomiting, fever, infection, fatigue and lethargy, rash, hepatic dysfunction (elevated liver enzymes), renal insufficiency, hematuria and dysuria, keratoconjunctivitis, anorexia, chills, myalgia, arthralgia, and diarrhea. Dyspnea and cough may occur; pulmonary edema is uncommon. Cardiac toxicity manifested by arrythmia, abnormal electrocardiograms and peripheral edema may occur but is infrequent. Neurologic toxicity is infrequent but may include anxiety, confusion, depression, dizziness, paresthesias, somnolence and abnormal thinking, and headache.

MISCELLANEOUS AGENTS

Cisplatin

PHARMACOLOGY

Cisplatin (*cis*-diamminedichloroplatinum [II]), an inorganic planar heavy metal coordination complex, was the first metal compound shown to have significant clinical anticancer activity. The antitumor activity correlates with the extent of DNA binding and the formation of bifunctional DNA intrastrand N_7 adducts at d(GpG) and d(ApG), which account for about 60% and 30% of total platinum binding to DNA, respectively; other intrastrand adducts such as d(GpXpG), interstrand crosslinks, monoadducts, and DNA-protein crosslinks account for the balance. The net effect is marked alteration of DNA conformation and inhibition of DNA replication. Cisplatin also binds avidly with accessible sulfur and nitrogen sites on a variety of nuclear and cytoplasmic proteins. Cisplatin can affect the transmembrane transport of essential amino acids, the function of sodium-potassium ATPase activity, and calcium channel function. Cisplatin also interferes with mitochondrial respiration, phosphate transport, and calcium accumulation. Interference with microtubule assembly has also been noted. The contribution of these other effects to cytotoxicity is unclear. The drug is most active in G_1, but behaves predominantly as a cell cycle nonspecific agent. Resistance has been attributed to alterations in transmembrane transport of the drug (reduced accumulation), increased intracellular content of sulfhydryl compounds (which bind the drug), and enhanced repair of DNA adducts.

Cisplatin is rapidly aquated and hydroxylated to various active species in the plasma; subsequently it becomes 90% protein bound. The drug is widely distributed with highest concentrations in the liver, kidneys, and large and small intestine. The drug is also distributed to pleural effusions and ascitic fluid, but CNS penetration is poor. Following intravenous bolus administration, the drug is eliminated in a triphasic manner with an initial half-life of 20–30 minutes, a β half-life of about 1 hour, and a terminal half-life of about 24 hours. The first 2 phases are thought to represent removal of non–protein-bound drug, while the γ phase reflects removal of protein-bound drug. About 25% of an administered dose is excreted from the body during the first 24 hours; of that, 90% is renally excreted (a result of both glomerular filtration and tubular secretion), and biliary excretion accounts for 10%. High-dose regimens have been reported to produce a higher systemic exposure of ultrafilterable platinum.

THERAPEUTIC USES

Cisplatin has an exceptionally broad spectrum of clinically useful antitumor activity. The drug is probably the most active single agent for nonseminomatous testicular cancer; the combinations of either cisplatin, bleomycin, and vinblastine (PVB) or cisplatin, etoposide and bleomycin (PEB) are curative in a large fraction of patients with disseminated disease. Cisplatin plus cyclophosphamide is commonly employed for metastatic ovarian carcinoma, producing objective response rates of 50% to 85%; doxorubicin and/or hexamethylmelamine are sometimes added to cisplatin and cyclophosphamide. Some patients with testicular cancer and ovarian cancer who have failed cisplatin-containing regimens at conventional doses have responded to high-dose cisplatin (total dose of 200 mg/m^2 per course). The value of intraperitoneal cisplatin in ovarian cancer patients with minimum residual disease setting is currently under investigation; some studies include systemic protection with intravenous sodium thiosulfate. Cisplatin is active against squamous or transitional cell cancers of various sites, including head and neck, cervix, esophagus, and urothelium. A large number of clinical trials have attempted to define the role of cisplatin-containing combinations against advanced disease or in the adjuvant setting. The combination of cisplatin and etoposide appears particularly active in small cell lung cancer. Combinations of cisplatin and etoposide or vinca alkaloids have modest activity in non–small cell lung cancer. The drug is also used in complex combinations for the treatment of osteogenic sarcoma and neuroblastoma. Cisplatin appears to function as a radiosensitizer, and ongoing clinical trials are exploring this potential application. Trials of regional drug administration, both intracavitary and intra-arterial, are also in progress.

DETAILS OF ADMINISTRATION

Cisplatin is commercially available (Platinol) in 10- and 50-mg vials containing sterile powder for injection along with 100 or 500 mg mannitol and 90 or 450 mg sodium chloride, respectively. Unopened vials should be stored at room temperature. The powder may be reconstituted by dissolving the contents of the vial with 10 or 50 ml sterile water for injection to yield a solution containing 1 mg/ml cisplatin, 1% mannitol, and 0.9% saline; this solution is stable at room temperature for 20 hours. The drug is unstable when admixed with dextrose-containing solutions. Further dilutions should be with 0.9% saline, because the stability of the solution is inversely related to the concentration of chloride ions. However, the diluted solution should not be refrigerated because precipitation may occur. The drug is also available as an aqueous solution (50- and 100-mg vials, 1 mg/ml). The drug should not be infused through syringe needles containing aluminum, because it reacts with this metal. Because of possible photoaquation, the drug should be protected from bright light such as direct sunlight.

As a single agent, cisplatin has been given over a broad range of doses (50–270 mg/m^2 per course) and in a wide variety of schedules, such as single-dose bolus, daily for 3 to 5 consecutive days, and continuous infusion for hours to days. Doses per course in excess of 120 mg/m^2 are not predictably safe unless the drug is accompanied by thiosulfate, hypertonic saline, WR 2721, diethyldithiocarbamate, or some other normal tissue protector; however, these latter approaches should be regarded as investigational.

When used singly, a single dose of 100–120 mg/m^2 or 20 mg/m^2 daily for 5 days every 3 weeks is appropriate. To minimize the chance of significant nephrotoxicity, the patient is liberally hydrated before treatment in order to ensure high urine flow at the time of drug administration. (See Chap. 31 for a detailed description of one particular cisplatin regimen.) Sufficient potassium chloride should be given with the infusion to correct any anticipated urinary losses. Serum magnesium levels should be monitored carefully and hypomagnesemia corrected. Many other schedules and hydration regimens are described in the literature; there is no preponderance of evidence establishing any of these as the best. In general, 1–2 liters of fluid is recommended over the 8–12 hours prior to administration. The intravenous fluids may be given alone or in combination with mannitol and/or furosemide at an initial rate to maintain a diuresis of 150–400 ml/hour during and for at least 4–6 hours after cisplatin, and then a diuresis of 100–200 ml/hour for the next 18–24 hours or until vomiting has stopped and oral fluids are tolerated. Administration of cisplatin by continuous infusion reduces nausea and vomiting, but has little effect on nephrotoxicity and neurotoxicity.

PRECAUTIONS AND DOSE MODIFICATIONS

Many physicians regard significant impairment in renal function as a contraindication to cisplatin administration. This may be overly cautious, since most acute cisplatin-induced decreases in renal function are transient. The dilemma is particularly difficult in cases where the drug is part of potentially lifesaving therapy. Clearly, decisions should be made individually. In situations in which responding patients are having progressive decreases in renal function with successive courses of treatment, carboplatin may be a reasonable substitute. The agent should be given with extreme caution to patients with impaired hearing, a preexisting peripheral neuropathy, or a past history of allergies to platinum.

DRUG INTERACTIONS

Combinations with agents excreted primarily by the kidneys, such as methotrexate, bleomycin, and ifosfamide must be administered with great care because of the possibility that cisplatin-induced renal damage will delay excretion of the other agents and increase toxicity. Because of the possibility of enhanced renal damage, aminoglycoside antibiotics and amphotericin B should be used with extreme caution in close temporal proximity to cisplatin therapy. In animals, the combination of cisplatin and ethacrynic acid produces significantly more ototoxicity than either agent singly. Sodium thiosulfate and mesna directly inactivate cisplatin; therefore, the combination should not be given together systemically. The strategy of using intravenous thiosulfate with intraperitoneal cisplatin is being explored to provide systemic protection.

TOXICITY

Cisplatin produces a dose-dependent impairment of renal tubular function, manifested as a rise in serum creatinine or blood urea nitrogen with a peak 10 to 15 days after therapy. Various hydration schedules with or without mannitol have been used effectively as prophylaxis. The acute nephrotoxicity is usually reversible, but repeated treatment and the attainment of high cumulative doses may produce a mild-to-moderate permanent impairment of renal function. Clinically significant hypocalcemia and hypomagnesemia may occur, requiring replacement therapy. Nausea and vomiting with cisplatin are characteristically severe and prolonged. Various combinations of antiemetics, generally including metoclopramide or ondansetron, a serotonin antagonist, effectively ameliorate this side effect (see Chap. 57). Thrombocytopenia and leukopenia are usually mild with conventional doses; anemia and Coombs'-positive hemolytic anemia have been reported. High-frequency hearing loss, tinnitus, and occasionally frank deafness may occur. The risk of peripheral neuropathy, manifested as paresthesias or sensory loss in a glove-and-stocking distribution or as frank muscular weakness, increases with increasing cumulative dose. Neuropathy may be very troublesome to the patient and may resolve very slowly or not at all. Anaphylactic reactions have been reported acutely with drug administration which respond to the usual measures, including epinephrine, antihistamines, and corticosteroids. Some patients exhibiting such reactions have been successfully retreated with cisplatin after pretreatment with antihistamines. Visual impairment (from both cortical blindness and retinal toxicity), focal encephalopathy, and seizures have occurred rarely. Possible cardiotoxicity including arrythmias and EKG abnormalities, have been reported, but are probably rare.

Carboplatin

PHARMACOLOGY

Carboplatin, diammine [1,1-cyclobutanedicarboxylato (2-)O,O′]-platinum (II) is a second-generation platinum complex developed as a possible clinical alternative to its highly active but nephrotoxic parent compound, cisplatin. The drug is ten times more water soluble than cisplatin; the carboxylato bonds are slowly hydrolyzed to yield transient aquated intermediates, the active species which bind to DNA and protein. At equipotent doses, its effects on DNA binding and crosslink formation are very similar to cisplatin.

The pharmacokinetics of carboplatin are different from that of cisplatin. After a bolus intravenous infusion, the elimination of total platinum from the plasma is triphasic; the initial half-life is 12 to 24 minutes, the β phase is 1.3–1.7 hours, and the γ half-life is 22–40 hours; these parameters do not change over the dose range of 75 to 450 mg/m^2. Relatively little of the intact drug is protein bound in plasma. During a 24-hour continuous intravenous infusion, the half-life of ultrafilterable platinum is about 170 minutes, and is independent of dose. A portion of the free platinum can be tightly bound to plasma proteins with an elimination half-life of 5 days. Pharmacokinetic studies during more prolonged continuous intravenous infusion indicate that although total platinum levels increase over the course of the infusion, free or active platinum levels decrease by a factor of two over a 4-day infusion. The major route of elimination is through the kidneys. Little metabolism of the drug occurs. The renal clearance of carboplatin correlates very well with creatinine clearance; nomograms have been constructed for use in patients with abnormal renal function. Carboplatin is also widely distributed in body fluids and achieves good penetration into third space fluids, and also distributes into cerebrospinal fluid (CSF : plasma ratio about 0.3).

THERAPEUTIC USES

Carboplatin has clear activity in a number of tumor types, including carcinomas of ovary, head and neck, small cell and non–small cell lung cancer, testicular cancer, bladder cancer, endometrial cancer, pediatric brain tumors, and relapsed and refractory acute leukemia. Compared to cisplatin, carboplatin produces more myelosuppression but much less nephrotoxicity, neurotoxicity, and vomiting. Randomized trials comparing cyclophosphamide in combination with either cisplatin or carboplatin in patients with advanced, suboptimally debulked, ovarian carcinoma suggest that antitumor efficacy is comparable. Patients with ovarian carcinoma who develop cisplatin-refractory disease rarely respond to salvage carboplatin using conventional doses. Randomized trials comparing cisplatin to carboplatin alone or in combination therapy are ongoing in other diseases. The drug is also being extensively investigated in many other tumor types and in high doses for possible incorporation into multiagent ablative regimens with bone marrow transplantation.

DETAILS OF ADMINISTRATION

Carboplatin is commercially available (Paraplatin) as a sterile lyophilized powder in glass vials containing 50, 150, and 450 mg with an equivalent amount of mannitol. The vials can be stored at room temperature and should be protected from light. These are reconstituted with 5 ml, 15 ml, and 45 ml, respectively, of either sterile water for injection USP, 5% dextrose in water, or 0.9% sodium chloride injection USP, yielding a final carboplatin concentration of 10 mg/ml. The reconstituted solution is chemically stable for at least 24 hours at room temperature, but the manufacturer recommends use within 8 hours because no antibacterial agent is included in the commercial formulation. The drug can be further diluted in 500 ml of 0.9% sodium chloride or 5% dextrose in water (0.5 mg/ml) and infused intravenously over 15 to 30 minutes without further hydration. Needles or IV sets that contain aluminum parts should not be used for the preparation or administration of carboplatin. The recommended single-agent dose in ovarian cancer patients with good marrow reserve is 360 mg/m^2 every 4 weeks; 300 mg/m^2 is recommended when combined with cyclophosphamide 600 mg/m^2. A variety of other dosing schedules have been used, including continuous infusion for 24 to 120 hours. High-dose regimens (>800 mg/m^2) are currently being explored.

PRECAUTIONS AND DOSE MODIFICATIONS

The dose should be reduced in the presence of abnormal renal function. The manufacturer recommends a dose of 250 mg/m^2 for patients with a creatinine clearance of 41–59 ml/min, and 200 mg/m^2 for patients with a clearance of 16 to 40 ml/min. A formula proposed by Calvert and colleagues adjusts the total dose of carboplatin based on creatinine clearance or glomerular filtration rate and a desired plasma concentration versus time product (AUC):

$$\text{total dose (units = mg)} = \text{AUC (units = mg/ml} \cdot \text{min)} \times [\text{GFR} + 25] \text{ (units = ml/min)}.$$

For previously untreated patients, the desired AUC is 6 to 8 mg/ml · min, whereas a desired AUC of 4 to 6 mg/ml · min is recommended for previously treated patients. More complicated nomograms have been constructed.

DRUG INTERACTIONS

No drug interactions have been reported.

TOXICITY

The principal toxicity of carboplatin is myelosuppression; thrombocytopenia is usually the most pronounced hematologic toxicity, and the platelet nadir typically occurs 3 weeks after dosing. In patients with ovarian cancer treated with carboplatin as first-line combination therapy, a granulocyte nadir below 1000/μl occurred in 82%; 35% required a platelet transfusion; and 16% had infection. Nausea and vomiting are seen frequently, but are severe in only one third of patients. Nephrotoxicity characterized by transient elevations in serum creatinine or blood urea nitrogen occurred in fewer than 20% of patients; electrolyte abnormalities can occur, particularly magnesium wasting (61%), while potassium, calcium and sodium wasting occur in 10–16% of patients. Hepatic enzyme elevations occur in 20–30% of patients, but bilirubin elevations are infrequent. Neurotoxicity is uncommon with conventional doses. High-dose regimens are complicated by hepatotoxicity and severe renal dysfunction. Hemorrhagic colitis, optic neuritis and interstitial pneumonitis have also been seen in a few patients treated with high doses.

Asparaginase

PHARMACOLOGY

L-Asparaginase is an enzyme isolated from a number of microbial sources; the molecular weight ranges from 141,000–144,000 according to the source, and is composed of four subunits, each with one active site. The preparation most commonly used clinically is derived from *Escherichia coli*. The enzyme hydrolyzes asparagine into aspartic acid with the release of ammonia. Thus, in certain tumor cells dependent on exogenous asparagine, asparaginase rapidly inhibits asparagine-dependent protein synthesis, with delayed inhibition of DNA and RNA synthesis. The inhibitory action is greatest in cells in the G_1 phase of the cell cycle. Asparagine is a nonessential amino acid in humans because normal cells contain asparagine synthase. Tumor cell resistance is also mediated by high asparagine synthase levels.

Asparaginase is inactive orally, and is administered by intramuscular injection or by intravenous infusion over 30 minutes. After intravenous administration, the apparent volume of distribution is slightly larger than plasma volume, and the drug has minimal distribution out of the vascular compartment. The plasma half-life is independent of dose and the terminal half-life varies between 8 and 30 hours. Metabolism is independent of hepatic and renal function. Urinary and biliary excretion is minimal. Plasma concentration is proportional to dose over a very wide range. The development of hypersensitivity greatly increases the clearance rate. Daily administration results in a cumulative increase in plasma levels. Plasma levels after intramuscular injection are about 50% of that achieved after intravenous administration.

THERAPEUTIC USES

Asparaginase is used in combination therapy for remission induction in pediatric acute lymphoblastic leukemia. To minimize the development of resistance and the chance of serious toxicity, it is not normally used for maintenance therapy.

DETAILS OF ADMINISTRATION

Each vial of the commercial preparation (Elspar) contains 10,000 IU of lyophilized asparaginase in 80 mg of mannitol. The drug should be stored under refrigeration. For intravenous injection, the vial may be reconstituted with 5 ml of either 0.9% sodium chloride injection or 5% dextrose in water. The solution may appear either clear or slightly cloudy; the vial should not be used if gross precipitation is noted. Further dilution in physiologic saline or dextrose is possible, as these solutions are relatively stable at room temperature. For intramuscular administration, a maximum volume of 2 ml should be used for individual injections at separate sites. The manufacturer recommends storage for no more than 8 hours because the solution has no antibacterial preservative. Asparaginase should not be infused through a final filter because of potential binding to the filter material.

For patients who become allergic to the *E. coli* form of

asparaginase, asparaginase derived from *Erwinia caratovora* may be substituted. An investigational formulation of asparaginase derived from *E. carotovora* is available under the Group C mechanism from the Division of Cancer Treatment, NCI, as a 10,000 IU vial containing 0.6 mg sodium chloride and 20 mg dextrose. The product is stable for 4 years under refrigeration and for 2 years at room temperature. Once reconstituted at concentrations up to 35 IU/ml with 5% dextrose or isotonic saline, it is stable for 20 days under refrigeration or at room temperature.

If given intravenously, asparaginase should be given over a period of not less than 30 minutes through the side arm of a freely running infusion of sodium chloride or 5% dextrose in water. Because of the frequency of hypersensitivity reactions, corticosteroids, epinephrine, and oxygen should be available during administration.

Asparaginase should be used in combination with other agents, usually vincristine and prednisone for remission induction. The usual pediatric dosage is 1000 IU/kg intravenously daily for 10 consecutive days, and is typically started on day 22 after vincristine (given days 1, 8 and 15) and prednisone (given days 1–15). An alternate regimen is 6000 IU/m^2 intramuscularly every 3 days for 9 doses starting day 4 (in this regimen, vincristine is given weekly for 4 doses starting day 1, and prednisone by mouth is given daily for 28 days). Other schedules also appear active. Asparaginase as a sole induction agent should only be used when a combined regimen is inappropriate or in cases refractory to other therapy; the dose for these unusual situations is 200 IU/kg intravenously daily for 28 days. The drug should only be used in hospitalized patients under close supervision. Appropriate agents for treatment of acute hypersensitivity reactions must be available. Hematopoietic, hepatic, renal, pancreatic, and CNS function should be determined prior to and regularly during asparaginase therapy.

PRECAUTIONS AND DOSE MODIFICATIONS

Dosing appears to be independent of major organ function. The drug is contraindicated in patients with a history of anaphylaxis to the drug derived from the same bacterial source. The manufacturer suggests that pancreatitis or a history of pancreatitis is also a contraindication.

DRUG INTERACTIONS

When asparaginase is administered immediately before or with methotrexate, it may diminish or abolish the cytotoxic effect of methotrexate. This effect persists as long as plasma asparagine levels remain depressed. Concomitant administration of asparaginase and vincristine may produce cumulative neuropathy. The toxicity seems to be less pronounced when asparaginase is administered after vincristine, instead of before or concurrently with the drug. Concurrent administration with prednisone may enhance hyperglycemia; concurrent mercaptopurine and/or prednisone, however, may reduce the incidence of hypersensitivity.

TOXICITY

Because asparaginase is a bacterial product, hypersensitivity reactions are common, occurring in about 20% to 35% of patients, and are manifested most commonly by urticarial skin rashes but also by chills, fever, and anaphylaxis. Hypersensitivity develops most commonly during the second or subsequent weeks of therapy and is more common in patients receiving higher doses, multiple courses, and intravenous (as opposed to intramuscular) administration. Patients who respond to *E. coli* asparaginase but develop allergic reactions may be treated relatively safely with the *Erwinia* preparation, although patients may subsequently develop hypersensitivity reactions to the latter preparation. Therefore, maintenance therapy is not recommended. Bone marrow suppression is mild. Anorexia, nausea, or vomiting occur in most patients, and weight loss may also occur. Decreases in circulating levels of the clotting factors synthesized in the liver are common during therapy, but this rarely results in clinically significant bleeding. A variety of other liver function abnormalities occur in most patients (including elevations of alkaline phosphatase, serum glutamic-oxaloacetic transaminase [SGOT], and bilirubin); although not usually clinically significant, liver toxicity has resulted in occasional fatalities. Liver biopsies show fatty changes. Hepatic protein synthesis is depressed, and hypoalbumineia may occur. Clinically significant pancreatitis, with resulting impairment of insulin secretion and exocrine function, has been observed; pancreatitis may be fulminant and fatal. Azotemia is common, and asparaginase occasionally produces renal functional impairment with oliguric renal failure. Various CNS manifestations (depression, lethargy, somnolence, disorientation, recent memory loss, headache, electroencephalographic changes) are also occasional side effects of therapy, but have occurred principally in adults. CSF levels of both asparagine and glutamine have decreased after intravenous dosing.

MODIFIED L-ASPARAGINASE PRODUCTS

Asparaginase has been chemically modified to eliminate glutaminase activity (present in some *E. coli* preparations, and to reduce the immunogenicity of the preparation. For example, conjugation of the enzyme to polyethylene glycol (PEG) has been investigated for the past several years. In clinical trials, PEG-asparaginase has a more extended half-life, a reduced incidence of hypersensitivity reactions, and appears to have comparable activity compared to the unmodified preparations. Further studies are ongoing to characterize the role of these modified products.

Mitotane

PHARMACOLOGY

Mitotane (o,p′-DDD) is structurally related to the insecticide chlorophenothane (DDT). The drug causes adrenal cortical atrophy by inhibiting mitochondrial function. It blocks adrenocortical hormone synthesis in normal and malignant cells. It also appears to have peripheral effects on glucocorticoid metabolism. The drug is cell cycle phase nonspecific.

Following oral administration, approximately 40% of mitotane is absorbed. The drug is degraded slowly in the liver and kidney and is extensively distributed in fat. The primary metabolites are oxidation products. Mitotane has a very long terminal half-life; plasma concentrations and adipose tissue levels remain detectable for 6 to 9 weeks and 20 months after the drug is discontinued, respectively. Ten to 20% of the drug is excreted in the urine as water-soluble metabolites. Biliary excretion accounts for less than 20% of an administered dose.

THERAPEUTIC USES

Mitotane is used in the palliative treatment of inoperable adrenocortical carcinoma (see Chap. 34).

DETAILS OF ADMINISTRATION

Mitotane is commercially available in a 500-mg tablet (Lysodren). It should be stored in a light-resistant container, preferably at temperatures below 40°C. The usual recommended starting dose is 2 to 6 g daily, administered in 3 to 4 divided doses. The dose is then increased incrementally to 9 to 10 g daily. In patients who have minimal toxicity, the dosage may be increased until tolerable adverse effects occur, because the probability of response may be related to dose (see Chap. 34). There is substantial variation in the maximum tolerated dose (2–20 g daily).

PRECAUTIONS AND DOSE MODIFICATIONS

It is probably advisable to decrease the dose in the presence of significant hepatic or renal functional impairment, although no pharmacologically validated guidelines exist for determining proper dose under these circumstances.

DRUG INTERACTIONS

Corticosteroid metabolism may be altered by mitotane, requiring higher replacement doses. Mitotane induces hepatic microsomal enzymes; it can, therefore, potentially increase the metabolism of drugs such as barbiturates, warfarin, and phenytoin. CNS depression may be pronounced when the drug is administered concomitantly with other CNS depressants.

TOXICITY

Gastrointestinal intolerance (anorexia, nausea, vomiting, and diarrhea), and CNS toxicity (lethargy, dizziness, vertigo) may be dose limiting. The development of adrenal insufficiency may necessitate glucocorticoid and sometimes mineralocorticoid replacement. At times of physiologic stress (*e.g.*, infection, bleeding, surgery) patients treated with mitotane should be assumed to have adrenal insufficiency and should be treated with replacement doses of glucocorticoids appropriate for stress situations. Neurologic and behavioral monitoring during therapy is necessary to anticipate such drug effects as depression, lethargy, and visual disturbances, as well as evidence of possible neurologic sequelae of long-term administration. A maculopapular rash occurs in about 15% of patients. Genitourinary toxicity in the form of hemorrhagic cystitis, hematuria, or albuminuria have occurred infrequently. Both hypertension and orthostatic hypotension have been occasionally reported.

Hydroxyurea

PHARMACOLOGY

Hydroxyurea appears to enter cells by passive diffusion, and inhibits ribonucleotide reductase; it is thought to inactivate a tyrosyl radical on the catalytic subunit of the enzyme, an effect which can be partially reversed by ferrous iron. The subsequent depletion of deoxyribonucleotides interferes with DNA synthesis and repair. The drug exerts cytotoxicity on cells in S phase, and may cause accumulation of cells at the G_2/M phase. Prolonged drug exposure enhances its cytotoxicity. There is recent evidence that hydroxyurea may eliminate amplified drug resistance genes and oncogenes located in extrachromosomal sites.

Hydroxyurea is well absorbed from the gastrointestinal tract; peak serum levels of 0.3–2.0 mM are seen about 1 hour after doses of 40–80 mg/kg are given. The elimination half-life is 3.5–4.5 hours. Animal studies using [^{14}C]-labeled drug indicated that about 50% of an oral dose is degraded in the liver and is excreted as respiratory carbon dioxide and in the urine as urea. The extent and significance of hydroxyurea metabolism in humans is unknown. Hydroxyurea can be degraded by urease, an enzyme found in intestinal bacteria. Renal excretion of intact drug occurs, but cumulative urinary excretion has varied enormously (9.5% to 95%) in several studies. Hydroxyurea readily enters the CNS (plasma : CSF ratios range from 4 : 1 to 9 : 1) and third space fluids (plasma : ascites ratios range from 2 : 1 to 7.5 : 1).

THERAPEUTIC USES

Hydroxyurea is a good alternative to busulfan in patients with chronic myelogenous leukemia (CML); because it is effective and well tolerated, many regard it as the drug of choice for control of the leukocytosis in CML. It has been used in conjunction with radiation therapy for certain squamous cancers, notably head and neck and cervix carcinomas, where it appears to potentiate the effect of radiation therapy. The drug has shown some evidence of activity in melanoma and refractory ovarian cancer, but it has no established role in the treatment of these cancers.

DETAILS OF ADMINISTRATION

Hydroxyurea is commercially available (Hydrea) for oral use in 500-mg capsules. The drug is stable at room temperature, but the capsules should be kept in a tightly sealed container with a desiccant included. If the patient is unable to swallow the capsule, its contents may be emptied into a glass of water and taken immediately. The patient should be advised that some inert materials in the capsule may not dissolve and may float on the surface. All dosages should be based on the patient's actual or ideal weight, whichever is less.

The usual dose for patients with CML is 20 mg to 30 mg/kg orally as a single daily dose. When used as a single agent for solid tumors, a similar dose schedule can be used. Alternatively, an intermittent schedule of 80 mg/kg in a single dose every third day is also feasible, and is the most common schedule for simultaneous administration with radiation therapy. In this situation, hydroxyurea should begin at least 7 days before initiation of the irradiation and should continue during the radiation therapy and indefinitely thereafter, as tolerated.

An investigational intravenous formulation is available from the Division of Cancer Treatment, NCI as a lyophilized powder containing 2 g hydroxyurea with anhydrous citric acid and sodium phosphate. The vial is reconstituted with 18.6 ml sterile water for injection, and may be further diluted up to 500 ml with 5% dextrose in water or 0.9% saline for administration as an intravenous infusion.

PRECAUTIONS AND DOSE MODIFICATIONS

The effect of hepatic or renal dysfunction on the dose of hydroxyurea is not known. In view of the relative importance of the renal route in drug disposition, it is reasonable to decrease the initial dose in the presence of renal failure until tolerance has been established.

DRUG INTERACTIONS

By decreasing dCTP levels, hydroxyurea increases the anabolism of cytarabine to its 5′-triphosphate derivative and enhances its subsequent incorporation into DNA. The drug is thought to be a radiation sensitizer. There is potential for antagonism between 5-FU and hydroxyurea in cells in which formation of FdUMP is primarily from fluorouridine diphosphate through the ribonucleotide reductase pathway. However, the combination of hydroxyurea or floxuridine with leucovorin may lead to enhanced cytotoxicity by decreasing the intracellular pools of deoxyuridine monophosphate (the normal substrate that competes with FdUMP for binding to thymidylate synthase). If the cancer cell is capable of converting 5-FU to floxuridine, the same rationale for adding hydroxyurea may pertain.

TOXICITY

The drug is generally very well tolerated. The major dose-limiting toxicity is hematologic, particularly leukopenia, with a median onset of 10 days. Anemia also occurs, while thrombocytopenia is occasionally seen. Resolution of myelosuppression follows rapidly on discontinuation of drug. Nausea, vomiting, stomatitis, and diarrhea occur less frequently. A maculopapular rash and facial erythema may occur. Hydroxyurea therapy may temporarily impair renal tubular function, accompanied by elevations of serum blood urea nitrogen, creatinine and uric acid. Moderate drowsiness may occur with high doses; other neurologic toxicities including headache, dizziness, disorientation, and seizures are extremely rare. Elevated liver function tests may be seen; occasionally, hepatic dysfunction may be severe. When given with radiation, increased tissue reactions may occur; some patients have radiation recall of erythema or hyperpigmentation in previously irradiated areas.

Procarbazine

PHARMACOLOGY

Procarbazine is a substituted hydrazine derivative (N-methylhydrazine) with a structure similar to that of some monoamine oxidase inhibitors. Procarbazine is a prodrug that undergoes complex metabolism. Following either chemical decomposition, auto-oxidation, or microsomal metabolism by the cytochrome P450 system, the drug forms numerous reactive intermediates including hydrogen peroxide, formaldehyde, and hydroxide radicals, which may directly damage DNA. Other unstable end products with monofunctional alkylating activity or the ability to covalently bind to RNA have been described. The drug inhibits DNA, RNA, and protein synthesis; effects on DNA synthesis are seen within several hours, while inhibition of RNA and protein synthesis occurs after a delay of 12–24 hours. Methylation of DNA and abnormal selective transmethylation of the N7 guanine on transfer RNA are observed. The drug may suppress mitosis by prolonging interphase; the drug has marked cytotoxicity in S and G_2 phases.

Procarbazine is rapidly and completely absorbed after oral administration; peak plasma concentrations occur within 1 hour, and the plasma half-life is approximately 10 minutes. The drug initially concentrates in the liver and kidneys, and it readily equilibrates between plasma and cerebrospinal fluid. About 75% of the metabolites are excreted in the urine within 24 hours; less than 5% is excreted as unchanged drug. Hence, both biotransformation and renal excretion play significant roles in clearance of both parent drug and metabolites.

THERAPEUTIC USES

The major use of procarbazine is in the initial treatment of advanced Hodgkin's disease as a component of MOPP therapy (in combination with mechlorethamine, vincristine, and prednisone). It has also been included in analogous regimens for the non-Hodgkin's lymphomas (COPP). Some evidence for activity in other tumor types (small cell lung cancer, melanoma, and brain tumors) has led to its incorporation into certain combinations for these diseases, but its role outside Hodgkin's disease has not been established.

DETAILS OF ADMINISTRATION

Procarbazine is available commercially (Matulane) in 50-mg capsules as the hydrochloride salt. The drug should be protected from water or moisture before administration to avoid decomposition. Used as a component in the MOPP regimen, the usual dosage is 100 mg/m^2 daily on days 1 to 14 of a 28-day cycle; this dose should not be attenuated during the first few days of treatment in anticipation of patient intolerance. Single-agent dosing has ranged from daily doses of 50 to 200 mg given continuously for 10 to 20 days. The dose may be taken at a single time or in divided doses. The manufacturer recommends that the initial dose be 2–4 mg/kg for the first week, with escalation to 4–6 mg/kg per day until there is evidence of hematologic toxicity. When the toxicity has resolved, the maintenance dose in adults is 1 to 2 mg/kg daily. In children, the manufacturer recommends 50 mg/m^2 daily for the first week, then daily doses of 100 mg/m^2 until maximum response or hematologic toxicity is seen. Upon resolution of toxicity, the maintenance dose is 50 mg/m^2 daily. The dose in obese or edematous patients should be based on estimated lean body mass.

PRECAUTIONS AND DOSE MODIFICATIONS

As with all cytotoxic agents, procarbazine must be administered with caution in patients with preexisting bone marrow compromise, or renal or hepatic impairment. There are no established guidelines for dose modification under these circumstances. Oral procarbazine can cause hemolysis in patients with glucose-6-phosphate deficiency.

DRUG INTERACTIONS

Since the drug may potentiate other CNS active drugs, concomitant administration with barbiturates, antihistamines, narcotic analgesics, opiates, hypotensive agents, or phenothiazines should be undertaken with great caution; additive CNS depression and respiratory depression have occurred. Furthermore, since procarbazine is a weak monoamine oxidase inhibitor, hypertensive crisis, tremor, excitation, cardiac palpitations, and angina may occur when sympathomimetics, tricyclic antidepressants, or foods with a high tyramine content (*e.g.*, dark beer, cheeses, red wine, or bananas) are ingested concomitantly. Procarbazine also interacts with alcohol, causing a disulfiram-like reaction (including severe gastrointestinal toxicity, nausea, vomiting, visual disturbances, and headache), as well as with cough and cold preparations that contain sympathomimetic drugs or alcohol. Patients should be instructed specifically about these interactions and must be warned to avoid these potentially dangerous substances.

TOXICITY

The usual dose-limiting toxicity is myelosuppression that affects all marrow elements, although thrombocytopenia tends to be predominant. The nadir occurs 4 to 6 weeks after the start of therapy when the drug is used singly. Gastrointestinal toxicities include nausea, vomiting, and diarrhea; although these effects may occasionally be dose limiting, tolerance may develop with continued administration. A flu-like syndrome may occur with initial therapy. Dermatologic reactions rarely occur; an allergic drug rash occurs in about 3% of patients, but responds to small doses of prednisone. A wide variety of neurologic symptoms may occur, including paresthesias, neuropathies, lethargy, dizziness, headache, ataxia; these symptoms may relate to inhibition of monoamine oxidase enzymes. Nightmares, depression, insomnia, nervousness, and hallucinations may occur in up to one third of patients, and may be dose-limiting in some patients. Tremors, convulsions, and coma are seen uncommonly, and mandate immediate cessation of therapy if they occur. Ophthalmalogic effects (nystagmus, diplopia, papilledema, and photophobia) and a hypersensitivity-type pneumonitis have been rarely noted.

Gallium Nitrate

PHARMACOLOGY

Gallium nitrate is a Group IIIa anhydrous heavy metal salt. Gallium was initially used medically for diagnostic scanning. Interest developed in using gallium as a possible antineoplastic agent when it was found that carrier-free ^{67}gallium citrate concentrated in a variety of malignant tissues. The mechanism of cytotoxicity is not precisely known. After intravenous administration, gallium is rapidly bound to plasma proteins, including transferrin. Gallium is thought to enter cells when the gallium-transferrin complex binds to the transferrin receptor and is then incorporated by active transport. Gallium competes with iron for normal iron binding sites in plasma and on cell membranes. Gallium is generally distributed throughout the intracellular compartments, including the nucleus and lysosomes. Gallium is a weak inhibitor of mammalian and viral DNA polymerases, and may inhibit calcium- and magnesium-dependent processes. Gallium also exerts an antihypercalcemic effect; the drug inhibits bone resorption in a dose- and time-dependent fashion. Gallium both decreases urinary excretion of calcium and inhibits calcium resorption from bone. Gallium also reduces the biochemical parameters associated with bone turnover in patients with bone metastases: bone resorption and turnover are inhibited, excretion of calcium and hydroxyproline in the urine is decreased, ionized calcium and phosphorus levels are reduced, and bone pain may decrease in about one third of patients.

Gallium nitrate is excreted primarily by the kidney. The pharmacokinetics have been described as biphasic, but individual studies report very different terminal half-lives (6 to 36 hours); renal excretion ranges from 15% to 72% within the first 24 hours. Abnormal renal function can significantly compromise drug elimination.

THERAPEUTIC USES

The drug is approved for the treatment of cancer-related hypercalcemia. In independent randomized trials, gallium was superior to both calcitonin and etidronate for acute control of modest to severe hypercalcemia. As an antineoplastic agent, gallium has activity in lymphoma, and some activity has been reported in refractory ovarian cancer, bladder cancer and prostate cancer.

DETAILS OF ADMINISTRATION

Gallium nitrate is commercially available (Ganite) as 500 mg in a 20-ml single-dose vial (25 mg/ml); the solution also contains sodium citrate dihydrate (29 mg/ml), and may contain sodium hydroxide for pH adjustment. The vials should be stored at room temperature. The daily dose should be diluted in 1000 ml 0.9% saline or in 5% dextrose injection for administration as a 24-hour intravenous infusion. Each of these solutions is stable for 48 hours at room temperature and for 7 days under refrigeration. The product contains no preservatives. The usual dose is 200 mg/m^2 daily for 5 days. The patient should be receiving adequate hydration throughout the treatment period.

As an antitumor agent, gallium nitrate has been given on several schedules. Continuous infusion appears to decrease the risk of nephrotoxicity, and doses of 300–350 mg/m^2 daily for 5–7 days are tolerated.

PRECAUTIONS AND DOSE MODIFICATIONS

The drug should not be given to patients with a serum creatinine above 2.5 mg/dl.

DRUG INTERACTIONS

The manufacturer warns against the use of nephrotoxic drugs, including aminoglycosides and amphotericin.

TOXICITY

When used to treat hypercalcemia, gallium nitrate is generally well tolerated. Hypocalcemia, hypophosphatemia, decreased serum bicarbonate, and symptomatic decreases in blood pressure may occur. As an antineoplastic agent, the major dose-limiting toxicity was renal impairment, characterized by elevations in blood urea nitrogen and serum creatinine. Renal toxicity is particularly evident with 30-minute infusion regimens, and can be partially circumvented with a continuous-infusion schedule; the latter is favored for future investigation. Other toxicities include bone marrow suppression, hypomagnesemia, tinnitus, decreased hearing, mucositis, optic neuropathy, metallic taste, nausea and vomiting, retinal hemorrhage, fever, and diarrhea.

Amsacrine

PHARMACOLOGY

Amascrine (AMSA), N-[4-acridinylamino)-3-methoxyphenyl] methanesulfonamide, is a synthetic aminoacridine derivative that intercalates between DNA base pairs, resulting in inhibition of DNA synthesis. AMSA induces protein-linked DNA strand breaks, presumably by stabilization of a cleavable complex between subunits of topoisomerase-2 and the 5′-terminus of a broken DNA strand. AMSA also produces DNA single-strand breaks. The drug is much more active in proliferating than in nonproliferating cells, and may cause cell cycle accumulation in G_2.

In humans, pharmacokinetics of [^{14}C]-labeled AMSA revealed a half-life of unchanged drug of 7.4 hours in patients with normal renal function, whereas it was prolonged to 17 hours in patients with impaired renal function. A prolonged terminal half-life of the total radiolabeled species was 46 hours. Pharmacokinetic studies using HPLC and fluorescence detection revealed a biphasic distribution, with an initial half-life of 10 to 15 minutes. The terminal disposition half-life for unchanged drug and total fluorescent species was 3 hours and 8–9 hours, respectively. Studies in animals treated with [^{14}C]-labeled AMSA indicated extensive drug localization in liver, primarily as metabolites, with rapid excretion in bile. The major metabolites were alkyl-thiol derivatives of acridine, which can be produced by non-enzymatic attack at C_9 by endogenous thiols; these metabolites can be excreted in either urine or bile. Microsomal activation of the drug results in metabolites which retain the ability to inhibit topoisomerase II. CNS penetration is minimal.

THERAPEUTIC USES

The drug is an investigational agent supplied by the Division of Cancer Treatment, NCI, and is also available under the Group C mechanism for the treatment of adult patients with refractory acute myelogenous leukemia. AMSA has activity in acute myelogenous and lymphoblastic leukemias, with single agent response rates of about 17%. The overall response rate in pediatric acute myelogenous and lymphoblastic leukemias is 35% and 15%, respectively. The drug also has a 20% response rate in adult patients with Hodgkin's and non-Hodgkin's lymphomas. The drug has been tested in front-line regimens in combination with cytarabine and thioguanine (AAT) versus standard treatment consisting of daunorubicin, cytarabine and thioguanine (DAT); while efficacy in terms of initial response rate may be comparable, it does not appear that the AMSA-containing combination offers a early therapeutic advantage. The drug is also being tested in various combinations as intensification and/or maintenance therapy for acute myelogenous leukemia in initial remission to determine its effect on overall patient survival. The combination of high-dose cytarabine with AMSA in patients with relapsed or refractory ANLL produces second complete remission rates of 60% or better, but it is not clear that the combination is superior to high-dose cytarabine alone; further, the toxicity of the two-drug combination is substantial. Although response rates of 15–25% were reported in Phase II studies of ovarian, cervical and endometrial cancer, the drug is not considered a useful addition to the therapeutic armamentarium in these solid tumors.

DETAILS OF ADMINISTRATION

AMSA is supplied in a Duopack containing two sterile liquids that must be aseptically combined prior to use. One vial contains 1.5 ml of a 50 mg/ml solution of AMSA in anhydrous N,N-dimethylacetamide. The other vial contains 13.5 mg of 0.0353 M L-lactic acid diluent. Both vials should be stored under refrigeration and are stable for at least 1 year. Once mixed together, the combined solution is 10% (v/v) (5 mg/ml AMSA and 0.0318 M L-lactic acid), which is stable at room temperature under normal light conditions for at least 48 hours. Glass syringes are recommended for reconstitution because the concentrated N,N-dimethylacetamide can dissolve certain plastic components. The combined solution is not stable with any chloride-containing solutions. Admixtures in 500 ml 5% dextrose, however, are stable for at least 48 hours. However, the final solution does not contain antibacterial preservatives and therefore should be discarded within 8 hours after preparation. Direct contact of AMSA solution with the skin and mucous membranes may cause skin sensitivity.

AMSA should be administered as a slow intravenous infusion over several hours. Close monitoring is required. Initial clinical studies in leukemia recommended doses of 70–90 mg/m^2 daily for 5 days. Currently, AMSA is generally administered at 120–150 mg/m^2 daily for 5 days or 225 mg/m^2 daily for 3 days for induction therapy. Doses of 75 mg to 90 mg/m^2 daily for 3 days are used in combination therapy for maintenance.

PRECAUTIONS AND DOSE MODIFICATIONS

Acute ventricular arrythmias have occurred in both adults and children receiving AMSA. Rapid infusion and hypokalemia may predispose to this complication. Severe myelosuppression and stomatitis have been seen in patients with renal and hepatic dysfunction who received full doses of AMSA. Although validated dose reduction guidelines are not available, some investigators have recommended 25–40% dose reductions in patients with a bilirubin $>$ 2 mg/dl and/or a serum creatinine $>$ 1.5 mg/ml.

DRUG INTERACTIONS

The hydrochloride salt of AMSA is poorly water soluble. The combined solution described above is physically incompatible with sodium chloride and other chloride-containing solutions.

TOXICITY

The dose-limiting toxicity of AMSA is myelosuppression, predominantly affecting granulocytes. The drug is relatively platelet-sparing. Phlebitis is common, although administration of the drug in 500 ml 5% dextrose may reduce the severity of vein irritation. The drug is a vesicant and care must be taken to avoid extravasation. Gastrointestinal toxic effects are common, and include nausea and vomiting, diarrhea, and mucositis; the latter is particularly common in patients receiving dose-intensive regimens. Cardiotoxicity has also been reported, manifested as a fall in ejection fraction, acute arrhythmias, and electrocardiographic abnormalities. The relative incidence of this toxicity compared with the anthracycline antibiotics is difficult to assess. In a review of the clinical literature involving 3200 patients, 2.3% of the patients treated with AMSA developed signs of cardiotoxicity, but almost all of these patients were heavily pretreated with anthracyclines, and some were hypokalemic. Less frequent toxicities include elevation in liver transaminases, alkaline phosphatase, and bilirubin. Alopecia is also a feature of treatment. The patient should be warned that the urine will turn orange during treatment. Neurotoxicity, including peripheral neuropathy, dizziness, headache, CNS depression and seizures, is uncommon.

PRACTICAL GUIDELINES FOR CHEMOTHERAPY ADMINISTRATION

Practical issues affecting the administration of intravenous antineoplastic agents fall into five major areas: techniques for the safe administration of antineoplastic agents, the prevention and management of morbidity, the care and maintenance of indwelling catheters, legal implications, and risk reduction to personnel during preparation and handling. The purpose of this chapter is to provide specific information about techniques and the requisite knowledge, judgment, and technical skills required to care for the devices that are used for vascular access and chemotherapy administration.[1–10]

Knowledge of the anatomy and physiology of veins and arteries, the therapies to be administered parenterally, and the management of complications is essential to safely administering chemotherapy. Technical proficiency should be acquired under the supervision of an experienced preceptor. Additionally, most institutions require that nurses demonstrate knowledge of and skill with drugs, proper reconstitution, administration, and normal dosage range as well as their physiologic effects and toxicities in a written and a practical examination before assuming responsibilities for drug administration.

Before venipuncture, an assessment of the patient should be conducted by the nurse, including a thorough allergy and medication history, and the patient's prior cancer treatments, if any. If the patient has had prior chemotherapy, any adverse reactions should be ascertained and well documented. All applicable laboratory studies should also be reviewed in detail. Ambulatory patients should be positioned comfortably in chairs with armrests or in special phlebotomy chairs. The purpose and duration of the infusion should be reiterated just before the venipuncture. The patient should be instructed to alert the nurse of any pain, burning, or changes in appearance or sensation of the IV site during the infusion. If the patient has undergone an axillary node dissection, the affected arm should be avoided. If it must be used, strict asepsis during venipuncture is absolutely essential. Use of the lower extremities should be avoided, since the risk of thrombophlebitis and embolism is increased.

Vein selection should be based on the type of cannula to be used, the purpose of the infusion, its duration, and the patient's general condition and activity level. Ideally, the vein that is selected should follow a straight course for a distance that is long enough to permit full insertion of the needle or catheter. The large, easily accessible veins found along the forearm, such as the cephalic, median, and basilic veins, provide safe, convenient venipuncture sites. The bones of the forearm provide a natural splint that eliminates the need for immobilizing the arm. The use of large veins reduces the risk of chemical thrombophlebitis when vascular irritants are to be infused. The choice of needle gauge should be based on the size of the vein.

Before venipuncture, the vein should be palpated for resilience. Thrombosed veins feel hard and cordlike. When prolonged intravenous therapy is anticipated, the distal aspect of veins should be used for venipuncture so that inadvertent thrombosis will not preclude future use of the proximal aspect. Extreme care must be exercised when irritating solutions or drugs are administered into veins that lie in the antecubital fossa or over the wrist joint. If administering vesicant solutions, these areas should be avoided, if at all possible, due to the extensive damage that can take place should an extravasation occur.

Whenever venipuncture is traumatic or the needle's position is in doubt, infuse a sterile solution of normal saline or water to ensure that the solution is not extravasating through a puncture in the posterior wall of the vein. If the entire bevel of the needle is in the vein, the fluid should infuse freely. If still in doubt, quickly pinching the tubing closest to the needle or pulling back gently with a syringe should give an immediate flashback of blood, ensuring that the needle is in the vein.

The selection of a specific intravenous cannula depends on the purpose and length of the infusion, as well as the size and condition of the patient's veins. Stainless steel scalp vein needles, centered and held by plastic wings, are associated with a low incidence of infection and thrombophlebitis and are employed for most short-term (<24 hour) infusions.[8,9] Steel scalp vein needles range from 25- to 16-gauge in diameter. The plastic wings of scalp vein needles provide stability and maximum control of the needle during insertion. The stability the wings provide also reduces the mechanical irritation to the vein after insertion. A short strip of tape should be placed over the plastic wings to anchor the needle. The tubing should be looped and taped independently to prevent a pull on the tubing from dislodging the needle. Scalp vein needles with self-sealing caps at the end of the tubing are available for use when intravenous therapy is intermittent. Armboards are useful for immobilizing the extremity when a long infusion is planned or sudden movements, such as vomiting, are anticipated. Tape placed over the needle and tubing should not be secured to the armboard, nor should it tightly constrict any part of the hand or arm.

Although peripheral intravenous catheters (plastic, Teflon, or silicone elastomer) can facilitate prolonged therapy, there is an increased risk of thrombophlebitis and infection. To minimize these risks, strict aseptic technique must be observed during insertion, and catheters must be anchored carefully. These catheters are employed for longer term therapy (>24 hours) than are scalp vein needles. They are also better tolerated by patients requiring more mobilization because they are less likely to infiltrate. When intermittent therapy is needed, sterile saline can be used to maintain these devices in patients for whom heparin is contraindicated. Once taught how to care for the IV, patients who might otherwise remain hospitalized for chemotherapy can often be treated as outpatients.

Chemotherapeutic agents that are to be administered daily or twice daily and do not cause local tissue damage are well suited for administration through both peripheral catheters and scalp vein needles. If an agent that is a tissue vesicant is to be administered, the area above the venipuncture site should not be obscured with tape until after the drug has been infused. This permits the site to be observed carefully for any subtle evidence of extravasation. If given peripherally, blood return should be checked frequently during the infusion, again to ensure venous patency.

Central Venous Catheters and Infusion Pumps

For patients in whom vascular access is difficult and for those requiring parenteral nutrition, frequent administration of blood products and/or drugs that are irritating to peripheral veins, use of central venous catheters, such as the Hickman, Groshong, and Broviac catheters, represents a major advance in supportive care. These catheters come in a variety of gauges and may be single-, double-, or triple-lumen. Composed of flexible and nonirritating silicone, these catheters are placed into the subclavian, cephalic, or external jugular vein and are tunneled subcutaneously to an exit site approximately 10 cm from the point of insertion. A Dacron cuff on the surface of the catheter is positioned about 2 cm from the exit site. This cuff elicits a fibroblastic reaction in the subcutaneous tissue, firmly securing the catheter and providing a mechanical barrier to microorganisms.[5,9–11] When a central line is to be used for hyperalimentation, drug administration, and blood withdrawal, a multilumen catheter must always be inserted so that one line can be used exclusively for parenteral nutrition. Numerous studies have shown these catheters to be practical and safe. Successful maintenance of indwelling catheters over a prolonged period is highly dependent on the use of aseptic procedures for care of the catheter and the exit site.[6,12] Therefore, patient and family education and participation are critical from the moment of insertion. The patient's understanding and willingness to participate in the daily care of the catheter must be thoroughly assessed.

When a patient is unable or unwilling to assume responsibility for the care of the catheter and the exit site, a totally implantable injection port (Infusaport, Port-a-cath, Mediport) provides a possible alternative to be explored.[5,10,12,13] The cosmetic advantage, convenience, and ease of maintenance make them quite acceptable to patients. Infusion ports consist of a reservoir that is implanted in a subcutaneous pocket under local anesthesia and a silicon catheter that is threaded through the subclavian vein to the superior vena cava. A 22-gauge non-coring Huber needle is used to penetrate a silicone diaphragm at the surface of the reservoir when drugs are to be infused. These ports may provide either a Hickman or Groshong-type tip and may have either a single or double lumen port available for infusion. Monthly flushing of the port is required when not in use.

Studies have shown that silver sulfadiazine and chlorhexadine catheter coatings and catheter cuffs impregnated with silver decrease the risk of catheter-related bacteremia.[14] Other innovations include increased use of peripherally inserted central catheters (PICC) and miniature port systems that can be implanted in the forearm (Passport). Both of these catheters are generally well tolerated by patients.

When an intravenous infusion of chemotherapy must be timed precisely, portable volumetric pumps that provide constant flow rates are useful.[5,10] Two classes of devices include powered syringe pumps and battery-powered peristaltic pumps.[11,14] While these pumps are well suited for ambulatory patients, they also require patient participation for successful use. Therefore, good vision, manual dexterity, and the ability to learn and follow instructions reliably are important considerations. The nurse must be well versed in pump care and maintenance in order to safely administer and monitor pump infusions.

Complications of Parenteral Therapy

Infection is the most serious complication of parenteral therapy. Almost all infections are preventable if insertion and maintenance techniques preserve sterility.[15] Most nosocomial infections develop at the puncture site in peripheral IVs, or at the exit site in a central venous catheter. These sites should be inspected regularly. Inevitably, the organisms involved are normal skin flora that have entered the body via the intravenous needle or catheter. In granulocytopenic patients, special attention must be paid to preserving the sterility of all in-line filters, stopcocks, tubing, and solutions, especially those rich in glucose.

The most common complications of intravenous therapy in peripheral veins are thrombophlebitis and infiltration with extravasation of the infusate. Whenever patients complain of pain during an infusion, the site should be carefully inspected. If no obvious sign of thrombophlebitis or infiltration are present, the infusion should be slowed and heat applied. If the discomfort is caused by venous spasm, heat will relieve pain by dilating the vessel and increasing the blood flow. Heat will not relieve pain caused by thrombophlebitis.

In addition to pain, thrombophlebitis produces erythema and tenderness along the length of the vessel. If the inflammation is severe, swelling, induration, and a tender palpable venous cord will also develop. Major factors contributing to the development of thrombophlebitis include cannula/catheter composition, site of insertion, trauma during insertion, blood flow, mechanical irritation, irritating diluents and drug additives, microparticulates, the duration of infusion, hypertonicity, highly acidic or alkaline pH, concentrations, and microbial contamination. The use of in-line final filters has been shown to reduce the incidence of thrombophlebitis caused by contaminated and particulate matter that is introduced during admixture procedures.

Local hypersensitivity ("flare") reactions, manifested by urticaria, erythematous streaking occurring within minutes with or without localized pruritus, and/or pain, have been reported with at least two agents: doxorubicin and daunorubicin. Pain associated with this type of reaction is often a dull ache over the course of the vein as opposed to localized burning or stinging. Although this type of reaction generally remains localized, at least one case of anaphylaxis has occurred with doxorubicin. Resolution of symptoms associated with hypersensitivity reactions generally occur spontaneously within 30–90 minutes, and the agent can be administered in a new vein without the reaction recurring.[8,16]

Mechlorethamine frequently produces venous discoloration and severe chemical phlebitis 1 to 3 days after administration even when administered as a slow bolus into a large vein. Dacarbazine (DTIC) and carmustine (BCNU), among others (Table 22-4), also cause irritation of the vascu-

TABLE 22–4. DRUGS REPORTED AS BEING IRRITANTS WHEN EXTRAVASATED

Bleomycin (Blenoxane)
Carmustine (BCNU)
Cisplatin (Platinol)
Dacarbazine (DTIC)
Etoposide (VP-16, Vepesid)
Mithramycin (Mithracin)
Paclitaxel (Taxol)
Streptozocin (Zanosar)
Teniposide (VM-16)
Thiotepa (TSPA)

lar endothelium and often produce venous spasm, severe pain, and evidence of thrombophlebitis during and following infusion. An attempt should be made to alleviate the pain by increasing the volume of fluid in which the agent is diluted and slowing the rate of infusion, because venous spasm can restrict blood flow and increase the risk of extravasation. Application of heat during the infusion can also reduce discomfort.

If the needle is dislodged or if the vein bursts during an infusion, infiltration and extravasation of the infusant into tissues can occur. Many chemotherapeutic agents, as well as other solutions that are hypertonic and/or highly acidic or alkaline, can cause serious tissue damage if extravasated. While pain and burning are often early indicators of an infiltration, even the most potent tissue vesicants can extravasate without producing immediate symptoms. Any evidence of infiltration (blanching, edema, unexplained slowing of the infusion, or loss of blood return) should be considered sufficient cause to interrupt an infusion when a solution containing chemotherapy is administered. Even if the agent is not a tissue vesicant, extravasation of the drug into tissues adversely affects drug absorption, reducing the potential therapeutic effect, and predisposes the area to infection.

Although generally safe, the use of indwelling catheters is associated with some complications. Catheter-related thrombosis and infection are two of the most common and clinically important complications associated with central catheters. When thrombi occur at the tip of the catheter, low doses of urokinase can lyse them, preserving catheter function.[17–19] Problems requiring catheter removal include catheter displacement, drug infiltration, mechanical damage, thrombophlebitis, cellulitis, and, occasionally, retrograde drug extravasation in the tunnel.[18–21]

The presence of a blood return or the absence of blanching and/or edema are not sufficient proof that all of the solution is entering the vein. If the posterior wall of the vessel has been punctured during venipuncture, some infusant can extravasate without obvious signs of infiltration. If enough of the needle's bevel remains in the vein, a good blood return may be apparent and blanching or edema may not be evident. Thus, since prevention of extravasation is key, the practitioner is wise to stop the infusion and restart elsewhere if the integrity of the IV is in question.[16,22]

Management of Extravasation

Numerous chemotherapeutic agents cause tissue toxicity when extravasated (Table 22-5). There are minimal data in humans linking the dose of drug extravasated and the degree of tissue damage. What is known is that recognizing extravasated tissue damage early and keeping the damaged area as minimal as possible are the two most significant factors of treatment.[20–24] Preclinical studies suggest that the degree of necrosis that occurs following extravasation of a given dose of a known tissue vesicant varies widely. The degree of tissue damage caused by drug extravasation in humans appears to be related to the concentration of the drug and the quantity of drug extravasated. However, management of local tissue toxicity following extravasation in humans is anecdotal and controversial. This factor should be considered when evaluating the potential of an antidote with efficacy in animal models.[2] Data supporting therapeutic efficacy should be divided into three major categories: therapeutic efficacy clinically suggested by case reports in the literature; efficacy suggested by animal studies without the benefit of clinical testing; and efficacy suggested by theoretical mechanism of action.

TABLE 22–5. DRUGS REPORTED AS BEING VESICANTS WHEN EXTRAVASATED

Amsacrine (M-AMSA)
Daunorubicin (Cerubidine)
Dactinomycin (Cosmagen)
Doxorubicin (Adriamycin)
Epirubicin
Estramustine phosphate (Estracyte)
Idarubicin
Mechlorethamine (Mustargen)
Mitomycin C (Mutamycin)
Vinblastine (Velban)
Vincristine (Oncovin)
Vindesine (Eldisine)

If an extravasation antidote is to be administered intravenously, every attempt should be made to aspirate any residual drug remaining in the needle, tubing, and tissues prior to the administration of the antidote. Specific antidotes that are recommended by the manufacturer include isotonic sodium thiosulfate for mechlorethamine extravasations, and heat combined with hyaluronidase (to promote drug absorption) for vincristine and vinblastine extravasations. The management of doxorubicin extravasation is generally recognized as one of the most troublesome problems in the administration of cancer chemotherapy, causing tissue damage that ranges from erythema, induration, and pain to extensive tissue necrosis requiring surgical debridement and split skin grafting, infection, and contractures. None of the proposed pharmacologic antidotes (sodium bicarbonate, corticosteroids, dimethyl sulfoxide, alpha tocoherol, N-acetylcystein, glutathione, lidocaine, diphenhdramine, cimetidine, propranolol, and isoproterenol) has demonstrated efficacy conclusively. Current data indicate that the immediate application of cold packs for 6 to 10 hours is an effective intervention in the mouse and pig.[15,25] Anatomical similarities between pig and human skin lend particular credence to the pig as a model. Therefore, a high index of suspicion, early detection and interruption of extravasating doxorubicin infusions, aspiration of residual drug, and careful observation with application of cold packs for 6 to 10 hours is the treatment of choice. Recently, more anecdotal reports have been generated concerning doxorubicin and mytomycin C extravasation studies using topical DMSO as an effective treatment.[20,21,23,24] These reports show great promise, but further research is needed. If an extravasation should occur, photos should be taken as soon as possible and with each follow-up appointment in order to keep abreast of tissue changes and treatment efficacy.

Prevention is still the best way to avoid local tissue toxicity. Therefore, only individuals who are skilled in IV therapy and familiar with the drugs and their toxic effects should administer these drugs. As clinical data become available, recommendations may change. Therefore, it is essential for those administering drugs that are tissue vesicants to remain current with the literature on the management of chemotherapy extravasation.[1,6,7,15,16,20–26]

Legal Implications of Expanded Roles in Chemotherapy

The state laws that govern intravenous therapy and the administration of parenteral drugs by registered nurses vary.[2] To permit nurses to assume responsibilities in this area, most states adopt consensus statements issued jointly by the state's medical society, nursing association, and the hospital association. While the content varies from state to state, these policy statements acknowledge intravenous therapy as an area where medical and nursing practice overlap, as well as describe the accountabilities and liabilities that are shared. Each employer must establish standards of practice that ensure that a nurse is qualified by knowledge, skill, and experience to administer intravenous chemotherapy.

The nurse must have a written order that specifies which patient is to be treated and the manner in which treatment is to be administered (*e.g.*, IV push, rapid infusion) that is signed and dated by a physician. The nurse can be held negligent if an incorrect drug or dosage is administered, even if the physician's order is incorrect. Negligence is defined as conduct that produces harm and falls below the standard of care for professional practice in a specific area. An oncology nurse is expected to act with the care and skill that any responsible and prudent nurse would employ under similar circumstances. Nurses have a legal responsibility to understand the purpose and effects of each chemotherapeutic agent that is prescribed. If there is any doubt about the accuracy of the drug, the dosage, or the manner in which the drug is to be administered, the order must be verified with the physician before it is carried out or the nurse will be liable for negligence if harm to the patient results.

Each institution should have standing physician orders/protocols describing actions the nurse should undertake in the event of a vesicant extravasation. Should an event take place, the nurse should immediately stop the infusion and act prudently according to the institutional protocol, and the physician should be notified immediately. All actions and patient responses should be thoroughly documented. In general, an oncology nurse will not be held liable for harm that results to a patient if the policies and procedures that have been developed as the standard of care for the institution have been followed.

Risk Associated with Handling of Antineoplastic Agents

A letter published in Lancet in 1979 reported that significant levels of mutagenic activity could be detected in the urine of nurses preparing chemotherapeutic agents and in the urine of patients receiving the drugs, while mutagenic activity could not be detected in the urine of unexposed workers in the same general environment. This report and data on the mutagenicity and carcinogenicity of many cancer chemotherapeutic agents have led to increasing concern about whether there is a significant cancer risk associated with the preparation of antineoplastic agents for intravenous administration. Although there is no evidence that handling antineoplastic drugs has caused cancer in any individual, concern about the potential occupational risk to pharmacists and nurses has prompted several studies that have attempted to determine whether mutagenic activity is a reliable assay of occupational exposure. Studies at the M.D. Anderson Hospital in Houston performed in a small group of pharmacists wearing protective apparel, who prepared drugs using laminar airflow cabinets, have found that mutagenic activity could not be detected in the urine when vertical laminar flow safety cabinets were used, whereas mutagenic activity *could* be detected when horizontal laminar flow cabinets were used. These data suggest that aerosolization of the agents during reconstitution represents a source of exposure and have led most institutions to recommend the use of class II vertical flow safety cabinets and gloves as precautionary measures to minimize the risk of exposure.

Although the precise risk of exposure to chemotherapeutic agents is unknown, available data dictate prudence in the preparation of injectable antineoplastic agents.[27–29] In the absence of definitive data, the following guidelines have been recommended by the Occupational Safety and Health Administration (OSHA), the American Society of Hospital Pharmacists (ASHP), the Oncology Nursing Society (ONS), and the Division of Safety of the National Institutes of Health (NIH).[23,27–29]

- A special preparation area should be set aside for the preparation of injectable agents. Drug reconstitution should be performed in a class II type B vertical flow biologic safety cabinet. The exhaust should be vented to the outdoors to limit possible exposure to personnel. This cabinet should be inspected periodically, as designated by OSHA guidelines.
- A disposable plastic-backed sheet of absorbent paper should be used to cover the work surface inside the cabi-

net to permit complete cleanup of inadvertent spills. The paper should be changed after any overt spills. Luer-lock equipment should be used to avoid possible leakage during preparation or administration.

- Non-powdered, thick latex gloves (chemotherapy gloves) should be worn and discarded if holes develop. A long-sleeved gown with elastic cuffs should be worn to protect the skin from drug contact. The gown should be lint-free and with low permeability.
- Drug ampules should be opened away from the face. The ampules should be wrapped with an alcohol pad at the anticipated breakpoint to minimize the risk of inhaling powders or aerosols and to protect against broken glass.
- When reconstituting a drug, the diluent should be injected slowly down the side of the vial. The vial should be vented with a device using a 0.22-μm hydrophobic filter. The needle should be kept from coming in contact with the solution, and air should be allowed back in the syringe to equalize pressure.
- A sterile alcohol swab should be placed over the needle as it is withdrawn from the vial to prevent aerosolization.
- The needle should be covered by a sterile alcohol swab or a sealed waste bottle when air bubbles are ejected from a filled syringe to prevent aerosolization.
- After reconstitution, the old needle should be replaced by a new one. A volume of air that is less than the volume of drug solution to be withdrawn should be introduced into the vial. When the reconstituted drug is withdrawn, excess solution should be injected into a waste bottle. Avoid overfilling syringes, bags, or bottles.
- IV tubing should be primed before adding cytotoxic drugs to the IV bag.
- The external surface of syringes and IV bottles should be wiped clean after reconstitution and/or admixture procedures and properly labeled as containing cytotoxic materials and dated.
- Contaminated needles and syringes should be disposed of in a leak-proof puncture-resistant container. Needles should not be recapped. Clipping of needles is not recommended because aerosols can be generated.
- Following completion of drug preparation, the interior of the safety cabinet should be washed with water followed by 70% alcohol. The cabinet should be decontaminated weekly or if a spill occurs.
- Protective clothing must be discarded in a separate waste container labeled as containing cytotoxic waste.
- Hands should be washed carefully after gloves are removed.

OSHA and ONS have also established guidelines regarding the safety of nursing personnel administering chemotherapy. Each institution should be aware of these guidelines and incorporate them into their policies and procedures for chemotherapy administration.

- Wash hands and don appropriate protective garb. Non-powdered, thick latex gloves (chemotherapy gloves) should be worn. These should be discarded if holes develop. A long-sleeved gown that is lint free, has low permeability, and with elastic cuffs should be worn. Gloves should overlap the cuffs of the gown.
- A disposable plastic-backed sheet of absorbent paper should be used to cover the work surface.
- A "back flow" method of priming tubing should be used if the pharmacist has not attached tubing to the IV bag. This ensures that no aerosolization or spill occurs.
- All tubing and syringes should have Luer-lock fittings and should be inspected for leakage. If any droplets are noted, they should be wiped with gauze.
- When administration of the chemotherapy is completed, the nurse should discard the protective garb in an appropriate container labeled as cytotoxic waste. Finally, hands should be washed.[28,29]

The disposal of antineoplastic drugs and contaminated materials presents another potential source of drug exposure to health care personnel. To ensure that all materials are handled properly, each syringe and IV bottle sent to a clinic or an inpatient unit should be labeled with instructions indicating the item should not be discarded with general waste. Cytotoxic drugs are categorized as regulated wastes. Needles, syringes, empty drug vials and ampules, gloves, used alcohol swabs, IV bags and tubing, and the like should be carefully packaged in leak-proof puncture-resistant containers labeled "cytotoxic waste only." These containers should be disposed of according to federal, state, and local requirements. Because the ultimate fate and effect of introducing these drugs into the environment by disposing of them with incineration and the use of landfills are not known, the NIH and OSHA are committed to further investigation into disposal options.

Every institution should have emergency spill kits with an appropriate policy in place to guide health professionals. Nurses and physicians should be instructed on the safe handling of chemotherapy for their own protection and that of their patients.

REFERENCES

1. Reymann P. Chemotherapy: Principles of administration. In Groenwald S, Frogge M, Goodman M, Yarbro C (eds). Cancer Nursing: Principles and Practice. Boston, Jones and Bartlett, 1993:294–327
2. Hubbard SM, Seipp CA. Administration of cancer treatments: Practical guide for physicians and nurses. In DeVita VT Jr, Hellman S, Rosenberg SA (eds). Cancer: Principles and Practice of Oncology. Philadelphia, JB Lippincott, 1985:2189–2223
3. Plummer AL. Principles and Practice of Intravenous Therapy. Boston, Little, Brown & Co, 1982

4. Knobf MK. Intravenous therapy guidelines for oncology practice. Oncol Nurs Forum 9:30–34, 1982
5. Current concepts in chemotherapy administration. Semin Oncol Nurs 3(2)1–161, 1987
6. Berman A, Chisholm L, de Carvalho M, et al. Cancer chemotherapy: Intravenous administration. Cancer Nursing 16:145–160, 1993
7. Wood L, Gullo S. IV vesicants: How to avoid extravasation. Am J Nurs 93(4):42–46, 1993
8. Tully JL, Friedlan GH, Baldini LM, Goldmann DA. Complications of intravenous therapy with steel needles and teflon catheters. Am J Med 70:702–706, 1981
9. Meguid MM, Eldar S, Wahga A. The delivery of nutritional support. A potpourri of new devices and methods. Cancer 55:279–289, 1985
10. Jenkins J. Parenteral chemotherapy. In Johnson BL, Gross J (eds). Handbook of Oncology Nursing. New York, John Wiley & Sons, 1985: 535–566
11. Carlson RW, Sikic BI. Continuous infusion or bolus injection in cancer chemotherapy. Ann Intern Med 99:823–833, 1983
12. Strum S, McDermed J, Korn A, Joseph C. Improved methods for venous access: The Port-a-Cath, a totally implanted catheter system. J Clin Oncol 4:596–603, 1986
13. Gyres J, Ensminger W, Neiderhuber JE. A totally implanted system for intravenous chemotherapy for blood sampling and chemotherapy administration. JAMA 251:2538–2541, 1984
14. Groeger JS, Lucas AB, Coit D. Venous access in the cancer patient. PPO Updates 3:1–14, 1991
15. Dorr RT, Alberts DS. Cold protection and heat enhancement of doxorubicin skin toxicity in the mouse. Cancer Treat Rep 69:431–437, 1985
16. Goodman M, Ladd L, Purl S. Integumentary and mucous membrane alterations. In Groenwald S, Frogge M, Goodman M, Yarbro C (eds). Cancer Nursing: Principles and Practice, Boston, Jones and Bartlett, 1993: 749–757
17. Legha SS, Haq M, Rabinowitz M et al. Evaluation of silicone elastomer catheters for long-term intravenous chemotherapy. Arch Intern Med 145:1208–1211, 1985
18. Anderson A, Krasnow S. Thrombosis: The major Hickman catheter complication in patients with solid tumor. Chest 95:71–75, 1989
19. Brown-Smith J, Stoner M, Barley Z. Tunneled catheter thrombosis: Factors related to incidence. Oncology Nursing Forum 17:543–549, 1990
20. Bertelli G, Dini D, Forno G, et al. Dimethylsulphoxide and cooling after extravasation of antitumor agents. Lancet 341:1098–1099, 1993
21. Tsavaris N, Komitsopoulou P, Karagiaouris P, et al. Prevention of tissue necrosis due to accidental extravasation of cytostatic drugs by a conservative approach. Cancer Chemother Pharmacol 30:330–333, 1992
22. Cancer chemotherapy guidelines and recommendations for the management of vesicant extravasation. Module V. Pittsburgh, Oncology Nursing Society, 1992
23. Recommended practices for personnel administering parenteral cytotoxic drugs. Recommendations for safe handling of parenteral antineoplastic drugs. Bethesda, MD, Division of Safety, National Institutes of Health, 1992. DHHS, PHS, NIH Publication No. 92-2621
24. Alberts D, Dorr R. Case report: Topical DMSO for mytomycin-C induced skin ulceration. Oncology Nursing Forum 18:693–695, 1991
25. Harwood KV, Bachur N. Evaluation of DMSO and local cooling as antidotes for doxorubicin extravasation in a pig model. Oncol Nurs Forum 14:39–43, 1987
26. Dorr RT. Antidotes to vesicant chemotherapy extravasations. Blood Rev:41–60, 1990
27. American Society of Hospital Pharmacists. ASHP Technical Assistance Bulletin on handling cytotoxic drugs in hospitals. Am J Hosp Pharm 42:131–137, 1985
28. Occupational Safety and Health Administration. Work Practice Guidelines for Personnel Dealing with Cytotoxic Drugs. Washington, D.C., US Department of Labor Publication 8-1.1, 1986
29. Oncology Nursing Society. Safe Handling of Cytotoxic Drugs. Pittsburgh, PA: Oncology Nursing Society, 1989

GENERAL REFERENCES

American Hospital Formulary Services Drug Information. Bethesda, MD, American Society of Hospital Pharmacists, 1993

Balis FM, Poplack DG. Central nervous system pharmacology of antileukemic drugs. Am J Ped Hematol Oncol 11:74–86, 1989

Bronner AK, Hood AF. Cutaneous complications of chemotherapeutic agents. J Am Acad Dermatol 9:645–663, 1983

Calabresi P, Chabner BA. Chemotherapy of neoplastic disease. In Gilman AG, Rall TW, Nies AS, Taylor P (eds). Goodman and Gilman's The Pharmacological Basis of Therapeutics. 8th ed. New York, Pergamon, 1990: 1202–1263

Chabner BA, Collins JM (eds). Cancer Chemotherapy: Principles and Practice. Philadelphia, JB Lippincott, 1990

Chabner BA, Myers CE. Antitumor antibiotics. In DeVita VT Jr, Hellman S, Rosenberg SA (eds). Cancer: Principles and Practice of Oncology. 4th ed. Philadelphia, JB Lippincott, 1993: 374–384

Chapman R. Effect of cytotoxic therapy on sexuality and gonadal function. Semin Oncol 9:84–94, 1982

Coleman CN, Tucker MA. Secondary cancers. In DeVita VT Jr, Hellman S, Rosenberg SA (eds). Cancer: Principles and Practice of Oncology. 3rd ed. Chap. 60. Philadelphia, JB Lippincott, 1989

Dorr RT, Von Hoff DD. Cancer Chemotherapy Handbook. New York, Elsevier North-Holland, 1993

Ginsberg SJ, Comis RL. The pulmonary toxicity of antineoplastic agents. Semin Oncol 9:34–51, 1982

Lokich JJ (ed): Cancer chemotherapy by infusion. Lancaster, England, MTP Press, 1987

NCI Investigational Drugs. Pharmaceutical Data, 1986. Washington, D.C., NIH Publication No. 86-2141, 1986

Olin BR, Hebel SK, Dombek CE (eds). Drug Facts and Comparisons. St. Louis, Wolters Kluwer Co, 1993.

Perry MC, Yarbro JW (eds). Toxicities of Chemotherapy. Orlando, Grune & Stratton, 1984

Pinedo HM, Longo DL, Chabner BA. Cancer Chemotherapy and Biological Response Modifiers. Annual 14. Amsterdam, Elsevier, 1993

Sherins RJ, Mulvihill JJ. Gonadal dysfunction. In DeVita VT Jr, Hellman S, Rosenberg SA (eds). Cancer: Principles and Practice of Oncology. 4th ed. Philadelphia, JB Lippincott, 1989: 2170–2180

Sulkes A, Collins JM. Reappraisal of some dosage adjustment guidelines. Cancer Treat Rep 71:229–233, 1987

Trissel LA. Handbook on Injectable Drugs. Bethesda, MD, American Society of Hospital Pharmacists, Inc, 1986

Von Hoff DD, Rozencweig M, Piccant M. The cardiotoxicity of anticancer agents. Semin Oncol 9:23–33, 1982

Warren RD, Bender RA. Drug interactions with antineoplastic agents. Cancer Treat Rep 61:1231–1241, 1977

Wittes RE, Adrianza ME, Parsons R et al. Compilation of Phase II results with single antineoplastic agents. Cancer Treatment Symposia 4:1–471, 1985

John S. Macdonald, Daniel G. Haller, Robert J. Mayer, Eds. *Manual of Oncologic Therapeutics*, Third Edition.

23. HORMONAL THERAPY OF CANCER

Charles L. Shapiro
Philip W. Kantoff

Steroid hormones are required for the growth and function of the breast, endometrium, and prostate. Cancers that arise in these tissues also depend on steroid hormones, and a variety of therapeutics are based on steroid hormone deprivation or steroid hormone antagonism. The specificity of these agents for their receptors allows these agents to be used with relatively low toxicity. Steroid hormones are being tested as cancer preventatives in high-risk populations.

MECHANISM OF STEROID HORMONE ACTION

Steroid hormones are derived from side chain modifications of the cholesterol molecule in the ovary, adrenal gland, and testes. The synthesis and release of steroid hormones is regulated by the pituitary gonadotropins luteinizing hormone (LH), follicle-stimulating hormone (FSH), and adrenocorticotropin hormone (ACTH). Pituitary gonadotropins are regulated in turn by the pulsatile release of hypothalamic releasing factors, and the plasma levels of steroid hormones, which exert a negative feedback on the release of pituitary gonadotropins and hypothalamic releasing factors.

The source of estrogen varies according to menopausal status. Before menopause the majority of the estrogen (as estradiol) is produced by the ovary in response to LH and FSH. Progesterone is produced by the corpus luteum of the ovary after ovulation. A smaller amount of estrogen in premenopausal women is derived from androstenedione, a weak androgen produced by the adrenal gland. Androstenedione is converted to estrogen in adipose and other peripheral tissues by an aromatase reaction. After menopause, ovarian estrogen production ceases, and the primary source of estrogen is the peripheral conversion of androstenedione to estrogen.

In men the principle source of androgen is from the testis in the form of testosterone. Weaker androgens are also produced by the adrenal gland, specifically androstenedione and dihydroepiandrostenedione. Testosterone and the weaker adrenal androgens are converted to the more potent androgen dihydrotestosterone (DHT) via the enzyme 5-alpha reductase in prostate and other androgen sensitive tissues. DHT is required for male secondary sex characteristics, and for the maintenance of spermatogenesis.

Tissue responsiveness to steroid hormones is mediated by specific receptors localized in the nucleus of the cell. Steroid hormone receptors and those for vitamin D, thyroid hormone, and retinoic acid share a similar structure and a common ancestry. The receptor protein is comprised of several distinct regions, or domains, which are critical to its function. These include a domain for binding the specific steroid hormone or ligand, and a highly conserved domain that binds deoxyribonucleic acid (DNA). Before binding steroid hormone, the receptor is inactive and complexed to a heat shock protein (HSP). After binding steroid hormone, the receptor is activated and disassociates from the HSP. The activated receptor binds to DNA via the DNA-binding domain, and this results in an increase in the activity of transcription factors that increase the transcription of certain target genes. These target genes are responsible for effects of steroid hormones.

The precise mechanism by which the activated receptor increases the transcription of target genes is unknown, as are the identities of all the relevant target genes. However, one important class of target genes whose expression is increased in response to steroid hormones includes growth factors and growth factor receptors. The production of growth factors and their receptors is postulated to regulate the normal growth of hormone responsive tissues and the aberrant growth of their neoplastic counterparts. The expression of a number of epithelial cell growth factors and their receptors increases in response to steroid hormones and promotes cell growth via autocrine and/or paracrine feedback loops (Table 23-1). Growth inhibitory factors are also produced in response to steroid hormones. For example, transforming growth factor-alpha (TGF-alpha) and related peptides stimulate the growth of human breast cancer cells. In hormone-sensitive breast cancer cells estrogens increase the expression of TGF-alpha and of the epidermal growth factor receptor (EGFR). TGF-alpha acts as a ligand for the EGFR, forming an autocrine pathway. Conversely, TGF-beta and related peptides are a family of growth inhibitory peptides found in normal breast epithelium. TGF-beta inhibits breast cancer cell growth and is produced in response to treatment with antiestrogens. Thus, the link between steroid hormones and growth factors provides a biologic rationale for the well established clinical observation that steroid hormone deprivation or steroid hormone antagonists may inhibit malignant epithelial growth.

The effects of hormone therapy are realized through steroid hormone deprivation or steroid hormone antagonism (Table 23-2). Because the source of estrogen varies before and after menopause, methods for estrogen deprivation dif-

TABLE 23–1. EPITHELIAL GROWTH FACTORS AND RECEPTORS THAT INCREASE IN RESPONSE TO STEROID HORMONES

RESPONDER	ACTION
GROWTH FACTOR	
Transforming growth factor-alpha	Stimulatory
Transforming growth factor-beta	Inhibitory
Insulin-like growth factor-1	Stimulatory
Platelet-derived growth factor	Stimulatory
Cathepsin D	Stimulatory
RECEPTOR	
Epidermal growth factor receptor	
Insulin-like growth factor-1 receptor	

fer in pre- and postmenopausal women. Ovarian estrogen may be diminished by surgical or irradiation-induced ovarian ablation, or alternatively with GnRH agonists. The GnRH agonists reversibly suppress ovarian function by decreasing pituitary secretion of LH and FSH via the down regulation of GnRH receptors.

The methods of ovarian ablation listed above do not work in postmenopausal women because most of their estrogen is derived from the adrenal gland via the peripheral aromatase reaction. Previously, adrenalectomy and hypophysectomy were used to lower estrogen levels in postmenopausal women; these procedures, however, have been replaced by the use of drugs that are less toxic and equally efficacious. Aminoglutethemide, which inhibits the aromatase reaction and adrenal steroid production, is one such drug. The latter effect may result in adrenal insufficiency, so corticosteroids are usually administered in combination with aminoglutethemide. Several newer aromatase inhibitors are being tested in phase II clinical trials.

TABLE 23–2. MECHANISM OF ACTION OF HORMONE THERAPY

THERAPY	MECHANISM OF ACTION
STEROID HORMONE DEPRIVATION	
Ovarian ablation	Reduces estrogen; effective in premenopausal women only
Orchiectomy	Reduces testosterone
GnRH agonist	Lowers LH levels; therapy reduces estrogen; effective in premenopausal women only
	Reduces testosterone in men
Progestins	Effective in endometrial and prostate cancers and primarily postmenopausal breast cancer, mechanism unknown
Aminogluthemide	Reduces estrogen; effective in postmenopausal women only; reduces production of adrenal androgens in men
Estrogen	Reduces estrogen; effective primarily in postmenopausal women
	Reduces testosterone in men
Androgens	Reduces estrogen; effective primarily in postmenopausal women
STEROID HORMONE ANTAGONISTS	
Tamoxifen	Antiestrogen; effective in both pre- and postmenopausal women
Flutamide	Antiandrogen; blocks androgen receptor

Tamoxifen is similar in structure to estrogen and is a competitive inhibitor of the estrogen receptor. Hence, it is the prototypic steroid hormone antagonist. Unlike estrogen, when tamoxifen binds to the estrogen receptor the activation of transcription factors and the increased expression of the growth-promoting target genes does not occur. Tamoxifen, however, is not a pure estrogen antagonist. In bone, liver, and endometrium tamoxifen has estrogen-like agonist activity. Tamoxifen, like estrogen, preserves bone mineral density, lowers total cholesterol and low density lipoproteins, and may cause endometrial hyperplasia. In some trials a small increase in the risk of endometrial cancer has also been observed in breast cancer patients receiving adjuvant tamoxifen.

Several other forms of endocrine therapy have activity in breast cancer. The progestational agents include megestrol acetate and medroxyprogesterone acetate. The mechanism of action of these drugs is not known. It is possible that some of their effects are mediated through the lowering of pituitary gonadotrophins or via the progesterone receptor. The estrogen diethylstilbestrol (DES) and androgens are also effective in breast cancer, but current usage of these drugs is limited due to their side effects.

In males, androgens are of testicular and adrenal origin. Testicular androgen deprivation is accomplished by orchiectomy, or by using GnRH agonists, which in effect accomplishes a chemical castration. DES also lowers testosterone by lowering the levels of pituitary gonadotropins. This drug is used infrequently due to its side effects, in particular, cardiovascular toxicity at doses of 3 mg/day or greater. Androgen deprivation results in the loss of libido, hot flashes (particularly with GnRH agonists), and gynecomastia (particularly with DES).

Antiandrogens such as flutamide block the stimulatory effect of DHT on the androgen receptor. Finasteride, an inhibitor of 5-alpha reductase, has proven activity in the treatment of benign prostatic hyperplasia (BPH), but its value in prostate cancer remains to be defined. Megestrol acetate also has activity in prostate cancer but the mechanism of action is uncertain. Other drugs such as aminoglutethemide, ketoconazole, and corticosteroids inhibit adrenal androgen production and are believed to possess antitumor activity in prostate cancer. Testicular androgen ablation in the form of an orchiectomy or a GnRH analogue is considered standard therapy for metastatic prostate cancer.

There is mounting evidence that combined androgen

blockade, *i.e.*, simultaneous ablation of testicular and adrenal androgens (generally accomplished by the combined use of chemical or surgical castration and an antiandrogen) is superior to either treatment alone in advanced prostate cancer.

STEROID HORMONES AS CANCER RISK FACTORS

Several risk factors implicate the importance of steroid hormones in the development of breast, endometrial, and prostate cancer. Early menarche and late menopause increase the risk of breast cancer, and obesity, late menopause, and polycystic ovarian disease increase the risk of endometrial cancer. In each of these situations there is prolonged and/or increased exposure to endogenous estrogens. Likewise, the prolonged use of oral contraceptives (OCP) or estrogen replacement therapy increases the risks of endometrial cancer and possibly of breast cancer. In particular, some studies suggest that the use of OCP for more than 4 years or prolonged use prior to the first pregnancy may increase the risk of breast cancer. Adding progestins to the estrogen replacement formulation decreases the risk of endometrial cancer, but it is uncertain whether this affects the risk of breast cancer.

Alcohol is another breast cancer risk factor. In cohort and case-control studies a dose-dependent effect of alcohol on the subsequent risk of breast cancer has been observed. The mechanism for this is unknown, but young age at the time of the exposure may be a critical factor. Recently, a link between alcohol intake and levels of circulating estrogens has been described. In a controlled study the estrogen levels in normal menstruating women were higher when they were drinking moderate amounts of alcohol daily, compared to when they were not drinking any alcohol. Perhaps alcohol increases breast cancer risk by raising the levels of endogenous estrogens. This observation requires additional study before it can be confirmed.

Age of pregnancy has a differential effect on breast cancer risk. A first full-term pregnancy before the age of 18 lowers the lifetime risk of breast cancer by 50%. In contrast, a first full-term pregnancy after the age of 35 is associated with a higher risk of breast cancer. The protective effects of early pregnancy might result from a pregnancy-induced maturation and differentiation of the breast epithelium that lowers the susceptibility of these cells to subsequent neoplastic transformation. Alternatively, after pregnancy sustained decreases in prolactin secretion and increases in sex-hormone-binding protein occur. Although these changes are well documented, it is still uncertain whether they affect the breast cancer risk.

The relationship between serum androgen levels and the development of prostate cancer is less well understood. Epidemiologic studies suggest a possible link between androgen levels and prostate cancer. Although androgens are clearly required for the growth of prostate cancer, it is less certain whether androgens are required for the development of prostate cancer. In populations at low risk for prostate cancer, such as the Japanese, endogenous levels of the 5-alpha reductase enzyme tend to be lower than in populations with higher rates of prostate cancer. This enzyme is responsible for converting testosterone to the more potent androgen DHT. Some reports have linked the level of serum testosterone with the likelihood of developing prostate cancer.

SELECTION OF PATIENTS FOR HORMONE THERAPY

Steroid hormone receptors for estrogen and progesterone are routinely measured in breast and endometrial cancers to select those patients who are likely to benefit from hormone therapy. The primary breast cancers of about 50% of premenopausal and 80% of postmenopausal women are positive for estrogen receptors. Estrogen receptor positivity correlates with response to tamoxifen or other hormone therapy. Other factors that predict for response to hormone therapy in breast cancer patients are a prior response to hormone therapy, a long disease-free interval between the primary diagnosis and the first relapse, and non-visceral sites of metastases, *e.g.*, liver.

Less than 10% of estrogen-receptor-negative tumors respond to tamoxifen, whereas between 50% and 60% of estrogen-receptor-positive tumors initially respond. Although the primary effects of tamoxifen are mediated through the estrogen receptor, it is plausible that within predominantly receptor-negative tumors there are also some estrogen-receptor-positive clones. It is possible that paracrine growth inhibitory factors produced by the receptor positive cells in response to tamoxifen inhibit the growth of nearby receptor negative cells. Others have suggested that there are mechanisms independent of the steroid hormone receptor, or alternatively that the responses observed in receptor-negative tumors is primarily due to falsely negative receptor assays. Further clarification of this is expected from ongoing adjuvant studies in which endocrine therapy is used in receptor-negative breast cancer patients.

Endometrial cancers also express estrogen and progesterone receptors, and progestational agents are often the initial treatment for recurrent endometrial cancers. The overall response rate to progestational agents is about 35%. Response is best correlated to the progesterone receptor content and the histologic tumor grade. Tamoxifen and other endocrine therapies have been used to treat endometrial cancers, but the response rates are generally lower than with progestational agents.

Hormone therapy remains the most effective treatment for metastatic prostate cancer, with approximately 80% of patients responding to such treatment. Markers for sensitivity or resistance to such therapy including a reliable test for androgen receptor content, are lacking. Although only 20% of patients do not respond to hormone therapy, there is a great variety amongst patients in terms of duration of response. Duration of response appears to correlate inversely with overall tumor burden as measured by bone scan. Duration of response also seems to correlate inversely with pretreatment serum testosterone level.

MECHANISMS OF RESISTANCE TO HORMONE THERAPY

The development of resistance to initially effective hormone therapy is frequently observed. Several mechanisms for resistance have been proposed. Before treatment, tumors may contain populations of hormone-sensitive and -resistant cells. Treatment with hormone therapy selects for the resistant cell populations by eliminating the sensitive cells. Another possibility is that acquired mutations in the genes for steroid hormone receptors, transcription factors, or the relevant target genes might confer resistance. Finally, it has been demonstrated experimentally that alterations in the metabolism of tamoxifen may result in the formation of less potent antiestrogen metabolites, or even estrogenic metabolites that could stimulate growth. It is not clear whether such pathways are relevant to hormone resistance in the clinic.

HORMONE THERAPY FLARE

Clinical and scintigraphic flare may occur within days to weeks after the initiation of hormone therapy. Clinical flare is characterized by the onset of one or more of the following signs or symptoms: diffuse musculoskeletal pain, fever, hypercalcemia, and increased size and erythema of skin metastases. The mechanism of flare is not well understood. It may represent a transient increase in tumor growth, or a host reaction to changes in the tumor induced by hormone therapy. Flare has been observed in about 3% of tamoxifen-treated breast cancer patients, as well as following the initiation of every form of hormone therapy. The signs and symptoms of flare usually subside within weeks to months, and most patients should be supported to manage the symptoms. The development of flare after GnRH analogs in prostate cancer patients can be effectively blocked by the simultaneous administration of an androgen receptor blocker, such as flutamide.

Scintigraphic flare is a transient worsening of the radionuclide bone scan with increased activity in existing lesions and the appearance of new lesions. Like clinical flare it typically occurs soon after the initiation of hormone therapy, but it also has been observed after other forms of systemic therapy. Scintigraphic flare may occur as part of the clinical flare, or it may occur without any clinical manifestations. Scintigraphic flare has been observed in between one and two thirds of breast cancer patients with skeletal metastases, and is often associated with a subsequent response to the therapy. The practical problem is that the radiographic picture of scintigraphic flare is often indistinguishable from disease progression. If scintigraphic flare is not recognized, potentially effective systemic therapy may be withdrawn prematurely.

HORMONE THERAPY WITHDRAWAL RESPONSE

After initial response to hormone therapy, stopping the drug can result in a subsequent antitumor response. This so-called withdrawal response has been observed in patients with breast and prostate cancer, although the mechanism of the effect is not well understood. In patients with prostate cancer, this phenomenon is seen with the withdrawal of antiandrogens but has not been observed with withdrawal of other agents. Most frequently the withdrawal response occurs in patients who have previously responded to hormone therapy. Rarely, if ever, are withdrawal responses observed in patients who failed to respond initially to hormone therapy.

STEROID HORMONES AS CANCER PREVENTATIVES

The possible efficacy of steroid hormones in cancer prevention is being investigated intensely. Tamoxifen and retinoids are being tested in several randomized controlled clinical trials in women at increased risk of developing breast cancer. Tamoxifen reduces the frequency of new contralateral breast cancers in women receiving adjuvant tamoxifen for breast cancer. This observation provided the major impetus for ongoing controlled randomized trials designed to test whether tamoxifen can reduce the incidence of breast cancer in women at high risk of developing this disease. These trials will also evaluate the effect tamoxifen has on the risks of cardiovascular disease and osteoporosis.

Vitamin A and related retinoids are important regulators of epithelial cell growth and differentiation. Retinoids have been shown to reduce the frequency of second tumors of the aerodigestive tract in patients with head and neck cancers, and they induce a high rate of complete remissions in patients with acute promyelocyctic leukemia (APL). The characteristic chromosomal translocation in APL is between chromosomes 15 and 17, and the retinoic acid receptor gene is located at the breakpoint of chromosome 17. The retinoid receptors share homology with other steroid hormone receptors. Like other steroid hormones, the actions of the retinoids may be mediated through the increased expression of inhibitory growth factors such as transforming growth factor-beta. Retinoids inhibit the growth of human breast cancer cell lines, and can prevent the development of chemically-induced mammary tumors. These observations have led to clinical trials designed to test retinoids as breast cancer preventatives.

A large national study is underway testing the utility of finasteride in the prevention of prostate cancer. The rationale for using finasteride is its ability to diminish tissue levels of DHT via the inhibition of 5-alpha reductase.

BIBLIOGRAPHY

Brown M. Estrogen receptor molecular biology. Hematology/Oncology Clinics of North America: New Directions in Breast Cancer 8:101–112, 1994

Crawford ED, Eisenberger MA, McLeod DG et al. A controlled trial of leuprolide with and without flutamide in prostatic carcinoma. N Engl J Med 321:419–424, 1989

Friess G, Prébois C, Vignon F. Control of breast cancer cell growth by steroids and growth factors: Interactions and mechanisms. Breast Cancer Res Treat 27:57–68, 1993

Geller J. Basis for hormonal management of advanced prostate cancer. Cancer Supp 71:1039–1045, 1993

Henderson BE. Endogenous and exogenous endocrine factors. Hematology/Oncology Clinics of North America. Diagnosis and Therapy of Breast Cancer 3:577–598, 1989

Henderson IC. Endocrine therapy of metastatic breast cancer. In Harris JR, Hellman S, Henderson IC, Kinne DW (eds). Breast Diseases. Philadelphia, JB Lippincott 1991:559–603

Horwitz KB. Mechanisms of hormone resistance in breast cancer. Breast Cancer Res Treat 26:119–130, 1993

Pritchard KI. The use of endocrine therapy. Hematology/Oncology Clinics of North America. Diagnosis and Therapy of Breast Cancer 3:765–805, 1989

Scher HI, Kelly WK. Flutamide withdrawal syndrome: Its impact on clinical trials in hormone-refractory prostate cancer. J Clin Onc 11:1566–1572, 1993

Sutherland DJ, Mobbs BG. Hormones and cancer. In Tannock IF, Hill RP (eds). The Basic Science of Oncology. 2nd ed. New York, McGraw-Hill 1992:207–231

John S. Macdonald, Daniel G. Haller, Robert J. Mayer, Eds. *Manual of Oncologic Therapeutics*, Third Edition.

IV. TREATMENT OF SPECIFIC DISEASES

24. NON–SMALL CELL LUNG CANCER

Daniel C. Ihde

When considered as a group, squamous (epidermoid) carcinoma, adenocarcinoma, and large cell carcinoma of the lung comprise approximately 80% of all cases of lung cancer in the United States. Despite some differences in their natural histories, therapeutic issues in these three pathologic types of bronchogenic carcinoma are quite similar; they will be dealt with together in this chapter and will be collectively referred to as non–small cell lung cancer (NSCLC). The three cell types of NSCLC share the potential for surgical cure in a significant minority of patients and show only modest responsiveness to current chemotherapeutic agents.

Among the various pathologic types of NSCLC, the etiology of squamous carcinoma is most clearly related to cigarette smoking. Adenocarcinoma is more common in women and is the most frequent type of lung cancer in never-smokers, although the majority of patients with adenocarcinoma are current or former smokers. Distant metastases at diagnosis are more common than in squamous carcinoma. Large cell carcinoma is a pathologic "diagnosis of exclusion" when features of squamous or adenocarcinoma cannot be detected in available pathologic material.

Squamous carcinoma is more frequently confined to the thorax at postmortem examination than other types of NSCLC and thus might be expected to be treated more successfully with locoregional forms of therapy. This is indeed the case, especially for the most localized tumors, because surgical resection is more often curative in patients with squamous carcinoma. After radiation therapy of NSCLC confined to the thorax, sites of failure are more often locoregional in squamous cancer, whereas distant metastases to the brain and other distant sites more commonly herald initial relapse in large cell and adenocarcinoma. There is no convincing evidence, however, that the cell types of NSCLC differ in their responsiveness to chemotherapy.

The 5-year survival of all patients with NSCLC is approximately 15%, without marked improvement over the past two decades. These bleak results are due to the lack of any substantially effective treatment for the occult or overt distant metastases that are present in most patients at the time of diagnosis. Within the past few years, there has been some indication that cisplatin-based chemotherapy may produce modest survival benefit in certain groups of patients with NSCLC. Nevertheless, treatment of the majority of patients remains a frustrating experience for patient and physician alike.

PRETREATMENT EVALUATION

Pathologic Evaluation

Squamous carcinoma was the most common type of NSCLC in the past, but the incidence of adenocarcinoma appears to be increasing and now exceeds squamous cancer in frequency in many institutions. The reason for this changing incidence is unclear, but it may be due to the increasing incidence of lung cancer in women. Review of diagnostic material by an experienced lung cancer pathologist in all cases of NSCLC is of major importance, since some subtypes of small cell lung cancer, which is managed very differently from NSCLC, may be mistaken for NSCLC.

Procedures for Obtaining Initial Pathologic Diagnosis

Methods by which the initial pathologic diagnosis of lung cancer is commonly obtained include fiberoptic bronchoscopy, sputum cytology, mediastinoscopy, and percutaneous needle aspiration. Sometimes the diagnosis will be established only at thoracotomy; this occurs most frequently in patients in whom surgical resection is possible. If the initial diagnosis is made from examination of pleural fluid or a pleural biopsy, or from biopsy of a metastatic site such as supraclavicular lymph node, bone, or liver, the patient has inoperable lung cancer. In patients who present with superior vena cava obstruction, radiation therapy has sometimes been administered without a pathologic diagnosis. This practice is not often necessary, since the dangers of judicious diagnostic procedures in these patients are much less than previously thought and treatments for NSCLC, small cell lung cancer, and lymphoma, the three most common causes of this syndrome, are so different.

Staging Procedures

Staging is critical in determining appropriate therapy for patients with NSCLC. This consists of a combination of clinical (physical examination, imaging studies) and limited operative (bronchoscopy, mediastinoscopy) maneuvers and formal thoracotomy with complete pathologic examination of biopsied or resected material. Because complete surgical resection represents the only hope of cure for all but a few NSCLC patients, only unequivocally positive results of any staging test should prevent thoracotomy with the intent of completely resecting the tumor.

Patients with NSCLC are first evaluated to determine if they are operable or inoperable. Extent of tumor dissemination, inability to tolerate thoracotomy and pulmonary resection for medical reasons, and refusal to undergo surgery all make a patient inoperable. At thoracotomy patients are found to be either resectable, meaning all tumor can be completely excised with pathologically negative margins, or unresectable.

Physical examination and chest radiograph are performed in all patients with lung cancer. The extent of further preoperative evaluation in potentially operable patients is usually guided by the philosophy of the operating surgeon. Bronchoscopy is frequently performed to assess proximal endobronchial tumor extension and the status of the contralateral lung. Computed tomography (CT) of the chest is much more sensitive than a chest film in detecting mediastinal lymph node metastases or direct mediastinal or chest wall invasion. The frequency of false-positive CT scans of the mediastinum depends on the radiologic criteria for positivity — the more sensitive, the less specific — and the frequency of benign causes of lymph node enlargement in the patient population. These factors may vary considerably in different institutions.

Mediastinoscopy or mediastinotomy should be used only if positive findings would prevent thoracotomy. Many thoracic surgeons omit these procedures for peripheral lesions (where mediastinal lymph node involvement is infrequent), when mediastinal nodes are not enlarged on CT scan, or if a decision on resectability of mediastinal metastases can be made only at thoracotomy. Some surgeons prefer to evaluate the brain and adrenal glands by CT scanning before thoracotomy. It has been shown that radionuclide scans of brain, liver, and bone infrequently detect metastases in the absence of symptoms or abnormal findings on physical examination or blood tests, so they should not be routinely performed.

STAGING SYSTEM AND PROGNOSTIC FACTORS

The international TNM staging system for lung cancer, presented in Table 24–1, is divided into the occult stage and Stages 0, I, II, IIIa, IIIb, and IV. Stage I and II tumors are usually surgically resectable. Cancer in which the primary tumor or metastatic lymph nodes extend beyond the visceral pleural reflection but are still regionally confined are assigned to Stage III. Stage IIIa tumors are less advanced and may sometimes be surgically resected, whereas Stage IIIb tumors are virtually always unresectable but may sometimes be given radiation therapy with curative intent. Patients with Stage IV, or distant metastatic, cancer are currently incurable. At diagnosis, approximately one third of NSCLC cases will have Stage I or II disease; one third will have Stage IIIa or IIIb; and the remainder will have Stage IV.

The major prognostic factors in NSCLC are the extent of tumor dissemination as assessed by detailed TNM staging, performance status, and weight loss. Patients with resectable tumors usually have excellent performance status. When thoracotomy reveals that surgical resection can be performed, careful sampling of multiple mediastinal lymph-node-bearing areas allows better delineation of the extent of nodal spread and further clarifies postoperative prognosis.

TREATMENT

Occult Stage

Presumed NSCLC in the occult stage is a tumor that is proven by the presence of malignant cells in bronchopulmonary secretions but is not visible radiographically or bronchoscopically. Treatment requires localization of the cancer. Endoscopy of the upper aerodigestive tract is performed to exclude a primary cancer in these sites. Detailed, selective fiberoptic bronchoscopy under general anesthesia often will reveal the primary tumor, which is then treated appropriately according to its stage. Tumors discovered in this fashion are generally early stage invasive or *in situ* carcinomas with a tendency to multicentricity. After treatment of the initial cancer, as in patients with surgically resected Stage I and II

TABLE 24–1. INTERNATIONAL TNM STAGING SYSTEM FOR LUNG CANCER

TUMOR (T)

TX	Occult carcinoma (malignant cells in sputum or bronchial washings but tumor not visualized by imaging studies or bronchoscopy)
Tis	Carcinoma in situ
T1	Tumor 3 cm or less in greatest diameter, surrounded by lung or visceral pleura, but not proximal to a lobar bronchus on bronchoscopy
T2	Tumor greater than 3 cm in diameter, or with involvement of main bronchus at least 2 cm distal to carina, or with visceral pleural invasion, or with associated atelectasis or obstructive pneumonitis extending to the hilar region but not involving the entire lung
T3	Tumor invading chest wall, diaphragm, mediastinal pleura, or parietal pericardium; or tumor in main bronchus within 2 cm of but not invading carina; or atelectasis or obstructive pneumonitis of entire lung
T4	Tumor invading mediastinum, heart, great vessels, trachea, esophagus, vertebral body, or carina; or ipsilateral malignant pleural effusion

NODES (N)

N0	No regional lymph node metastases
N1	Metastases to ipsilateral peribronchial or hilar nodes
N2	Metastases to ipsilateral mediastinal or subcarinal nodes
N3	Metastases to contralateral mediastinal or hilar, or to any scalene or supraclavicular nodes

DISTANT METASTASES (M)

M0	No distant metastases
M1	Distant metastases

STAGE GROUPINGS

Occult	TX	N0	M0
Stage 0	TIS	N0	M0
Stage I	T1-2	N0	M0
Stage II	T1-2	N1	M0
IIIa	T3	N0–2	M0
	T1–3	N2	M0
IIIb	T4	N0–3	M0
	T1–4	N3	M0
Stage IV	Any T	Any N	M1

Modified from American Joint Committee on Cancer. Lung. Manual for Staging of Cancer. 4th ed. Philadelphia, JB Lippincott, 1992:115.

tumors, there is an increased likelihood of subsequent development of a second primary NSCLC and other smoking-related cancers.

Clinically Resectable Cancer (Stages I and II)

Surgical resection is the treatment of choice for patients with Stage I and II NSCLC. Careful preoperative assessment of cardiopulmonary status and the patient's ability to tolerate lung resection is required. Lobectomy, pneumonectomy, segmentectomy or wedge resection, and sleeve resection each may be indicated in selected situations, based on the surgeon's intraoperative findings. The procedure of choice will remove all of the tumor with adequate margins of resection and maximum conservation of normal lung tissue. Postoperative mortality of 3% for lobectomy and 5% to 8% for pneumonectomy can be anticipated.

Following complete resection of patients with clinical Stage I NSCLC, 5-year survival of approximately 45% is reported. The corresponding figure in clinical Stage II patients is approximately 25%. In patients with pathologic Stage I or II tumors proven by extensive sampling of mediastinal lymph nodes with negative pathologic findings, even higher survival rates can be expected.

There is no proven role for postoperative adjuvant radiotherapy, chemotherapy, or immunotherapy after complete surgical resection. Radiotherapy will reduce local recurrences in Stage II tumors, but a randomized study in patients with squamous carcinoma does not suggest any survival benefit. Two randomized studies found that combination chemotherapy prolongs time to tumor recurrence in resected Stage II patients, but proof of increased survival will be required before adjuvant chemotherapy can be recommended as standard treatment.

In medically inoperable clinical Stage I and II patients with sufficient pulmonary reserve, chest irradiation with curative intent should be administered. Five-year survival of 15% to 20% has been reported in this setting.

Advanced Locoregional Cancer (Stages IIIa and IIIb)

In the United States, radiation therapy alone has been the usual treatment for most patients with advanced locoregional NSCLC; selected cases undergo surgical resection with or without chest irradiation. Five-year survival of 5% to 10% is observed for all Stage III cases, but much better results can be anticipated in selected subsets of patients.

Approximately half of NSCLC patients receiving chest irradiation obtain objective tumor regression, but 5-year survival of only 4% to 8% is reported in several series of patients completing radiation therapy that was administered with curative intent. Such irradiation is usually not begun in patients with poor performance status, malignant pleural effusion, or bulky tumors and poor pulmonary function, and is not completed in those with early development of progressive tumor or distant metastases. Potentially curative radiation therapy is customarily administered to a total dose of 5500 to 6000 cGy in continuous fractionation using megavoltage equipment. Precise definition of target volume with the minimum possible dose to critical adjacent normal structures is needed; this requires the use of a simulator. The best outcome occurs in patients with excellent performance status and lesser tumor volume and in those in whom surgical unresectability was demonstrated only at thoracotomy.

In the 4000 to 6000 cGy range, increasing tumor dose is associated with a higher rate of complete response and decreased frequency of local recurrence, but no definite improvement in survival, due to the high probability of occult distant metastases at the time of irradiation.

In NSCLC patients entering investigational studies of systemic therapy or in patients with poor prognostic features who are not candidates for attempted curative irradiation, chest radiation therapy may appropriately be deferred until the development of intrathoracic symptoms, provided that the patient is closely observed. Chest irradiation provides the best available palliation for symptoms due to locoregional NSCLC, and it is especially effective in ameliorating pain, hemoptysis, superior vena cava obstruction, and dyspnea and pneumonitis due to an incompletely obstructed bronchus. Atelectasis and vocal cord paralysis are less often relieved.

In the past few years, several randomized trials and a meta-analysis of all randomized trials have shown that Stage IIIa and IIIb NSCLC patients who are fully ambulatory with less than 5% weight loss and no malignant pleural effusion derive modest survival benefit when cisplatin-based chemotherapy is added to chest irradiation, compared with patients receiving chest irradiation alone. Two successive North American controlled studies found that a 5-week regimen of vinblastine and cisplatin preceding irradiation significantly improved median survival by approximately 3 months and, in the earlier trial, approximately doubled 3- and 5-year survival. This program may appropriately be presented as a reasonable treatment option to good-risk (as defined above) Stage IIIa/IIIb patients in clinical practice.

Surgical resection is integrated into the management of selected Stage IIIa NSCLC patients. In these cases, 5-year survival as high as 20% to 35% has been reported. Bulky peripheral primary tumors that directly invade adjacent structures but have no or only hilar nodal metastases can sometimes be resected with curative intent. Patients with only parietal pleural (not chest wall) involvement and those without nodal metastases have a better prognosis. T1 or T2 primary tumors with ipsilateral mediastinal or subcarinal lymph node involvement can also sometimes be successfully resected, particularly if the mediastinal metastases were not detected preoperatively by imaging studies or mediastinoscopy. Postoperative irradiation is often administered, but its survival benefit has not been demonstrated. Superior sulcus tumors often pursue a relatively indolent clinical course, with extensive local invasion but a decreased tendency for nodal and distant metastases. Preoperative irradiation followed by surgical resection can sometimes be curative. External-beam radiation therapy alone yields similar results in some institutions.

Cisplatin-based chemotherapy after surgical resection has increased time to tumor recurrence in two randomized trials including Stage IIIa NSCLC patients. No survival benefit was demonstrated, however; consequently, adjuvant chemotherapy after surgical resection cannot be recommended in clinical practice. A large U.S. Intergroup study is currently comparing postoperative irradiation with or without etoposide/cisplatin treatment in patients with completely resected Stage II and IIIa tumors. Over the past decade, numerous uncontrolled studies evaluated preoperative chemotherapy (sometimes with the addition of chest radiation therapy) in heterogeneously staged patients with marginally-resectable Stage IIIa and IIIb disease. Some trials reported higher-than-expected rates of surgical resection and, on occasion, absence of cancer in the operative specimen, but the survival impact of these approaches could not be determined. In 1994, two small randomized trials in Stage IIIa patients who were judged to be operative candidates reported improved survival with cisplatin-based preoperative chemotherapy, compared with patients who proceeded directly to surgery. Although these results are provocative, criteria for study entry were poorly defined. At present, the more relevant question in the minority of Stage IIIa patients who are operative candidates is probably whether surgery adds to the results of chemotherapy and chest irradiation, rather than whether chemotherapy improves survival after surgery.

Distant Metastases (Stage IV)

Prospects for prolonged survival are dismal in patients with distant metastatic NSCLC. Median survival of fully ambulatory patients is 6 months and is only 1 to 2 months for bedridden patients. Five-year survival is less than 1%. Given these facts, palliation of symptoms is a major goal of management. Radiation therapy plays an important role in this regard and is often useful for palliation of many intrathoracic symptoms, as already discussed, and of symptoms from distant metastases, particularly in brain and bone. Asymptomatic chest tumor is sometimes irradiated, but with careful follow-up radiation can be deferred unless symptoms develop. Malignant pleural effusions can be a vexing problem but are sometimes successfully managed with tube thoracostomy and instillation of sclerosing agents. Bronchial obstruction unresponsive to irradiation can occasionally be palliated with endoscopic laser therapy.

Single-agent chemotherapy of NSCLC yields only 5% to 20% response rates and does not affect survival. Recently, combination chemotherapy regimens, most containing cisplatin, have produced higher response rates (20% to 40%) in fully ambulatory patients, the group most likely to respond. However, complete responses are uncommon. Whether patient survival is improved with chemotherapy compared with patients given supportive care alone has been controversial, since all but two of the randomized clinical trials addressing this issue have been negative. A meta-analysis of all randomized trials comparing chemotherapy to supportive care (including palliative radiation therapy) was completed in 1994. Patients given cisplatin-based chemotherapy experienced a significant 27% relative reduction in mortality rate compared with those receiving only supportive care. This translated into an absolute improvement in median survival of 2 months. Patients receiving long-term alkylating agents without cisplatin, however, had a marginally significant relative increase of 26% in their death rate, compared with patients on supportive care alone.

Given these modest therapeutic benefits, no chemotherapy program can be recommended as standard treatment for NSCLC, and entry of eligible patients into investigational protocols is entirely appropriate. Outside a clinical trial setting, individual patients who are fully ambulatory may be offered a published cisplatin-based chemotherapy regimen provided that they (1) do not have major symptoms that could be successfully palliated with radiation therapy or other means, (2) have evaluable tumor lesions so that response to treatment can be assessed and therapy stopped if it proves ineffective, and (3) understand the limitations of chemotherapy but still desire it. Patients not opting for chemotherapy should be closely observed and their symptoms palliated as they arise.

BIBLIOGRAPHY

American Joint Committee on Cancer. Lung. In Beahrs OH, Henson DE, Hutter RVP et al (eds). Manual for the Staging of Cancer. 4th ed. Philadelphia, JB Lippincott, 1992:115–122

Dillman RO, Seagren SL, Propert KJ et al. A randomized trial of induction chemotherapy plus high-dose radiation versus radiation alone in Stage III non-small cell lung cancer. N Engl J Med 323:940–945, 1990

Ginsberg RJ, Kris MG, Armstrong JG. Cancer of the lung: Section 1. Non-small cell lung cancer. In DeVita VT, Hellman S, Rosenberg SA (eds). Cancer: Principles & Practice of Oncology. 4th ed. Phildelphia, JB Lippincott, 1993:673–723

Holmes EC, Livingston R, Turrisi A III. Neoplasms of the thorax. In Holland JF, Frei E III, Bast RC et al (eds). Cancer Medicine, 3rd ed. Philadelphia, Lea & Febiger, 1993:1285–1337

Komaki R, Cox JD, Hartz AJ et al. Characteristics of long-term survivors after treatment for inoperable carcinoma of the lung. Am J Clin Oncol (CCT) 8:362–370, 1985

Perez CA, Pajak TF, Rubin P et al. Long-term observations of the patterns of failure in patients with unresectable non-oat cell carcinoma of the lung treated with definitive radiotherapy: Report by the Radiation Therapy Oncology Group. Cancer 59:1874–1881, 1987Sause W, Scott C, Taylor S et al. Preliminary analysis of a Phase III trial in regionally advanced unresectable non-small cell lung cancer (abstr). Proc Am Soc Clin Oncol 13: 325, 1994

Shields TW. Surgical therapy for carcinoma of the lung. Clinics Chest Med 14(1):121–147, 1993

Stewart LA, Pignon JP, Parmar MKB et al. A meta-analysis using individual patient data from randomised clinical trials of chemotherapy in non-small cell lung cancer: Survival in the supportive care setting (abstr). Proc Am Soc Clin Oncol 13:337, 1994

John S. Macdonald, Daniel G. Haller, Robert J. Mayer, Eds. *Manual of Oncologic Therapeutics*, Third Edition.

25. SMALL CELL LUNG CANCER

Daniel C. Ihde

Approximately 20% of all cases of lung cancer in the United States are pathologically diagnosed as small cell lung cancer (SCLC), also sometimes called *oat cell carcinoma* or *high-grade neuroendrocrine carcinoma*. Like squamous carcinoma of the lung, SCLC is strongly associated with cigarette abuse. It differs markedly from all types of non-small cell lung cancer in its natural history, cell biology, and response to different types of therapy. Compared with other bronchogenic carcinomas, SCLC has a rapid clinical course with shorter duration of symptoms before diagnosis and median survival in the absence of treatment of only 2 months for disseminated and 4 months for localized disease. It is also distinguished by its propensity for covert or overt distant metastatic disease. Almost 70% of patients will have distant metastases in autopsies performed after postoperative deaths within 30 days of putatively curative surgical resection, and two thirds will have clinically detectable tumor beyond the supraclavicular fossae when modern staging procedures are used at the time of initial diagnosis. Because of this high probability of tumor dissemination, patients with SCLC can only rarely be cured with the localized therapeutic modalities of surgical resection or thoracic irradiation.

SCLC exhibits features of neuroendocrine or APUD (amine precursor uptake and decarboxylation) differentiation, including neurosecretory granules on electron micrographs, production of various polypeptide hormones both *in vitro* and *in vivo*, and a much higher frequency of certain paraneoplastic syndromes, including ectopic Cushing's syndrome, inappropriate secretion of antidiuretic hormone, and the Eaton-Lambert or myasthenia-like syndrome, than occurs in other types of lung cancer. Unfortunately, the ability to detect specific circulating biologic products has yet to prove useful in the early diagnosis or management of patients.

Finally, and most importantly for this discussion, patients with SCLC are markedly more responsive to chemotherapy and radiation therapy than are patients afflicted with other lung cancer cell types. Introduction of effective combination chemotherapy with or without chest irradiation into the management of SCLC has led to four- to five-fold improvement in median survival compared with survival of untreated patients. In a small fraction of patients, the tumor can be permanently eradicated.

PRETREATMENT EVALUATION

Pathologic Evaluation

Because SCLC is not usually diagnosed by surgical resection, the amount of pathologic material available for review is often limited. Because of the therapeutic implication of the diagnosis, it is imperative that diagnostic histologic or cytologic slides be reviewed by an experienced lung cancer pathologist. Although morphologic subtypes of this tumor have similar response to therapy and survival, some are less readily distinguished from non-SCLC. It is also important to ascertain that the pathologic material is of adequate quality, particularly in cases diagnosed by percutaneous needle aspiration, which can produce crush artifact that can be mistaken for SCLC.

Staging Procedures

Because all patients with SCLC should receive combination chemotherapy as part of their treatment, staging is not performed to identify a subset of patients who can be treated solely with locoregional therapy. However, assessing the extent of tumor dissemination is useful to establish prognosis, to document evaluable tumor lesions that can be used to assess response, and to identify patients with clinically localized disease in order to administer chest irradiation to this group.

Common sites of distant metastases in SCLC are the liver, bone, bone marrow, brain, lymph nodes, and subcutaneous tissue. A physical examination and chest film should be performed in all patients. Clinical circumstances dictate the extent of further staging evaluation. Imaging studies of liver, brain, or bone should be performed in the presence of suggestive symptoms or abnormalities on physical examination or blood tests. Bone marrow aspiration and biopsy should be obtained in the presence of cytopenias or an abnormal peripheral blood smear. In patients who have no evidence of distant metastases at this point and are candidates for thoracic radiation therapy, imaging studies of liver (often evaluated by including upper abdominal cuts in computed tomography [CT] of the chest) and bone, and brain and bone marrow examination, if not previously obtained, are needed. If any of these studies are positive, there is no need for further evaluation, as the patient has extensive-stage tumor. Chest CT scan is also helpful in defining portals for thoracic radiation therapy. In the unusual SCLC patient in whom surgical resection is being considered, mediastinoscopy or mediastinotomy, as appropriate, should precede thoracotomy, since mediastinal node involvement is common and resection is contraindicated in its presence.

STAGING SYSTEM AND PROGNOSTIC FACTORS

Except in the few SCLC patients who undergo attempts at surgical resection, detailed delineation of intrathoracic tumor extent is rarely pathologically documented, and the TNM staging system used in non-small cell lung cancer is not often employed. A two-stage system of limited and extensive stage disease is more commonly used. Limited disease is defined as tumor confined to the hemithorax of origin and regional lymph nodes that can be encompassed in a tolerable radiation therapy port. Extensive disease is tumor beyond these bounds. Ipsilateral pleural effusion and supraclavicular adenopathy have been both included and excluded from limited stage by various authorities. The requirement that limited disease must be safely treatable with irradiation introduces physiologic as well as anatomical factors into this staging system.

The three most important prognostic factors in SCLC are tumor extent, usually assessed as limited or extensive stage, performance status, and weight loss. Performance status is probably most important, although relatively few patients with limited disease have markedly impaired functional status. Assessment of performance status before initiation of therapy is extremely important, since the morbidity and mortality of optimal doses of combination chemotherapy are greatly increased in fully bedridden patients and tumor responses lasting over a year are virtually nonexistent in this group. Abnormal serum levels of lactate dehydrogenase, carcinoembryonic antigen, and sodium have been shown to provide additional prognostic information, and are especially useful in the analysis of clinical trial results.

TREATMENT

Principles of Chemotherapy

Similar to other cancers in which chemotherapy yields major improvement in survival and some cures, responses to chemotherapy occur quickly in SCLC, and the major survival benefits of treatment accrue to patients whose tumors exhibit complete clinical disappearance. It is uncommon to observe further improvement in response status after 12 weeks of chemotherapy in the SCLC patient. Several early randomized trials demonstrated that combination chemotherapy is more effective than single-agent treatment in SCLC, in terms of both response rate and survival.

Moderately intensive drug doses associated with nadirs of leukopenia in the range of 1000 to 2000 cells/μl yield superior results to regimens producing more modest myelosuppression, although the two-drug regimen of etoposide and cisplatin appears to be an exception to this statement. However, initial administration of even more intensive drug regimens requiring hospitalization of most patients is not associated with greater therapeutic benefit. Although so-called non–cross-resistant drug regimens are often given in alternating fashion to patients with SCLC, there is little evidence that survival is improved by this strategy. Both controlled and uncontrolled clinical data now demonstrate that there is little benefit to administering chemotherapy for more than 3 to 6 months in patients with SCLC, even those whose tumors have not completely responded to treatment.

Chemotherapy programs used in SCLC generally include two to four drugs selected from known active single agents such as cyclophosphamide, doxorubicin, vincristine, methotrexate, etoposide, cisplatin, or a nitrosourea such as lomustine (CCNU). Several frequently employed regimens that have been documented to produce high response rates and a fraction of long-term survivors in limited stage disease are listed in Table 25–1. Although few prospective randomized trials have been performed to compare one of these or other published combination programs to another, there is little evidence to suggest that any one of these regimens is greatly superior to the others. Rather, the delivery of a regimen that is known to be effective without unnecessary compromises in specified drug doses and schedules is usually more important in achieving optimal therapeutic results than which specific regimen is selected.

In contrast to its effectiveness in newly diagnosed cases, chemotherapy infrequently yields objective tumor responses in patients with relapsed SCLC; it is almost never of benefit in patients whose tumor progresses while the initial chemotherapy program is still being administered. As duration of chemotherapy programs has been shortened, it has been found that patients who have a "chemotherapy-free interval" before receiving drugs for recurrent cancer do not have quite such dismal prospects for response, but long-term survival after treatment for progressive SCLC is still almost nonexistent.

The major toxicities produced by all combination chemotherapy programs used in SCLC are those related to myelosuppression, specifically neutropenia-associated fever, infection, and bleeding. Nausea, vomiting, and alopecia are seen with many drugs. Toxicities peculiar to specific drugs, such as congestive heart failure with doxorubicin and neuropathy with vincristine and cisplatin, are also observed. With current commonly used chemotherapy regimes, treatment-associated death rates of 1% to 4% in limited and 3% to 8% in extensive stage disease can be anticipated. Although this potential for major morbidity and mortality emphasizes that chemotherapy for SCLC should be administered only by physicians experienced in avoiding and managing drug-related toxicity, the survival benefits of chemotherapy greatly exceed survival detriments produced by its toxicities.

Treatment of Limited-Stage Disease

Combination chemotherapy is the cornerstone of management of limited-stage SCLC. Overall (complete plus partial) response rates of 80% to 95%, complete response rates of 40% to 70%, median survival of 12 to 20 months, 2-year sur-

TABLE 25–1. EFFECTIVE COMBINATION CHEMOTHERAPY REGIMENS COMMONLY USED IN SMALL CELL LUNG CANCER

REGIMEN AND DRUGS	DOSE (mg/M²)*	SCHEDULE
VP-16/CISPLATIN REGIMEN (q3 Weeks)		
Etoposide (VP-16)	80	Days 1–3
Cisplatin	80	Day 1
VAC REGIMEN (q3 Weeks)		
Vincristine	1 (2 mg maximum)‡	Days 1, 8, 15 in first cycle; Day 1 only thereafter
Doxorubicin (Adriamycin)	40	Day 1
Cyclophosphamide	1000	Day 1
VAC–VP-16/CISPLATIN REGIMEN		
Cycle of VAC as above alternating every 3 weeks with cycle of VP-16/ cisplatin as above		
CAVp REGIMEN (q3 Weeks)		
Cyclophosphamide	1000	Day 1
Doxorubicin (Adriamycin)	45	Day 1
Etoposide (VP-16)	50	Days 1–5
CAVVp REGIMEN (q3 Weeks)		
Cyclophosphamide	1000	Day 1
Doxorubicin (Adriamycin)	50	Day 1
Vincristine	1.5 (2 mg maximum)‡	Day 1
Etoposide (VP–16)	60	Days 1–5
CMCV REGIMEN (q4 Weeks)		
Cyclophosphamide	700	Day 1
Methotrexate	20, PO	Days 18, 21
Lomustine (CCNU)	70, PO	Day 1
Vincristine	1.3 (2 mg maximum)‡	Days 1, 8, 15, 22 in first cycle; Day 1 only thereafter

*Administered intravenously unless otherwise noted.
‡2-mg maximum specified in the original protocols.

vival of 10% to 40%, and 5-year survival (with probable cure of the original SCLC) of 6% to 12% can be expected when chemotherapy, often with chest irradiation, is delivered according to the principles just outlined. Patients living 5 years do not experience normal survival, however, and are at increased risk for development of additional smoking-related cancers. Until recently, the major debate on optimal treatment for limited SCLC concerned the magnitude of survival benefit resulting from the addition of chest irradiation to combination chemotherapy.

Compared to other histologic types of lung cancer, SCLC responds much more readily to chest irradiation, with overall response rates of up to 90%. In patients treated with radiation therapy alone, however, distant metastases usually ensue within a few months. In the 1970s, controlled and uncontrolled clinical studies demonstrated that chemotherapy plus chest irradiation improved survival compared with radiation therapy alone in limited-stage SCLC. Moreover, some early studies using chemotherapy alone resulted in survival that was not distinguishable from that attained with combined modality therapy. Randomized trials comparing combined modality treatment with chemotherapy alone have shown conclusively that combined therapy reduces the failure rate at the primary tumor site but is associated with more hematologic, pulmonary, and esophageal toxicity.

Over the past few years, 13 randomized trials with prolonged follow-up data comparing combination chemotherapy with chest irradiation to the same chemotherapy given alone have been performed. The majority demonstrated improved overall survival for the combined modality program, which was statistically significant in at least three trials and was usually more evident beyond 1 year of follow-up. A recent meta-analysis of all these studies confirmed that combined modality therapy was associated with a 14% relative reduction in the death rate and a 5.4% absolute improvement in 3-year survival compared with chemotherapy alone. The optimal timing of irradiation — concurrently with chemotherapy, "sandwiched" between chemotherapy cycles in an alternating fashion, or sequentially (with delay of chemotherapy for administration of irradiation) — has not been resolved, although sequential programs are clearly less toxic.

Large uncontrolled trials of thoracic radiotherapy begun concurrently with the first of four cycles of etoposide/cisplatin recently reported excellent survival results, with 2-year survival rates of 30% to 40% and only modest pulmonary toxicity. For limited-stage SCLC patients who are fully ambulatory without major compromises in pulmonary function, this combined modality program appears as good or better than any other. However, there is no doubt that the survival benefits of adding irradiation to chemotherapy have been modest, emphasizing that the major factor needed to improve survival for most SCLC patients remains better systemic therapy.

In limited-stage SCLC patients receiving effective chemotherapy with or without chest irradiation, superior outcomes usually occur in the minority of patients whose tumors are surgically resected prior to chemotherapy. It is unclear whether this improved outcome is due to resection per se, or to the fact that patients who can undergo resection necessarily have lesser tumor bulk and thus have a better prognosis than most patients receiving chemotherapy. Tumor resection in such patients without mediastinal node involvement at thoracotomy is appropriate. Postoperatively, a standard combination chemotherapy program should be administered, probably with chest irradiation. Surgical resection of the primary tumor after response to initial chemotherapy has also been under evaluation in uncontrolled trials, but a recent large randomized North American study could not document any survival advantage from attempted surgical resection followed by radiation therapy in patients responding to chemotherapy, compared with patients receiving radiation therapy alone.

Treatment of Extensive-Stage Disease

There is almost universal agreement that chest irradiation has no impact on survival in patients with extensive-stage disease. Therefore, combination chemotherapy alone is customarily administered, with results inferior to those obtained in limited disease. Overall response rates of 65% to 85%, complete response rates of 15% to 30%, median survival of 7 to 11 months, 2-year survival of 0% to 5%, and only anecdotal 5-year survival can be anticipated when combination chemotherapy programs are employed in disseminated SCLC. Almost all patients with poor performance status at the time of diagnosis have extensive-stage tumor. Combination chemotherapy regimens associated with the best outcomes are appropriate only for patients who are physiologically fit to tolerate them. Recently, single-agent chemotherapy programs with only modest toxicity have been shown to yield survival durations in elderly patients that are not markedly compromised compared with those of patients receiving combination chemotherapy. Whether single-agent and combination programs are of equivalent efficacy in extensive-stage patients is unresolved. However, single-agent etoposide or teniposide is certainly reasonable treatment for patients judged to be at excessive risk of toxicities from chemotherapy because of poor performance status, advanced age, marked organ dysfunction, or other factors.

Radiation therapy plays a major palliative role in the management of SCLC, particularly in patients with extensive-stage and recurrent disease. It can be extremely useful in short-term control of brain metastases; palliation of symptoms from pathologic bone fractures, painful bony metastases, and spinal cord compression; and in treatment of bronchial obstruction or superior vena cava syndrome unresponsive to or recurring after chemotherapy. Chemotherapy and chemotherapy with chest irradiation yield similar results in the initial treatment of superior vena cava syndrome.

Prophylactic Cranial Irradiation

SCLC is the type of lung cancer most likely to metastasize to the brain, and early studies of both chest irradiation and chemotherapy documented that the brain was a frequent site of relapsing tumor in responding patients. Therefore, prophylactic cranial irradiation, either concurrently with initial therapy or after response, was administered to many patients in the 1970s and was later proved in prospective randomized clinical trials to diminish the frequency of clinically detectable brain relapse. However, no survival benefit has been demonstrated. More recent studies have shown that the clinical benefit of prophylactic brain radiation therapy is confined to patients with a complete response to chemotherapy. Administration of prophylactic cranial irradiation would not be controversial, were it not for the fact that some authors have described neuropsychologic impairments, sometimes of major degree, in long-term survivors with SCLC. A contribution of prophylactic brain radiation therapy to these deficits is possible. Currently, prophylactic cranial irradiation should be restricted to patients in complete response and given in low doses per fraction, preferably only after chemotherapy has been completed. It is critical that the patient be fully informed of the potential risks and benefits of prophylactic irradiation before it is initiated.

BIBLIOGRAPHY

Bork E, Ersbøll J, Dombernowsky P et al. Teniposide and etoposide in previously untreated small-cell lung cancer: A randomized study. J Clin Oncol 9: 1627–1631, 1991

Holmes EC, Livingston R, Turrisi A III. Neoplasms of the thorax. In Holland JF, Frei E III, Bast RC et al (eds). Cancer Medicine. 3rd ed. Philadelphia, Lea & Febiger, 1993:1285–1337.

Ihde DC. Drug therapy: Chemotherapy of lung cancer. N Engl J Med 327:1434–1441, 1992

Ihde DC, Pass HI, Glatstein E. Cancer of the lung: Section 2. Small cell lung cancer. In DeVita VT, Hellman S, Rosenberg SA (eds). Cancer: Principles and Practice of Oncology. 4th ed. Philadelphia, JB Lippincott, 1993:723–758

Johnson DH, Kim K, Turrisi AT et al. Cisplatin & etoposide + concurrent thoracic radiotherapy administered once versus twice daily for limited-stage small cell lung cancer: Preliminary results of an intergroup trial (abstr). Proc Am Soc Clin Oncol 13: 333, 1994

Lad T, Thomas P, Piantadosi S. Surgical resection of small cell lung cancer: A prospective randomized trial (abstr). Proc Am Soc Clin Oncol 10: 244, 1991

Pignon JP, Arriagada R, Ihde DC et al. A meta-analysis of thoracic radiotherapy for small-cell lung cancer. N Engl J Med 327:1618–1624, 1992

Richardson GE, Tucker MA, Venzon DJ et al. Smoking cessation after successful treatment of small cell lung cancer is associated with fewer smoking-related second primary cancers. Ann Intern Med 119:383–390, 1993

Williams CJ, McMillan I Lea R et al. Surgery after initial chemotherapy for localized small cell carcinoma of the lung. J Clin Oncol 5:1579–1588, 1987

John S. Macdonald, Daniel G. Haller, Robert J. Mayer, Eds. *Manual of Oncologic Therapeutics*, Third Edition.

26. BREAST CANCER

Peter M. Ravdin
C. Kent Osborne

Clinical studies and work in the basic sciences since the late 1960s have led to dramatic changes and improvements in the treatment of breast cancer. The current basic paradigm for breast cancer is a malignancy that arises within the breast, but for many women becomes a systemic disease (with widespread micrometastases) early in its course. Thus, current therapy and research efforts focus on the following:

1. Prevention of breast cancer
2. Screening of women at risk so as to detect occurrences as early as possible
3. Definitive local therapy to the primary site
4. Adjuvant therapy to eradicate systemic disease when micrometastatic
5. Therapy for macroscopic recurrence of disease.

Significant advances have been made in definition of women at risk for breast cancer for screening and participation in prevention trials. Clinical trials of surgical alternatives for primary breast tumors have shown that for most women radical surgeries are not indicated, and lesser, more cosmetically and physically acceptable procedures are as efficacious. More accurate techniques are available for the identification of patients at risk for relapse after apparently successful surgery. Better chemotherapeutic and endocrine therapies are available to prevent or delay disease recurrence, and to treat disease if it recurs.

Selection of the strategies to be applied to lessen a woman's risk of dying of breast cancer depends on many factors, including her age, menopausal status, past medical history, general health, genetics, and the physical, histopathologic, and biochemical details of her breast tumor tissue.

BREAST CANCER PREVENTION (TREATMENT OF CANCER AT A PRECLINICAL STAGE)

There is no clinically proven method for preventing breast cancer. There is some indirect evidence that tamoxifen may be able to prevent breast cancer, and this has led to the initiation of a clinical trial comparing tamoxifen to placebo in a population of women at higher than average risk for breast cancer. This study was initiated when it became apparent that in women with a history of breast cancer, tamoxifen lessened the risk of developing a new breast cancer (by about 40%) in the opposite breast. Whether women without a history of breast cancer will benefit is unclear, and there are negative aspects of taking tamoxifen (*e.g.*, increased hot flashes and vaginal dryness, and possibly increased risks of thrombosis and endometrial cancer) that may lead to no net benefit.

Thus, at this time there is no clinically proven preventative, but we are able to identify women who are at special risk for developing breast cancer. The strongest risk factors are family history, a past history of breast cancer, and a history of a breast biopsy showing nonmalignant but high risk histopathology such as DCIS (ductal carcinoma in situ, or atypical hyperplasia). The addition of mammography to self examination of the breasts, and annual health checkups can reduce, but not eliminate, the risk of dying of breast cancer.

INITIAL EVALUATION AND STAGING FOR THE BREAST CANCER PATIENT

The standard evaluation for new patients with breast cancer is shown in Table 26–1. Mammography is required to look for evidence of tumor multicentricity or of bilateral involvement. Bone scans are cost-effective only in patients with more advanced disease, or in those with suspicious symptoms or an elevated alkaline phosphatase. Routine liver or brain scans are not indicated in the absence of clinical symptoms or signs suggesting tumor involvement.

After a thorough pretreatment evaluation, the patient with breast cancer can be clinically staged on the basis of the characteristics of the primary tumor, physical examination of the axillary lymph nodes, and the presence of distant metastases. However, clinical staging of the axilla is inaccurate. Because of the prognostic significance of the axillary nodes, the pathologic stage (stage of disease after surgery) is more significant than the clinical stage. The pathologic staging classification recommended by the American Joint Committee on Cancer (AJCC) is shown in Table 26–2.

PROGNOSTIC FACTORS

Several tumor characteristics that have important prognostic significance need to be considered when designing an optimal treatment strategy for the individual patient.

Axillary Lymph Nodes

Axillary lymph node status is the most important predictor of disease recurrence and survival. Seventy percent of patients with negative nodes survive 10 years. Prognosis worsens as the number of positive lymph nodes increases. About 40% of

TABLE 26–1. INITIAL PATIENT EVALUATION

History and physical examination
Complete blood count, liver function tests, serum calcium
Mammography
Chest film
Bone scan* (and bone films of suspicious areas)

*Not indicated in patients with clinical Stage I or II disease unless bone pain or elevated alkaline phosphatase is present.

patients with one to three positive nodes survive 10 years, whereas only 15% of those with four or more nodes survive with surgical treatment alone. Node involvement serves as a marker for the presence of distant micrometastases and alerts the physician to the high risk of recurrence.

Histopathology

The histologic subtype of invasive breast cancer is of little prognostic importance. Uncommon subtypes such as mucinous, papillary, or tubular carcinoma may have a better prognosis. Tumor size is an important prognostic factor; patients with negative axillary lymph nodes and tumors ≤1 cm in diameter have a recurrence rate of only 9% at 10 years. Histologic features of tumor differentiation, such as nuclear grade, also have prognostic implications. Unfortunately, assessment of breast cancer histology is poorly reproducible among pathologists.

Estrogen and Progesterone Receptors

Estrogen receptors (ER) and progesterone receptors (PR) are cellular proteins present in hormone-responsive target tissues. About 60% to 70% of primary breast cancers contain measurable ER, and 40% to 50% have PR. Postmenopausal women more frequently have receptor-positive tumors than premenopausal women do, and the receptor concentration tends to be higher. Receptor content may change over the course of the disease. Tissue should be obtained, if possible, at the time of a recurrence to assess receptor status accurately.

Patients with receptor-positive primary tumors have a lower rate of recurrence and longer survival than those with receptor-negative tumors. The presence of receptor positivity may be useful in selecting patients who might benefit most from adjuvant endocrine therapy.

TABLE 26–2. PATHOLOGIC STAGING SYSTEM

PRIMARY TUMOR (T)

TX	Primary tumor cannot be assessed
T0	No evidence of primary tumor
Tis*	Carcinoma in situ: Intraductal carcinoma, lobular carcinoma in situ, or Paget's disease of the nipple with no tumor
T1	Tumor 2 cm or less in greatest dimension
	T1a—0.5 cm or less in greatest dimension
	T1b—More than 0.5 cm but not more than 1 cm in greatest dimension
	T1c—More than 1 cm but not more than 2 cm in greatest dimension
T2	Tumor more than 2 cm but not more than 5 cm in greatest dimension
T3	Tumor more than 5 cm in greatest dimension
T4†	Tumor of any size with direct extension to chest wall or skin
	T4a—Extension to chest wall
	T4b—Edema (including peau d'orange) or ulceration of the skin of the breast or satellite skin nodules confined to the same breast
	T4c—Both (T4a and T4b)
	T4d—Inflammatory carcinoma

REGIONAL LYMPH NODES (N)

NX	Regional lymph nodes cannot be assessed (*e.g.*, previously removed)
N0	No regional lymph node metastasis
N1	Metastasis to movable ipsilateral axillary lymph node(s)
N2	Metastasis to ipsilateral axillary lymph node(s) fixed to one another or to other structures
N3	Metastasis to ipsilateral internal mammary lymph node(s)

DISTANT METASTASIS (M)

MX	Presence of distant metastasis cannot be assessed
M0	No distant metastasis
M1	Distant metastasis (includes metastasis to ipsilateral supraclavicular lymph node(s)

STAGE GROUPING

Stage 0	Tis	N0	M0
Stage I	T1	N0	M0
Stage IIA	T0	N1	M0
	T1	N1	M0
	T2	N0	M0
Stage IIB	T2	N1	M0
	T3	N0	M0
Stage IIIA	T0	N2	M0
	T1	N2	M0
	T2	N2	M0
	T3	N1,N2	M0
Stage IIIB	T4	Any N	M0
	Any T	N3	M0
Stage IV	Any T	Any N	M1

*Paget's disease associated with a tumor is classified according to the size of the tumor.

†Chest wall includes ribs, intercostal muscles, and serratus anterior muscle but not pectoral muscle.

From the American Joint Committee on Cancer. Staging for Breast Carcinoma, 3 ed. American Cancer Society, Inc., 1989

Approximately 50% of patients with ER-positive advanced breast cancer benefit from endocrine therapy, whereas the response rate in patients with ER-negative tumors is less than 10%. Tumors with high ER content are more likely to be hormone-dependent. PR analysis adds to the predictive accuracy of ER. Tumors that are positive for both receptors have a 60% response rate; ER-positive, PR-negative tumors have a response rate of only 30%.

Cell Proliferative Indices and DNA Ploidy

Several studies suggest that assessment of cell proliferative potential may have important prognostic significance. Determination of the S-phase fraction by the tritiated thymidine labeling index or by flow cytometry can identify patients with different risks for recurrence. High S-phase fraction tumors are associated with a worse prognosis. DNA content (ploidy) also has prognostic significance. Diploid tumors have a lower risk for recurrence than aneuploid tumors.

Other reported prognostic factors, including HER-2 oncogene expression, cathepsin D, the epidermal growth factor receptor (EGF-R), altered P53 suppressor gene, histologic evidence of extensive angiogenesis in the tumor, micrometastases in the axillary lymph nodes, expression of various proteolytic enzymes, the pS2 estrogen-regulated protein, and the stress-response proteins, remain experimental.

TREATMENT

Primary Breast Cancer

Therapeutic goals in the patient with primary operable breast cancer are twofold. First, optimal control of disease in the breast and regional tissues should be obtained while providing the patient with the best possible cosmetic result. Second, systemic therapy should be considered, except in patients with a very low risk of recurrence, to inhibit growth of micrometastases.

Clinical trials have shown that for most breast cancer patients surgical procedures that are more physically and cosmetically acceptable than the classical radical mastectomy give the patient equivalent disease-free and overall survival. The most commonly performed primary surgeries done since the early 1980s are the modified radical mastectomy and the partial mastectomy (lumpectomy, quadrantectomy) with axillary dissection.

Patients treated by total mastectomy or with breast conservation surgery must have a level I and II axillary dissection. Adequate tissue can be obtained while preserving the pectoralis minor muscle and the lateral pectoral nerve. A level III dissection should be considered in patients with clinically positive nodes to obtain optimal local control.

The initial diagnostic biopsy must be done with the possible definitive treatment approaches in mind. In patients desiring breast preservation, an excisional biopsy, if required, should combine the function of biopsy and definitive lumpectomy in the same procedure. A needle-aspiration biopsy is often helpful in establishing a diagnosis in such patients. The physician can then discuss treatment alternatives with the patient before definitive surgery. The optimal surgical approach is determined by the stage of disease, tumor size and location, breast size and configuration, the presence of multicentricity clinically or mammographically, available surgical and radiotherapeutic expertise, and patient wishes.

SPECIFIC PROCEDURES

Radical Mastectomy. This procedure involves en bloc removal of the breast, pectoral muscles, and axillary contents. This operation is not indicated today except perhaps for the removal of very large, fixed tumors. Extended radical mastectomy, which includes removal of the internal mammary nodes, is no longer performed.

Modified Radical Mastectomy. The breast and axillary contents are removed through a horizontal incision, and the pectoralis muscles are preserved. The cosmetic result is improved by the more normal appearance of the upper chest wall.

Partial Mastectomy, Axillary Dissection, and Breast Irradiation. This breast-preserving procedure involves excision of the tumor with an adjacent rim of normal breast tissue. Lumpectomy is a modification that entails excision of gross tumor only. An axillary dissection through a separate incision is required for accurate staging and local control. Radiation therapy is used to treat the remaining breast tissue to reduce the chance of local recurrence. Treatment consists of external-beam radiation therapy plus an optional boost to the local tumor site with either external-beam or interstitial radiation.

Breast Reconstruction. Patients who desire but are not candidates for breast preservation can obtain an acceptable cosmetic result with immediate or delayed reconstruction after mastectomy.

Postmastectomy Radiation Therapy. Once routine, postoperative radiation following modified radical mastectomy is now reserved for patients with a high risk of local recurrence. Risk factors include tumors greater than 5 cm in diameter with positive axillary nodes; tumor involvement at the margin of surgical resection; invasion of the pectoral fascia or muscle; or extranodal extension into the axillary fat. In patients with a high risk for distant micrometastases, radiation therapy, if necessary, should be delayed until the completion of adjuvant chemotherapy. The risk for arm lymphedema is increased by postoperative radiation therapy to the axilla.

Prophylactic Mastectomy. Contralateral prophylactic mastectomy in a patient with primary breast cancer is not indicated except in unusual circumstances. Close follow-up with breast self-examination, regular physician examination, and annual mammography is indicated.

TREATMENT RECOMMENDATIONS

Carcinoma in situ: Intraductal Carcinoma. Optimal therapy has not yet been defined. Lumpectomy, partial mastectomy, and total mastectomy, with or without axillary dissection, have been used for this highly curable stage of disease. Total mastectomy (with reconstruction) may be required for large or multicentric lesions. The need for axillary dissection in these patients is questionable; less than 5% will be found to have lymph node metastases. The use of breast irradiation in patients treated with breast preservation should be considered. Clinical trials now suggest that such therapy may reduce the rate of local recurrence (about one half of these recurrences are demonstrated to have an invasive histology). Systemic adjuvant therapy should not be given to patients with pure intraductal cancer, since they are cured by local treatment alone.

Stage I and IIA Breast Cancer. Partial mastectomy (or lumpectomy) plus axillary dissection and breast irradiation is appropriate for some women desiring breast preservation. Patients with small breasts or relatively large tumors, or those with evidence of tumor multicentricity are not appropriate candidates for this procedure. In addition, radiation of large pendulous breasts is more difficult, and the cosmetic result may be suboptimal. Tumor location within the breast is less important, although the nipple–areola complex may have to be sacrificed (with later reconstruction) in those with central or subareola masses.

For other patients with Stage I and II disease, modified radical mastectomy is the preferred treatment. Breast reconstruction should be offered to women desiring the best possible cosmetic result.

Stage IIB (T2-3a, N0-1, M0). The general approach to these patients is similar to that for Stages I and IIA. Cure or long-term control is possible, especially if the axillary lymph nodes are pathologically negative. Because of the large tumor size, breast preservation is not an option for most patients. Modified radical mastectomy with reconstructive surgery provides a better cosmetic result. Postoperative radiation should be considered in select patients at high risk of local recurrence.

Stage III. Patients with Stage III or inflammatory disease have a high rate of local and distant recurrence and a poor survival. A combined-modality approach using systemic therapy in addition to surgery and radiation is required. Aggressive combination chemotherapy should be initiated after biopsy confirmation of the disease. Initial chemotherapy serves two purposes: (1) to reduce tumor bulk, which may facilitate more effective local treatment, and (2) to immediately attack distant micrometastases, which are present in nearly all patients with these stages. About 70% of patients will have significant tumor regression, with about 20% to 25% having a clinical complete response. Chemotherapy should be continued in responding patients until maximal reduction in tumor size is obtained (usually 3 to 6 months of treatment). Surgery and radiation therapy are then introduced in a sequence determined by the extent of tumor regression observed with chemotherapy. After local therapy, chemotherapy may be reinstituted for several additional months. With this approach, about 30% to 40% of patients with Stage III disease will remain disease-free at 5 years. The prognosis is worse with inflammatory breast cancer. In elderly patients or other patients for whom aggressive chemotherapy is contraindicated, systemic hormonal therapy with tamoxifen may be considered, especially if the tumor contains high levels of ER or PR.

Systemic Treatment (Adjuvant Therapy). About 50% of all patients with operable primary breast cancer survive 10 years after surgery without developing recurrent disease and presumably do not have viable distant micrometastases at the time of diagnosis. Identification of patients with established micrometastases who may benefit from adjuvant therapy is a challenge. Currently, no tests or tumor marker studies are available to accurately identify patients who are destined to relapse. However, several prognostic indicators can be used to classify patients according to their relative risk for recurrence (Table 26–3). The most important factor is the axillary lymph node status. Although patients with negative nodes have a relatively good prognosis, certain subsets such as those with receptor-negative, poorly differentiated, or large tumors, and those with aneuploid DNA content or high S-phase fraction have a relatively high recurrence rate and should be considered for adjuvant therapy. Patients with small, mammographically detected invasive cancers ≤ 1 cm in diameter should probably not receive adjuvant therapy since they have an excellent prognosis and since adjuvant therapy has not yet been shown beneficial in this subset.

Adjuvant Chemotherapy. Adjuvant chemotherapy delays recurrence and improves survival of women with positive axillary nodes. Additional follow-up is required to deter-

TABLE 26–3. FACTORS ASSOCIATED WITH DECREASED RISK FOR RECURRENT DISEASE

Axillary lymph nodes	Negative
ER/PgR status	Positive
Tumor size	≤2 cm
Histopathology	Low nuclear grade
Proliferative index	Low S-phase fraction
Histologic type	Pure tubular papillary or mucinous

mine whether a fraction of patients has actually been cured. The major benefit is observed in premenopausal patients, where adjuvant chemotherapy has been estimated to cause a proportional 25% reduction in mortality at 10 years. Adjuvant chemotherapy may also be beneficial in certain postmenopausal subsets, although the data are less convincing. Studies suggest that adjuvant chemotherapy may also be beneficial in delaying recurrence in both pre- and postmenopausal patients with negative axillary nodes, but who have a higher risk for recurrence based on negative ER status, larger tumor size, or other adverse prognostic factors. Whether treatment prolongs survival of these patients requires longer follow-up of these trials.

Studies have demonstrated that combination chemotherapy is superior to single-agent treatment. In addition, shorter duration treatment may be just as effective as prolonged treatment; with the widely used CMF (cyclophosphamide, methotrexate, 5-fluorouracil [5-FU]) regimen repeated every 28 days, 6 cycles of treatment are as effective as 12. Physicians should be cautious in extrapolating these results to other drug regimens or schedules for which optimal duration remains to be defined.

Several popular chemotherapy regimens have been used for adjuvant therapy of breast cancer (Table 26–4). There are insufficient data to strongly recommend one regimen over another. Arbitrary modifications or dose alterations of regimens with proven benefit are to be avoided. Data do suggest that maximal drug dosage should be used unless significant toxicity or poor patient tolerance necessitates dose reduction. Although there is a suggestion that more dose-intensive adjuvant therapy regimens are more effective, very intensive regimens requiring stem cell rescue (either from the bone marrow or the peripheral blood) are still investigational.

The toxicity of adjuvant chemotherapy is acceptable and depends on the drug regimen as well as the judicious use of preventive measures. Acute reversible toxicity includes nausea, vomiting, mucositis, diarrhea, alopecia, and myelosuppression. These side effects may be more severe with doxorubicin, although scalp cooling may minimize hair loss, and antiemetics may minimize nausea and vomiting. The potential for cardiac toxicity should be considered with regimens containing doxorubicin. Fortunately, fatal toxicities are rare in this population of generally healthy women.

Chronic or delayed toxicities from adjuvant chemotherapy have been few, although they still must be considered largely unknown. A serious side effect in premenopausal women is ovarian dysfunction, which varies from reversible amenorrhea to complete medical castration with sterility, atrophic vaginitis and dyspareunia, and the theoretical risk of premature osteoporosis and cardiovascular disease. No increased risk of second malignancy has yet been observed in breast cancer patients treated with adjuvant cytotoxic chemotherapy.

Adjuvant Endocrine Therapy. More recent studies have evaluated the role of adjuvant therapy with the antiestrogen tamoxifen, because of the low toxicity and ease of administration of this agent. Most adjuvant studies have used 10 mg to 20 mg of tamoxifen, twice a day, for 1 or 2 years after local treatment. Delayed recurrence and modest improvement in survival are observed; in contrast to cytotoxic chemotherapy, the greatest benefit is seen in postmenopausal patients. There

TABLE 26–4. ADJUVANT CHEMOTHERAPY REGIMENS FOR BREAST CANCER

ACRONYM	DRUGS	DOSE (mg/M^2)	CYCLE FREQUENCY	DURATION
CMF	Cyclophosphamide	100, PO days 1 to 14	Every 28 days	6 cycles
	Methotrexate	40, IV days 1 and 8		
	5-Fluorouracil	600, IV days 1 and 8		
CMF	Cyclophosphamide	600, IV day 1	Every 21 days	12 cycles
	Methotrexate	40, IV day 1		
	5-Fluorouracil	600, IV day 1		
CMFVP	Cyclophosphamide	60, PO daily	NA	1 year
	Methotrexate	15, IV weekly		
	5-Fluorouracil	400, IV weekly		
	Vincristine	0.625, IV weekly for 10 weeks		
	Prednisone	30, PO daily for 14 days		
		20, PO daily for 14 days		
		10, PO daily for 14 days		
AC	Cyclophosphamide	600, IV day 1	Every 21 days	4 cycles
	Doxorubicin	60, IV day 1		
CAF	Cyclophosphamide	100, PO days 1 and 14	Every 28 days`	6 cycles
	Doxorubicin	30, IV days 1 and 8		
	5-Fluorouracil	500, IV days 1 and 8		
FAC	5-Fluorouracil	500, IV days 1 and 8	Every 21 days	6 cycles
	Doxorubicin	50, IV day 1		
	Cyclophosphamide	500, IV day 1		

is a correlation between clinical benefit with tamoxifen and positive ER and PR status. A 21% proportional reduction in mortality at 10 years has been estimated for tamoxifen treatment in these patients. The optimal duration of treatment is under investigation, but many current research studies prescribe the drug for 5 years. Whether tamoxifen benefits ER-negative patients is controversial, although if it does so, its effects in this population are less than in ER-positive patients. Both node-negative and node-positive patients appear to benefit from the antiestrogen.

The long-term side effects of tamoxifen are largely unknown. Some data suggest a slightly increased risk of thromboembolic phenomenon and of endometrial cancer. Preliminary data suggest that tamoxifen may protect against postmenopausal bone loss and that it may alter blood lipid profiles in a favorable way.

Ovarian ablation as adjuvant endocrine therapy has been studied in premenopausal patients with mixed results. A meta-analysis of these trials suggests that it may be an effective adjuvant therapy, causing a proportional (about 30%) reduction in mortality at 10 years. A direct comparison of oophorectomy with long-term tamoxifen (≥ 5 years) in premenopausal patients has not been done.

Adjuvant Chemoendocrine Therapy. Studies have shown that the addition of tamoxifen to standard chemotherapy regimens such as PF (melphalan and 5-FU) or CMF may improve the disease-free and total survival in postmenopausal women with hormone receptor-positive tumors. Because the improved results could be attributed to the endocrine agent itself, firm recommendations await the results of ongoing studies. Preliminary results from two completed studies are contradictory; one study suggests an advantage for the addition of doxorubicin-based chemotherapy to tamoxifen in postmenopausal node-positive patients, whereas the addition of CMFVP to tamoxifen in another study showed no benefit. This question requires further study.

Continued research is necessary to more accurately define the subsets of patients for whom adjuvant treatment is appropriate and to define the optimal regimen and duration of therapy. However, based on results of completed trials, patients outside a clinical trial can be managed on an individual basis as outlined in Table 26–5.

Treatment of Local-Regional Recurrence. Local regional recurrence of breast cancer on the chest wall or in adjacent lymphatics is relatively common. Usually, local recurrence is a harbinger of widespread disease. In a small subset of patients, however, distant metastases are not present and local therapy may be curative. Treatment includes a combination of surgery, radiation therapy, and systemic treatment. If distant metastases are absent, wide excision followed by radiation therapy is indicated. If the lesion is unresectable, radiation alone should be used. The value of chemotherapy or endocrine therapy in patients rendered disease free by local treatment has not been established, but it is advocated by some physicians in selected patients. If the local recurrence is extensive or if distant metastases are present, the patient should be treated with systemic therapy as outlined in the following section. Ipsilateral breast recurrence after treatment by lumpectomy and irradiation is not a harbinger of widespread metastasis. Such patients usually require total mastectomy. The value of additional systemic therapy in this setting is unknown.

TABLE 26–5. RECOMMENDATIONS FOR ADJUVANT THERAPY

NODE-POSITIVE

Premenopausal: combination chemotherapy, regardless of ER status

Postmenopausal: tamoxifen if ER-positive and consider additional chemotherapy if at high risk ER+; consider chemotherapy if ER-negative

NODE-NEGATIVE*

Premenopausal: combination chemotherapy for both ER-positive and ER-negative high-risk patients; consider tamoxifen for ER-positive patients

Postmenopausal: tamoxifen if ER-positive; consider chemotherapy for high-risk ER-positive or ER-negative patients

*Observation alone should be considered in node-negative patients with other low-risk factors: small tumors (≤1 cm) or ≤2 cm and well differentiated with positive estrogen and/or progesterone receptors.

Advanced Disease Metastatic breast cancer is not curable by current treatment modalities, although temporary regession of disease is attainable in about two thirds of the patients. Clinical complete remission is observed in 10% to 20% of patients, but these remissions are rarely of long duration. Median survival is less than 2 years. Palliation of symptoms and prolongation of useful, high-quality life become the major therapeutic goals.

Surgery and radiation therapy play a limited role in patients with metastatic disease. Surgical biopsy of lesions is often required for histologic diagnosis or for determination of hormone receptor status. Mastectomy may be required, even in patients presenting with metastases, to prevent local complications. Surgical treatment of spinal cord compression or impending pathological bone fracture is indicated in some patients. Radiation therapy is often helpful in patients with localized pain from a metastatic lesion or in the treatment of brain metastases and spinal cord compression.

Systemic treatment by endocrine manipulation or with cytotoxic drugs is the major treatment modality for patients with advanced breast cancer. A general strategy for the treatment of patients with metastatic disease is shown in Figure 26–1. Patients are divided into two groups based on receptor status and clinical criteria. Patients with negative receptors or those with positive receptors who have aggressive, life-threatening disease should receive combination chemother-

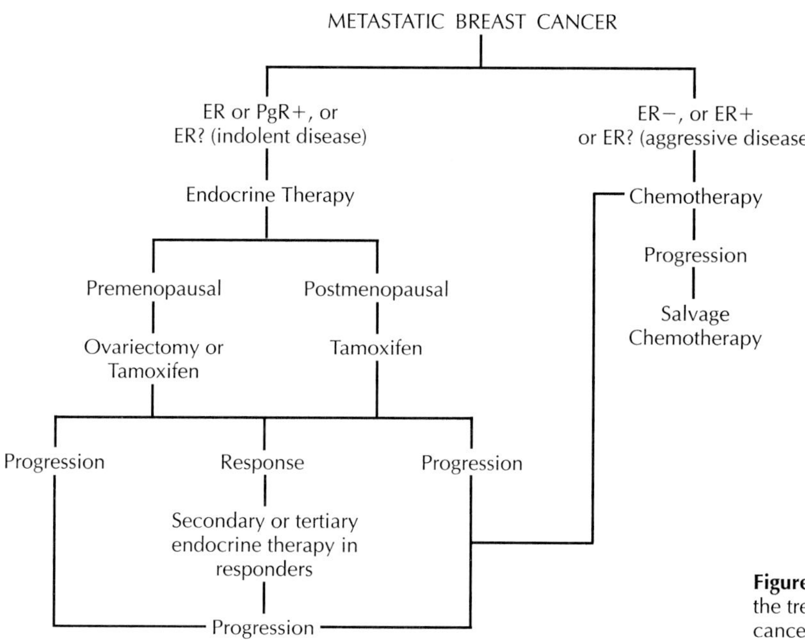

Figure 26–1. General approach to the treatment of metastatic breast cancer.

apy initially. If the disease responds to treatment and then progresses in a more indolent fashion later, endocrine therapy might be considered, especially for ER- or PR-positive tumors.

Patients with ER- or PR-positive tumors or those with unknown receptor status with indolent disease characterized by long disease-free interval and the lack of extensive visceral involvement are best treated initially with endocrine therapy. Premenopausal patients can be treated with either surgical ovariectomy or with the antiestrogen tamoxifen. The new gonadotropin-releasing hormone analogues can induce "medical castration." Additional study will be required to determine if they are as effective as existing therapies. Patients initially treated with tamoxifen who have had a tumor response may respond to castration later, at the time of progression. Tamoxifen is the most popular first-line endocrine therapy for postmenopausal patients because of the lack of toxic side effects.

Some physicians argue that a trial of endocrine therapy is indicated in select patients with indolent disease even if the tumor is receptor-negative. Although the chance of response is less than 10%, little will be lost with a 6- to 8-week trial of tamoxifen, particularly in elderly patients who may not tolerate chemotherapy.

Time to response may be quite prolonged with endocrine therapy, and treatment should not be abandoned prematurely. Disease progression should not be confused with a "tumor flare," which may cause transiently increased bone pain, swelling or erythema of superficial lesions, or hypercalcemia during the first week or two of treatment. This phenomenon frequently predicts for a subsequent response if therapy is continued.

In general, patients who do not respond to initial endocrine therapy have hormone-resistant tumors and should be switched to chemotherapy. However, 15% to 20% of patients failing initial hormone therapy may respond to a second-line hormonal therapy. This approach might be considered for patients who still demonstrate indolent disease and who have receptor-positive tumors. Patients who respond to endocrine therapy and then progress later should be treated with sequential endocrine therapy until they demonstrate hormone-refractory or aggressive visceral disease. A subset of patients can be controlled for more than 5 years with this approach.

SPECIFIC ENDOCRINE THERAPIES (SEE ALSO CHAPTER 23)

Ablative Therapies. Ablative treatments involve the destruction or surgical removal of endocrine organs such as the ovaries, adrenals, or the pituitary gland. In unselected patients with advanced breast cancer, the response ranges from 20% to 40%. The response rate is higher in patients with ER- or PR-positive tumors. Adrenalectomy and hypophysectomy are rarely indicated today because of the associated morbidity and mortality and because of the availability of other effective additive hormone treatments. Ovariectomy remains the preferred first- or second-line endocrine therapy in premenopausal women.

TABLE 26–6. RELATIVE TOXICITY OF HORMONE THERAPIES

SIDE EFFECT	TAMOXIFEN	PROGESTINS	AMINOGLUTETHIMIDE	ESTROGENS	ANDROGENS
Flushing	+	−	+	−	+
Nausea,vomiting	+	+	+	+++	+
Fluid retention	−	++	−	+++	+
Thromboembolic	+/−	+/−	−	++	−
Weight gain	−	++	−	+	+
Virilization	−	−	−	−	+++
Rash	−	−	++	−	−
Lethargy/depression	+/−	+/−	++	−	−
Expense	+	++	++	−	+

+, sometimes occurs

++, occasionally significant

+++, major issue

+/−, may be associated

−, absent

Additive Therapies. The antiestrogen tamoxifen is effective in both pre- and postmenopausal patients. Response rates are similar to other primary endocrine therapies. A major advantage of tamoxifen is the low-toxicity profile (Table 26–6). Standard doses are 20 mg to 40 mg per day. The drug and its active metabolites have a prolonged half-life of at least 7 days.

Progestins are also effective as first-, second-, or third-line treatment in postmenopausal patients. Megestrol acetate, 40 mg 4 times a day, is the most popular agent and has few side effects.

Aminoglutethimide lowers serum estrogen concentration by inhibiting adrenal steroid synthesis and by inhibiting the enzyme aromatase. It is effective only in postmenopausal patients (natural or surgical) and has been used as first- or second-line treatment. Depending on the dosage used, it may or may not require additional therapy with hydrocortisone. Toxicity is most frequent during the first 2 weeks of therapy and includes skin rash, lethargy, depression, dizziness, and ataxia. The drug is well tolerated chronically. Preliminary data suggest that administration of the drug on a twice daily schedule may be just as effective as four times per day.

High-dose estrogen is effective secondary or tertiary therapy in postmenopausal patients. Diethylstilbestrol, 15 mg daily, or ethinyl estradiol, 3 mg daily, are the most common preparations. Side effects are more common with estrogen therapy.

Androgens have more toxicity, primarily related to virilization. However, these drugs are effective and are used sequentially in patients responding to other agents. Fluoxymesterone, 10 mg twice a day, is a commonly used agent.

Corticosteroids are useful in the short-term palliation of symptoms in the terminally ill patient and as adjunctive therapy in patients with central nervous system metastases.

CYTOTOXIC CHEMOTHERAPY

Chemotherapy is indicated for patients refractory to hormonal manipulation and for those with aggressive disease. Combination chemotherapy is superior to single-agent treatment; response rates range from 50% to 70% and response durations range from 6 to 12 months. Several chemotherapy regimens have been used with similar results (Table 26–7). Regimens containing doxorubicin may have slightly higher response rates, but they offer no significant survival advantage. Toxicity depends on the individual agents used and includes myelosuppression, alopecia, nausea, vomiting, and mucositis. Cardiomyopathy is observed with doxorubicin, usually at total doses exceeding 500 mg/m^2. Optimal duration of treatment in responding patients is under investigation.

Salvage chemotherapy for patients progressing on initial treatment is disappointing. Response rates are low (20% to 40%) and durations short (4 to 10 months). Combination regimens have not been shown to be superior to single agents. Doxorubicin, vinblastine, mitomycin C, and mitoxantrone are the most active agents. Very high dose therapy with or without autologous bone marrow support remains experimental and should not be performed outside of a clinical trial. A number of new agents have been recently described that have excellent activity as single agents (*e.g.*, taxol, taxotere, navelbine). The use of these agents alone and in combination with other agents is being investigated.

Chemoendocrine Therapy. Randomized trials do not support the use of an endocrine agent combined with chemotherapy. There is no significant advantage in or duration of survival with combined therapy compared with the sequential use of the two modalities. Identification of patients with hormone-sensitive tumors is obscured by this approach.

TABLE 26-7. COMMONLY USED CHEMOTHERAPY REGIMENS FOR ADVANCED BREAST CANCER

ACRONYM	DRUGS	DOSE (mg/M²)	RESPONSE RATE (%)*	MEDIAN DURATION OF RESPONSE (MONTHS)*
CMF	Cyclophosphamide	100, PO days 1 to 14	49–59	5–8
	Methotrexate	40, IV days 1 and 8		
	5-Fluorouracil	600, IV days 1 and 8 repeat every 28 days		
FAC	5-Fluorouracil	500, IV days 1 and 8	50–75	6–10
	Doxorubicin	50, IV day1		
	Cyclophosphamide	500, IV day 1; repeat every 21 days		
CAF	Cyclophosphamide	100, PO days 1 to 14	60–80	10–12
	Doxorubicin	30, IV days 1 and 8		
	5-Fluorouracil	500, IV days 1 and 8		
TAXOL	Paclitaxel	175, IV repeat every 21 days	30	6

*Range of values reported in the literature

BIBLIOGRAPHY

Bonadonna G, Valagussa P. Adjuvant systemic therapy for resectable breast cancer. J Clin Oncol 3:259–275, 1985

Breitmeyer JB, Henderson IC. Adjuvant chemotherapy of breast cancer. Surgical Clinics of North America 70:1081, 1990

Carter CL, Allen C, Henson DE. Relation of tumor size, lymph node status, and survival in 24,740 breast cancer cases. Cancer 63:181–187, 1989

Clark GM, Dressler LG, Owens MA et al. Prediction of relapse or survival in patients with node-negative breast cancer by DNA flow cytometry. N Engl J Med 320:627–633, 1989

Consensus Statement: Treatment of Early-Stage Breast Cancer. National Institutes of Health Consensus Development Panel. J Natl Cancer Institute Monographs 11:1–5, 1992

Early Breast Cancer Trialists' Collaborative Group. Systemic treatment of early breast cancer by hormonal, cytotoxic, or immune therapy. Lancet 339:1–15, 71–85, 1992

Fisher B. Reappraisal of breast biopsy prompted by the use of lumpectomy: Surgical strategy. JAMA 253:2585–2588, 1985

Fisher B, Costantino J, Redmond C et al. A randomized clinical trial evaluating tamoxifen in the treatment of patients with node-negative breast cancer who have estrogen-receptor-positive tumors. N Engl J Med 320:479–484, 1989

Fisher B, Redmond C, Poisson R et al. Eight-year results of a randomized clinical trial comparing total mastectomy and lumpectomy with or without irradiation in the treatment of breast cancer. N Engl J Med 320:822, 1989

Gail MH, Brinton LA, Byar DP et al. Projecting individualized probabilities of developing breast cancer for white females who are being examined annually. J Natl Cancer Inst 81:1879–1886, 1989

Nemoto T, Vana J, Bedwani RN et al. Management and survival of female breast cancer: Results of a national survey by the American College of Surgeons. Cancer 45:2917–2924, 1980

Osborne CK, McGuire WL. Endocrine therapy of metastatic breast cancer. In Kreiger DT, Bardin CW (eds). Current Therapy in Endocrinology 1983–1984. St. Louis, CV Mosby, 1983:334–341

Rosner D, Lane WW. Node-negative minimal invasive breast cancer patients are not candidates for routine systemic adjuvant therapy. Cancer 66:199–205, 1990

John S. Macdonald, Daniel G. Haller, Robert J. Mayer, Eds. *Manual of Oncologic Therapeutics*, Third Edition.

27. HEAD AND NECK CANCERS

Charlotte D. Jacobs
Harlan Pinto

Cancers of the head and neck are a heterogeneous group with variable presentation, staging, treatment, and expected outcome. There are, however, general principles of management that apply to all sites. Most of the material in this chapter refers to squamous cancers, except when noted otherwise.

EPIDEMIOLOGY

Squamous cancers account for approximately 5% of neoplasms in the United States. They usually occur in the 50- to 60-year age group, and the incidence is three times higher in males than in females. Southern Chinese are at a high risk for nasopharyngeal cancer, and Chinese-Americans have an incidence of this cancer 25 times greater than the general population.

ETIOLOGY

The major cause of head and neck cancer is tobacco, and the relative risk increases with number of cigarettes smoked per day. Alcohol produces a synergistic effect. Other known agents that have a direct association with head and neck cancers include the following:

- Cigars and pipe tobacco — lip and oral cavity
- Chewing tobacco — oral cavity
- Betel nut (mixed with tobacco and lime) — buccal mucosa and floor of mouth
- Syphilis — tongue
- Nickel exposure — nasal cavity and paranasal sinus
- Woodworking — nasopharyngeal
- Prolonged sun exposure — lip
- Plummer-Vinson syndrome — hypopharyngeal and esophageal cancers.

Infection with Epstein-Barr virus and consumption of salted fish have been associated with nasopharyngeal cancer.

PATHOLOGY

Ninety-five percent of all head and neck carcinomas are of the squamous cell type, classified as well-differentiated, moderately well-differentiated, poorly differentiated, or undifferentiated. Spread is predominantly local or to regional nodes, and the probability of positive nodes is related to primary site, size of primary, and tumor differentiation. Late dissemination occurs to lung, liver, or bone. Metastases are more common from nasopharyngeal or hypopharyngeal primaries and from advanced local disease.

PRETREATMENT EVALUATION

Proper staging is crucial for planning appropriate treatment, and stage is the single most important factor in determining prognosis. Precise localization of the primary tumor and assessment of regional spread are key. Because metastases are rare at presentation, a limited metastatic evaluation only is advised.

Diagnostic Biopsy

Biopsies should be of full thickness and should be obtained from the non-necrotic portion of the tumor, areas at the edge of the tumor, and adjacent normal mucosa. Open biopsy of a neck node is contraindicated if squamous cell cancer is suspected (see the following section, Evaluation of an Unknown Primary). Fine-needle aspiration is useful for unknown primaries presenting in the neck, as well as salivary gland and thyroid cancers. The incidence of false-negative results can be high among inexperienced pathologists.

Endoscopy

Panendoscopy, including laryngoscopy, bronchoscopy, and esophagoscopy, should be performed before therapy planning. This allows the surgeon to palpate the extent of the primary lesion; to perform additional biopsies of suspicious areas; and to rule out simultaneous second primaries in the lung, esophagus, or other head and neck sites. A three-dimensional description of the tumor and a diagram are made.

Radiographic Studies

In patients with cancers that may encroach on the alveolus, bony invasion is evaluated with a mandible series. Occlusal or Panorex views of the mandible are often more useful studies. Computed tomography (CT) and magnetic resonance imaging (MRI) are complementary for evaluation of the nasopharynx, oral cavity, and oropharynx. CT is superior for evaluating laryngeal lesions (particularly thyroid cartilage invasion), bony erosion of the base of the skull, and metastatic adenopathy. MRI is useful in determining vascular fixation and to distinguish inflammation from tumor, particularly for nasopharynx, nose, and paranasal sinus cancers. Patients with cancers of the piriform sinus, posterior pharynx, or postcricoid area should have a barium swallow if esophagoscopy was not performed to rule out esophageal extension or second primaries. Before treatment, a chest film may reveal underlying pulmonary disease or metastatic spread. Because of the low incidence of metastatic spread at presentation, bone scan and liver CT are only indicated if a patient has symptoms of bone or liver disease or elevated alkaline phosphatase transaminases, bilirubin, or lactic dehydrogenase.

Laboratory Studies

A complete blood count (CBC) and chemistry profile, including liver function tests, are part of the initial evaluation. Epstein-Barr virus (EBV) antibody titers are increased in patients with nasopharyngeal cancer, and the level correlates with disease activity. Some physicians use IgA to viral capsid antigen and IgG to early antigen to follow disease activity.

Other Tests

Patients who are candidates for partial laryngectomy and who have suspected compromise of pulmonary function should have pulmonary function tests before surgery. Patients should undergo a thorough dental evaluation before treatment, and nonsalvageable teeth should be extracted. Postradiation extractions are associated with increased risk of osteoradionecrosis. Fluoride treatments should be prescribed. Patients who require resection of the palate, maxilla, nose, or ear should be seen preoperatively by a posthodontist so an appliance will be ready in the immediate postoperative period. Patients with head and neck cancer are often nutritionally deficient because they have difficulty eating. Attempts should be made to bring the patient into positive nitrogen balance to reduce postoperative complications and improve tolerance to radiation therapy and/or chemotherapy.

Evaluation of an Unknown Primary

If a patient with a history of smoking and/or alcohol use presents with an enlarged neck node, infection has been ruled out, and head and neck cancer is suspected, an incisional lymph node biopsy is contraindicated. First, a history and physical examination (including indirect laryngoscopy) should be performed. Evaluation includes a chest film, and CT scan may be helpful. Fine-needle aspiration may be used to confirm a malignancy and sometimes to determine histologic subtype. If no primary is found, the patient should undergo quadruple endoscopy (nasopharyngoscopy, direct laryngoscopy, bronchoscopy, and esophagoscopy), and if no cancer is seen, random biopsies of the piriform sinus, base of tongue, nasopharynx, and tonsils (the most common sites of unknown primaries) should be performed. If a primary is still not found, the patient should be prepared for a neck dissection, with frozen-tissue confirmation of squamous cancer before neck dissection. Patients should not undergo lymph node biopsy initially for several reasons: (1) a search for the primary site is still necessary; (2) this may increase the risk of metastatic spread; (3) biopsy makes subsequent neck dissection more difficult.

STAGING SYSTEM

The TNM Staging System is used for classification of head and neck cancers. This system defines extent of primary tumor (*T*), status of regional lymph nodes (*N*), and absence or presence of metastatic spread (*M*). The T, N, and M categories are grouped into stages that determine treatment and prognosis. The staging system described below was adopted by the American Joint Committee on Cancer in 1992.

Primary Tumor (T)

For each of the head and neck regions, the definition of the T classification varies.

- **oral cavity** (lip, buccal mucosa, alveolar ridge, retromolar trigone, floor of mouth, hard palate, and anterior two thirds of the tongue) and **oropharynx** (soft palate, uvula, faucial pillars, tonsillar fossa, tonsil, base tongue, and pharyngeal wall).
  - T1 Greatest diameter ≤2 cm
  - T2 Greatest diameter >2 cm to 4 cm
  - T3 Greatest diameter >4 cm
  - T4 Invades adjacent structures
- **hypopharynx** (piriform sinus, postcricoid area, posterior pharyngeal wall)
  - T1 Limited to one subsite
  - T2 Invades more than one subsite or adjacent site, without fixation of hemilarynx
  - T3 Invades more than one subsite or adjacent site, with fixation of hemilarynx
  - T4 Invades adjacent structures (cartilage, soft tissues of neck)
- **supraglottic larynx** (false cords, arytenoids, epiglottis, aryepiglottic folds)
  - T1 Limited to one subsite, normal cord mobility
  - T2 Invades more than one subsite, normal cord mobility
  - T3 Limited to larynx with vocal cord fixation and/or invades postcricoid area, preepiglottic tissues, or piriform sinus
  - T4 Invades through thyroid cartilage and/or extends beyond larynx
- **glottis** (true vocal cords, including anterior and posterior commissures)

T1	Limited to vocal cord, normal mobility
T2	Extends to supraglottis and/or subglottis, and/or impaired mobility
T3	Limited to larynx, vocal cord fixation
T4	Invades through thyroid cartilage and/or extends beyond larynx

- **nasopharynx**

T1	Confined to one subsite
T2	Involves more than one subsite
T3	Invades nasal cavity and/or oropharynx
T4	Invades skull and/or cranial nerves

- **paranasal sinuses**

T1	Limited to antral mucosa, no erosion or bony destruction
T2	Erosion or destruction of infrastructure
T3	Invades skin of cheek, posterior wall of maxillary sinus, floor or medial wall orbit, anterior ethmoids
T4	Invades orbit, cribriform plate, posterior ethmoids or sphenoids, nasopharynx, soft palate, pterygomaxillary or temporal fossae, or base of skull

- **Cervical Nodes (N)**

N0	No nodal metastasis
N1	Single ipsilateral node ≤3 cm in greatest dimension
N2a	Single ipsilateral node >3 cm to ≤6 cm
N2b	Multiple ipsilateral nodes ≤6 cm
N2c	Bilateral or contralateral nodes ≤6 cm
N3	Node >6 cm

- **Distant Metastasis (M)**

Following appropriate evaluation, the M status is defined as follows:

MX	Not assessed
M0	Not known distant metastasis
M1	Distant metastasis

- **Stage Grouping**

Depending on T, N, and M, a patient is grouped into one of the following stages:

Stage I	T1, N0, M0
Stage II	T2, N0, M0
Stage III	T3, N0, M0
	T1 or T2 or T3, N1, M0
Stage IV	T4, N0 or N1, M0
	Any T, N2 or N3, M0
	Any T, any N, M1

TREATMENT

Standard therapeutic modalities for primary treatment of head and neck cancers include surgery and/or radiation therapy. Adjunctive therapies or those used for recurrent disease include chemotherapy, hyperthermia, and laser therapy. Treatment decisions are based on site, stage, pathology, age, coexisting disease, and patient acceptance. It is ideal for a patient to be evaluated first by a team of head and neck surgeons, radiation therapists, medical oncologists, posthodontist, speech therapist, and nutritionist.

SURGICAL GUIDELINES

Resection of the Primary Tumor

The extent of surgical resection is dictated by the tumor stage. In general, resection may be used alone for small lesions or as part of a combined-modality approach for advanced disease. The primary lesion should be widely excised with negative margins. If there is any question as to adequacy of margins, frozen-section examination should be done. Primary closure of the surgical defect is preferable and often possible, but local or regional skin flaps, such as the pectoral myocutaneous, should be used when required.

ORAL CAVITY

A composite resection includes the primary, part of the mandible (if necessary), and cervical nodes. For patients in whom tumor approaches, but does not grossly involve, adjacent bone, a partial mandibulectomy may be performed. Gross bone invasion demands segmental mandibular resection, the extent of which depends on the degree of clinical involvement.

OROPHARYNX

If the lesion extends below the level of the arytenoids, a total laryngectomy is recommended because of aspiration.

SUPRAGLOTTIC LARYNX

A supraglottic laryngectomy can be performed if the cancer is confined to the supraglottic region and the forced expiratory volume (FEV) is more than 60%. A total laryngectomy should be done if (1) tumor extends to the commissures, arytenoids, thyroid cartilage, or glottis; or (2) there is impaired mobility or fixation of vocal cords.

LARYNX

Hemilaryngectomy is appropriate for T1–2 failures of radiation. A total or near total laryngectomy is required for more advanced disease.

Neck Dissection

For patients with known neck disease, a standard radical or modified radical neck dissection should be performed. A radical neck dissection includes the superficial and deep cervical fascia with its enclosed lymph nodes, the sternocleidomastoid and omohyoid muscles, the internal and external jugular veins, the spinal accessory nerve, and the submaxillary gland. Often the spinal accessory nerve can be spared. For patients with cancers of the oral cavity, oropharynx, and supraglottic larynx in whom there are no clinically positive nodes and for whom surgical management of the neck is chosen, a functional neck dissection can be performed. This leaves the sternocleidomastoid, the internal jugular vein, and the spinal accessory nerve intact.

Surgical Complications

In addition to the immediate problems with postoperative infections and bleeding, long-term problems include the following:

1. Cosmetic deformities — reconstruction should be performed as early as possible.
2. Speech impediment — a speech therapist should be part of the team.
3. Aspiration pneumonia — this is most marked with base-of-tongue cancers and partial laryngeal surgery.
4. Shoulder droop and pain — this may result from spinal accessory nerve dysfunction following neck dissection.

RADIATION THERAPY GUIDELINES

Teletherapy

Treatment with a linear accelerator (4–6 MeV energy) is preferred. Cobalt-60 units are acceptable if they operate at 80 SSD (source-to-skin distance). The patient is treated while in the sitting, lateral decubitus, or supine position. The head should be resting on a head holder or immobilized with a bite block or individually-fitted mask. Laser localization is desirable, and a simulator should be used for localization and verification.

A combination of lateral opposed fields, anterior and lateral wedged fields, or isocentric multiple fields is used for the primary tumor site. A single anterior field with a midline block can be used to treat the neck, and lower neck fields should match the primary field at the skin. With carcinomas of the piriform sinus, glottic and supraglottic areas, the tracheostome must be treated, and a midline bar should not be used. The mediastinal T also should be treated when multiple and/or low neck nodes are positive.

Tumor doses are expressed in cGy (rad), calculated at the center of the tumor volume when lateral opposed ports are used. For mediastinal fields, the depth is calculated at 5 cm or one third of the thoracic diameter. The accepted dose rate is 180 cGy to 200 cGy per day (200 cGy for T1–2 larynx cancers). The dose to tumor volume for primary treatment is approximately 6600 cGy to 7000 cGy in 6 to 7 weeks. The dose to a tumor bed following resection is 5500 cGy in 5 to 5 ½ weeks for negative margins, 6000 cGy for close margins, and 6600 cGy — 7000 cGy for positive margins. The maximum dose to the spinal cord should be no more than 4000 cGy when 200 cGy fractions are used. Great care should be used with opposed lateral fields and anterior fields without a midline bar to avoid overlap. Postoperative radiation should begin as soon as healing is satisfactory (about 2 weeks).

Brachytherapy

Interstitial implantation of radioactive sources is a means of obtaining high localized radiation dose to the tumor bed while minimizing normal tissue injury. The most commonly used permanent implant source is iodine 125. The most commonly used removable brachytherapy source is Iridium 192 seeds. The dose rate for removable implants is between 40 cGy to 100 cGy per hour. In previously untreated patients, the total dose of iodine 125 for 1 year is approximately 12,000–15,000 cGy. Removable interstitial doses, used to boost a local area after 5500 cGy external beam, should be limited to 2500 cGy to 3000 cGy.

Hyperthermia

Ultrasound or microwaves to heat tumors to 44°C with or without external radiation are used to treat locally recurrent disease.

Toxicities of Radiation Therapy

The toxic effects of radiation therapy include the following:

1. Xerostomia and loss of taste are very troublesome. Dental cavities are frequent, and fluoride mouthwash should be used regularly.
2. Mucositis may necessitate delays in treatment. The tongue and buccal mucosa must be protected from x-ray dental scatter.
3. Otitis media should be managed with decongestants but may require tube placement.
4. Osteoradionecrosis of the mandible can often be prevented by appropriate dental extractions before radiation. Treatment is with antibiotics (penicillin), but in severe cases, hyperbaric oxygen and/or resection may be required.
5. Laryngeal edema may follow radiation to the larynx, and a small percentage of patients may develop cartilage necrosis or a compromised airway. Conservative treatment includes antibiotics and/or steroids. Persistent edema following radiation should make one highly suspicious of tumor recurrence.
6. Lhermitte's syndrome, which is characterized by electric sensations in the spine, arms, or legs on neck flexion, requires no treatment.
7. A small percentage of patients develop hypothyroidism, heralded by an elevation of thyroid-stimulating hormone.

CHEMOTHERAPY GUIDELINES

Single Agents

The most active single agents are methotrexate and cisplatin. Methotrexate is generally given intravenously at 40–60 mg/m^2 weekly. There is no evidence that large doses of methotrexate are superior to standard doses. Because of renal excretion, the patient should have a normal serum creatinine. Toxicities include mucositis, myelosuppression, hepatotoxicity, nephrotoxicity, and severe fatigue. Elderly patients or those with poor nutritional status are more likely to have severe reactions. CBC and platelets should be monitored weekly; liver function tests and serum creatinine should be monitored at least monthly. The cytotoxic effects of the drug can be reversed with leucovorin, a reduced folate.

Cisplatin is an effective drug whose major route of excretion is renal, and its use should be limited to patients with a creatinine clearance that is more than 50 ml/minute. The standard dose is 100 mg/m^2 every 3 weeks. Because of nephrotoxicity, a 24-hour infusion or mannitol diuresis is recommended. Typical standing orders are as follows: 12 hours before administration of cisplatin, prehydrate with 2 liters dextrose, 5% in 0.5 normal saline plus 20 meq of potassium chloride. Three hours before administration of cisplatin, increase to 300 ml/hour. Just before administration of cisplatin, mannitol (12.5 g) is given by rapid intravenous injection, followed by cisplatin (100 mg/m^2) in saline infused over 30 minutes to a concentration of 1 mg/ml. Follow this with a continuous infusion of mannitol (10 g/hour for 6 hours) with concurrent dextrose, 5% in 0.5 normal saline plus 20 meq potassium chloride per liter at 200 ml/hour for 6 hours. Furosemide may be repeated if there is an inadequate diuretic response to mannitol. Toxicities include nephrotoxicity, mild myelosupression, moderately severe nausea and vomiting, hypomagnesemia, ototoxicity, and neurotoxicity. Patients should have renal function and blood counts monitored closely throughout treatment. Response rates of 20–30% are expected in patients with recurrent disease.

Response rates in excess of 15% for recurrent disease have been reported with several other drugs, including bleomycin, 5-fluorouracil (5-FU), adriamycin, cyclophosphamide, hydroxyurea, carboplatin, ifosphamide, and taxol.

Combination Chemotherapy

Multiple combinations have been reported for recurrent head and neck cancers, with complete and overall response rates higher than those of single agents. Two commonly used regimens are:

Cisplatin, 50 mg/m^2 on day 6; methotrexate, 40 mg/m^2 on days 1 and 15; bleomycin, 10 mg on days 1, 8, 15.

Cisplatin, 100 mg/m^2 on day 1; 5-FU, 1000 mg/m^2 by continuous infusion for days 1–4.

Intra-arterial Chemotherapy

Intra-arterial chemotherapy has been used to improve drug delivery to local disease. With currently available implantable drug delivery systems, chemotherapy can be safely delivered if performed by a team familiar with this technique. This approach has not yet been shown superior to and less toxic than systemic chemotherapy.

THERAPEUTIC PLAN

Standard Therapy

The treatment plan must be individualized based on stage, site, and the patient's general health. The goal should be cure with acceptable morbidity. For T1 and T2 cancers, in general, surgery or radiation therapy is acceptable with equivalent outcome. Small floor of mouth cancers that encroach on the mandible are better managed with surgery because of the risk of osteoradionecrosis. Brachytherapy has been particularly successful for base of tongue and tonsil primaries.

Most T3 and resectable T4 cancers require combined surgery and radiation. Exceptions include small T3 glottic cancers, which some prefer to treat with single modality, and nasopharynx cancer, which is managed with radiation alone. Radiation therapy used before or after surgery gives equivalent results, although there may be fewer surgical complications if radiation is used following surgery. For larynx cancer, chemotherapy and radiation are an alternative to laryngectomy and radiation.

The decision of whether to treat the neck with clinical stage N0 is based on the likelihood of occult disease in the neck. In general, cancers larger than a small T1 (>1.5 cm), have high enough risk that the neck should be treated with either radiation or neck dissection. Exceptions include the vocal cord and paranasal sinuses, for which the incidence is low. For an N1 neck ≤3 cm, radiation alone can control disease, but for larger or multiple nodes, a modified or radical neck dissection should be performed as well. The exception is nasopharyngeal cancer, in which most large nodes can be treated with radiation alone because of its radiosensitivity. Lymph nodes with extracapsular spread and/or carotid artery fixation are associated with poor prognosis.

For patients with an unknown squamous primary, a neck dissection is recommended, followed by radiation to a large head and neck field encompassing the nasopharynx, base of tongue, piriform sinus, tonsils, and neck.

Role of Chemotherapy

The standard role of chemotherapy is for palliation of recurrent or metastatic disease. Methotrexate and cisplatin as single agents each produce response rates of approximately 30% (mostly partial responses) lasting 4 to 6 months. Although drug combinations appear to produce higher response rates (up to 70%), there is no evidence to date that combination chemotherapy prolongs survival compared with single-agent chemotherapy, although it is more costly and toxic.

Chemotherapy is also being evaluated as part of a combined modality approach for previously untreated patients as (1) induction therapy for resectable patients, (2) concurrent therapy with radiation for unresectable patients, and (3) an organ-sparing therapy.

INDUCTION CHEMOTHERAPY

Chemotherapy has been used before surgery in attempts to reduce tumor size and to decrease local or distal recurrence. When using chemotherapy in this manner, the optimal response is obtained after two to three cycles. Reported response rates vary from 70% to 90% overall with 20% to 50% complete responses. Two commonly used induction regimens are as follows:

1. Cisplatin (100 mg/m^2) as noted above, plus 5-FU (1 g/m^2 dissolved in 2 liters of dextrose, 5% in 0.5 normal saline infused over 24 hours), daily for 5 days, repeated every 3 weeks. Additional toxicities from 5-FU include mucositis, diarrhea, alopecia, and cardiac ischemia.
2. Cisplatin (100 mg/m^2) and 5-FU as outlined above plus leucovorin (50 mg/m^2 po q 6 hrs) daily for 5 days. The regimen is repeated every 3 weeks.

Although several trials have shown a significant reduction in metastatic rate, no trial to date has shown that the addition of induction chemotherapy to surgery and/or radiation has improved curability. This approach is still considered experimental.

Another role that has been investigated for induction chemotherapy is that of organ preservation, that is, decreasing morbidity by substituting chemotherapy for surgical resection. Using induction cisplatin-5FU followed by radiation, the Department of Veterans Affairs Laryngeal Cancer Study Group was able to preserve the larynx in 66% of patients with advanced cancer. There was a decrease in disease-free survival in this group compared to the laryngectomy-radiation group, but salvage laryngectomy effected the same overall survival.

CONCURRENT RADIOTHERAPY AND CHEMOTHERAPY

Bleomycin (5 mg intramuscularly twice weekly), 5-FU, and mitomycin C have been used concurrently with radiotherapy in attempts to improve radiation efficacy and reduce local recurrence in patients with advanced, unresectable disease. Randomized trials have shown minimal decrease in recurrence rate. Combinations of agents with concurrent radiation are being evaluated and appear promising. Increased local radiation reactions, however, have been noted with concurrent chemotherapy. Superior survival has been demonstrated for rapidly alternating combination chemotherapy and radiation compared to radiation alone.

MAINTENANCE CHEMOTHERAPY

Adjuvant chemotherapy following primary surgery and/or radiation has not been extensively tested in head and neck cancer. Although adjuvant chemotherapy has reduced metastatic rate in a few trials, this has not resulted in improved survival.

THERAPEUTIC OUTCOME

Cure for squamous cancers of the head and neck is measured in terms of 5-year survival, although most relapses occur in the first 3 years following therapy. Survival in this group of patients is significantly shortened by second primaries and other health problems. Follow-up should consist of a thorough head and neck examination every 1 to 2 months for the first year, with progressively longer intervals up to 5 years. A chest film should be obtained yearly. Reports of disease-free survival and survival differ with primary site, TNM classification, treatment modality, number of patients, and follow-up. Approximate disease-free survival rates are presented in Table 27–1.

These results are usually better in patients with negative neck nodes and decrease with increasing amounts of neck disease.

PREVENTION

Future efforts in head and neck cancer should be directed toward early detection and prevention. Unfortunately, the incidence and survival rates in this disease have not changed

TABLE 27–1. DISEASE-FREE SURVIVAL RATES FOR HEAD AND NECK CANCER

DISEASE SITE	STAGE	SURVIVAL RATE (%)
Oral tongue	T1, T2	70–85
	T3, T4	30–40
Floor of mouth	T1, T2	65–80
	T3, T4	20–45
Tonsil	T1, T2	60–75
	T3, T4	20–35
Piriform sinus	T3, T4	25
Glottic larynx	T1, T2	80–90
	T3, T4	25–40
Supraglottic larynx	T1, T2	60–85
	T3, T4	25–40
Base of tongue	T1, T2	50–60
	T3, T4	25–40
Nasopharynx	T1, T2	70–75
	T3	55
	T4	≤10

significantly despite screening and smoking cessation programs. In addition, these patients develop second primaries at an annual rate of 4–7%. Chemoprevention with retinoids is a promising new approach. Retinoids can reduce oral leukoplakia and, in a randomized trial, significantly reduced the incidence of second primaries. To date, toxicity and noncompliance have limited optimal use of these agents.

SALIVARY GLAND CANCERS

Cancers of the salivary gland account for less than 5% of head and neck neoplasms. The majority arise in the parotid gland, and approximately 25% of parotid tumors are malignant. Of those originating in the submaxillary gland and minor salivary glands (palate, nasal cavity, and paranasal sinuses), half are malignant. These cancers usually present as painless masses and infrequently produce pain from nerve involvement.

Pathology

The most common histologic subtype is mucoepidermoid (low grade or high grade). Others include acinic cell, malignant mixed, adenoid cystic, adenocarcinoma, poorly differentiated, squamous, and anaplastic carcinoma. The diagnosis can be made by needle biopsy if the pathologist is familiar with this technique. Excisional biopsy alone is usually contraindicated because it makes the definitive surgical procedure more difficult. Diagnosis is best made at time of parotidectomy. These cancers spread by direct extension, and some, like adenoid cystic, have a propensity to spread along nerve sheaths. Lymph node spread is found in up to 30% of high-grade cancers (adenocarcinoma, squamous, undifferentiated, anaplastic, and high-grade mucoepidermoid).

Pretreatment Evaluation

The most common site of metastatic spread is lung, and a chest film should be done before surgery. A CT scan with contrast or MRI can help evaluate parotid masses but seldom differentiates benign from malignant lesions.

Staging System

The TNM staging system for salivary gland cancers is presented in Table 27–2.

TABLE 27–2. TNM STAGING SYSTEM FOR SALIVARY GLAND CANCERS

The N and M definitions are the same as for squamous cancers.

T DEFINITIONS

T1	≤2cm in greatest dimension
T2	2 cm to 4 cm
T3	4 cm to 6 cm
T4	>6cm

a, no local extension; b, local extension

STAGES

Stage I	T1a, T2a, N0, M0
Stage II	T1b, T2b, T3a, N0, M0
Stage III	T3b, T4a, N0, M0
Stage IV	T4b, any N, M0
	Any T, N2, N3, M0, M1

Therapeutic Plan

Surgery is the treatment of choice for salivary gland neoplasms. For parotid cancers that are low-grade and involve only the superficial lobe, a superficial parotidectomy may be performed. For all others, a total parotidectomy is recommended. The facial nerve often can be preserved, but if it is involved and needs to be sacrificed, a nerve graft may preserve function. At the time of surgery if periparotid nodes are positive, a radical neck dissection should be performed. Because of the high incidence of occult neck disease, patients with high-grade tumors should have a prophylactic neck dissection. Treatment of minor salivary gland cancers includes a wide excision. Most would recommend postoperative radiation for patients with high-grade cancers, positive margin, perineural invasion, deep lobe involvement, and regional lymph node metastases, at a minimum dose of 5000 cGy to 5500 cGy or 6600 cGy for positive margins. Primary radiotherapy is reserved for inoperable patients, and neutrons may be useful in this situation. Chemotherapy has been used mainly for palliation of recurrent disease. The best single agents are cisplatin, doxorubicin, 5-FU, and methotrexate. Overall, responses have been noted in up to 30% of patients, but most series are small. Combination chemotherapy can improve response rates, but toxicity is increased. In some patients with recurrent disease, particularly adenoid cystic carcinoma, the tempo of disease is so slow that patients do not need to be treated for prolonged time periods.

Outcome

The major factors that influence outcome are histology, site of tumor, and tumor size. Local control is achieved in approximately 80% of low-grade cancers and approximately 30% of high-grade cancers. Twenty percent of patients with high-grade neoplasms develop distant metastases in lung or bone. Five-year survival for parotid cancers range from 30% in undifferentiated neoplasms to 92% in acinic cell cancer, but since salivary gland cancers can recur at 10 and 15 years, 5-year survival rates are unreliable. Because of the small number of patients with salivary gland cancers, multicenter efforts will be necessary to demonstrate the impact of new therapeutic approaches.

BIBLIOGRAPHY

American Joint Committee on Cancer. Manual for Staging of Cancer, 4th ed. Philadelphia, JB Lippincott, 1992

Bailet JW, Mark RJ, Abemayor E et. al. Nasopharyngeal carcinoma: treatment results with primary radiation therapy. Laryngoscope 102:965–972, 1992

Carrau RL, Myers EN, Johnson JT. Paranasal sinus carcinoma — diagnosis, treatment, and prognosis. Oncology 6:43–50, 1992

Department of Veterans Affairs Laryngeal Cancer Study Group. Induction chemotherapy plus radiation compared with surgery plus radiation in patients with advanced laryngeal cancer. N Engl J Med 324:1685–1690, 1991

Dimery IW, Hong WK. Overview of combined modality therapies for head. J Natl Cancer Inst 85:95–111, 1993

Jacobs CD, Goffinet DR, Fee WE. Head and neck squamous cancers. Current Problems in Cancer 14:1–7, 1990

Johnson JT, Hao SP, Myers E, Wagner R. Outcome of open surgical therapy for glottic carcinoma. Ann Otol Rhinol Laryngol 102:752–755, 1993

Merlano M, Vitale V, Rosso R et. al. Treatment of advanced squamous cell carcinoma of the head and neck with alternating chemotherapy and radiotherapy. New Engl J Med 327:1115–1121, 1992

Rodgers LW, Stringer SP, Mendenhall WM et. al. Management of squamous cell carcinomas of the floor of mouth. Head and Neck 15:16–19, 1993

Spiro IJ, Wang CC, Montgomery WW. Carcinoma of the parotid gland. Cancer 71:2699–2705, 1993

Vokes EE, Weichselbaum RR, Lippman SM, Hong WK. Head and neck cancer. N Engl J Med 328:184–194, 1993

Wang CC, Montgomery WW. Deciding on optimal management of supraglottic carcinoma. Oncology 5:41–49, 1991

Young RC. Cancer prevention. Arch Otolaryngol Head Neck Surg 119:732–734, 1993

28. GASTROINTESTINAL CANCERS

Sandra Schnall
John S. Macdonald

Cancers of the gastrointestinal (GI) tract are the most common neoplasms in the Western world. They represent approximately 20% of all malignancies diagnosed annually in the United States. There are variations in the epidemiology and etiology of these cancers, leading to different treatment regimens and therapeutic approaches. Pretreatment evaluations now may include molecular techniques, in conjunction with radiographic and pathological studies, to help determine prognostic indicators and treatment planning.

ESOPHAGEAL CARCINOMA

Carcinoma of the esophagus accounts for approximately 1% of all cancers and 7% of all GI tumors. It is estimated that in 1993 there will be 11,300 new cases of esophageal carcinoma diagnosed in the United States and, approximately 10,200 deaths. There is a male predominance, with a male to female ratio of 5:1. Esophageal cancer is not increasing, and the overall incidence in both males and females has remained constant in the United States.

In other parts of the world, such as northern China, Iran, and parts of India, the age-adjusted incidence of esophageal carcinoma is much higher. This is likely a reflection of exposure to different etiologic factors. In the United States, squamous cell carcinoma of the esophagus is most commonly associated with cigarette smoking and/or alcohol consumption. However, in the Middle East and Asian countries, nitrosamines in the food chain, vitamin deficiency, or hot burning liquids capable of producing thermal burns have been implicated.

There are a few medical conditions that may predispose to esophageal carcinoma. These include achalasia, Plummer-Vinson syndrome, tylosis palmaris, Barrett's esophagus, and lye-induced strictures.

The most common pathology is still squamous cell carcinoma, reported in up to 90% of esophageal tumors. However, other cell types, particularly adenocarcinomas, appear to be increasing in relative incidence. Adenocarcinomas are most common in the distal esophagus and often are associated with Barrett's epithelium. Other neoplasms, including carcinoid tumors, small cell carcinomas, leiomyosarcomas, melanomas, and lymphomas occur uncommonly.

Presentation

The most common presenting symptoms of esophageal carcinoma, dysphagia and weight loss, are seen in 90% of patients. These may be progressive, and patients may note difficulty swallowing solid foods before they experience difficulties with soft or liquid products. More advanced symptoms include odynophagia, regurgitation, hematemesis, cough (*i.e.*, tracheoesophageal fistula), hoarseness, or symptoms of a superior vena cava syndrome.

The morbidity and mortality associated with esophageal carcinoma reflects the pattern of spread. Due to the absence of a serosa on the esophagus, the tumor may spread into the mediastinal tissues (the trachea, pleura, and great vessels) early in the disease. Involvement of the lymphatics occurs early. The lymphatics arise in the mucosa and external muscular coat and drain longitudinally, with many intercommunications between channels. Due to the complexity of the lymphatic network, skip lesions with long intervening segments of normal esophagus are common. Metastatic foci most commonly involve the liver, lung, or bone; however, metastasis to the adrenals, brain, and stomach may also be seen.

Evaluation

Mass lesions of the esophagus are often easily identified with a barium swallow. Patients usually do not experience symptoms (*e.g.*, dysphagia) until more than 50% of the lumen is occluded. Upper endoscopy confirms the presence of esophageal tumors in those with an abnormal barium swallow. Brushings and biopsies during endoscopy help obtain tissue confirmation. Due to an increased incidence of synchronous tumors in other areas of the aerodigestive tract, laryngoscopy and bronchoscopy should also be performed. Bronchoscopy also will help identify any direct invasion into the tracheal tree.

Routine laboratory data including a chemistry package and complete blood count (CBC) should be obtained. A computed tomographic (CT) scan of the chest and abdomen helps identify the extent of the tumor locally, helps identify adenopathy, or detects evidence of metastatic spread to the liver or the lungs. A bone scan may be indicated if the patient complains of bony pain or has an elevated alkaline phosphatase.

Endoluminal ultrasound has added another dimension to evaluation of esophageal tumors. It gives excellent information on the depth of penetration of the tumor through the esophageal wall in up to 90% of patients. It has less accuracy in identifying lymph node metastases, however.

Staging System

The most widely used TNM staging system for esophageal cancers is outlined on Table 28–1. The TNM system recognizes localized (stage I), locally advanced (stage II), and more disseminated (stage III) disease.

TABLE 28–1. TNM STAGING FOR ESOPHAGEAL CANCER

PRIMARY TUMOR

T0	No demonstrable tumor
T1S	Carcinoma in situ
T1	Tumor involves 5 cm or less of esophageal length with no obstruction or complete circumferential involvement or extraesophageal spread
T2	Tumor involves more than 5 cm of esophagus and produces obstruction with circumferential involvement of the esophagus but no extraesophageal spread
T3	Tumor with extension outside the esophagus involving mediastinal structures

REGIONAL LYMPH NODES (N)

Cervical esophagus (cervical and supraclavicular lymph nodes)

N0	No nodal involvement
N1	Unilateral involvement (moveable)
N2	Bilateral involvement (moveable)
N3	Fixed nodes

Thoracic esophagus (nodes in the thorax, not those of the cervical, supraclavicular, or abdominal areas)

N0	No nodal involvement
N1	Nodal involvement

DISTANT METASTASES (M)

M0	No metastases
M1	Distant metastases. Cancer of thoracic esophagus with cervical, supraclavicular, or abdominal lymph node involvement is classified as M1.

STAGE I

T1, N0, M0

STAGE II

T1, N1, M0
T1, N2, M0
T2, N0, M0
T2, N1, M0
T2, N2, M0

STAGE III

Any M1
Any T3

Adapted from American Joint Committee on Cancer. Manual for Staging of Cancer. 3rd ed. Philadelphia, JB Lippincott, 1988

Therapy

The treatment of esophageal carcinoma is evolving steadily. For many years the standard therapy for localized disease was esophagectomy. The overall 5-year survival rate after surgical resection alone is at best approximately 20%. The pattern of recurrence is characterized by both local and distant failure. Early dissemination has been attributed to the lack of serosa. Radiation and/or chemotherapy were previously recommended for palliative treatment of advanced tumors.

Because of the poor results with surgery alone, combined modality approaches are being evaluated. They include preoperative radiation therapy alone, preoperative chemotherapy alone, or preoperative radiation therapy in conjunction with chemotherapy. Many Phase II (nonrandomized) trials and a few Phase III (prospectively randomized) trials have been completed to date.

Studies evaluating preoperative radiation therapy alone do not show that this approach is superior to surgery alone. At total dose levels ranging from 3300 to 5500 cGy, toxicity was acceptable. However, improved survival was not detected when compared to surgery alone.

Because the overall poor survival noted with surgery with or without radiation therapy was often secondary to disseminated tumor, trials evaluating preoperative chemotherapy were developed. Single-agent chemotherapy as well as combination chemotherapy has been employed. The most active agents are bleomycin, cisplatinum, 5-fluorouracil (5-FU), vinblastine, and mitomycin-C. In randomized and nonrandomized trials, no improvement was noted in the expected 12-month median survival with surgery alone.

The first trials using combined modality therapy prior to esophagectomy were conducted at Wayne State University in the 1970s. Subsequent trials by the Southwest Oncology Group (SWOG) and at Wayne State used combinations of radiation therapy, 5-FU, and cisplatin (Table 28–2). Eighteen of 71 cases (25%) demonstrated a complete pathologic response (CR) to this therapy documented by the absence of tumor in the resected esophagus. The median survival time of all patients was 12–14 months, but for the complete responders it was 32 months. These early data suggest that patients rendered disease-free preoperatively with radiation and chemotherapy may have prolonged survival.

Forstiere and coworkers recently published the results of a 3-week intensive preoperative chemoradiation regimen for the treatment of local–regional esophageal carcinoma. Patients received a bolus of vinblastine and continuous infusion cisplatin and 5-FU over a 21-day period with concurrent radiation therapy. On day 42, patients underwent a transhiatal esophagectomy. The results were improved compared to historical controls receiving surgery alone. Thirty-two percent of patients with residual tumor in the resected specimen were long-term survivors, with a median survival of 26

TABLE 28–2. COMBINED-MODALITY THERAPY FOR ESOPHAGEAL CARCINOMA

5-FU, 1000 mg/m^2 per day, IV continuous infusion on days 1 to 4; repeat on days 29 to 32
Cisplatin, 75 mg/m^2, IV day 1 and day 29 only
Radiation therapy, 3000 cGy delivered in 15 fractions, days 1 to 19

↓

Evaluation ⟶ No distant metastases

↓

Surgery

months. The patients attaining a pathologic CR had a 70-month median survival.

Herskovic and colleagues published data demonstrating that patients receiving combined modality therapy with radiation therapy (5000 cGy) and chemotherapy (5-FU and cisplatin) had improved survival and decreased distant metastasis compared to cases receiving radiation alone (6400 cGy).

A major question that must be answered is whether surgical resection adds any significant benefit for patients after combined therapy with radiation and chemotherapy. A large scale Intergroup trial currently is underway addressing this issue (INT 0113). Patients are randomized to receive either the standard treatment of surgery alone or three cycles of preoperative cisplatin and 5-FU followed by esophagectomy. Postoperatively these cases receive two additional cycles of chemotherapy. A second Intergroup trial begun in 1994 compares chemotherapy and radiation therapy given concurrently versus chemotherapy followed by radiation therapy.

Off-protocol patients with localized esophageal tumor may be reasonably offered preoperative radiation therapy with chemotherapy (Table 28–2), although surgical resection alone must still be considered standard therapy.

The treatment of stage III (metastatic disease) is palliative. Chemotherapy of advanced esophageal carcinoma has been uniformly disappointing. The fluorouracil/cisplatinum regimen outlined in Table 28–3 is a reasonable approach, with response rates of approximately 30%. Palliative radiation therapy may produce response rates of up to 70% in some series and may decrease dysphagia from obstructing tumor. In general, patients are given 4000 cGy in 20 fractions. Combined modality therapy (Table 28–2) may also be a reasonable approach to localized advanced disease in patients with a good performance status.

Other supportive care approaches may also be of value. There has been much interest in endoscopic laser therapy to help alleviate esophageal obstruction. Another maneuver, designed to improve nutrition, is the placement of a percutaneous endoscopic gastrostomy (PEG). After adequate patency of the esophagus (with either laser or radiation therapy) has been achieved, a PEG may be placed for ongoing alimentation. A surgical feeding gastrostomy may be placed if one is unable to insert a PEG. Total parenteral hyperalimentation (TPN) also may be used, but enteral alimentation is the treatment of choice. Nutritional support should not be used in the patient for whom no effective palliative antitumor therapy is planned. Such patients are best managed with analgesics and hospice care.

TABLE 28–3. CHEMOTHERAPY REGIMEN FOR ESOPHAGEAL CANCER

	OVERALL RESPONSE RATE (%)
Cisplatin, 75 mg/m^2 on day 1 5-FU, 1000 mg/m^2 per day, continuous infusion, days 1 to 4	30–50

CARCINOMA OF THE STOMACH

Worldwide there is geographic variation in the incidence of gastric carcinoma. It is much more common in Japan and some South American countries than in the United States. These variations may reflect certain ethnic dietary habits. Low consumption of fresh vegetables and fruit and a high intake of salt, smoked foods, and nitrates correlates with an increased incidence of this tumor. Neither smoking nor drinking has been convincingly associated with the risk of gastric carcinoma. The incidence of gastric carcinoma has decreased significantly in the United States in this century, but the incidence has been relatively stable since the mid-1970s. The reason for the decrease is poorly understood. It is estimated that there will be 24,000 new cases of gastric carcinoma in the United States in 1993 and approximately 13,000 cancer-related deaths.

Special notation must be made of adenocarcinoma at the gastroesophageal (GE) junction. Despite a decreased incidence of tumors in the body of the stomach, an increase in lesions of the gastric cardia and GE junction has been noted, especially in young Caucasian males. The reason for this increase is poorly understood, but the increased incidence of proximal gastric cancer has led to the level overall incidence of all stomach carcinomas since the mid-1970s.

Medical and genetic conditions may predispose to gastric tumors. Individuals with blood group A, those who have undergone a gastric resection for benign disease, have *Helicobacter pylori* infection, or have a history of Barrett's esophagus, may have an increased risk for stomach or cardioesophageal junction carcinomas. There has been some association with certain occupations, including coal mining, nickel refining, and rubber processing. There also appears to be an increased incidence of stomach cancers in asbestos workers.

More than 90% of neoplasms in the stomach are adenocarcinomas. Other histologies are leiomyosarcoma, lymphoma, and carcinoid tumors. Most adenocarcinomas are ulcerative masses greater than 1 cm with heaped edges or borders. Endoscopically, they may resemble a benign ulcer. Scirrhous adenocarcinomas produce a desmoplastic reaction that typically shows no ulcerated mass but may infiltrate the muscle wall of the stomach, yielding a stiff and fibrotic organ that leads to the clinical picture of linitis plastica.

Presentation

At the time of presentation, most patients with gastric carcinoma have locally advanced or metastatic tumors. The initial symptom often is vague dyspepsia (heartburn) that may or may not respond to H_2 blockers, and abdominal fullness. If the tumor involves the GE junction or gastric cardia, dysphagia may be an early presenting complaint. As the disease progresses, unexplained weight loss is common. Although GI blood loss is associated with gastric tumors, a massive or exsanguinating GI bleed is not commonly associated with adenocarcinomas. Such an event is more commonly associated with leiomyosarcomas, esophageal varices, or benign gastric ulcers.

Gastric tumors may spread by direct extension to the omentum, liver, pancreas, or other surrounding organs. The lymphatic spread is commonly to local abdominal lymph nodes. It may also spread to Virchow's node (left supraclavicular) or Irish's node (left axilla). The most common site of hematologic metastasis is to the liver, although pulmonary, bone, and even leptomeningeal tumors have been reported. Intraabdominal spread of tumor may also occur. There are several defined syndromes, such as the Kruckenberg tumor, which results from metastases to the ovary; Blumer's shelf, involving metastases to the peritoneal reflexion), and Sister Joseph nodules, which are periumbilical peritoneal metastatic foci.

Evaluation

Pretreatment evaluation of gastric carcinomas should include a thorough physical examination, including attention to the sites noted in the previous section. Any evidence of spread to these areas (*e.g.*, supraclavicular fossa, rectal shelf, ovary, or umbilicus) implies surgically incurable tumor, although palliative gastric resection may still be appropriate.

Although fiberoptic endoscopy is now the most commonly used diagnostic technique, a double-contrast upper GI study may help identify an ulcerated lesion. The barium study may also show areas of the gastric wall with abnormal movement or aperistalsis, possibly suggesting a linitis plastica lesion. Endoscopy offers the ability to obtain a tissue diagnosis. Usually at least six biopsies are performed, one from each of the quadrants of the ulcer and two from the center. Cytologic brushings may also yield a diagnosis.

Further staging helps to obtain a treatment plan. A CT scan is less sensitive than an upper GI in detecting the primary lesion, but it will help determine the extramural extent of the tumor, as well as sites of metastatic disease including lymph nodes, liver, or evidence of peritoneal carcinomatosis.

Endoscopic ultrasound has also been used in staging gastric carcinomas to determine the depth of tumor infiltration through the gastric wall and to assess nodal involvement. It should, however, be used in conjunction with CT and endoscopy.

A new avenue of evaluation uses molecular techniques. DNA-ploidy, S-phase fraction, and oncogene expression have been investigated as tools for better understanding tumor biology and helping to identify indicators of prognosis. Early investigation in gastric carcinoma shows non-random chromosome abnormalities on the short arm of chromosome 11. Up to 11% of patients studied also have overexpression of the HER2/NEU oncogene. RAS oncogene mutations, however, have not been detected in gastric carcinomas. DNA analyses by flow cytometry show most proximal tumors to be aneuploid, whereas only 50% of the distal gastric tumors are aneuploid. These abnormal molecular parameters are similar in both Western and Asian populations.

Staging

The TNM classification and staging system is shown in Table 28–4. Stage I, II, and III tumors represent progressively local tumor, whereas stage IV disease represents distant metastasis.

Treatment

The primary treatment of gastric carcinoma is surgery. The most common approach is a radical subtotal gastrectomy. In this procedure, 80% to 85% of the stomach, the first portion of the duodenum, the omentum, and the draining nodes are resected. Monthly parenteral vitamin B_{12} must be provided postoperatively after gastric resection. Complications of surgery include a dumping syndrome, manifested by vomiting, abdominal fullness, tachycardia, and weakness. This likely develops as a result of the loss of the gastric antrum and, therefore, of the reservoir function of the stomach. Treatment is a low carbohydrate diet and antiperistaltic agents.

The overall survival for gastric carcinoma after resection is shown in Table 28–5. Most patients do poorly; therefore, efforts utilizing other treatment modalities must be explored.

TREATMENT OF ADVANCED DISEASE

For locally advanced disease, (*i.e.*, patients who are unable to be resected), external beam radiation therapy may be palliative in reducing pain, relieving obstruction, and perhaps relieving bleeding. Palliative total gastrectomy probably should not be considered an option, as the morbidity of the procedure likely outweighs any palliative benefit to the patient. Partial gastrectomy for distal lesions may be palliative. It is doubtful that chemotherapy alone is useful in treatment of locally advanced gastric carcinoma; however, chemotherapy in conjunction with radiation may yield significant benefit. Two trials have been completed that randomized patients to radiation therapy alone versus radiation therapy with chemotherapy. In one study, those who received 5-FU and radiation therapy had a median survival of 12 months versus a median survival of 5.9 months for those with radiation therapy alone. Similarly, a study by the GI Tumor Study Group (GITSG) demonstrated prolonged disease-free survival in cases treated with radiation therapy plus chemotherapy (methyl-CCNU plus 5-FU) versus those treated with chemotherapy alone.

TABLE 28–4. TNM STAGING FOR STOMACH CANCER

PRIMARY TUMOR

TX	Primary tumor cannot be assessed
T0	No evidence of primary tumor
Tis	Carcinoma in situ: intraepithelial tumor without invasion of the lamina propria
T1	Tumor invades lamina propria or submucosa
T2	Tumor invades muscularis propria or subserosa
T3	Tumor penetrates serosa (visceral peritoneum) without invasion of adjacent structures
T3	Tumor invades adjacent structures

REGIONAL LYMPH NODES (N)

NX	Regional lymph node(s) cannot be assessed
N0	No regional lymph node metastasis
N1	Metastasis in perigastric lymph node(s) within 3 cm of the edge of the primary tumor
N2	Metastasis in perigastric lymph node(s) more than 3 cm from the edge of the primary tumor, or in lymph nodes along the left gastric, common hepatic, splenic, or celiac arteries

DISTANT METASTASIS (M)

MX	Presence of distant metastasis cannot be assessed
M0	No metastasis
M1	Distant metastasis

STAGE I
T1, N0–1, M0
T2, N0, M0

STAGE II
T1, N2, M0
T2, N1, M0
T3, N0, M0

STAGE III
T2, N2, M0
T3, N1–2, M0
T4, N0–1, M0

STAGE IV
T4, N2, M0
ANY M1

Adapted from American Joint Committee on Cancer. Manual for Staging of Cancer. 3rd ed. Philadelphia, JB Lippincott, 1988

Current combined modality trials for locally advanced gastric carcinoma are evaluating a "sandwich technique," in which radiation therapy is given between courses of chemotherapy. Another approach to locally advanced disease is neoadjuvant therapy, which will be described later in this section. If no protocol is available, treatment of locally advanced gastric adenocarcinoma should include either combined modality therapy with 5-FU plus radiation therapy or a neoadjuvant approach.

Treatment of advanced (metastatic) gastric carcinoma is usually chemotherapy-based. Radiation therapy has a role in palliative treatment of obstructing painful lesions. Single-agent chemotherapy does not often yield a high response rate (Table 28–6). Response rates are generally of brief duration and do not have significant impact on survival.

Combination chemotherapy regimens have been widely tested in advanced stomach cancer. Several Phase II and Phase III trials have been reported. The more commonly used regimens are listed in Table 28–7. In the past the most widely applied program has been the 5-FU, doxorubicin, mitomycin-C (FAM) regimen. A review of about 300 patients treated with FAM in eight separate series documented an overall response rate of 35% but a complete response rate of less than 5%. FAM should not be considered a first-line therapy.

Several new combinations show some promise in advanced gastric carcinoma. The EAP regimen (Table 28–7) was initially reported to produce a response rate greater than 50%, with 15% complete responses. The median survival was 9 months. However, subsequent trials failed to confirm this initial data. EAP was also associated with significant toxicity and, occasionally, death from myelosuppression. It may now be possible to give EAP-like regimens more safely with growth factor support.

Due to the toxicity of EAP and the presumed efficacy of etoposide the ELF (Table 28–7) regimen was designed. It was hoped that ELF would be a less toxic but still effective regimen. However, approximately 29% of patients receiving ELF experience grade 3 to 4 myelosuppression.

FAMTX (Table 28–7) was designed to take advantage of methotrexate's ability to modulate the activity of 5-FU. The response rates with this regimen are similar to those achieved with EAP (Table 28–8). FAMTX does, however,

TABLE 28–5. GASTRIC CANCER: PROGNOSIS BY STAGE

STAGE	5-YEAR SURVIVAL (%)
I	85
II	45–55
III	17
IV	<5

TABLE 28–6. SINGLE-AGENT ACTIVITY IN GASTRIC CARCINOMAS

DRUG	NO. OF RESPONSES/ NO. OF PATIENTS	RESPONSES (%)
Doxorubicin	17/68	25
5-Fluorouracil	84/392	21
Mitomycin-C	63/211	30
Hydroxyurea	6/31	19
BCNU	6/33	18
Chorambucil	3/18	17
Mechlorethamine	3/23	13
Methyl-CCNU	3/37	8
Cisplatin	8/36	22
Traizinate	4/26	15
Methotrexate	3/28	11

TABLE 28–7. COMBINATION TREATMENT REGIMENS IN GASTRIC CANCER

FAM
5-FU, 600 mg/m^2 IV on days 1, 8, 29, 36
Doxorubicin, 30 mg/m^2 IV on days 1, 29
Mitomycin-C, 10 mg/m^2 IV on day 1
Repeat every 8 weeks

FAP
5-FU, 300 mg/m^2 IV on days 1 to 5
Doxorubicin, 50 mg/m^2 IV on day 1
Cisplatin, 60 mg/m^2 IV on day 1
Repeat every 5 weeks

EAP
Etoposide, 120 mg/m^2 on days 4, 5, 6
Doxorubicin, 20 mg/m^2 on days 1, 7
Cisplatin, 40 mg/m^2 on days 2, 8
Repeat every 4 weeks

FAMTX
Methotrexate, 1500 mg/m^2 on day 1* followed after 1 hour by: 5-FU, 1500 mg/m^2 on day 1
Doxorubicin, 30 mg/m^2 on day 15
Repeat every 4 weeks

ELF
Etoposide, 120 mg/m^2 days 1, 2, 3
Leucovorin, 300 mg/m^2 days 1, 2, 3
5-FU, 500 mg/m^2 days 1, 2, 3
Repeat every 3–4 weeks

*Leucovorin rescue 15 mg/m^2 PO q 6 hours × 48 hours

require careful monitoring of the methotrexate levels, with leucovorin rescue. A trial comparing FAMTX with EAP showed a median survival of approximately 7 months for both regimens. FAMTX has less severe myelosuppressive toxicity than etoposide-based regimens.

ADJUVANT THERAPY OF GASTRIC CANCER

Patients who are at high risk for relapse after surgical resection are those with T3 or T4 lesions or those with any nodal involvement. Most patients in the United States fall into this high-risk group.

Table 28–9 summarizes selected adjuvant chemotherapy trials in the United States. These prospective randomized studies compare postoperative chemotherapy with a surgical control arm. In the United States only one study suggested benefit. The GITSG demonstrated benefit for patients treated postoperatively with 5-FU and methyl-CCNU. Two similar studies performed by the Eastern Cooperative Oncology Group (ECOG) and the Veterans Administration Surgical Oncology Group (VASOG), however, showed no benefit for 5-FU and methyl-CCNU. Because methyl-CCNU is leukemogenic it has no role in adjuvant therapy. Two studies that examined the role of FAM as a surgical adjuvant demonstrated no overall survival benefit for the regimen as adjuvant therapy.

Due to the risk of local regional failure, radiation therapy must also be considered as adjuvant treatment. Few studies have evaluated radiation therapy alone as adjuvant treatment to surgery. A few studies have explored 5-FU chemotherapy with radiation therapy. The data to date have shown no survival advantage for radiation in poor-risk gastric carcinomas.

A current Intergroup trial (INT 0116) is evaluating 5-FU and leucovorin plus radiation therapy versus surgery alone for patients with resected gastric cancer. This study is planned to accept 350 cases and should be completed in 1995.

An interesting approach to the management of gastric carcinomas has been the introduction of neoadjuvant therapy with chemotherapy or combined modality therapy. Given for several cycles prior to definitive local regional therapy, chemotherapy allows treatment of potential metastatic foci as well as the primary tumor, at a time when the patient is best able to tolerate toxicity. A variety of regimens including EAP have been evaluated as neoadjuvant therapy in Phase II trials. In two trials, although the toxicity was tolerable, the median survival was only 15 to 18 months. A current trial at Memorial Sloan-Kettering Cancer Center is using FAMTX as neoadjuvant therapy. This study also incorporates intraperitoneal chemotherapy to test an approach aimed at the treatment of subclinical peritoneal metastasis. To evaluate neoadjuvant therapy adequately, prospective Phase III studies must be performed. Currently there is no advantage to adjuvant or neoadjuvant therapy for gastric carcinomas. Every effort should be made to enroll eligible patients on available protocols.

TABLE 28–8. COMBINATION CHEMOTHERAPY FOR GASTRIC CANCER

REGIMEN	NO. OF PATIENTS	NO. OF COMPLETE RESPONSES	NO. OF PARTIAL RESPONSES	MEDIAN SURVIVAL (MO.)
FAM	302	7 (2%)	104 (34%)	6.5 (8 series)
EAP	55	8 (15%)	23 (42%)	9
FAMTX	55	5 (9%)	20 (36%)	10
ELF	51	7 (12%)	21 (41%)	11
FAP	68	3 (4%)	24 (35%)	9.0 (3 series)

SMALL BOWEL MALIGNANCIES

Malignant and benign small bowel tumors are rare. It is estimated that about 3600 cases of small intestine tumors will be diagnosed in the United States in 1993. These tumors account for approximately 1%–3% of all GI malignancies despite the fact that the small bowel accounts for 75% of the length of the entire GI tract. It is not clear why malignancy spares the largest absorptive surface of the GI tract. Small bowel carcinomas are most commonly noted in the duodenum, less commonly in the jejunum, and least commonly in the ileum.

Patients with small bowel tumors are often in the 7th decade of life. Several disorders predispose a patient to the

TABLE 28–9. GASTRIC CANCER: PROSPECTIVE RANDOMIZED ADJUVANT TRIALS WITH CONTROLS TREATED BY SURGERY ALONE

TREATMENT	STUDY GROUP	NO. PATIENTS RANDOMIZED	SURVIVAL BENEFIT
SINGLE AGENTS			
Thiotepa	VASOG	194	NS
Fluorodeoxyridine	VASOG	276	NS
Mitomycin; thiotepa	SCSG-J	209	NS
Mitomycin	SCSG-J	472	NS
TWO-DRUG COMBINATIONS			
5-FU + mitomycin	SCSG-J	460	NS
5-FU + methyl-CCNU	VASOG	134	NS
5-FU + methyl-CCNU	ECOG	160	NS
5-FU + methyl-CCNU	GITSG	142	p<.03
5-FU + doxorubicin	NCCTG	120	NS
THREE-DRUG COMBINATIONS			
FAM	SWOG	212	Ongoing
FAM	MAOP	281	NS

5-FU, 5-fluorouracil; FAM, 5-FU + doxorubicin + mitomycin; ECOG, Eastern Cooperative Oncology Group; GITSG, Gastrointestinal Tumor Study Group; MAOP, Middle Atlantic Oncology Group; NCCTG, North Central Cancer Treatment Group; SCGS-J, Stomach Cancer Study Group - Japan; SWOG, Southwest Oncology Group; VASOG, Veterans Administration Surgical Oncology Group

development of a small bowel malignancy. These include adenomatous polyps, a history of Crohn's disease, a long-standing history of adult celiac disease (non-tropical sprue), a history of Peutz-Jeghers syndrome, and a history of Von Recklinghausen's neurofibromatosis. There are many different types of benign and malignant small bowel tumors. The most common malignant tumors are adenocarcinoma, sarcoma, lymphoma, and carcinoid tumors.

Presentation

There is no specific symptom complex that is diagnostic of small bowel tumors. The presentation is dependent upon the type of tumor, as well as its site. There is often a delay of about 6–8 months from initial onset of symptoms until definitive diagnosis, due to the nonspecificity of complaints. Symptoms may include pain (most commonly), or symptoms of impending obstruction such as colic, bloating, distention, vomiting, and weight loss. Clinically, the patient may have anemia secondary to bleeding; however, this is more associated with sarcomas than carcinomas.

Evaluation

A plain abdominal radiograph is often of minimal help in diagnosing a small bowel tumor. Other than the evidence of a small bowel obstruction there are no diagnostic clues. An upper GI with small bowel study can help make a diagnosis in 50%–80% of patients, and this rate improves with the use of enteroclysis. CT scan of the abdomen is accurate in detecting small bowel tumors in 80% of cases. It may also give information of extraluminal extent, hepatic involvement, and adenopathy. A barium enema may be helpful in diagnosing small bowel lymphoma, especially if there is evidence of reflux into the terminal ileum. An upper endoscopy is positive if the tumor is in the duodenum, proximal to the ligament of Treitz.

On physical examination hepatomegaly due to metastatic disease may be noted. The carcinoembryonic antigen (CEA) level (in adenocarcinoma) often does not elevate until late in the course of the disease. A useful marker for carcinoid tumors, however, is the urinary 5-HIAA, especially when there are hepatic metastases.

Staging

There is no established staging system. The same staging systems that are commonly used in large bowel carcinomas, such as the Dukes' classification, have generally been applied to small bowel cancers. The most important prognostic factor is resectability. The overall 5-year survival rates after surgery range from 10% to 20%.

Treatment

Curative therapy for small bowel malignancies is surgery, except in the case of lymphomas. Patients with a suspected small bowel carcinoma should be evaluated for resection. Resection of the tumor should encompass the mesentery and nodal drainage of the involved area of the small bowel whenever possible. In patients with unresectable disease, particularly those with obstructive symptoms, bypass of the affected area of the small bowel may be of considerable symptomatic benefit and may result in prolonged survival.

Radiation therapy may provide significant palliation for patients with pain and high-grade obstruction who cannot undergo resection. However, there are no studies that suggest that radiation is curative. It is clear that patients tolerate extensive radiation of the small bowel poorly; symptoms resulting from radiation enteritis are common, especially with high doses. Therefore, care should be taken to limit radiation to the area of tumor and to avoid, as much as possible, the normal small bowel.

Chemotherapy strategies for small bowel tumors are similar to those with similar histologic subtypes at other sites. Adenocarcinomas are treated like large bowel cancers, including modulated 5-FU regimens. There are no data, however, on adjuvant therapy after surgical resection in small bowel tumors. Lymphomas can be treated with standard systemic chemotherapy regimens appropriate for the grade of the lymphoma. Sarcomas and carcinoid tumors are best served by complete surgical resection.

COLORECTAL CARCINOMA

Colorectal carcinoma is one of the most common malignancies in Western nations. It is estimated that in 1993 there will be approximately 150,000 new cases of colorectal carcinoma diagnosed in the United States and approximately 57,000 deaths.

Worldwide, colorectal carcinoma is much more prevalent in industrialized societies (except Japan). Males generally have a slightly higher incidence, with a male to female ratio of 1.4:1. Men and women over the age of 50 are the population at highest risk. The risk steadily increases up to the 8th decade of life.

Several etiologic factors may affect the development of colorectal carcinoma (Table 28–10). These include dietary, genetic, medical, and anatomic factors. It has long been postulated that colorectal carcinoma may be caused by environmental factors. Certain mutagenic compounds in the human feces are thought to be produced by bowel microflora and are believed to be carcinogenic. These include fecalpentenes and 3-ketosteroids. Free bile acids in the colon are also thought to induce gut lumen proliferation.

Dietary factors have long been associated with colon cancer, especially dietary fat, cholesterol, and fiber. It has been observed that in populations where diets are high in fat colon carcinoma rates are much higher. Case control studies have been performed and a significant correlation has been made between fat intake and the risk of colon carcinoma in many, but not all, of these studies.

The interest in dietary fiber in colon carcinoma was first observed by Burkitt in 1971. He noted that when fiber was removed from diets, the risk of colorectal carcinoma increased. Dietary fiber has since been the focus of many studies on the etiology of colorectal carcinoma, but the mechanism of action is complex and still incompletely understood. Information to date leads to a compelling association but not a direct causal relationship between decreased dietary fiber and colorectal carcinoma.

TABLE 28–10. RISK FACTORS FOR COLORECTAL CARCINOMA

DIETARY/ENVIRONMENTAL
Fat
Fiber
Cholesterol
Bile acids
GENETIC/FAMILIAL
Familial adenomatous polyposis syndrome (FAP)
Peutz-Jeghers syndrome
Hereditary nonpolyposis colorectal cancer (HNPCC)
Lynch I syndrome
Hereditary adenocarcinomatosis syndrome: Lynch II syndrome
Family history of colorectal carcinoma
PRE-EXISTING DISEASE
Inflammatory bowel disease
Colorectal cancer

Several medical and genetic risk factors also place a patient at risk for colorectal carcinoma. The familial polyposis syndromes represent several inherited disorders associated with adenomatous polyps and a risk of colorectal carcinoma. They include the familial adenomatous polyposis syndrome (FAP), the hereditary nonpolypolis colon cancer syndrome (HNPCC), and the flat adenoma syndrome (FAS). FAP is fortunately rare. It is inherited as an autosomal dominant trait with 90% penetrance. Virtually all persons affected will develop polyps by late adolescence and eventually will develop colorectal carcinoma if not treated with a prophylactic colectomy.

Some families have a high frequency of colorectal carcinoma without a history of adenomatous polyps. This has been termed the HNPCC syndrome, first described by Lynch and Lynch. The Lynch I syndrome is inherited as an autosomal dominant trait with greater than 90% penetrance. Patients often develop colorectal carcinoma at an early age, commonly in the more proximal large bowel. The Lynch II syndrome, also an autosomal dominant disorder, is indicated by families with early development of multiple colon adenocarcinomas as well as extracolonic adenocarcinomas in the colon, ovary, pancreas, breast, endometrium, and stomach.

In patients with a family history of sporadic colon cancer, there is a 2- to 3-fold greater chance of developing large bowel tumors. The tumors occur in the third to fifth decade of life. Approximately 20–25% of patients who develop colorectal carcinoma by the age of 50 will have a sibling who will also develop disease at approximately the same stage of life.

Despite these "familial" syndromes, over 70% of patients with colorectal carcinoma have no family history or syndrome as a risk factor. Colorectal carcinomas are more common in patients who have had a prior adenomatous polyp or villous adenoma. Risk factors for the presence of carcinoma in polyps increase with the size, number, and pathology of the polyps.

Patients with a history of inflammatory bowel disease are also at approximately 30-fold higher risk of developing colorectal carcinoma. A history of ulcerative colitis involving the bowel for more than 10 years is associated with a colon cancer risk of about 4% per year. The relative risk is lower with ulcerative proctitis than with a pancolitis. Patients with Crohn's disease are also at risk but not as frequently as those with ulcerative colitis.

Patients who have undergone therapy for a large bowel adenocarcinoma are at greater risk to develop a second colonic tumor and have an approximately three-fold increased risk. Patients who have undergone radiation therapy for cervical, endometrial, or genitourinary carcinomas may be at an enhanced risk of developing a colorectal tumor.

The major histologic type of large bowel cancer is adenocarcinoma, which accounts for 90–95% of all tumors. Certain subtypes exist such as mucinous/colloid carcinomas or signet ring cell carcinomas. Other variants include squamous cell, adenosquamous, and undifferentiated carcinomas, and also carcinoid tumors, sarcomas, and lymphomas.

Screening

Due to the prevalence of colorectal carcinoma, there is considerable interest in screening populations for early detection. Three technologies are currently available: digital rectal examination (DRE), flexible sigmoidoscopy, and fecal occult blood testing. The DRE is a traditional part of any annual physical exam and is a simple low-cost procedure. A flexible sigmoidoscopy will visualize up to 65 cm of the proximal distal bowel and can detect polyps and tumors at an early stage. Current recommendations are that persons of the ages 50–75 have a flexible sigmoidoscopy every 3 to 5 years. The fecal occult blood test is an inexpensive method of testing blood in the stool. Unfortunately, it is associated with a very high false positive rate (90%) and a false negative rate of up to 20–30%. There are several types of products for fecal testing available in the United States. Although recent studies have suggested that fecal occult blood testing may be a useful screening test for colorectal tumors, the conclusions are still controversial. It is likely that most cancers in the United States, as well as polyps, will be missed by this technique alone.

Presentation

Symptoms most commonly associated with colorectal carcinoma include bright red blood per rectum, crampy abdominal pain, or a change in bowel habits, either constipation or diarrhea. Clinically silent GI bleeding may cause a patient to present with symptoms of anemia. Rectal tumors may present with local regional pain or a sensation of incomplete rectal evacuation.

The site of tumor growth may also influence the presenting complaints. Left-sided lesions may cause obstructive symptoms, as the stool is more solid and less easily passed through a narrowed lumen. Left-sided lesions also may present with gross blood in the stool. Right-sided lesions may present at a more advanced status, as they remain clinically silent for longer periods of time. Right-sided lesions present with symptoms related to anemia, crampy abdominal pain, or abdominal distention. This is unfortunate, as there has been a relative increase in right-sided colon tumors in the last 40 years.

Patients with advanced colon carcinoma may present with weight loss, jaundice, and hepatomegaly from hepatic metastases. Approximately 10% of patients will present with symptoms secondary to involvement of contiguous organs such as a fecal vaginal discharge and air or feces in the urine.

Evaluation

Pretreatment evaluation of colorectal carcinoma directs primary therapy and may define prognosis. After a thorough history and physical examination, if colorectal carcinoma is suspected, a colonoscopy or an air-contrast barium enema should be scheduled. These tests are often complementary. Colonoscopy is somewhat more sensitive than barium studies and offers the advantage of a histopathologic diagnosis. Barium studies are useful to evaluate colonic architecture and are less expensive than colonoscopy. It is important, however, that the entire bowel be examined, as synchronous lesions may occur in 20–60% of patients.

A CT scan of the abdomen and pelvis is an appropriate adjunct to the preoperative evaluation of colorectal carcinoma. It may help evaluate the depth of penetration through the bowel wall, detect any enlarged nodes, and perhaps delineate sites of metastatic disease (*e.g.*, liver or omentum).

Laboratory evaluation should include a CBC and a chemistry panel. A microcytic anemia may indicate chronic blood loss and, abnormal liver function tests may indicate evidence of hepatic tumor involvement. A preoperative carcinoembryonic antigen (CEA) level may be of prognostic value if elevated. A preoperative CEA level greater than 5 ng/ml in a nonsmoker is a poor prognostic sign. The usefulness of serial CEA levels for detection of early relapse has recently been questioned by Moertel and colleagues.

More recently, the introduction of monoclonal antibodies directed against CEA or other colon-specific antigens may facilitate detection of relapsed tumor. The antibodies are conjugated with a radioactive isotope, most commonly indium 111 or technetium 99, and are administered to the patient, followed by scintigraphy. Although it has not yet been shown to improve survival in relapsed patients, this technique should be thought of as a diagnostic tool that may have value in the future.

The molecular genetics of colorectal carcinoma is truly in evolution. Families with FAP have been analyzed, and a gene strongly associated with FAP has been identified on the 5th chromosome at band q21-22. Tumor suppressor genes on chromosome 18 (DCC, deleted in colon cancer gene) and on chromosome 17 (the p53 gene) also have been associated with colorectal carcinoma. Additional molecular genetic abnormalities in colorectal carcinoma are enhanced expression of the C-myc proto-oncogene and activation of and mutation of K-ras. Recently, a gene on chromosome 2 has been associated with familial nonpolyposis colon cancer. Analysis of DNA content as measured by flow cytometry may be important in assessing prognosis in some cases of colorectal cancer.

Staging

The most commonly used staging for colorectal carcinoma is still the Astler-Coller modification of the original Dukes' staging system (Table 28–11). The Dukes' system correlates prognosis with pathologic stage to define the extent of invasion of colon and rectal tumors. However, there is an attempt to increase the use of TNM staging system in colorectal cancer. Table 28–11 correlates the TNM stage with the modified Astler-Coller staging system.

Treatment

The primary treatment of colorectal carcinoma is surgical resection. The overriding principle in surgical management is to resect an adequate segment of bowel containing the area of malignancy and the adjacent mesentery with lymph nodes. The appropriate surgical procedure is directed by the location of the tumor. For other than rectal carcinomas, the procedures are variations of right, left, or transverse colectomies. For rectal cancer an anterior resection may be performed if the tumor is located proximal enough to allow tumor resection with adequate margins and low rectal anastomosis. The ability to perform anterior resection with end-to-end anastomosis has been considerably facilitated by the widespread use of stapling devices. If, however, a rectal cancer is located so far distally that an anastomosis is not possible, an abdominal-perineal resection must be performed. This procedure sacrifices the rectum and patients have a permanent colostomy. Surgeons are beginning to explore endoscopic-assisted resections for large bowel cancers. It should be emphasized that the appropriate role for this technique in large bowel tumors has not been defined.

THERAPY FOR ADVANCED COLORECTAL CARCINOMA

Because almost 50% of patients with colorectal carcinoma will develop a recurrence, the treatment of advanced disease is an important clinical problem. The most common sites of dissemination are the liver and abdominal cavity.

Of the large number of single agents tested to date, none have significantly greater activity than the fluorinated pyrimidines, of which the most common and only commercially available are 5-FU and FUDR. Various schedules, routes, and intervals of 5-FU have been tried. The oral use of 5-FU has virtually been abandoned in colorectal carcinomas, due to erratic GI absorption and poor response rates. Intravenous 5-FU is by far the most widely used route of drug administration.

5-FU can be given as a bolus of 500–600 mg/m^2 5 days a week monthly, or once weekly, with myelosuppression as the dose-limiting toxicity in both modalities. Alternatively, 5-FU may be given as a continuous infusion at 1 gm/m^2 per day for 5 days with resultant stomatitis and diarrhea rather than

TABLE 28–11. DUKES' CLASSIFICATION: ASTLER-COLLIER MODIFICATION

		TNM STAGE	5-YEAR SURVIVAL %
INITIAL EXTENSION			
A	Mucosa only	I (T1–2, N0, M0)	95
B1	Within wall		85–90
B2(m)	Microscopically through wall	II (T3–4, N0, M0)	60–70
B2(g)	Grossly through wall		50
B3	Involves adjacent structures		30
LYMPH NODES POSITIVE FOR TUMOR			
C1	Within wall	III (T2, N1–2, M0)	40–50
C2(m)	Microscopically through wall	(T3, N1–2, M0)	
C2(g)	Grossly through wall	(T4, N1–2, M0)	15–25
C3	Involves adjacent structures		10–20
D	Distant metastatic disease	IV (T any, N any, M1)	5

Adapted from American Joint Committee on Cancer. Manual for Staging of Cancer. 3rd ed. Philadelphia, JB Lippincott, 1988 hematologic toxicity. Continuous low-dose 5-FU given at 200–300 mg/m^2 per day via indwelling catheter and portable infusion pump may produce the hand/foot syndrome as toxicity. The response rates for these 5-FU regimens vary between less than 20% (intravenous bolus therapy) and 30–40% (infusional therapy).

Agents other than the fluorinated pyrimidines, including BCNU, CCNU, methyl-CCNU, and mitomycin-C, have been used in the past and produce only a 10–15% response rate. The poor response rates with single agents may be due to a variety of reasons. Colonic mucosa normally expresses the p170 protein encoded by the multidrug resistent (MDR) gene, which may explain the resistance of colon cancers to many natural–product-derived drugs.

Newer agents being evaluated in colon cancer are new fluorinated pyrimidines, thymidylate synthase inhibitors, Taxol and its analalogue Taxotere, and the topoisomerase I inhibitors CPT-11 and topotecan.

Combination chemotherapy programs in advanced colorectal carcinoma have most commonly used 5-FU in conjunction with other agents including methyl-CCNU and vincristine. Attempts at using mitomycin-C and/or cisplatin have proved fruitless in improving survival compared to 5-FU alone.

One approach to the chemotherapy of colon cancer that has been useful is the biochemical modulation of 5-FU (Table 28–12). The method of 5-FU modulation of most clinical interest has entailed the use of folinic acid (leucovorin). Intracellular reduced folates enhance 5-FU cytotoxicity by stabilizing the covalent ternary complex of thymidylate synthase (TS) and FdUMP. Numerous studies have been performed using various doses of 5-FU with leucovorin, as well as varying the time schedule. The combination of 5-FU and leucovorin appears to provide enhanced efficacy when compared to 5-FU alone, including an improved quality of life. Toxicity is often limited to mild leukopenia when administered weekly and mucositis/enteritis when administered daily. Another mechanism of 5-FU modulation is with methotrexate (MTX). MTX inhibits purine metabolism, causing accumulation of 5-phosphoribosyl-1-pyrophosphate (PRPP) and increased conversion of 5-FU to its active metabolites. Several MTX doses and schedules have been reported. Mucositis and leukopenia are the most common toxic effects. Other attempts to enhance 5-FU have used the pyrimidine synthesis inhibitor PALA to deplete intracellular pools of uridine triphosphate and to enhance formation of FUTP. Initial studies using high doses of PALA resulted in extreme toxicity. Recent studies using lower doses have been better tolerated (Table 28–12). Response rates up to 40% have been reported.

Recent studies have focused on interferon α to modulate the anti-tumor affects of 5-FU. The exact mechanism of interferon activity is not known, although interferon has been shown to enhance conversion of 5-FU to FdUMP, reduce cellular levels of thymidylate synthase, and inhibit thymidine salvage pathways. The most widely used regimen is listed on Table 28–13. Response rates are demonstrated to be 25%–40% in several studies. Toxicities include leukopenia, mucositis, diarrhea, fevers, chills, and myalgias. Current trials are combining 5-FU with leucovorin and interferon in a double biochemical modulation strategy.

The Southwest Oncology Group (SWOG) recently completed a seven-arm trial comparing 5-FU alone to various attempts at 5-FU modulation. This study suggests that there are no major differences in survival benefit for modulation versus bolus 5-FU and that continuous infusion regimens appear to have response rates equivalent to leukovorin-containing regimens. Final analysis of this study is pending.

Special mention must be made of the role of regional chemotherapy. The liver is a dominant site of metastatic dis-

TABLE 28–12. 5-FU MODULATION: SCHEDULE AND DOSES

5-FU	MODULATION	SCHEDULE
	LEUKOVORIN	
600 mg/m^2 IVP	500 mg/m^2 2 hr infusion	Weekly × 6
425 mg/m^2 IVP	20 mg/m^2 IVP	Days 1–5 every 4 weeks
	METHOTREXATE	
650 mg/m^2	200 mg/m^2 *	Weekly with leukovorin
650 mg/m^2	200 mg/m^2 †	Weekly with leukovorin
	PALA	
2600 mg/m^2 CI × 24h	250 mg/m^2 †	Weekly
	IFN	
750 mg/m^2	9 million units SQ	5 days loading, then 5-FU weekly IFN 3 times per week

IVP, intravenous push; CI, continuous infusion; SQ, subcutaneously

*given 24 hours prior to 5-FU

†given 1 hour prior to 5-FU

TABLE 28–13. ADJUVANT STUDIES IN DUKES' B & C COLON CANCER

REGIMEN	NO. PATIENTS	DURATION OF THERAPY (WKS)	GROUP
Control vs. levamisole vs. 5-FU + levamisole	401	52	NCCTG
Control vs. levamisole vs. 5-FU + levamisole	1296	52	Intergroup
Control vs. 5-FU + heparin via portal vein	224	7 days	NCCTG
Control vs. 5-FU + heparin via portal vein	1158	7 days	NSABP

NCCTG, North Central Cancer Treatment Group; NSABP, National Surgical Adjuvant Breast and Bowel Project

ease, and high concentrations of chemotherapy can be administered directly through the hepatic artery or portal vein. The availability and reliability of portable pumps in conjunction with permanent access ports make this therapy relatively easy to perform. FUDR has been the most commonly used agent at doses of 0.15–0.3 mg/kg per day for 14 days each month. The average hepatic response rate is approximately 40%. Although response rates are greater than in systemic therapy, the overall survival is not significantly improved. Careful attention must be given to liver toxicity. If liver function studies (transaminases, alkaline phosphatase, or bilirubin) significantly increase, the dose must be held and resumed at a lower dose once the liver function studies return to normal. Infusion of dexamethasone with FUDR may decrease the liver toxicity. If sclerosing cholangitis develops, the therapy must be abandoned.

Out of a protocol setting, modulated 5-FU therapy (*e.g.*, with leucovorin) is an appropriate treatment for patients with advanced colon carcinoma.

ADJUVANT CHEMOTHERAPY FOR COLON CARCINOMA

Patients with Dukes' B2 and C colon carcinoma are at high risk for relapse after surgery alone (Table 28–11). As in metastatic colon carcinoma, 5-FU remains the most widely used therapy.

Combination chemotherapy has been explored as adjuvant therapy for colon carcinoma. The GITSG showed no benefit for 5-FU/vincristine/methyl-CCNU (MOF) with or without the methanol-extracted residue of BCG. The NSABP tested the MOF combination in its CO1 trial, with an initial 67% 5-year survival demonstrated for MOF versus 58% percent for the control arm. Over time, however, the survival advantage to MOF has lessened.

In the last several years several studies have demonstrated a significant benefit for adjuvant therapy. Levamisole is an antihelminthic agent that has been used alone and in combination with 5-FU. Levamisole has a broad range of immunomodulary properties. Two Phase III studies comparing adjuvant levamisole plus 5-FU versus surgery alone have been completed in the United States (Table 28-13). The Intergroup trial (INT 0089) demonstrated in Dukes' C (Stage III) cases a 41% decrease in relapse and a 33% decrease in death from cancer in the 5-FU plus levamisole treatment arm. These results have continued to be maintained at a median of 5 years of follow-up. Levamisole alone was ineffective as adjuvant therapy in Dukes' C carcinomas. 5-FU plus levamisole was of no benefit in Dukes' B cases.

Another interesting adjuvant approach has been the evaluation of the role of portal vein infusion of 5-FU versus control (see Table 28–13). Two trials have been conducted in the United States. The study by the NSABP revealed a significant improvement in disease-free survival (74% versus 64%) and a trend toward improved survival (81% versus 73%). However, there was no reduction in hepatic metastasis, making it likely that portal vein 5-FU had a systemic adjuvant effect.

Ongoing trials include a NSABP study evaluating 5-FU/leucovorin with and without interferon. There also is a study of specific immunotherapy with autologous tumor vaccine being completed by the ECOG.

At present, outside of a clinical trial, the standard of care for patients with Dukes' B3 and C colon carcinoma is the use of 5-FU and levamisole (Table 28–14).

TREATMENT OF RECTAL CARCINOMA

As in colon carcinoma, the primary therapy for rectal carcinoma is surgery.

For advanced and metastatic tumors, chemotherapy approaches are similar to those used in colon carcinoma. If possible, local recurrence can be treated with external beam radiation therapy or brachytherapy.

Adjuvant therapy for rectal carcinoma, however, differs from that for colon carcinoma. There is evidence to support the role of radiation therapy in preventing local recurrence of rectal cancer. Radiation has been used both pre- and postoperatively. Although older studies have suggested that preoperative irradiation may downstage tumors and decrease local recurrences, the major adjuvant studies of the last 20 years have used postoperative radiation. Postoperative radiation therapy has the advantage of allowing an accurate pathologic staging before therapy.

TABLE 28–14. 5-FU AND LEVAMISOLE: ADJUVANT THERAPY

5-FU 450 mg/m² IVP × 5 then on day 28 start 450 mg/m² weekly
Levamisole 50 mg po three times a day × 3 days every other week
Treatment: 1 year

In 1991, the NCCTG published data from a Phase III study evaluating 5000 cGy radiation therapy alone versus radiation therapy with chemotherapy (5-FU plus methyl-CCNU). The combination of radiation with 5-FU and methyl-CCNU reduced the recurrence of both local and distant disease in rectal carcinomas by 34%. An Intergroup study recently demonstrated that 5-FU alone was equal to 5-FU plus methyl-CCNU when compared with radiation in patients with resected rectal cancers. This same study also demonstrated that 5-FU by continuous infusion was superior to bolus 5-FU as a radiation sensitizer.

Another Intergroup trial (INT 0114) has recently completed accrual. This study evaluated radiation therapy with either 5-FU, 5-FU with leucovorin, 5-FU with levamisole, or 5-FU with leucovorin and levamisole. The results of this study are pending and will define the role of leucovorin and levamisole in resected rectal cancer.

In managing a patient with resected rectal cancer at high risk for recurrence, the first option should be a clinical trial. If none is available, therapy with resection, 5-FU, and radiation should be considered a standard approach.

CARCINOMA OF THE ANAL REGION

Anal carcinomas account for 2–4% of all tumors of the GI tract. In the United States, anal carcinomas occur more frequently in females than in male patients. Carcinomas of the anal margin however, are more common in men, whereas women have a higher incidence of carcinomas of the anal canal. Overall, epidermoid carcinoma of the anal region develops in a population in the 6th and 7th decade of life, although this age distribution may change if the incidence of this disease continues to increase in male homosexuals.

The human papilloma virus (HPV) appears to be an important etiologic factor in the development of anal carcinoma. The most common HPV serotypes associated with anal tumors are 16 and 18 or types 31, 33, and 35. Even before the AIDS epidemic, there was an increased risk of anal carcinoma in homosexual men. There appears to be an additional risk, however, with HIV-infected individuals in conjunction with HPV. In women with a history of genital warts, anal carcinoma is associated with herpes simplex virus type I infection, as well as with *Chlamydia trachomatis*. Additional risk factors for anal carcinoma include prior local radiation therapy, cigarette smoking, and immunosuppression (*e.g.*, post–organ transplant).

The majority of anal region carcinomas are of the squamous cell variety (63%). They occur in the anal canal, the rectum, or the perianal skin. These tumors have been classified as keratinizing or nonkeratinizing squamous cell carcinomas. The keratinizing tumors have a somewhat better prognosis, as they tend to occur in the more distal anus and perianal skin and tend to be smaller at the time of detection. Likewise, nonkeratinizing tumors occur in the anal canal, frequently in the area of the pectinate line, and tend to be larger and have a somewhat poorer prognosis. Most investigators currently feel, however, that prognosis may depend more on stage than histologic type. Other histologic subtypes include transitional carcinoma (cloacogenic), basaloid carcinoma, adenocarcinoma, small cell carcinoma, or melanomas.

Presentation

Patients often present early with symptoms localized to the anal region. They often note rectal bleeding, which initially may be attributed to hemorrhoids or fissures and can therefore cause delay in diagnosis. Pain and a sensation of a mass or incomplete bowel evacuation are also common presenting symptoms. Other complaints include pruritus, anal discharge, or change in bowel habits.

Evaluation

The pretreatment evaluation of anal carcinomas should be based on the knowledge of the natural history and pattern of spread. Initially there is infiltration of the anal canal and sphincter. Advanced local growth may involve the prostate and vagina. Nodal metastasis to inguinal lymph nodes may occur either synchronous with diagnosis or later. Distant metastases to the liver and lungs are rare.

A physical examination should include a rectal exam with anoscopy. An incisional biopsy is needed to confirm the diagnosis. Suspicious inguinal lymph nodes should be biopsied to differentiate metastatic foci versus inflammatory changes. A formal lymph node/groin dissection is usually not necessary, however. A CT scan of the abdomen and pelvis helps define local extension of tumor and may detect evidence of distant nodal or visceral involvement. Transanal/rectal sonography has also been suggested as a useful diagnostic tool, especially to help determine depth of tumor invasion.

Chromosome evaluation of anal carcinoma is now being explored. Preliminary studies have demonstrated abnormalities in chromosomes 11 and 13. More cases, however, need to be studied to verify these data.

Staging

A variety of staging systems have been applied to anal carcinomas. Some stratify for tumor size versus depth of invasion. Table 28–15 separates patients by degree of local invasion and the presence of nodal metastasis.

Treatment

The absence of data from randomized trials makes recommendations for treatment difficult in certain circumstances. A major determinant of appropriate treatment is the location of the primary tumor.

Superficial perianal skin carcinomas (as of the anal margin), outside the anal verge, can be treated with wide local excision with good results. A 1-cm margin using primary closure is usually appropriate. Local failure rates are high if the margin of the tumor involves the anal canal. Radiation therapy may be considered for some patients who are judged unresectable or who are medically inoperable. Due to the high incidence of radionecrosis, external beam radiation therapy is probably better than radiation implants in this circumstance. Concurrent radiation therapy and chemotherapy is an interesting approach but is still considered investigational. Carcinomas with deep infiltration of the anal margin, may need to be approached with an abdominal-perineal (AP) resection.

Treatment of anal canal carcinoma traditionally has been surgical, often including an AP resection. However, small localized tumors may be handled with wide excision alone. Tumors that involve the dentate line, are greater than 2 cm, or involve greater than ½ the bowel circumference are probably best served by a combined modality treatment. This integrated approach improves overall survival and may allow radical surgery to be avoided.

In the last several years, there have been several large series using combined modality therapy with radiation plus chemotherapy after local resection. These results appear to be superior to either modality alone and produce less morbidity than an AP resection. Table 28–16 demonstrates a typical combination chemotherapy/radiation schema. This combined modality therapy is given concurrently and is highly effective. However, some patients will still require an AP resection. At completion of therapy, the patient should undergo rebiopsy of the tumor site. Transrectal ultrasound may also be of use in revealing residual tumor. If there is a pathologic complete response, no surgery is warranted. However, if there is residual tumor, an AP resection is recommended. Fortunately more than 70% of patients obtain a complete response and are long-term survivors. Toxicity associated with this combined modality therapy may include anal mucositis, pruritus, and even an oral mucositis. Some newer regimens are substituting cisplatin for mitomycin-C. Preliminary data show equivalent results.

Patients with synchronous involved inguinal nodes (at diagnosis) have a worse prognosis, with survival initially felt to be very poor. However, current recommendations for limited surgical nodal sampling, combined chemotherapy, and radiation therapy with boost doses to the involved groin can achieve adequate local control rates. The long-term survival rate is reported to be approximately 58%.

Surgical salvage may be done for isolated recurrences. The development of metachronous inguinal lymph nodes is less ominous. Patients often can be treated with nodal dissection and further chemotherapy. Additional radiation therapy depends on prior treatment doses and fields.

Metastatic anal carcinoma is rare. Most patients have local/regional recurrences. Chemotherapy either as a single agent or in combination has been used in the treatment of metastatic disease. These agents have included doxorubicin, bleomycin, velban, cisplatin and high-dose methotrexate. The BOM regimen (bleomycin, vincristine, and high-dose methotrexate) has produced a response rate of approximately 25% among 12 patients. However, this response was of short duration.

Other histologic types of tumors of the anal region (*e.g.*, melanoma, adenocarcinoma, and small cell carcinomas) are treated as they would be at other sites.

TABLE 28–15. STAGING SYSTEM FOR LOCALIZED CARCINOMA OF THE ANAL REGION

STAGE		PROPORTION OF PATIENTS IN EACH STAGE	5-YEAR SURVIVAL (%)
A	Invasion to mucosa and submucosa	N = 106	N = 114
B	Sphincter muscle involved	4 (4%)	4/4 (100%)
B1	Invasion to internal sphincter	24 (23%)	20/26 (77%)
B2	Invasion to external sphincter	13 (12%)	10/13 (77%)
B3	Invasion beyond sphincter into adjacent tissue	29 (27%)	15/31 (48%)
C	Lymph node involvement	36 (34%)	19/40 (48%)

Adapted from American Joint Committee on Cancer. Manual for Staging of Cancer. 3rd ed. Philadelphia, JB Lippincott, 1988

TABLE 28–16. COMBINED-MODALITY THERAPY OF ANAL CARCINOMA

5-FU 1000 mg/m² per day, as continuous infusion on days 1 to 4; repeat on days 28 to 31
Mitomycin-C, 15 mg/m² IV bolus on day 1 only
External radiation therapy, 3000 cGy to 5000 cGy

BIBLIOGRAPHY

General

Boring CC, Squires TS, Tong T. Cancer statistics 1993. Cancer Journal for Clinicians 43(1):7–26, 1993

Kelsen D. Neo-adjuvant therapy of gastrointestinal cancers. Oncology 7(9):25–32, 1993

Tepper JE. Combined radiotherapy and chemotherapy in the treatment of gastrointestinal malignancies. Seminars in Oncology 19(4):96–101, 1992

Esophagus

Coia LR. Esophageal cancer: Is esophagectomy necessary? Oncology 3(4):101–115, 1989

Forastiere AA, Orringer MB, Perez-Tamayo C, et al. Pre-operative chemoradiation followed by transhiatal esophagecteomy for carcinoma of the esophagus: Final report. J Clin Oncol 11:1118–1123, 1993

Gill PG, Denham JW, Jamieson GG et al. Patterns of treatment failure and prognostic factors associated with the treatment of esophageal carcinoma with chemotherapy and radiotherapy either as sole treatment or followed by surgery. J Clin Oncol 10:1037–1043, 1992

Herskovic A, Martz K, Al-Sarraf M et al. Combined chemotherapy and radiotherapy compared with radiotherapy alone in patients with cancer of the esophagus. N Engl J Med 326:1593–1598, 1992

Gastric Carcinoma

Ajani JA, Ota DM, Jackson DE. Current strategies in the management oflocoregional and metastatic gastric carcinoma. Cancer 67:260–265, 1991

Alexander HR, Grem JL, Pass HI et al. Neoadjuvant chemotherapy for locally advanced gastric adenocarcinoma. Oncology 7(5):37–53, 1993

Blot WJ, Devesa SS, Kneller RW, Fraumeni JF. Rising incidence of adenocarcinoma of the esophagus and gastric cardia. JAMA 265:1287–1289, 1991

Douglass HO Jr. Gastric cancer: Current status of adjuvant therapy. Oncology 3(4):61–77, 1989

Kelsen D, Antig UT, Saltz L et al. FAMTX versus etoposide, doxorubicin, and cisplatin: A random assignment trial in gastric cancer. J Clin Oncol 10:541–548, 1992

Parsonnet J, Friedman GD, Danier MS et al. Helicobacter pylori infection and the risk of gastric carcinoma. N Engl J Med 325:1127–1131, 1991

Wilke H, Preusser P, Fink U et al. New developments in the treatment of gastric carcinoma. Seminars in Oncology 17:61–70, 1990

Small Bowel

Ashley SW, Wells SA. Tumors of the small intestine. Seminars in Oncology 15:116–128, 1988

Colorectal Carcinoma

Alquist DA, Weiand HS, Moertel CG et al. Accuracy of fecal occult blood screening for colorectal neoplasia. JAMA 269:1262–1267, 1993

Bodmer WF, Bailey LJ, Bodmer J et al. Localization of the gene for familial adenomatous polyposis on chromosone 5. Nature 328:2–4, 1987

Brachman DG, Schilsky RL. Adjuvant chemotherapy and radiation therapy in colorectal cancer. PPO Update 6(3):1–12, 1992

Burkett DP. Epidemiology of cancer of the colon and rectum. Cancer 28:3, 1971

Cohen AM, Minsky BD, Schilsky RC. Colon cancer. In Devita VT, Hellman S, Rosenberg SA (eds). Cancer: Principles and Practices of Oncology, 4th ed. Philadelphia, JB Lippincott, 1993:929–977

Doerr RJ, Abdel-Nabi H, Krag O et al. Radioloabeled antibody imaging in the management of colorectal cancer. Ann Surg 214:118–124, 1991

Hansen R. Systemic therapy in colorectal cancer. Arch Int Med 150:2265–2269, 1990

Kim JA, Triozzi PL, Martin EW Jr. Radioimmunoguided surgery for colorectal cancer. Oncology 7(2):55–64, 1993

Kinzler KW, Vogelstein B. The colorectal cancer gene hunt: Current findings. Hospital Practice. November 15, 1992:51–58

Krook JE, Moertel CG, Gunderson LL et al. Effective surgical adjuvant therapy for high risk rectal carcinoma. N Engl J Med 324:709–715, 1991

Lynch HT, Albano WA, Lynch JF et al. Recognition of the cancer family syndrome. Gastroenterology 84:672–673, 1993

Moertel CG, Fleming TR, Macdonald JS et al. Levamisole and fluorouracil for adjuvant therapy of resected colon carcinoma. N Engl J Med 322:352–358, 1990

Posner MR, Steele G. Adjuvant treatment of colorectal adenocarcinoma. Current Problems in Cancer 12(4):221–272, 1993

Schneebaum S, Arnold MW, Martin EW. Adjuvant treatment for rectal cancer: Current status. Oncology 7(3):83–101, 1993

Wolmark N, Rockette H, Wickerham DL et al. Adjuvant therapy of Duke's A, B, and C adenocarcinoma of the colon with portal-vein fluorouracil hepatic infusion: Preliminary results of the National Surgical Adjuvant Breast and Bowel Project Protocol C-02. J Clin Oncol 8:1466–1475, 1990

John S. Macdonald, Daniel G. Haller, Robert J. Mayer, Eds. *Manual of Oncologic Therapeutics*, Third Edition.

29. CANCERS OF THE PANCREAS AND HEPATOBILIARY SYSTEM

Michael A. Friedman

Cancers of the pancreas and hepatobiliary system remain among the most refractory and challenging of malignancies. Too often, these tumors are diagnosed at an advanced stage, produce symptoms that are poorly palliated, and rapidly result in death. The majority of patients die within the first year, and more than 90% die within 5 years. Arising deep within the abdomen or in the retroperitoneum, these tumors initially produce vague symptoms, often misdiagnosed by both patient and physician, and often directly invade critical vascular and visceral anatomical sites. This growth pattern accounts for many of the symptoms associated with the diseases as well as the difficulties in treatment and the low cure rates.

PRETREATMENT EVALUATION

Only those patients presenting with early jaundice or incidentally found to have a tumor at laparotomy are conventionally considered curable. Most tumors of the pancreas arise in the head of the pancreas. A subset of these tumors (especially in the periampullary area) present with persistent jaundice and are amenable to radical surgical resection with the possibility of cure. Patients with hepatobiliary tumors often present a similarly subtle clinical picture early, and gross disease later. However, because of the difficulty in identifying signs or symptoms specifically related to the malignant process, patients often first undergo a diagnostic workup to rule out cholelithiasis, hepatitis, benign peptic ulcer disease, and so forth.

The most crucial steps in the initial workup are pathologic confirmation of the presence of malignancy and, secondarily, identification of the histologic type of tumor. For carcinomas of the pancreas, liver, and biliary system, ultrasound or computed tomographic (CT)-guided fine-needle aspiration of either the primary tumor or a metastatic site (lymph node or liver) is a usual method of obtaining pathologic material directly. An additional useful test is endoscopic retrograde cholangiopancreatography (ERCP), which can provide cytologic washings. ERCP can confirm the histologic diagnosis as well as the anatomical localization of an abnormality. Such efforts to confirm the exact histologic type of malignancy are necessary in order to identify those rarer histologies, such as islet cell or microadenocarcinoma of the pancreas, or lymphoma of the liver or retroperitoneum, which have a different natural history, require different therapy, and have a better outcome than the far more common adenocarcinoma.

Serologic tests are usually of limited value, liver function abnormalities are totally nonspecific, and carcinoembryonic antigen is only slightly more helpful. Alpha-fetoprotein may be of value in identifying primary liver cancer.

Having made the diagnosis, the physician must next determine the extent of disease (potential resectability). The fact that most patients' tumors are unresectable should not deter the physician from carefully evaluating each patient with the hope that a particular individual might benefit from a curative surgical intervention. In order to stage the tumor clinically, noninvasive techniques are initially employed. Ultrasonography is less expensive and discriminating than CT scanning with contrast or magnetic resonance imaging, but all can detect gross metastases. To better define local tumor extent, ERCP, biliary or transhepatic cholangiography, and, finally, angiography are employed. The more invasive tests are reserved for those patients who are not obviously incurable. These tests evaluate the size and location of tumor and suggest possible complications arising from a surgical attempt to extirpate the tumor. Additionally, cholecystography and radionuclide scans may assist in the evaluation of those patients with hepatobiliary tumors. Even with these sophisticated radiographic procedures, in some patients laparotomy will still be required to confirm the diagnosis, to define the extent of disease, and to consider an attempt to resect the tumor for cure. Resection is often a formidable technical procedure and should be performed only in cases that have received accurate and complete preoperative evaluation.

STAGING SYSTEM

No staging system for pancreatic tumors is satisfactory (or completely accepted). Nonetheless, the American Joint Committee on Cancer provides an acceptable system.[1] Only a small minority of patients have tumors confined to the pancreas (Stage I) or adjacent viscera (Stage II) without regional lymphatic involvement. Such localized tumors can be treated with total resection, but patients have a relatively poor chance of survival. Stage III patients (regional lymphatic metastases) have a dismal prognosis and are not conventionally considered candidates for a curative resection. Stage IV disease is yet more widely disseminated, and local means of therapy (surgery or radiation) are usually inappropriate.

TREATMENT

Cancer of the Pancreas

The majority of patients with carcinoma of the pancreas present with unresectable (*i.e.*, incurable) malignancy. However, up to 20% of carefully screened patients can undergo a laparotomy with the expectation of a radical resection. Of those patients who undergo such a resection, perhaps 20% will be cured, resulting in an overall 4% or 5% cure rate. Of course, radical surgery (such as a Whipple procedure) is associated with an appreciable operative mortality (at least 5% of patients) and morbidity. The median survival for all patients treated with radical surgery alone is approximately 11 months. Preliminary data suggest that the addition of radiation therapy and 5-fluorouracil (5-FU) may be beneficial.[2] Supervoltage radiation is delivered to a field of 400 cm^2 or less and to a total dosage of 4000 cGy. Each treatment is given in a schedule of 200 cGy/day, five times per week, and after 2000 cGy a 2-week rest period intervenes and then the final 2000 cGy is administered. Concurrent with the initiation of each 2000-cGy course, 5-FU 500 mg/m^2/day is given intravenously (IV) on 3 consecutive days. A 1-month rest period after the completion of radiation is followed by weekly 5-FU (500 mg/m^2) therapy for a total treatment time of 2 years. Patients undergoing this combined-modality approach had a median survival of approximately 21 months. The 2-year survival for this combination therapy group is 46%, with about 25% of the patients alive at 5 years with no evidence of disease. Clearly, this very aggressive treatment is appropriate for a minority of patients (those with localized disease). Toxicities include the malaise, hematotoxicity, mucositis, and diarrhea typically associated with aggressive chemotherapy/radiation combinations.

For those patients whose disease is not resectable because of local contiguous involvement, the most appropriate consideration for treatment is a combination of radiation therapy and chemotherapy for local palliation. Conventional external irradiation results in a median survival of approximately 16 weeks. The combination of radiation and chemotherapy (such as that described for adjuvant patients above) yields a median survival of 40 weeks. While a variety of other chemotherapies have been suggested as potentially useful with radiation therapy, no comparative trial has demonstrated the superiority of any treatment over 5-FU plus radiation.[3] A special consideration for those patients with unresectable local disease (but no metastases) is brachytherapy or intraoperative radiation at the time of the documentation of unresectability. However, intraoperative radiation is not generally available and can be given only at selected centers where surgical and radiation facilities are specially designed and coordinated to provide this sort of care.

For the majority of pancreatic cancer patients who present with extensive disease not amenable to either of the previously described two approaches, systemic chemotherapy can be considered.

The clinician's frustration with conventional chemotherapy agents alone or in combinations remains unrelieved. Investigators have attempted to combine drugs thought to have efficacy, such as 5-FU, mitomycin C, streptozotocin, and doxorubicin. Objective partial response rates range between 5% and 35%, with median survivals ranging from 9 to 26 weeks. In occasional individual patients substantial subjective and objective benefit will be gained, but complete responses are rare and cures nonexistent. There is little to recommend one particular chemotherapy or combination over another,[4] and for many patients, 5-FU, vigorously employed, is the most appropriate choice. However, for all stages of this disease therapeutic choices are so poor that investigational options are quite reasonable.

Cancer of the Biliary System

Surgical resection is the mainstay of therapy for cancer of the gallbladder or extrahepatic biliary system. When possible, total resection of an early gallbladder cancer (confined to the mucosa) can result in 80% survival at 5 years. The prognosis for apparently localized extrahepatic biliary tumors is worse. In both situations, meaningful palliation may be achieved by mechanical biliary drainage or diverting procedures or by localized radiation therapy. Conventional chemotherapy has not been extensively evaluated but is usually of very little value.

Cancer of the Liver

Patients at risk for developing hepatocellular cancer often have underlying liver disease with deranged metabolic function and may not be suitable candidates for resection. Up to 80% of the liver can be removed (trisegmentectomy), but the mortality and morbidity postoperatively can be substantial. However, properly selected cases can benefit from a partial hepatectomy. Localized cancer is often discovered incidentally, but with complete resection perhaps 25% of patients can be cured. Unfortunately, this approach is appropriate for only 10% or less of patients.

Most patients are not candidates for complete tumor resection, and these patients may benefit from such regional approaches as percutaneous hepatic artery embolization or ligation, which produces ischemic necrosis of the tumor. This may result in dramatic tumor shrinkage, but unfortunately the response is usually temporary. Side-effects include pleuroperitonitis, fever, hepatic pain, and laboratory evidence of hepatocellular necrosis. After a few days to weeks of discomfort, patients may experience meaningful palliation.

Chemotherapy has generally been disappointing. When given by hepatic intra-arterial infusion, the fluoropyrimidines result in modest effects, but this therapy requires either prolonged hospitalization (percutaneous administration) or surgical placement of a catheter. Many patients are too ill for such treatment.[4]

Systemic chemotherapy is likewise only modestly effective. Doxorubicin (40–80 mg/m^2 IV every 3 weeks) results in median survival of only 12 to 20 weeks. Other agents, such as 5-FU or mitomycin, are inconsistently effective when given systemically.[5] For patients with an estimated survival of 1 month or more, the use of single-agent doxorubicin is appropriate.

External irradiation (300 cGy/day for 7 days) can result in palliation without severe organ toxicity, and up to 20% of patients will experience tumor shrinkage, while more than 50% will have diminished local symptoms.[6]

GENERAL SYMPTOMATIC MANAGEMENT OF PANCREATIC AND HEPATOBILIARY CANCER

The relief of symptoms is paramount for proper patient management. Epigastric or dorsal pain may be the major problem faced by the patient, and therefore proper analgesia is an overriding consideration. In selected cases consideration should also be given to the use of percutaneous techniques such as splanchnic nerve blocks (injection of the celiac plexus) or other neurosurgical interruption of pain sensation from the upper abdomen. This sort of severe pain often indicates nonresectability when it is a presenting feature.

Nutrition is a second (nearly universal) consideration. Often, patients complain of diarrhea, steatorrhea, weight loss, and malnutrition. This malnutrition may be due to anorexia from tumor or analgesics; or to mechanical blockage from intraabdominal tumor, adhesions, or ascites; or to the effects of digestive system failure such as the inability of bile salts to reach intestinal contents; or exocrine failure of the pancreas. The therapy of this complicated constellation of problems must be individualized. Many patients respond to small, frequent feedings, the careful use of antiemetics, and digestive enzyme replacement. Enzyme replacement tablets such as pancreatin (Viokase) should be given vigorously — six to eight tablets per meal. The replacement of the lost lipase enzyme activity is especially important, and patients should generally limit intake of saturated fatty acids and consider the use of medium-chain triglyceride preparations to provide necessary calories without increasing steatorrhea. Ideally, 1500 to 6000 calories per day are required by a patient, and these should be supplied chiefly by carbohydrates and protein. Occasionally, patients will experience fat-soluble vitamin deficiencies, and these can be replenished with appropriate vitamin supplementation. Finally, enzymes produced by the pancreas tend to be more effective in an alkaline environment, and in patients with disturbed digestive tracts after surgery or influenced by malignancy, the use of antacids or cimetidine can enhance enzyme effect.

Obstruction is a major anatomical feature of these diseases and may produce substantial pain, discomfort, and physiologic derangement. Biliary obstruction alters the metabolism of bile salts, with diminished access to the digestive system, jaundice, pruritus, and pain in either the right upper quadrant or the retroperitoneum. Surgical attempts to restore biliary continuity are usually associated with a diagnostic or therapeutic intervention. Transhepatic percutaneous drainage, which decompresses liver and biliary tree, is less traumatic. For patients with biliary tumors, the use of external irradiation or iridium wire implants can occasionally result in useful palliation of obstructive symptoms (with or without surgical intervention). Secondly, obstruction of a tubular viscus, such as the stomach, duodenum, or small intestine, by tumor invasion is a painful and potentially life-threatening complication. Gastric or duodenal tube enterostomies, placed percutaneously or at the time of surgery, provide necessary drainage for otherwise intractable obstruction and also permit feeding of the patient without the expensive, cumbersome difficulties of intravenous nutritional support.

Obviously, those patients who undergo resection of the pancreas as part of a curative procedure require a chronic metabolic intervention to deal not only with the loss of the exocrine digestive functions of the pancreas but also with the surgically induced endocrinopathy (glucose intolerance). Patients with a complete pancreatectomy require careful insulin replacement.

REFERENCES

1. American Joint Committee on Cancer. Manual for Staging of Cancer, 4th ed. Philadelphia, JB Lippincott, 1992
2. Gastrointestinal Tumor Study Group. Further evidence of effective adjuvant combined radiation and chemotherapy following curative resection of pancreatic cancer. Cancer 59:2006–2010, 1987
3. Gastrointestinal Tumor Study Group. Therapy of locally unresectable pancreatic carcinoma: A randomized comparison of high-dose (6000 rads) radiation alone, moderate-dose radiation (4000 rads + 5-fluorouracil), and high-dose radiation + 5-fluorouracil. Cancer 48(8):1705–1710, 1981
4. O'Connell MJ. Current status of chemotherapy for advanced pancreatic and gastric cancer: A review article. J Clin Oncol 3(7):1032–1039, 1985
5. Friedman MA. Primary hepatocellular cancer — Present results and future prospects. Int J Rad Oncol Biol Phys 9:1841–1850, 1984
6. DiBisceglie AM, Rustgi VK, Hoofnagle JH et al. NIH Conference: Hepatocellular cancer. Ann Intern Med 108:390–401, 1988

John S. Macdonald, Daniel G. Haller, Robert J. Mayer, Eds. *Manual of Oncologic Therapeutics*, Third Edition.

30. GENITOURINARY CANCERS

Alan Yagoda

KIDNEY TUMORS

Renal cell carcinoma accounts for 2.3% of all cancers (2.7% in males and 1.8% in females) with 27,600 new cases and 11,300 deaths annually in the United States. The male to female ratio is approximately 2:1, and the average age at presentation, 55 to 60 years,[1] is decreasing because of the use of ultrasonography and computed tomographic (CT) scans for non-urological problems.[2,3] Not only have these diagnostic tests increased the detection rate by more than 18% but, of more importance, most cancers found are small stage I lesions that can be cured by partial, simple, radical, or laparoscopic nephrectomy.[2–6] Renal cell cancers are associated with congenital and acquired polycystic disease after long-term chronic dialysis, and rarely may arise within a renal cyst. Uncommon tumors include those originating from the distal tubules, adult Wilms' and multilocular cystic nephroma (a benign variant of Wilms' found in women in the third and fourth decade), and every histologic subtype of soft tissue sarcomas from stromal tissue, renal capsule, or Gerota's fascia.

It is increasingly clear that Wilms', von Hippel-Lindau, familial, and sporadic renal cancers are associated with loss of a tumor suppressor gene involving the short arm of chromosome 3 (3p).[7] Abnormalities include translocation of t(3:8), t(3:6), or t(3:11) with the breaking point at 3p13-p14, deletion of 3p13-tel, and loss of heterozygosity between 3p13-p21; such changes are absent in oncocytoma. Another abnormality, increased copies of chromosome 7 and 17, has been reported in papillary cystadenocarcinomas.[7] Renal cancers display increased expression of epidermal growth factor and c-myc, and some also express p53, c-Ha-raf, c-fos, and c-fms. One member of the multidrug resistance gene family (mdr1), which is present in the apical membrane of normal proximal tubules, is over-expressed, producing increased production of the plasma membrane p-glycoprotein 170 in 80% of unpretreated renal cancers. Immunohistochemical techniques point to the proximal tubule as the origin of over 90% of all renal cancers[8]; 30% demonstrate a phenotype consistent with derivation from the convoluted portion, 18% from the straight portion, and 50% possess the fetal antigens URO[8] and URO[10]. Less than 5% originate from the distal portion of the nephron and collecting duct; these include Bellini duct carcinoma, oncocytoma, chromophobe cell carcinoma (malignant variant of oncocytoma), and papillary cystadenocarcinoma.

The most frequent histology in more than 75% of cases is clear cell carcinoma, with the remaining cell types being granular, mixed, and spindle.[1] The latter, also called sarcomatoid or hypernephroma with sarcomatous degeneration, is a very aggressive high-grade cancer that expresses keratin, thereby indicating renal and not mesenchymal soft tissue lineage. Multicentric renal tumors are found in 7% to 13% of nephrectomy specimens. Tumor emboli within the renal vein occur in 20% and inferior vena cava in about 15% of cases, of which 50% are subhepatic, 40% intrahepatic, and 10% atrial. Hematogenous dissemination via such emboli and the extreme vascularity of renal cell tumors partially explain the frequent metastatic pattern to lung (60%), bone (35%), brain (12%), and liver, thyroid, and other sites. Local recurrence is uncommon unless tumor has penetrated the renal capsule into the retroperitoneal and adrenal areas or inadequate surgery was performed.[5] Regional lymph node metastases are found in 15% to 30% with subsequent involvement of pulmonary hilar and mediastinal nodes.

Presenting signs include gross or microscopic hematuria in about 40% to 70% of cases, sometimes precipitated by use of anticoagulants, aspirin, or nonsteroidal anti-inflammatory drugs (NSAIDs); abdominal mass or flank pain in 20% to 40%; weight loss and cachexia in 30% to 50%; and intermittent fever, malaise, night sweats, eosinophilia, increased sedimentation rate, leukemoid reaction, and anemia in 5% to 30%.[1] The "classic triad" of gross hematuria, flank pain, and a palpable abdominal mass is seen in 10% to 17% of cases. Hypercalcemia (due to prostaglan-dins or parathormone production), polycythemia, hepatic dysfunction ("hypernephroma hepatopathy"), Cushing's syndrome, feminization and masculinization (due to gonado-tropins), and hypertension, all of which may be attributed to a paraneoplastic process, can be observed in up to 25% of cases. Metastases are present at diagnosis in 40% of patients.

Pretreatment Evaluation

Work-up consists of complete blood and platelet counts, biochemical screening profile, prothrombin and partial thromboplastin times, chest x-ray (frequently followed by CT scan), and abdominal CT scan; the latter has replaced nephrotomography, intravenous pyelography, and ultrasonography.[2] These tests should define the presence of anemia, clotting abnormalities, and pulmonary, liver, nodal and local organ involvement; extent of the primary tumor; presence of inferior vena cava invasion; and also the presence of two kidneys.

Sonograms are useful in detecting benign cysts (accuracy is greater than 97%), and help in distinguishing a benign lesion, angiomyolipoma, by the fat content pattern of increased echogenicity. Intraoperative ultrasonography can be useful in localizing intrarenal lesions and planning for parenchymal-sparing surgery. Magnetic resonance imaging (MRI) with paramagnetic contrast agents is helpful when iodinated contrast cannot be given for CT enhancement. It is also useful for detecting lesions 1.5 cm and smaller, tumor compression versus invasion of adjacent organs, adrenal masses, and, with accuracy approaching 91%, patency or tumor thrombosis in the inferior vena cava.[2] Venography and renal angiography have a very limited role but still are employed to define small, potentially resectable intrarenal and cystic-appearing tumors, and to plan for partial nephrectomy, "bench" surgery, inferior vena cava tumor embolectomy, and to stop bleeding by therapeutic embolization of renal tumors.[2,3] Urinary cytology for renal cell cancer is worthless and is done only to exclude another urinary tract tumor originating from the renal pelvis, ureter, bladder, or other organ as the cause of hematuria. Tissue diagnosis usually is obtained by CT- or ultrasonographic-guided percutaneous biopsy; current techniques are safe and almost never produce a "tumor track."[2] Bone scans are obtained prior to surgery; radionuclide abnormalities must be evaluated by x-rays. Osteolytic metastasis are not always detected by scan, and a skeletal survey may be required. Any patient complaining of symptoms referable to the central nervous system or spinal cord requires a neurologic examination and CT scan or MRI of the suspected area. Monoclonal biologic markers are being evaluated for diagnosis and scanning.[8]

Staging System

The American Joint Committee on Cancer (AJCC) TNM classification, outlined in Table 30–1, includes four stages:

TABLE 30–1. RENAL CELL CANCER STAGING SYSTEM (AJCC)

T	**PRIMARY TUMOR**
TX	Cannot be assessed
TO	No tumor clinically
T1	Tumor < 2.5 cm
T2	Tumor > 2.5 cm
T3	Tumor extends into vein or Gerota's fascia
	T3a in perinephric tissue, adrenals
	T3b in renal vein, vena cava below the diaphragm
	T3c in vena cava above the diaphragm
T4	Tumor extends beyond Gerota's fascia
N	**REGIONAL LYMPH NODES**
NX	Cannot be assessed
NO	No lymph node clinically
N1	Single node < 2 cm
N2	Single node > 2 cm and <5 cm; multiple nodes, all < 5 cm
N3	Node > 5 cm
M	**DISTANT METASTASIS**
MX	Cannot be assessed
MO	No metastasis
M1	Distant metastasis

Stage I	T1 — 2.5 cm or less; confined to kidney and capsule
Stage II	T2 — invasion of perinephric fat but within Gerota's fascia
Stage III	T1-2,N1 or T3,N0-1 — involvement of one regional lymph node, renal vein, or vena cava
Stage IV	T4 or N2-3 or M1, extension beyond Gerota's fascia or distant metastases.

Laterality does not affect N classification. Although the AJCC system predicts differences in survival, a major limitation is the grouping together of renal vein, lymphatics, and inferior vena cava involvement, because renal vein invasion without perinephritic fat or regional lymph node metastasis does not significantly affect survival; prognosis is similar to Stage I, with a survival rate of 60% to 90%.[9] The AJCC and International Union Against Cancer (UICC) Staging System are very similar.

Pathologic stage is the most important prognostic factor affecting survival, followed by grade and tumor ploidy. Grade 1 and 2 diploid cancers have 5- and 10-year survivals of 82% and 62%, respectively, compared to aneuploid tumors, which have survivals of 62% and 37%, respectively. Aneuploidy increases from 40% to 77% for Stage I versus Stages II–IV.[10,11] Renal cell tumors are heterogeneous, evidenced by 57% having at least one population of aneuploid cells; 10% of diploid cases versus 77% of aneuploid tumor cases ($p<0.001$) died within the time frame of the study.[12] In general, metastases revealed concordance with the primary tumor, and excision of metastatic diploid lesions seemed to affect survival.

Treatment

Radical nephrectomy, which involves removal of Gerota's fascia and its contents, has been the standard approach for locoregional renal cell carcinoma (stages I-III); the impact of lymphadenectomy on survival, however, is uncertain. Five-year survivals are 70% to over 80% for stage I, and 60% to 70% for stage II. Peritoneal laparoscopic nephrectomy is being done with minimal morbidity and excellent preliminary results, and, in selected cases, will probably replace currently used surgical techniques. Retroperitoneal laparoscopic surgery, which is now being done for benign renal problems, will also have a role. When renal cell carcinoma invades the renal vein and inferior vena cava, tumor embolectomy is performed to remove all residual disease; the need for this procedure should not deny patients surgical resection, since survival may not necessarily be compromised with this presentation.

Partial nephrectomy is performed in selected cases presenting with small Grade I renal cell carcinoma, which usually contains small areas of calcification and is frequently diploid; results with tumor enucleation, even as for those as small as 0.6 cm, have been disappointing, with recurrence in

85%. Partial nephrectomy, sometimes with renal hypothermia, also is undertaken in patients having a single or horseshoe kidney in whom a chronic dialysis program cannot be obtained, and with a history of calculi, chronic pyelonephritis, ureteral reflux, or systemic medical problems (*e.g.*, diabetes, nephrosclerosis, collagen vascular disease, von Hippel-Lindau). In rare instances when synchronous or metachronous tumors occur bilaterally, renal dialysis is required; transplantation, with its required immunosuppressive agents, is not considered a viable option.

Nephrectomy or selective renal arterial embolization has been performed to stop life-threatening uncontrollable hematuria and flank pain in patients with metastases; however, it should not be done with the expectation of inducing remission in metastatic sites, which occurs in 0.8%, an incidence less than the mortality rate for surgery. Moreover, surgery has never demonstrated a benefit in remission rates or survival when performed prior to starting immunotherapy for metastatic disease, despite evidence suggesting more responses with such agents in nephrectomized cases. Of note, some recent data have described survival advantage in selected patients with metastases undergoing nephrectomy following successful neoadjuvant therapy with interferon or interleukin-2 (IL-2). In some patients presenting with one or two metastatic lesions, particularly diploid ones, that show no significant tumor progression without the appearance of new lesions, surgical resection can be considered. Although 5-year survivals approach 60% to 75% for stage I and 47% to 65% for stage II, the rate decreases for Stage III to 20% to 50% for node-negative and 5% to 15% for node-positive disease. The rate is less than 5% for stage IV. Median survival for patients with metastatic disease is 7 months, with a range of 2 to 13 months.[13]

There is no evidence to suggest a survival benefit with preoperative or postoperative radiation therapy, hormones, and adjuvant chemo- and immunotherapy. Immunotherapy has not lived up to its promise. Alpha-interferon, usually in doses of 5 to 18 $\times 10^6$ U/m^2 daily or three times weekly, produces an overall response in about 15%; the rate increases to 25% to 35% in asymptomatic patients with minimal nodal and pulmonary metastases.[14] Complete tumor regression is very uncommon, and there is no evidence that survival has been improved in advanced disease or when interferon is given adjuvantly. Various doses and schedules of IL-2, alone or with lymphokine-activated killer (LAK) cells and tumor-infiltrating lymphocytes (TIL), have a similar rate, although approximately 3% to 5% will achieve a relatively long-lasting complete remission (CR).[14] These agents have been combined with many other cytokines, cytotoxics, and cis-retinoic acid, but there is no statistical evidence at this time of true success. New approaches being evaluated include monoclonal antibodies, standard and genetically engineered vaccines, autolymphocyte therapy, and gene insertion therapy.

Hormonal and cytotoxic chemotherapy, singly or in combination regimens, are mostly ineffective. In 83 trials of investigational and experimental agents in 4093 patients culled from 161 publications between 1983 and 1993, CR were noted in 1.3% and partial remissions (PR) in 4.7%.[15] Some agents frequently employed are vinblastine, nitrosoureas, and floxuridine or fluorouracil. The consistent therapeutic failure of cytotoxic agents in renal cell cancers probably is multifactorial, *i.e.*, it probably involves overexpression of both p-170 and glutathione-S transferase, and down-regulation of topoisomerase-2. However, trials adding agents that modulate such gene products have been discouraging thus far. Even combining various cytotoxic drugs with immunologic drugs have been disappointing; no randomized studies have proven such combinations statistically superior to interferon or IL-2 used singularly.

Follow-up

Physicians need to be aware of the frequent metastatic pattern of renal cell carcinoma to the brain and spinal cord. Although early diagnosis is important to minimize or prevent a decrease in the quality of life, survival following irradiation and corticosteroids is generally short, 1 to 3 months. Hypercalcemia may be controlled for a limited period of time, but is usually a terminal event, with a median survival of 4 to 6 weeks. Osseous painful metastases usually can be controlled with radiation therapy. Weight-bearing sites should be irradiated prophylactically to avoid fracture; many patients will require an orthopedic procedure for prophylactic stabilization.

After radical nephrectomy for cure, patients require proper follow-up, which should include a chest film and physical examination every 2 to 3 months during the first year, with a CT scan 2 months following surgery to establish the postsurgical anatomy and again at 4- to 6-month intervals. Complete blood and platelet counts, sedimentation rate, and biochemical screen should be obtained at 3- to 4-month intervals during the first 2 years. It is important to remember that metastases from renal cancer can appear 30 years or more after diagnosis.

UROTHELIAL TRACT TUMORS

Bladder tumors, which account for 4.2% of new cancers diagnosed annually in the United States, rank fourth in males, with 38,000 cases (6%) and ninth in females, with 13,200 cases (2.3%). Although mortality from urothelial neoplasms is only 2% of the total cancer deaths, it ranks ninth in males with 7000 cases (2.5%) and twelfth in females with 3600 cases (1.4%). It is the fifth leading cause of cancer death in men older than 75 years of age. The initial presentation of potentially curable superficial papillary tumors (Ta) in 60% to 75% of patients, tumors invading the lamina propria (T1) in 10% to 20%, and carcinoma in situ (Cis) in less than 10% accounts for the large difference between incidence and mortality rates. While about 30% of Ta cases presenting with one lesion and 70% with two lesions will develop another lesion within 3 years, no more than 5% to 15% will have Cis.[16] However, the Cis recurrence rate is more than 75% in patients presenting with Cis, and Cis is seen concurrently with papillary or invasive transitional cell carcinoma (TCC) in more than 90%.[16,17] The median and mean ages for bladder cancer are 68 and 64 years, respectively; the Caucasian to African American ratio is 2:1, and the male to female ratio is 2.9:1. The higher male incidence is thought to be due to exposure in the workplace to chemical carcinogens (*e.g.*, polycyclic aromatic hydrocarbons, beta-naphthylamine, aniline dyes, arylamines, o-toluidine, and benzidine), and to smoking (tobacco contains 4-aminobiphenyl and 2-aminonaphthylene).[18] Cigarette smoking, which probably has a promoting effect, is felt to be responsible for almost half of the bladder tumors in men, and for 56% to 82% in men and 37% to 62% in women of renal pelvis and ureteral carcinomas. Smoking cessation of more than 10 years reduces the risk almost 70%.[17,19] Bladder mucosal abnormalities are found at autopsy in almost 50% of smokers compared to less than 4% of nonsmokers. Cyclophosphamide, phenacetin, and high concentrations of nitrates in drinking water from nitrogen fertilizers and pesticide contamination have also been implicated as etiologic agents, as well as in calculus disease and chronic infection (*e.g.*, schistosoma haematobium, cystitis cystica, and cystitis glandularis).[18] The elapsed time from carcinogenic exposure to tumor formation ranges from 2 to 45 years.

Abnormalities have been described in chromosomes 1, 3p, 4, 6p, 7, 9q, 11p (in 40%), 14q, 17p (in 65%), and 18q; in loss of ABH expression (chromosome 9); presence of Le^x; activation of mutated p53 ras; increased expression of mdr1 receptor/p-glycoprotein; and alterations in the retinoblastoma gene.[16,20,21] More than 50% of Grade I and II Ta lesions exhibit loss of heterozygosity in the proximal 9q or 9p area, 63% of invasive tumors are ABH^- compared to 4% of ABH^+, 13% of untreated cancer cells express mdr1 mRNA compared to 32% to 55% of chemotherapy-treated primary and metastatic masses, respectively, and 3 of 18 p53 negative tumors progressed compared to 13 of 15 p53 positive. Although chromosome 9q tumor suppressor gene inactivation may well be the first event for Ta, some data suggest a different pathway for Cis, namely chromosome 17p induced p53/ras change.[17,20] Monoclonal antibodies, T138 and T43, also are predictive for invasiveness and, of much more significance, the metastatic phenotype.[21]

Since the whole urothelial lining — renal pelvis, ureter, urinary bladder, urethra, and prostatic ducts — is exposed to urinary excreted carcinogens, tumors tend to recur in time and space ("polychronotropism," "field-effect").[16,17] For example, patients who survive an invasive renal pelvis tumor are 21 times more likely to develop another urothelial tract tumor. Between 5% and 40% of cystectomy specimens containing muscle-invasive transitional cell carcinoma (TCC) will have Cis in the ureter, urethra, and prostatic ducts.[22] Additionally, complete responders (CR) to intravesical bacillus Calmette-Guerin (BCG) therapy also have an increasing incidence of Cis of the urethra and prostatic ducts. Cystoprostatectomy is the treatment of choice when Cis invades the prostatic ducts and parenchyma because of the uncertainty of intravesical agents bathing the involved mucosal surface, and of the inadequacy of complete cystoscopic visualization.[22-24] Although Cis can progress to an invasive lesion, most muscle-invading tumors probably originate de novo in the background of an unstable bladder mucosa that has already given rise to recurrent Cis.[17,23]

Over 90% of urothelial carcinomas were reported previously as TCC, but the percentage of mixed histologies in phase 2 trials has risen to 10% to 35%. Squamous cell carcinoma accounts for 6% to 8%, and adenocarcinoma and urachal carcinoma for 2% to 5%.[16] Squamous cell carcinoma is more frequently found in patients having lithiasis and adenocarcinoma in those having a history of cystitis glandularis. Clear cell, carcinosarcoma, small cell, carcinoid, and soft-tissue sarcomas are uncommon in adults, and embryonal rhabdomyosarcoma occurs mostly in children. An unusual type, yet extremely chemotherapeutically responsive, is lymphoepithelioma-like TCC. Most TCC originate in the lateral and posterior bladder wall, while adenocarcinoma is found in the dome and trigone; tumors can occur within a bladder diverticula. Urachal cancer, which originates from embryologic remnant of the gut, the urachus, is similar to colonic adenocarcinoma and therefore produces carcinoembryonic antigen (CEA), which can serve as an excellent biologic marker for response and recurrence.[16] These tumors, as well as CEA-positive TCC, respond poorly to chemotherapy, while those histologically positive for beta human chorionic gonadotropin, present in about 10% of TCC specimens, are more responsive.

The lamina propria and its extremely small layer, the muscularis mucosa, separates the 3- to 7-layer avascular mucosa from bladder muscle, the muscularis propria. Adipose tissue surrounds bladder muscle, with the parietal peritoneum covering only the cephalad portion, and nerves, blood vessels, and lymphatics permeate all tissues except the mucosa, thereby explaining lymphatic and hematogenous patterns of dissemination with high-grade lesions. Metastases can involve the hypogastric and internal and external lymph chains, which then drain to the aortic bifurcation and retroperitoneum. Common sites for metastasis include lymph nodes in 28% to 74%, lung in 29%, bone in 25%, and liver in 15%. Renal pelvis and ureteral tumors, 75% of which are aneuploid and high-grade, extend directly into the renal pelvis and down the ureter, as well as to regional lymph nodes and surrounding tissues. Urethral cancers, which invade the surrounding structures, drain to the inguinal lymph nodes.

The most frequent sign is gross hematuria in about 75% of cases, usually microscopic at first. Dysuria and increased urinary frequency from tumor-induced bladder irritability occur in 25%. Urinary obstruction and anuria, which are poor-risk factors, are seen with trigone lesions. Although such symptoms often are attributed to urinary tract infections or prostatitis, recurrent complaints require a urine examination for blood and cytology.

Pretreatment Evaluation

Transurethral cystoscopy under anesthesia with bimanual palpation and appropriate biopsies and transurethral resections (TURs) of visual abnormalities, as well as sampling of normal-appearing mucosa, are mandatory for diagnosis.[22] The diagnostic yield for urinary cytology is more often positive for high- than low-grade lesions — 94% and 34% respectively — and after cystoscopy.[16,23] While DNA cytometry is not yet accepted for screening because of low specificity in low-risk patients (positive in less than 50% with papilloma compared to over 82% with Tis, Ta, T1 or T2), aneuploidy is an excellent predictor of treatment failure and disease progression after intravesical therapy and after irradiation. Tetraploidy may be present for up to 2 years after radiotherapy.[16,23] Following TUR, progression occurred in 35% of 54 aneuploid lesions compared to 0% of 175 diploid cases, while other Ta and T1 studies report 60% to 87% recurrence for aneuploid versus 2% to 34% for diploid tumors.[22–24] Other tests include intravenous urography to evaluate the upper tracts and bladder, and a contrast pelvic and abdominal CT scan; MRI occasionally is used to better define local soft tissue involvement, particularly following cystectomy and nephroureterectomy. For renal pelvis tumors, retrograde pyelogram and differential washings from each ureter for cytologic examination are performed. Before surgery, chest film, blood count, and automated biochemical screen are obtained, but radionuclide bone scans are not part of the preoperative work-up because abnormalities are found in less than 10% of asymptomatic patients. Since pelvic and abdominal lymph node metastasis is an extremely poor prognostic sign, predictive for subsequent dissemination in over two thirds of cases, CT-guided fine-needle aspiration and, recently, laparoscopic surgery may be necessary to exclude such involvement. A positive aspiration may preclude surgery but a negative one does not.

Staging System

Although the Jewett-Strong-Marshall (JSM) Staging System has been used in the United States, the AJCC (Table 30–2) is gaining more acceptance. In the JSM system, Stage 0 indicates superficial mucosal tumors, both Cis and exophytic papillary (Ta) lesions, while lamina propria invasion is Stage A (T1). Stage A includes no induration on bimanual examination with a freely mobile mass that disappears after resection. Stage B1 (T2) denotes a mobile induration of the bladder on bimanual examination that disappears after resection of a tumor involving less than half, and B2 (T3a) more than half of the bladder muscle; however, B2 lesions have induration or nodularity persisting after TUR. Since depth of invasion may depend completely on the extent of the TUR,[22,24] and survival rates for high-grade aneuploid Stage B1 and B2 lesions are similar, many pathologists combine both into a single B Stage. Grade 1 well-differentiated diploid lesions, which are a good-risk prognostic feature, tend to be mostly B1. Stage C indicates perivesical fat invasion, while D1 means adjacent organ extension or nodes below the sacral promontory and D2 above the pelvis. Staging for renal pelvis tumors is similar to that for the urinary bladder, except that renal parenchymal involvement is included in T3. Urethral staging categorizes tumor extending into the corpus spongiosum, prostate, or periurethral muscle as T2, and invasion of the corpus cavernosum, anterior vagina, bladder neck, or beyond the prostatic capsule as T3. In the UICC system, involvement of Virchow's supraclavicular node is N^+ for renal pelvis malignancies but M^+ for bladder tumors.

Grading of urothelial cancer depends on the definition used for superficial exophytic papillomas, which some pathologists feel are non-cancerous since less than 5% ever exhibit local progression.[16,22] Broder's Grade 0 signifies such

TABLE 30–2. BLADDER CANCER STAGING SYSTEM (AJCC)

T	**PRIMARY TUMOR**
TX	Cannot be assessed
T0	No tumor clinically
Tis	Carcinoma in situ: "flat tumor" (JSM = 0)
Ta	Noninvasive papillary carcinoma (JSM = 0)
T1	Tumor in subepithelial connective tissue (JSM = A)
T2	Tumor in superficial (inner half) muscle (JSM = B1)
T3	Tumor in deep muscle or perivesical fat
	T3a in deep (outer half) muscle (JSM = B2)
	T3b in perivesical fat (JSM = C)
	i. microscopically
	ii. macroscopically (extravesical mass)
T4	Tumor in adjacent structures
	T4a in prostate, uterus, or vagina (JSM = D1)
	T4b in pelvic or abdominal wall
N	**REGIONAL LYMPH NODES***
NX	Cannot be assessed
N0	No lymph node clinically
N1	Single node < 2 cm
N2	Single node > 2 cm and <5 cm; multiple nodes, all < 5 cm
N3	Node > 5 cm
M	**DISTANT METASTASIS**
MX	Cannot be assessed
M0	No metastasis
M1	Distant metastasis (JSM = D2)

JSM, Jewett-Strong-Marshall System

*Regional nodes are only within the true pelvis (JSM = D1 for N1-3); all other juxtaregional are distant nodes (JSM = D2, or M1).

lesions as benign tumors, Grade 1 tumors as well-differentiated, Grade 2 as moderately differentiated, and Grade 3 as anaplastic or poorly differentiated. Other systems place papilloma into the Grade 1 well-differentiated group, thereby indicating that such tumors must be considered a low grade cancer, and separate Grade 3 and 4 into poorly differentiated and anaplastic, respectively.

Low-grade superficial tumors have a mortality approaching 0%, compared to 90% for deeply invasive high-grade lesions.[23,24] For Grade 3 tumors, the median time is about 30 months to local recurrence, 12 months to distant metastasis, and 15 months to death; median survival for Grade 2 is 30 months. However, the staging error approaches 50% for Stages B1-2 and C lesions. For example, one study reported the T:P (clinical to pathological) error was 33% for B1 tumors (mostly understaged), 59% of B2, 35% of C (23% overstaging), and 50% of D1. Lymph node metastases increase from less than 5% for T0, Cis, and T1 lesions to about 18% for T2 and T3a, and 35% to 44% for T3b and T4.[25,26] CT scan can help in staging by defining nodal involvement but is accurate in only 44% to 70%, at best; laparoscopic evaluation may be somewhat more sensitive. Cis lesions usually are accurately staged with an error of less than 8%. This high clinical staging error, 35% to 55% for T2-4, has a significant impact on results of neoadjuvant radiation and chemotherapy trials for invasive bladder cancer.

Treatment

Therapy for superficial lesions (T0, Tis, T1, and low-grade T2) is endoscopic resection and fulguration with cystoscopy repeated every 3 months; low-grade papillomas can be followed at much less frequent intervals.[22–24] Intravesical therapy is used prophylactically to prevent new lesions and delay or prevent development of both metastasis and muscle invading tumors, and therapeutically to eradicate an existing lesion and non-visualized disease evidenced by a positive cytology. The most effective intravesical treatment is weekly BCG given for 6 weeks, with CR achieved in 47% to 85% of cases.[22–24] Randomized BCG studies find disease-free survival in 85% compared to 64% of patients treated by TUR alone.[22] At 10 years, 50% given BCG remained continuously disease-free or experienced one recurrence, and only 25% progressed within 5 years. Furthermore, there was a marked delay in time to cystectomy and improved survival in BCG responders compared with TUR. Some urologists feel one cycle of BCG is suboptimal and at least two are needed for CR. A recent trial in Ta and T1 cases has determined that three additional weekly treatments at 3 months increase CR from 73% to 87%, and three more weekly treatments at 6 months improve long-term disease-free status from 50% to 83%.[22,24] Attachment of BCG to mucosal fibronectin and integrin appears essential for its action, which involves IL-1, -2, -6, -10 and -12, tumor necrosis factor, interferon, and lymphokine activated and natural killer (NK) cells. Another agent, although less efficacious for high grade lesions, is thiotepa, 60 mg/60 ml weekly for 6 consecutive weeks. Approximately 30% to 40% of patients will respond, particularly those with low-grade papillary lesions.[22] Since this drug has a low molecular weight, it is absorbed systemically after intravesical administration, and can produce severe myelosuppression. Mitomycin-C, 20 mg to 40 mg/20 ml to 40 ml, has a complete response rate of about 40%, even in BCG and thiotepa failures, and nearly the same efficacy has been observed with doxorubicin, 20 mg to 60 mg, and epirubicin.[22] In six randomized BCG versus mitomycin-C studies, two found significant advantages with BCG, and all trials have consistently shown BCG to be superior to thiotepa, adriamycin, interferon, and keyhole limpet hemocyanin.[22,23] The latter immunogic agent is undergoing further studies, as is bropiramine, an oral interferon inducer. One double-blind study of mega-dose vitamin A (40,000 units), B6 (100 mg), C (2 g) and E (400 units), with 90 mg of zinc, described heightened NK activity and reduced tumor recurrences in 25% to 45% of Ta, T1, and T2 lesions. Other studies are testing this hypothesis. Radical cystectomy is considered for diffuse or recurrent Cis lesions after BCG failure, a procedure resulting in a 5-year survival rate of >90%.[23,24]

While the 5-year survival for T1 is 72% overall, the 5- and 10-year rates are lower for Grade 3–4 lesions, 60% and 50%, respectively. T1 treated by TUR alone will progress to muscle invasion in 30%, but with successful chemotherapy muscle invasion decreases to 20% and with BCG treatment to 14%.[24] Vascular or lymphatic permeation, which occurs in 18% of T1 specimens, is a poor-risk factor since all will develop T2-3 cancers within 1 to 2 years. Median progression for TUR-treated cases is 6 months compared to 30 months for BCG responders; cystectomy is indicated within 3 to 6 months in BCG failures.[23,21]

Standard therapy for muscle invasive tumors is radical cystectomy with locoregional lymphnodal resection, proximal urethrectomy, and distal ureterectomy, in addition to resection of the prostate and seminal vesicles in men, and of the uterus, fallopian tubes, ovaries, and anterior vaginal wall in females.[25,26] Operative mortality has decreased dramatically from more than 14% to less than 2%. The standard ileal conduit requiring external ostomy appliances is being replaced by non-refluxing continent ileal and colonic pouches (e.g., Indiana, Kock, Camay, Mainz), which can hold large urine volumes with pressures up to 40 cm H_2O, and need self-catheterization only 2 to 3 times daily. Of importance to oncologists is that such pouches can increase methotrexate toxicity because of reabsorption, and catheterization may be required during drug administration. A continent neopouch can be directly attached to the urethra in men with tumors not involving the bladder base, trigone, or urethra; the short urethra in females impedes such procedures. Partial cystectomy should be performed in selected cases having no Cis history and a single lesion outside the trigone, preferably low in grade and stage, which can have 2-

cm clean margins at resection.[26] Since 59% to 80% of cases will have residual or recurrent disease, this operation should comprise less than 15% of cystectomy procedures. Salvage cystectomy is a viable option in radiation failures, but partial cystectomy is to be avoided because of subsequent fibrosis, which leads to a small bladder capacity, severely affecting quality of life.[27] For renal pelvis and ureteral cancers, a nephroureterectomy with an ipsilateral bladder cuff at the ureteral insertion is performed.

The literature previously indicated a 5-year overall survival of no more than 40% for all grades of muscle invasive disease,[26] but recent data find 60% to 88% for pathologically staged T2, 50% to 78% for T3a, 15% to 48% for T3b, and 5% to 25% for T4.[25] The higher percentage would be found for low-grade lesions having good-risk features.[28] The presence of pelvic nodes indicates an extremely poor prognosis, regardless of T stage. Previously, it was accepted that less than 5% to 10% of all N+ cases survived 5 years,[26] but re-examination finds a rate of 19% to over 35% for N1 lesions, unusually low-grade low T stage tumors, and a median time to relapse of 23 to 43 months.[28] N2–3 cases still have a very poor 5-year survival, 0% to 9%, with 50% relapsing within 4 to 6 months and over 70% dying in one year.[26]

Radiation therapy, 50 Gy to 68 Gy in 4 to 7.5 weeks, produces 5-year survival in about 20% to 30% of T2–4 cases; the rate increases to 40% to 60% for low-grade low-stage tumors.[27] A major difficulty in evaluating the efficacy of irradiation is the high clinical staging error resulting in a fair number of cases having N+ disease. Although no data suggest survival benefit with pre-, intra-, and postoperative irradiation, hyperthermia, or chemotherapy, concomitant cisplatin increases CR in 61% to 88% of cases and reduces loco-regional failure from 55% to 33%.[27]

The most active agents[29] are cisplatin (DDP) with response (CR and partial remission [PR]) in 30%, carboplatin in 13% (274 cases),[30] iproplatin in 18% (39 cases),[31] methotrexate (MTX) in 30%, trimetrexate in 17% (51 cases),[32] adriamycin (ADM) in 17%, epirubicin in 28% (36 cases), pirarubicin in 19% (57 cases), vinblastine (VLB) in 16%, taxol in 42% (26 cases),[33] mitomycin in 13% (29 cases), ifosfamide in 28% (101 cases), and gallium nitrate in 30% (54 cases).[34,35] Although carboplatin data suggest less activity than DDP, a cooperative group study finds statistically equivalent rates for carboplatin (14%), iproplatin (18%), and DDP (9%).[31] In general single agents induce PR for 3 to 5 months; CR is uncommon.[29]

While many chemotherapy regimens in non-randomized trials report superior results compared to single agents[29]—CR in 10% to 35% and PR in 10% to 30% — only M-VAC[36] (Table 30–3) has been proven statistically superior, $p<0.0001$, to cisplatin[37] (36% and 13.5 months for M-VAC versus 11% and 8.2 months for cisplatin), and to CISCA (65% and 82 weeks for M-VAC versus 46% and 40 weeks for CISCA).[38] Approximately 15% of M-VAC–treated advanced

TABLE 30–3. CHEMOTHERAPY FOR UROTHELIAL TRACT CANCER*

M-VAC[21]	Methrotrexate 30 mg/m² on d1,15,22 + vinblastine 3 mg/m² on d2,15,22 + adriamycin 30 mg/m² on d2 + cisplatin 70 mg/m² on d2, per month
MCV[12]	Methotrexate 30 mg/m² on d1,15,22 + vinblastine 3 mg/m² on d2,15,22 + cisplatin 70 mg/m² on d2 + cisplatin 70 mg/m² every 3 weeks during radiation therapy
CMV[14]	Cisplatin 100 mg/m² on d2 + vinblastine 4 mg/m² on d1,8 + methotrexate 30 mg/m² on d1,8, every 3 weeks.
MVCarb[15]	Methotrexate 30 mg/m² on d1 + vinblastine 3–4 mg/m² on d1 + carboplatin 300–350 mg/m² on d1, every 3 weeks
Trimetrexate[17]	8 mg/m² on d1–5† every 3 weeks
Taxol[18]	250 mg/m² on d1 by CI†† on d1+ G-CSF = 5 μg/kg on d3–13 SC every 3 weeks
Gallium[19,20]	300 mg/m² on d1–7 by CI every 3 weeks
GaFU[26]	Gallium nitrate 300 mg/m² on d1–5 by CI + 5-fluorouracil 1000 mg/m² on d1–5 by CI, every 3 weeks
VIG[27]	Vinblastine 0.11 mg/kg on d1,2 + ifosfamide 1200 mg/m² on d1–5 in a 4-hour infusion + mesna 240 mg/m² on d1–5 at 0, 4, and 8 hours + gallium nitrate 300 mg/m² on d1–5 by CI + G-CSF 5 μg/kg on d6–12, every 3 weeks
IFN-FU[24]	5-Fluorouracil 750 mg/m² on d1–5 by CI + 5-fluorouracil 750 mg/m² weekly, every 5 weeks + interferon 9 miu/m² on d1–5 then, TW1 SC, every 3 weeks
C-IFN-FU[25]	5-Fluorouracil 500 mg/m² on d1–5 by CI + interferon 5 miu/m² on d1–5,8,10,12,15,17,19 SC + cisplatin 25 mg/m² on d1,8,15 every 3 weeks
MVMJ[15]	Methotrexate 50 mg/m² on d1,15 + folinic acid 15 mg on d2,16 PO + vinblastine 3 mg/m² on d1, + mitoxantrone 10 mg/m² on d1 + carboplatin 200 mg/m² on d1 every month

*Major dose modifications exist for all single agents and combinations, and the original study must be checked before using the initial maximum doses listed.

†D1–5 = daily each day for 5 days

††CI = continuous 24-hour infusion.

TCC cases survive 5 years, and death in some after CR of 2 to 3 years is from development of a new urothelial primary and brain metastasis. M-VAC seems to be ineffective against Tis and TCC liver metastasis, squamous cell carcinoma, adenocarcinoma, and prevention of de novo urothelial tract cancers.[36] Although GM- and G-CSF with M-VAC prevent or can favorably modulate myelosuppression, there is (not surprisingly with the non-hematologic toxicities of ADM, DDP, and MTX) no evidence that M-VAC dose intensity is more efficacious.[29] High-dose MTX with leucovorin rescue also has been ineffective. New ADM derivatives, which produce almost similar responses with less cardiac toxicity, have been substituted in some combinations (*e.g.*, epirubicin for ADM in M-VEC). Since the contribution of ADM in M-VAC has been questioned, CMV and CMV-like regimens have been developed,[29] and in patients with suboptimal renal or auditory function, DDP has been replaced by carboplatin (MVCarb, M-VACarb).[30] Promising investigational regimens include interferon (IFN) and 5-fluorouracil (FU) (30% PR in 30 cases),[39] and both plus DDP (7% CR and 54% PR in 31 cases),[40] gallium nitrate and FU (50% in 14 cases),[41] and VIG or vinblastine, ifosfamide, gallium nitrate (68% in 25 cases with 5 CR+ 12 PR, 5 of whom achieved CR with surgery),[42] and MVMJ (MTX, VLB, mitoxantrone, carboplatin).[30] Regimens for squamous cell and adenocarcinoma variants, which usually combine FU and DDP or mitomycin, or CMV, sometimes with bleomycin, have demonstrated some antitumor activity with PR in 20% to 40%.[29]

The benefit of neoadjuvant treatment is that chemosensitivity can be determined in vivo, which not only can guide future therapy but also can be of prognostic signifiance, and downstaging can convert an "unresectable" to a "resectable" lesion. In contrast, adjuvant therapy bypasses the inaccuracies of clinical staging, and more clearly defines the poor-risk patient who may benefit from chemotherapy. Many phase 2 non-randomized neoadjuvant and adjuvant trials have reported improved survival compared to historical controls. M-VAC used neoadjuvantly in 111 cases induced pathological CR in 22% to 43%, a 5-year survival of 54% for patients achieving downstaging compared to 12% for those failing chemotherapy, and a select number in whom bladder preservation was possible.[43] In 147 cases from 8 institutions given neoadjuvant cisplatin-based chemotherapy, significant downstaging of clinical T2–4 lesions to pathological P0 and Pis, and Pa occurred in more than 50% and up to 35% of cases, respectively.[44] Such results translated in a survival benefit at 3 years of 80% versus 25%, respectively, and since nonresponders had a death rate more rapid than previously described, downstaging by chemotherapy seems to distinguish a good-risk group. Randomized trials of 1 and of 2-drug combinations have been ineffective. There are more than 6 neoadjuvant and 3 adjuvant randomized multidrug chemotherapy trials describing improved survival, but all entered too few cases to support a compelling statistically significant survival benefit.[43] Prospective randomized trials now are evaluating the benefit, if any, of neoadjuvant M-VAC followed by cystectomy in 300 cases, CMV with cystectomy or radiotherapy in over 900 cases, and adjuvant versus neoadjuvant M-VAC in 150 cystectomy cases.

Another neoadjuvant approach being investigated in 250 cases, which evaluates bladder preservation in addition to survival, combines 2 cycles of MCV followed by radiation therapy, 40 Gy, with cisplatin. Nonresponders undergo immediate cystectomy, while those exhibiting significant tumor downstaging receive an additional 25 Gy; salvage cystectomy is permitted at the time of locoregional progression.[27] In the pilot phase 2 study, not only did 74% achieve CR and 72% survive more than 3-years, but 70% achieved bladder preservation.[27] Other radiation/chemotherapy protocols have evaluated CMV and mitomycin plus FU.

Follow-up

Urine cytology and cystoscopy at 3- to 4-month intervals is needed for patients achieving CR of superficial disease after intravesical therapy. In the first year following successful treatment of invasive urothelial tract cancer by surgery or radiation therapy, patients should have chest films at 2- to 3-month intervals, urine cytology after upper tract cancers, and urethral cytology if urethrectomy was not performed at cystectomy. Abdominal and pelvic CT scans should be obtained within 3 months after radical cystectomy to serve as a baseline for future examinations at 4- to 6-month intervals during the next 2 years. Onset of osseous discomfort requires x-rays and scans to evaluate for possible metastasis; if found, radiation therapy should be given. Weight-bearing areas may benefit from a prophylactic orthopedic procedure to prevent fractures. Patients with disseminated disease who obtain CR, particularly in lung metastasis, require follow-up brain CT scans since up to 18% may develop sanctuary central nervous system lesions. Despite radiation therapy, however, survival after discovery of brain metastasis is less than 3 months.

PROSTATE CANCER

Prostate tumors, with 200,000 new cases in 1994, is the leading cancer in men in the United States, representing 31.6% of all male neoplasms. Approximately one out of 11 men eventually will develop this tumor, and autopsies in men over 50 years of age find a 30% incidence (range 14% to 46%) of latent or established cancers, of which 10% would have been clinically significant. African Americans, who have the highest incidence in the world (79 per 100,000), have a rate 1.7 times that for white Americans; Japanese men have the lowest, 4 per 100,000. Prostate cancer is the third leading cause of cancer mortality, with 38,000 deaths (overall 7.1%, and in men 13.4%) annually. Risk factors include age, race, testosterone levels, family history (probably representing a subset of familial genetically determined tumors), and, possibly, dietary fat, vasectomy, and 5-alpha reductase activity.[45] Since various growth factors (epidermal, nerve, basic fibroblast, keratinocyte, transforming-alpha) influence prostate cells in culture, variations in paracrine and autocrine cytokines may also be of importance since they affect mesenchymal–epithelial interactions resulting in induction of ductal, acinar, and seminal vesicle (SV) tumors.[46]

Prostate specific antigen (PSA), coupled with the transrectal ultrasonographic (TRUS)-directed spring-loaded biopsy gun, has resulted in the marked increase in incidence, and has produced a major lead-time bias, manifested by a larger number of cases presenting with very early stage tumors.[47] PSA, which is a 34,000-dalton kallikrein-like serine protease, is recognized as an effective screening procedure, despite some questions concerning an overall impact on survival. A PSA should be obtained in African American men beginning at age 40, and in others after 50. Each gram of benign prostate hypertrophied (BPH) tissue contains 0.3 mg/ml, while each gram of adenocarcinoma can increase the serum PSA by up to 3.5 ng/ml. In men with BPH having a negative digital rectal examination (DRE), the positive predictive value (PPV) of a PSA greater than 10 ng/ml is 31% compared to 9% for those with a PSA less than 4 ng/ml. The PSA level and an annual increase (PSA velocity or PSAV) greater than 0.8 ng/ml are strong indicators of cancer; however, 0.4 ng/ml/year in those presenting with a level greater than 4 ng/ml may be more appropriate with enhanced sensitivity of 63% and specificity of 62%. For example, in 47% who had a PSAV greater than 0.75 ng/ml a cancer was found, versus only 11% of men with a lower slope.[48] Since the extent of BPH has an effect on PSA levels, particularly the transitional zone,[49] prostate volume measured by TRUS divided into PSA (PSA density or PSAD) apparently is more accurate. A PSAD greater than 0.15 is highly suggestive of malignancy.[48] The impact of BPH can be minimized with finasteride, a 5-alpha reductase (Proscar), which reduces the size of the prostate by 20% and the PSA by 50% at one year; most of the PSA decreases by 3 months.[50] Using a PSAD greater than 0.15 after finasteride leads to increased sensitivity (81% to 99%), with a minimal decrease in specificity (86% to 83%). While further PSA refinements are being tested, particularly the PSAD in relationship to volume changes in the transitional zone (PSAT), and PSA isomers (free PSA), the importance of a digital rectal examination (DRE) as a screening procedure is emphasized by the fact that most tumors arise in the peripheral (70%) zone of the prostate, and are most frequent in the apex or caudal portion.[49] Such tumors begin as a single nodule or are diffuse multifocal lesions which invade through the prostate capsule, because of their peripheral origin, and within the prostate's perineural and vascular spaces, followed by extension to periprostatic tissue, bladder, rectum, and seminal vesicles (SV). Distant metastases involve bone in over 90% of cases, but soft tissue lesions can be observed at initial presentation in up to 30% and after hormone failure in 10% to 20%,[51] and are prominent at autopsy in the lung, nodes, liver, peritoneum, and central nervous system and meninges. Regional nodes are found in the periprostatic obturator area, followed by external iliac and hypogastric chains, and common iliac and periaortic chains.

Studies have clearly indicated the prognostic importance of staging pelvic lymphadenectomy, since 40% to 50% of men with positive lymph nodes progress in less than 2 years, and by 5 years, 75% develop distant metastases versus less than 20% of node-negative patients.[47,48] Flow cytometry, which can determine ploidy status is of prognostic significance, but has not yet been incorporated into the staging system.[49,52,53] For example, less than 10% of Stage T1b or A2 node positive diploid tumors progress at 5 years versus about 70% with aneuploid cells. Of note, 88% of aneuploid tumors exhibit changes in chromosome 8 and/or 7. Over 90% of cases with SV invasion have aneuploid tumors, which may explain the much poorer prognosis and the high prevalence of N+ disease (80% for Gleason scores of 8 to 10). Tumors with Gleason scores of 2 to 4 are almost all diploid compared to those with a score of 7, which are only 25% diploid.[52] Diploid tumors consistently have a lower rate of nodal metastasis, a delay in time to relapse, and a better prognosis.[53]

Transitional cell carcinoma of the primary prostatic ducts is being described more often in patients who have had urothelial tract tumors, particularly after successful therapy for superficial bladder cancer. Such primary ductal cancers respond to chemotherapy regimens effective for bladder cancer, and are unresponsive to hormonal manipulation. Additionally, the number of secondary ductal and small cell carcinomas are increasing, mostly as a mixed component with the acinar glandular adenocarcinoma. Such tumors usually are high grade, and have a preference for nodal, liver, and lung metastasis, especially after hormones. In patients under 50 years of age who present with a poorly differentiated prostate cancer that is marginally- or non-responsive to hormones, the pathology should be reviewed to look for transitional, ductal and small cell elements. Rare prostate carcinomas include endometroid, which arises from the verumontanum; carcinosarcoma; signet cell; comedo; sarcomas originating from the gland, capsule or spermatic cord; and tumors of the periurethral gland. The latter and small cell carcinomas have an extremely poor prognosis, with few surviving 1 to 2 years. A newly recognized premalignant lesion is the grade 3 PIN (prostatic intraductal neoplasia); PIN-1 and -2 may not be of clinical significance. The presence of PIN-3, which is usually multifocal, has been reported to be associated with a 39% invasive prostate cancer incidence within a mean of 18 months compared to 15% of cases without PIN-3.

Presenting signs and symptoms include a palpable prostatic nodule (>50%), dysuria, complaints relating to cystitis or prostatitis, urinary retention, dribbling, frequency, decreased urinary stream, hermatospermia, and terminal hematuria. One must remember that BPH, with its transitional zone enlargement at the bladder base, usually produces these signs, which then lead patients to seek medical advice.[49] However, the PSA has changed these statistics. In one study, transurethral resection (TUR) for BPH now rarely diagnosed T1a cases; more than 20% of cases had no palpable disease, including 11% of T2 and T3.[47] However, the PSA led to a diagnosis of T1 in 76% of men treated with radiation therapy, T2 in 57%, and T3 in 56%. Advanced signs are pain associated with osseous metastases, fatigue, general malaise, uremia due to urethral obstruction at the bladder base, systemic bleeding from disseminated intravascular coagulation, weight loss, and cachexia. The American College of Surgeons reported a Stage C and D incidence of 43% in 1947, which by 1990, before PSA screening, had decreased to 33%. It has been estimated that in 1994 more than 58% of newly diagnosed cases will present with disease localized to the prostate, and further change can be expected with PSA screening — only 18% are anticipated to present with distant disease in 1994.

Pretreatment Evaluation

PSA and DRE are the most sensitive and cost-effective clinical diagnostic tests. The PSA increases less than 0.4 ng/ml after DRE, in contrast to marked changes in the serum acid phosphatase (SAP); most investigators have abandoned SAP because of gross inaccuracies in delineating the status of both early and late disease. A PSA greater than 10 ng/ml or 4.1 to 10 ng/ml with a PSAD of 0.15, should lead to a six-quadrant TRUS-directed biopsy in those presenting with no palpable masses; any palpable mass must be biopsied. The PPV of a PSA greater than 4 ng/ml is 35%, which is actually higher than that for mammography (10% to 25%) for breast screening. An SV biopsy should be performed when an abnormality is discovered on DRE, TRUS, or CT scan, since the presence of a high grade tumor statistically suggests the presence of N+ disease, thereby precluding surgery. The decision to perform some tests is related to the PSA level and Gleason score. For example, T2b with a PSA less than 4 ng/ml and a Gleason score of 5 has a 67% likelihood of organ-confined disease compared to 31% for Gleason's 8; if the PSA is 4 to 10 ng/ml organ-confined disease will be found in 56% compared to 22%, respectively. A PSA greater than 20 ng/ml in a clinical T2b case has only a 1% to 11% chance of having organ-confined disease.[48]

Although almost all patients have a bone scan as part of the initial work-up, many investigators perform this test only in those with a PSA greater than 10 ng/ml; bone scans are probably falsely negative in 10% of T1a,b,c and T2a,b,c cases.[47] One study described only one positive scan in 306 cases with a PSA of less than 20 ng/ml. Accuracy of the TRUS to delineate the extent of intraglandular, capsular, and SV involvement is limited — for example, in one prostatectomy study, it accurately predicted extracapsular disease in 66% and local disease in only 46%. Lymphangiography has been abandoned as a staging procedure because metastases frequently do not disturb the nodal architecture, and the hypograstic nodes are not visualized. CT scans, which most physicians use for nodal evaluation before surgery, are very imprecise; some radiation oncologists still use them for radiation therapy treatment planning.[47] Body MRI also is inaccurate, correctly predicting extracapsular disease in 77% but local lesions in 57% of cases undergoing prostatectomy. Endorectal and surface coil MRI are being investigated, and preliminary data suggest somewhat better sensitivity and specificity, particularly for capsular, SV, and nerve bundle involvement. However, about 30% to 50% of clinical T1–2 lesions will be found pathologically to be T3, indicating the immense staging error with currently available techniques.[48,54,55] In a highly selected prostatectomy series involving 995 cases between 1982 and 1991, before PSA, only 37% of clinically staged T1–2 cases had organ–confined disease, while 48% had capsular penetration, 7% had SV invasion, and 8% had positive nodes.[48] Although such tests should be performed for a PSA greater than 10 to 20 ng/ml, newer staging techniques include monoclonal antibody scanning (7E11-C5.3 or ^{111}In-CYT-356),[56] laparoscopic staging, and an enhanced reverse transcriptase polymerase chain reaction assay using PSA primers (RT–PCR-PSA)[57] or prostate-specific membrane antigens (PSMA). PCR-PSA, which can detect one prostate cell in half a million peripheral blood cells, has a PPV of 80% for organ-confined disease, and 100% sensitivity for identifying margin-positive disease in unpretreated cases, with a specificity of 94% in 65 cases. Both PCR-PSA and PSMA will probably become strong molecular tools for staging and for determining those who truly have organ-confined disease and should undergo surgery. Laparoscopic surgery is undergoing extensive investigation, but may well be replaced by molecular tests.

The standard and hypersensitive PSA can become abnormal 6 to 11 months before documentation of hormone failure, and is an important diagnostic tool to follow response and progression of disease, particularly after surgery and radiation therapy. Additional preoperative tests include blood urea nitrogen, creatinine, alkaline phosphatase, biochemical screen, blood and platelet counts, prothrombin and partial thromboplastin times, electrocardiogram, and a chest film. Abnormalities on bone scans require evaluation by x-rays, MRI, or biopsy. Some urologists continue to perform intravenous urography and/or abdominal and pelvic CT scans.

Staging System

The 1992 uniform AJCC/UICC Staging System (Table 30–4), which incorporates PSA combined with new imaging techniques not previously available,[55] is rapidly replacing

TABLE 30–4. PROSTATE CANCER STAGING SYSTEM (AJCC)

T	**PRIMARY TUMOR**
TX	Cannot be assessed
T0	No evidence of primary tumor*
T1	Clinically inapparent tumor not palpable or visible by imaging† (WJ = A)
	T1a Tumor in <5% of resected tissue (WJ = A1)
	T1b Tumor in ≥5% of resected tissue (WJ = A2)
	T1c Tumor identified by biopsy because of an elevated PSA (WJ = D0 because of increased SAP, not PSA)
T2	Clinically apparent tumor confined within prostate§ (WJ = B)
	T2a Involves less than half a lobe (WJ = B1)
	T2b Involves more than half a lobe (WJ = B2)
	T2c Involves both lobes (WJ = B3)
T3	Tumor extends through prostatic capsule‖ (WJ = C)
	T3a Unilateral extracapsular extension (WJ = C1)
	T3b Bilateral extracapsular extension (WJ = C1)
	T3c Invades seminal vesicle(s) (WJ = C2)
T4	Tumor is fixed or invades adjacent structures (WJ = C3)
	T4a In bladder neck, external sphincter, or rectum (WJ = C3)
	T4b In levator muscles and/or fixed to pelvic wall (WJ = C3)
N	**REGIONAL LYMPH NODES††**
NX	Cannot be assessed
N0	No metastasis (WJ modification = D0 if SAP increased)
N1	Single node < 2 cm (WJ = D1)
N2	Single node ≥ 2 cm and <5 cm; multiple nodes but all < 5 cm (WJ = D1)
N3	Node ≥ 5 cm (WJ = D1)
M	**DISTANT METASTASIS¶**
MX	Cannot be assessed
M0	No metastasis
M1	Distant metastasis
	M1a Nonregional lymph node (WJ = D1)
	M1b Bone (WJ = D2)
	M1c Other site(s) (WJ = D2)

WJ, Whitmore-Jewett Staging System

*No tumor identified by any staging procedure including biopsy, if performed

†Tumor incidentally identified by biopsy

††Regional are only within the true pelvis, *i.e.*, below the bifurcation of the common iliac arteries; all others are distant metastasis or M1a

§Tumor found in one or both lobes by needle biopsy, but not palpable or visible by imaging, is still classified as T1c

‖Invasion into the prostate apex or into, but not beyond, the prostatic capsule is T2 and not T3

¶When more than one site is present, the most advanced category is used.

the Whitmore-Jewett system, which classifies as A, B, C, and D. T1c is a new staging addition based on a PSA-driven positive biopsy, which is performed despite completely negative clinical findings by DRE and all other imaging studies.[54] The subsequent pathological findings do not upgrade the final clinical stage, *i.e.*, tumor found in both lobes (old T2c or B3), SV (T3c or B3), or periprostatic fat (T3a or C), remains T1c.[55] Single tumor nodules with volumes 0.2 cm^3 or less are considered latent and clinically insignificant (T1a or A1), with almost all having Gleason scores of 4/5 or less. Of these over 80% are diploid, and 62% may originate in the transition zone.[52] Only the largest single nodule is considered, and multiple nodules are not summed to give an overall volume.[54] Nodules from 0.2 to 0.5 cm^3 with a Gleason score of 6 or less approach biologic significance because 13% will have capsular penetration. Those nodules greater than 0.5 cm^3 generally have Gleason scores of 7 or more, and exhibit a 10-year progression rate of 15% after prostatectomy. Such tumors should be considered indolent but clinically significant.[48,54] Because 80% to 90% of T1c cancers are larger than 0.2 to 0.5 cm^3 and have a high grade, they seem to be prognostically analogous to a palpable cancer.[55] Diffuse multifocal tumors found in more than 5% of the biopsied chips, with the biopsy performed because of BPH and not an abnormal PSA or PSAD, are T2b or A2.[55] Such cancers are frequently high grade, have a volume greater than 0.2 cm^3, and are more frequently aneuploid. Thus, such cases have a poorer prognosis than T2a or B1, evidenced by disease-related death in 50% to 80%, and lymph node metastasis in 30% discovered at prostatectomy.

Tumors confined within the capsule are T2 or B; those involving a single lobe are T2a or B1. More diffuse cancers within one or both lobes are T2b or B2, and T2c or B3, respectively. In the old classification, the T2a or B1 defined a clinically insignificant indolent low grade tumor nodule less than 1.0 or 1.5 cm, whereas the new T2a means a tumor found in half of one lobe. Low-grade lesions should be considered B1, while high grade lesions would be B2 and would suggest a sampling error. One problem with the new classification is that there is no way to define the presence of capsular invasion without extension through the capsule into the surrounding periprostatic tissue. While such cases remain T2, the extent of capsular penetration is of clinical significance, with more than 40% exhibiting disease progression at 8 years.[54] Stage T3a for unilateral and T3b for bilateral (C1) signifies extracapsular extension into periprostatic tissues, and T3c (C2) into the SV(s). SV invasion, which is usually accompanied by lymph node metastasis, particularly for Gleason scores of 7 and more, has an ominous prognosis, with an 85% to 100% risk of disease progression within 6 years after prostatectomy.[54] Another T2 problem, which may lead to "reverse stage migration," is the biopsy finding of bilobar disease (T2c in the old classification) in men who do not have bilobar findings on DRE or TRUS. Such cases now will be categorized as T1c, T2a, or T2b, thereby indicating a better prognosis.[47] Stage D denotes disseminated disease, with D1 meaning regional nodes (Tany, N1–3), bladder or rectum (T4a), or pelvic tissue (T4b); D2 bone and other organs; and D0 an SAP elevation without clinical evidence of nodal or osseous disease. Some studies have found that a single node, or those smaller than 2 mm, did not affect survival after prostatectomy, and that the most important factor is the presence of aneuploidy.

The AJCC/UICC Histopathologic Grading for adenocarcinoma includes well- (G1), moderately- (G2), and poorly-differentiated or undifferentiated (G3-4) tumors.[57] However, most prefer the Gleason classification, which recognizes the heterogeneity of prostatic lesions based on primary and secondary differentiation "patterns," each of which receives a grade of 1 to 5, resulting in a final score of 2 to 10. Tumors with scores less than 4 are equivalent to G1, 5 to 7 are G2, and 7/8 or more are G3.[52]

Treatment

The best approach to organ-confined curable prostate cancer remains controversial. Much has been written concerning the role of surveillance, but most European studies are based on an aspiration biopsy, which is difficult to evaluate, and the majority of cancers found are low grade. In contrast, 60% to 80% of biopsied tumors in the United States are high grade, and as such, probably benefit by up to 2 years with surgery or radiation therapy. Prior university and cancer center data describe a higher survival rate of 10 to 15 and more years with prostatectomy compared to radiation therapy,[58] yet a national radiation survey has suggested almost similar results.[47] At this time most urologists feel prostatectomy is best for those under 70 years of age. Conformal three-dimensional irradiation, particularly with dose escalation to 75 to 80 Gy, may favorably change such statistics for T1,2 lesions.[47] Radiation therapy is the treatment of choice for men over 70 years, and for those with significant medical problems. However, no good survival data exist that demonstrate a survival benefit to irradiating N^+ lesions. Salvage prostatectomy can be performed after radiation failure, but morbidity is markedly increased, and cryosurgery is now being tried in such cases. The impact of radiation therapy on margin-positive prostatectomy cases (T3 or C), which despite better patient selection is reported in up to 50% of cases, is primarily in better local control. Since there is little proof that such treatment influences survival, many physicians prefer to wait for symptoms or to administer hormones. PSA can be an excellent monitor of radiation. When the initial and 6-month levels were compared, the crude rate of recurrence was more than 14% compared to 34% when the level failed to decrease by 50%. Actuarial 4-year relapse free survival was 84% for those having a normal PSA at 6 months compared to 60% for those with persistently elevated levels.[59] Local failure in those men having a positive prostate biopsy years after radiation therapy occurred in 53% versus 9% with a negative biopsy, and up to 75% of T1 cases had a rising PSA at 5 years compared to 23% at 10 years in a surgical series.[48,58] Neoadjuvant hormonal treatment will decrease the prostate, but nodes remain positive in 30%. While change in prostate size can markedly decrease toxicity from irradiation and surgery, long-term survival may not be affected. Early results at 3 years for the combination of radiation therapy and four monthly LHRH doses produced a local control rate of 84% compared to 71% for nonhormonally treated cases ($p = 0.003$). Disease-free survival was 46% versus 26% ($p = 0.0001$); however, the incidence of distant metastasis was unchanged. Although one trial seems to show an 18-month improved PSA level when finasteride was used for very early PSA relapse, many questions still need answers. (Finasteride is being compared against a placebo in 16,000 high-risk men as a cancer preventive agent.) Interstitial implants have not produced equivalent survival statistics, and although conformal techniques with palladium are being evaluated, follow-up is too short (less than 5 years). Hyperthermia with implants and cryosurgery are too new to produce long-term data.

The new nerve-sparing technique for radical prostatectomy preserves normal sexual function in up to 70% to 90% of men less than 50 years, 50% to 70% in those between 50 and 60, and 10% to 25% for ages greater than 70 years.[58] Mortality has decreased to 1% to 3%, and with experienced surgeons, some stress incontinence is reported in only 5% to 15% after 3 to 12 months, and it is severe in less than 3%. An artificial urinary sphincter or collagen injection may ameliorate most problems. Surgery, external radiation therapy, and implants produce 5-year survival rates for T1, 2 disease of 90%, 85%, and 68% and 10-year rates of 70%, 60%, and 44%, respectively. The poor survival for large T3b,c, T4, N2,3 or C, D0 and D1 cancers has led to a large number of randomized trials of immediate hormonal manipulation with either irradiation or surgery. Patients with very symptomatic D2 disease survive approximately 112 weeks compared to those with asymptomatic cases, who survive about 160 to 170 weeks. However, survival data vary for each treatment modality due to patient selection factors such as tumor grade and ploidy, stage, and mode of staging of regional nodes (surgical versus clinical). There may be a role for surgery in those having a very limited number of nodes, particularly with diploid tumors. The one series showing benefit used immediate hormonal manipulation after surgery, but early results of two randomized trials question any survival difference compared to hormone therapy alone.

Hormonal treatment for advanced disease is luteinizing hormone-releasing hormone (LHRH) agonists (*i.e.*, leuprolide, bruserelin, goserelin), or orchiectomy, with or without an antiandrogen (*i.e.*, flutamide or cyproterone acetate). Although some randomized trials have demonstrated no statistical superiority of "total androgen blockade," others have described a 7-month survival benefit, ranging from approximately 130 to 140 weeks for the single modality treated group to 150 to 170 weeks for the combination; survival is even more impressive for good-risk minimal disease cases (5 years).[60] Another function of antiandrogens is to minimize the transient "flare" reaction typically observed within 5 to 14 days after starting LHRH. Although castration results in less symptomatology, troublesome toxicities include hot flashes and sweating in 60%, impotence in 100%, and nipple tenderness and gynecomastia in up to 40%. Breast irradiation probably does not prevent gynecomastia, and hot flashes may never dissipate; very-low-dose estrogens have been reported to diminish the latter. Because flutamide is formulated with lactose, diarrhea and other symptoms relating to lactase deficiency occur in affected individuals. Death from flutamide hepatic toxicity has been reported. The administration of exogenous female hormones (*i.e.*, diethylstilbesterol), singly or with progestins, should be avoided since they lead to feminization with the complaints listed above, as well as to personality change, weight gain, edema, and a significant incidence of thromboembolic and cardiac complications. Serum testosterone will decrease to castrate levels, but not uncommonly may increase again to slightly above castrate levels 6 to 12 months later. None of the randomized trials employing cytotoxic agents added to initial hormone manipulation have found any improvement in survival. If an orchiectomy has not been performed, LHRH should be continued because studies have found that survival is slightly longer in those receiving chemotherapy, possibly because of continued suppression of some hormone-sensitive cells. When a rapid decrease in serum testosterone levels is required, because of spinal cord compression or severe osseous pain after starting LHRH, intravenous diethylstilbesterol disphosphate, 1000 mg daily, or oral ketoconazole, 400 mg every 8 hours, may be helpful.

Hormonal manipulation will induce remission in up to 80% of patients, depending on the criteria employed, but CR is very rare. Typically, the prostate and soft-tissue lesions regress, bone pain rapidly decreases in days, and marked subjective improvement is observed with weight gain and a sense of well-being. With good responses, the PSA decreases to normal values, the alkaline phosphatase shows a transient increase (indicating bone healing) but should eventually return to normal, and bone scans may exhibit increased activity secondary to healing followed by improvement at 1 year. Bone films will demonstrate more osteoblastic activity, sometimes at initially normal sites on bone scan, during the healing process; increased osteolytic activity is indicative of disease progression. If pain is increasing, disease is probably progressing, unless there is evidence of fracture or compression. The median duration of hormone response is 9 to 18 months, and patients die 9 to 18 months after treatment failure. Further hormone manipulation will produce objective improvement in less than 10% (LHRH after orchiectomy) and 25% (flutamide after LHRH) of cases. Remissions are of very short duration, and the addition of flutamide after LHRH has no impact on survival, which remains 11 months. Flutamide, which initially acts as an antagonist, may also function as an agonist. Withdrawal in men originally started on total androgen blockade can induce PR in 29% to 40%, lasting 2 to 10 months.[61] The cardinal question, as yet unanswered, is whether early hormone manipulation, particularly in an asymptomatic patient with an increasing PSA, prolongs overall survival or simply lengthens the disease-free interval.

When one excludes stabilization of disease as a response category, cytotoxic agents, singly and in combination, are inactive, with CR and PR in 6.5% of 3184 and 8.7% of 961 cases.[51] Many trials are now PSA-driven, but the percentage of PSA decrease required to be significant has varied; many investigators require greater than a 75% decrease since reaching such levels seems to impact on survival. Marginal efficacy (10% to 15%) has been noted with adriamycin (45 to 60 mg/m^2 every 3 weeks or 20 mg/m^2 weekly), mitomycin-C, vinblastine by infusion, cisplatin and iproplatin, oral etoposide, and trimetrexate (methotrexate and edatrexate are inactive).[51] CR is never observed, and PR averages 3 to 5 months. Survival ranges from 5 to 6 months for those with a poor performance status (PS) and bidimensional disease to 11 to 15 months for those entering trials with a good PS and an early PSA change.

Prednisone given 10 to 20 mg daily has demonstrated not only symptomatic improvement in hormone-resistant cases but remissions in 20%, evidenced by PSA changes. Ketoconazole given 1200 mg daily acts by inhibiting P 450-III enzymes, which not only suppresses adrenal androgenic steroid production but is present in some prostate cancer cells. However, the drug may also function via modulation of retinoic acid metabolism, as suggested by a new derivative, liarozole. Response occurs within 2 to 3 weeks, and may depend on bioavailability, which requires maintaining gastric acidity. Ketoconazole can induce gastrointestinal and liver toxicity. Estramustine, 10 mg/kg daily, is a nor-nitrogen mustard linked to estradiol, and functions as both an estrogen and a mitotic spindle and mdr1 inhibitor. Eighty percent of untreated and about 20% (range 14% to 37%) of hormone-resistant cases will respond. In 83 men given the drug in combination with 3 to 6 mg/m^2 of vinblastine weekly, 32% to 48% responded;[51] oral etoposide and taxol seem to exhibit similar activity. Suramin, a reverse transcriptase inhibitor, affects various growth factors (epidermal, basic fibroblastic, insulin-like, IL-2), protein kinase C and G, and topoisomerase-2.[62] In 178 cases, a greater than 50% and 75% decrease in the PSA occurred in 43% and 43%, respectively, and PR was noted in 22% of bidimensional cases. Some remissions have persisted for more than 1 to 2 years. While new fixed and "adaptive control" schedules have minimized toxicity, yet have assured appropriate serum levels, a recent question has been raised concerning the possibility that some responses may be due to required steroid replacement.

When small cell lesions are present, cisplatin- and etoposide-based regimens should be started. Appropriate treatment of secondary ductal tumors has not been defined, but cisplatin and adriamycin, or medroxyprogesterone acetate has been used.

Follow-Up

The PSA should be obtained 1 to 2 months after starting hormones to document response and for the patient's psychological comfort. Another PSA within 3 months is needed to evaluate the extent of the nadir, and thereafter at 3- to 4-month intervals during the first year. Monthly PSA determinations may be needed for those not showing a significant nadir. Since the median duration of hormone response is 12 months (range 9 to 18 months), more frequent determinations may be appropriate after 1 year. It is best to have two PSA determinations when it increases above the nadir to minimize laboratory error and document PSA progression; at that time, a serum testosterone should be obtained to ensure castrated levels. Another bone scan may be relevant at 6 months in those cases presenting minimal or suspicious scans, since the true extent of initial osseous involvement may become more apparent because of a "flare reaction," indicating osteoblastic healing of unknown metastases. Radionuclide monoclonal scans may also be helpful when they become available. Alkaline phosphatase, skeletal surveys, and bone scans in advanced disease are of limited value. The presence of ductal components may lead to a negative radionuclide scan, and osteolytic lesions may only be discovered on x-rays. Weight bearing areas need to be watched, and radiation therapy or an orthopedic procedure to avoid fractures may be required.

Patients demonstrating progressive disease require good medical management with appropriate analgesics and radiation to painful sites. Although the PSA may not be a completely reliable monitor of tumor progression because of tumor heterogeneity, an increasing PSA is enough to predict progression in more than 70% of cases. Anemia, with hemoglobin of 8 to 9 g/dl, is mostly due to ineffective erythropoiesis rather than low erythropoietin levels, and frequent transfusion may be required; erythropoietin replacement seldom helps. Some patients, particularly terminal ones, present with recurring thromboembolic, phlebitic, or intravascular coagulation problems, and hypercalcemia. All of these require appropriate treatment with standard medical management, but most patients with such problems die within 4 to 8 weeks. A very frequent and major quality-of-life problem is spinal cord compression. Any symptom, even a minor one, relating to such difficulties should be vigorously pursued and needs urgent evaluation by neurologic and imaging techniques. Steroids and irradiation should be instituted early for evidence of epidural disease to prevent paralysis; surgery may be required. Numbness of the chin (mental nerve syndrome) may be indicative of base of brain or meningeal involvement, and should be treated appropriately, although the latter usually is a terminal event. Lastly, steroids (*e.g.*, prednisone, 10 to 25 mg daily) can be very useful in terminal patients to alleviate pain, osseous discomfort, weight loss, depression, and to induce euphoria, and a sense of well-being.

PENILE TUMORS

Proper hygiene and early circumcision have made penile carcinoma rare in the United States, accounting for only about 0.5% of male cancers; the prevalence is much higher in India, Brazil, and China. While smegma and human papilloma virus type 16 have been incriminated as carcinogens,[63] venereal disease has not. Recent data have described clonal numerical and structural chromosome abnormalities, particularly loss on 13, and to a lesser extent on 17, 22, and Y. Precancerous lesions include leukoplakia, frequently associated with chronic irritation and development of squamous cell tumors; erythroplasia of Queyrat (raised red velvet lesions found on the dorsum of the glans in uncircumcised males); Paget's disease; Bowen's disease (intraepithelial carcinoma); and Buschke-Loewenstein tumors, which either coexist with cancer or undergo malignant degeneration. Malignant tumors include carcinoma in situ and, most commonly, squamous cell (epidermoid) carcinoma. Rare cancers are basal cell carcinoma; soft-tissue sarcomas (especially fibrosarcoma), which occur most often in the shaft; and Kaposi's sarcoma. Metastatic tumors from bladder, prostate, rectosigmoid, and other sites have also been reported.

Presenting signs include phimosis of recent onset, penile mass or ulcer, bleeding, urethral obstruction, and an inguinal mass. Fear of penectomy often leads to delay in diagnosis. Whereas penile soft-tissue sarcomas metastasize primarily via the blood stream, squamous cell carcinoma drains via the lymphatics to inguinal and deep iliac nodes. The first drainage site, the sentinel node, is superiomedial to the saphenofemoral junction in the groin. Palpable inguinal lymph nodes generally are found at presentation but pathologically are positive in only 35% to 60% of cases. When biopsy of the sentinel node is negative, 0% to 20% of patients will have inguinal or deep pelvic node involvement compared to up to 55% with a positive sentinel node.[64] Lymphatic communication at the base of the penis explains the frequency of bilateral iliac node dissemination.

Pretreatment Evaluation

Following clinical examination of the penis and regional lymph nodes, a penile biopsy is obtained. Other diagnostic tests are blood count, screening chemistry, intravenous urogram, chest films, and pelvic CT that includes the inguinal area to assess involvement of deeper nodes. Bipedal lymphangiography is rarely performed since the introduction of

CT scans and MRI. After penectomy or biopsy, urologists usually wait 3 weeks after antibiotic therapy before removing the sentinel node. If bone pain or hypercalcemia is present, a radionuclide bone scan and parathormone level should be obtained.

Staging System

The AJCC Staging System is outlined in Table 30–5. The Jackson Staging System, which is still used by many urologists, defines tumor limited to the glans and prepuce as Stage I, tumors invading the shaft or corpora alone as Stage II and with regional lymph nodes as Stage III, and any primary lesion with inoperable lymph node involvement and distant metastasis as Stage IV. In the UICC TNM classification, Tis signifies carcinoma in situ (usually including Bowen's disease and erythroplasia of Queyrat, since 10% to 20% of these patients develop invasive disease); T1 signifies superficial or exophytic masses and lesions less than 2 cm; T2 are 2 cm to 5 cm tumors; T3 are greater than 5 cm masses; and T4 means invasion of adjacent structures. Because lymph node enlargement is commonly observed at presentation in 50% of cases, a distinction is made between clinically appearing benign versus fixed malignant papable nodes. Thus, the UICC classification subdivides N1 and N2 into "a" and "b," which signify nodes not considered clinically to contain cancer (a) versus those deemed strongly suspicious for tumor (b).

TABLE 30–5. PENILE CANCER STAGING SYSTEM (AJCC)

T	**PRIMARY TUMOR**
TX	Cannot be assessed
T0	No tumor clinically
Tis	Carcinoma in situ
Ta	Noninvasive verrucous carcinoma
T1	Tumor in subepithelial connective tissue
T2	Tumor in corpus spongiosum or cavernosum
T3	Tumor in urethra or prostate
T4	Tumor in adjacent structures
N	**REGIONAL LYMPH NODES**
NX	Cannot be assessed
N0	No lymph node clinically
N1	Single superficial inguinal lymph node
N2	Multiple or bilateral superficial inguinal lymph nodes
N3	Deep inguinal or pelvic lymph node(s), unilateral or bilateral
M	**DISTANT METASTASIS**
MX	Cannot be assessed
M0	No metastasis
M1	Distant metastasis

Treatment

Therapy for carcinoma in situ and limited superficial lesions of the glans is complete local incision using standard surgical techniques or the Mohs method, but small exophytic noninvasive tumors of the prepuce can be successfully treated by circumcision. Although low-volume superficial disease has also been treated effectively by neodymium YAG laser with excellent cosmetic and functional results, 8% to 50% of cases experience local recurrence.[65] Interferon, which is also active against a human papilloma virus–associated benign lesion, condyloma acuminatum, has been curative in a patient with verrucous carcinoma of the penis (Ta), and is under investigation for therapy of superficial lesions.[66] For erythroplasia of Queyrat, topical 5-fluorouracil twice daily has been effective; radiation therapy has not. Tumors of the mid- or proximal corpora carvernosa require total penectomy, but those of the glans and distal shaft can be treated by partial penectomy if 2- to 3-cm clean margins can be obtained. When invasion is suspected, deep excision or partial amputation can be performed in selected cases since the incidence of recurrence is extremely low. In contrast, intraepithelial carcinomas and Bushke-Loewenstein tumors frequently require penectomy because of a significantly higher incidence of local recurrence. Partial penectomy is performed for melanoma of the skin of the distal penis, while total penectomy with node dissection is required for deeply invasive lesions because nodal metastases often are found at initial diagnosis. Soft-tissue sarcoma requires total penectomy but not lymph node dissection since metastases occur primarily via the bloodstream.

The low incidence of nodal metastases and the absence of data to indicate that prophylactic node dissection for clinically negative disease increases survival justify penectomy without routine ilioinguinal node dissection for Stage I disease.[64] Additionally, prophylactic radiation therapy for suspected but not documented inguinal involvement is of unproven benefit in decreasing subsequent groin metastasis. Approximately two thirds of cases with corpus cavernosum involvement will have proven nodal extension. Despite data indicating that locally invasive penile lesions with clinically significant enlarged inguinal nodes generally will be proven to have metastatic involvement, controversy still persists concerning the role of lymphadenectomy for all patients in this setting. For Stage III disease with clinically positive unilateral lymph node enlargement, bilateral pelvic and inguinal node dissection is performed, since a positive node on the contralateral side is found in at least 25% of patients. The 5-year survival rate in such cases can approach more than 50%. Morbidity of an ilioinguinal dissection, however, is not insignificant, and includes skin flap necrosis, lymphedema, and wound infection in 10% to 50% of cases; postoperative radiation therapy can markedly increase such problems.

Radiation therapy in doses of 65 Gy to 70 Gy, which produce much less functional and psychological sequelae, can be curative in selected cases with early stage disease, producing 5-year survival rates similar to surgery.[67] Although penile interstitial implants with ^{192}Ir, ^{137}Ce, or ^{226}Ra, have been effective for tumors less than 5 cm, lesions greater than 4 cm generally are not offered external beam irradiation because of increasing morbidity from tissue necrosis and urethral strictures. In patients who have unresectable, recurrent, or metastatic masses, significant palliation can be achieved with doses of 40 to 60 Gy.

Whereas 50% to 70% of penile cancers without lymphadenopathy are cured by surgery or radiation therapy, 5-year survival decreases to 40% to 50% for men with unilateral groin and pelvic involvement, and 10% to 30% with more extensive loco-regional disease. Less than 10% having bilateral pelvic adenopathy survive 5 years.

Methotrexate (30 to 40 mg/m^2 per week), bleomycin, and cisplatin (70 to 100 mg/m^2 every 3–4 weeks) induce complete and partial remissions in less than 20% to 40%.[68] Responses generally are of short duration, lasting only 2 to 8 months. New promising regimens employ monthly cycles of cisplatin (100 mg/m^2 on day 1) plus 5-fluorouracil (960 mg/m^2 by continuous infusion for 5 consecutive days), and cisplatin (20 mg/m^2 intravenously) plus interferon (5×10^6 U/m^2 subcutaneously for 5 days).[69,70] Various combinations of methotrexate, bleomycin, and cisplatin have also been reported to induce higher rates of response.[71] All of these regimens, including those combining interferon with cis-retinoic acid, which report remissions in 30% to 65% of cases, seem to be more efficacious. They have been evaluated in very limited numbers of patients, resulting in wide 95% confidence intervals; thus, such regimens have not yet truly been proven superior to single-agent treatment. Little progress will be made for this uncommon tumor until a global effort that will provide adequate numbers for randomized studies is undertaken.

Adjuvant and neoadjuvant therapies are being investigated because of limited survival for advanced loco-regional disease following surgery or radiation therapy. Although tumor recurrence rates lower than usually reported and possible improvement in survival have been described, no definite benefit has yet been proven.[71,72] Randomized studies are needed.

Follow-up

During the first year, physical examination and chest x-rays should be performed every 2 to 3 months, and an abdominal/pelvic CT scan obtained every 4 months. CT scans should be performed when recurrence is suspected. Lymph node dissection for loco-regional relapse should be undertaken in patients who have not previously undergone this procedure. For patients with advanced but resected disease, blood counts, calcium and renal tests, chest films and CT scans, and bone scans should be followed.

REFERENCES

1. Cronin RE. Renal cell carcinoma. Amer J Med Sci 302:249–256, 1991
2. Bosniak MA. The small (<3 cm) renal parenchymal tumor: Detection, diagnosis, and controversies. Radiology 179:307–317, 1991
3. Thompson IM, Peck M. Improvement in survival of patients with renal cell carcinoma: Role of serendipitously detected tumor. J Urol 140:487–490, 1988
4. Provet J, Tessler A, Brown J, et al. Partial nephrectomy for renal cell carcinoma: Indications, results and implications. J Urol 145:472–476, 1991
5. deKernion JB, Mukamel E. Selection of initial therapy for renal cell carcinoma. Cancer 60:539–549, 1987
6. McDougall EM, Clayman RV. Advances in laparoscopic surgery: Part II. Innovations and future implications for urologic surgeons. Urology 43:585–593, 1994
7. Gnarra JR, Glen GM, Latif F, et al. Molecular genetic studies of sporadic and familial renal cell carcinoma. Urol Clin North Am 20:207–216, 1993
8. Bander ET. Immunodiagnosis of renal cell carcinoma. Immunology Series 53:469–483, 1990
9. Hermanek P, Schrott KM. Evaluation of new tumors, nodes, and metastasis classification of renal cell carcinoma. J Urol 144:238–242, 1990
10. Ljungberg B, Forsslund G, Stenling R, et al. Prognostic significance of the DNA content in renal cell carcinoma. J Urol 135:422–426, 1986
11. Rainwater LM, Hosaka Y, Farrow GM, et al. Well differentiated clear cell renal carcinoma: Significance of nuclear deoxyribonucleic acid patterns studied by flow cytometry. J Urol:137:15–20, 1987
12. Ljungberg B, Stenling R, Roos G. Prognostic value of deoxyribonucleic acid content in metastatic renal cell carcinoma. J Urol 136:801–804, 1986
13. Elson PJ, Witte RS, Trump DL. Prognostic factors for survival in patients with recurrent or metastatic renal cell carcinoma. Cancer Res 48:7310–7313, 1988
14. Wirth M. Immunotherapy for metastatic renal cell carcinoma. Urol Clin North Am 20:283–296, 1993
15. Yagoda A, Abi-Rached B, Petrylak DP. Chemotherapy for advanced renal cell carcinoma: 1983-1993. Semin Oncol (in press)
16. Brodsky GL. Pathology of bladder carcinoma. Hematol Oncol Clin North Am 6:59–80, 1992
17. Jones PA, Droller MJ. Pathways of development and progression in bladder cancer: new correlations between clinical observation and molecular mechanisms. Semin Urol 11:177–192, 1993
18. Shirai T. Etiology of bladder cancer. Semin Urol 11:113–126, 1993
19. McLaughlin JK, Silverman DT, Hsing AW, et al. Cigarette smoking and cancers of the renal pelvis and ureter. Cancer Res 52:254–257, 1992
20. Cordon-Cardo C, Dalbagni G, Sarkis AS, et al. Genetic alterations associated with bladder cancer. In: DeVita VT Jr, Hellman S, Rosenberg SA, eds. Important Advances in Oncology-1994. Philadelphia, JB Lippincott 1994; pp 71–83
21. Fradet Y, Cordon-Cardo C. Critical appraisal of tumor markers in bladder cancer. Semin Urol 11(3):145–153, 1993

22. Fleischmann J, Goldberg G. Management of superficial transitional cell carcinoma of the bladder. Semin Urol 11(4):193–204, 1993
23. Badalament RA, Ortolano V, Burgers JK. Recurrent or aggressive bladder cancer: indications for adjuvant intravesical therapy. Urol Clin North Am 19:485–498, 1992
24. Herr H, Jaske G. pT1 bladder cancer. Eur Urol 20:1–8, 1991
25. Frazier HA, Robertson JE, Dodge RK, et al. The value of pathologic factors in predicting cancer-specific survival among patients treated with radical cystectomy for transitional cell carcinoma of the bladder and prostate. Cancer 71:3993–4001, 1993
26. Whitmore WF. Management of invasive bladder neoplasms. Semin Urol 1:4–10, 1983
27. Zeitman AI, Shipley WU, Kaufman DS. The combination of cisplatin based chemotherapy and radiation in the treatment of muscle-invading transitional cell cancer of the bladder. Int J Radiat Oncol Biol Phys 27:161–170, 1993
28. Lerner SP, Skinner E, Skinner DG. Radical cystectomy in regionally advanced bladder cancer. Urol Clin North Am 19:713–724, 1992
29. Yagoda A. The role of cisplatin-based chemotherapy in advanced urothelial tract cancer. Semin Oncol 16(suppl 6):98–104, 1989
30. Mottet-Auselo N, Bons-Rosset F, Costa P, et al. Carboplatin and urothelial tumors. Oncology 50 (suppl 2):28–36, 1993
31. Trump DL, Elson R, Madajewicz S, et al: Randomized phase II comparison of carboplatin and CHIP in advanced trasitional cell carcinoma of the urothelium: the Eastern Cooperative Oncology Group. J Urol 144:1119–1122, 1990
32. Witte RS, Elson P, Khandakar J, et al. An Eastern Cooperative Oncology Group phase II trial of trimetrexate in the treatment of advanced urothelial carcinoma. Cancer 73:688–691, 1994
33. Roth BJ, Dreicer R, Einhorn LH, et al. Placitaxel in previously treated, advanced trasitional cell carcinoma of the urothelium: a phase II trial of the Eastern Cooperative Oncology Group (abstr 704). Proc Am Soc Clin Oncol 13:230, 1994
34. Seligman PA, Crawford ED. Treatment of advanced transitional cell carcinoma of the bladder with constant infusion gallium nitrate. J Natl Cancer Inst 83:1582–1584, 1991
35. Seidman AD, Scher HI, Bajorin DF, et al. Gallium nitrate. an active agent in refractory transitional cell carcinoma of the bladder. Cancer 68:2651–2655, 1991
36. Sternberg C, Yagoda A, Scher HI, et al. Methotrexate, vinblastine, doxorubicin, and cisplatin for transitional cell carcinoma of the urothelium: efficacy and patterns of response and relapse. Cancer 64:2448–2458, 1989
37. Loehrer PJ, Einhorn LH, Elson PJ, et al. A randomized comparison of cisplatin alone or in combination with methotrexate, vinblastine, and doxorubicin in patients with metastatic urothelial carcinoma: a cooperative group trial. J Clin Oncol 10:1066–1073, 1992
38. Logothetis CJ, Dexeus FH, Finn L, et al. A prospective randomized trial comparing M-VAC and CISCA chemotherapy for patients with metastatic urothelial tumors. J Clin Oncol 8:1050–1062, 1990
39. Logothetis CJ, Dexeus F, Sella A, et al. Fluorouracil and recombinant human interferon alfa-2a in the treatment of metastatic chemotherapy-refractory urothelial tumors. J Natl Cancer Inst 83:285–288, 1991
40. Logothetis C, Dieringer P, Ellerhorst J, et al. A 61% response rate with 5-fluorouracil, interferon-alpha 2b and cisplatin in metastatic chemotherapy refractory transitional cell carcinoma (abstr 1323). Proc Am Assoc Cancer Res 33:221, 1992
41. Schultz P, Bajorin DE, Kelly WK, et al. Combination gallium nitrate and 5-fluorouracil for platinum-resistant metastatic transitional cell carcinoma of the bladder (abstr 1209). Proc Am Assoc Cancer Res 34:203, 1993
42. Einhorn LH, Roth BJ, Dreicer R, et al. Vinblastine, ifosfamide and gallium (VIG) combination chemotherapy in urothelial carcinoma (abstr 702). Proc Am Soc Clin Oncol 9, 1994
43. Scher H. Chemotherapy for invasive bladder cancer: neoadjuvant vs. adjuvant. Semin Oncol 17:555–564, 1990
44. Splinter TA, Scher HI, Denis L, et al. The prognostic value of the pathological response to combination chemotherapy before cystectomy in patients with invasive bladder cancer. European Organization for Research on Treatment of Cancer Genitourinary Group. J Urol 147:606–608, 1992
45. Pienta KJ, Esper PS. Risk factors for prostate cancer. Ann Intern Med 118:1300–1305, 1993
46. Cunha GR. Role of mesenchymal-epithelial interactions in normal and abnormal development of the mammary gland and prostate. Cancer 74:1034–1044, 1994
47. Hanks GE. Treatment of early stage prostate cancer: Radiotherapy. In: DeVita VT Jr, Hellman S, Rosenberg SA (eds). Important Advances in Oncology—1994. Philadelphia: JB Lippincott, pp 225–239
48. Partin AW, Pound CR, Clemens JQ, et al. Serum PSA following anatomical radical prostatectomy: The John Hopkins experience after ten years. Urol Clin North Amer 20:713–721, 1993
49. McNeal JE, Redwine EA, Freiha FS. Zonal distribution of prostate adenocarcinoma: Correlation with histological pattern and direction of spread. Amer J Surg Pathol 12:897–906, 1988
50. Gormley GJ, Ng J, Cook T, et al. Effect of finasteride on prostate-specific antigen density. Urology 43:53–59, 1994
51. Yagoda A, Petrylak D. Cytotoxic chemotherapy for advanced hormone-resistant prostate cancer. Cancer 71:1098–1109, 1993
52. Greene DR, Wheeler TM. Clinical relevance of the individual cancer focus. Cancer Inves 12:425–437, 1994
53. Ring RS, Karp FS, Olsson CA, et al. Flow cytometric analysis of localized adenocarcinoma of the prostate: The use of archival DNA analysis in conjunction with pathological grading to predict clinical outcome following radical prostatectomy. Prostate 17:155–164, 1990
54. Epstein JI, Walsh PC, Carmichael M, et al. Pathologic and clinical findings to predict tumor extent of nonpalpable (stage T1c) prostate cancer. JAMA 271:368–374, 1994
55. Ohori M, Wheeler TM, Scardino PT. The new American Joint Committee on Cancer and International Union Against Cancer TNM classification of prostate cancer: Clinicopathologic correlations. Cancer 73:104–114, 1994
56. Abdel-Nabi H, Wright GL, Gulfo JV, et al. Monoclonal antibodies and radioimmunoconjugates in the diagnosis

and treatment of prostate cancer. Semin Urol 10:45–54, 1992

57. Katz AK, Olsson C, Raffo AJ, et al. Molecular staging of prostate cancer with the use of an enhanced reverse transcriptase-PCR assay. Urology 43:765–775, 1994
58. Walsh PC, Partin AW. Treatment of early stage prostate cancer: Radical prostatectomy. In: DeVita VT Jr, Hellman S, Rosenberg SA (eds). Important Advances in Oncology–1994. Philadelphia, JB Lippincott: pp 211–224
59. Chauvet B, Felix-Faure C, Lupsacka N, et al. Prostate-specific antigen decline: A major prognostic factor for prostate cancer treated with radiation therapy. J Clin Oncol 12:1402–1407 1994
60. Denis L. Role of maximal androgen blockade in advanced prostate cancer. Prostate 5(Suppl):17–22, 1994
61. Scher HI, Kelley WK. Flutamide withdrawal syndrome: Its impact on clinical trials in hormone-refractory prostate cancer. J Clin Oncol 11:1566–1572, 1993
62. Scher HI, Kelley WK. Suramin: A novel growth factor antagonist in the clinic. Principles and Practice of Oncology Updates 7:1–15, 1993
63. Sarkar FH, Miles BJ, Plieth DH. Detection of human papillomavirus in squamous neoplasm of the penis. J Urol 147:389–392, 1992
64. Klein EA: Partial and total penectomy for cancer. Urol Clin North Am 18:161–169, 1991
65. Malloy TR, Wein AJ, Carpiniello VL. Carcinoma of the penis treated with neodymium YAG laser. Urol 31:26–29, 1988
66. Pyrhonen S, Maiche AG, Mantysajavi R: Verrcucous carcinoma of the penis successfully treated with interferon. Br J Urol 68:102–104, 1991
67. Jones WG, Fossa SD, Hamers H, et al. Penis cancer: A review by the Joint Radiotherapy Committee of the European Organization for Research and Treatment of Cancer. J Surg Oncol 40:227–231, 1989
68. Gagliano RG, Blumenstein BA, Carwford ED, et al. Cis-diamminedichloroplatinum in the treatment of advanced carcinoma of the penis: A Southwest Oncology Group study. J Urol 141:66–67, 1989
69. Shammas FV, Dos S, Fossa SD. Cisplatin and 5-fluorouracil in advanced cancer of the penis. J Urol 147:630–632, 1992
70. Hussein AM, Benedetto P, Sridhar KS. Chemotherapy with cisplatin and 5-fluorouracil for penile and urethral squamous cell carcinomas. Cancer 65:433–438, 1990
71. Pizzocaro G, Piva L. Adjuvant and neoadjuvant vincristine, bleomycin and methotrexatre for inguinal metastases from squamous cell carcinoma of the penis. Acta Oncol 27:823–824, 1988
72. Fisher HAG, Barad JH, Horton J, et al. Neoadjuvant therapy with cisplatin and 5-fluorouracil for Stage III squamous cell carcinoma of the penis. J Urol 143:352A, 1990 (Abstract)

John S. Macdonald, Daniel G. Haller, Robert J. Mayer, Eds. *Manual of Oncologic Therapeutics*, Third Edition.

31. GERM CELL TUMORS

Scott Saxman
Craig Nichols

Although only 5500 new cases of germ cell tumors (GCT) are diagnosed in the United States annually, these are important diseases because they represent the most common solid tumor in men between ages 15 and 35 years and because of their high degree of curability. Overall, GCT account for 1% of all malignancies in males and affect whites far more commonly than other races. GCT may arise from many midline structures, but >90% are testicular in origin. Approximately 10% of men with testicular cancer have a history of cryptorchidism. Because of the advent of cisplatin-based chemotherapy, improvement of surgical techniques, and availability of accurate tumor markers, testicular cancer is now the most curable adult neoplasm. Overall cure rates for patients with disseminated testicular cancer exceed 80%, and patients with local or local/regional disease are cured nearly 100% of the time.

HISTOLOGY

Primary neoplasms of the testis can arise from Sertoli's or Leydig's cells, but >95% of testicular malignancies are of germinal (spermatogenic) origin. Germ cell tumors are divided into seminoma and a variety of other histologies collectively referred to as nonseminomatous germ cell tumors (NSGCT) (Table 31–1). Many of these tumors have a mixture of several histologies. For clinical purposes, if any of the nonseminomatous elements are present the patient should be categorized as having a nonseminomatous tumor. Cytogenetics can be a useful tool, particularly in patients with extragonadal GCT. The most consistent abnormality is one or more copies of the isochrome of the short arm of chromosome 12, seen in >80% of germ cell tumors and not found in any other neoplasm.

Seminoma

Pure seminoma is the most common single histology, accounting for 40% of patients with GCT. Seminoma is further categorized as typical or classic, which accounts for 85% of all seminomas and most commonly occurs in the fourth decade of life. Anaplastic seminoma accounts for 10% of all seminomas and may have greater metastatic potential. Stage for stage, however, there is no difference in treatment or survival between these two subgroups. Spermatocytic seminoma is a disease of older men and is treated with radical orchiectomy alone because metastases are rare.

Nonseminomatous Germ Cell Tumors

NSGCT are divided into four major categories, which may occur in pure form or more commonly in combination with seminoma or other nonseminomatous histologies. Embryonal carcinoma is believed to represent the most primitive cell type, which can further differentiate into endodermal sinus tumor, choriocarcinoma, and teratoma. Endodermal sinus tumor (EST, also known as yolk sac tumor) is the malignant counterpart of the embryonic yolk sac and is rarely found in pure form in the adult testis. EST is the most common testicular tumor in infants and children up to age 3 and is a common component of GCT arising in the mediastinum. Choriocarcinoma in the testis is histologically identical to gestational choriocarcinoma but is much more biologically aggressive. Choriocarcinoma is extremely rare in pure form and is unusual because of its ability to metastasize widely to the lungs or central nervous system without involving the retroperitoneum. Choriocarcinomas are also extremely hemorrhagic with hemoptysis being a prominent clinical feature in some patients. Teratomas contain tissues derived from all three germ layers (ectoderm, mesoderm, endoderm) that form fetal or adult body structures. In the ovary, mature teratoma has a benign clinical course. Teratoma in the testis, however, implies that a malignancy is present, and even fully mature teratomas have metastatic potential. The term teratocarcinoma refers to tumors that have both teratoma and embryonal cell elements.

PRETREATMENT EVALUATION AND STAGING

Signs and Symptoms

The majority of patients present with a firm testicular mass or nodule discovered by them or their sexual partners. The mass is often painless but can be accompanied by a dull ache or "heaviness" in the scrotum. The testis should be examined by palpating it between the thumb and first two fingers, carefully separating the epididymis from the testis. The normal testis is freely movable and homogeneous in consistency. The suspect testis should be compared to the contralateral testis; differences in size, contour, or consistency should raise the suspicion of malignancy. Occasionally patients can present with signs or symptoms of metastatic disease, such as shortness of breath from pulmonary metastasis, cervical adenopathy, or back pain from retroperitoneal involvement. Acute testicular pain is unusual but can lead to

TABLE 31–1. HISTOLOGY

SEMINOMA
Anaplastic
Classic
Spermatocytic
NONSEMINOMA
Teratoma
Mature
Immature
With malignant transformation (*i.e.*, sarcoma, carcinoma)
Embryonal cell carcinoma
Yolk sac (endodermal sinus tumor)
Choriocarcinoma

the misdiagnosis of epididymitis, testicular torsion, or orchitis. This can be especially problematic because the patient with acute pain rarely allows the physician to do a thorough testicular examination. Thus, patients treated for suspected epididymitis should be re-examined when their pain resolves. If they do not improve with 2 to 4 weeks of antibiotics, they should be evaluated for testicular cancer. Ultrasonography is useful in the evaluation of patients with suspected testicular cancer. Ultrasonography can determine whether a palpable scrotal mass is intratesticular or extratesticular and can determine whether the testis is homogeneous. A hypoechogenic mass within a testicle is highly suspicious for malignancy.

Once testicular cancer is suspected, the testis and spermatic cord should be removed *in toto* through the inguinal canal (radical orchiectomy). A transcrotal biopsy or orchiectomy should never be attempted because malignant cells may contaminate the scrotum and complicate future curative therapy.

Staging

Serum tumor markers are extremely valuable in the diagnosis, staging, and monitoring of GCT patients. Alpha-fetoprotein (AFP) is an embryonic protein with a serum half-life of 5 to 7 days. AFP is produced by embryonal carcinoma or yolk sac tumors but is never elevated in patients with pure seminoma. A patient who has a testicular tumor that is pure seminoma pathologically but has an elevated AFP should be recategorized and treated as having NSGCT. The beta-subunit of human chorionic gonadotropin (HCG) is produced by syncytiotrophoblastic cells and has a half-life of 24 to 36 hours. HCG levels are elevated in patients with choriocarcinoma and approximately 50% of patients with embryonal cell carcinoma. Also, 5% to 10% of patients with pure seminoma have modest elevations of HCG. In all, about 80% of patients with metastatic disease will have elevations of one or both of these proteins. These markers are clinically useful in several ways: (1) detecting small volume disease when radiographic imaging techniques may be normal, (2) evaluating tumor response during chemotherapy, and (3) monitoring patients after surgery or chemotherapy. Rising tumor markers are virtually diagnostic of recurrent disease.

Evaluation of a patient with testicular cancer must include computed tomography (CT) of the abdomen and chest as well as serum HCG and AFP. Other radiographic procedures are of minimal value and should be undertaken only as symptoms or physical examination dictate. There are several staging systems for testicular cancer in common usage. Most systems recognize three stages (Table 31–2). Each stage may be clinical or pathologic, depending on the extent of the surgical evaluation. Because the lymphatic drainage of the testes is to the retroperitoneal lymph nodes, a key feature of the staging evaluation is determining whether the disease is confined to the retroperitoneum (Stage II) or has spread beyond it (Stage III).

TABLE 31–2. STAGING

Stage I: Tumor confined to the testis with or without involvement of the epididymis or spermatic cord
Stage II: Tumor with metastasis limited to retroperitoneal lymph nodes
Stage III: Tumor spread beyond retroperitoneal lymph nodes

TREATMENT

Nonseminomatous Germ Cell Tumors

It has long been known that GCT are chemosensitive. Before the advent of modern chemotherapy, patients were treated with dactinomycin alone or in combination with vinblastine and bleomycin with an overall response rate of 50% and a cure rate of 5%. In the mid-1970s, cisplatin was incorporated into the treatment of GCT and drastically improved the overall curability of this disease. Since that time, randomized clinical trials have been completed that further define the appropriate dose and schedule of cisplatin as well as the role of other chemotherapeutic agents. The two most commonly used regimens are summarized in Table 31–3. Because treatment differs according to the stage of disease, each stage is discussed separately.

STAGE I

Approximately one third of patients with NSGCT present with clinical Stage I disease. Two treatment options exist for patients in this group. Historically patients have been pathologically staged and treated with retroperitoneal lymph node dissection (RPLND). The traditional RPLND involved removal of lymphatic, neural, and connective tissue bilaterally, from the bifurcation of the common iliac artery inferiorly to the crus of the diaphragm superiorly. The major long-term complication is retrograde ejaculation with subsequent infertility. To eliminate this problem, urologic surgeons can now prospectively locate the sympathetic nerve fibers, then per-

TABLE 31–3. CHEMOTHERAPY REGIMENS

BEP
Bleomycin 30 Units IV days, 1, 8, 15
Etoposide 100 mg/m² IV days 1–5
Cisplatin 20 mg/m² IV days 1–5

Cycles repeated every 21 days for three cycles (good risk) or four cycles (poor risk)

VAB-6
Vinblastine 4 mg/m² IV day 1
Cyclophosphamide 600 mg/m² IV day 1
Dactinomycin 1.0 mg/m² IV day 1
Bleomycin 30 units IV day 1
Bleomycin 20 units/m² continuous infusion days 1–3
Cisplatin 120 mg/m² IV with mannitol diuresis day 4

Repeated every 4 weeks for three cycles
No bleomycin is given during the third cycle

VeIP (VIP) GIVEN AS SALVAGE THERAPY
Cisplatin 20 mg/m² IV days 1–5
Ifosfamide 1.2 g/m² IV days 1–5
Vinblastine 0.11 mg/kg IV days 1 and 2
or
Etoposide 75 mg/m² IV days 1–5 (if patient received vinblastine as initial chemotherapy)

Cycles repeated every 21 days for four cycles
Mesna should be given with ifosfamide to prevent hemorrhagic cystitis

form a modified lymphadenectomy. When done appropriately by experienced surgeons, little morbidity and almost no mortality are associated with a nerve-sparing RPLND, and most patients retain ejaculatory capacity and fertility. The cure rate with surgery alone for patients with pathologically confirmed Stage I disease approaches 90%. These patients do not need further therapy and can be followed with chest x-ray and serum markers monthly for the first year and every other month the second year. About 20% to 25% of patients with clinical Stage I disease are found to be Stage II pathologically; they are discussed later.

Because 75% of patients with clinical Stage I disease will not have lymph node involvement, the other option for selected patients is surveillance without RPLND. Patients chosen for surveillance should not have any poor prognostic features for extratesticular involvement, which includes invasion of the epididymis or tunica albuginea by the primary tumor, microscopic evidence of lymphatic or vascular invasion, or a significant percentage of embryonal cell carcinoma. Patients who elect surveillance must be followed monthly with serum markers and chest x-ray for the first year, and every other month for the second year. Because many of these patients relapse in the retroperitoneum, CT scans must be performed every 2 months for the first year and every 4 months thereafter. If patients are selected and followed appropriately, the overall survival is similar to that for patients undergoing RPLND.

STAGE II

Approximately 30% of patients with NGCT present with clinical Stage II disease. The advent of effective chemotherapy has made the treatment of these patients somewhat controversial. It is generally agreed that patients whose retroperitoneal disease is > 3 cm should be treated primarily with chemotherapy followed by RPLND if there are residual radiographic abnormalities. Patients with disease < 3 cm are usually treated with RPLND initially. For patients who fall between these parameters, either option is reasonable and is usually based on several factors, including the number of enlarged nodes, presence or absence of suprahilar disease, and surgical expertise.

Patients with pathologically proven Stage II disease have an overall relapse rate of roughly 30%. Both number and size of the retroperitoneal involvement influence the risk of relapse. Therapy for these patients is optional. A randomized trial has demonstrated that two cycles of adjuvant chemotherapy given after RPLND is equivalent to close observation followed by standard chemotherapy in the patients who have relapse. Patient education and close medical supervision are critical for those who choose observation. They should receive monthly chest x-ray and serum markers and should be treated immediately at the time of recurrence. Patients who are unable or unwilling to comply should be given chemotherapy. Patients with Stage II disease who are not completely resectable or who have persistently elevated markers after RPLND should be treated the same as patients with Stage III disease.

STAGE III

The remaining one third of patients with NSGCT present with Stage III disease. The lungs are the most common site of metastatic disease (usually in association with retroperitoneal disease), but liver, bone, and brain can also be involved. Because this is such a heterogeneous group, these patients have been further categorized as good risk (minimal or moderate disease) or poor risk (advanced disease), depending on the number and size of pulmonary metastases (Table 31–4). Other prognostic factors include age, performance status, and degree of elevation of HCG, AFP, and serum lactate dehydrogenase. All of these patients are treated with chemotherapy, which should begin promptly after the diagnosis is made. Often, severely ill patients are treated without histologic confirmation, since the clinical scenario of a young male with a testicular mass, pulmonary metastasis, and elevated markers is virtually pathognomonic for GCT.

Cisplatin is the most active drug in patients with GCT. In the initial studies at Indiana University patients were treated with four cycles of cisplatin, bleomycin and vinblastine (PBV) followed by maintenance vinblastine for 21

TABLE 31–4. INDIANA UNIVERSITY STAGING SYSTEM FOR DISSEMINATED DISEASE

MINIMAL
1. Elevated markers only
2. Cervical nodes (± nonpalpable retroperitoneal nodes)
3. Unresectable, nonpalpable retroperitoneal disease
4. Fewer than five pulmonary metastases per lung field and largest <2 cm (± nonpalpable retroperitoneal disease)

MODERATE

5. Palpable abdominal mass only
6. Moderate pulmonary metastases: 5–10 metastases per lung field and largest <3 cm *or* solitary pulmonary metastasis of any size >2 cm (± nonpalpable retroperitoneal disease)

ADVANCED

7. Advanced pulmonary metastases: >10 pulmonary metastases per lung field *or* multiple pulmonary metastases with largest >3 cm (± nonpalpable retroperitoneal disease) *or* primary mediastinal nonseminomatous germ cell tumor
8. Palpable abdominal mass plus supradiaphragmatic disease
9. Liver, bone, or central nervous system metastasis

Minimal and moderate = good risk; advanced = poor risk.

months. The 5-year survival rate of 64% represented a major advance in the treatment of metastatic GCT. To determine the role of maintainance vinblastine, the Southeast Cancer Study Group randomized patients achieving a complete response with PBV to either 21 months of vinblastine or no further therapy. Survival was the same in both arms, confirming that maintainence vinblastine was unnecessary. A subsequent Phase III trial compared PBV with a regimen containing identical doses of cisplatin and bleomycin, but replacing vinblastine with etoposide (BEP). This study demonstrated that when etoposide is substituted for vinblastine, there is equal efficacy with less toxicity. BEP is now the standard chemotherapeutic regimen for the initial therapy of patients with GCT.

Because of the nephrotoxicity associated with cisplatin, patients must be vigorously hydrated with 3 to 4 liters of normal saline per day. Because most of these patients are young and otherwise healthy, congestive heart failure from fluid overload is rare. Cisplatin is also extremely emetogenic, so patients must receive aggressive antiemetic therapy. Ondansetron with dexamethasone has been shown to be superior to older regimens.

Patients with good-risk disease should be treated with three cycles of chemotherapy, while poor-risk patients require four cycles. More than four cycles do not enhance curability and may promote the development of cisplatin resistance. Chemotherapy should be given every 21 days, regardless of the blood counts. Patients who are leukopenic at the beginning of a chemotherapy cycle should have their blood counts checked daily. If the granulocyte count does not rise by the fifth day, the last dose of etoposide should be withheld. Cisplatin should be given for all 5 days. Serum markers should be obtained at the beginning of each cycle. There should be approximately a one-log reduction in the HCG level with each cycle of chemotherapy. A rate of decrease less than this may indicate the presence of resistant disease. Complete response is the goal in these patients; however, many patients have residual radiographic abnormalities with normal serum markers at the completion of treatment. If possible, these patients should undergo complete surgical resection of all residual abnormalities. Pathologically, the resected tissue will be (1) necrotic debris or fibrosis, (2) teratoma, or (3) viable GCT. It is critical that the tissue be carefully examined for all of these elements. Patients with necrosis/fibrosis or teratoma do not require any further therapy and only need close observation, with a relapse rate of <10%. Patients with residual GCT should be treated with two more cycles of chemotherapy and have a higher relapse rate (30–35%). Patients who do not normalize their markers after four cycles of chemotherapy or who progress during chemotherapy have a poorer prognosis and should be treated with a salvage regimen.

Occasionally, patients are treated without undergoing orchiectomy. Because the testis is a sanctuary site from chemotherapy, it should be removed after the chemotherapy has been completed to prevent local recurrence.

Seminoma

The majority of patients with seminoma present with early-stage disease, and because of its exquisite sensitivity to radiation, nearly all of these patients are cured. Bipedal lymphangiography is often helpful in detecting occult nodal metastasis and planning radiation therapy dosage and ports. Patients with Stage I disease are treated to a total dose of 2500 cGy given in daily fractions over 3 to 4 weeks, using opposed anterior and posterior fields to include the ipsilateral iliac nodes and the retroperitoneal lymph nodes bilaterally. Patients with lymph node involvement are treated in exactly the same manner, but a total dose of 3000 cGy is given to patients with abnormalities on a lymphangiogram, and patients with enlarged nodes on a CT scan are treated with 3500 cGy. Radiation to the mediastinum is contraindicated and can compromise curative chemotherapy should the patient relapse. Shielding of the contralateral testis limits its radiation exposure and can maintain fertility. Bulky retroperitoneal disease (>5 cm) or Stage III disease is treated with the same chemotherapy as used in nonseminomatous disease. However, because teratoma is not seen in patients with pure seminoma, residual radiographic abnormalities are most often scar tissue or necrosis and do not require surgical resection.

Toxicity of Cisplatin Combination Chemotherapy

Because the majority of patients with testicular cancer are cured of their disease, the short- and long-term toxicities of chemotherapy are important considerations. Ways to minimize toxicity have been the focus of several randomized trials. Cisplatin is highly emetogenic, and severe electrolyte imbalances were once common in these patients. The advent of new antiemetic agents has greatly lowered the incidence of severe nausea and vomiting. Myalgias and peripheral neuropathies are unusual now that etoposide has replaced vinblastine as initial therapy. Ifosfamide, currently used as salvage therapy, can cause hemorrhagic cystitis. This can usually be prevented by the prophylactic use of the urothelial protective agent mesna. Vascular complications such as the Raynaud's phenomenon, transient ischemic attacks, and myocardial infarctions have been described, but the incidence is low and it is unclear whether they are treatment-related.

FERTILITY

Most patients with testicular cancer are oligospermic or azoospermic at the time of diagnosis. Nearly all patients will become azoospermic after 3 or 4 courses of chemotherapy. There is little information on fertility after chemotherapy, but retrospective analysis suggests that at least 40% to 50% of these patients will regain reproductive potential.

PULMONARY

Rarely bleomycin can cause severe and even fatal pneumonitis. Risk factors for this complication include advanced pulmonary disease, age >45, renal insufficiency, previous mediastinal irradiation, and total cumulative dose of the drug. The lungs should be auscultated before each dose of bleomycin, and the drug discontinued if the patient develops basilar crackles, a dry cough, or shortness of breath. Bleomycin can also cause radiographic pulmonary nodules that can be confused with progressive or recurrent disease.

LEUKEMIA

Several reports have implicated etoposide as a risk factor for the development of myelodysplasia or acute leukemia. A recent review of all patients with GCT receiving standard-dose etoposide at Indiana University demonstrated a small but definite risk for the development of secondary leukemia. This rare association does not alter the risk-to-benefit ratio of etoposide in patients with GCT.

Salvage Therapy

Patients who fail after first-line chemotherapy are still curable using salvage regimens. A combination consisting of cisplatin, ifosfamide, and either vinblastine or etoposide (depending on which drug was given during initial therapy) (see Table 31–3) can result in up to 30% of patients achieving long-term disease-free status. High-dose chemotherapy, usually consisting of etoposide and carboplatin followed by autologous bone marrow rescue, has been evaluated in patients who relapse after salvage chemotherapy. Overall, 15% of these patients are long-term survivors. The role of bone marrow rescue as initial salvage therapy is being evaluated. Occasionally, patients are seen who have failed salvage chemotherapy but still have apparently localized disease. Such patients may benefit from aggressive surgical resection of all disease with curative intent. Patients with refractory disease occasionally experience palliation with daily oral etoposide.

Follow-up After Surgery or Chemotherapy

The majority of patients with GCT who relapse do so in the first 2 years following therapy. Patients should be followed with monthly chest r-ray and markers during the first year and every 2 months the second year. Patients should then be followed approximately every 4 months for the third year, twice the fourth year, and yearly thereafter. Because tumors can arise in the remaining testis, patients should be taught to do testicular self-examination and told to report any changes immediately.

Extragonadal Germ Cell Tumors

GCT of all histologic subtypes occasionally arise in midline structures, including the retroperitoneum, mediastinum, and pineal gland. Pineal gland tumors are most often seen in children and are usually seminomas (dysgerminomas). Pineal gland GCT are treated with cranial or craniospinal radiation therapy. Patients with presumed retroperitoneal GCT should have a testicular sonogram to exclude the possibility of an occult testicular primary tumor. This is especially important since the testis is a sanctuary site for chemotherapy, and relapses can occur if it is not removed. Primary retroperitoneal GCT are midline masses. If the adenopathy is predominantly one-sided, the ipsilateral testis should be removed. Mediastinal NSGCT are associated with Klinefelter syndrome and with hematologic malignancies, particularly acute megakaryocytic leukemia. The surgical and chemotherapeutic management of extragonadal GCT is identical to that of advanced testicular cancer. The overall curability of these tumors is lower, and salvage chemotherapy is far less effective than in patients with testicular primary tumors.

Ovarian Germ Cell Tumors

Ovarian GCT are rare, accounting for only 2% to 3% of all ovarian cancers. The histologic patterns are the same as for testicular GCT. In the past, patients with ovarian NSGCT have been treated surgically with dismal results. Collected experience from small published studies indicates that chemotherapy is effective with most patients achieving long-term survival. Although there are no randomized studies, Phase II trials in ovarian GCT and experience with testicular cancer suggest that BEP is the preferred therapy for all patients, regardless of stage. Ovarian dysgerminoma is the counterpart of testicular seminoma in males. The Gynecologic Oncologic Group's experience with this rare tumor suggests that most patients have long-term survival after platinum-based chemotherapy, which is now the treatment of choice. Radiation therapy should be reserved for patients with locally persistent disease after chemotherapy.

GCT: Recent and Current Areas of Investigation

Cisplatin has been tested in a randomized fashion in high doses (40 mg/m^2/day for 5 days) and found to be more toxic with no improved efficacy. Carboplatin is a platinum analog that has less nephrotoxicity and ototoxicity than cisplatin. Early reports of a randomized study comparing cisplatin and carboplatin in good-risk patients suggest that carboplatin is inferior to cisplatin in response and overall survival. Several other studies have now confirmed that carboplatin is inferior in both good-risk patients and patients with advanced disease, so carboplatin should not be substituted for cisplatin. To evaluate the role of bleomycin, Indiana University and the Eastern Cooperative Oncology Group (ECOG) compared three cycles of BEP to the same regimen without the bleomycin (EP) in patients with good-risk disease. Patients treated with the EP regimen had a significantly higher relapse rate with no difference in toxicity between the two arms. Other studies suggest that bleomycin could be deleted if four cycles of chemotherapy are given. However, the negligible toxicity of 9 weeks of bleomycin makes it likely that the fourth course of EP would add to the overall toxicity. Most recently, ECOG compared cisplatin plus etoposide with either bleomycin (BEP) or ifosfamide (VIP) in advanced-stage patients. The preliminary results of this trial demonstrate that the regimens are therapeutically equivalent but that VIP has significantly more hematologic toxicity. Therefore, despite these efforts to improve survival or eliminate toxicity, BEP continues to be the standard therapy for patients with testicular GCT.

Current studies are investigating the activity of Phase II drugs such as paclitaxel and vinorelbine in patients with otherwise refractory disease. Indiana University is also studying the role of daily oral etoposide for 3 months in patients achieving remission with salvage chemotherapy. Newer technology is also being applied and studied, including DNA flow cytometry as a predictor of disease response and recurrence, and positron-emission tomography scanning to differentiate between viable GCT and necrosis in patients with residual radiographic abnormalities after chemotherapy.

BIBLIOGRAPHY

Bosl GJ, Geller NL, Bajorin D. Identification and management of poor risk patients with germ cell tumors: The Memorial Sloan-Kettering Cancer Center experience. Semin Oncol 15:339–344, 1989

Broun ER, Nichols CR, Kneebone P et al. Long-term outcome of patients with relapsed and refractory germ cell tumors treated with high-dose chemotherapy and autologous bone marrow rescue. Ann Intern Med 117:124–128, 1992

Einhorn LH. Treatment of testicular cancer: A new and improved model. J Clin Oncol 8:1777–1781, 1990

Einhorn LH, Williams SD, Loehrer PJ et al. Evaluation of optimal duration of chemotherapy in favorable-prognosis disseminated germ cell tumors: A Southeastern Cancer Study Group Protocol. J Clin Oncol 7:387–391, 1989

Nichols CR, Breeden ES, Loehrer PJ et al. Secondary leukemia associated with a conventional dose of etoposide: Review of serial germ cell tumor protocols. J Natl Cancer Inst 85:36–40, 1993

Nichols CR, Saxman S, Williams DS et al. Primary mediastinal nonseminomatous germ cell tumors. A modern single institution experience. Cancer 65:1641–1646, 1990

Nichols CR, Williams SD, Loehrer PJ et al. Randomized study of cisplatin dose intensity in poor-risk germ cell tumors: A Southeastern Cancer Study Group and Southwest Oncology Group Protocol. J Clin Oncol 9:1163–1172, 1991

Saxman S. Salvage therapy in recurrent testicular cancer. Semin Oncol 19:143–147, 1992

Williams SD. Chemotherapy of ovarian germ cell tumors. Hematol Onc Clin N Am 5:1261–1269, 1991

Williams SD, Birch R, Einhorn LH et al. Treatment of disseminated germ cell tumors with cisplatin, bleomycin and either vinblastine or etoposide. N Engl J Med 316:1435–1440, 1987

Williams SD, Stablein DM, Einhorn LH et al. Immediate adjuvant chemotherapy versus observation with treatment of relapse in pathological Stage II testicular cancer. N Engl J Med 317:1433–1438, 1987

John S. Macdonald, Daniel G. Haller, Robert J. Mayer, Eds. *Manual of Oncologic Therapeutics*, Third Edition.

32. GYNECOLOGIC CANCERS

Tate Thigpen

Cancers of the female genital tract include a variety of neoplasms that originate in virtually every portion of the tract. Three lesions, however, account for over 90% of all cases: celomic epithelial carcinoma of the ovary, carcinoma of the cervix, and endometrial carcinoma. Sufficient data exist to provide a rational guide to management of at least two other types of neoplasm: uterine sarcoma and germ cell carcinoma of the ovary. These five lesions are the focus of the following discussion.

CELOMIC EPITHELIAL CARCINOMA OF THE OVARY

Cancer of the ovary includes several types of malignancy: celomic epithelial carcinomas, germ cell neoplasms, and stromal tumors. The celomic epithelial carcinomas (henceforth referred to as ovarian carcinoma) account for almost 90% of these and are the most common cause of death due to gynecologic cancers in the United States. These lesions are the subject of the great majority of clinical trials of ovarian cancer, which are the basis of the current clinical approach to the disease.

General Considerations

The etiology of ovarian carcinoma is not known, but there is an association between uninterrupted ovulation and the disease.[1] Familial factors are also evident from the identification of hereditary ovarian cancer syndrome, hereditary breast-ovarian syndrome, and Lynch II syndrome (colon carcinoma in association with ovarian cancer).[2] The hallmarks of these syndromes are occurrence at a younger age (median 45–52 years versus 59 years for other cases) and first-order relatives with the disease.

The most significant prognostic factors for ovarian carcinoma are age,[3] histologic type and grade,[4] extent of disease (stage), and volume of residual disease (Table 32–1).[5–8] Older patients have a poorer prognosis than do younger patients. Those with serous or endometrioid tumors have a better prognosis than do those with mucinous or clear-cell lesions. More poorly differentiated tumors are associated with a poorer prognosis. The most important determinant of prognosis, however, is the extent of disease at the time of diagnosis. This is expressed in the International Federation of Gynecology and Obstetrics (FIGO) staging system[9] (Table 32–2).

The FIGO staging system reflects certain important characteristics of ovarian carcinoma. First, the most common route of spread is via peritoneal dissemination; Stage III includes patients who have disseminated disease confined to the peritoneal cavity. Second, among patients with Stage III disease, the volume of disease is an important determinant of response to chemotherapy and survival (those with nodules smaller than 2 cm have a higher response rate and a longer survival time); Stage III is subdivided according to volume of disease at the time that the abdomen is opened. Third, ovarian carcinoma most often presents at an advanced stage (Stage III or IV) because of the lack of early manifestations and an effective screening test. Although much has been written about the potential role of CA-125 and transvaginal ultrasonography as potential screening techniques, neither has proven efficacy as a screen.[10]

Patients usually present with nonspecific symptoms, such as a heavy sensation in the pelvis or increasing abdominal girth because of ascites. Although physical examination and various imaging techniques are employed in the evaluation, all patients without demonstrated Stage IV disease require an exploratory laparotomy to establish the diagnosis and extent of disease.

Management of Advanced Disease

Patients with advanced disease, unless Stage IV is already established, undergo exploratory laparotomy, which, in addition to establishing the extent of disease, affords the first step in therapy. The laparotomy should be done through an incision sufficient to permit the exploration of the entire peritoneal cavity. In the absence of gross disease outside the pelvis, multiple biopsies should be taken to rule out microscopic disease. Finally, based on considerations noted above, an aggressive attempt at surgical cytoreduction should be undertaken.[11]

The mainstay of the treatment of advanced disease is chemotherapy. A number of chemotherapeutic agents are active against ovarian carcinoma: platinum compounds, alkylating agents, taxol, doxorubicin, hexamethylmelamine, 5-fluorouracil, methotrexate, and tamoxifen (Table 32–3).[12] The standard of care for first-line therapy currently is a combination of taxol 135 mg/m^2 over 24 hours followed by cisplatin 75 mg/m^2 with the combination repeated every 3 weeks for six cycles (Table 32–4).[13] This combination should yield regressions of 50% or greater in 75% of patients with large-volume disease, complete regression of disease in

TABLE 32–1. PROGNOSTIC FACTORS IN CELOMIC EPITHELIAL CARCINOMA OF THE OVARY [3–8]

FACTOR	IMPACT
Age	Survival is worse in older patients
Grade	Patients with high-grade lesions have poorer survival, at least those with limited disease
Histologic type	Patients with clear-cell and mucinous lesions, stage for stage, have poorer survival
Stage	Survival worsens as extent of disease (FIGO stage) increases
Volume of disease	Stage III patients with larger-volume disease have a poorer survival

FIGO = International Federation of Gynecology and Obstetrics.

40% to 50% of such patients, a pathologically complete response (patient is disease-free at second-look laparotomy at the conclusion of chemotherapy) in 20% to 25%, a progression-free survival of 15 to 20 months, and an overall survival of 20 to 25 months.

Other combinations that have been used, with somewhat less success, include cisplatin plus cyclophosphamide, carboplatin plus cyclophosphamide, and cisplatin plus doxorubicin plus cyclophosphamide.[14] The frequency of pathologically complete response, the duration of response, and the overall survival will be significantly better in patients with small-volume disease, than in those with large-volume disease (Table 32–5).[5–8]

TABLE 32–2. FIGO STAGING SYSTEM FOR OVARIAN CARCINOMA

STAGE	DESCRIPTION
I	Growth limited to the ovaries
A	One ovary, no ascites, capsule intact, no tumor on external surface
B	Two ovaries, no ascites, capsule intact, no tumor on external surface
C	One or both ovaries with surface tumor, ruptured capsule, or ascites or peritoneal washings with malignant cells
II	Pelvic extension
A	Involvement of uterus and/or tubes
B	Involvement of other pelvic tissues
C	IIA or IIB with factors as in IC
III	Peritoneal implants outside pelvis and/or positive retroperitoneal or inguinal nodes
A	Grossly limited to true pelvis, negative nodes, microscopic seeding of abdominal peritoneum
B	Implants of abdominal peritoneum 2 cm or less, nodes negative
C	Abdominal implants greater than 2 cm and/or positive retroperitoneal or inguinal nodes
IV	Distant metastases

From The new FIGO stage grouping for primary carcinoma of the ovary (1985). Gynecol Oncol 25:383, 1986.

FIGO = International Federation of Gynecology and Obstetrics.

TABLE 32–3. ACTIVITY OF SYSTEMIC AGENTS IN CELOMIC EPITHELIAL CARCINOMA OF THE OVARY

DRUG	PATIENTS (RESPONSE RATE %)	
AVAILABLE AGENTS		
Alkylating agents	1408	(33%)
Cisplatin	190	(32%)
Carboplatin	82	(24%)
Taxol	189	(29%)
Doxorubicin	102	(33%)
5-Fluorouracil	126	(29%)
Methotrexate	34	(18%)
Mitomycin	49	(16%)
Hexamethylmelamine	215	(24%)
INVESTIGATIONAL AGENTS		
Prednimustine	36	(28%)
Dihydroxybusulfan	26	(27%)
Galactitol	39	(15%)
HORMONES AND BIOLOGIC AGENTS		
Progestins	176	(12%)
Antiestrogens	42	(19%)
Alpha interferon	21	(19%)
Gamma interferon	14	(29%)

From Thigpen T. Chemotherapy of cancers of the female genital tract. In Perry M (ed): The Chemotherapy Source Book. Baltimore, Williams & Wilkins, 1992:1039–1065.

TABLE 32–4. GYNECOLOGIC ONCOLOGY GROUP PROTOCOL 111, A COMPARISON OF CISPLATIN PLUS EITHER CYCLOPHOSPHAMIDE OR TAXOL

RESPONSE	CIS/CYCLO*	CIS/TAXOL†
Complete response	37 (33%)	52 (54%)
Partial response	32 (29%)	22 (23%)
No response	42 (38%)	22 (23%)
Not evaluated	6 (5%)	6 (5%)
Response rate	69 (62%)	74 (77%)
Total	117 (100%)	102 (100%)

From McGuire WP, Hoskins WH, Brady MF et al: A phase III trial comparing cisplatin/cytoxan and cisplatin/taxol in advanced ovarian cancer. Proc ASCO 12:255, 1993.

*Cisplatin 75 mg/m^2 plus cyclophosphamide 750 mg/m2 intravenously every 3 weeks.

†Taxol 135 mg/m^2 intravenously over 24 hours followed by cisplatin 75 mg/m^2 intravenously every 3 weeks.

Clinical response with cisplatin/taxol is superior (p = .02).

TABLE 32–5. RECOMMENDATIONS FOR MANAGEMENT OF PREVIOUSLY UNTREATED PATIENTS

DISEASE STATUS	RECOMMENDATION
Limited disease	
Low risk	Total abdominal hysterectomy, bilateral salpingo-oophorectomy, and observation
High risk	Same surgery as for low risk followed by adjuvant platinum-based chemotherapy
Advanced disease	
Small volume	Maximum surgical cytoreduction followed by taxol/cisplatin
Large volume	Taxol/cisplatin

Management of Limited Disease

As in advanced disease, exploratory laparotomy is essential to determine whether disease is truly confined to the ovaries (Stage I) or pelvis (Stage II).[4,15] Information from the laparotomy characterizes the patient as being at low risk for recurrence (Grade 1 or 2, intracystic disease, no extraovarian disease, no ascites, and negative peritoneal cytology results) or at high risk (Grade 3, extracystic disease, extraovarian disease, ascites, or positive peritoneal cytology results) (Table 32–6).[4] Patients at low risk have a cure rate that exceeds 90% with total abdominal hysterectomy, bilateral salpingo-oophorectomy, and omentectomy alone and require no additional therapy. Those at high risk have a recurrence rate that may reach as high as 40% and should receive additional therapy after surgical resection. Accepted therapy is either intraperitoneal chromic phosphate or intravenous platinum-based chemotherapy, although more recent data suggest that platinum-based chemotherapy is superior.[16]

TABLE 32–6. RISK GROUPS OF PATIENTS WITH LIMITED OVARIAN CARCINOMA

GROUP	CHARACTERISTICS
Low risk	Grade 1 or 2 disease
	Intact capsule
	No tumor on external surface
	Negative peritoneal cytology results
	No ascites
	Growth confined to ovaries
High risk	Grade 3 disease
	Ruptured capsule
	Tumor on external surface
	Positive peritoneal cytology results
	Ascites
	Growth outside ovaries

If any high-risk factors are present, the patient is considered high risk.

From Young RC, Walton L, Ellenberg SS et al. Adjuvant therapy in stage I and stage II epithelial ovarian cancer. Results of two prospective randomized trials. N Engl J Med 322:1021–1027, 1990.

Salvage Therapy

For patients who have a recurrence after initial therapy, appropriate management is determined by response to initial treatment (Table 32–7).[17] Patients who initially respond to platinum-based chemotherapy and then have a recurrence more than 6 months after completion of initial treatment should be considered "platinum-sensitive." Such patients respond well to repeat treatment with platinum-based therapy. However, those who have progressive disease on platinum-based treatment, who exhibit persistent disease at the end of initial platinum-based therapy, or whose disease recurs within 6 months respond infrequently to repeat platinum-based treatment and should be considered "platinum-resistant." Such patients should be treated with taxol if they have not received it as a part of initial therapy. Other agents reported to yield at least some responses include ifosfamide, hexamethylmelamine, 5-fluorouracil, and tamoxifen.

Currently, data do not support the use, outside of clinical trials, of either intraperitoneal therapy or high-dose chemotherapy with autologous bone marrow support as a part of either first-line or salvage treatment.

Management of the High-Risk Patient

Much attention has recently been directed to individuals at high risk for the development of ovarian carcinoma. The overall lifetime risk for the development of ovarian carcinoma for women in the United States is approximately 1.4% (1 in 70). Reasonable evidence supports an enhanced risk for women who have one first-order relative (mother or sibling) with the disease; this approximates 5%.[2] For women with two or more first-order relatives with ovarian carcinoma, the risk is considerably higher (estimates range from 10% to more than 50%, but the actual risk is not yet clear).[2,13]

As noted earlier, no screening test of proven efficacy is available. Some authors have suggested a role for the tumor marker CA-125 and for transvaginal ultrasonography, but definitive evidence of their effectiveness as screening tests is lacking.[10] In the absence of an effective screening test, some have suggested that women at high risk should undergo pro-

TABLE 32–7. PLATINUM-SENSITIVE AND PLATINUM-RESISTANT PATIENTS

Platinum-sensitive	Initial response to platinum
	Platinum-free interval >6 months
Platinum-resistant	Progression on platinum
	Stable disease on prior platinum
	Relapse <6 months after prior platinum

phylactic oophorectomy.[18,19] Although that approach has appeal, recent reports of celomic epithelial carcinomas of the peritoneal surface in women who have undergone prophylactic oophorectomy raise questions about whether it is truly effective. Six such cases have been reported among 324 high-risk women who have undergone prophylactic oophorectomy, for an overall incidence of 1.8%.[19] Although that rate is lower than would be anticipated in a high-risk group, further follow-up is needed before any conclusions can be drawn.

At present, no dogmatic recommendations can be made. Issues regarding the use of CA-125 and transvaginal ultrasonography for screening and prophylactic oophorectomy in women at high risk for developing ovarian cancer should be discussed with patients, but they cannot be recommended for widespread application based on currently available data.

SQUAMOUS CELL CARCINOMA OF THE UTERINE CERVIX

Cancer of the uterine cervix includes a variety of histologies. The most common is squamous cell carcinoma, which accounts for more than 85% of all cases. This common histologic type is the focus of this portion of the discussion.

General Considerations

The etiology of squamous cell carcinoma of the uterine cervix is not fully understood, but certain facts are clear and clinically relevant. The process exhibits the epidemiology of a venereal disease.[20] Associated factors include lower socioeconomic status, onset of coitus at an early age, frequent coitus, multiple sexual partners, and coitus with an uncircumcised partner or one who practices poor genital hygiene. There is also an intimate connection between the disease and human papillomavirus (HPV).[21]

Squamous cell carcinoma of the uterine cervix is associated with a well-described premalignant state, which is variously described as cervical intraepithelial neoplasia (CIN 1–3) or a squamous intraepithelial lesion (SIL: low-grade [LGSIL] and high-grade [HGSIL]).[22] These lesions can be detected by cervical cytology, which constitutes the most effective screening test for cancer. The process by which cells go from mild to severe dysplasia and carcinoma in situ to frankly invasive cancer usually takes years; hence, there is a significant window of opportunity for early diagnosis and cure of the vast majority of women with the disease.

Once invasive cancer is present, the most important prognostic feature is the extent of disease at the time of diagnosis as expressed in the FIGO staging system (Table 32–8).[23] This clinical staging system is the basis for selection of treatment. An appropriate evaluation of patients to determine stage should include careful history and physical examination, including a thorough pelvic and rectal examination, complete blood count, tests to evaluate hepatic and renal status, urinalysis, flexible sigmoidoscopy, barium enema, intravenous pyelogram, and computed tomographic scan of the abdomen and pelvis. A histologic diagnosis of malignancy is a mandatory part of this assessment and may require cytologic smears, colposcopy, conization, punch biopsies of four quadrants of the cervix, dilatation and curettage, and cystoscopy. The extent of the workup is determined by the findings of each procedure but must yield sufficient information to stage the patient accurately.

TABLE 32–8. FIGO STAGING SYSTEM FOR CERVICAL CANCER

STAGE	DESCRIPTION
0	Carcinoma in situ
I	Cervical carcinoma confined to uterus (disregard extension to corpus)
IA	Invasive carcinoma diagnosed by microscopy only
IA1	Minimal microscopic stromal invasion
IA2	Invasive component <5-mm depth from base of epithelium and ≤7-mm horizontal spread
IB	Larger than IA2
II	Invasion beyond uterus but not to pelvic wall or lower third of vagina
IIA	No parametrial invasion
IIB	Parametrial invasion
III	Extension to pelvic wall and/or involvement of lower third of vagina or hydronephrosis or nonfunctioning kidney
IIIA	Lower third of vagina only
IIIB	Pelvic wall involvement, hydronephrosis, or nonfunctioning kidney
IVA	Involvement of mucosa of bladder or rectum
IVB	Extension beyond true pelvis

From Beahrs OH, Henson DE, Hutter RVP et al. Manual for Staging of Cancer, 3rd ed. Philadelphia, JB Lippincott, 1988:151–153.

Management of Limited Disease

Patients found to have disease confined to the cervix, evidenced by microscopy only, and limited in invasion to 5 mm or less in depth, taken from the base of the epithelium, and 7 mm or less in horizontal spread have Stage 0 (carcinoma in situ), Stage IA1 (minimal microscopic stromal invasion), or Stage IA2 (more invasive up to the limits described). The definitive treatment for these lesions is total abdominal hysterectomy, although nonsurgical candidates can be treated with radiotherapy.[24] Selected patients, in particular those with carcinoma in situ and those with minimally invasive lesions (less than 1 mm in depth), can be managed with more conservative measures such as conization, provided all margins are clear (Table 32–9).[25]

TABLE 32–9. MANAGEMENT RECOMMENDATIONS FOR CERVICAL CANCER

DISEASE STATUS	RECOMMENDATIONS
Preinvasive or IA	Total abdominal hysterectomy; lesser procedures in selected cases of preinvasive disease
Stage IB/IIA	Radiotherapy with or without surgery, except in selected cases appropriate for radical hysterectomy; role of chemotherapy undetermined
Stage IIB/III/IVA	Radiotherapy; randomized trials support the use of concomitant hydroxyurea
Stage IVB or recurrent	Systemic therapy: platinum compounds, ifosfamide, doxorubicin

Management of Locoregionally Advanced Disease

Patients with Stage IB to Stage IVA disease have more advanced disease that is still confined to the pelvis. In addition to the prognostic impact of the extent of disease within the pelvis, an equally important prognostic factor is the status of the para-aortic lymph nodes.[26] As a result, management of patients with uninvolved para-aortic nodes is discussed stage by stage, followed by consideration of the management of those with involved para-aortic nodes (Table 32–10).

The choice of therapy for patients with para-aortic node–negative Stage IB or IIA disease is perhaps the least clear. Either pelvic radiotherapy or radical hysterectomy constitutes reasonable treatment. With either approach, 5-year survival should exceed 80% in carefully staged patients. Current research is directed toward evaluation of combined modality regimens using either combinations of surgery and radiotherapy or platinum-based chemotherapy integrated with either surgery or radiotherapy.[27,28]

For patients with more advanced locoregional disease (Stages IIB–IVA), solid evidence from randomized trials supports the enhanced efficacy of concomitant chemotherapy and radiotherapy. Gynecologic Oncology Group (GOG) studies have demonstrated the superiority of hydroxyurea 4 g/m^2 twice weekly during radiotherapy over radiotherapy alone and equivalence for hydroxyurea plus radiotherapy and radiotherapy concomitant with 5-fluorouracil plus cisplatin. Benefit for combined treatment appears to be greatest in patients with Stage IIIB or IVA disease. The standard of care, based on considerations of efficacy and toxicity, is hydroxyurea plus radiotherapy.[26,29,30]

In patients with positive para-aortic nodes, the survival rate is considerably lower.[31] The standard approach to these patients is radiotherapy with extension of the port to include the para-aortic node area. Five-year survival approximates 10% to 15%. To date, there have been no good randomized studies of systemic therapy in combination with radiotherapy, although the rationale for such an approach is excellent.

TABLE 32–10. ACTIVE DRUGS IN CERVICAL CARCINOMA

DRUG	RESPONSE (%)	
Alkylating agents		
Cyclophosphamide	38/251	15%
Chlorambucil	11/44	25%
Melphalan	4/20	20%
Ifosfamide	25/157	15%
Dibromodulcitol	23/102	29%
Galactitol	7/36	19%
Heavy metal complexes		
Cisplatin	190/815	23%
Carboplatin	27/175	15%
Antibiotics		
Doxorubicin	45/266	20%
Porfiromycin	17/78	22%
Antimetabolites		
5-Fluorouracil	29/142	20%
Methotrexate	17/96	18%
Baker's Antifol	5/32	16%
Plant alkaloids		
Vincristine	10/55	18%
Vindesine	5/21	24%
Other agents		
ICRF-159	5/28	18%
Hexamethylmelamine	12/64	19%

From Thigpen T. Chemotherapy of cancers of the female genital tract. In Perry M (ed): The Chemotherapy Source Book. Baltimore, Williams & Wilkins, 1992:1039–1065.

Management of Advanced or Recurrent Disease

Patients who present with disease outside the pelvis (Stage IVB) or whose disease recurs after initial therapy for limited disease are candidates for systemic therapy. A number of chemotherapeutic agents have moderate activity,[12] but four drugs in particular have consistently yielded single-agent response rates in excess of 20%: the platinum compounds, ifosfamide, dibromodulcitol, and doxorubicin.

A number of studies of combination chemotherapy have been reported; virtually all of these are uncontrolled trials in selected patients and are difficult to interpret. Combinations of continuing interest include ifosfamide plus a platinum compound with or without bleomycin,[32,33] a platinum compound plus 5-fluorouracil,[34] doxorubicin-platinum–based combinations,[35] and a combination of a platinum compound plus dibromodulcitol.[36] No data are yet available to show that any combination is superior to single-agent therapy. GOG is conducting an ongoing randomized trial of cisplatin alone or with either ifosfamide or dibromodulcitol; the trial is incomplete with no data yet available.

In summary, the current treatment of choice for patients with advanced or recurrent disease is single-agent chemotherapy. The most extensively studied and apparently most active drug is cisplatin 50 to 100 mg/m^2 intravenously every 3 weeks with an overall response rate of 23%, a clinical complete response rate of 8%, and a median duration of response of 4 to 8 months.

ENDOMETRIAL CARCINOMA

Endometrial carcinoma, with over 30,000 new cases each year, is the most common invasive malignancy of the female genital tract. Although the cure rate is high at 66%, a significant proportion of patients develop recurrence and eventually die of their disease. This discussion focuses on the facts necessary to develop a rational approach to management.

General Considerations

Endometrial carcinoma is a disease primarily of menopausal and postmenopausal women; the median patient age is 61 years. Personal risk factors include obesity, nulliparity, late menopause, diabetes, hypertension, immunodeficiency, and exogenous estrogens.[37] The most common presenting manifestation is dysfunctional uterine bleeding. Such bleeding in postmenopausal women results from malignancies approximately 20% of the time; a majority of these are endometrial carcinoma. Over 90% of endometrial carcinomas present with dysfunctional bleeding.

Endometrial carcinoma may be any one of five different histologic types. The most common type, accounting for 70% of patients with endometrial carcinoma, is pure adenocarcinoma.[38] Most of the remaining patients have adenocarcinoma mixed with either squamous metaplasia (adenoacanthoma) or squamous carcinoma (adenosquamous carcinoma). When corrected for stage and grade, the three most common cell types appear to have little influence on prognosis or approach to therapy.

Endometrial carcinoma arises from the glandular component of the endometrium. Malignant changes may be preceded by endometrial hyperplasia with dysplastic changes (adenomatous hyperplasia).[39] Early growth within the uterine cavity yields an exophytic, friable mass with spontaneous bleeding. Both vertical and horizontal spread occurs with involvement of the myometrium and the cervix. Spread beyond the uterus occurs as a result of lymphatic spread to parametrial, pelvic, inguinal, and para-aortic nodes; hematogenous dissemination to distant sites such as the lungs, liver, and bones; and peritoneal implantation from either transtubal spread or vertical penetration of the entire thickness of the uterine wall.

Recurrence after initial treatment is most commonly extrapelvic in such locations as lungs, liver, bone, abdominal cavity, and lymph nodes. A majority of failures occur within 2 years of initial treatment.

Prognostic Factors

The most important prognostic factor is the extent of the disease at presentation. Because a majority of patients will have Stage I disease initially, one must consider additional factors that separate Stage I patients into low-risk and high-risk groups.

STAGE

The extent of disease at the time of initial presentation is reflected in the staging system evolved by FIGO (Table 32–11).[40] Stage I disease is by far the most common stage at presentation (75%) with an excellent 5-year survival rate of 76%. Survival decreases dramatically as initial extent of disease increases, but the overall 5-year rate is 66%, as a result of the frequency of Stage I disease. From a practical standpoint, Stages I and II are considered limited disease, whereas Stages III and IV are regarded as advanced disease.

TABLE 32–11. FIGO STAGING SYSTEM FOR ENDOMETRIAL CARCINOMA

STAGE	DESCRIPTION
0	Carcinoma in situ; histologic findings suspicious for malignancy
I	Carcinoma confined to corpus
IAG123	Tumor limited to endometrium
IBG123	Invasion to <½ myometrium
ICG123	Invasivion to >½ myometrium
II	Carcinoma involving corpus and cervix but not extending outside uterus
IIAG123	Endocervical glandular involvement only
IIBG123	Cervical stromal invasion
III	Carcinoma extending outside uterus but not outside true pelvis
IIIAG123	Tumor invades serosa or adnexae or positive peritoneal cytology
IIIBG123	Vaginal metastases
IIICG123	Metastases to pelvix or para-aortic lymph nodes
IV	Carcinoma extending outside true pelvis or involving bladder or rectal mucosa
IVAG123	Tumor invasion of bladder and/or bowel mucosa
IVB	Distant metastases including intra-abdominal and/or inguinal lymph nodes

From FIGO. Corpus cancer staging. Int J Gynecol Obstet 28: 190, 1989. FIGO = International Federation of Gynecology and Obstetrics.

FACTORS IN LIMITED DISEASE

Patients with limited disease may be broadly separated into those at low risk for recurrence and those at high risk, based on a number of features of the primary lesion and its regional spread.[38,41] The factors of importance include six pathologic features, which provide a reasonably precise grouping patients into prognostic categories to form the basis of a rational approach to management: histologic grade, depth of myometrial invasion, involvement of pelvic and/or para-aortic lymph nodes, peritoneal cytology, adnexal spread, and involvement of the cervix (Table 32–12).

Using these pathologic features, patients at low risk for recurrence are those with all of the following features: either a Grade 1 lesion without deep myometrial invasion or Grade 2 lesion with no myometrial invasion, negative peritoneal cytology results, no stromal invasion of the cervix, and no extrauterine spread. Those at high risk for recurrence include all other clinical Stage I and all clinical Stage II patients who exhibit one or more of the following factors: a Grade 3 lesion, a Grade 1 or 2 lesion with myometrial invasion, a Grade 1 lesion with deep myometrial invasion, positive pelvic and/or para-aortic lymph nodes, positive peritoneal cytology, stromal invasion of the cervix, or extrauterine spread.

FACTORS IN ADVANCED DISEASE

Patients who present with advanced (Stage III or IV) or recurrent disease can be grouped into two prognostic categories according to the site of involvement. Those with locoregional disease only (confined to the pelvis) account for about 40% of these patients and may have a distinctly better prognosis than those with distant disease with or without locoregional involvement.

TABLE 32–12. RISK GROUPS BASED ON PATHOLOGIC VARIABLES IN PATIENTS WITH EARLY ENDOMETRIAL CARCINOMA

RISK CATEGORY	PATHOLOGIC FEATURES
High*	Grade 3 lesion Grade 1 or 2 lesion with deep myometrial invasion Positive pelvic and/or para-aortic lymph nodes Positive peritoneal cytology result Stromal invasion of the cervix Extrauterine spread
Low†	Grade 1 or 2 lesion without deep myometrial invasion Negative peritoneal cytology result No stromal invasion of the cervix No extrauterine spread

From Boronow RC, Morrow CP, Creasman WT et al. Surgical staging in endometrial cancer: I. Clinical-pathologic findings of a prospective study. Obstet Gynecol 63:825–832, 1984.

*One or more factors are present.

†All factors are present.

Diagnosis and Evaluation

Patients with dysfunctional uterine bleeding should have a thorough evaluation for possible endometrial carcinoma. The key to this evaluation is obtaining an adequate tissue sample of the endometrium. The Papanicolaou smear, although the simplest technique, suffers from a low diagnostic accuracy of only 40%. Aspiration techniques in the ambulatory setting yield a better accuracy of 70%, but a negative result does not rule out endometrial carcinoma. A more accurate and complete evaluation is provided by dilatation and fractional curettage, which also allows for assessment for endocervical involvement.

Pretreatment evaluation delineates the clinical stage of the disease and the additional pathologic features that have been discussed. The results allow an accurate determination of prognostic category and hence the appropriate therapy. In certain categories, such as patients with clinical Stage I disease, additional information about significant pathologic factors obtained at the time of the initial surgery must also be considered in the final management decision.

Management of Limited Disease

Patients with limited (clinical Stage I or II) disease constitute the vast majority of patients with endometrial carcinoma and have an excellent chance of cure. The appropriate approach to an individual patient depends on the patient's risk status (Table 32–13). Virtually all patients with limited disease should have surgical resection of the primary disease unless the operative risk is deemed unacceptably high. The surgical procedure should include not only the standard total abdominal hysterectomy and bilateral salpingo-oophorectomy but also assessment of peritoneal cytology and pelvic and para-aortic lymph nodes to determine the patient's risk of recurrence.

TABLE 32–13. MANAGEMENT RECOMMENDATIONS FOR LIMITED ENDOMETRIAL CARCINOMA

DISEASE STATUS	RECOMMENDATIONS
Low risk	Total abdominal hysterectomy, bilateral salpingo-oophorectomy
High risk	Same surgery as for low risk followed by adjuvant therapy; no form of adjuvant therapy, however, shown to be of benefit

LOW-RISK PATIENTS

Patients at low risk for recurrence have greater than 90% chance of remaining disease-free beyond 5 years when treated with surgery alone.[41] No evidence exists that more radical surgery, adjuvant radiotherapy, or adjuvant systemic therapy will improve the results with surgery alone. The appropriate approach is therefore total abdominal hysterectomy and bilateral salpingo-oophorectomy with additional measures at surgery to ensure that none of the high-risk features is present.

HIGH-RISK PATIENTS

Patients at high risk for recurrence have been treated with a myriad of approaches combining surgery and radiotherapy, including surgery preceded by radium and/or external beam radiotherapy, surgery followed by radium and/or external beam radiotherapy, and surgery both preceded and followed by radiotherapy. Dose and schedule for radiotherapy have varied widely. No concurrently controlled studies and no good uncontrolled data currently available show conclusive benefit from radiotherapy in combination with surgery in terms of survival, although preoperative radiotherapy does appear to reduce the incidence of vaginal recurrence (from 12% to 2%).[42] Standard treatment for the high-risk patient, however, is considered to be a combination of surgery and radiotherapy. Systemic adjuvant therapy is not warranted at the present time.

Management of Advanced or Recurrent Disease

The management of patients with advanced (clinical Stage III or IV) or recurrent endometrial carcinoma is determined by whether the disease is confined to the pelvis and/or abdomen or includes distant spread (Table 32–14).

TABLE 32–14. MANAGEMENT RECOMMENDATIONS FOR ADVANCED OR RECURRENT ENDOMETRIAL CARCINOMA

DISEASE STATUS	RECOMMENDATIONS
Locoregional disease	If confined to uterus, ovaries, and fallopian tubes—radical hysterectomy and pelvic node dissection followed by pelvic radiotherapy; for other patients—radiotherapy
Disseminated disease	Systemic therapy: progestins for well-differentiated or receptor-positive patients; doxorubicin plus cisplatin for others

LOCOREGIONAL DISEASE

Careful evaluation should be done to rule out distant spread to such sites as the lungs, liver, abdominal cavity, and bone before assigning a patient to the group with locoregional involvement only. If a patient indeed has only locoregional disease, the mainstay of treatment is radiotherapy with or without surgery. Patients in this group with the best prognosis are those with disease confined clinically to the uterus, ovaries, and/or fallopian tubes. Such patients are generally managed with a radical hysterectomy and bilateral pelvic lymphadenectomy followed by postoperative pelvic radiotherapy. Five-year survival is reported to be 50%. For patients with parametrial extension, vaginal involvement, or other pelvic extension, radiotherapy is the initial treatment modality. Five-year survivals are reported to be between 25% and 50%.

DISSEMINATED DISEASE

Patients with evidence of disseminated disease are candidates for systemic therapy with either hormones or chemotherapy, neither of which has been adequately studied in endometrial carcinoma (Table 32–15). For *hormonal therapy*, the most commonly employed systemic therapy has been progestational agents. Recent series demonstrate response rates of 20% to 24% with oral preparations.[44,45] Median duration of response is 3 or 4 months; median survival, 9 or 10 months. A randomized trial looking at standard versus high-dose progestin therapy showed no advantage to giving higher doses.[45] Standard therapy would thus be considered to be either medroxyprogesterone 200 mg/day orally or megestrol acetate 160 mg/day orally.

A number of factors thought to be predictive of response to hormonal therapy have been evaluated.[46] Two factors that appear to be most predictive are the histologic grade (the better the differentiation, the greater is the frequency of response) and hormone-receptor status (positive estrogen and progesterone receptor assays yield higher response rates) (Table 32–16).[12]

Among other hormonal therapies, only tamoxifen has been studied in endometrial carcinoma. There is some indication that the drug is active, although further studies are needed to confirm this activity.[47]

TABLE 32–15. ACTIVE SINGLE DRUGS IN ENDOMETRIAL CARCINOMA

DRUG	PATIENTS	RESPONSE (%)
Medroxyprogesterone acetate	609	20%
Tamoxifen	52	24%
Doxorubicin	161	26%
Cisplatin	124	24%
Carboplatin	52	31%

From Thigpen T. Chemotherapy of cancers of the female genital tract. In Perry M (ed): The Chemotherapy Source Book. Baltimore, Williams & Wilkins, 1992:1039–1065.

TABLE 32–16. RECEPTOR STATUS AND RESPONSE TO PROGESTIN THERAPY

SERIES	ER+ PR+	ER− PR−
Creasman	3/5 (60%)	1/8 (12%)
Ehrlich	7/8 (80%)	1/16 (7%)
Benraad	5/6 (83%)	0/5 (0%)
Martin	13/13 (100%)	1/7 (14%)
McCarty	4/5 (80%)	0/8 (0%)
Thigpen	4/10 (40%)	3/25 (12%)
Total	36/47 (77%)	6/69 (9%)

ER = estrogen receptor; PR = progestin receptor.

From Thigpen T, Vance R, Lambath B et al. Chemotherapy for advanced or recurrent gynecologic cancer. Cancer 60:2104, 2116, 1987.

TABLE 32–17. GYNECOLOGIC ONCOLOGY GROUP PROTOCOL 107: A RANDOMIZED TRIAL OF DOXORUBICIN WITH OR WITHOUT CISPLATIN

RESPONSE STATUS*	DOXORUBICIN	DOXORUBICIN/ CISPLATIN
Complete response	10 (8%)	23 (21%)
Partial response	25 (20%)	25 (23%)
Stable disease	60 (47%)	46 (42%)
Increasing disease	32 (25%)	16 (15%)
Total	127 (100%)	110 (100%)

*The overall response rate of 44% with the combination is significantly superior to the 28% with doxorubicin. The progression-free interval with the combination is also superior.

From Thigpen T, Blessing J, Homesley H et al. Phase III trial of doxorubicin +/− cisplatin in advanced or recurrent endometrial carcinoma: A Gynecologic Oncology Group study. Proc ASCO 12:261, 1993.

Because endometrial carcinoma has been widely regarded as a "benign" neoplasm not requiring cytotoxic drugs, *chemotherapy* has been studied intensively only in the last 2 decades. The only active drugs identified to date are doxorubicin[48,49] and the platinum compounds,[50–52] each with response rates in excess of 20%, median durations of response ranging from 4 to 7 months, and median survivals of 9 to 12 months (Table 32–17).

Despite the lack of an abundance of active drugs, trials of combination chemotherapy for endometrial carcinoma have been conducted. Most of these trials are single-arm studies of relatively small numbers of patients, trials that permit no definitive conclusions about the relative merits of the combination versus single-agent therapy. A recently completed randomized trial comparing doxorubicin alone with doxorubicin plus cisplatin showed superior response rate and progression-free survival for patients receiving the combination regimen.[53] The treatment of choice for patients with advanced or recurrent disease no longer responsive to hormonal agents is therefore a combination of doxorubicin 60 mg/m^2 plus cisplatin 50 mg/m^2 intravenously every 3 weeks (see Table 32–17).

Summary

The proper clinical approach to endometrial carcinoma rests on attention to early diagnosis. Any patient with dysfunctional uterine bleeding must be evaluated with uterine tissue sampling and, in most instances, dilatation and fractional curettage. Once a diagnosis of endometrial carcinoma has been made, careful clinical staging is essential, with attention to significant pathologic factors in patients with clinical Stage I disease: histologic grade, depth of myometrial penetration, status of pelvic and para-aortic lymph nodes, peritoneal cytology, cervical involvement, and extrauterine spread.

Patients with limited (clinical Stages I and II) disease will be managed with surgery and/or radiotherapy. Patients at low risk for recurrence require total abdominal hysterectomy and bilateral salpingo-oophorectomy only and should have a 5-year survival rate that exceeds 90%. High-risk patients are currently managed with a combination of surgery plus radiotherapy with the specifics of the regimen varying from institution to institution. Systemic therapy has no proven role in early disease.

Patients with advanced or recurrent disease should be evaluated to determine whether disease is confined to pelvis alone or involves extrapelvic sites. In the former case, radiotherapy with or without surgery has the potential to yield long-term survivors. In the latter case, systemic therapy is required. Active systemic agents include progestins, antiestrogens, doxorubicin, and the platinum compounds. Current recommendations are to use hormonal agents first and then to employ cytotoxic drugs. The chemotherapy of choice is doxorubicin plus cisplatin.

UNCOMMON GYNECOLOGIC MALIGNANCIES

A number of uncommon malignant neoplasms originate in the female genital tract. Some of these are sufficiently uncommon that little meaningful information about appropriate management is available. For others, however, well-done single-arm trials provide a framework for rational decision making. These include uterine sarcomas and germ cell neoplasms of the ovary.

Uterine Sarcomas

Sarcomas of the uterus account for less than 5% of all corpus cancers. There is a clear association between prior exposure to radiation and the frequency of the disease.[54] These lesions include mixed mesodermal sarcomas, leiomyosarcomas, endometrial stromal sarcomas, and certain rare histologic types; but the first two of these, which represent 90% of the cases, are the only types for which meaningful data are available.[55]

Although some of these lesions can be indolent (*e.g.*, low-grade leiomyosarcomas), most are more aggressive. Extent of disease is the most important determinant of outcome (Table 32–18). Although there is no formal staging system, a modification of the staging system for endometrial carcinoma is used. Patients who have disease limited to the corpus (Stage I disease) have the best outcome, but recurrence rate in even this limited disease group approximates 50%. Such high recurrence rates underline the importance of developing effective systemic therapy.

The most common presenting manifestation is vaginal bleeding, which occurs in up to 95% of patients. Biopsy is required to establish the histologic diagnosis. Evaluation of patients should be directed to the most likely sites of spread: other pelvic structures, pelvic and para-aortic lymph nodes, other abdominal structures, and the lungs.

The initial management of the patient depends on the extent of disease (Table 32–19). Patient with disease limited to the corpus (Stage I) or the corpus plus the cervix (Stage II) should undergo surgical resection of disease (total abdominal hysterectomy). Patients who present with disease extending to other pelvic structures (Stage III) or to distant sites (Stage IV), except in carefully selected circumstances in which all disease can be resected or in which surgical resection offers significant palliation, will require systemic therapy.

The remainder of the discussion focuses on the role of chemotherapy in uterine sarcomas. Because the two common histologic types appear to respond differently to chemotherapy, each is presented as a separate patient population. Within each population, there are two distinct groups in which chemotherapy has been studied: patients with advanced or recurrent disease and those requiring adjuvant treatment of Stage I or II disease following complete surgical resection.

ADVANCED OR RECURRENT DISEASE

Of drugs studied as *single agents* in uterine sarcomas, two have been identified as active in mixed mesodermal sarcomas: ifosfamide and cisplatin (Table 32–20). Ifosfamide at a dose of 1.5 g/m^2/day for five days every 4 weeks produced five complete and four partial responses among 28 patients with no prior chemotherapy.[56] Cisplatin 50 mg/m^2 every 3 weeks was studied in patients with prior chemotherapy (18% response rate in 28 patients) and in patients with no prior chemotherapy (19% response rate in 63 patients).[57,58] At a higher dose ranging from 75 to 100 mg/m^2 every 3 weeks in 12 patients, one complete and four partial responses were observed (42%).[59] Doxorubicin demonstrated relatively little activity in two trials of patients with mixed mesodermal sarcomas: four responses among 41 patients (9%) with a dose of 60 mg/m^2 every 3 weeks[60] and no responses among nine patients with a range of doses from 50 to 90 mg/m^2 every 3 weeks.[61]

Among patients with leiomyosarcomas (see Table 32–20), the most active single agent appears to be doxorubicin (seven responses among 28 patients treated with 60 mg/m^2 every 3 weeks).[60] Ifosfamide demonstrated moderate activity (four partial responses among 28 patients),[56] as did etoposide (one complete and two partial responses among 28 patients).[62]

Only two randomized trials of *combination chemotherapy* have been completed. The first compared doxorubicin with

TABLE 32–18. STAGING SYSTEM FOR UTERINE SARCOMAS

STAGE	DESCRIPTION
I	Confined to the uterine corpus
II	Confined to corpus plus cervix
III	Beyond the uterus but confined to the pelvis
IV	Outside the pelvis

TABLE 32–19. MANAGEMENT RECOMMENDATIONS FOR UTERINE SARCOMA

DISEASE STATUS	RECOMMENDATIONS
Stage I/II resected	Total abdominal hysterectomy, bilateral salpingo-oophorectomy, adjuvant therapy; no adjuvant therapy has been shown to be effective
Stage III/IV	Except in carefully selected cases, amenable to surgical resection, chemotherapy; for MMT, ifosfamide or cisplatin; for LMS, doxorubicin

*MMT = mixed mesodermal sarcoma; LMS = leiomyosarcoma.

TABLE 32–20. ACTIVE AND POSSIBLY ACTIVE DRUGS IN UTERINE SARCOMA

DRUG	MMT (%)	LMS (%)
Doxorubicin	4/50 (8%)	7/28 (25%)
Ifosfamide	9/28 (32%)	4/28 (14%)
Cisplatin	22/103 (21%)	2/52 (4%)
VP-16	2/31 (6%)	3/28 (11%)

MMT = mixed mesodermal sarcoma; LMS = leiomyosarcoma.

From Thigpen T. Chemotherapy of cancers of the female genital tract. In Perry M (ed): The Chemotherapy Source Book. Baltimore, Williams & Wilkins, 1992:1039–1065.

TABLE 32–21. GYNECOLOGIC ONCOLOGY GROUP PROTOCOL 21: DOXORUBICIN WITH OR WITHOUT DTIC IN ADVANCED OR RECURRENT UTERINE SARCOMA

HISTOLOGIC TYPE	DOXORUBICIN	DOXORUBICIN + DTIC
Leiomyosarcoma	7/28 (25%)	6/20 (30%)
Mixed mesodermal sarcoma	4/41 (10%)	7/31 (23%)
Other sarcomas	2/11 (18%)	3/15 (20%)

DTIC = dimethyl triazinoimidazole carboxamide.

From Omura GA, Major FJ, Blessing JA et al. A randomized study of Adriamycin with and without dimethyl triazinoimidazole carboxamide in advanced uterine sarcomas. Cancer 52:626–632, 1983.

or without dimethyl triazinoimidazole carboxamide (DTIC) with no significant differences noted between the two regimens (Table 32–21).[60] The study was designed before the apparent differences in response to chemotherapy for leiomyosarcomas and mixed mesodermal sarcomas were observed; hence, there are an insufficient number of each histologic type to permit analysis.

The second trial studied doxorubicin with or without cyclophosphamide.[61] No significant differences were noted between the two regimens. The overall response rate for the combined data was similar to that seen in the first randomized trial.

In conclusion, there is currently no evidence to support the use of combination chemotherapy for advanced or recurrent uterine sarcomas. Patients with mixed mesodermal sarcomas should be managed with either ifosfamide or cisplatin, whereas patients with leiomyosarcomas should receive doxorubicin.

LIMITED DISEASE

There is no defined role for adjuvant chemotherapy for Stage I disease after complete surgical resection. The one meaningful study completed to date randomized patients to either doxorubicin 60 mg/m^2 every 3 weeks for eight cycles or no further therapy.[63] No significant differences in recurrence rate, progression-free interval, or survival were noted between the two arms for either the overall patient population or the two major histologic subsets. In the overall population, the median survival was 73.7 months for the doxorubicin arm and 55.0 months for no further therapy.

The relatively low frequency of the disease makes it difficult to accrue a sufficient number of patients to complete a study in a reasonable period of time. Additionally, the difference in response to chemotherapy for the two major histologic types further complicates the problem of low disease incidence. There is no evidence that adjuvant chemotherapy is of any value in uterine sarcomas. It is unlikely that there will be additional data in the near future.

Germ Cell Neoplasms of the Ovary

Less than 5% of ovarian cancer consists of germ cell carcinomas, which are classified into two broad groups: dysgerminomas and nondysgerminomas.[64] The staging system is that used for celomic epithelial carcinomas. Management begins with exploratory laparotomy to determine extent of disease and to permit surgical resection. Subsequent treatment is determined by histology and findings at laparotomy, which categorize patients as those with completely resected Stage I to Stage III disease and those with incompletely resected Stage III and Stage IV disease.

TUMOR MARKERS

Ovarian germ cell tumors produce alpha-fetoprotein or beta-human chorionic gonadotropin in a majority of cases. Alpha-fetoprotein elevations have been noted in patients with endodermal sinus tumors, immature teratomas, mixed germ cell tumors, embryonal carcinomas, and polyembryomas; whereas elevated human chorionic gonadotropin is seen with choriocarcinomas, embryonal carcinomas, polyembryomas, mixed cell tumors, and, less commonly, dysgerminomas. These markers are useful in assessing response to chemotherapy and in following patients in complete remission for evidence of recurrence.

STAGES I TO III COMPLETELY RESECTED

Patients with completely resected Stage I, II, or III endodermal sinus tumors, mixed cell tumors, embryonal car-

TABLE 32–22. GYNECOLOGIC ONCOLOGY GROUP ADJUVANT CHEMOTHERAPY STUDIES IN OVARIAN GERM CELL CARCINOMA: PATIENTS DISEASE-FREE AT A MEDIAN FOLLOW-UP OF 16 MONTHS AFTER THERAPY

THERAPY	EST AND MCT	IMMATURE TERATOMA
No adjuvant	34/165 (21%)	36/56 (64%)
VAC	53/82 (65%)	59/70 (84%)
BEP	30/31 (97%)	18/19 (95%)

VAC: Vincristine 1.5 mg/m^2 IV (max 2 mg) q2wk × 12
Actinomycin D 350 μ/m^2 IV daily × 5 days q4wk × 6
Cyclophosphamide 150 mg/m^2 IV daily × 5 days q4wk × 6

BEP: Bleomycin 20 units/m^2 IV (max 30 units) weekly × 9
Etoposide 100 mg/m^2 IV daily × 5 q3wk × 3
Cisplatin 20 mg/m^2 IV daily × 5 q3wk × 3

EST = endodermal sinus tumor; MCT = mixed cell tumor.

From Slayton RE, Park RC, Silverberg SG et al. Vincristine dactinomycin and cyclophosphamide in the treatment of malignant germ cell tumors of the ovary: A Gynecologic Oncology Group study (a final report). Cancer 56:243–248, 1985; and Williams S, Blessing J, Slayton R et al. Ovarian germ cell tumors: adjuvant trials of the Gynecologic Oncology Group (GOG). Proc ASCO 8:150, 1989.

TABLE 32–23. GYNECOLOGIC ONCOLOGY GROUP TRIALS OF COMBINATION CHEMOTHERAPY IN INCOMPLETELY RESECTED STAGE III AND STAGE IV GERM CELL CARCINOMAS OF THE OVARY

HISTOLOGY AND THERAPY	CR	PR	DISEASE FREE
Immature teratoma			
VAC	—	—	4/8 (50%)
PVB	2/9 (22%)	2/9 (22%)	12/24 (50%)
Endodermal sinus tumor and mixed cell tumor			
VAC	—	—	3/14 (21%)
PVB	13/24 (54%)	8/24 (33%)	31/58 (53%)
Dysgerminoma			
PVB	3/4 (75%)	1/4 (25%)	7/8 (88%)
Choriocarcinoma			
PVB	2/3 (67%)	1/3 (33%)	2/3 (67%)

VAC: Vincristine 1.5 mg/m^2 IV (max 2 mg) q2wk × 12
Actinomycin D 350 μg/m^2 IV daily × 5 days q4wk × 6
Cyclophosphamide 150 mg/m^2 IV daily × 5 days q4wk × 6

PVB: Vinblastine 12 mg/m^2 IV q3wk × 4
Bleomycin 20 units/m^2 IV (max 30 units) weekly × 12
Cisplatin 20 mg/m^2 IV daily × 5 q3wk × 3 or 4

CR = complete response; PR = partial response.

From Williams SD, Blessing JA, Moore DH et al. Cisplatin, vinblastine, and bleomycin in recurrent ovarian germ cell tumors: A trial of the Gynecologic Oncology Group. Ann Intern Med 3:22–27, 1989.

cinomas, choriocarcinomas, and immature teratomas have a sufficiently high recurrence rate that adjuvant therapy is warranted. Both vincristine, actinomycin D, and cyclophosphamide (VAC) and bleomycin, etoposide, and cisplatin (BEP) have been tested in adjuvant trials (Table 32–22).[65,66] Comparison with historical data on no adjuvant therapy shows a steady increase in the percentage of patients remaining disease-free at 16 months of follow-up as treatment progresses from no adjuvant therapy through VAC to BEP. These data support adjuvant BEP as the treatment of choice for patients with completely resected Stages I to III disease of specific histologies: immature teratoma Grades 2 and 3, endodermal sinus tumor, mixed cell tumor, embryonal carcinoma, and choriocarcinoma. For other histologies, data are insufficient to permit definitive conclusions.

STAGE III INCOMPLETELY RESECTED AND STAGE IV DISEASE

Two chemotherapy regimens are active in patients with advanced or recurrent disease: VAC and cisplatin, vinblastine, and bleomycin (PVB) (Table 32–23).[67] The cisplatin-based combination yields higher response rates and a greater percentage of patients who remain disease-free for extended periods and is the current treatment of choice for advanced or recurrent disease.

REFERENCES

1. Cassagrande JT, Pike MC, Russ RK et al. Incessant ovulation and ovarian cancer. Lancet 2:170, 1979
2. Lynch HT, Watson P, Lynch JF et al. Hereditary ovarian cancer: Heterogeneity in age at onset. Cancer 71:573–581, 1993
3. Thigpen T, Brady M, Omura G et al. Age as a prognostic factor in ovarian carcinoma: The Gynecologic Oncology Group experience. Cancer 71:606–614, 1993
4. Young RC, Walton L, Ellenberg SS et al. Adjuvant therapy in stage I and stage II epithelial ovarian cancer. Results of two prospective randomized trials. N Engl J Med 322:1021–1027, 1990
5. Omura G, Blessing J, Ehrlich C et al. A randomized trial of cyclophosphamide and doxorubicin with or without cisplatin in advanced ovarian carcinoma. Cancer 57: 1725–1730, 1986
6. Ehrlich C, Einhorn L, Williams S et al. Chemotherapy for stage III–IV epithelial ovarian cancer with cis-dichlorodiammine-platinum (II), Adriamycin, and cyclophosphamide: A preliminary report. Cancer Treat Rep 63:281–288, 1979
7. Greco F, Julian C, Richardson R et al. Advanced ovarian cancer: Brief intensive combination chemotherapy and second-look operation. Obstet Gynecol 58:199–205, 1981
8. Young R, Howser D, Myers C et al. Combination chemotherapy (CHex-UP) with intraperitoneal maintenance in advanced ovarian adenocarcinoma. Proc ASCO 22:465, 1981

9. The new FIGO stage grouping for primary carcinoma of the ovary (1985). Gynecol Oncol 25:383–385, 1986
10. Van Nagell JR, DePriest PD, Gallion HH et al. Ovarian cancer screening. Cancer 71:1523–1528, 1993
11. Hoskins WJ. Surgical staging and cytoreductive surgery of epithelial ovarian cancer. Cancer 71:1534–1540, 1993
12. Thigpen JT. Chemotherapy of cancers of the female genital tract. In Perry M (ed): The Chemotherapy Source Book. Baltimore, Williams & Wilkins, 1992:1039–1065
13. McGuire WP, Hoskins WJ, Brady MF et al. A phase III trial comparing cisplatin/cytoxan and cisplatin/taxol in advanced ovarian cancer. Proc ASCO 12:255, 1993
14. McGuire WP. Primary treatment of epithelial ovarian malignancies. Cancer 71:1541–1550, 1993
15. Day TG, Smith JP. Diagnosis and staging of ovarian carcinoma. Semin Oncol 2:217, 1975
16. Bolis G, Colombo N, Favalli G et al. Randomized multicenter clinical trials in stage I epithelial ovarian cancer. Proc ASCO 11:225, 1992
17. Thigpen JT, Vance RB, Khansur T. Second-line chemotherapy for recurrent carcinoma of the ovary. Cancer 71:1559–1564, 1993
18. Piver MS, Baker TR, Jishi MF et al. Familial ovarian cancer: A report of 658 families from the Gilda Radner Familial Ovarian Cancer Registry (1981–1991). Cancer 71:582–588, 1993
19. Piver MS, Jishi MF, Tsukada Y et al. Primary peritoneal carcinoma after oophorectomy in women with a family history of ovarian cancer. Cancer 71:2751–2755, 1993
20. Keighley E. Carcinoma of the cervix among prostitutes in a women's prison. Br J Vener Dis 44:254–255, 1968
21. Boon ME, Susanti I, Tasche MJA et al. Human papillomavirus-associated male and female genital carcinomas in a Hindu population: The male as a vector and victim. Cancer 64:559–565, 1989
22. Richart RM, Wright TC. Controversies in the management of low-grade cervical intraepithelial neoplasia. Cancer 71:1413–1421, 1993
23. Beahrs OH, Henson DE, Hutter RVP et al. Manual for Staging of Cancer, 3rd ed. Philadelphia, JB Lippincott, 1988:151–153
24. Grigsby PW, Perez CA. Radiotherapy alone for medically inoperable carcinoma of the cervix: Stage IA and carcinoma-in-situ. Int J Radiat Oncol Biol Phys 21:375–378, 1991
25. Kolstad P. Folow-up study of 232 patients with stage IA1 and 411 patients with stage IA2 squamous cell carcinoma of the cervix (microinvasive carcinoma). Gynecol Oncol 33: 265–272, 1989
26. Stehman F, Bundy B, Keys H et al. A randomized trial of hydroxyurea versus misonidazole adjunct to radiation therapy in carcinoma of the cervix. Am J Obstet Gynecol 159:87–94, 1988
27. Averette HE, Nguyen HN, Donato DM et al. Radical hysterectomy for invasive cervical cancer. Cancer 71:1422–1437, 1993
28. Marcial VA, Marcial LV. Radiation therapy of cervical cancer. Cancer 71:1438–1445, 1993
29. Hreshchyshyn M, Aron B, Boronow R et al. Hydroxyurea or placebo combined with radiation to treat stages IIIB and IV cervical cancer confined to the pelvis. Int J Radiat Oncol Biol Phys 5:317–322, 1979
30. Whitney C. Personal communication
31. DiSaia P, Bundy B, Curry S et al. Phase III study on the treatment of women with cervical cancer, stage IIB, IIIB, and IVA (confined to the pelvis and/or periaortic nodes), with radiotherapy alone versus radiotherapy plus immunotherapy with intravenous Corynebacterium parvum: A Gynecologic Oncology Group study. Gynecol Oncol 26:386–397, 1987
32. Lara P, Garcia-Puche J, Pedraza V. Cisplatin-ifosfamide as neoadjuvant chemotherapy in stage IIIB cervical uterine squamous-cell carcinoma. Cancer Chemother Pharmacol 26:S36–S38, 1990
33. Buxton E, Meanwell C, Hilton C et al. Combination bleomycin, ifosfamide, and cisplatin chemotherapy in cervical cancer. J Natl Cancer Inst 81:359–361, 1989
34. Bonomi P, Blessing J, Ball H et al. A phase II evaluation of cisplatin and 5-fluorouracil in patients with advanced squamous cell carcinoma of the cervix: A Gynecologic Oncology Group study. Gynecol Oncol 34:357–359, 1989
35. Omura GA, Hubbard J, Hatch K. Limited tolerance for high dose cisplatin plus doxorubicin after radiotherapy for female pelvic cancer: A Gynecologic Oncology Group pilot study. Am J Clin Oncol 8:347–349, 1985
36. Omura GA, Hubbard J, Hatch K et al. Chemotherapy of cervix cancer with mitolactol and cisplatin: A phase I pilot study of the Gynecologic Oncology Group. Am J Clin Oncol 15:185–187, 1992
37. MacMahon B. Risk factors for endometrial cancer. Gynecol Oncol 2:122, 1974
38. Creasman WT, Morrow CP, Bundy BN et al. Surgical pathological spread patterns of endometrial cancer (a Gynecologic Oncology Group study). Cancer 60:2035–2041, 1987
39. Kurman RJ, Kaminski PF, Norris HJ. The behavior of endometrial hyperplasia: A long-term study of "untreated" hyperplasia in 170 patients. CA Cancer J Clin 56:403, 1985
40. FIGO. Corpus cancer staging. Int J Gynecol Obstet 28:190, 1989
41. Boronow RC, Morrow CP, Creasman WT et al. Surgical staging in endometrial cancer: 1. Clinical-pathologic findings of a prospective study. Obstet Gynecol 63:825–832, 1984
42. Moss WT, Brand WN, Battifora H. Radiation Oncology — Rationale, Technique, Results, 5th ed. St Louis, CV Mosby,1979:492
43. Barber HR, Braunschwig A. Treatment and results of recurrent cancer of corpus uteri in patients receiving anterior and total pelvic exenteration 1947–1963. Cancer 22:949–955, 1968
44. Thigpen T, Blessing J, DiSaia P et al. A randomized comparison of adriamycin with or without cyclophosphamide in the treatment of advanced or recurrent endometrial carcinoma. Proc Am Soc Clin Oncol 4:115, 1985
45. Thigpen T, Blessing J, Hatch K et al. A randomized trial of medroxyprogesterone acetate 200 mg versus 1000 mg daily in advanced or recurrent endometrial carcinoma: A Gynecologic Oncology Group study. Proc ASCO 10: 185, 1991
46. Thigpen T, Blessing J, DiSaia P. Oral medroxyprogesterone acetate in advanced or recurrent endometrial carcinoma: Results of therapy and correlation with estrogen and proges-

terone receptor levels. The Gynecologic Oncology Group experience. In Baulieu EE, Slacobelli S, McGuire WL (eds): Endocrinology of Malignancy, Park Ridge, NJ, Parthenon, 1986:446

47. Thigpen T, Vance R, Lambuth B et al. Chemotherapy for advanced or recurrent gynecologic cancer. Cancer 60:2104, 2116, 1987
48. Thigpen T, Buchsbaum H, Mangan C et al. Phase II trial of Adriamycin in the treatment of advanced or recurrent endometrial carcinoma: A Gynecologic Oncology Group study. Cancer Treat Rep 63:21–27, 1979
49. Thigpen T, Blessing J, DiSaia P et al. A randomized comparison of Adriamycin with or without cyclophosphamide in the treatment of advanced or recurrent endometrial carcinoma. Proc Am Soc Clin Oncol 4:115, 1985
50. Thigpen T, Blessing J, Homesley H et al. Phase II trial of cisplatin as first-line chemotherapy in patients with advanced or recurrent endometrial carcinoma: A Gynecologic Oncology Group study. Gynecol Oncol 33:68–70, 1989
51. Thigpen T, Blessing JA, Lagasse LD et al. Phase II trial of cisplatin as second-line chemotherapy in patients with advanced or recurrent endometrial carcinoma (a Gynecologic Oncology Group study). Am J Clin Oncol 7:253–256, 1984
52. Thigpen T. Systemic therapy with single agents for advanced or recurrent endometrial carcinoma. In Alberts D, Surwit E (eds): Endometrial Carcinoma. Boston, Martinus Nijhoff, 1989
53. Thigpen T, Blessing J, Homesley H et al. Phase III trial of doxorubicin +/− cisplatin in advanced or recurrent endometrial carcinoma: A Gynecologic Oncology Group study. Proc ASCO 12:261, 1993
54. Meredith RF, Eisert DR, Kaka Z et al. An excess of uterine sarcomas after pelvic irradiation. Cancer 58:2003, 1986
55. Major FJ, Blessing JA, Silverberg SG et al. Prognostic factors in early uterine sarcoma: A Gynecologic Oncology Group study. Cancer 71:1702–1709, 1992
56. Sutton GP, Blessing JA, Rosenheim N et al. Phase II trial of ifosfamide and mesna in mixed mesodermal tumors of the uterus (A Gyncologic Oncology Group study). Am J Obstet Gynecol 161:309–312, 1989
57. Thigpen T, Blessing JA, Beecham J et al. Phase II trial of cisplatin as first-line chemotherapy in patients with advanced or recurrent uterine sarcomas (a Gynecologic Oncology Group study). J Clin Oncol 9:1962–1966, 1991
58. Thigpen T, Blessing JA, Orr JW Jr et al. Phase II trial of cisplatin in the treatment of patients with advanced or recurrent mixed mesodermal sarcomas of the uterus: A Gynecologic Oncology Group study. Cancer Treat Rep 70:271–274, 1986
59. Gershenson DM, Kavanagh JJ, Copeland LJ et al. Cisplatin therapy for disseminated mixed mesodermal sarcoma of the uterus. J Clin Oncol 5:618–621, 1987
60. Omura GA, Major FJ, Blessing JA et al. A randomized study of Adriamycin with and without dimethyl triazinoimidazole carboxamide in advanced uterine sarcomas. Cancer 52:626–632, 1983
61. Muss HB, Bundy BN, DiSaia PJ et al. Treatment of recurrent or advanced uterine sarcoma: A randomized trial of doxorubicin versus doxorubicin and cyclophosphamide (a phase III trial of the Gynecologic Oncology Group). Cancer 55:1648–1653, 1985
62. Slayton R, Blessing J, Angel C et al. Phase II trial of etoposide in the management of advanced or recurrent leiomyosarcoma of the uterus: A Gynecologic Oncology Group study. Cancer Treat Rep 71:1303–1304, 1987
63. Omura GA, Blessing JA, Major F et al. A randomized clinical trial of adjuvant adriamycin in uterine sarcomas: A Gynecologic Oncology Group study. J Clin Oncol 3:1240–1245, 1985
64. Gershenson DM, Malone JM Jr: Chemotherapy for malignant germ cell tumors of the ovary. In Deppe G (ed): Chemotherapy of Gynecologic Cancer, 2nd ed. New York, Wiley-Liss, 1990:217–239
65. Slayton RE, Park RC, Silverberg SG et al. Vincristine, dactinomycin and cyclophosphamide in the treatment of malignant germ cell tumors of the ovary: A Gynecologic Oncology Group study (a final report). Cancer 56:243–248, 1985
66. Williams S, Blessing J, Slayton R et al. Ovarian germ cell tumors: adjuvant trials of the Gynecologic Oncology Group (GOG). Proc ASCO 8:150, 1989
67. Williams SD, Blessing JA, Moore DH et al. Cisplatin, vinblastine, and bleomycin in recurrent ovarian germ cell tumors: A trial of the Gynecologic Oncology Group. Ann Intern Med 3:22–27, 1989

John S. Macdonald, Daniel G. Haller, Robert J. Mayer, Eds. *Manual of Oncologic Therapeutics*, Third Edition.

33. SOFT TISSUE AND BONE SARCOMAS

Anthony D. Elias
Karen Antman

The malignant tumors of muscle, fat, bone, and fibrous tissues and those of neuroectodermal origin constitute the sarcomas. They are frequently studied in animal model systems. However, because of the numerous histologic subtypes, myriad of primary sites, and relative rarity of sarcomas, their local and systemic management is best handled by multimodality specialty teams. Approximately 7900 new sarcomas are diagnosed in the United States each year, constituting 1% and 15% of adult and pediatric malignancies, respectively. Approximately 50% to 60% of these patients will develop and die of disseminated disease within 5 years of diagnosis. Local-regional and systemic management of these tumors frequently presents clinical and diagnostic dilemmas.

PATHOGENESIS

The study of sarcoma patients has been central to the discovery of cancer families, some of which have germ line mutations of tumor suppressor genes. Two such tumor suppressor gene syndromes have now been recognized. The retinoblastoma gene is dysfunctional in the rare retinoblastoma syndrome; an abnormal or absent gene product (RB1) has also been described in sporadic and retinoblastoma-associated osteosarcomas, small cell lung cancer, breast cancer, leiomyosarcoma, and synovial cell sarcoma. Although detectable mutations at the DNA level are less common, up to 70% of sarcomas had altered RB1 gene protein levels.[1] The Li-Fraumeni syndrome has been associated with germ line p53 mutations.[2] This cancer syndrome is characterized by an autosomal dominant inheritance of susceptibility to multiple types of cancers, including sarcomas, breast cancer, glioma, and adrenocortical carcinomas, among others. Because the inactivation of p53 has also been observed in multiple tumor histologies, it may be one of the rate-limiting steps in the transformation of many tissues. The gene, NF1, associated with classic von Recklinghausen's disease (multiple neurofibromas) is located on 17q. Malignant transformation *de novo* or arising from a pre-existing neurofibroma occurs with a lifetime risk of 10%. The neurofibromasarcomas arising from neurofibromas were found to have additional deletions or mutations of 17p, particularly in the region of the p53 gene (17p12–13.1).[3] Thus, it may be that the initial alteration on the NF1 gene leads to benign neurofibromas, but secondary hits to the p53 gene locus may allow malignant transformation. How frequent are familial/genetic cancers? While risk of cancer in the siblings of children with sarcomas is increased, no definite increase in risk was demonstrated for the patients' mothers or second-degree relatives. It appears likely that the vast majority of sarcomas represent new mutational events. Nevertheless, a thorough family history should be taken from all young cancer victims to assess the risk for close relatives.

A translocation between chromosome 11 and 22 is seen in both Ewing's sarcoma and peripheral neuroectodermal tumors (PNETs). These two sarcomas also share a similar pattern of oncogene expression. These observations have resulted in improved therapy for PNETs. Originally treated rather unsuccessfully on protocols for neuroblastoma, PNETs are currently treated with regimens for Ewing's sarcoma with a substantially higher response rate. Synovial sarcomas characteristically carry an X:18 translocation. Many other sarcomas possess distinct abnormalities characteristic for the histologic subtypes.

Other Risk Factors

Radiation and chemical exposures increase the risk of developing a sarcoma. Approximately 5% of new sarcoma diagnoses are associated with a history of radiotherapy. Radiation from thorium dioxide (Thorotrast) is associated with visceral angiosarcomas; external beam radiotherapy is associated with an increased risk (overall 0.46 events per million per year) of secondary osteosarcoma, fibrosarcoma, or malignant fibrous histiocytoma (MFH) at a median of 10 to 15 years (range 2–25 years) following exposure.[4] The dose of radiation is generally high, but may be only several Grays (Gy) in radium watch painters. Chemical exposure with polyvinyl chloride, arsenic, and wood preservatives are associated with hemangiosarcomas of the liver. Dioxin (Agent Orange), alkylating agents for prior childhood malignancies, and agricultural herbicides may result in a higher incidence of soft tissue sarcomas and lymphomas, although the evidence is conflicting. Asbestos is clearly related to mesothelioma. Although avian, feline, and simian sarcoma viruses exist, evidence of a viral etiology for human sarcomas is lacking. Cytomegalovirus (CMV) and human immunodeficiency virus have been associated with Kaposi's sarcoma, but a direct causal relationship between virus and Kaposi's sarcoma has not been established.

Sarcomas may be classified into two major groups: those arising in bone and those in soft tissue. Soft tissue sarcomas are further subdivided into somatic sarcomas (extremities and retroperitoneum) and visceral sarcomas (gastrointestinal and gynecologic). A miscellaneous group includes Kaposi's sarcoma and mesothelioma.

BONE SARCOMAS

Osteosarcoma is a spindle cell tumor that produces malignant osteoid. The classic central medullary osteosarcoma is a high-grade malignancy. Several variants such as parosteal, periosteal, and low-grade interosseus osteosarcoma represent lower-grade malignant lesions that are histologically and radiographically distinct from classic osteosarcoma. About 1000 new cases occur each year in the United States, with a male-to-female ratio of 1.5 : 1. The age distribution is bimodal, with the first peak in the second and third decades and the second in the sixth decade. The tumor arises in the growth plates of the long bones (distal femur, proximal tibia, and humerus) during the adolescent growth spurt (ages 10–25) or in older adults in sites of prior radiotherapy, pre-existing bone lesions, or Paget's disease. Primary lesions in the axial skeleton occur in less than 10% of pediatric patients but in 30% to 50% of adults, in whom they generally carry a worse prognosis. Extraosseous presentations are rare, but they occur in older adults. The major prognostic variables for osteosarcoma include grade (low or high), invasion through the bone cortex to involve soft tissue, and presence or absence of metastases. A significant soft tissue component may decrease the possibility of limb-sparing surgery.

Pretreatment Evaluation of Osteosarcoma

Patients with possible osteosarcoma should be referred to an experienced multimodality sarcoma service prior to biopsy. Preoperative staging should preferably be done prior to biopsy and should include bone scan, chest film, computed tomography (CT) of the chest. Evaluation of the primary tumor is performed using bone scan and magnetic resonance imaging (MRI) paying particular attention to the entire length of the involved bone and the area across the joint to look for "skip" lesions. In some cases, CT scan can complement MRI to evaluate the extent of primary tumor. A baseline angiogram may delineate the extent of invasion but, more important, defines the vascular anatomy for limb-sparing surgery and allows evaluation of response to preoperative chemotherapy by assessment of tumor blush.

The biopsy should be performed by the surgeon who is prepared to do the definitive resection. Because the radiographic picture can be virtually diagnostic, a needle biopsy may be adequate to confirm the clinical impression. An improperly placed biopsy site, particularly for proximal tibula lesions, may render limb-sparing surgery impossible. In patients referred for definitive treatment to M.D. Anderson Hospital, only 19% of biopsies were appropriately located.[5] Similarly, of patients referred to Massachusetts General Hospital, a major error in diagnosis occurred in 60%, and 18% had to have suboptimal treatment because of incorrectly placed biopsies.[6]

Treatment of Osteosarcoma

Surgical treatment of osteosarcoma should include either amputation or limb-sparing surgery. Wide excision (including a cuff of several centimeters of pathologically normal tissue combined with adjuvant chemotherapy) usually achieves local control in 90% to 97% and survival similar to that for amputation in selected patients.[7] Following limb-sparing procedures, functional results are excellent in 60% to 75% of patients. Treatment complications may occasionally necessitate amputation. Of 62 patients with no tumor recurrence, 14 required subsequent amputation for infection, dislocation, or fracture.[5]

Patients with significant neurovascular involvement or a soft tissue component, or anticipated poor function generally require amputation. Limb-sparing surgery is more successful for the non–weight-bearing upper-extremity lesions. Fractures remain important complications in athletic individuals. If the tumor develops before the adolescent growth spurt, leg length disparities can be partially averted by the use of expandable prostheses.

Osteosarcoma tends to be markedly radioresistant. Preoperative radiotherapy for osteosarcoma has not been shown to improve the rate of successful limb-sparing surgery, but it may increase the local complication rate.[7] Postoperative radiotherapy for close or positive surgical margins may increase the likelihood of local control.

Adjuvant Chemotherapy for Osteosarcoma

Early trials of adjuvant chemotherapy were prompted by the less than 20% 5-year disease-free survival of surgically treated osteosarcoma patients. Although these studies produced an actuarial disease-free survival of 50% to 80%, the results were challenged by retrospective analysis of the Mayo Clinic data from 1963 to 1974, which revealed that disease-free survival for cohorts of patients treated with surgery alone improved from 13% for patients treated between 1963 and 1968 to 42% for patients treated between 1972 and 1974.[8]

Three small randomized trials subsequently compared multiagent adjuvant chemotherapy with observation. Adjuvant vincristine and high-dose methotrexate were not significantly better than observation alone in the Mayo Clinic study.[9] However, the other two studies from the Pediatric Oncology Group (POG) and University of California at Los Angeles (UCLA) showed markedly improved 2-year disease-free survival after five and six doxorubicin and cisplatin-based drug adjuvant regimens.[7,10] Moreover, the UCLA study demonstrated survival benefit. Based on these randomized trials, intensive multiagent chemotherapy has been established as the standard of care. The regimens and outcomes are shown in Table 33–1. The optimal combination of agents and schedule is not yet established.

TABLE 33–1. RANDOMIZED TRIALS OF ADJUVANT CHEMOTHERAPY FOR OSTEOSARCOMA WITH AN OBSERVATION CONTROL ARM

		OBSERVATION			THERAPY			
INSTITUTION	REGIMEN	N	%DFS	%S	N	%DFS	%S	p
Mayo Clinic	MV	18	44	62	20	40	80	NS
POG	MABCDP	18	17		18	66		<.001
UCLA	MABCD	28	39	65	27	59	86	.005

M = high-dose methotrexate; P = cisplatin; V = vincristine; A = doxorubicin; C = cyclophosphamide; B = bleomycin; D = actinomycin D; DFS = disease-free survival; S = survival (2–5 years); POG = Pediatric Oncology Group; UCLA = University of California at Los Angeles.

Preoperative chemotherapy has many theoretical advantages over postoperative adjuvant chemotherapy. Preoperative chemotherapy may increase the feasibility of limb-sparing surgery with preservation of muscle groups and better function. Early systemic treatment without the month-long delay required for healing postoperatively may more effectively eradicate microscopic metastatic deposits and decrease the potential for viable tumor spread. The delay in surgery also allows the surgeon to obtain the correct size of prosthesis if a knee-joint replacement is contemplated. Response to preoperative chemotherapy can be evaluated histologically and/or angiographically, and the regimen modified, if the response is suboptimal. Tumor necrosis of >90% in tumors resected after preopreative chemotherapy is associated with better survival and local control.[11] Resolution of tumor vascularity on angiography correlates with histologic necrosis. For patients with <90% tumor necrosis, the postoperative use of other effective agents may increase disease-free survival of this poor-prognosis group to 40%, although more effective agents are still needed. Potential risks of preoperative chemotherapy include increased local and distant failure rates for the few patients with a poor response to therapy. Any evidence of progression should lead to prompt resection. A POG study comparing pre- with postoperative adjuvant chemotherapy has been completed and is undergoing analysis. The current POG intergroup trial is evaluating the role of ifosamide and a biological response modifier liposomal muramyl tripeptide.

The rationale for intra-arterial therapy is to increase local drug concentrations to the tumor. With doxorubicin, there is no advantage to intra-arterial therapy.[12] Intra-arterial cisplatin does produce a greater pathologic response than intravenous cisplatin, with a low risk of vasculitis.[5] Although local control is usually obtained, the increased local tumor response may no longer correlate with the response of micrometastatic disease, which ultimately kills patients. Thus, using intra-arterial chemotherapy to enhance local concentrations at the potential expense of systemic concentrations may not prove a worthwhile objective.

Metastatic Osteosarcoma

Between 20% and 40% of patients who undergo complete resection of pulmonary metastases are cured. Statistics may be more favorable if surgery and chemotherapy can be combined, especially when patients present with metastatic disease at diagnosis.

Most patients who develop metastases have already received adjuvant chemotherapy. If there had been an interval of 6 months or longer since the last adjuvant treatment, readministration of the same drugs might achieve palliation. The most active single agents are doxorubicin, high-dose methotrexate, cisplatin, and ifosfamide. Cyclophosphamide, melphalan, mitomycin C, and dacarbazine have response rates about 15%. Palliation with standard agents is less common if progression occurred within 6 months. These patients would be candidates for new agents.

Ewing's Sarcoma

Ewing's sarcoma, a disease predominantly affecting adolescents (range 5–30 years), is easily distinguished from osteosarcoma. Patients complain of fever, weight loss, malaise, and poorly localized bone pain in the area of the primary lesion. Flat bones and the diaphyses of long bones are involved, frequently with a prominent soft tissue component. Like in PNET, the cell of origin is unknown, but cytogenetics reveal an 11/22 translocation in most cases. Up to a third of patients present with clinically detectable metastases involving the lung, bone, and bone marrow. Poor prognostic features include pelvic, humoral, or rib primaries, age >16 years, a high level of lactate dehydrogenase, and extensive soft tissue involvement. Although 60% disease-free survival may be observed in patients who present with localized disease treated with multimodality therapy, fewer than 30% of those with metastases survive. Pretreatment evaluation should include chest x-ray and CT scan of the primary and lungs, bone scan, and bone marrow aspirate and biopsy.

Ewing's sarcoma is a systemic disease at presentation,

since >90% die if treated with surgical resection alone. The additions of doxorubicin to adjuvant vincristine, actinomycin-D, and cyclophosphamide (VACA) provided a survival advantage. Recently a survival advantage for VACA alternating with ifosfamide and etoposide was reported compared with VACA alone (80% vs. 56% at 3 years). Despite greater toxicity, the magnitude of this effect supports the recommendation that the alternating regimen represents state of the art therapy.[35] Radiotherapy to about 6000 cGy delivered to the primary tumor during the fourth or fifth cycle of chemotherapy controls the local disease in most patients, with good functional results. Surgical resection may enhance the likelihood of local control beyond that of radiotherapy alone.

Thus, resection seems appropriate if the Ewing's sarcoma arises in an expendable bone or if biopsy after radiotherapy and chemotherapy reveals residual viable tumor. Dose intensity has shown promising results in some European trials using high-dose chemotherapy consolidation with autologous marrow support following conventional-dose induction therapy.

Other Bone Sarcomas

Chondrosarcoma, fibrous sarcoma, malignant giant cell tumors of the bone, and malignant fibrous histiocytoma are less responsive to chemotherapy, and their treatment is usually similar to that for soft tissue sarcomas.

SOFT TISSUE SARCOMAS

Soft tissue sarcomas cause a mass, swelling, or pain in the trunk or extremities. Retroperitoneal tumors generally present late with weight loss or deep-seated pain. Gynecologic and gastrointestinal sarcomas most frequently present with bleeding. Approximately 40% present in the lower extremity, 30% in the trunk and retroperitoneum, and 15% each in the upper extremity and the head and neck.

Biopsy

Any mass with measurable growth or any mass greater than 5 cm in diameter must be regarded with suspicion, particularly if it is firm, deep, or fixed. Biopsy should be undertaken by the surgeon who is prepared to perform the definitive resection; the biopsy site must be carefully selected to allow subsequent resection and radiation of the tumor bed with maximum function preservation. An incisional biopsy (or excisional biopsy for lesions <3 cm in diameter) is recommended.

The principal prognostic and management variables are presented by the tumor grade, size, margins of resection, and histologic subtype. The tumor grade as measured by the number of mitoses per 10 high-power fields (hpf), degree of cellularity, cell necrosis, and anaplasia serves as an accurate measure of biological aggressiveness by correlating with proliferative thrust, likelihood of metastasis, and survival. Size is an independent prognostic factor that correlates with both local and distant failure and reflects a composite of several factors: natural history, tumor growth rate, anatomical localization, and the ability of the tumor to traverse fascial planes into other tissue compartments (*i.e.*, intramuscular, intracompartmental, or extracompartmental involvement). The margins of resection and the location of tumor determine whether optimal local-regional therapy can be delivered. Although multiple histologic subtypes are recognized, with few exception— such as rhabdomyosarcoma, the biological behavior of soft tissue sarcoma appears similar enough that the histologic subtype contributes little to clinical decisions. The American Joint Committee Staging System is shown in Table 33–2.[13]

Initial evaluation staging should include plain film and MRI or CT scan of the primary tumor. MRI appears to be superior to the CT scan in the definition of soft tissue planes and tumor margins. A positive bone scan adjacent to a deep extremity tumor suggests but is not diagnostic of bone involvement, decreasing the feasibility of limb-sparing surgery. A chest radiograph and, if normal, a chest CT scan should be performed. A CT scan of the liver, abdomen, and pelvis should be obtained for visceral sarcomas but is needed for extremity sarcomas only if hepatic function is abnormal.

Surgical Considerations

Definitive resection requires either a wide surgical excision with 2 to 4 cm of pathologically documented margins of normal tissue, or pre- or postoperative radiotherapy with conservative resection that includes pathologically documented tumor-free margins. The biopsy site should be excised with the definitive resection *en bloc*. If microscopically involved margins are documented, re-excision is preferable. Common surgical mistakes include "shelling out" or removal of tumor in pieces after surprise diagnosis. Both procedures result in seeding of the entire surgical field and a high local failure rate. Wide re-excision should then be performed, followed by high-dose radiotherapy. Radiation alone should not be relied on to sterilize a field after clearly inadequate surgery. At surgery, the *en bloc* resection must be oriented with delineation of the margins so that the pathologist can accurately determine the resection margins. The extent of the surgical field should be marked with clips to guide subsequent therapy. With optimal approaches, local control rates are 90% to 95%, 50% to 75%, and 30% to 50% for extremity, truncal, and retroperitoneal sarcomas, respectively. For truncal and retroperitoneal sarcomas, local control is hampered by technical difficulties in obtaining adequate surgical margins and the poor tolerance of adjacent normal tissues of high-dose radiotherapy. Surgical expertise is paramount. Jaques and colleagues reported that in the Memorial Sloan-Kettering

TABLE 33–2. AJCC STAGING SYSTEM FOR SOFT TISSUE SARCOMAS

PRIMARY TUMOR (T)	
TX	Minimum requirements to assess the primary tumor cannot be met.
T0	No demonstrable tumor
T1	Tumor <5 cm in diameter
T2	Tumor ≥5 cm in diameter
TUMOR GRADE (G)	
G1	Well-differentiated
G2	Moderately well differentiated
G3	Poorly differentiated
NODAL INVOLVEMENT (N)	
NX	Minimum requirements to assess the regional nodes cannot be met
N0	No histologically verified metastases to lymph nodes
N1	Histologically verified regional lymph node metastasis
DISTANT METASTASIS (M)	
MX	Minimum requirements to assess the presence of distant metastasis cannot be met
M0	No (known) distant metastasis
M1	Distant metastasis present
STAGE GROUPING	
STAGE I	
IA	G1, T1, N0, M0
IB	G1, T2, N0, M0
STAGE II	
IIA	G2, T1, N0, M0
IIB	G2, T2, N0, M0
STAGE III	
IIIA	G3, T1, N0, M0
IIIB	G3, T2, N0, M0
IIIC	G1–3, T1–2, N0, M0, neurovascular bundle involvement
STAGE IV	
IVA	G1–3, T1–2, N1, M0
IVB	G1–3, T1–2, N0–1, M1

AJCC = American Joint Committee on Cancer

Cancer Center experience with retroperitoneal sarcomas, fully 55% of the patients deemed inoperable at other centers had complete resection with acceptable operative morbidity. Complete resection was associated with improved survival.[14]

The majority of patients with extremity primaries are suitable for function-preserving surgery. The local control rate of >90% and overall disease-free survival of 60% are similar to that seen after amputation or radical resection. Preoperative chemotherapy or radiotherapy may improve the potential for limb-sparing surgery in borderline resectable tumors. If tumor recurs locally, resection is possible, although half of all patients require amputation.

Radiotherapy

The National Cancer Institute (NCI) conducted a randomized trial that demonstrated that limb-sparing surgery and radiotherapy result in equivalent survival to amputation.[15] Although there is no direct comparison of conservative surgery with or without radiotherapy, local recurrence rates with radiotherapy are generally between 0% and 15%, whereas the local failure rate in a trial from the Mayo Clinic in which radiotherapy was not used was 30% (Table 33–3). Thus, pre- or postoperative radiotherapy would be recommended when pathologically documented tumor margins are less than 2 to 4 cm in all directions. Occasionally, complete resection is not possible because of involvement of vital structures. The use of brachytherapy, heavy-particle radiotherapy, hyperthermia, or radiation-enhancing agents may improve the local control. The delivery of radiotherapy after resection of visceral or retroperitoneal sarcomas remains controversial in that adequate dose delivery is rarely possible. There are conflicting reports on whether intraoperative radiotherapy (IORT) accompanied by external beam radiotherapy can improve disease-free survival.

Preoperative radiotherapy is advocated by some investigators despite the potential for delayed wound healing. Treatment volumes are smaller, and the viability of the tumor at surgery might be reduced, theoretically reducing the chance for dissemination during surgery. Preoperative radiotherapy may increase the ability to attain complete resection and/or limb-sparing surgery for borderline, operable large sarcomas. Advantages for postoperative radiotherapy are that it can treat the entire surgical field and let the pathologists assess a nonirradiated specimen. There is no direct randomized comparison of pre- and postoperative radiotherapy: either seems appropriate. An initial dose of 5000 cGy in 200-cGy fractions should be delivered to the entire compartment and surgical field with at least a 5-cm margin. A boost using a shrinking field technique to the tumor bed includes an additional 1000 cGy and a boost of 600 cGy more to the scar. At least one third of the circumference of the extremity should be spared, (*i.e.*, 2 or 4 cm on the forearm or thigh, respectively), to prevent lymphedema.

Adjuvant Chemotherapy

Although local control of sarcomas has improved with advances in surgery and radiotherapy, 40% to 60% of patients with high-grade tumors die of metastatic disease despite primary control. Although randomized trials clearly establish a role for adjuvant chemotherapy in management of osteosarcoma, Ewing's sarcoma, and rhabdomyosarcoma, the role of adjuvant therapy for soft tissue sarcomas remains controversial.[16]

Table 33–4 summarizes randomized adjuvant soft tissue sarcoma trials with observation control arms. Seven studies used single-agent doxorubicin, and five used combination

TABLE 33–3. RANDOMIZED ADJUVANT TRIALS: SOFT TISSUE SARCOMAS COMBINATION CHEMOTHERAPY AND SINGLE-AGENT DOXORUBICIN STUDIES IN ORDER OF PATIENT NUMBER

INSTITUTE	DRUGS	MEDIAN MO FU	STAGE	N	% DFS –	% DFS +	% S –	% S +
EORTC	ACVD	44	I–IVA	468	61	61	68	74
NCI	ACM	85	IIA–IVA	104				
Extremities		60		67	28	54*	60	54
Trunk		36		22	47	77*	61	82
Retroperitoneal		24		15	49	92	100*	47
Bordeaux	ACVD	40	IIB–IVA	59	37	65*	43	83*
MD Anderson	ACVAd	>120	IIB/IIIB	47	83	76	NA	NA
Mayo Clinic	AVDAd	64	I–IVB	61	68	65	70	70
GOG	A	60	FIGO I–II	156	45	60	47	60
Scandinavian	A	22	III/IVA	139	44	40	55	52
UCLA	A	28	III	119	52	56	70	80
ISTSS	A	20	IIB–IVA	86	55	73	49	67
Rizzoli Institute	A	106	III/IVA	76	25	56*	49	63
DFCI/MGH	A	>46	IIB–IVA	46	62	67	72	71
ECOG	A	>59	IIB–IVA	36	55	66	52	65

MO = months; FU = follow-up; DFS = disease-free survival; S = survival; EORTC = European Organization for the Research and Treatment of Cancer; NCI = National Cancer Institute; GOG = Gynecologic Oncology Group; UCLA = University of California at Los Angeles; ISTSS = Intergroup Soft Tissue Sarcoma Study; DFCI = Dana Farber Cancer Institute; MGH = Massachusetts General Hospital; ECOG = Eastern Cooperative Oncology Group; A = doxorubicin; C = cyclophosphamide; V = vincristine; D = actinomycin D; M = methotrexate; Ad = actinomycin; FIGO = International Federation of Gynecology and Obstetrics; + = treated; – = control.

chemotherapy. Overall, one study from Bordeaux of 59 patients continues to show a significant survival advantage for therapy.[17] Three other studies of extremity lesions demonstrate significant disease-free, but not overall, survival advantages.[18–21] In the NCI study, whereas the extremity-lesion subset enjoyed a disease-free survival benefit, the retroperitoneal primary subset experienced a significant survival disadvantage for the chemotherapy-treated arm. The regimen used was toxic: 14% had doxorubicin-induced congestive heart failure, and there was an 18% withdrawal rate due to gastrointestinal and hematologic toxicity.[19]

Although many of the studies demonstrate a trend toward

TABLE 33–4. RANDOMIZED ADJUVANT TRIALS IN EXTREMITY SOFT TISSUE SARCOMAS (STUDIES LIMITED TO EXTREMITY SARCOMAS AND SUBSET ANALYSIS OF STUDIES THAT INCLUDED SARCOMAS IN OTHER SITES) IN ORDER OF PATIENT NUMBER

INSTITUTE	DRUGS	N	% LC –	% LC +	% DFS –	% DFS +	% S –	% S +
EORTC	CAVD	233	90	90	52	67	74	79
NCI	ACM	67	86	97	28	54*	54	60
Mayo Clinic	AVDAd	48	75	67	67	88	83	63
MD Anderson	ACVAd	43	65	90	35	54	36	65
Scandinavian	A	139	91	91	55	52	44	40
UCLA	A	119	90	90	52	56	70	80
Rizzoli	A	76	75	88	25	56*	49	63
ISSG	A	41	NA	NA	58	78	39	81
DFCI/MGH	A	26	94	100	71	90	81	89
ECOG	A	18	100	100	63	70	63	61

% LC = percent with local control; for explanations of the other abbreviations see the footnote to Table 34–3.

*$p < .05$

improved survival or disease-free survival, in three studies (Eastern Cooperative Oncology Group, Scandinavian, and Mayo Clinic), the survival time of the treatment arm is slightly less than that of controls. Several trials had promising results at the initial report, but with subsequent late relapses the advantages of chemotherapy waned. The association of therapy with 10% serious morbidity and mortality, particularly related to myelosuppression and cardiac toxicity, offset the potential improvement in disease-free survival. At present, adjuvant chemotherapy should not be considered standard outside a prospective randomized trial. Adjuvant chemotherapy randomized trials using a doxorubicin and ifosfamide combinatin should be considered for patients with high-grade large (>5 cm) lesions who have adequate local regional control. Fractionated-dose doxorubicin and greater sophistication in managing myelosuppression might decrease therapeutic risks. Thus, an assessment of the therapeutic index should be re-explored.

Therapy for Metastatic Sarcoma

SURGICAL RESECTION OF PULMONARY NODULES

The presence of metastatic pulmonary disease, either at presentation or relapse, does not preclude cure.[22] A number of studies have reported a 10% to 40% disease-free survival after resection of limited numbers (<5–15) of pulmonary metastases. Patients should meet the following criteria:

1. The primary site must be controlled.
2. The patient must be a candidate for surgery.
3. No extrapulmonary metastases may be present.
4. The pulmonary disease must be completely resectable.

Survival statistics are generally higher for osteosarcoma and somewhat lower for soft tissue sarcoma. Surgical resection of Ewing's sarcoma metastases has not seemed worthwhile. Prognostic variables in some, but not other, studies include longer survival for those with a disease-free interval of more than 1 year, a doubling time of more than 20 days, fewer than five pulmonary nodules, and resection of all gross disease with clean margins.[22] The NCI study had no long-term survivors with soft tissue sarcomas that had a doubling time of less than 20 days.[22] Involvement of parietal pleura or mediastinal structures usually precludes resection.

The surgeon is generally able to find about twice the number of pulmonary metastases detected by CT scan. Most surgeons are unwilling to consider resection when more than ten lesions are visible on CT scan. Although some surgeons advocate a period of observation to calculate tumor doubling time and to see if extrapulmonary metastases develop, others advocate scheduling surgery as soon as possible to prevent tumor growth. Whether video-assisted thoracoscopy (VATS) will provide adequate surgical exposure for complete metastatectomy will be studied in a prospective trial. Some patients who have developed additional nodules can be salvaged by repeated thoracotomy.

Guidelines for the combination of chemotherapy before or after thoracotomy have not been established. Preoperative therapy at least allows an evaluation of response. One reasonable approach but never rigorously studied is to administer a course or two of chemotherapy preoperatively and, if a response is observed, to continue postoperative chemotherapy. Few data are available on surgical resection of metastatic disease involving other sites, such as bone or liver. These are generally treated palliatively with chemotherapy. For patients with very-low-grade indolent tumors, localized therapy of metastatic lesions using surgery or radiotherapy can provide excellent palliation.

CHEMOTHERAPY FOR ADVANCED SARCOMA

Table 33–5 summarizes randomized evaluations of chemotherapy in soft tissue sarcoma. Only two single agents have more than a 20% response rate. Single-agent doxorubicin (and its analog, epirubicin) have response rates of 15% to 35%. A dose-response relationship has been observed with higher response rates at doses greater than 50 mg/m^2 every 3 weeks. Doxorubicin is less cardiotoxic when administered by divided doses over 3 or 4 days.

Ifosfamide yields response rates of 20% to 40% in previously treated patients. It produced less myelotoxicity and doubled the response rate of cyclophosphamide. In Europe the dose schedule most commonly used is 5 g/m^2 delivered over 24 hours.[23] In the United States, fractionated doses of 6 to 10 g/m^2 divided over 4 or 5 days with mesna uroprotection is most often used.

Dimethyl triazinoimidazole carboxamide (DTIC) has a single-agent response rate of 17%. Nausea is decreased by continuous-infusion administration. The ECOG and the Gynecologic Oncology Group trials demonstrated improved response rates for doxorubicin and DTIC over doxorubicin alone.[24–26] However, in both studies, nausea and vomiting were increased in the group receiving DTIC. Other commercially available agents have borderline activity. Phase II trials of taxol are not yet reported.

The two leading combination chemotherapy regimens are cyclophosphamide, doxorubicin, and DTIC (CYADIC) and mesna, Adriamycin, and ifosfamide ± DTIC (MAID).[27] With aggressive dosing, response rates of 40% to 57% and 11% complete response have been observed. With less intensive dose schedules in cooperative group trials, lower activity has been observed.

Three randomized trials have compared doxorubicin-containing therapy with or without ifosfamide. In the CALGB/SWOG trial, ifosfamide was added to full-dose doxorubicin and DTIC.[28] Ifosfamide markedly increased toxicity and response rates. However, disease-free and overall survival times were not affected. In the two other reported randomized trials from EORTC[29] and ECOG,[30] the planned doxorubicin dose was reduced when combined in the ifosfamide arm. There were no noted advantages in response rate or in disease-free or overall survival. Other randomized

TABLE 33–5. RANDOMIZED TRIALS OF IN MEASURABLE SOFT-TISSUE SARCOMA*

	GROUP	REGIMEN	N	% CR	% RR	MS	COMMENTS
STUDIES COMPARING THE ADDITION OF DTIC							
Omura	GOG	A	80	6	16		Uterine sarcoma only
		AD	66	11	24		
Lerner	ECOG	A	34	3	18		Leiomyosarcomas only
		AD	32	3	44		
Borden	ECOG	A q3wk	93	6	19		A 15 mg/m^2 wk
		A qwk	92	4	16		A 70 mg/m^2 q 3 wk
		AD	95	6	30		
Benjamin	SWOG	ACVD	221	14	52		
		ACVAd	224	12	40		
STUDIES EVALUATING THE ADDITION OF CYCLOPHOSPHAMIDE							
Schoenfield	ECOG	A	66	6	27		A 70 mg/m^2
		ACV	70	4	19		A 50 mg/m^2
		CVAd	64	2	11		A 0 mg/m^2
Baker	SWOG	AD	79	14	32		
		ADC	95	13	35		
		ADAd	98	9	24		
		AC	54	2	20		
STUDIES EVALUATING DOSE AND SCHEDULE							
Baker	SWOG	AD	135	7	19		Bolus
		AD	143	10	18		Continuous infusion
Brennan/Casper	MSKCC	A	38	N/A = adjuvant therapy			Bolus
		A	44	N/A = adjuvant therapy			Continuous infusion
Bodey	SWOG	ADCV	27	15	67		A 50 mg/m^2 C 500 mg/m^2
		ADCV	24	33	71		A 80 mg/m^2 C 800 mg/m^2
Pinedo	EORTC	ADCV	71	20	38		Full dose rate
		ADCV	74	5	14		Half dose rate
STUDIES EVALUATING IFOSFAMIDE							
Bramwell	EORTC	I	68	2	18		5 g/m^2
		C	67	1	8		1.5 g/m^2
Antman	CALGB/SWOG	AD	170	2	17	13	
		ADI	166	4	*32	12	Older patients, more toxicity
Santoro	EORTC	A	212	4	24	12	
		AI	202	6	27	12	
		ACD	135	8	28	12	
Edmonson	ECOG	A	90	2	20	9	
		AI	88	3	*34	12	Younger patients did better
		MAP	84	7	32	9	

I = ifosfamide; A = doxorubicin; D = dacarbazine; C = cyclophosphamide; M = mitomycin C; P = cisplatin; Ad = actinomycin D; V = vincristine; N = # evaluable patients; CR = complete response; RR = % responding; MS = median survival; GOG = Gynecologic Oncology Group; ECOG = Eastern Cooperative Oncology Group; SWOG = Southwest Oncology Group; MSKCC = Memorial Sloan-Kettering Cancer Center; EORTC = European Organization for Research and Treatment of Cancer; CALGB = Cancer and Leukemia Group B.

*Updated from Cancer Treatment Symposia 3:110, 1985.

trials have established that cyclophosphamide and vincristine add nothing to single-agent doxorubicin, in part because of the dose compromise of doxorubicin necessitated by additive myelosuppression.

Thus, combination chemotherapy is likely to produce increased tumor response rates over single-agent sequential therapy at the expense of increased toxicity. For clinical situations in which response may be important, such as preoperative therapy or adjuvant or quasi-adjuvant settings, combination therapy would be recommended. For situations in which metastatic disease exists, sequential single-agent therapy can be recommended. Because doxorubicin is more easily administered and tolerated than ifosfamide, it is generally used first. These patients would also be candidates for novel agents.

Special Problems

Rhabdomyosarcoma, a malignancy of striated muscle, has three histologic variants. Embryonal rhabdomyosarcoma usually arises in genitourinary or orbital sites in 2- to 6-year-old children; alveolar rhabdomyosarcoma in extremity lesions in adolescents; and pleomorphic rhabdomyosarcoma in adults over 40 years of age. Many of the pleomorphic rhabdomyosarcomas would be reclassified as malignant fibrous histiocytoma by recently trained pathologists. Twenty percent of rhabdomyosarcoma patients will have lymph node metastases (rarely with orbital primary tumors). Most patients have apparently localized disease at diagnosis. Without intensive chemotherapy, 80% will relapse in distant sites, usually lung, lymph nodes, and bone marrow. Clinical evaluation should include x-ray film of the primary, CT scan of the chest, bone scan, and bilateral bone marrow aspirates and biopsies. For parameningeal primary tumors, head CT and spinal fluid examination are recommended. The most important prognostic factor is the presence of metastases, which reduces the 5-year survival to 20% to 30% despite intensive multimodality therapy. Other adverse findings include nodal involvement, large lesions, invasion through fascial planes, and inability to completely resect known disease.

Where extensive surgery would be disfiguring, (*i.e.*, orbital tumors), lesions may be biopsied and treated with radiotherapy and chemotherapy; otherwise, complete resection is attempted. Variations of the VACA chemotherapy regimen are used. Unlike in Ewing's sarcoma, the addition of doxorubicin has not increased survival in randomized studies of rhabdomyosarcoma. In general, organ preservation is possible with primary chemotherapy. Good-prognosis patients can probably be treated with less intensive two-agent chemotherapy. For patients with advanced disease, the addition of ifosfamide, etoposide, and cisplatin is being explored.

Visceral Sarcomas

Gastrointestinal sarcomas are generally leiomyosarcomas that present with pain and bleeding. Obstruction, intussusception, perforation, and fistula formation are rare. Gastrointestinal sarcomas arise in the stomach (62%), small intestine (29%), or colon (10%). Liver, lung, and intraperitoneal seeding are the most frequent metastatic sites. The 5-year survival is 35% to 50%. Subtotal excision results in poor prognosis. The response rate to chemotherapy appears equivalent to that of soft tissue sarcomas in other locations.

Gynecologic sarcomas represent 1% of gynecologic malignancies and 1% to 6% of uterine tumors. Uterine sarcomas are histologically either homologous or heterologous (*i.e.*, derived from mesenchymal tissue normally present or absent in the uterus, respectively). Tumors that contain both sarcomas and epithelial elements are called mixed mesodermal sarcomas. Uterine smooth muscle tumors constitute a continuum of lesions from benign (fibroids) to malignant high-grade leiomyosarcomas. Leiomyosarcomas have more than ten mitoses per 10 hpf (or 5–10 mitoses per 10 hpf with anaplasia, pleomorphism, or epithelial histology). Well-differentiated lesions with 2 to 4 mitoses per 10 hpf are "of uncertain malignant potential." "Metastasizing leiomyoma" and "intravenous leiomyomatosis," are benign lesions, often associated with pregnancy, which may spontaneously regress or may respond to hormonal therapy. The incidence of degeneration of leiomyomata to malignancy is low (less than 0.13%). In postmenopausal women, leiomyosarcomas will increase in size, whereas fibroids should involute.

Endometrial stromal cell tumors include three variants: benign stromal nodules, low-grade endometrial stromal meiosis, and high-grade endometrial stromal sarcoma. The differential diagnoses include lymphoma or small cell carcinoma of the cervix. Single cells or small clumps of cells surrounded by reticulum fibers on reticulum stain indicate a stromal sarcoma.

Presenting symptoms of uterine sarcomas include heavy, irregular vaginal bleeding and an abdominal mass or pain. The pelvic examination may be normal in 20%. Although dilatation and curettage is diagnostic for endometrial stromal cell sarcomas, it may yield negative results in leiomyosarcoma and may be misleading in mixed müllerian tumors in that only one type of tissue may be obtained. Preoperative staging should include CT scans of the chest, abdomen, and pelvis. Total abdominal hysterectomy and bilateral salpingo-oophorectomy is the treatment of choice for local disease. Pre- or postoperative radiotherapy decreases the local recurrence rate but does not affect survival and frequently precludes delivery of adequate doses of subsequent chemotherapy.

Kaposi's Sarcoma

Kaposi's sarcoma (multiple idiopathic hemorrhagic sarcoma), when it presents as an indolent tumor of the lower extremities of men of Mediterranean origin, is generally treated with surgical resection or radiotherapy. If it is systemic, low doses of vinblastine or doxorubicin are frequently effective. Secondary tumors, especially lymphomas, are common. Kaposi's sarcoma in renal transplant patients and other immunocompromised hosts may respond to a decrease in immunosuppressive therapy. A highly aggressive form of Kaposi's sarcoma is associated with acquired immunodeficiency syndrome (AIDS). AIDS-associated Kaposi's sarcoma frequently involves lymph nodes, mucous membranes, and viscera. When Kaposi's sarcoma occurs in the absence of opportunistic infection, prognosis is more favorable, with a median survival of 29 months. Radiotherapy may be used for localized lesions with good local control. A variety of chemotherapy agents have been used, including etoposide, vinblastine, DTIC, bleomycin, actinomycin D, and doxorubicin, but with exacerbation of host immunosuppression. Alpha-interferon has also been effective. Therapy directed against the AIDS-associated Kaposi's sarcoma does not alter the course of AIDS and eventual death from opportunistic infection.

Mesothelioma

About 50% to 75% of mesotheliomas are associated with asbestos exposure that occurs 20 to 40 or more years prior to diagnosis.[31] Patients present with chest pain, shortness of breath, and unilateral pleural effusion, frequently with the physical finding of scoliosis. There is no standard therapy, although a number of institutions have investigational programs. Of 52 patients treated with extrapleural pneumonectomy, low-dose chemotherapy, and radiotherapy, survival was 70% at 1 year and 48% at 2 years.[32] Patients with histologically documented clean margins, epithelial histology (as opposed to sarcomatoid or mixed variants), and negative mediastinal nodes had more favorable outcomes (45% 5-year survival). Decortication with partial debulking may provide palliation. Chest tube sclerosis can preclude surgical approaches.

Drugs with activity include doxorubicin, ifosfamide, and mitomycin C. Trials evaluating edatrexate and taxol demonstrate activity, but are ongoing. In a randomized study, in measurable disease cisplatin plus mitomycin C and cisplatin and doxorubicin produced a 25% response rate each. In both arms, median times to failure and survival were about 4 and 8 months, respectively.[33]

In patients with peritoneal mesothelioma, intraperitoneal doxorubicin and cisplatin after debulking surgery and followed by total abdominal radiotherapy has resulted in 5-year disease-free survival in four of six patients entered in a pilot study. Currently about 20% of 20 patients entered in a much less restricted study remain disease-free with 2- to 3-year follow-up.[34]

REFERENCES

1. Cance WG, Brennan MF, Dudas ME et al. Altered expression of the retinoblastoma gene product in human sarcomas. N Engl J Med 323:1457–1462, 1990
2. Malkin D, Li FP, Strong LC et al. Germ line p53 mutations in a familial syndrome of breast cancer, sarcomas, and other neoplasms. Science 250:1233–1238, 1990
3. Menon AG, Anderson KM, Riccardi VM et al. Chromosome 17p deletions and p53 gene mutations associated with the formation of malignant neurofibrosarcomas in von Recklinghausen neurofibromatosis. Proc Natl Acad Sci USA 87:5435–5439, 1990
4. Taghian A, de Vathaire F, Terrier P et al. Long-term risk of sarcoma following radiation treatment for breast cancer. Int J Radiat Oncol Biol Phys 21:3361–3367, 1991
5. Murray JA, Jessup K, Romsdahl M et al. Limb-salvage study in osteosarcoma: Early experience at MD Anderson Hospital and Tumor Institute. Cancer Treat Symp 3:131–137, 1985
6. Mankin HJ, Lange TA, Spanier S. The hazards of biopsy in patients with malignant primary bone and soft-tissue tumors. J Bone Joint Surg [Am] 64:1121–1127, 1982
7. Eilber F, Guiliano A, Eckhardt J et al. Adjuvant chemotherapy for osteosarcoma: A randomized prospective trial. J Clin Oncol 5:21–26, 1987
8. Taylor WF, Ivins JC, Dahlin DC et al. Trends and variability in survival from osteosarcoma. Mayo Clin Proc 53:695–700, 1978
9. Edmonson J, Green S, Ivins J et al. A controlled pilot study of high-dose methotrexate as postsurgical adjuvant treatment for primary osteosarcoma. J Clin Oncol 2:152–156, 1984
10. Link M, Goorin A, Miser A et al. The effect of adjuvant chemotherapy on relapse-free survival in patients with osteosarcoma of the extremity. N Engl J Med 314:1600–1606, 1986
11. Winkler K, Beron G, Delling G et al. Neoadjuvant chemotherapy of osteosarcoma: Results of a randomized cooperative trial (COSS-82) with salvage chemotherapy based on histological tumor response. J Clin Oncol 6:329–337, 1988
12. Jaffe N, Robertson R, Ayala A et al. Comparison of intra-arterial cis-diamminedichloroplatinum II with high-dose methotrexate and citrovorum factor rescue in the treatment of primary osteosarcoma. J Clin Oncol 3:1101–1104, 1985
13. American Joint Committee on Cancer. Manual for Staging of Cancer, 2nd ed. Philadelphia, JB Lippincott, 1983:115
14. Jaques DP, Coit DG, Hajdu SI et al. Management of primary and recurrent soft-tissue sarcoma of the retroperitoneum. Ann Surg 212:51–59, 1990
15. Rosenberg SA, Tepper J, Gladstein E. The treatment of soft-tissue sarcomas of the extremities: Prospective randomized evaluation of (1) limb-sparing surgery plus radiation therapy compared with amputation and (2) the role of adjuvant chemotherapy. Ann Surg 196:305–315, 1982
16. Elias AD, Antman KH. Adjuvant chemotherapy for soft-tissue sarcoma: An approach in search of an effective regimen. Semin Oncol 16:1–7, 1989
17. Ravaud A, Nguyen BB, Coindre JM et al. Adjuvant chemotherapy with CyVADIC in high-risk soft tissue sarcoma: A randomized prospective trial. In Salmon SE (ed): Adjuvant Therapy of Cancer VI, Philadelphia, WB Saunders, 1990:556–566
18. Chang A, Kinsella T, Glatstein E et al. Adjuvant chemotherapy for patients with high-grade soft-tissue sarcomas of the extremity. J Clin Oncol 6:1491–1500, 1988
19. Baker AR, Chang AE, Glatstein E et al. National Cancer

Institute experience in the management of high-grade extremity soft tissue sarcomas. In Ryan JR, Baker LH (ed): Recent Concepts in Sarcoma Treatment, Dordrecht, the Netherlands, Kluwer Academic, 1988:123–130

20. Gherlinzoni F, Bacci G, Picci P, Campana R et al. A randomized trial for the treatment of high-grade soft-tissue sarcomas of the extremities: Preliminary observations. J Clin Oncol 4:552–558, 1986
21. Gherlinzoni F, Picci P, Bacci G et al. Late results of a randomized trail for the treatment of soft tissue sarcomas (STS) of the extremities in adult patients. Proc ASCO 12:468 (1633), 1993
22. Todd TR. Pulmonary metastatectomy: Current indications for removing lung metastases. Chest 103 (suppl): 401S–403S, 1993
23. Bramwell V, Mouridsen H, Santoro G et al. Cyclophosphamide vs ifosfamide: Final report of a randomized phase II trial in adult soft tissue sarcoma. Eur J Cancer Clin Oncol 23:311–321, 1987
24. Lerner H, Amato D, Stevens C et al. Leiomyosarcoma: The Eastern Cooperative Oncology Group experience with 222 patients. Proc Am Assoc Cancer Res 24:142 (C-561), 1983
25. Borden EC, Amato D, Enterline HT et al. Randomized comparison of Adriamycin regimens for treatment of metastatic soft tissue sarcomas. J Clin Oncol 5:840–850, 1987
26. Omura GA, Major FJ, Blessing JA et al. A randomized study of Adriamycin with and without dimethyl trazenoimidazole carboxamide in advanced uterine sarcomas. Cancer 52:626–632, 1983
27. Elias A, Ryan L, Sulkes A et al. Response to mesna, doxorubicin, ifosfamide, and dacarbazine in 108 patients with metastatic or unresectable sarcoma and no prior chemotherapy. J Clin Oncol 7:1208–1216, 1989
28. Antman KH, Crowley J, Balcerzak SP et al. An Intergroup Phase III randomized study of doxorubicin and dacarbazine with or without ifosfamide and mesna in advanced tissue and bone sarcomas. J Clin Oncol 11:1276–1285, 1993
29. Santoro A, Rouesse J, Steward W et al. A randomized EORTC study in advanced soft tissue sarcomas: Adriamycin vs Adriamycin and ifosfamide vs CYVADIC. Proc ASCO 9:309 (1196), 1990
30. Edmonson JH, Ryan LM, Blum RH, et al. Randomized comparison of doxorubicin alone versus ifosfamide plus doxorubicin or mitomycin, doxorubicin, and cisplatin against advanced soft tissue sarcomas. J Clin Oncol 11:1269–1275, 1993
31. Antman KH. Natural history and epidemiology of malignant mesothelioma. Chest 103 (suppl 4):373S–376S, 1993
32. Sugarbaker DJ, Strauss GM, Lynch TJ et al. Node status has prognostic significance in the multimodality therapy of diffuse, malignant mesothelioma. J Clin Oncol 11: 1172–1178, 1993
33. Chahinian AP, Antman K, Goutsou M et al. Randomized phase II trial of cisplatin with mitomycin or doxorubicin for malignant mesothelioma by the Cancer and Leukemia Group B. J Clin Oncol 11:1559–1565, 1993
34. Weissmann L, Osteen R, Corson J et al. Combined modality therapy for intraperitoneal mesothelioma. Proc ASCO 9:274 (1063), 1990
35. Grier H, Krailo M, Link M et al. Improved outcome in nonmetastatic Ewing's sarcoma (EWS) and PNET of bone with the addition of ifosfamide (I), and etoposide (E) to vincristine (V), adriamycin (Ad), cyclophosphamide (C), and actinomycin (A): A Children's Cancer Group (CCG) and Pediatric Oncology Group (POG) report. Proc ASCO 13:421 (abstract 1443), 1994

John S. Macdonald, Daniel G. Haller, Robert J. Mayer, Eds. *Manual of Oncologic Therapeutics*, Third Edition.

34. ENDOCRINE SYSTEM

Robert E. Wittes
John S. Macdonald

THYROID CANCER

The thyroid cancers are a heterogeneous group of disorders encompassing an extraordinarily broad spectrum of clinical behavior. In the United States in 1993, 12,700 new thyroid cancers were diagnosed; there were 1100 deaths from the disease. Because of the relative rarity of these cancers, optimal approaches to many aspects of diagnosis and treatment have not been clearly defined. At the same time, the large number of thyroid nodules in the general population (prevalence estimated at about 4% of adults) means that questions about the diagnosis of thyroid neoplasia arise commonly in the practice of medicine.

The most important predisposing factor for the development of thyroid cancer is radiotherapy in infancy or childhood for various benign conditions, including thymic or tonsillar enlargement and skin diseases. The dose-response curve is relatively linear, yielding three or four cases per year per cGy per million people up to about 1270 rem of absorbed dose. Women appear to be at greater risk than men. The carcinogenic effect of radiation persists three to four decades after exposure.

Classification

Most histologic classifications of the thyroid cancers recognize the subtypes described in the following discussions.

PAPILLARY

Accounting for about two thirds of all thyroid cancer and about 80% of patients under the age of 40 years, this category includes both pure papillary carcinoma and mixtures of papillary and follicular histologies. Curiously, mixed tumors tend to behave more or less like pure papillary tumors, even when there is a significant admixture of follicular elements. Papillary cancers commonly occur in a multifocal distribution within the gland with a high incidence of cervical lymph node metastases at presentation (50–75%). About 40% of these lesions have characteristic laminated calcific spherules (psammoma bodies) whose radiologic appearance suggests the diagnosis.

The disease usually has an indolent natural history; overall survival at 10 years is approximately 80%. Indeed, lesions that are small and confined to the thyroid at diagnosis carry a negligible mortality rate. On the other hand, tumors that are very large or that invade adjacent structures from the capsule carry a significantly poorer prognosis. Surprisingly, the presence of positive regional nodes at diagnosis does not significantly worsen the prognosis. When papillary carcinoma metastasizes distantly (20% of cases), the most common site is the lungs; even with distant metastases, however, survival may be measured in decades. Occult papillary carcinoma is an incidental finding in about 5% to 10% of thyroid glands examined at autopsy.

FOLLICULAR

Pure follicular carcinoma, which constitutes about 15% of all thyroid cancers, occurs in a somewhat older population than papillary carcinoma and behaves in a more aggressive fashion. In many patients the distinction between follicular carcinoma and benign follicular adenoma cannot be made cytologically; it is only certain in the presence of capsular or blood vessel invasion or of metastases. Follicular carcinoma metastasizes to regional nodes much less frequently than papillary cancer does. Its most common distant metastatic site is bone, and the metastases are usually lytic. In fact, the amount of blastic activity is often so slight that the bone scan results may be negative even in the presence of radiologically evident bone destruction.

HÜRTHLE CELL

A rare variant of follicular carcinoma, constituting 6% of all thyroid cancers, Hürthle cell tumors tend to occur in older patients. Hürthle cell adenomas carry an excellent prognosis; however, large (>2 cm) malignant tumors have a recurrence rate as high as 60%.

MEDULLARY

Medullary tumors are of parafollicular (C-cell) origin; about 50% are familial. When detected in conventional fashion by physical examination, they almost always involve both lobes. They may also be accompanied by tumors in other endocrine glands (multiple endocrine neoplasia [MEN], Type 2A). The sporadic cases usually present with unilateral involvement. Unlike papillary cancer, cervical node involvement seems to carry adverse prognostic significance. Medullary carcinoma tends to form dense, irregular calcifications in the primary tumor and in metastases. The tumor secretes calcitonin, which is therefore a useful marker in following the course of the disease with treatment. Histology frequently shows amyloid in the tumor.

Determination of calcitonin levels, with or without pentagastrin stimulation or calcium infusion, has successfully been used in screening relatives of affected individuals; such programs have detected tumors (or C-cell hyperplasia) at an earlier stage than can conventional screening techniques, when tumors are small, unilateral, and without evidence of metastases. In MEN 2A, a genetic abnormality mapping to the centromeric region of chromosome 10 has been identified. Evidence is mounting that the ret oncogene in this location is the specific gene associated with MEN 2A. There is no doubt that in the future, molecular diagnostic techniques will be used in early diagnosis of medullary cancer or MEN 2A.

ANAPLASTIC

Anaplastic tumors, which compose about 7% of all thyroid tumors, are of the small cell and large (spindle and giant) cell varieties. They are among the most aggressive and rapidly fatal of cancers and are characterized by explosive local growth. Until recently, they have been notoriously resistant to all forms of treatment.

OTHER

Many other tumor types (*e.g.*, soft-tissue sarcoma, lymphoma, epidermoid carcinoma) occur rarely as primary tumors in the thyroid. The thyroid can also serve as a site of metastasis for malignant tumors of other sites.

Approach to Patient With History of Previous Irradiation to Neck

Because the use of radiotherapy for a number of benign conditions was common practice until recently, identifying and screening previously irradiated patients for the presence of thyroid cancer is a significant medical problem. Studies of asymptomatic patients with a history of childhood irradiation revealed that about 25% had abnormalities on physical examination or scan; of those who were then surgically explored, 33% or more proved to have thyroid cancer. To give the medical community reasonable guidance, a workshop cosponsored by the National Institutes of Health (NIH) and the Food and Drug Administration (FDA) issued the following recommendations:

1. The patient with no visible or palpable abnormalities should be followed with a clinical evaluation at least every 2 years. If scans are performed, focal abnormalities that do not correspond to palpable abnormalities need not be investigated further.
2. The patient with a discrete nodule on palpation should be surgically explored, whether the nodule is "hot" or "cold" on scan, even though hot nodules are only rarely malignant. Small, soft nodules (<1.5 cm) may be observed while the patient is given L-thyroxine (T_4) suppression for 6 months; exploration follows failure to resolve.
3. The patient with diffuse thyroid enlargement without focal abnormalities on physical examination should be studied with tests of thyroid function, antithyroid antibodies, and a scan. If the patient does not have thyrotoxicosis, T_4 suppression is instituted for 6 months. At that time, if a nodule is apparent on physical examination, the patient is explored surgically; otherwise, the patient is maintained on T_4 and re-evaluated at intervals.

These recommendations were published before the general acceptance of fine-needle aspiration as a key diagnostic technique (see following discussion).

Evaluation of the Solitary Nodule

About 20% of patients coming to surgery with solitary nodules prove to have cancer. Solitary nodules in men are about three times more likely than women to be malignant. Nodules in children are more likely to be malignant (about 50% are cancer) than in adults, simply because benign causes of thyroid nodules are relatively much less common in children. Finally, as noted above, previous radiotherapy markedly increases the risk that a nodule may be cancerous.

The aim should be to make a diagnosis as expeditiously and inexpensively as possible. As always, the first step is taking a careful history. Does the patient have a personal history of radiotherapy in infancy or childhood, or a history of previous invasive cancers or thyroid disease? Is there a family history of thyroid cancer or endocrine tumors elsewhere? The physical examination delineates the thyroid nodule itself, its consistency, its fixation to surrounding structures, and the status of the cervical lymph nodes. Does the thyroid nodule move with swallowing, as it should? If not, it is probably extrathyroidal. Does the patient have trouble swallowing or exhibit any sign of hoarseness or recent voice change? If so, indirect laryngoscopy should assess movement of the vocal cords, since impairment of recurrent laryngeal nerve function may be a sign of extracapsular spread of tumor.

The various laboratory tests of thyroid function, as well as determination of serum thyroglobulin levels and antithyroid antibodies, are all nonspecific; elevated serum calcitonin levels, however, strongly suggest C-cell hyperplasia or medullary carcinoma. Serum histaminase may also be elevated in medullary carcinoma.

From this point, opinions about the optimal approach diverge. The relative roles of ultrasonography and scintiscans for imaging are unsettled. If carefully performed and correlated with the anatomical features of the gland, the scintiscan can give valuable information about whether a palpable nodule is functional. However, scans are not very useful for diagnosis, because the majority of clinically significant thyroid nodules, whether benign or malignant, are less functional than normal tissue and therefore appear cold on scintiscan. Scintiscans are mainly helpful in identifying the small number of nodules that are hyperfunctional and therefore not serious candidates for malignancy. Scintiscans should, where possible, be performed with ^{99m}Tc-pertechnetate or ^{123}I, because the amount of radiation absorbed by the thyroid with these isotopes is much less than that absorbed with ^{131}I or other alternatives.

Ultrasonography reliably distinguishes cystic, solid, and mixed lesions; this may be useful, since pure cysts smaller than 4 cm are almost never malignant. Otherwise, the sonogram cannot differentiate malignant from benign lesions.

Ultimately, the diagnosis of cancer must rest on histologic or cytologic evaluation. Most thyroidologists advocate the liberal use of fine-needle aspiration. Enthusiasm for this technique has greatly increased in recent years. The University of California at Los Angeles group has suggested that fine-needle aspiration, followed by scan when the cytology is suspicious but not diagnostic of malignancy, is the most cost-effective way of evaluating thyroid nodules. As with any technique, its reliability increases in the hands of the most experienced clinicians and pathologists.

In a recent study by Piromalli *et al.*, 216 patients underwent surgical excision of thyroid masses after fine-needle aspirations. There were two false-positive results and three false-negative ones. Thus, sensitivity and specificity were 95% and 97.5%, respectively. Because of such encouraging results for fine-needle aspiration and because thyroid cancer itself is indolent, many clinics use negative fine-needle aspiration results to defer further invasive studies in favor of careful follow-up.

With the use of fine-needle aspiration, a decrease in the number of thyroid explorations and an increase in the percentage of cancers diagnosed in explored patients are seen. Patients with negative fine-needle aspiration results are generally placed on T_4 suppression and followed carefully. Lesions that do not resolve after an adequate period of suppression should be re-evaluated for biopsy. What constitutes an adequate period of observation is not clear; although 6 months is commonly used, some recent data suggest that the incidence of regression of nonmalignant thyroid nodules over 56 months of observation is no greater with T_4 than with placebo.

Despite the generally high diagnostic accuracy of fine-needle aspiration, a negative result should not necessarily discourage exploratory surgery if the clinical context is suspicious enough (*e.g.*, a young male with a rapidly growing, hard, and irregular nodule).

Federman (1984) has outlined a diagnostic approach that relies heavily on scintiscan findings and the patient's radiotherapy history, age, and gender as the major determinants of cancer risk. He advocates surgical exploration and/or aspiration biopsy for (1) all patients with history of radiotherapy, (2) all women less than 30 years of age, and (3) all men, again irrespective of radiotherapy history.

Staging

Although various staging systems have been proposed, none is in common use.

Treatment

The primary treatment for thyroid cancer is surgery, but there is no agreement about the optimal approach. Advocates of total thyroidectomy point to the frequent multifocal distribution of thyroid cancer within the gland. They also contend that the removal of all functioning thyroid tissue prepares the patient for subsequent therapy of any metastatic disease with ^{131}I.

Advocates of less extensive procedures, such as lobectomy or subtotal thyroidectomy, cite the serious potential complications of radical surgery (hypoparathyroidism, damage to the recurrent laryngeal nerve); they also note that radical surgery does not seem to be associated with reduction of overall mortality from the disease, even though local control rates are somewhat better with more extensive operations. They further point out that ablation of functioning thyroid tissue can be accomplished with ^{131}I without jeopardizing the parathyroids or the ninth nerve. Brennan (1989) advocates a lobectomy for most confined nodules, and a near-total thyroidectomy for lesions larger than 2 to 3 cm; this operation leaves a rim of thyroid tissue to spare the ipsilateral ninth nerve and parathyroids.

Most surgeons favor a modified neck dissection sparing the sternocleidomastoid and the accessory nerve for patients with clinically positive or suspicious nodes; the clinically negative neck is generally left alone. Other points of view abound in the literature.

For medullary carcinoma, many surgeons favor at least a near-total thyroidectomy, along with a neck dissection if nodes are clinically or histologically positive. Retrospective reviews have suggested that the more extensive surgery is associated with higher survival rates.

After surgery, the issue of clinical importance is whether any cancer remains and, if so, what to do about it. As noted above, for patients with papillary or follicular carcinoma, many advocate ablation of all functioning thyroid tissue, either by resecting it all at the primary operation or by administering radioactive iodine (RAI) postoperatively. The purpose of ablation is to increase circulating thyroid-stimulating hormone (TSH) levels, with subsequent increase in the uptake of RAI in any remaining thyroid tissue or metastases, which can then be detected on scintiscans and treated with therapeutic doses of RAI. The use of RAI to treat residual or metastatic disease is widespread practice; although the effect of RAI on survival is not entirely clear, it seems certain that in properly selected patients, the use of postoperative RAI and T_4 can significantly decrease the recurrence rate.

Many prefer ablation on a selective basis for patients at high risk; at the Memorial Sloan-Kettering Cancer Center, for example, Leeper (1985) favored ablation for patients in the following groups: patients younger than 20 years old; those 20 to 40 years old with known persistent, recurrent, or residual disease; and those over 40 years old with follicular or nonoccult papillary cancer. DeGroot (1979) suggests ablation for all patients except those with small unifocal lesions confined to the thyroid.

If ablation with RAI is elected, certain procedures should be observed. Administration should be scheduled no sooner than 4 weeks postoperatively, or when the patient has been off triiodothyronine (T_3) for at least 4 weeks or off T_4 for at least 6 weeks. Iodinated contrast agents should not be used during this time. The patient must avoid food, food additives, and medicines that have a high iodine content; these include certain breads, vitamins, all seafood, kelp, iodinized salt, certain antiseptics, and cough medicines.

RAI may be administered only by qualified and specially licensed physicians and therefore is not described in detail here. The ablative dose is usually preceded by a 1-mCi tracer dose with a total-body scan. If uptake is detected outside the thyroid, the patient is given a cancerocidal dose of RAI, as described below. Otherwise, 50 to 75 mCi usually suffices for ablation, which is deemed successful if at the time of rescanning 6 weeks later, less than 0.3% of the administered tracer dose remains in the thyroid at 48 hours, or if the TSH becomes elevated and the patient becomes clinically hypothyroid. Under these circumstances, the rescanning procedure may reveal previously undetected metastatic disease. Possible medical complications of a radioiodine dose of this magnitude include sialoadenitis, with permanent cessation of salivary flow in some patients, and a small risk of the later development of acute leukemia.

Once ablation is successful, patients are placed on T_4 suppression in order to keep TSH levels as low as possible. Serum thyroglobulin determinations may be useful in following patients in whom postoperative levels are low or undetectable and antithyroglobulin antibodies are absent. Subsequent scans may be done if serum thyroglobulin levels become persistently elevated or recurrent disease becomes clinically apparent.

Metastatic Disease

The most common varieties of differentiated thyroid cancer develop metastases with fair frequency. Lung metastases from papillary cancer are often only very slowly progressive and may be stable for long periods. Because adenocarcinomas from other primary sites (*e.g.*, lung and ovary) may also have papillary features, the histologic diagnosis of metastatic papillary adenocarcinoma does not necessarily signify origin in the thyroid. The presence of mucin in a metastatic adenocarcinoma points strongly away from thyroid as the primary site.

Bone metastases from follicular carcinoma may be the first clinical manifestation of this tumor; the primary tumor may be occult and may become apparent only after careful imaging studies. Alternatively, a bone metastasis described by the pathologist as "follicular adenocarcinoma compatible with thyroid origin" may be secondary to a tumor resected from the thyroid years ago, at which time it may have been mistakenly diagnosed as a benign follicular adenoma.

The preferred initial therapy for metastatic thyroid cancer is RAI in full therapeutic doses. Before this treatment is given, one should be certain that the metastases are thyroidal in origin and that they take up RAI in sufficient quantity to make the therapy potentially useful. As noted above, they will not do this unless normal thyroid function has been ablated. Note also that the level of iodine uptake for medullary and anaplastic histologies is too low to attain therapeutic levels.

In preparation for therapy, thyroid replacement with T_4 or T_3 is discontinued, and after 4 to 6 weeks elapse and a hypothyroid state has been induced, tracer is administered to establish that the metastatic tumor significantly concentrates RAI; at this time, dosimetry may be performed to permit the radioiodine dose to be tailored to the individual patient. Some centers prefer to administer a fixed total dose of ^{131}I (about 300 mCi) to all patients. Patients to be treated with RAI are placed in a single room, and the usual irradiation precautions for the institution are implemented. A few days after isotope administration, T_4 replacement is restarted and the patient is discharged from isolation and followed.

Leeper (1985) has reported a 48% cure rate of patients with metastatic disease treated with ^{131}I; failures tend to occur in older patients with either bulky disease and bony metastases or with poor ^{131}I uptake. Retreatment is often necessary. Leeper has also observed that careful dosimetry permits a significantly higher dose to be given safely to many patients than would be given by a fixed-dose procedure.

Side-effects of therapeutic doses of ^{131}I are those attributable to radiation: nausea and vomiting, transient bone marrow suppression, pulmonary fibrosis, rare late leukemia, and sialoadenitis.

External beam radiotherapy may be used for locally persistent or recurrent disease that does not take up radioactive iodine. The Memorial group has recently achieved excellent control rates in the neck using combined external radiotherapy (200 cGy/fraction, five times a week for 5 weeks) and doxorubicin (10 mg/m^2 intravenously, 90 minutes before the first administration of radiotherapy and weekly thereafter). This regimen is apparently much less effective at distant metastatic sites. In a small pilot study in spindle and giant cell carcinoma, a modification of this regimen (hyperfractionated radiotherapy, two treatments per day, three times a week, plus doxorubicin) has produced an apparent three- to fourfold improvement in median survival (12 months versus 3–4 months). Clearly, these results require confirmation.

Experience with systemic chemotherapy is limited; the relative rarity of the disease and its clinical heterogeneity have frustrated attempts at systematic study. On the basis of the relatively small amount of available information, a reasonable regimen is the combination of cisplatin (40 mg/m^2) and doxorubicin (60 mg/m^2) given every 3 weeks; in a randomized trial involving 84 evaluable patients, this combination yielded a somewhat higher response rate (26%) than doxorubicin alone (17%) and, perhaps more significantly, produced a number of patients with complete responses (12%), several of whom survived for more than 2 years. A trial published in 1990 by Kobler et al. evaluated the combination of cisplatin, vincristine, and mitoxantrone in a small number of patients. The overall response rate was 67% with 27% complete responders. These results are of interest but require confirmation in larger studies.

TUMORS OF THE ADRENAL GLAND

Tumors of the adrenal gland are rare; about 150 to 300 adrenocortical tumors and about 400 pheochromocytomas (of which about 10% are malignant) occur in the United States each year. By contrast, various series have reported the existence of clinically inapparent adrenal adenomas in 1.4% to 8.7% of autopsies; the physiologic or clinical significance of this finding is unclear. As with many endocrine glands, the cytologic distinction between benign and malignant adrenal tumors is often not reliable; evidence of vascular invasion or metastasis is required.

The differential diagnosis of an adrenal mass includes cortical adenoma and carcinoma, pheochromocytoma, neuroblastoma, ganglioneuroma, cysts, myelolipoma, adenolipoma, and metastases from other primary malignancies. The patient's age, the clinical setting, the size of the mass, and the presence or absence of associated signs or symptoms are important in orienting the diagnostic approach. Cortical adenomas are generally small (<6 cm diameter) and characteristically secrete a single steroid activity, usually glucocorticoid, occasionally aldosterone, and rarely androgens. The clinical onset of Cushing's syndrome from adrenal adenomas is gradual, and surgical resection is almost always curative. However, adrenalectomy for aldosterone-producing adenomas may not always resolve hypertension. Androgen-producing tumors carry the worse prognosis, probably because they may frequently be misdiagnosed as adenomas when they are in fact adrenocortical carcinomas.

Carcinomas tend to present with large tumors and to secrete multiple classes of steroids, usually glucocorticoids and androgens, and less commonly mineralocorticoids or estrogens. This tendency can result in a clinical picture of mixed endocrine hyperfunction (*e.g.*, Cushing's syndrome plus virilization). Carcinomas often produce marked elevations of urinary 17-hydroxysteroids (17 OH) and 17-ketosteroids (17 KS) and characteristically have a rapid onset and progression of symptoms. The percentage of cortical carcinomas that are "nonfunctional" has varied widely in reported series (4–76%), probably according to how meticulously investigators have attempted to document endocrine function. Because postpubertal males cannot be virilized, functional adrenocortical carcinomas may be underdiagnosed in males, since these tumors frequently produce androgenic steroids. Nonfunctional tumors produce little clinical effect early and therefore present only after they have attained substantial size.

Adrenal tumors are very uncommon causes of hypertension in adults. However, it is appropriate to look for evidence of mineralocorticoid excess when hypertension and otherwise unexplained hypokalemia coexist. Pheochromocytoma might reasonably be suspected in patients with sustained or paroxysmal hypertension and a history of sweating, tachycardia or palpitations, anxiety, or headaches. The disease should also be suspected in patients who have malignant or refractory hypertension or who experience hypertensive episodes on induction of anesthesia, surgery, or childbirth. The presence of a family history consistent with MEN 2A or B is obviously a red flag.

When arising from adrenal tumors, disorders of sex hormone secretion are usually associated with large tumors that are either palpable or easily imaged with conventional techniques. Neuroblastoma and ganglioneuroma are characteristically tumors of early childhood and are not considered here (see Chap. 45).

The prognosis of malignant adrenal tumors appears to depend chiefly on the extent of disease at the time of diagnosis; not surprisingly, patients with relatively small, resectable tumors have a much better chance of cure than those with large invasive and/or metastatic tumors. For cortical carcinoma, various studies have alleged the prognostic importance of other factors, such as degree of cellular pleomorphism (pleomorphic worse than differentiated) and steroid secretory status (nonfunctional worse than functional), but these have not been confirmed in large, independent series. Even though metastatic disease implies a very poor prognosis, individual patients can have significant palliation from therapy and can live for years with well-controlled disease.

Diagnostic Evaluation

The possibility of an adrenal tumor generally arises in either of two clinical circumstances: (1) The patient presents with a mass compatible with an adrenal tumor; the mass itself may be the presenting sign or it may be clinically inapparent and detected incidentally in the course of imaging the abdomen for some other purpose. (2) The patient presents with a syndrome of hormonal overproduction compatible with adrenal hyperfunction (Table 34–1). When the adrenal mass is the presenting feature, the physician must assess its anatomical characteristics, extent, and physiologic activity, if any. Alternatively, evidence of hormonal hypersecretion may draw attention to the possibility of an adrenal tumor, the existence of which is then established by biochemical studies and imaging techniques. Whatever the presentation, the anatomical extent and character of the lesion are obviously

TABLE 34–1. DISORDERS OF HORMONAL HYPERSECRETION FROM ADRENAL TUMORS

SYNDROME	TUMOR	DIFFERENTIAL DIAGNOSIS
Cushing's syndrome	Cortical adenoma or carcinoma	Cushing's disease Ectopic ACTH secretion Exogenous glucocorticoids
Virilism	Cortical adenoma or carcinoma	Ovarian tumors Exogenous androgens Polycystic ovaries Other ovarian stomal disorders Late-onset congenital adrenal hyperplasia
Feminization	Cortical adenoma or carcinoma	Gonadal tumors Exogenous estrogens Gonadotropin-producing tumors Drugs
Hypertension	Pheochromocytoma Cortical adenoma	Essential hypertension Renovascular

ACTH = adrenocorticotropic hormone.

crucial information, since the primary treatment is most often surgical. No less important, however, is the physiologic characterization of a steroid-producing tumor or a pheochromocytoma; although the technical details of the surgical procedure do not depend on the hormonal secretion patterns of a tumor, the necessary medical supportive care before, during, and after operation may critically depend on the tumor's physiology.

For the patient with an incidentally discovered adrenal mass, Copeland (1983) has suggested an approach based on the size and character of the lesion and its biochemical functioning. In brief, for lesions greater than 6 cm in diameter, if the lesion is solid on computed tomographic (CT) scan, the patient receives the biochemical assessment outlined in Table 34–2 and is explored surgically. However, if the lesion is cystic on CT scan, fine-needle aspiration may be performed. If clear fluid is obtained, the evaluation is terminated; if bloody fluid is obtained, biochemical assessment and surgery follow.

TABLE 34–2. BIOCHEMICAL SCREENING STUDIES FOR PATIENTS WITH AN ADRENAL MASS AND NO CLINICAL STIGMATA OF HORMONAL HYPERSECTION

Twenty-four-hour urine collection
- Metanephrines (or vanillylmandelic acid), catecholamines
- 17-Hydroxysteroids
- 17-Ketosteroids
- 17-Ketogenic steroids (if 17-hydroxysteroids and 17-ketosteroids are within normal limits)

Low-dose dexamethasone suppression test

If hypertensive, serum potassium on a high-sodium (≥200 mEq) and low-potassium (≤100 mEq) diet

For lesions 6 cm or less in diameter, if biochemical assessment reveals activity, the patient is explored surgically. If the tumor is nonfunctional and cystic, fine-needle aspiration is performed. Cysts yielding clear fluid are not investigated further; those yielding bloody fluid are evaluated in the same way as solid lesions. If the tumor is nonfunctional and solid, the CT scan is repeated at intervals (2, 6, and 18 months). If the lesion shows no growth during this period of observation, it is declared to be of no clinical consequence; if it shows growth, the patient is assessed biochemically and explored surgically.

This approach seems reasonable in the setting of no history of invasive malignancy. For cases in which it seems clinically possible that the adrenal mass is a manifestation of metastatic disease from another primary site, particularly breast or lung, clinical judgment should dictate the desirability of a formal adrenal evaluation.

Patients presenting with a large, clinically apparent abdominal mass compatible clinically and radiologically with a tumor of adrenal origin can reasonably be evaluated according to the approach given above for lesions larger than 6 cm in diameter. However, the biochemical evaluation can often be targeted in these cases, because the hormonal secretion patterns of large tumors is usually clinically apparent by the time they are discovered.

For patients presenting with signs of hormonal excess, the task is to document that excess and/or nonsuppressibility of normally suppressible hormonal function. The techniques used for this documentation often point to the anatomically responsible site (Table 34–3). Clinically significant mineralocorticoid excess with no other hormonal abnormalities is nearly always due to either a benign adrenal adenoma (Conn's syndrome) or bilateral adrenal hyperplasia and is not considered further here. As noted, carcinomas

TABLE 34–3. SCREENING FOR SYNDROMES OF HORMONAL EXCESS

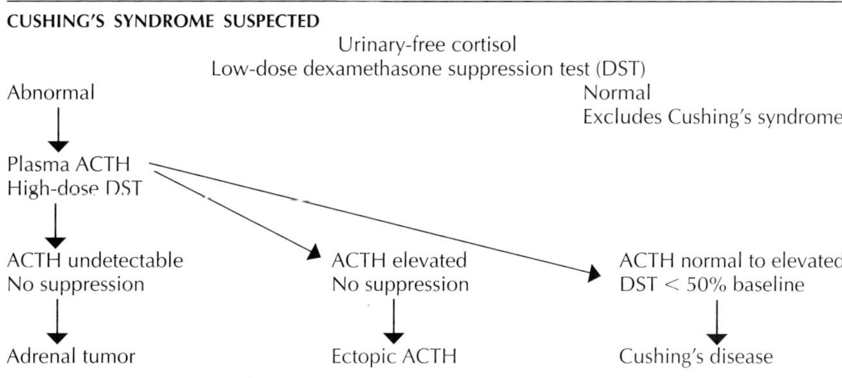

PHEOCHROMOCYTOMA SUSPECTED

Urinary metanephrines (or vanillylmandelic acid), urinary catecholamines

Plasma catecholamines (in fasting patients after 30 minutes of recumbent rest)

If these are equivocal in presence of hypertension and pheochromocytoma is still suspected, glucagon stimulation test is indicated

If catecholamines are elevated and diagnosis of pheochromocytoma is equivocal, clonidine suppression test is indicated

SEX-HORMONE OVERPRODUCTION SUSPECTED

Urinary 17 KS, DHEA, DHEA-S

Plasma testosterone

Urinary estrogens

ACTH = adrenocorticotropic hormone; 17 KS = 17-ketosteroids; DHEA = dehydroepiandrosterone; DHEA-S = dehydroepiandrosterone sulfate.

are more common adrenal causes of virilism (relatively common) and feminization (rare) than are adenomas; high levels of 17 KS or 17 KS steroids generally point to an adrenal rather than a gonadal source. This finding is not uniformly reliable, however, and several recent reports have documented the existence of testosterone-secreting, virilizing adrenal adenomas in which urinary 17 KS were not high. The finding of feminization in adult males with no other obvious cause should prompt a search for an adrenal tumor, particularly if 17 KS and estrogen levels are high.

Once hormonal excess is verified, the responsible tumor must be located. No currently available imaging technique reliably distinguishes benign from malignant adrenal tumors. Tumor localization is currently best accomplished with CT scanning and magnetic resonance imaging (MRI). T2-weighted MRI may be of particular value in distinguishing adrenal carcinomas, adenomas, and metastatic disease by the brightness of the image. For adrenocortical tumors, selective arteriography is sometimes useful preoperatively to delineate a tumor's extent and vascular supply. In difficult cases in which CT and ultrasonography have failed to localize a putative adrenal tumor, selective venous sampling may help; this is usually done bilaterally and simultaneously, before and after adrenocorticotropic hormone (ACTH) infusion. Radionuclide scanning with an ^{131}I-labeled cholesterol (6-iodomethyl norcholesterol) may also help localize functional tumors.

For patients with suspected pheochromocytoma and a negative abdominal CT scan, the chest film should be scrutinized for paratracheal masses, because these tumors can rarely be primary in the posterior mediastinum. If the chest film is negative, abdominal arteriography after alpha-adrenergic blockade may be necessary (see below). If all else fails, catheterization of the inferior vena cava with sampling at multiple levels may reveal the localization of the primary tumor, metastases, or recurrent disease. Recent data suggest that ^{131}I-metaiodobenzylguanidine (^{131}I-MIGB) provides excellent images of small lesions; it may also be useful for the screening of kindreds for MEN 2, although the recent identification of a MEN 2 gene on chromosome 10 may obviate the use of this and other screening tests to identify MEN 2 kindreds.

Staging

The most commonly used staging system for adrenocortical carcinoma is presented in Table 34–4.

TABLE 34–4. STAGING CRITERIA FOR ADRENOCORTICAL CARCINOMA

DEFINITION	CRITERIA
T1	Tumor ≤5 cm, invasion absent
T2	Tumor >5 cm, invasion absent
T3	Tumor outside adrenal in fat
T4	Tumor invading adjacent organs
N0	No positive lymph nodes
N1	Positive lymph nodes
M0	No distant metastases
M1	Distant metastases
STAGE	**TNM CRITERIA**
I	T1, N0, M0
II	T2, N0, M0
III	T1 or T2N1M0, T3N0M0
IV	Any T, any N if M1 or T3T4N1

Treatment

ADRENOCORTICAL TUMORS

The initial treatment of choice, whenever possible, is surgical excision. Even subtotal resection of tumor bulk reduces the body burden of functioning cancer and can provide significant palliation. In cases of benign adenoma, excision should be curative.

Patients with Cushing's syndrome from an adrenal tumor should be assumed to have a suppressed pituitary-adrenal axis. Thus, when undergoing either bilateral adrenalectomy or unilateral adrenalectomy with plans for postoperative mitotane, these patients need both perioperative and long-term glucocorticoid replacement; patients undergoing a unilateral adrenalectomy for a hyperfunctioning tumor need only perioperative replacement. Suitable perioperative coverage is provided by hydrocortisone, 100 mg intravenously every 8 hours, on the day of operation. The daily dose is tapered gradually over the next 5 days to maintenance levels of cortisone acetate, 25 mg orally every morning and 12.5 orally every night.

Patients who have residual functional disease after surgery or recurrent or metastatic disease not amenable to surgical resection should be treated with mitotane (o,p′-DDD). The usual starting dose is 8 to 10 g daily, although many patients are not able to continue treatment at this level because of side-effects (nausea, vomiting, diarrhea, depression, and somnolence). Some advocate beginning therapy at a lower dose (*e.g.*, 2 g/day) and escalating weekly to tolerance. The maximum tolerated dose has varied from 2 to 18 g daily; patients should probably receive the maximum dose that they can tolerate without unacceptable side-effects. About 70% respond with decreased steroid secretion, and in about 30% to 40% tumor size is significantly reduced.

Nonresponders can be treated with metyrapone (750 mg orally every 4 hours) or aminoglutethamide (250 mg orally every 6 hours initially, with stepwise dose increase to a total of 2 g/day or until dose-limiting side-effects occur). Because metyrapone inhibits 11-beta hydroxylation, patients receiving long-term treatment should be monitored for the development of hypertension. Patients receiving any of these inhibitors of adrenal steroid synthesis may require administration of replacement doses of glucocorticoid and mineralocorticoid and should be assumed to have adrenal insufficiency during times of stress. Plasma cortisol should be used to monitor adrenal function in the presence of mitotane, because the drug alters the hepatic metabolism of glucocorticoids, rendering urinary 17 OH an unreliable measure.

The rarity of adrenocortical carcinoma has precluded the systematic study of cytotoxic agents. Combinations including alkylating agents or doxorubicin have produced responses in isolated cases, but data are too sparse to provide meaningful clinical guidance. Whether newer and novel agents, such as suramin, will be beneficial is yet unknown.

PHEOCHROMOCYTOMA

The cornerstone of treatment is surgical resection, with appropriate medical support to control blood pressure and intravascular volume during and after surgery.

Seven to ten days before operation (and before any invasive localization tests) pheoxybenzamine, 10 to 20 mg three or four times a day, or prazosin, 2 to 5 mg orally twice a day, is instituted to induce alpha-adrenergic blockade. Beta-adrenergic blockade may also be required if arrhythmias are present, and many clinicians advocate its use in all patients to prevent catecholamine-induced tachyarrhythmias during surgery. Beta-adrenergic blockade can be achieved with propranolol; the starting dose of 10 mg orally four times a day can be titrated upward until the pulse rate is normal. If beta-adrenergic blockade is used, it should be induced only after alpha-adrenergic blockade is well established, since loss of beta-adrenergic–related vasodilation could lead to increasing hypertension if alpha-adrenergic blockade is not highly effective.

Although the rationale for alpha-adrenergic blockade is clear, it has an operational disadvantage in that the operating team is not alerted to the fall in blood pressure that occurs with successful resection of functioning tumor. Similarly, they cannot see the acute rise in blood pressure that often accompanies palpation of a small tumor that is otherwise difficult to detect.

Preoperatively the blood volume should be expanded with 1 to 2 units of blood within a day of surgery. Adequate blood replacement during surgery is essential to prevent volume depletion and hypotension. Intraoperative hypertension can be controlled with phentolamine or nitroprusside; hypotension is usually best treated with volume replacement.

The treatment of inoperable malignant pheochromocytomas is often frustrating. Alpha-adrenergic blockade, along with other antihypertensive agents, can control blood pressure in many patients. Beta-adrenergic blockade may suppress arrhythmias. Metyrosine, 0.25 to 1 g orally four times a day, can block catecholamine biosynthesis and is a useful adjunct. The selective delivery of radiotherapy via therapeutic doses of ^{131}I-MIBG has produced some evidence of tumor reduction and decreased catecholamine secretion in early trials.

Predictably, not much is known about the activity of individual cytotoxic agents. In a small pilot trial at the NIH recently reported by Keiser and coworkers (1985), the combination of cyclophosphamide, 750 mg/m^2 intravenously on day 1; vincristine 1.4 mg/m^2 intravenously on day 1; and dacarbazine, 600 mg/m^2 intravenously on days 1 and 2, given in 3- or 4-week treatment cycles, has produced impressive evidence of an antitumor effect, in tumor shrinkage (partial responses in 3/3 of cases) and blood pressure control. Patients treated with cytotoxic chemotherapy should probably have adequate alpha-receptor blockade before treatment, since release of catecholamines with tumor lysis has been described.

BIBLIOGRAPHY

Baxter JD, Tyrrell JB. The adrenal cortex. In Felig P, Baxter JD, Broadus AE et al (eds). Endocrinology and Metabolism, 2nd ed. New York, McGraw-Hill, 1987:599–650

Bertagna C, Orth DN. Clinical and laboratory findings and results of therapy in 58 patients with adrenocortical tumors admitted to a single medical center (1951 to 1978). Am J Med 71:855–875, 1981

Bravo EL, Gifford RW Jr. Pheochromocytoma: Diagnosis, localization and management. N Engl J Med 311:1298–1303, 1984

Brennan MF. Cancer of the endocrine system. In DeVita VT Jr, Hellman SE, Rosenberg SA (eds): Cancer: Principles and Practice of Oncology, 3rd ed. Philadelphia, JB Lippincott, 1989

Burrows GN. The thyroid: Nodules and neoplasms. In Felig P, Baxter JD, Broadus AE et al (eds). Endocrinology and Metabolism, 2nd ed. New York, McGraw-Hill, 1987:473–507

Copeland PM. The incidentally discovered adrenal mass. Ann Intern Med 98:940–945, 1983

DeGroot LJ. Thyroid neoplasia. In DeGroot LJ, Cahill GF Jr, Martini L et al (eds). Endocrinology, Vol. 1. Orlando, Grune & Stratton, 1979:509–521

DeGroot LJ, Reilly M, Pinnameneni K et al. Retrospective and prospective study of radiation-induced thyroid disease. Am J Med 74:852–862, 1983

Federman D. Thyroid. In Rubenstein E, Federman DD (eds). Scientific American Medicine. New York, Scientific American, Inc. 1984:21–24

Gharib H, James EM, Charbonneau JW et al. Suppressive therapy with levothyroxine for solitary thyroid nodules. A double-blind controlled clinical study. N Engl J Med 317:70–75, 1987

Graze K, Spiler IJ, Tashjian AH et al. Natural history of familial medullary thyroid carcinoma. Effect of a program for early diagnosis. N Engl J Med 299:980–985, 1978

Haq MM, Legha SS, Samaan et al. Cytotoxic chemotherapy in adrenal cortical carcinoma. Cancer Treat Rep 64:909–913, 1980

Hutter AM, Kayhoe DE. Adrenal cortical carcinoma: Results of treatment with o,p′-DDD in 138 patients. Am J Med 41:581–592, 1966

Information for Physicians. Irradiation-related thyroid cancer. DHEW Publication No (NIH) 77-1120. Prepared by the Division of Cancer Control and Rehabilitation, National Cancer Institute, Bethesda, MD, 1977

Keiser HR, Goldstein DS, Wade JL et al. Treatment of malignant pheochromocytoma with combination chemotherapy. Hypertension 7 (suppl I):I-18, 1–24, 1985

Kober F, Heiss A, Keminger K et al. Chemotherapy of highly malignant thyroid tumors. Wien Klin Wochenschr 102:274, 1990

Leeper RD. Thyroid cancer. Med Clin North Am 69:1079–1096, 1985

Luton JP, Cerdas S, Billand L et al. Clinical features of adrenocortical carcinoma, prognostic factors, and the effect of mitotane therapy. N Engl J Med 322:1195–1201, 1990

Miller JM. Evaluation of thyroid nodules. Med Clin North Am 69:1063–1077, 1985

Piromalli D, Martell G, Del Prato I et al. The role of fine needle aspiration in diagnosis of thyroid nodules: Analysis of 795 consecutive cases. J Surg Oncol 50:247–250, 1992

Richie JP, Gittes RF. Carcinoma of the adrenal cortex. Cancer 45:1957

Roubidoux M, Dunnick NR. Adrenal cortical tumors. Bull NY Acad Med 67:119, 1991

Schneider AB, Recant W, Pinsky SM et al. Radiation-induced thyroid cancer. Ann Intern Med 105:405–412, 1986

Shimaoka K, Shoenfeld DA, DeWys WD et al. A randomized trial of doxorubicin versus doxorubicin plus cisplatin in patients with advanced thyroid carcinoma. Cancer 56: 2155–2160, 1985

VanHerle AJ (moderator). The thyroid nodule. Ann Intern Med 96:221–232, 1982

John S. Macdonald, Daniel G. Haller, Robert J. Mayer, Eds. *Manual of Oncologic Therapeutics*, Third Edition.

35. NEUROENDOCRINE TUMORS

David Kelsen
Leonard Saltz

Neuroendocrine tumors are rare neoplasms characterized histologically by the presence of neurosecretory granules. Neuroendocrine tumors of gastrointestinal origin include carcinoid tumors, which arise from the neuroendocrine tissues of the gut, and islet cell tumors, which arise in the pancreatic islets of Langerhans. Other rarer neuroendocrine tumors include medullary thyroid carcinomas, paragangliomas, pheochromocytomas, Merkel's cell tumors, and pituitary adenomas. Histologically, typical carcinoid and islet cell tumors are relatively bland and monotonous small cell tumors with homogeneous nuclei under light microscopy. Cells often appear in orderly rows or "ribbons," and the mitotic rate is low. Less well-differentiated neuroendocrine tumors vary from "atypical," with increased variability in cell size and increased mitotic rate, to "poorly differentiated" neuroendocrine tumors. The extreme other end of the spectrum — one end being the classic, well-differentiated carcinoid or islet cell tumor — is undifferentiated small cell carcinoma, a high-grade neuroendocrine tumor that has an aggressive growth pattern, scant cytoplasm, and a high mitotic rate.

Neuroendocrine tumors are carcinomas, and therefore stain positively for cytokeratins. The hallmark of a neuroendocrine tumor is the presence of neurosecretory granules, which are demonstrated by a positive chromogranin, synaptophysin, or Grimelius stain. Neuron-specific enolase is a less specific stain and usually should not, by itself, be accepted as proof of a neuroendocrine tumor. Stains for specific hormones may be helpful for further tumor characterization. Electron microscopy, when available, may be helpful in establishing the presence of neurosecretory granules. Unless an identifying hormone is demonstrated, microscopy cannot differentiate between islet cell and carcinoid tumors.

Even metastatic classic carcinoid and islet cell tumors are indolent. In one series of carcinoid patients, the median survival from time of diagnosis was 38 months with individuals surviving up to 17 years.[1] Another series reported a 5-year survival from the time of diagnosis of 65%.[2] As the degree of tumor atypia or anaplasia increases, however, so does the aggressiveness of the disease. Although neuroendocrine tumors are uncommon, the fact that many of them are benign (and thus curable by surgery) and the devastating clinical picture caused by hormonal secretion (*e.g.*, profound hypoglycemia due to an insulin-secreting islet cell tumor) make them important entities. In addition, some neuroendocrine tumors appear in genetically linked combinations; thus, family members of the patient may have early, asymptomatic, and highly curable forms of the disease.

The diagnosis of a neuroendocrine tumor may be suspected in three different settings: (1) the patient exhibits symptoms due to a substance produced by the tumor; (2) the patient has unexplained hepatomegaly (frequently with a nonfunctional islet cell or carcinoid); and (3) the patient is being screened as the relative of a proband. In the first group, although neuroendocrine tumors can produce more than one polypeptide or amine, the clinical presentation is usually dominated by one complaint (*e.g.*, flushing or diarrhea from a carcinoid tumor, symptoms of hypoglycemia from insulin overproduction, or intractable gastric ulceration from a gastrin-producing islet cell tumor). In the second group, a tip-off to possible neuroendocrine tumor (probably not producing a hormone) is that many of these patients are almost asymptomatic, despite huge enlargement of the liver. Patients in the third group are almost always asymptomatic by definition.

ISLET CELL TUMORS

Insulinomas

Among the more common pancreatic endocrine tumors are insulinomas (insulin-producing islet cell tumors). They are usually seen in adults in the fourth to sixth decades of life. The tumor's onset can be insidious, and symptoms actually due to hypoglycemia may be mistakenly attributed to neurologic or psychiatric disorders. The classic complaints of fatigue, weakness, tremulousness, or hunger usually increase during a fast. The diagnosis of insulinoma is confirmed by the finding of an elevated serum insulin level relative to hypoglycemia. In most patients, this finding is obtained after a 24-hour fast, but occasionally a 72-hour fast is needed. Although there is a sex difference in the absolute level of hypoglycemia seen during fasting (with women having a lower level than men), the 24-hour value for normal subjects of either sex is rarely, if ever, below 60 mg/dl.[3] However, not all patients with proven insulinomas develop levels below 60 mg/dl at 24 hours; a longer period of fasting should be initiated, and comparison of simultaneous serum glucose and insulin concentrations should be performed. An increase in the insulin level, or its failure to fall with declining glucose levels, establishes the presence of organic hyperinsulinism. This can be expressed as the insulin-to-glucose ratio. If at 72 hours hypoglycemia has not occurred, a period of vigorous exercise (which normally raises the glucose level) may be useful. Stimulation tests may be used but are rarely needed today because of the accuracy of the insulin-to-glucose ratio.

The symptoms caused by insulinoma have four general characteristics: periodicity (occurring at about the same time of day, although the intervals between attacks may be irregular); repetitiveness (the symptoms in any given patient are constant); presence of hypoglycemia during a symptomatic episode; and finally, rapid resolution of symptoms with glucose administration.

For preoperative localization, computed tomography (CT) and transabdominal ultrasonography are relatively insensitive in identifying small-volume disease. Angiography has traditionally been the diagnostic procedure of choice; with careful attention to catheter placement, up to 80% of tumors can be identified. Insulinomas are intensely vascular, and a tumor blush may persist well into the venous phase. Differential sampling of venous blood may also help in tumor localization and in separating diffuse pancreatic islet cell disease from a localized process. Recently, however, endoscopic ultrasonography has been demonstrated to be a highly sensitive technique for the localization of small pancreatic endocrine tumors in patients with negative CT scans, with sensitivity and specificity superior to those of angiography.[4]

Gastrin-Producing Islet Cell Tumors

Gastrinomas are responsible for the Zollinger-Ellison syndrome, which consists of fulminant peptic ulcer disease caused by excessive production of gastrin. Although ulceration may occur in atypical locations, most patients with gastrinoma have typical duodenal ulcers. Diarrhea or steatorrhea are other common symptoms and may, in some cases, be the only presenting symptom. In addition, asymptomatic gastrinoma may be found during screening for multiple endocrine neoplasia syndrome Type I (MEN I). Although precise numbers are not available, it appears that approximately two thirds of cases are sporadic, and one third familial. Most of the sporadic gastrinomas are malignant, whereas many of MEN-linked tumors are benign, usually small, and often in multiple locations. The most common site remains the pancreas, but extrapancreatic gastrinomas have been reported with increasing frequency. Other primary sites include the duodenal wall, stomach, and jejunum.[5] For the subset of patients with full-blown Zollinger-Ellison syndrome, the primary site is found in only 50% of patients.

Once the diagnosis of gastrinoma is suspected, a serum gastrin and basal acid output (BAO) should be obtained. An elevated serum gastrin and BAO more than 15 mEq/hour for a patient not having undergone prior gastric resection (>5 mEq/hour for those having had gastric surgery) are highly suspicious for the diagnosis of Zollinger-Ellison syndrome; a secretin stimulation test is usually confirmatory but is not necessary if the BAO is more than 15 and the serum gastrin level is higher than 1000 pg/ml.

Once the diagnosis has been confirmed, locating the tumor may be difficult. Angiography is useful in determining the primary site in only 10% to 30% of patients. Differential venous gastrin levels have also been used with varying success. Endoscopic ultrasonography appears to be a better technique and can be useful even in very small tumors. Intraoperative ultrasonography may also be a major technical advance.

Recent investigations using a radiolabeled somatostatin analog for whole-body scintigraphy appear promising for localization of gastrinomas and other islet cell tumors. Investigations using a somatostatin analog with a tyrosine residue conjugated to ^{123}I demonstrated that the majority of neuroendocrine tumors express high concentrations of somatostatin receptors on their surfaces.[6] Preliminary diagnostic studies used this iodinated compound to demonstrate the feasibility of somatostatin receptor imaging with whole-body scintigraphy.[7] More recently, the somatostatin analog octreotide has been linked to diethylinetriamine pentaacetic acid (DTPA), a chelating agent that binds ^{111}In.[8] ^{111}In-octreotide scintigraphy appears to be a powerful new tool for the localization of small islet cell tumors. It is superior to ^{123}I scanning in that the indium-labeled analog is more stable and is excreted renally, rather than hepatically, thereby permitting more detailed imaging of the liver, pancreas, and duodenum. Insulinomas, because they often lack the Type II somatostatin receptor recognized by octreotide, are not as well imaged by somatostatin analog-receptor imaging as are the other types of islet cell tumors.

Glucagonomas

The clinical syndrome seen in patients with glucagon-producing tumors includes diabetes, a characteristic skin rash (necrolytic migratory erythema), painful glossitis, and hyperaminoaciduria. The rash is often seen in the perioral and perigenital regions, and in the fingers, legs, and feet. Thromboembolic phenomena are common in patients with glucagonomas. Glucagonomas are usually large at presentation; localization is not usually a problem. An elevated glucagon level (the average in previously reported cases is 2100 pg/ml) is diagnostic.

VIP-omas

Islet cell tumors producing vasoactive intestinal polypeptide (VIP) produce a syndrome of profuse diarrhea, hypokalemia, and hypochlorhydria. The volume of diarrhea may be up to 6 to 8 l/day. In addition to diarrhea and electrolyte abnormalities, facial flushing, hypercalcemia, and a large, distended gallbladder may be seen, also as a result of the polypeptide. Persistent diarrhea after 48 hours of fasting is highly suspicious for a VIP-oma. Although the pancreas is the usual site of the primary tumor, neurogenic locations (ganglioneuroblastomas) have been reported, mostly in children. An elevated VIP level is diagnostic, but a specific and sensitive radioimmunoassay is required. Somatostatin receptor imaging would be expected to be useful in localization of small tumors.

Somatostatin-Producing Islet Cell Tumors

Somatostatin-producing islet cell tumors are very rare. Clinically, patients with somatostatinoma have hypochlorhydria, diabetes, weight loss, and malabsorption. Most tumors are in the pancreas. The diagnosis is confirmed by high blood levels of somatostatin. Surgical resection, if possible, is curative.

CARCINOID TUMORS

Carcinoids are neuroendocrine tumors that may produce the amine serotonin or, more rarely, other substances such as 5-hydroxytryptamine, bradykinin, adrenocorticotropic hormone (ACTH), and kallikrein. Histologically, they are indistinguishable from islet cell tumors: small, round cells growing in ribbon-like structures. The appendix is the most common site for this disease, with most appendiceal carcinoids acting in a clinically benign fashion.[10] Other sites of origin include the rectum, small bowel, bronchus, esophagus, stomach, and pancreas.

Many carcinoids are nonfunctional; that is, they do not appear to release measurable amounts of serotonin or other substances, although they may be found to have such substances intracellularly by histochemical techniques. Carcinoids may first be found as asymptomatic hepatomegaly or as a mass on a chest film. Because serotonin is rapidly metabolized by the liver, patients with intra-abdominal primary tumors do not develop the carcinoid syndrome until after liver metastases have occurred. Functional carcinoids of the bronchus or of any area not drained by the portal system may cause the syndrome before metastases occur.

The diagnosis of carcinoid tumor is based on histologic findings; an elevated 5-hydroxyindoleacetic acid (5-HIAA) is confirmatory but not necessary. If 5-HIAA is produced, however, its absolute level is of prognostic importance. In a study of untreated patients, those with a 24-hour excretion of 5-HIAA of 49 mg or less lived a median of 29 months; those with levels between 50 and 149 mg, a median of 21 months; and those with levels greater than 150 mg, a median of 13 months.[9] The range of survival times is extremely variable, from only a few months to more than 25 years. The carcinoid syndrome involves flushing, wheezing, diarrhea, and hypotension. Carcinoid heart disease involves an endomyocardial fibrosis, primarily of the tricuspid and pulmonic valves. It can be the direct cause of death in these patients.[10]

TREATMENT OF NEUROENDOCRINE TUMORS

Surgery remains the treatment of choice for localized neuroendocrine tumors. Approximately 90% of insulinomas are benign and cured by surgical resection.[11] Even in the presence of regional lymph node metastases, prolonged disease-free survival has been reported for both midgut and bronchial carcinoids.[10,12,13] For appendiceal carcinoids, if the tumor is less than 2 cm in diameter, appendectomy alone is adequate. If the tumor is large (>2 cm), a more aggressive cancer operation is indicated (hemicolectomy). For patients with liver metastasis from functional carcinoids or islet cell tumors, surgical debulking may ameliorate the carcinoid syndrome or the effects of polypeptide hormones from islet cell carcinomas.[14] Bypass of unresectable obstructing tumors may also give long-term palliation. In selected patients with severe carcinoid heart disease, valve replacement is indicated. Moertel has noted that mesenteric arterial occlusion has occurred in some patients, probably because of marked fibrosis as seen in the endocardium.[15] Resection of infarcted bowel is indicated in these patients. Hepatic embolization has also been used successfully; careful medical management of these patients is important, as massive release of hormone following embolization of the hepatic artery may induce a carcinoid crisis. The major acute symptom of toxicity of hepatic artery embolization is pain (seen in 60–90% of patients). Although the embolization is otherwise fairly well tolerated, a morality rate of 4% to 5% has been reported in several series.[16–18]

Medical management of mild carcinoid syndrome includes use of antiserotonin agents (cyproheptadine), and antidiarrheals.[15] Cyproheptadine (Periactin), 4 to 8 mg three to four times daily, is useful in controlling diarrhea in selected patients. In patients with bronchial carcinoids, prednisone, 10 to 20 mg/day, has occasionally been found to be of benefit. Diphenoxylate hydrochloride (Lomotil), one or two tablets two to four times per day, is also useful in controlling the diarrhea associated with both carcinoid and some islet cell tumors. The usefulness of all of these agents, and their dosages, is quite unpredictable, and what works well for one patient may be useless for another. Diarrhea is usually easier to control than wheezing or flushing.

More recently, the long-acting somatostatin analog octreotide (Sandostatin) has become available for general use.[19,20] It produces rapid resolution (within minutes to hours) of the symptoms of many islet cell or carcinoid tumors. For routine use, octreotide is self-administered as a subcutaneous injection. Treatment is usually started as 50 μg twice daily and then rapidly increased to 150 μg three times daily. A large majority of patients (77%) have had prompt relief of symptoms associated with the carcinoid syndrome. Similar effects have also been noted in certain functional islet cell tumors (*e.g.*, VIP-oma). Unfortunately, resistance to the analog does develop, but control may continue for many months in some patients (median 6–12 months). Because of the inconvenience of thrice-daily injections and the considerable cost of octreotide, simpler, cheaper therapies are usually attempted first, before octreotide therapy is begun. A long-acting depot octreotide injection is about to enter clinical trials.

Octreotide has few side-effects. Cholelithiasis has been noted in some patients, and serial sonograms of the gallbladder should be performed in patients receiving octreotide for long periods of time.

Octreotide is also effective in aborting a carcinoid crisis. Carcinoid crisis may occur in patients with high 5-HIAA and/or a history of carcinoid syndrome. It may be stimulated by invasive procedures, induction of anesthesia, chemotherapy, trauma, or alcohol ingestion. It is characterized by the sudden onset of profound hypotension, usually accompanied by tachycardia. Management requires prompt recognition, rapid volume expansion with intravenous fluids, and intravenous administration of octreotide, 50 to 100 μg, to be repeated in 1 or 2 minutes if no significant response is achieved.[21] It is imperative that standard pressors (*e.g.*, dopamine, Levophed) not be administered, as these may further stimulate serotonin release from the tumor and exacerbate hypotension. Patients at risk for carcinoid crisis should receive prophylactic octreotide, 150 to 250 μg subcutaneously 30 minutes prior to procedures. A rescue, intravenous dose should accompany the patient to procedures.

For insulinomas, if the tumor is malignant and has metastasized beyond the possibility of surgical care, medical management includes dietary changes such as smaller, more frequent meals or increased carbohydrates, intravenously if needed, if hyperglycemia is severe. Diazoxide in doses of 300 to 800 mg daily inhibits release of insulin and also has a peripheral hyperglycemic effect; a benzothiadiazide diuretic should be given with diazoxide. Propranolol and glucocorticoids have also been used, usually in the doses outlined above. Octreotide must be used with extreme caution, because some patients may have tumors that do not express the type of somatostatin receptor recognized by octreotide. In these cases, octreotide may blunt the normal glucagon response and thereby further exacerbate hypoglycemia.

In the setting of acute severe Zollinger-Ellison syndrome, the primary management should be medical. Continuous nasogastric suction should be started, fluid and electrolyte status should be monitored, and replacement should be given as needed. Intravenous H_2 blockers (*e.g.*, cimetidine or ranitidine) should be started promptly and supplemented with anticholinergics. The dosage of the H_2 blocker employed should be titrated to the acid secretory rates, symptoms, and healing of ulcer disease. Ranitidine, 150 mg three or four times daily, will control most patients with Zollinger-Ellison syndrome. Some patients may require 50 mg intravenously, four times daily; rarely is 300 mg, three times daily, needed. Most patients will be controlled by cimetidine 2.4 g daily (600 mg four times daily; *i.e.*, twice the normal maximum dose), but some patients may need 5 or 6 g/day. Omeprazole, 20 to 360 mg in three divided doses, is also effective. Once the patient is stabilized, surgery can be performed if necessary for perforation, obstruction, or uncontrollable bleeding. In general, it is best to avoid surgery at this time; once the emergency is over, more definitive surgical procedures, if indicated, can be scheduled. Resection of all functional tumor, defined as return of gastrin levels to normal with negative stimulatory tests, is possible in approximately 20% of patients, including those with MEN I. Even if not curative, resection of all gross disease may make medical management easier and may improve survival.

Long-term therapy options for patients with Zollinger-Ellison syndrome include continued medical management with octreotide, H_2 blockers, omeprazole, and anticholinergics, and resection of the primary tumor where possible. Elective total gastrectomy is usually reserved for poorly motivated patients in whom compliance with medical management is uncertain. Chemotherapy may be useful in gastrin-producing islet cell tumors, but responses are usually only partial. A patient with known Zollinger-Ellison syndrome should continue to receive H_2 blockers, omeprazole, and/or octreotide at the time of chemotherapy or surgery. The results of surgery appear to be poorer in the MEN I subgroup.

The majority of glucagon-producing tumors are malignant, and most patients have metastases at the time of diagnosis. If the tumor has not metastasized, surgical resection is curative. Even if the tumor has spread, debulking of functional tissue may help control symptoms. Systemic antineoplastic therapy is discussed below.

Observation

Although many patients with metastatic, unresectable neuroendocrine tumors will eventually require aggressive chemotherapy, many others will have indolent tumors with prolonged periods of stability and a long natural history. Many physicians have followed patients with documented unresectable metastases for many months, and occasionally many years, before any antineoplastic treatment was required.[20] Our usual practice is to obtain CT scans every 3 or 4 months in order to ascertain the pace of the disease. Expectant observation is frequently the most beneficial, and certainly least toxic, approach. Patients for whom this course is chosen should not have evidence of rapid tumor progression and should be asymptomatic or have symptoms controlled by medical management and/or judicious surgery.

Chemotherapy of Neuroendocrine Tumors

There is no standard chemotherapy of proven efficacy for carcinoid tumors. Indications for chemotherapy include refractory hormonal symptoms, pain or symptoms referable to bulk disease, or unequivocal substantial progression of disease under observation. Existence of metastases does not in itself constitute an indication for treatment, since the disease may remain stable for months to years. However, once substantial disease progression starts, a more aggressive course is usually observed, and initiation of chemotherapy may be warranted. At this point many patients have entered investigational chemotherapy trials. Trials reporting survival from the start of chemotherapy have indicated median survivals averaging 12 to 24 months.

Single agents with reported modest clinical activity include doxorubicin, 5-fluorouracil (5-FU), cyclophosphamide, dacarbazine, and streptozocin (STZ). STZ has far less activity in carcinoid than in islet cell tumors. Combination chemotherapy regimens have not been shown to be superior to single agents but are more toxic; their use is most appropriate in the setting of a clinical trial. Objective tumor responses to octreotide are essentially anecdotal, although short-term tumor stabilization has been reported, and patients receiving octreotide in a nonrandomized trial appeared to survive longer than historical controls.[22] In addition, alpha-interferon has recently been shown to cause objective reductions in hormone production at a rate comparable to that of octreotide. However, actual objective reduction in tumor size is uncommon with alpha-interferon. The doses of interferon used in these studies ranged from 3×10^6 to 6×10^6 international units given intramuscularly or subcutaneously on a daily schedule.[23] A more recent trial using higher doses on a thrice-weekly schedule was disappointing in that objective response rates were low, responses were of short duration, and toxicity was substantial.[24]

Most combination chemotherapy regimens have been based on STZ. Several randomized trials have compared single-agent with combination chemotherapy. In an Eastern Cooperative Oncology Group (ECOG) study of patients with carcinoid tumors, 5-FU plus STZ was compared with doxorubicin alone.[25] There were 86 patients in each arm of the trial. There were no significant differences in objective response rates (21% vs. 22%), in median durations of response (31 vs. 26 weeks), or in survival (64 vs. 48 weeks). Another randomized ECOG study compared STZ plus 5-FU with STZ plus cyclophosphamide in patients with carcinoid tumors.[26] A total of 89 evaluable patients were studied; an additional 28 patients were entered into the trial but were inevaluable for response for a variety of reasons. There were no differences in response rates (33% vs. 26%), in durations of response (7 vs. 6 months), or in survival (11.2 vs. 12.5 months).

On the other hand, in islet cell tumors, an ECOG trial compared STZ alone with a combination of STZ plus 5-FU in a total of 82 evaluable patients.[27] Responses were seen in 15 of 42 patients (36%) receiving STZ alone, and 25 of 40 (63%) receiving the two-drug combination; the difference was statistically significant. The median durations of survival were 16.5 and 26 months, respectively. A subsequent ECOG trial in islet cell tumors randomized patients to receive either STZ plus 5-FU or STZ plus doxorubicin.[28] Patients receiving STZ plus doxorubicin had a higher response rate (69% vs. 45%), a longer median length of time to tumor progression (20 vs. 6.9 months), and longer survival (26.5 vs. 17 months) than patients receiving STZ plus 5-FU. The reason for the poorer results achieved with STZ plus 5-FU in the more recent study as compared with the earlier study is not clear.

Thus, although histologically similar, carcinoid tumors appear to have a poorer response to streptozocin-based chemotherapy than do islet cell tumors. In carcinoids, there is little evidence that any one of these combination regimens is superior to another or to single agents such as doxorubicin. The major toxicities of all of the STZ combination trials are severe nausea and vomiting; myelosuppression, and renal damage. Drug-related deaths were seen in 2% to 4% of patients in each of the ECOG studies, usually due to renal toxicity or to sepsis with myelosuppression. Although moderate activity is seen in carcinoid tumors with conventional chemotherapy, response durations are short, complete regressions are unusual, and many patients do not respond at all. Every effort should be made to place these patients in a research study. In the absence of an investigational trial, it is reasonable to treat these patients with single-agent doxorubicin.

Symptomatic islet cell patients not responding to octreotide or other measures and/or those with clearly progressing tumor may be palliated with STZ-doxorubicin (STZ 500 mg/m^2 intravenously daily for 5 days, every 6 weeks, and doxorubicin 50 mg/m^2 intravenously day 1 and day 21). Patients with relative contraindications to doxorubicin can be treated with STZ, 500 mg/m^2 intravenously, and 5-FU, 400 mg/m^2 intravenously, daily for 5 days; each cycle is repeated in 5 weeks. The major side-effects are nausea and vomiting, myelosuppression, and nephrotoxicity. Careful attention to dosage attenuation for myelosuppression and renal toxicity is mandatory.

Irradiation

Although neuroendocrine tumors had been thought to be relatively radioresistant, a few recent reports indicate that palliation of painful metastases can be achieved with irradiation.[29]

REFERENCES

1. Davis Z, Moertel CG, Mellrath CD. The malignant carcinoid syndrome. Surg Gynecol Obstet 137:636–644, 1973
2. Andaker L et al. Follow-up of 102 patients operated on for gastrointestinal carcinoid. Acta Chirurg Scand 151:469–473, 1985
3. Merimee JJ, Tyson JE. Stabilization of plasma glucose during fasting. N Engl J Med 291:1765, 1974

4. Rosch T, Lightdale CJ, Botet JF et al. Localization of pancreatic endocrine tumors by endoscopic ultrasonography. N Engl J Med 326:1721–1726, 1992
5. Wolfe MM et al. Extrapancreatic, extraintestinal gastrinoma. N Engl J Med 306:1533, 1982
6. Reubi JC, Kvols LK, Waser B et al. Detection of somatostatin receptors in surgical and percutaneous needle biopsy samples of carcinoids and islet cell carcinomas. Cancer Res 50:5969–5977, 1990
7. Lamberts SWJ, Bakker WH, Reubi JC et al. Somatostatin-receptor imaging in the localization of endocrine tumors. N Engl J Med 323:1246–1249, 1990
8. Krenning EP, Bakker WH, Kooij PPM et al. Somatostatin receptor scintigraphy with Indium 111-DTPA-D-Phe-1-octreotide in man: Metabolism, dosimetry, and comparison with iodine-123-Tyr-3-octreotide. J Nucl Med 33:652–658, 1992
9. Moertel CG, Dockerty MB, Judd ES. Carcinoid tumors of the vermiform appendix. Cancer 21:270, 1968
10. Ross E, Roberts W. The carcinoid syndrome: Comparison of 21 necropsy subjects with carcinoid heart disease to 15 necropsy subjects without carcinoid heart disease. Am J Med 79:339, 1985
11. Brennen M. Cancer of the endocrine system. In DeVita VT, Hellman S, Rosenberg SA (eds). Cancer: Principles and Practice of Oncology, 3rd ed. Philadelphia, JB Lippincott, 1989:1325
12. Juan R et al. Medical and surgical options in the management of patients with gastrinoma. Gastroenterology 84:1524, 1983
13. McCaughan B, Martini N, Bains M. Bronchial carcinoids: Review of 124 cases. J Thorac Cardiovasc Surg 89:8, 1985
14. Martin J et al. Surgical treatment of functioning metastatic carcinoid tumors. Arch Surg 118:537, 1983
15. Moertel C. Treatment of the carcinoid tumor and the malignant carcinoid syndrome. J Clin Oncol 1:727, 1983
16. Allison D, Jordan H, Hennessy O. Therapeutic embolization of the hepatic artery. A review of 75 procedures. Lancet 1:595, 1985
17. Ajani J, Carraso H, Chamsabave C et al. Islet cell tumors metastatic to the liver: Effective palliation by sequential hepatic artery embolization. Ann Intern Med 108:340, 1980
18. Mitty H, Warner R, Newman L et al. Control of carcinoid syndrome with hepatic artery embolization. Radiology 155:623, 1985
19. Gordon P, Coni R, Maton P et al. Somatostatin and somatostatin-analogue (SMS 201-995) in treatment of hormone-secreting tumors of the pituitary and gastrointestinal tract and non-neoplastic diseases of the gut. Ann Intern Med 110:35, 1989
20. Nordheim I, Oberg K, Theodorsson-Norheim E et al. Malignant carcinoid tumors. Ann Surg 206:115, 1987
21. Kvols LK, Martin JK, Marsh HM et al. Rapid reversal of carcinoid crisis with a somatostatin analogue. N Engl J Med 313:1229–1230, 1985
22. Saltz L, Trochanowski B, Buckley M et al. Octreotide as an antineoplastic agent in the treatment of functional and nonfunctional neuroendocrine tumors. Cancer 72:244–248, 1993
23. Oberg K, Funa K, Alm G. Effects of leukocyte interferon on clinical symptoms and hormone levels in patients with midgut carcinoid tumors and carcinoid syndrome. N Engl J Med 309:129, 1983
24. Moertel CG, Rubin J, Kvols LK. Therapy of metastatic carcinoid tumor and the malignant carcinoid syndrome with recombinant leukocyte A interferon. J Clin Oncol 7:865–868, 1989
25. Engstrom P, Lavin P, Moertel C. Streptozocin plus fluorouracil versus doxorubicin therapy for metastatic carcinoid tumor. J Clin Oncol 2:1255, 1984
26. Moertel C, Hanley J. Combination chemotherapy trials in metastatic carcinoid tumors and the malignant carcinoid syndrome. Cancer Clin Trials 2:327, 1979
27. Moertel C, Hanley J, Johnson L. Streptozocin alone compared with streptozotocin plus fluorouracil in the treatment of advanced islet-cell carcinoma. N Engl J Med 303:21, 1980
28. Moertel CG et al. Streptozocin-doxorubicin, streptozotocin-fluorouracil, or chlorozotocin in the treatment of advanced islet cell carcinoma. N Engl J Med 326:519–523, 1992
29. Schupak KD, Wallner KE. The role of radiation therapy in the treatment of locally unresectable or metastatic carcinoid tumors. Int J Rad Oncol Biol Phys 20:489–495, 1991

John S. Macdonald, Daniel G. Haller, Robert J. Mayer, Eds. *Manual of Oncologic Therapeutics*, Third Edition.

36. MANAGEMENT OF MELANOMA

Lynn M. Schuchter
DuPont Guerry

Malignant melanoma is now the eighth most common cancer in the United States; 10 years ago it was the twentieth. The incidence rate of melanoma is rising faster than that of other cancer except lung cancer in women.[1] It is estimated that by the year 2000, 1 in 90 individuals will develop melanoma. In many studies, the incidence is doubling every 6 to 10 years. The explanation for this remarkable rise is unclear but likely lies in a cohort effect related to sun exposure in the young. Only a small proportion of the increase can be attributed to diagnostic changes; none is yet attributable to the predicted increase in solar radiation at ground level due to the stratospheric ozone depletion. Although the population-based mortality rate has also been increasing for decades, this may have stabilized lately as a result of a sharply decreased case fatality rate: from almost 90% in the early 1920s to less than 20% today. Earlier diagnosis is the primary advance that has led to this improvement in survival.

EPIDEMIOLOGY AND RISK FACTORS

There is persuasive evidence that excessive sun exposure is a major cause of cutaneous melanoma. This is based primarily on data showing a higher incidence and mortality of melanoma associated with residence at lower latitudes and on more than 30 case-control studies that link sun exposure with melanoma incidence.[2] Studies done in midlatitudes relate melanoma risk most directly to intermittent, intense sun exposure associated with sun vacations and participation in outdoor sports and recreational activities. In particular, measures of damaging sun exposure acquired in childhood (*e.g.*, blistering sunburns) have been associated with the increased incidence of melanoma in adults. Individuals with poor ability to tan, fair skin, red or blond hair, blue eyes, freckling, and a history of nonmelanoma skin cancers are all at increased risk.[3] Patients with a personal or family history of melanoma are also at increased risk. Some protective effect may derive from chronic sun exposure by outdoor occupations. Congenital nevi occur in 1% of the U.S. population. The lifetime risk of developing melanoma in a small congenital nevus is very small; in a giant congenital nevus the risk is about 5%.[3]

Among the strongest associations with melanoma risk are an increased number of common acquired nevi and the presence and number of atypical or dysplastic nevi. Atypical nevi are both markers of melanoma risk and potential (nonobligate) precursors of melanoma.[4,5] These lesions can occur in two well-described settings. The familial atypical mole and melanoma syndrome is an autosomal dominantly inherited syndrome defined by the occurrence of melanoma in two or more first- or second-degree relatives and the presence of large numbers of atypical nevi. Family members of patients who have melanoma with atypical nevi have a significantly increased risk of developing melanoma with a lifetime risk that approaches 100%.[6] Hereditary melanoma accounts for 10% of all melanomas. Atypical nevi also occur outside the context of familial melanoma. Prevalence estimates in the general population range from 5% to 20%.[7] The melanoma risk associated with sporadic (nonfamilial) atypical nevi is less than that in familial melanoma kindreds. The point estimates of the adjusted relative risk for melanoma in multiple studies range from 2.1 to 16.[8–11]

Clinical features of atypical nevi include considerations of size, border, and color. Atypical nevi are large, more than 5 mm in diameter, and have a border that characteristically is ill-defined or fuzzy. These nevi are usually brown or tan with a mottled appearance, often with a pink-blue. They are macular or flat throughout or have a macular component (resembling "sunny-side" fried eggs). Significant asymmetry and substantial heterogeneity in color, focal black areas, or gray areas suggestive of partial regression should prompt a biopsy to rule out melanoma. Atypical nevi occur at any site and are most common on the trunk. They are often found on sites of low sun exposure, the buttocks, and the female breasts. Management of individuals who have atypical nevi relies on periodic professional and self-examination of the skin, supplemented in those with multiple lesions by cutaneous photography summarized in Table 36–1. Excisional biopsy is reserved for lesions that are changing, new in comparison to previous examination, or suspicious for melanoma.

CLINICAL CHARACTERISTICS

Melanomas often arise in a pre-existing mole (a congenital, common acquired, or atypical nevus). Although melanomas can be located anywhere on the body, they occur most commonly on the backs of both sexes and the lower extremities of women. Typical morphologic characteristics of melanoma are represented by the ABCD mnemonic: *asymmetry*, a lesion that is neither round nor oval; an irregular *border*, with notching or scalloped edges; heterogeneity of *color*, with a range of hues from black and blue-black to various shades of brown, pink, and white. Occasionally melanomas are entirely pink or red (amelanotic melanomas). Their *diameter* is generally larger than 6 mm. Most early melanomas are

TABLE 36–1. MANAGEMENT GUIDELINES FOR INDIVIDUALS WITH ATYPICAL NEVI

Thorough examination of the skin to include scalp and external genitalia
Baseline overview and close-up color photography for patients with many lesions or at high risk*
Excisional biopsy of representative lesion for histologic confirmation (optional)
Excisional biopsy of any changing, new, or suspicious lesions
Regular follow-up examination every 6–12 months
Patient education in the recognition of signs of early melanoma, periodic self-examination, and instruction in sun protection and sun avoidance
Screening of first-degree relatives

*A member of the melanoma-prone kindred or an individual with atypical nevi and a previous history of melanoma

asymptomatic, although patients often give a history of change.

Cutaneous melanomas can be divided into four clinicopathologic types. Superficial spreading melanoma (SSM) is the most common form of cutaneous melanoma, accounting for 70% of cases, and has the typical features described above. The lesions of superficial spreading melanoma may occur anywhere on the skin, most commonly on the trunk and extremities. Nodular melanoma (NM) presents as an elevated or polypoid lesion with no flat component. It has the same anatomical distribution as SSM and the same epidemiologic association with intermittent, intense sun exposure. Lentigo maligna melanoma (LMM) is a disease of older individuals and is most directly related to long-term exposure to sunlight. Thus, it occurs most commonly in sun-damaged skin of the face, neck, and back and is related to such outdoor occupations as fishing and farming. It is not associated with precursor nevi. LMMs account for only 4% to 10% of melanomas. Acral lentiginous melanoma (ALM) is a distinct histologic and epidemiologic variant of melanoma arising in the palms, soles, and nail beds. It has no association with sun exposure or precursor nevi and is the most common form of melanoma in African and Asian Americans (although its incidence is likely the same in all races). ALM is characterized by irregular, brown-black, indolently spreading stains on palms and soles. A pigmented nail streak associated with extension of pigment into the skin of the paronychium or eponychium (Hutchinson's sign) is highly suspicious for subungual melanoma.

Staging

The most recent modifications to the tumor, node, metastasis (TNM) classification for the staging of melanoma were adopted by the American Joint Committee on Cancer (AJCC) in 1988 (Table 36–2).[12] Modifications were necessary because 85% of newly diagnosed melanoma patients present with clinically localized disease, and designating all of these as Stage I did not reflect their heterogeneity in survival. Therefore, Stage I and Stage II represent localized melanoma and are divided into subsets based on tumor thickness. Stage III disease is intransit metastases (recurrence between the primary site and regional lymph node basin) or nodal metastases. Stage IV disease represents distant metastases.

Microstaging

An additional substantive advance in the treatment of melanoma has been the elucidation of clinical and histologic prognostic factors for patients with melanoma AJCC Stages I and II.[13,14] Numerous reports have confirmed that tumor thickness (as measured in millimeters from a reference point in the epidermis to the deepest tumor cell) is one of the most important prognostic factors in patients with primary melanoma. Table 36–3 summarizes the 5-year survival rates associated with various tumor thicknesses. Early melanomas (melanoma in situ and thin invasive melanomas <1 mm) have a greater than 90% long-term survival.

Invasive melanomas have been divided into a nontumorigenic step, the invasive radial growth phase and a subsequent tumorigenic step, the vertical growth phase. The former (about one third of primary invasive melanomas) are apparently not capable of metastasis. The latter's likelihood of metastasis is measured in a prognostic model more accurate than thickness in which independent prognostic factors are tumor thickness, mitotic index, tumor-infiltrating lympho-

TABLE 36–2. NEW STAGING SYSTEM FOR MELANOMA ADOPTED BY THE AMERICAN JOINT COMMITTEE ON CANCER

STAGE	CRITERIA
IA	Localized melanoma ≤0.75 mm or Level II (T1N0M0)
IB	Localized melanoma 0.76–1.5 mm or Level III* (T2N0M0)
IIA	Localized melanoma >1.5–4 mm or Level V* (T3N0M0)
IIB	Localized melanoma >4 mm or Level V* (T4N0M0)
III	Limited nodal metastases involving only one regional lymph node basin, or fewer than five in-transit metastases without nodal metastases (any T, N1M0)
IV	Advanced regional metastases (any T, N2M0) or any patient with distant metastases (any T, any N, M1 or M2)

*When the thickness and level of invasion criteria do not coincide within a T classification, thickness should take precedence.

TABLE 36–3. SURVIVAL BY TUMOR THICKNESS

THICKNESS (MM)	5-YEAR SURVIVAL
<0.85	99%
0.85–1.69	94%
1.70–3.65	78%
>3.65	42%

cytes (more are better), regression (unfavorable), tumor location (extremities are better than axial), and patient gender (women do better).[15] In other data sets, tumor ulceration and satellites are unfavorable attributes. Simple, accurate, reliable, and clinically useful multivariable prognostic models are anticipated.[16]

MANAGEMENT OF PRIMARY LESION

The management of primary melanoma begins with recognition (which begins with a thorough cutaneous examination of any patient) and biopsy. The biopsy should be excisional with a narrow margin of normal-appearing skin and should include a portion of underlying subcutaneous fat for accurate microstaging. A punch biopsy in the thickest part of the lesion is an acceptable alternative first step for diagnostically or cosmetically problematic lesions. Techniques that might confound microstaging — superficial shave biopsies and any destructive procedure — are grossly inadequate. Expert pathology, ideally by a pathologist with a particular interest in pigmented lesions, is mandatory. The aim of definitive therapy is control of the primary tumor, including prevention of local recurrence. This is accomplished by surgical excision (generally re-excision, although a single-step procedure is adequate in biologically early lesions), with the dimensions of the procedure dictated primarily by the microstage of the primary tumor and secondarily by anatomical and cosmetic considerations.

Two recent prospective randomized studies have addressed the issue of optimal margins of excision for melanomas. In a study conducted by the World Health Organizational Melanoma Program, 612 patients with primary melanomas less than 2 mm in thickness were randomly assigned to undergo surgical excision of their primary lesion with either a 1- or 3-cm margin.[17] Survival in both groups was identical. In the intergroup study, 486 patients with lesions of intermediate thickness (those 1–4 mm) were randomized to 2- or 4-cm re-excision margins. Overall, there was no statistically significant difference in survival, rate of distant metastases, or incidence of local recurrences between the two groups.[18]

These two studies provide the basis for a current set of recommendations on the margins of excision[19] for invasive melanomas smaller than 4 mm. Melanoma in situ should be excised with at least a 0.5-cm margin, and for invasive melanomas that are less than 1 mm in thickness, a 1-cm margin is optimal. For melanomas that range between 1 and 4 mm in thickness, a 2-cm margin is recommended and allows for primary closure in 90% of cases. In anatomical locations where a 2-cm margin will require the use of a skin graft, a 1-cm margin is acceptable for the subset of the patients with tumors between 1 and 2 mm in thickness. Lesions that are larger than 4.0 mm in thickness may require minimal margins wider than 2 cm to reduce the local recurrence rate. While optimal margins have not been addressed in prospective studies, the present standard is 3 cm.[20] Surgical margins should be histologically uninvolved, and this must be meticulously addressed in melanomas with neurotropism.[21] Various surgical techniques of primary closure have largely replaced the split-thickness skin graft. The use of the narrower margin has allowed for better cosmetic and functional results without compromising overall survival or local control.

The frequency of follow-up visits varies depending on the risk of the primary lesion and the presence of atypical moles. Patients with primary tumors less than 1 mm thick should be followed at 3- to 6-month intervals for 2 or 3 years, with the shorter interval chosen for those with unfavorable prognostic factors or with atypical nevi. Thereafter, yearly follow-up has been recommended.[22] Patients with primary tumors at higher risk should be followed more closely, *e.g.*, 3-monthly for 1 year, 4-monthly for 2 years, 6-monthly for 2 years, and yearly thereafter.

At each follow-up visit, particular attention should be paid to the cutaneous examination (for metastases, changing atypical nevi, and new primary tumors) and palpation of regional lymph nodes (treatment of locoregional recurrences is associated with a significant long-term survival rate). Liver function tests, lactate dehydrogenase, and a chest x-ray film complete routine screening for visceral disease, both at the time of definitive treatment and in follow-up. Additional investigations should be done when prompted by abnormalities. Patient education is an extremely important part of the follow-up. This should include educating patients of the early warning signs of melanoma, how to perform a monthly self-skin examination, and the importance of sun protection and sun avoidance. A detailed family history should be obtained to establish whether the patient belongs to a melanoma-prone family.

MANAGEMENT OF REGIONAL LYMPH NODES

Surgical excision of regional lymph nodes remains the most effective modality in terms of overall survival and local disease control. Surgery can be performed at the time of clinically evident disease (therapeutic lymph node dissection) or before there is clinical evidence of regional lymph node involvement (elective or prophylactic lymph node dissection).

Once regional lymph nodes are clinically involved (AJCC Stage III), standard practice is a therapeutic lymph node dissection. The overall survival at 10 years of patients with regional lymph node involvement who have undergone lymphadenectomy is approximately 25% but varies depending on the number of lymph nodes involved.[23]

Despite the publication of numerous retrospective and prospective randomized trials, the role of elective lymph node dissection (ELND) in the management of patients with AJCC Stage I and Stage II disease remains under debate. This topic has recently been reviewed in detail.[24–26] The application of ELND is controversial because a significant percentage of patients with Stage I and Stage II disease do not have nodal metastases, and therefore are unlikely to benefit from the procedure, which may unnecessarily expose patients to both short- and long-term morbidities. Those who favor ELND suggest that delaying the lymphadenectomy until patients develop clinical evidence may permit the spread of melanoma to multiple nodes and distant sites prior to detection and therefore affect overall survival. Overall, the existing data fail to demonstrate a statistically significant benefit to ELND in the absence of clinical nodal disease.[27,28] Two large, prospective randomized trials designed with the limitations of the previous prospective trials in mind have recently been completed. These studies include patients with intermediate-thickness melanomas, a subset of patients who would most likely benefit from ELND. One hopes that the results from these randomized studies will resolve the controversy.

A new approach that involves selective lymphadenectomy using intraoperative lymphatic mapping may be a useful strategy to identify patients who have microscopic nodal disease. Morton et al. have developed a technique that involves injecting the intradermal site adjacent to the primary tumor with a vital blue dye, followed by a biopsy of the initial node that collects the dye, the "sentinel node."[29] The sentinel nodes are most likely to harbor micrometastases. Using immunohistochemical staining techniques, this node is examined for micrometastases. If it is positive, a formal node dissection is done. This approach may be able to identify patients at high risk for nodal involvement. Additional prospective studies need to be carried out with this new approach to evaluate its diagnostic utility and impact on survival.

Postsurgical Adjuvant Therapy

The risk of relapse of patients with thick primary melanomas (>4 mm) or regional lymph node involvement is high. Despite decades of clinical investigation, no systemic adjuvant therapy has been proved to improve overall survival. Most recently, interferon (IFN) has been evaluated in the adjuvant setting. Preliminary results on 252 patients randomized to observation versus high-dose interferon alfa-2b for 48 weeks have been reported.[30] Although the relapse-free survival of IFN-treated patients was longer than that of untreated patients (the median relapse-free survival of patients receiving IFN was 1.61 years, and in controls was 0.9 years, $p = .7$), there was no impact on overall survival. Based on these results, IFN cannot be accepted as standard clinical treatment for patients with Stage II or III disease. The results of ongoing randomized studies should define the role of adjuvant IFN therapy.

Active specific immunization using melanoma vaccines is undergoing extensive evaluation in the adjuvant setting. A number of vaccine design strategies have been developed using whole melanoma cells (autologous cells and allogeneic cells), melanoma cell lysates, purified antigens including gangliosides, recombinant proteins, immunogenic peptides, genetically modified melanoma cells, and anti-idiotype antibodies.[31–33] Preliminary results are encouraging but far from conclusive. Several randomized, Phase III clinical trials using various vaccine preparations will establish the effectiveness of currently available vaccines, and Phase I studies are just beginning with the newer preparations in patients with metastatic disease.

Regional Limb Perfusion

The goal for regional limb perfusion is to deliver a high concentration of cytotoxic agents to an extremity, with little systemic toxicity. Such an approach with or without hyperthermia has been used for years for indications ranging from adjuvant therapy of subclinical micrometastases to palliation of multiple in-transit metastases. Multiple drugs have been used either alone or in combination and have included melphalan, nitrogen mustard, dacarbazine, and cisplatin. The drug most commonly studied and most effective has been melphalan, with response rates often exceeding 80% when combined with hyperthermia. No significant impact on overall survival has been established.[34] There is renewed interest in regional perfusion because of a recent report of a 90% response rate with hyperthermia and the combination of tumor necrosis factor, IFN gamma and melphalan.[35] However, this therapy is associated with significant regional and systemic toxicity, and its role remains undefined.

MANAGEMENT OF METASTATIC MELANOMA

Melanoma, which has escaped beyond the region of the primary, is an incurable neoplasm in the vast majority of cases. The goal of treatment of patients with Stage IV disease is to palliate and provide, where possible, some significant prolongation of reasonable-quality survival. The specific therapeutic plan for an individual patient will therefore depend on such host factors as age and performance status, and such tumor attributes as tumor burden, number of metastatic sites, specific organ involvement, and pace of tumor growth.

Because it is difficult to argue that there is any standard therapy for disseminated disease, a significant proportion of patients should be considered for clinical research protocols.

The most common first site of visceral metastasis is in the lungs, which emphasizes the role of routine chest radiographs in follow-up. Of visceral sites, the pulmonary site alone has the best survival expectation (a median of 1 year). The brain is the next most common site of initial nonregional metastatic disease (15–20%) and is a common site as the disease evolves. Given the symptomatic importance of brain involvement and its potential for response to radiation therapy (or neurosurgery in selected cases with solitary brain involvement), patients with nonregional metastatic disease of any other site should have magnetic resonance imaging or contrast-enhanced computed tomographic scanning of the brain (whether or not neurologic symptoms are present). Metastases of liver, gastrointestinal tract, and bone are less common at presentation, but subsequent symptomatic involvement of these organ systems is frequently of clinical importance. Surgery should also be considered for solitary metastases.[19] Mean survival of patients with metastatic melanoma is 5 to 6 months, and less than 20% of patients survive 1 year.

Systemic therapies for the treatment of metastatic melanoma include chemotherapy, biological therapy, and various combinations. Patients with involvement of skin, subcutaneous sites, and nodal disease respond most frequently to systemic therapies.

Chemotherapy

Dacarbazine (DTIC) remains the only agent approved by the Food and Drug Administration for the treatment of advanced melanoma. The overall response rate to DTIC is 15% to 20%.[36] The ineffectiveness of single-agent chemotherapy has led to the exploration of combination regimens. The most active of these may be that including tamoxifen, DTIC, carmustine, and cisplatin, with reported response rates ranging from 40% to 50% (predominantly partial responses).[37] In clinical studies that have used similar chemotherapy combinations without tamoxifen, the response rate has ranged from 10% to 30%.[38,39] Tamoxifen as a single agent has minimal activity against metastatic melanoma, so the mechanism of the additive effect of tamoxifen is unclear. Preclinical studies have demonstrated that tamoxifen can enhance the growth inhibitory effects of cisplatin and modulate the pharmacokinectics of carmustine.[36] Tamoxifen has also been evaluated as a modulator of DTIC. In a multicenter randomized trial reported by Cocconi, DTIC alone was compared with DTIC and tamoxifen in patients with metastatic melanoma. A response advantage with the combination, 28% response rate versus 12% with single-agent DTIC was noted.[40] However, other studies have failed to confirm an improvement in overall response rate or survival with the combination of DTIC and tamoxifen. Ongoing randomized trials should address the role of tamoxifen as a modulator of combination chemotherapy.

Biologic Response Modifiers

The promise of these agents and modalities has yet to be realized. An overview of the results of IFN alpha therapy has recently been summarized.[41] The overall response rate is 16%. No optimal schedule or dosage of IFN has been defined. Patients with lower tumor burdens have shown the greatest response rates. Clinical studies using interleukin 2 (IL-2) alone (high-dose and low-dose) or in combination with lymphokine-activated killer (LAK) cells have been completed in patients with metastatic melanoma, and the results are disappointing with an overall response rate ranging from 10% to 25% at the cost of substantial toxicity.[42,43] Whether the addition of gene-altered tumor-infiltrating lymphocytes (TIL) or other cytokines will have clinical utility remains to be determined.[44] Monoclonal antibodies have been developed against melanoma-associated antigens and may have application in diagnosis and therapy. The most extensively studied of the monoclonal antibodies is R24, an immunoglobulin 3 directed against the disialoganglioside GD3.[33] Toxicity has been mild to moderate, and durable responses have been observed in a small number of patients.

Combination of Chemotherapy and Biologic Response Modifiers

In an effort to improve the overall response rate, numerous studies have evaluated the addition of biological response modifiers to chemotherapy. Preliminary results of a series of Phase I and Phase II studies using combinations of IL-2, IFN-alpha, and cisplatin, either alone or with combination chemotherapy regimens, have reported response rates ranging from 25% to 75%.[45,46] The responses have been of brief duration, and therapy is associated with substantial toxicity. This approach has yielded encouraging results, but confirmatory studies are needed.

CONCLUSION

Although the worldwide incidence of cutaneous melanoma continues to increase, physician awareness, public education, and screening programs have resulted in a greater percentage of melanoma patients diagnosed with early and more curable disease. Surgery remains the mainstay of the treatment of melanoma.

What is standard therapy for patients with disseminated melanoma? There is none. The range of treatment options include simple observation of certain patients with minimal disease, surgical excision of solitary metastases, radiation therapy to some lesions, therapy with single- or multiple-agent chemotherapy regimens, participation in a clinical trial, and palliative care. Although therapy of disseminated disease has made only incremental progress, important advances in cataloging the molecular mechanisms of tumor cell growth and in molecular immunology, coupled with explosive growth of the technology of gene transfer, hold the promise of therapeutic advances.

REFERENCES

1. Boring CC, Squires TS, Tong T. Cancer statistics. CA 43:7, 1993
2. Elwood JM, Koh H. Etiology, epidemiology, risk-factors, and public health issues of melanoma. Curr Opin Onc 6:179–187, 1994
3. Rhodes AR, Sober AJ, Day CL et al. The malignant potential of small congenital nevocellular nevi. an estimate of association based on a histologic study of 234 primary cutaneous melanomas. Am Acad Dermatol 6:230–241, 1982
4. Greene MH, Clark WH, Tucker MA, et al. Current concepts: acquired precursors of cutaneous malignant melanoma. N Engl J Med 312:91–97, 1985
5. Clark WH Jr, Reimer RR, Greene M et al. Origin of familial malignant melanomas from heritable melanocytic lesions: "The B-K mole syndrome." Arch Dermatol 114: 732–738, 1978
6. Greene MN, Clark WH Jr, Tucker MA et al. High risk of malignant melanoma in melanoma prone families with dysplastic nevi. Ann Intern Med 102:458–486, 1985
7. Kraemer KH, Greene MH, Tarone R, et al. Dysplastic naevi and cutaneous melanoma risk. Lancet 2:1076–1077, 1983
8. Halpern AC, Guerry D IV, Elder DE et al. Dysplastic nevi as risk markers of sporadic (non-familial) melanoma. Arch Dermatol 127:995–999, 1991
9. MacKie RM, Freudenberger T, Aitchison TC. Personal risk factor chart for cutaneous melanoma. Lancet 2:487–490, 1989
10. Holly EA, Kelly JW, Shpall SN et al. Number of melanocytic nevi as a major risk factor for malignant melanoma. J Am Acad Dermatol 17:459–468, 1987
11. Augustsson A, Ulrika S, Rosdahl I et al. Common and dysplastic naevi as risk factors for cutaneous malignant melanoma in a Swedish population. Acta Derm Vereol (Stockh) 71:518–524, 1991
12. Ketcham AS, Mofft FL, Balch CM. Classification and staging. In Balch CM, Houghton AW, Milton GW et al (eds). Cutaneous Melanoma. Philadelphia, JB Lippincott, 213–220, 1992
13. Clark WH Jr et al. The histogenesis and biological behavior of primary human malignant melanomas of the skin. Cancer Res 29:705–727, 1969
14. Breslow A. Tumor thickness level of invasion and node dissection in Stage I cutaneous melanoma. Ann Surg 182:572–575, 1975
15. Clark WH Jr, Elder DE, Guerry D et al. Model predicting survival in stage I melanoma based upon tumor progression. J Natl Cancer Inst 81:1893–1904, 1989
16. Schuchter LM, Schultz DJ et al. A simple prognostic model predicting ten year survival in patients with stage I melanoma. Proc ASCO, 11:343, 1992
17. Veronesi U, Cascinelli N. Narrow excision (1 cm margin): a safe procedure for thin cutaneous melanoma. Arch Surg 126:438–441, 1991
18. Balch CM, Urist MM, Karakousis CP et al. Efficacy of 2 cm surgical margins for intermediate thickness melanoma (1 to 4 mm). Ann Surg 218:262–269, 1993
19. Ross MI. Surgery and other local-regional modalities for all stages of melanoma. Current Option Oncol 6:197–203, 1984
20. Timmons MJ. Malignant melanoma excision margins: Marking a choice. Lancet 340:1393–1395, 1992
21. Kibbi AG, Mihm MC. Malignant melanoma with desmoplasia and neurotropism. J Dermatol Surg Oncol 13:1204–1208, 1987
22. National Institutes of Health Consensus Development Conference Statement on Diagnosis and Treatment of Early Melanoma, January 27–29, 1992. Am J Dermatol 15:34–43, 1993
23. Morton DL, Wanek L, Nizze JA et al. Improved long-term survival after lymphadenectomy of melanoma metastatic to regional lymph nodes. Ann Surg 214:491–501, 1991
24. Sutherland CM, Mather FJ. Prophylactic lymph node dissection for malignant melanoma: What to do while we wait. J Surg Oncol 51:1–4, 1992
25. Ross MI. The Case for elective lymphadenectomy. Surg Oncol Clin North Am 1:205–222, 1992
26. Crowley NJ. The Case Against Elective Lymphadenectomy. Surg Oncol Clin North Am 1:223–243, 1992
27. Veronesi U, Adamus J, Bandiera D et al. Inefficacy of immediate node dissection in Stage I melanoma of the limbs. N Engl J Med 297:627–630, 1977
28. Sim F, Taylor W, Pritchard D et al. Lymphadenectomy in the management of Stage I malignant melanoma: A prospective randomized study. Mayo Clin Proc 61:697–705, 1986
29. Morton DL, Wen DR, Wong JM. Technical Details of Intra-Operative Lymphatic Mapping for Early Stage Melanoma. Arch Surg 127:392–399, 1992
30. Kirkwood J, Hunt M, Smith T et al. A randomized controlled trial of high-dose IFN alfa-2b for high-risk melanoma: The ECOG trial EST-1684. Proc Am Soc Clin Oncol 12:390, 1993
31. Beretta G. Randomized study of prolonged chemotherapy, immunotherapy, and chemoimmunotherapy as an adjuvant to surgery in stage I and II malignant melanoma (trial 6). Proceedings of Second International Conference on the Immunotherapy of Cancer. April 28–29, 1980; Bethesda, Md, p 8
32. Mitchell MS. Allogeneic vaccines: rationale, results and possible mechanisms of action. In Bystryn J-C, Ferrone S, Livingston P (eds). Specific Immunotherapy of Cancer with Vaccines. Washington, DC, New York Academy of Sciences, 1993
33. Houghton AN, Mintzer D, Cordon-Cardo C et al. Mouse monoclonal IgG_3 antibody detecting GD3 ganglioside: A phase I trial in patients with malignant melanoma. Proc Natl Acad Sci USA 82:1242, 1985
34. Coit DG. Hyperthermic limb perfusion for malignant melanoma: A review. Cancer Invest 10:277–284, 1992
35. Liendard DP, Eualeaka P, DeMotte J et al. High-dose recombinant tumor necrosis factor alpha in combination with interferon gamma and melphalan in isolation perfusion of

the limbs for melanoma and sarcoma. J Clin Oncol 10:52–60, 1992
36. Kirkwood JM, Agarwala SS. Systemic cytotoxic and biologic therapy of melanoma. PPO Updates 7:1–16, 1993
37. De Prete SA, Maurer LH, O'Donnell J. Combination chemotherapy with cisplatin, carmustine, dacarbazine, and tamoxifen in metastatic melanoma. Cancer Treat Rep 68:1403, 1984
38. McClay EF, Mastrangelo MJ, Bellet RE. Combination chemotherapy and hormonal therapy in the treatment of malignant melanoma. Cancer Treat Rep 71:465, 1987
39. McClay EF, Mastrangelo MJ, Berd D, Bellet RE. Effective combination chemo/hormonal therapy for malignant melanoma: Experience with three clinical trials. Int J Cancer 50:553, 1992
40. Cocconi G, Bella M, Calbresi F, et al. Treatment of metastatic malignant melanoma with dacarbazine plus tamoxifen. N Engl J Med 327:516, 1992
41. Kirkwood JM, Ernstoff MS. Cutaneous melanoma. In DeVita VT Jr, Hellman S, Rosenberg SA (eds). Biologic Therapy of Cancer. Philadelphia, JB Lippincott, 1991: 311–333
42. Dutcher JP, Creekmore S, Weiss GR et al. Phase II study of high dose interleukin-2 and lymphokine activated killer cells in patients with metastatic malignant melanoma. J Clin Oncol 7:477–485, 1989
43. Parkinson DR, Abrams JS, Wiernik PH et al. Interleukin-2 therapy in patients with metastatic malignant melanoma: A phase II study. J Clin Oncol 8:1650–1656, 1990
44. Rosenberg SA. The immunotherapy and gene therapy of cancer. J Clin Oncol 10:180–199, 1992
45. Falkson CI, Falkson G, Falkson HC. Improved results with the addition of interferon alfa-2b to dacarbazine in the treatment of patients with metastatic malignant melanoma. J Clin Oncol 9:1403, 1991
46. Richards JM, Mehta N, Ramming K, et al. Sequential chemoimmunotherapy in the treatment of metastatic melanoma. J Clin Oncol 8:1338, 1992

John S. Macdonald, Daniel G. Haller, Robert J. Mayer, Eds. *Manual of Oncologic Therapeutics*, Third Edition.

37. NONMELANOMA SKIN CANCER

Arthur J. Sober
Robert E. Wittes

Tumors arising from the epithelial cells of the skin are the most common malignancies of human beings; more than 700,000 new cases are estimated to occur annually in the United States. At present, the most important etiologic factor is probably chronic exposure to ultraviolet radiation. Residence at equatorial latitudes, lightness of skin and hair color, blue or gray eyes, freckling, easy burning and poor tanning, and a history of outdoor occupation all indicate increased risk. Thus, skin cancer is much more common in Caucasians than African Americans, has an increasing incidence with age, and favors solar-exposed areas of skin, such as the head and neck, and the dorsa of the hands.

Other risk factors include industrial exposures to tar products and ingestion of arsenic from contaminated water, medicines (Fowler's solution), or herbicides and pesticides. Skin cancers also occur as sequelae of occupational or therapeutic exposure to ionizing radiation, chronic infections, burns, trauma, and immunosuppression. They are also associated with some well-established premalignant conditions of the skin (actinic keratoses, Bowen's disease, and erythroplasia of Queyrat), as well as with certain heritable disorders (xeroderma pigmentosum, albinism, and the basal cell nevus syndrome).

Nonmelanoma skin cancers are the most curable malignant tumors of human beings. Most tend to remain localized for their entire natural history. Although basal cell carcinomas (BCC) are clearly capable of metastasizing, they do so only rarely (only about 400 cases of metastatic BCC have been reported) and then only very late in the course of inadequately controlled local disease. Squamous cell carcinoma (SCC) behaves more variably. The usual SCC arising in light-exposed areas of skin damaged by chronic ultraviolet exposure has a low incidence of metastasis. By contrast, the propensity of SCC for metastasis in other settings may be appreciably higher. SCC after irradiation metastasizes in about 20% to 25% of cases; tumors in the setting of chronic infection, ulcers, or draining sinuses, about 30%; and SCC arising from Bowen's lesions or from erythroplasia of Queyrat, about 20% to 40%. In addition, SCC appearing *de novo* from normal skin or from mucosal surfaces (lip, vulva, anus) appears to be more aggressive clinically than SCC arising from pre-existing lesions. SCC causes approximately 2000 deaths annually in the United States.

The relative rarity of metastasis from skin cancer, however, does not mean that these tumors are clinically inconsequential. Patients who develop skin cancer have an increased likelihood of developing additional skin tumors, either synchronously or metachronously, so that skin cancer is a medical problem requiring continued surveillance at 6- to 12-month intervals and often periodic therapy. Also, if inadequately treated, skin cancers are capable of great mischief. A locally uncontrolled skin cancer on the skin of the face, for example, may cause horrific misery by invading and destroying contiguous normal structures, such as the bones of the face, the cranial vault, and even the brain. As with other epithelial tumors, early diagnosis and adequate definitive treatment yield the optimal therapeutic result.

PRETREATMENT EVALUATION

Every clinician should be familiar with the characteristic appearance of BCC and SCC; representative color photos of good quality are available in standard texts. Nevertheless, even the seasoned observer can be fooled by atypical presentations: The pigmented BCC masquerading as malignant melanoma, sebaceous gland hyperplasia or trichoepithelioma that looks like a BCC, or eczematoid "rashes" that turn out to be *in situ* SCC. As at other sites, therefore, biopsy confirmation is necessary, either before or at the time of definitive therapy. The type of biopsy (incisional or excisional) and the technique to be used depend on the lesion's location, size, and character. Physical examination should include complete examination of all skin surfaces and clinical assessment of regional nodes; significant adenopathy in the nodes draining the area of SCC is an indication for node biopsy. In view of the great rarity of distant metastases at the time of initial presentation, screening radiographs and scans are not indicated in the absence of clinical symptoms.

STAGING

No generally accepted staging system exists.

TREATMENT

The goal of therapy ought to be the expeditious removal of all viable tumor in a manner that ensures a satisfactory cosmetic result. Surgical excision, radiation, electrodessication and curettage, cryotherapy, and microscopically controlled "fresh-tissue" surgery are the available modalities. Selection of the approach in a particular case is a matter of expert judgment and depends on such parameters as the location, type, size, number, and depth of the lesion(s); the character of the underlying skin; the type of prior treatment; the expertise of the treating physician; and the wishes of the patient.

Surgical excision is applicable to a wide variety of presentations. It is particularly appropriate for large tumors in many locations, for tumors that remain after radiotherapy, and for tumors occurring in scars, ulcers, or draining sinuses. If the tumor is large and located in an area where the surgical defect cannot be closed primarily, a flap or skin graft may be necessary.

Curettage is most useful for small (<10 mm diameter) BCC that are located on flat surfaces or tumors having depth no greater than the dermis or, at most, the upper subcutaneous layer. This procedure, with or without electrodesiccation of the base, can be used to good advantage for single or multiple lesions. Cryotherapy is useful in generally the same clinical circumstances as curettage.

Radiotherapy is particularly appropriate for lesions on the face, where surgery is either technically difficult or likely to yield a cosmetically unsatisfactory result (nose, lip, eyelid, canthus). Radiotherapy is not generally satisfactory once tumor has invaded underlying bone or cartilage. When possible, radiotherapy is usually reserved for patients over the age of 60.

For tumors such as the morphea-type BCC, whose anatomical limits are difficult to define, and any cases that have recurred despite previous therapy, the technique of fresh-tissue (Mohs') surgery probably offers the best chance of cure. This involves painstaking resection of residual tumor with ongoing histologic monitoring of lateral and deep margins; the process continues until there is no further histologic evidence of malignancy in the resected specimens. In addition to recurrent tumors, this technique is especially useful for lesions located on the scalp, behind the ear, and in the inner canthus or nasolabial folds.

Experimental agents for the treatment of basal cell carcinoma include intralesional interferon and laser therapy with hematoporphyrin derivative.

Patients treated for skin cancer need careful follow-up to verify the adequacy of treatment and to monitor the occurrence of new cancers. In a patient with a new BCC the likelihood of a second occurrence of BCC after 1-year follow-up is 20%; multiple previous BCC raise the likelihood of additional tumors by 1 year to 40%. Young patients in particular should be advised about the risks of sun exposure and should be counseled to limit sun exposure during the time when the sun's rays are most direct (11 AM to about 2:30 PM) and to use potent sunscreens (at least SPF 15) when sun exposure is unavoidable.

Not much is known about chemotherapy for disseminated disease; the rarity of metastasis from skin primaries has confined reports on the efficacy of individual drugs or regimens to a series of anecdotes. It appears that cisplatin has antitumor activity; this agent singly, or in combination with bleomycin or doxorubicin, has produced major regressions of tumor in selected cases, some of which have been for impressive durations. For palliation of symptoms from metastatic tumor in critical locations, radiotherapy should be considered.

TREATMENT OF PREMALIGNANT LESIONS OF SKIN

Actinic keratoses can be removed by excision, curettage, or cryotherapy. For patients with multiple lesions, topical 5-fluorouracil (5-FU) is effective; 1% to 5% 5-FU cream or gel is applied twice daily for 10 to 21 days or longer until marked erythema and crusting develop in the treated skin; the lesions are then allowed to slough and re-epithelialize. Masoprocol twice daily for 28 days is a recently released alternative.

Bowen's disease (squamous cell carcinoma in situ) may be approached in a similar fashion; here, however, if 5-FU is employed, it must be of longer duration and under occlusion. In addition, the physician should be alert to the frequent association of Bowen's disease occurring on covered areas of skin with internal malignancies. The basis for this association is not entirely clear; the presence of a common etiologic factor such as arsenic appears likely. In any case, these patients should be carefully screened on presentation and followed carefully.

Leukoplakia occurring in the setting of chronic tobacco usage should probably be treated with one of the techniques noted above, if the lesion is single and discrete. For multiple or widespread lesions, a recent study has shown that the use of isotretinoin (13-cis-retinoic acid), 1 mg to 2 mg/kg/day for 3 months, significantly decreases the number and size of leukoplakia lesions in such patients. Whether isotretinoin will also decrease the rate of development of invasive cancer is unknown at present. Recurrence rates after isotretinoin treatment are also presently unknown. Because of the potential side-effects, this agent is best employed by physicians experienced in its use. Pregnancy is an absolute contraindication.

BIBLIOGRAPHY

Carter DM, Lin AN. Basal cell carcinoma. In Fitzpatrick TB, Eisen AZ, Wolff K et al. (eds). Dermatology in General Medicine, 4th ed. New York, McGraw-Hill, 1993:840–847,

Farmer ER, Helwig EB. Metastatic basal cell carcinoma: A clinico-pathologic study of seventeen cases. Cancer 46:748–757, 1980

Guthrie TH Jr, McElveen LJ, Porubsky ES et al. Cisplatin and doxorubicin: An effective chemotherapy combination in the treatment of advanced basal cell and squamous carcinoma of the skin. Cancer 55:1629–1632, 1985

Haynes HA, Mead KW, Goldwyn RM. Cancers of the skin. In DeVita VT Jr, Hellman SH, Rosenberg SA (eds). Cancer: Principles & Practice of Oncology, 3rd ed. Philadelphia, JB Lippincott, 1989

Hong WK, Endicott J, Itri LM et al. 13-Cis-retinoic acid in the treatment of oral leukoplakia. N Engl J Med 315:1501–1505, 1986

Schwartz RA, Stoll HL Jr. Squamous cell carcinoma. In Fitzpatrick TB, Eisen AZ, Wolff K et al (eds). Dermatology in General Medicine, 4th ed. New York, McGraw-Hill, 1993:821–833

John S. Macdonald, Daniel G. Haller, Robert J. Mayer, Eds. *Manual of Oncologic Therapeutics*, Third Edition.

38. PRIMARY CENTRAL NERVOUS SYSTEM TUMORS

Howard A. Fine

Once thought to be rare, primary tumors of the central nervous system (CNS) are now recognized as a significant cancer problem in the United States. Approximately 15,000 new cases of malignant brain tumors are diagnosed in the United States each year (7.3 per 100,000 population), accounting for 1% to 2% of all malignancies in this country. Although the majority of patients who develop primary brain tumors are over the age of 40, these tumors represent a major cause of morbidity and mortality in younger patients. They rank next to leukemia as the major cause of cancer-related deaths in children less than 15 years old and are the third leading cause of cancer-related mortality in men between the ages of 15 and 54, and the fourth in women between the ages of 15 and 34. Furthermore, recent data suggest an increasing incidence of primary brain tumors. In particular, the incidence of primary CNS lymphomas in immunocompetent patients has tripled, with an even greater increase in immunodeficient patients and a four- to fivefold increase in astrocytomas in the elderly.

PATHOGENESIS

The etiology of most primary brain tumors remains largely unsolved, although several environmental stimuli have been implicated as risk factors. The most well-documented of these is ionizing radiation. It is clear that children with a history of cranial radiation therapy are at significantly increased risk of developing primary brain tumors. The highest risk is for the development of meningiomas, whereas the risk of glial tumors is probably double that of the general population. Exposure to vinyl chloride has also been linked to the development of primary brain tumors, however, this association and the data on other occupational exposures remain uncertain. Several congenital genetic disorders are clearly associated with an increased risk of primary brain tumors, including neurofibromatosis I and II, tuberous sclerosis, Turcot's syndrome, Rendu-Osler-Weber syndrome, and the Li-Fraumeni syndrome. Viruses have been implicated in the pathogenesis of gliomas in animals, although the correlation has not yet been made in humans. The Epstein-Barr virus, however, can be found in the vast majority of primary CNS lymphoma cells in immunodeficient patients, and genomic deoxyribonucleic acid (DNA) from the SV40 polyoma virus has been identified in choroid plexus tumors of infancy.

PRESENTING SIGNS AND SYMPTOMS

Headache is the most common presenting symptom of patients with primary brain tumors. Patients commonly complain that their headache is worse on wakening and generally improves during the course of the day. This may represent increased cerebral edema secondary to the prone position assumed during the night and the redistribution of fluid to the lower body on rising. Despite this common pattern, however, all types and patterns of headaches can be seen and are a rather nonspecific symptom. Approximately half of the patients with primary brain tumors present with either subtle mental status changes, seizures, hemiparesis, or combination of the above. Nausea and vomiting, dysphasia, and visual problems are much less commonly seen as presenting symptoms. Most large clinical trials have reported that the longer duration of symptoms, the better is the ultimate prognosis. This probably reflects a slower growth rate of the tumor.

In addition to physical findings corresponding to the above-mentioned symptoms, historically one could detect papilledema in 50% of all patients at presentation. With the greater accessibility to sensitive neuroradiographic imaging modalities (*i.e.*, computed tomographic [CT] scan, magnetic resonance imaging [MRI]) tumors are now being discovered earlier, so that the diagnosis can be made well before there is a significant elevation in intracranial pressure. Thus, the incidence of papilledema is probably significantly lower now than in the past.

DIAGNOSIS

Advances in neuroimaging and neurosurgery have made the diagnosis of primary brain tumors significantly easier over the last decade. The ready accessibility to CT scanning and MRI in most places in the United States has allowed for the discovery of intracranial space-occupying lesions in a more timely fashion than ever before. Specific types of primary brain tumors have certain radiographic features that suggest their nature. For instance, a homogeneously enhancing dural-based lesion that does not appear to be infiltrating the brain is highly suggestive of a meningioma. Conversely, a highly infiltrative, heterogeneously enhancing mass with areas of cystic formation and necrosis associated with mass effect and edema is suggestive of a malignant glioma. A low attenuating mass within the substance of the brain and associated with calcification is commonly an oligodendroglioma, whereas multifocal ring-enhancing lesions in a perventricular distribution in an immunocompromised host are likely to be lymphoma. The anatomical distribution of the tumor, as much as its radiographic characteristics, may also be a clue to the diagnosis. For instance, a contrast-enhancing lesion in the pontine-cerebellar angle involving cranial nerve VIII is likely to be an acoustic neuroma, whereas an infiltrating, enhancing lesion in the cerebellar vermis of a child is likely to be a medulloblastoma.

MRI is generally more sensitive for discovering small or multiple lesions than is a CT scan. MRI is also more accurate for determining heterogeneity within a tumor mass as well as tumor extension. MRI is particularly superior to the CT scan for visualizing infratentorial structures (*i.e.*, midbrain, brain stem) and posterior fossa abnormalities, since the bony structures encasing these anatomical sites commonly cause significant distortion on CT images.

No matter how characteristic a lesion may appear on CT scan or MRI, however, most radiographically defined lesions should be histologically confirmed by biopsy. One possible exception to this rule is an elderly patient who presents with a severe and rapid neurologic decline and is found to have a large enhancing necrotic-appearing mass. Physicians often choose not to subject this type of patient to a surgical procedure but rather to offer palliative radiation therapy, or supportive care, on the assumption that this represents a glioblastoma. The second clinical scenario in which biopsy may not be obtained is in a young child with a heterogeneously enhancing, infiltrative, brain stem lesion. Surgeons and radiotherapists often forego biopsy of these lesions secondary to the danger of invading sensitive areas and causing significant neurologic damage, when, in fact, the lesion is likely to be an intrinsic brain stem glioma. Nevertheless, the indications for not making a histologic diagnosis are becoming small. The reason is that in the past, open biopsy of brain tumor lesions was associated with significantly high mortality and morbidity. Furthermore, many tumors were totally inaccessible through open biopsies because of their deep location in the brain (thalamic or pineal region tumors) or their proximity to exquisitely sensitive structures (brain stem). This all changed with the advent of the technology known as stereotaxis.

Stereotaxis involves the placement of a fixed frame onto the patient's skull, followed by a CT scan or MRI with the frame in place. The frame functions as a reference point in space, relative to the patient's cranium, so that localization of the tumor seen in the two-dimensional radiographs can be converted to three-dimensional coordinates. A surgical device is then attached to the stereotactic frame, and the biopsy needle can be advanced to the tumor, based on the stereotactic coordinates. The coordinates are chosen not only to localize the tumor, but to allow for a pathway to the tumor that avoids important intracerebral structures.

Advances in pathology have also allowed for a more accurate diagnosis of primary brain tumors. The discovery of several cell lineage–specific antibodies has led to the development of immunohistochemical techniques that help the pathologist determine an accurate histologic diagnosis. Among those most commonly utilized are stains for glial fibrillary acidic protein, a glial-specific marker; synoptophysin, a marker of neuroendocrine differentiation; Leu-7, a marker of oligodendroglioma differentiation; and leukocyte common antigen, a marker of lymphoid cells. Molecular biology techniques are also becoming increasingly useful. For instance, techniques such as Southern analysis and polymerase chain reaction are useful for evaluating whether lymphoid cells are monoclonal or polyclonal by examining the pattern of rearrangement of the immunoglobulin gene. Electron microscopy is also occasionally useful, especially for differentiating between primary and metastatic tumors.

GENERAL PATIENT MANAGEMENT ISSUES

The management of patients with a malignant brain tumor can be a difficult task. The problems these patients face cross many subspecialty lines, including neurosurgery, neurology, and internal medicine. The types of neurologic problems seen in these patients are variable and depend on the size, histology, and anatomical location of the tumor, while their medical problems are often a result of their neurologic disability and side-effects from therapeutic interventions. For these reasons, each patient has individual management issues. Nevertheless, several noteworthy management problems are common to most patients with intracranial lesions.

Cerebral Edema

Most intracerebral tumors cause the normally tight endothelial connections (blood brain barrier) to become leaky, thus resulting in increased intracerebral fluid, a condition known as vasogenic edema. The mechanism by which tumors induce vasogenic edema remains largely unknown; however, the consequence of the edema is an increase in intracranial pressure. Vasogenic edema is greatest in the immediate area of the tumor and disperses as it moves away from the primary tumor site. This edema and resultant increased intracranial pressure can result in neurologic compromise. For example, if a patient has a tumor in the right frontal lobe, anterior to the motor strip (in the parietal lobe), the patient still might be hemiparetic on the left side secondary to extension of vasogenic edema posteriorly.

In addition to causing focal neurologic dysfunction, vasogenic edema causes headaches and nausea as well as increased seizure activity. Thus, decreasing cerebral edema is of primary importance. In the acute setting, this can effectively be done by administering an intravascular hyperosmotic agent such as mannitol. Mannitol can be given as 25- to 50-mg boluses every 15 to 30 minutes. The only major contraindication to mannitol is compromised cardiac function. Mannitol administration can cause a rapid increase in intravascular volume, thereby causing acute congestive heart failure. If patients are being given multiple doses of mannitol, serum osmolarity needs to be frequently checked in order to prevent hyperosmolarity. The major disadvantage of mannitol is that it needs to be administered frequently and it rapidly loses effectiveness over several days.

The only drugs shown to control vasogenic edema effectively over extended periods of time are the glucocorticoids. In general, dexamethasone has been the glucocorticoid of choice. There appears to be a dose-response relationship between the amount of dexamethasone and neurologic improvement. This improvement may take as long as 4 to 7 days to be clinically apparent, as opposed to the acute response often seen with mannitol. Anecdotal experience also suggests that frequent daily dosing (two to four times per day) is more effective than once-a-day dosing. Unfortunately, along with the greater efficacy of higher and more frequent dosing is a greater incidence of glucocorticoid-associated toxicities. These include increases in appetite and weight gain, resulting in a cushingoid appearance. The weight gain can be profound enough to interfere with the patient's ability to ambulate. Glucocorticoids also cause psychiatric problems, most often emotional lability. In its most severe form, glucocorticoids can induce frank psychosis. If the steroids can be tapered to lower doses, this usually remits.

Steroid myopathy is another dexamethasone-related problem that can result in profound ambulatory problems. This myopathy most commonly effects the proximal muscle groups, particularly of the lower extremities. Elderly patients appear especially susceptible to this problem. Dexamethasone can also cause glucose intolerance, possibly through increased hepatic gluconeogenesis. For this reason, the hyperglycemia often does not respond to diet or oral hypoglycemic agents and thus may necessitate insulin.

Potentially, the most serious glucocorticoid-related problem is immunosuppression. Although glucocorticoids can effect the entire immune system, cellular immune responses are most profoundly diminished. This makes patients much more susceptible to viral infections, such as herpes, as well as intracellular parasites, such as tuberculosis. In particular, brain tumor patients maintained on high doses of glucocorticoids have a significantly increased chance of developing *Pneumocystis carinii* pneumonia (PCP). Interestingly, PCP most commonly occurs when steroid doses are reduced. Thus, for patients on chronically high doses of glucocorticoids, prophylaxis for PCP (trimethoprim-sulfamethoxazole [Bactrim], 1 double-strength tablet three times per week) should be considered.

The need to decrease cerebral edema balanced by the need to minimize the risk of glucocorticoid-related toxicities makes dexamethasone dosing one of the most important and challenging management issues in patients with brain tumors. In general, when a patient is found to have symptomatic cerebral edema, dexamethasone is initiated at a dose between 2 and 24 mg/day in two to four divided daily doses. Maximal symptomatic benefit (abatement of headache, nausea, and neurologic dysfunction is usually observed) in 4 to 7 days, at which point the dexamethasone dose is slowly decreased by increments of 1 to 4 mg every 4 to 14 days. Decisions on dexamethasone (Decadron) dosing should be based almost entirely on clinical assessment of the patient rather than on CT scans or MRI. For instance, if MRI shows a significant amount of edema but the patient is asymptomatic, there is no compelling reason to start dexamethasone. Alternately, if the MRI shows only a minimal amount of edema in the left temporal lobe but the patient becomes aphasic, a therapeutic trial of dexamethasone is clearly indicated.

Seizures

The management and prevention of seizures are paramount in patients with primary brain tumors. Not only can seizures disrupt the patient's life (in most states patients with generalized seizures are not allowed to drive) and unpleasant for family members to observe, but they can also cause significant morbidity in patients with brain tumors. In patients without space-occupying intracranial lesions, the usual post-seizure neurologic dysfunction (*i.e.*, "Todd's paralysis") lasts for only several hours. In patients with primary brain tumors, however, the deficit can be profound, long-lasting (days to weeks), and occasionally permanent. Furthermore, in patients with large amounts of intracerebral edema, death can ensue following a prolonged generalized seizure, presumably secondary to supratentorial cerebral herniation (although the mechanism is unknown, it is possibly due to increased intracerebral edema related to seizure activity). Thus one must try to completely prevent or at least reduce the frequency and/or intensity of seizures in patients with brain tumors.

Most patients are placed on antiseizure medications either after the radiographic demonstration of an intracranial mass or before the diagnostic neurosurgical procedure. The most common drug used is phenytoin followed by carbamazepine and phenobarbitol. Some neurologists feel carbamazepine should be the first-line drug for temporal lobe or focal seizures. If a patient experiences a seizure while on one of these drugs, the physician should attempt to increase the dose of the drug in order to obtain a high therapeutic serum level. Drug levels can be pushed higher than "therapeutic levels" as long as the patient is not experiencing any drug-related side-effects (*i.e.*, dizziness, nausea, somnolence, ataxia). If a patient is still having seizures with a high therapeutic dose of a single drug, then a second drug is usually added. Using this general approach, seizures are usually well controlled in patients with brain tumors. For the occasional patient with persistent seizure, the help of an experienced neurologist is invaluable.

A question that commonly arises is whether all patients with brain tumors require antiseizure medications, especially if they have never experienced a seizure. It is generally thought that for patients who have tumors anywhere in the supratentorial cortex, the likelihood of a seizure is high enough to make the use of antiepileptic therapy worthwhile, given how well therapy is generally tolerated. Alternatively, patients with infratentorial lesions, such as those in the brain stem or cerebellum, are at low risk of a seizure; thus it is reasonable not to treat them expectantly with antiseizure medication.

A final practical question that is often raised is whether a patient can ever be safely withdrawn from antiepileptic therapy. Although most patients will probably need to be kept on these medications for most of their lives, there is a subgroup of patients for whom withdrawal of antiseizure medication is probably reasonable. These are patients who have tumors in remission (at least radiographically) and who are seizure-free for a long time (1 year). For this small subgroup of patients, we routinely obtain an electroencephalogram (EEG). If the EEG shows no signs of a seizure focus, we slowly wean the patient off the antiepileptic agent.

THERAPY OF PRIMARY BRAIN TUMORS

One of the most important concepts in the treatment of a patient with a primary brain tumor is that staging, treatment options, and eventual prognosis depend greatly on the specific histology and grade of the tumor. Although there are many types of primary brain tumors (Table 38–1), many are benign lesions seen almost exclusively by neurosurgeons. For the purposes of this chapter, we discuss treatment strategies only for the most common primary brain tumors seen by medical oncologists.

TABLE 38–1. MAJOR PATHOLOGIC CATEGORIES OF PRIMARY CNS TUMORS

TUMORS OF NEUROEPITHELIAL ORIGIN
Astrocytoma
Low-grade
Anaplastic
Glioblastoma multiforme
Oligodendrogliomas
Low-grade
Anaplastic
Mixed oligo/astrocytoma
Neuronal tumors
Gangliogliomas (cytomas)
Neuroblastoma
Pineal cell tumors
Pinealocytoma
Pinealoblastoma
Ependymal and choroid plexus tumors
Ependymoma
Choroid plexus papilloma
Primitive neuroendocrine tumors (PNET)
Medulloblastoma
Cortical PNET
TUMORS OF MENINGEAL ORIGIN
Meningioma
Menigeal sarcoma
NERVE SHEATH TUMORS
Schwannoma (neurinoma)
Neurofibroma
PRIMARY CNS LYMPHOMA
PRIMARY CNS GERM CELL TUMORS
Dysgerminoma
Mixed germ cell
Teratoma
PITUITARY TUMORS

Astrocytomas

Astrocytomas are the most common primary brain tumors in adults. The management, and ultimately the prognosis, of patients with astrocytomas is intimately related to the grade of the tumor. The grading of astrocytomas, however, is difficult to understand because of the many grading systems currently in use. Furthermore, even within a given grading system, there is much interobserver variability among pathologists.

In general there are two major grading schemas: a three-tier system and a four-tier system. Within these systems are two distinctly different prognostic subgroups, low-grade astrocytomas (Grades I/III, or Grades I–II/IV) and high-grade astrocytomas (Grades II–III/III, Grades III–IV/IV). Although the median survival of patients with low-grade astrocytomas is significantly better than those with high-grade tumors (4–10 years vs. 8–18 months, respectively), low-grade astrocytomas are not benign lesions. The majority of patients with these tumors ultimately die of their disease. Because most adults who are stricken with low-grade astrocytomas are young, these tumors can hardly be called benign.

Unfortunately, because of the rarity of these tumors and their long natural history, few prospective randomized trials have tested different treatment options in these patients. Based mostly on retrospective data, current recommendations for patients with low-grade astrocytomas are for maximal surgical debulking. If a complete gross resection is achieved, postsurgical treatment is probably not indicated, and the patient can be conservatively followed with MRI every 6 to 12 months. If, on the other hand, the tumor cannot be completely removed, postsurgical therapy with involved-field radiation therapy to approximately 5400 cGy is considered standard treatment. There is no proven role for postirradiation chemotherapy in these patients.

There are considerably more data on the treatment of patients with high-grade astrocytomas than on treatment of those with low-grade tumors. The first fact that the treating physician should be aware of is that several prognostic variables are strongly predictive of the relative survival of patients with high-grade astrocytomas. Poor prognostic variables include older age (greater than 60), poor performance status, and Grade III/III or IV/IV histology. Although high-grade astrocytomas are often considered to be a homogeneous group of tumors, in fact, data from many of the large prospective trials have shown that patients with anaplastic astrocytomas (Grades II/III or III/IV) have significantly longer survivals than those with glioblastoma multiforme (Grades III/III or IV/IV), 26–36 vs. 8–10 months, respectively).

The role of surgery in the management of high-grade astrocytomas remains unclear. Some neurosurgeons believe that maximal surgical debulking is optimal, whereas others believe that aggressive surgery offers no benefits over biopsy alone. Although retrospective reviews of several studies suggest that the amount of postsurgical residual tumor as assessed by CT scan is inversely related to survival, this does not necessarily mean that maximal surgical debulking increases survival. Nevertheless, a large debulking surgical procedure (when it can be done safely) allows for a decompression of intracerebral mass effect and supplies a large enough amount of tissue for accurate histologic diagnosis and grading. Regardless of the extent of surgery, however, patients with high-grade astrocytomas will require postsurgical adjuvant treatment because of the diffusely infiltrative nature of the tumor.

Several large, prospective, randomized trials have conclusively demonstrated that postsurgical radiation therapy can more than double the median survival of these patients. Based on a number of nonrandomized studies, current recommendations for radiation therapy of high-grade astrocytomas have been generated and call for radiation to be delivered in 180- to 200-cGy fractions over the course of 6 to 7 weeks, to a total dose of approximately 6000 cGy. Although there have been no prospective randomized trials evaluating the optimal volume of irradiated tissue, several studies suggest that involved-field radiation is equivalent to whole-brain radiation for tumor control yet associated with significantly less long-term neurologic morbidity.

The role of postirradiation chemotherapy in the treatment of patients with high-grade astrocytomas has been a controversial area for some time. More than 20 randomized trials have been conducted to evaluate whether postirradiation chemotherapy increases survival, compared with radiation therapy alone. The results of these randomized trials have been mixed, largely because of the relatively small number of patients in each of the trials, thereby limiting the statistical power of each of the studies to detect a significant therapeutic difference. The trials have also been plagued by heterogeneous patient populations and lack of control for major prognostic factors. A recent meta-analysis of many of the randomized trials, however, suggests that postirradiation chemotherapy for patients with anaplastic astrocytomas does indeed increase median survival. Alternately, it appears as though postirradiation chemotherapy for patients with glioblastoma is less effective and in fact probably benefits only a small minority of patients. These are patients with the best prognostic factors, including young age, good performance status, and minimal postsurgical residual disease.

Traditional postirradiation chemotherapy for high-grade astrocytomas has included a nitrosourea, most often single-agent carmustine (BCNU) given at a dose of 80 mg/m^2/day for 3 consecutive days or 200 mg/m^2 on day 1 with cycles repeated every 6 weeks. A recent randomized trial comparing this regimen of BCNU versus the commonly utilized three-drug combination of procarbazine, lomastine (CCNU), and vincristine (PCV: CCNU 110 mg/m^2 on day 1; procarbazine 60 mg/m^2 days 8 to 21; vincristine 1.4 mg/m^2 days 8 and 28) in the postirradiation setting demonstrated no significant survival difference. A subroup analysis, however, revealed that patients with anaplastic astrocytomas treated with PCV had nearly twice the median survival, compared with the patients treated with BCNU. Although conclusions drawn from a subgroup analysis need to be viewed with caution, this survival difference was impressive enough that standard treatment of patients with anaplastic astrocytomas following radiation therapy now includes the three-drug combination PCV.

Despite this aggressive trimodality approach (surgery, radiation therapy, and chemotherapy), almost all patients with high-grade astrocytomas have tumor progression at some point. Retrospective analyses demonstrate that nearly all of these tumors will recur within a 2-cm margin of the original tumor site. This propensity for local recurrence has prompted new strategies designed to deliver high-dose focal radiation to the immediate tumor site. Several Phase II studies have been conducted to evaluate the role of conformal radiation therapy as a "boost" to standard external beam radiation therapy and chemotherapy as part of the initial treatment of these tumors. Most of the data come from studies of brachytherapy.

Brachytherapy is a technique whereby afterloading catheters are stereotactically placed in the residual tumor bed following standard external beam radiation therapy. The catheters are then loaded with a radioactive source (*i.e.*, ^{125}I seeds) and removed several days later. This technique allows for a high dose of local radiation to be delivered within the contours of the tumor bed with a rapid drop-off of radiation dose as one approaches the normal tissue. A similar strategy can be applied by using various methods that deliver focal external beam radiation. Such techniques include proton beam therapy and radiosurgery.

Radiosurgery is a technique whereby noncoplanar converging arcs of radiation are delivered with the arcs intersecting and converging (the "isocenter") on the residual tumor volume. There are various techniques for delivering high doses of focal radiation based on three-dimensional imaging.

Despite the technical differences in the methodology, all these techniques aim for the same biologic endpoint, which is to deliver a high dose of focal radiation to the residual tumor along with a margin of normal tissue. Normal brain tissue is therefore spared the destructive effect of high-dose radiation.

Early Phase II data suggest that patients with glioblastoma treated with focal radiation boost (either brachytherapy or radiosurgery) survive longer than those treated merely with conventional methods. Unfortunately, these focal radiation techniques are associated with a high incidence of symptomatic radiation necrosis, often requiring high doses of steroids for edema control and often necessitating reoperation to remove necrotic tissue. Thus, quality of life needs to be evaluated in considering focal radiation for the treatment of patients with high-grade astrocytomas. Currently, the Brain Tumor Cooperative Group is conducting a randomized trial of brachytherapy *versus* conventional therapy, and the Radiation Therapy Oncology Group is planning a trial that will compare radiosurgery to conventional therapy. Perhaps these prospective randomized trials will help elucidate the role of focal radiation in the treatment of glioblastoma.

RECURRENT HIGH-GRADE ASTROCYTOMAS

Regardless of the type of primary therapy patients receive, most have tumor recurrence. Occasionally, the tumors recur in a focal pattern such that repeat surgical resection might be possible. Although it is unclear whether surgical resection in this subgroup of patients is clearly beneficial, it appears to be a reasonable option for young, healthy patients. Focal radiation techniques are also potentially applicable for patients with locally confined recurrent disease, assuming that the recurrence is in a relatively silent area of the brain in which radiation necrosis will not cause significant neurologic morbidity.

Most patients with recurrent disease require systemic treatment because of the diffusely infiltrative nature of the tumor. Although single-agent nitrosoureas and the PCV regimen are considered first-line standard therapies, it is clear that the response to these agents is generally suboptimal. The actual response rate to these drugs is not known because there have been no prospective Phase II trials (in the post-CT scan era) to evaluate the activity of nitrosoureas for recurrent gliomas. Anectodal experience suggests, however, that patients with anaplastic astrocytomas have a higher response rate than those with glioblastoma. This does appear to be the case in the few well-conducted Phase II trials of newer investigational agents. Nevertheless, even for patients who do respond to systemic chemotherapy, the time to tumor progression is relatively short. Median survival of patients with glioblastoma following the recurrence of their disease is usually less than 6 months.

Along with nitrosoureas and procarbazine-based regimens, other standard chemotherapeutic agents that have some activity are cisplatin, carboplatin, cyclophosphamide, and interferon alpha and beta. Preliminary results also suggest that high-dose tamoxifen may have some activity. Again, however, even in patients who do respond to second-line therapy, the time to tumor progression is short.

Because of the paucity of truly effective agents in the treatment of these tumors, physicians are encouraged to attempt to enroll most patients on well-designed clinical trials. However, past experience has taught us that there is a subgroup of patients for whom further therapy should not be offered. They include patients with poor performance status, advanced physiologic age, and severe neurologic deficits and whose whose disease has failed to respond to multiple therapeutic agents. These patients should be offered comfort measures only.

Oligodendrogliomas

Another type of glioma that commonly afflicts adults is oligodendroglioma. Oligodendrogliomas constitute approximately 6% to 10% of all gliomas in adults. These are usually low-grade tumors that commonly present with new seizures in adults or follow a long history of "idiopathic" seizures. Radiographically, these tumors most commonly look like low-grade astrocytomas, except that more than half are calcified. Optimal treatment for most oligodendrogliomas is maximal surgical resection. If the tumor can be grossly removed, most patients can expect an excellent prognosis.

One subgroup of oligodendrogliomas recurs multiple times or has anaplastic features at the time of presentation. Despite aggressive local measures, these tumors cause local cerebral destruction and dissemination throughout the cranial-spinal axis. Occasionally, malignant or anaplastic oligodendrogliomas may systemically metastasize. They tend to be significantly more radioresistant than astrocytomas; thus, the role of radiation therapy remains unclear.

Recent data have demonstrated that anaplastic oligodendrogliomas are highly chemosensitive. In particular, the regimen of "intensive PCV" (CCNU 130 mg/m^2 on day 1, procarbazine 75 mg/m^2 on days 8 to 21, vincristine 1.4 mg/m^2 on days 8 and 29) has been shown in retrospective and prospective Phase II studies to have objective radiographic response rates of nearly 70% to 80%. Some of these responses are complete and can be long-lasting. Because of this dramatic new development, the treatment of anaplastic oligodendrogliomas is undergoing reassessment. A planned multinational randomized trial will be evaluating the use of intensive PCV in the initial management of oligodendrogliomas. All physicians are encouraged to enroll patients on this trial. For patients for whom the trial is not available, treatment of recurrent anaplastic oligodendroglioma with intensive PCV appears to be indicated. For those who cannot tolerate PCV or who have recurrent tumor following the treatment, it appears that other alkylating agents — such as thiotepa and cyclophosphamide — are active.

For the initial management of anaplastic oligodendroglioma, it is reasonable to treat patients with maximal surgical debulking followed by involved-field radiation followed by intensive PCV if patients are not eligible for a clinical trial. Several centers are investigating the use of high-dose chemotherapy followed by autologous bone marrow transplantation in the setting of recurrent oligodendroglioma, given the chemosensitivity of this tumor.

Primary CNS Lymphoma

Primary CNS lymphoma (PCNSL) is defined as a malignant lymphoma limited to the CNS in a patient with no history of lymphoma. Although patients with immunodeficiency are at greatest risk of developing PCNSL, immunocompetent patients can also be afflicted. Among the immunodeficient patient population at risk for PCNSL are patients with congenital immunodeficiencies, such as the Wiskott-Aldrich syndrome, and those with acquired immunodeficiency, such as organ allograft recipients and patients with the acquired immunodeficiency syndrome (AIDS). For patients with no known immunodeficiency who develop PCNSL, there are no known risk factors, despite the fact that the incidence of the disease has tripled in the last decade. This, along with the rapidly growing prevalence of the disease in the immunocompromised population (mostly because of the increasing incidence of AIDS) has led to the prediction that by the turn of the century, PCNSL will be the most common primary brain tumor in adults.

The Epstein-Barr virus has been implicated in the pathogenesis of PCNSL in immunodeficient patients, because Epstein-Barr virus genomic DNA can be found incorporated in lymphoma cell chromosomes in more than 90% of examined cases.

The pathophysiology of PCNSL also differs significantly from that of astrocytomas. PCNSL tends to be a diffuse tumor at presentation, with a high propensity for the lymphoma cells to spread along cerebrospinal fluid (CSF) pathways. This is in contrast to the local migration of malignant astrocytes along white fiber tracks. Radiographically, the disease also differs from gliomas in that more than 90% of the tumors are either iso- or hyperdense, compared with the usual hypodensity seen in gliomas. Nearly all of these tumors are contrast-enhancing, although approximately 10% of PCNSL in the AIDS population are nonenhancing. The typical radiographic appearance of this disease is one of a periventricular enhancing mass, or masses, with less associated edema than might be expected for metastases or glioma. In approximately 25% of immunocompetent and approximately 50% of immunodeficient patients, the tumor is multifocal. Patients can also initially present with CSF dissemination or spinal cord involvement, or occasionally (5% to 10%) with lymphomatous involvement of the vitreous humor. In addition to the increased frequency of multiple radiographic lesions at presentation, 50% of the enhancing lesions in AIDS patients are ring-enhancing.

The evaluation and staging of patients with PCNSL include a CT scan or MRI of the head and gadolinium-enhanced MRI of the spine to rule out drop metastases. If there is no significant increase in intracranial pressure and no lesion in the posterior fossa, a lumbar puncture with removal of CSF is indicated to rule out lymphomatous meningitis. A slit-lamp examination of the eyes is indicated to rule out vitreous involvement. Evaluation for systemic lymphoma in a patient who presents with a CNS lymphoma should involve a complete physical examination as well as routine blood tests (*i.e.*, complete blood count, blood urea nitrogen and creatinine, electrolytes, and liver function tests) and a chest radiograph. If these examinations reveal no obvious pathology, then further systemic evaluation, such as bilateral bone marrow biopsies, CT scans, and gallium scans, are not indicated.

The role of surgery for PCNSL is clearly limited to biopsy to establish a histologic diagnosis. More extensive surgery is not indicated, since, as previously mentioned, this is a diffusely infiltrative disease that has often spread throughout the entire cranial spinal axis by the time of diagnosis. The therapeutic approach following surgery for PCNSL is significantly different, depending on whether the patient is immunocompetent or immunodeficient. For immunocompetent patients, historically the standard treatment was whole-brain radiation. Although complete responses are seen in more than 80% of the cases, tumors generally recur within 1 year. Median survival of these patients is between 10 and 16 months.

The literature is filled with anecdotal reports of various chemotherapeutic agents causing partial or complete responses in patients with recurrent PCNSL. The most common agent that has been used is high-dose methotrexate. Unfortunately, these patients ultimately have a relapse and die of their disease. However, given the apparent activity of systemic chemotherapy, recent efforts have been devoted to the use of chemotherapy as part of the initial treatment regimen. Table 38–2 illustrates three prospective Phase II studies that evaluate the use of preirradiation chemotherapy in the treatment of PCNSL in immunocompetent patients. As can be seen from the median survival in these trials, there appears to be a significant increase in survival over that seen historically with conventional radiation therapy.

The use of chemotherapy before, rather than after, radiation therapy is based on several reasons. First, it has been demonstrated by using positron-emission tomography that the blood-brain barrier is variously disrupted by the tumor before therapy. Once the tumor is effectively treated, however, the blood-brain barrier repairs itself, thereby limiting the amount of drug that can enter the brain parenchyma. Theoretically, this could limit the effectiveness of postirradiation chemotherapy. Another reason for believing that preirradiation chemotherapy is superior to postirradiation therapy is that one can effectively evaluate the activity of the chemotherapy drugs by obtaining serial MRI or CT scans after each cycle of chemotherapy. If radiation therapy is delivered first, usually no radiographically evaluable disease is left to monitor the effectiveness of chemotherapy. Finally, some retrospective data suggest that many chemotherapeutic agents, such as methotrexate and cisplatin, cause more neurotoxicity when given after radiation therapy than when administered before it. For all of these reasons, most of the ongoing Phase II trials are evaluating the use of preirradiation

TABLE 38–2. PROSPECTIVE PREIRRADIATION CHEMOTHERAPY TRIALS IN PCNSL

	PATIENT NUMBERS	MEDIAN AGE (YEARS)	CHEMOTHERAPY	RESPONSE	RADIATION THERAPY (MONTHS)
MGH (Gabbai)	13	62	Methotrexate (3.5 g/m^2 × 3)	Complete response: 9/13 (69%) Partial response: 4/13 (31%)	3000 cGy (12/13 patients)
University of Oregon (Neuwelt)	16	53.7	Blood-brain barrier disruption Cyclophosphamide/ methotrexate + procarbazine	Complete response: 13/16 (81%) Partial response: 3/16 (19%)	5000 cGy (9/16)
MSKCC (DeAngelis)	31	58	Methotrexate (IV + intra-Ommaya) + cytarabine	Complete response: 0 Partial response: 17/22 (77%) Stable disease: 5/22	4000 cGy + 1 boost

MGH = Massachusetts General Hospital; MSKCC = Memorial Sloan-Kettering Cancer Center.

chemotherapy. The Radiation Therapy Oncology Group is currently planning a national Phase II study of the use of preirradiation chemotherapy. All physicians with immunocompetent patients with newly diagnosed PCNSL are encouraged to enroll patients on this or other clinical trials.

In the absence of an available clinical trial, some type of preirradiation chemotherapy in a young, healthy individual is probably warranted. Given the lack of data for the optimal chemotherapy regimen, a simple one consisting of high-dose methotrexates seems appropriate. However, the delivery of high-dose methotrexate in a patient with an intracranial space-occupying lesion is a potentially dangerous and difficult treatment. The reason for this is that in order to avoid nephrotoxicity, patients given high-dose methotrexate must receive significant amounts of intravenous hydration. However, hydration in patients with intracranial tumors often results in increased intracerebral edema followed by increased intracranial pressure and potential for herniation and death. Therefore, the delivery of high-dose methotrexate in a patient with primary CNS lymphoma needs to be done with mannitol diuresis and close observation of the fluid balance of the treated patient. Physicians are encouraged to refer patients with this tumor to centers with experience in the treatment of CNS tumors.

Unfortunately, the encouraging results seen with chemotherapy for immunocompetent patients with PCNSL have not been duplicated in patients with AIDS. Recent evidence demonstrates that regardless of the type of therapy, AIDS patients with PCNSL have a median survival of approximately 3 months. This is because the median CD4 lymphocyte count in AIDS patients who develop PCNSL is less than 50/mm^3. Thus, AIDS patients who develop this tumor are at the end-stage of their disease. Even if patients are effectively cured of their tumor, they rapidly succumb to opportunistic infections and death. Therefore, the current recommendation for most AIDS patients with PCNSL is whole-brain radiation to decrease neurologic morbidity and no chemotherapy outside of a research protocol.

Another important aspect of the management of AIDS patients with newly found, multiple intracranial ring-enhancing lesions is the consideration of the diagnosis of toxoplasmosis versus PCNSL. The radiographic appearance of intracerebral toxoplasmosis is indistinguishable from that of PCNSL; thus, it is reasonable to presumptively treat an AIDS patient with such a radiographic presentation with antitoxoplasmosis therapy for 7 to 10 days (particularly if they have antitoxoplasmosis immunoglobulin G in their serum). If the patient clinically and radiographically responds, then one can assume the diagnosis is toxoplasmosis and treat for an appropriate period of time. If, however, the patient neurologically declines or there is no change in the radiographic lesions, then the patient should undergo a stereotactic biopsy to confirm the diagnosis.

Meningiomas

Meningiomas are common neoplasms of the meningeal surfaces of the CNS. There are several different histologic subgroups of meningiomas, although none has significant prognostic importance. Meningiomas can generally be cured if they can be fully surgically resected. Unfortunately, many meningiomas occur in areas of the brain that are not accessible for complete neurosurgical resection. These tumors inevitably recur within a time span of 1 to 20 years. If a meningioma cannot be fully resected, anecdotal experience suggests that involved-field radiation therapy may delay the time to tumor progression, although it will certainly not cure the tumor. There is increasing interest in high-dose focal radiation (*i.e.*, radiosurgery) for residual meningioma following surgical resection, although, again, the data are too preliminary to establish the effectiveness of this approach.

In patients with multiple recurrent and inoperable meningiomas, some preliminary data suggest that they may be amenable to hormonal manipulation. It is known that meningiomas harbor estrogen and, even more commonly, progesterone receptors. In the past, clinical trials have tested the effectiveness of tamoxifen, but these studies have generally been disappointing. A recent study, however, suggests that an antiprogesterone agent, RU-486 may indeed be capable of halting the growth of meningiomas or even of causing tumor regression. An ongoing national trial is evaluating the effectiveness of RU-486 in the treatment of recurrent meningiomas.

A small subgroup of meningiomas have malignant features at presentation. Histologically, they have characteristics suggestive of sarcomas and behave like other malignant tumors by diffusely infiltrating brain parenchyma. These tumors inevitably recur despite maximal surgical debulking and aggressive radiation therapy. Despite attempts to use various chemotherapeutic agents that are active in sarcomas, such as doxorubicin (Adriamycin) and dacarbazine (DTIC), currently there is no known active agent for the treatment of malignant meningiomas.

REFERENCES

General

Burch JD, Craib KJ, Choi BC et al. An exploratory case-control study of brain tumors in adults. J Natl Cancer Inst 78:601–609, 1987

Ron E, Modan B, J.D. B et al. Tumors of the brain and central nervous system after radiotherapy in childhood. N Engl J Med 319:1033–1039, 1988

Walker AE, Robins M, Weinfeld FD. Epidemiology of brain tumors: The national survey of intracranial neoplasm. Neurology 35:219, 1985

Astrocytomas

Ammirati M, Vick N, Liao YL et al. Effect of the extent of surgical resection on survival and quality of life in patients with supratentorial glioblastoma and anaplastic astrocytomas. Neurosurgery 21:201–206, 1987

Eagan RT, Scott M. Evaluation of prognostic factors in chemotherapy of recurrent brain tumors. J Clin Oncol 1:38–44, 1983

Fine HA, Dear KBG, Loeffler JS et al. Meta-analysis of radiation therapy with and without adjuvant chemotherapy for malignant gliomas in adults. Cancer 71:2585–2597, 1993

Hochberg FH, Pruitt A. Assumptions in the radiotherapy of glioblastomas. Neurology 30:907–991, 1980

Leibel SA, Scott CB, Pajak TF. The management of malignant gliomas with radiation therapy: Therapeutic results and research strategies. Semin Radiat Oncol 1:32–49, 1991

Levin VA, Silver P, Hannigan J et al. Superiority of post-radiotherapy adjuvant chemotherapy with CCNU, procarbazine, and vincristine (PCV) over BCNU for anaplastic gliomas: NCOG 6G61 final report. Int J Radiat Oncol Biol Phys 18:321–324, 1990

Loeffler JS, Alexander EI, Wen PY et al. Results of stereotactic brachytherapy used in the initial management of patients with glioblastoma. Natl Cancer Inst 82:1918–1921, 1990

Loeffler JS, III EA, Shea WM et al. Radiosurgery as part of the initial management of patients with malignant gliomas. J Clin Oncol 10:1379–1385, 1992

MacDonald DR, Cascino TL, Clifford S et al. Response criteria for Phase II studies of supratentorial malignant glioma. J Clin Oncol 8:1277–1280, 1990

Maholey MS, Whaley RA, Blue M et al. Central neurotoxicity following intracarotid BCNU chemotherapy for malignant gliomas. J Neuro-oncol 3:297–314, 1986

Prados MD, Gutin PH, Phillips TL et al. Interstitial brachytherapy for newly diagnosed patients with malignant gliomas: The UCSF experience. Int J Radiat Oncol Biol Phys 24:593–597, 1992

Stewart DJ. The role of chemotherapy in the treatment of gliomas in adults. Cancer Treat Rev 16:129–160, 1989

Walker MD, Green SB, Byar DP et al. Randomized comparisons of radiotherapy and nitrosoureas for the treatment of malignant gliomas after surgery. N Engl J Med 303:1323–1329, 1980

Meningiomas

Barbaro NM, Gutin, PH, Wilson CB et al. Radiation therapy in the treatment of partially resected meningiomas. Neurosurgery 20:525–528, 1987

Grunberg M, Weiss I, Spitz C et al. Treatment of meningioma with the oral anti-progestational agent mifepristone (RU486). Proc Am Soc Clin Oncol 371, 1991

Rubinstein AB, Schein M, Reichenthal E. The association of carcinoma of the breast with meningiomas. Surg Gynecol Obstet 169:334–336, 1989

Primary CNS Lymphoma

Baumgartner JE, Rachlin JR, Beckstead JH et al. Primary central nervous system lymphomas: Natural history and response to radiation therapy in 55 patients with acquired immunodeficiency syndrome: J Neurosurg 73:206–211, 1990

DeAngelis LM, Yahalom J, Thaler HT et al. Combined modality therapy for primary CNS lymphoma. J Clin Oncol 10:635–643, 1992

Eby NL, Grufferman S, Flannelly CM et al. Increasing incidence of primary brain lymphoma in the U.S. Cancer 62:2461–2465, 1988

Ervin T, Canellos GP. Successful treatment of recurrent primary central nervous system lymphoma with high-dose methotrexate. Cancer 45:1556–1557, 1980

Gabbai AA, Hochberg FH, Linggood R. High dose methotrexate therapy of primary brain lymphomas. J Neurosurg 70:190–194, 1989

Hochberg FH, Miller DC. Primary central nervous system lymphoma. J Neurosurg 68:835–852, 1988

Loeffler JS, Ervin TJ, Mauch P et al. Primary lymphomas of the central nervous system: Patterns of failure and factors that influence survival. J Clin Oncol 3:490–494, 1985

MacMahon EME, Glass JD, Hayward SD et al. Epstein-Barr in AIDS-related primary central nervous system lymphoma. Lancet 338:969–981, 1991

Neuwelt EA, Goldman DL, Dahlborg SA et al. Primary central nervous system lymphoma treated with osmotic blood-brain barrier disruption: Prolonged survival and presentation of cognitive function. J Clin Oncol 9:1580–1590, 1991

O'Neill BP, Illig JJ. Primary central nervous system lymphoma. Mayo Clin Proc 64:1005–1020, 1989

Remick SC, Diamond C, Migliozzi JA et al. Primary central nervous system lymphoma in patients with and without the acquired immune deficiency syndrome. Medicine 69:345–360, 1990

Oligodendroglioma

Cairncross G, MacDonald D, Ludwin S et al. Phase II study of chemotherapy for anaplastic oligodendroglioma (preliminary report). A National Cancer Institute of Canada Clinical Trials Group (NCIC CTG) study. Proc Am Soc Clin Oncol 12:175, 1993

MacDonald DR, Gasper LE, Cairncross JG. Successful chemotherapy for newly diagnosed aggressive oligodendroglioma. Ann Neurol 27:573–574, 1990

John S. Macdonald, Daniel G. Haller, Robert J. Mayer, Eds. *Manual of Oncologic Therapeutics*, Third Edition.

39. ACUTE LEUKEMIAS

Bruce D. Cheson

DIAGNOSIS

The acute leukemias result from a neoplastic proliferation of hematopoietic cells blocked at an undifferentiated, or partially differentiated, stage of maturation. Eventual replacement of normal blood elements by cells capable of continued proliferation results in clinical and laboratory evidence of anemia, leukopenia, and thrombocytopenia. Acute leukemias generally arise *de novo*; secondary leukemias may result from exposure to toxins, such as benzene, or chemotherapy drugs, such as alkylating agents, and generally follow a myelodysplastic phase. Recently, acute myeloid leukemia (AML) associated with etoposide or doxorubicin therapy has been described with a characteristic chromosome abnormality involving 11q23.

An elevated white blood cell (WBC) count often alerts the physician to the diagnosis of acute leukemia, but the WBC count is normal in 15% and low in almost a third of patients. In the leukopenic patient, it is essential to rule out other causes of apparent bone marrow failure, including aplastic anemia, myelodysplastic syndromes, myeloproliferative disorders (*e.g.*, idiopathic myelofibrosis), ineffective myelopoiesis (folate or B_{12} deficiency), and immune-mediated neutropenia (systemic lupus erythematosus, acquired immunodeficiency syndrome, or drug-induced leukopenia). For patients presenting with leukocytosis, other diseases in the differential diagnosis include infection, chronic leukemias, leukemoid reactions (tuberculosis, neoplasms), inflammatory conditions, and steroid therapy.

Careful evaluation of the peripheral blood smear by an experienced observer is essential; blasts can be identified in 85% of patients at presentation. A bone marrow aspirate should be accompanied by a biopsy to assess cellularity, to provide an estimate of fibrosis, and to allow for adequate evaluation in cases of an insufficient aspirate (dry tap), which may be encountered with a hypercellular bone marrow completely replaced by blasts or extensive fibrosis.

CLASSIFICATION

Acute leukemias are heterogeneous with respect to clinical manifestations, response to therapy, anticipated complications, and prognosis. Accurate classification of acute leukemia is necessary because effective therapies differ for the various leukemias. The simplest scheme divides them into acute lymphocytic leukemias (ALL) and AML. Although useful, this distinction is obviously insufficient.

The French-American-British (FAB) classification categorizes the various subtypes of AML and ALL, and the myelodysplastic syndromes on the basis of morphology and histochemical stains. The cytochemical stains used to identify these subclasses include peroxidase (M1-5), nonspecific esterase (M4, M5), and periodic acid–Schiff (ALL-L1) (Table 39–1).

Cytogenetics and cellular phenotyping with monoclonal antibodies have identified several clinically important subgroups.

TREATMENT OF ACUTE MYELOID LEUKEMIA

The treatment of AML, and acute leukemia in general, involves toxic therapy that should be administered only by experienced physicians with readily available supportive care (*i.e.*, blood components, intravenous antibiotics, and specialized nursing care).

When to Treat

The majority of patients with AML have progressive or symptomatic disease at presentation and require treatment as soon as the initial evaluation has been completed.

Preinduction Management

Accurate classification of leukemia and identification of medical, social, and psychological problems that need management should be determined prior to treatment. The baseline laboratory evaluation should include the following:

1. Hematologic studies are done as noted above (complete blood count, differential, bone marrow aspirate, and biopsy).
2. Serum chemistries and electrolytes: Normal electrolytes minimize the risk of certain drug side-effects, such as anthracycline cardiotoxicity. Blood urea nitrogen and serum creatinine determinations identify patients with leukemia renal infiltration and those at increased risk for side-effects from drugs, such as aminoglycoside antibiotics and amphotericin B. Abnormal hepatic function may indicate leukemic infiltration or infection. In addition, modification of doses of drugs such as anthracyclines and vincristine may be necessary.
3. Coagulation profile: Patients with acute promyelocytic leukemia (AML-M3) are at an increased risk for disseminated intravascular coagulation (DIC). A decreasing fib-

TABLE 39–1. FRENCH-AMERICAN-BRITISH CLASSIFICATION OF ACUTE MYELOID LEUKEMIA AS MODIFIED BY THE NCI-WORKSHOP

DESCRIPTION	DESIGNATION
Acute myeloid leukemia lacking myeloid differentiation, with reactivity with myeloid antigens or ultrastructural evidence of peroxidase + blasts	M0
Acute myeloid leukemia without maturation	M1
Acute myeloid leukemia with maturation	M2
Promyelocytic leukemia	M3
Acute myelomonocytic leukemia	M4
Acute monocytic leukemia	M5
Erythroleukemia	M6
Acute megakaryocytic leukemia	M7

NCI = National Cancer Institute

rinogen and other evidence of DIC (*e.g.*, split products) should prompt the initiation of treatment. Therapy includes aggressive platelet transfusions, as often as two or three times per day. Heparin can be administered at 50 to 100 units/kg intravenously every 6 hours or in continuous infusions of 7.5 to 15 units/kg/hour, until the coagulation profile becomes normal; however, the utility of heparin therapy has not been proved. DIC can also be treated with intensive administration of fresh-frozen plasma and platelet support without the risks of heparin, although the risk of transmissible diseases makes this approach less desirable.

4. Blood typing is done to ensure ready availability of red blood cells.
5. Human leukocyte antigen (HLA) typing should be performed on admission, if the patient has adequate lymphocytes for study, to identify family members who may be preferred blood donors and facilitate the identification of optimal platelet donors. For patients less than 55 years of age, this test also determines who may be future candidates for allogeneic bone marrow transplantation.
6. A baseline chest x-ray film should be obtained to aid in the interpretation of subsequent radiographs.

Central venous access should be obtained as soon as possible. A Hickman, Broviac, Groshong, or similar catheter, preferably with multiple lumens, should be implanted to minimize venipunctures and to facilitate infusions of drugs and blood products. Such catheters should be implanted by experienced physicians and used only by trained personnel (including the patient) to reduce infectious complications and to increase catheter longevity.

Sources of infection should be identified and treated. Surveillance cultures may predict an eventual bacterial pathogen, but they are not cost-effective because broad-spectrum antibiotics are routinely administered in the febrile, neutropenic patient.

Whether to delay chemotherapy until an infection is successfully treated should be influenced by the status of the leukemia, the severity of the infection, and the number of circulating neutrophils. In a patient with stable disease and more than 1000/μl neutrophils, treatment may be delayed until the infection is under control, since the neutrophils may provide antimicrobial activity. Patients with fewer than 500/μl neutrophils and progressive leukemia should be treated as soon as possible because the circulating neutrophils are inadequate for host defense.

The value of protected environments is controversial. Although survival may be improved for patients with aplastic anemia, no clear advantage has been shown for AML. The frequency of infections and the number of febrile days may be decreased, but systemic antibiotics are still required in all patients, and there is no influence on survival. Myeloid growth factors appear to expedite recovery of normal neutrophils.

The use of gowns, masks, sterile food and water, oral nonabsorbable antibiotics, and similar precautions cannot be recommended as standard practice. Only total compliance with such a program may be of benefit, and any component alone (*e.g.*, low-bacteria diets) is of little value. Reverse isolation provides no more than a reminder of the importance of handwashing.

Although patients lose a large proportion of body weight during induction therapy, systemic hyperalimentation is not recommended. Once remission is achieved, weight is regained; until that time, oral supplements usually suffice.

Although uncommon in AML, urate nephropathy may occur, particularly in patients with an elevated WBC count. This problem can be prevented with allopurinol, 300 mg/day orally. This drug can be myelosuppressive and should therefore be discontinued when the bone marrow becomes hypocellular.

The oral cavity is a potential source of infections, and a program of good oral hygiene, including regular use of a soft brush to prevent gingival trauma, is essential.

Therapeutic Approach

Therapy for acute leukemia is initially directed at inducing a complete remission and subsequently maintaining it.

INDUCTION THERAPY

The most important factor in determining survival of AML patients is a complete remission. To achieve a complete remission, combinations of the most active drugs are administered in myelotoxic doses with the goal of bone marrow ablation and eventual repopulation by normal cells.

The most active agents for induction therapy are cytarabine (ara-C) and the anthracyclines (daunorubicin and idarubicin, which appear to have similar efficacies).

Treatment programs usually consist of 7 days of cytarabine (100–200 mg/m^2) administered by continuous infusion through a mechanical pump to ensure consistent drug delivery, with 3 days of an anthracycline (*e.g.*, daunorubicin, 45–60 mg/m^2/day; idarubicin 10–13 mg/m^2/day). Results appear similar if the anthracycline is administered during the first 3 or last 3 days of the cytarabine. Related drugs (*e.g.*, mitoxantrone, amsacrine) have not been shown to be as effective. Representative chemotherapy programs are presented in Table 39–2.

High doses of cytarabine (1–3 g/m^2 every 12 hours for 6 days) given during induction therapy have not improved complete remission rates, except perhaps in certain phenotypic subsets of patients (*e.g.*, CD34+). However, it is associated with substantially greater toxicity, particularly cerebellar dysfunction, ranging in severity from incoordination to coma. This effect is usually, although not always, reversible and is more common in patients over 50 years of age and those with renal dysfunction. As a result, the recommended dose for older patients is 1 to 2 g/m^2, which appears to be as active as the higher dose. Other common toxicities include conjunctivitis, which may be prevented by the prophylactic use of corticosteroid eye drops. Therefore, high-dose cytarabine (HiDAC) should not be routinely used in induction.

An Australian study suggested that the addition of etoposide (75 mg/m^2 for 7 days) during induction had no effect on response rate and induced more stomatitis; nevertheless, the duration of complete remissions appeared to be longer. A repeat bone marrow aspiration and biopsy should be performed during the first week of therapy to determine the extent of antileukemic effect, and again when there is evidence of marrow recovery with increasing neutrophils and platelets in the peripheral blood. An unexplained delay (approximately 3 weeks) in return of blood counts should alert the physician to the possibility of leukemic recurrence, and examination of the bone marrow to confirm this impression is indicated. If the bone marrow remains hypocellular, the patient should be observed with a repeat sampling at weekly intervals. A leukemic infiltrate in a cellular sample is an indication to consider a second course of therapy.

Recent data suggest that the use of myeloid growth factors (e.g., granulocyte [G-CSF] or granulocyte-macrophage colony-stimulating factor [GM-CSF]) beginning within 3 or 4 days of discontinuing induction therapy may accelerate the recovery of normal myelopoiesis; however, whether the use of growth factors improves survival is controversial. Delaying the administration of growth factor until marrow hypoplasia occurs eliminates its benefit. The use of growth factors before chemotherapy to "prime" blasts may have a detrimental effect.

Current induction regimens achieve complete remissions in 65% to 85% of patients, and 15% to 30% of patients may be cured. Complete remission rates are inversely related to age: for less than 20 years, they are 70% to 85%; for 20 to 40 years, 60% to 75%; for 40 to 60 years, 40% to 50%; and for over 60 years, only 25% to 40%. The cytogenetic abnormalities t(15;17), inv 16, t(8;21) are associated with a more favorable prognosis, whereas abnormalities such as −5 and −7 are associated with a poor outcome. An antecedent hematologic disorder, particularly a myelodysplastic syndrome, generally confers a worse prognosis.

Younger patients die more often during induction therapy from refractory disease than do older patients, who have a greater than 30% risk of dying as a complication of therapy. Attenuated doses of drugs (*e.g.*, daunorubicin decreased from 45 to 30 mg/m^2, and cytarabine from 100 to 70 mg/m^2) have been reported to reduce treatment-related mortality in older patients. Unfortunately, remission rates have not been enhanced with such programs.

Identification of various subgroups of patients and subtypes of disease may permit more case-specific treatment, and risk-oriented approaches are being considered. For example, a hypercellular bone marrow with a preponderance of blasts on day 6 may help distinguish the patient who requires immediate intensification of therapy from one who has a hypocellular bone marrow and a high likelihood of achieving a complete remission without receiving additional drugs.

Seventy-five percent of complete remissions are achieved after a single course. Approximately 20% of patients who fail to achieve a complete remission with a single induction

TABLE 39–2. CURRENT INDUCTION REGIMENS FOR ADULT AML

SOURCE	DRUG	DOSE (mg/m^2)	ROUTE	DAYS OF ADMINISTRATION
CALGB	Daunorubicin	45	Intravenous	1–3
	Cytarabine	200	Continuous Intravenous infusion	1–7
ECOG	Idarubicin	12	Intravenous	1–3
	Cytarabine	25	Intravenous push	1
		100	Continuous Intravenous infusion	1–7
Berman et al	Idarubicin	12	Intravenous	1–3
	Cytarabine	200	Continuous Intravenous infusion	1–5

AML = acute myeloid leukemia; CALGB = Cancer and Leukemia Group B; ECOG = Eastern Cooperative Oncology Group.

course yet exhibit antileukemic activity (chemotherapy-induced aplasia with a return of blasts) achieve a complete remission with a second course of the same regimen. However, such responses may be less durable than those occurring after a single course. Patients unable to achieve a complete remission with a second induction attempt are "failures" and should be considered for alternative approaches. Patients with M3 leukemia may enter remission slowly and without bone marrow aplasia, and caution should be exercised so as not to administer a second course of therapy unnecessarily.

Management of Infection

During remission induction, the two major causes of mortality are infection and bleeding. Rapid diagnosis and treatment of infections are imperative, even if a surgical procedure, such as open lung biopsy, is required to make a correct diagnosis. Prophylactic platelet transfusions immediately before, during, and after the operation will minimize the risk of bleeding.

A daily physical examination is necessary to diagnose early signs of infection. A perineal examination may detect evidence of a perirectal abscess. This infection should be treated with systemic antibiotics and local measures (*e.g.*, sitz baths and local hygiene). Surgical drainage is occasionally warranted.

To minimize the risk of bacteremia or perirectal abscess, it is critical that use of rectal thermometers and enemas be avoided and that rectal examinations be performed only on admission or when an abscess is suspected.

Management of Hemorrhage

Thrombocytopenia is the leading cause of bleeding. Platelet infusions are more effective in the prophylactic setting than during active bleeding. Patients who are elderly or have a rapid fall in platelet count are more likely to bleed at a similar level of platelets than younger, healthier patients who have prolonged, persistent thrombocytopenia. For the elderly group, attempts should be made to maintain an adequate (>20,000/μl) platelet count. In younger patients, however, clinical judgment is warranted to minimize platelet alloimmunization by excessive transfusions. Daily funduscopic examinations are necessary, and platelets should be administered at the first sign of retinal or other serious hemorrhages.

Central Nervous System Leukemia

Less than 5% of patients present with central nervous system (CNS) involvement. The risk is greater in patients with M4 and M5 histologies and those with a WBC count greater than 100,000/μl. Patients with chromosomal abnormalities involving del(16)(22) and inv(16)(p13;q22), despite a high complete remission rate, tend to have a high frequency of CNS relapse, often with chloromas (myeloblastomas), rather than the generally more common leptomeningeal disease.

CNS leukemia should be suspected with symptoms of headache, blurred vision, altered mentation, cranial nerve palsy, unexplained fever, or papilledema.

Each AML patient should undergo a lumbar puncture to determine if blasts are present. The precise timing of the lumbar puncture is controversial. One concern is that a lumbar puncture in the presence of blasts may contaminate the CNS, establishing CNS disease, although few data support such an event. Postponement until circulating blasts are absent from the periphery is recommended because any trauma from the procedure may create a false interpretation of established CNS leukemia. If prophylactic (or therapeutic) intrathecal chemotherapy is to be given, a dose should be administered at the time of the initial lumbar puncture, because this reduces by one the number of subsequent lumbar punctures to which the patient may be subjected. An exception is the rare patient in whom an active CNS infection is suspected.

CNS leukemia should be managed with intrathecal therapy, through either a lumbar puncture or an Ommaya reservoir. Although the latter requires a surgical procedure, it is preferable in patients who will require repeated sampling of CSF and administration of drug over weeks to months, especially if other factors (*e.g.*, obesity, scoliosis) make the lumbar puncture difficult to perform.

Commonly used drugs include methotrexate (10–15 mg) or cytarabine (100 mg) in 10 ml of a sterile, preservative-free diluent. Therapy is administered twice weekly until the CNS has cleared, and if a systemic complete remission is achieved, monthly thereafter. Combinations of either of these drugs with an additional one, such as hydrocortisone (20 mg), may increase the CNS response rate and duration. Radiation therapy may be of additional benefit in eradicating CNS disease. Patients receiving treatment with high-dose, systemic cytarabine may exhibit eradication of CNS disease without the need for concurrent intrathecal therapy.

The role of CNS prophylaxis is not established in AML. Although intrathecal methotrexate or cytarabine may reduce the frequency of CNS relapse, there is no clear influence on survival.

POSTREMISSION THERAPY

Postremission therapy is necessary for durable remissions, although the optimal approach has not yet been defined. The median duration of unmaintained remissions is 4 to 8 months, compared with 18 or more months with postremission therapy.

The various forms of postremission therapy include consolidation, maintenance, and intensification, and are described below. Consolidation and maintenance programs have received the most attention and appear to yield similar results, although consolidation is more convenient and makes lengthy delivery of chemotherapy unnecessary. The optimal duration of each treatment remains to be determined, as does the value of combinations of these programs.

Consolidation. Consolidation refers to therapy given shortly after induction and usually involves the same drugs used in the induction regimen, at similar doses but for an abbreviated duration and repeated two to four times at approximately monthly intervals, usually in an inpatient setting. Another approach includes active agents that were not in the induction regimen. The relative efficacy of these strategies is under evaluation. Dose intensity appears to be important in consolidation. In a recent Cancer and Leukemia Group B study, 596 patients who achieved a complete remission with a 7 + 3 program were randomized consolidation with cytarabine at 3 g/m^2 over 3 hours every 12 hours for six doses), 400 mg/m^2/day by continuous infusion for 5 days, or 100 mg/m^2/day for 5 days. Patients who received the HiDAC experienced a significantly longer disease-free and overall survival.

Intensification. Intensification refers to treatment several months after induction of a complete remission with myelosuppressive doses of either agents used during remission or other active drugs. Such programs are generally used in combination with maintenance therapy and are substituted, for example, for months 3 and 9 of maintenance therapy. A role for such therapy remains to be established.

Maintenance. Maintenance involves monthly courses of outpatient treatment designed to maintain a WBC count of at least 1000/μl and platelet count of 75,000/μl or more. Programs may last from 6 to 8 months to 1 to 3 years, although comparative studies have not demonstrated an advantage to the longer duration. Standard maintenance regimens include cytarabine 25 mg/m^2 every 6 hours for 5 to 10 days with one or more of the following: prednisone, vincristine, daunorubicin, or 6-thioguanine. It is not clear that maintenance has additional benefit for patients who have received intensive consolidation therapy.

Whatever post–remission approach is used, blood counts must be monitored to prevent death from hypoplasia during remission. Blood counts must be obtained at least weekly; patients with neutropenic fevers should be hospitalized and given systemic antibiotics, even before culture results are available.

Bone Marrow Transplantation

The optimal timing of allogeneic bone marrow transplantation is controversial; there appears to be no advantage to transplantation during the first complete remission, compared with during the early first relapse. The role of autologous bone marrow transplantation in first remission is being evaluated.

Acute Promyelocytic Leukemia

AML-M3 is distinct in its morphology, cytogenetics, molecular biology, response to therapy, and prognosis. Most patients present with a bleeding diathesis, such as DIC. The blasts exhibit the t(15;17)(q22;q12), and the breakpoint on chromosome 17 is in the intron of the α-retinoic acid receptor gene.

Acute promyelocytic leukemia (APL) is generally treated with standard induction therapy; however, the role of an anthracycline appears to be more important than in other forms of AML. Patients may gradually enter a complete remission without experiencing bone marrow aplasia. This feature is important to recognize, to avoid administering a second, unnecessary course of induction therapy.

All-trans retinoic acid (ATRA) has been reported to achieve complete remissions in more than 80% of patients with relapsed or previously untreated APL. How best to integrate this agent into a standard chemotherapy induction regimen is currently being investigated. ATRA therapy may be associated with a potentially fatal pulmonary "retinoic acid syndrome," frequently, but not invariably, accompanied by an elevated WBC count. Treatment with corticosteroids may be successful. ATRA does not cure patients with APL, and the addition of some form of chemotherapy is essential. An international study is comparing standard induction and consolidation with ATRA as induction, followed by chemotherapy consolidation in previously untreated patients with APL.

TREATMENT AT RELAPSE

Patients who fail chemotherapy can be categorized into two clinically meaningful groups: those who never achieve a complete remission with induction or who experience relapse within a few months (primary refractory), and those who experience a prolonged disease-free period before relapse (relapsed). Failure to distinguish between these groups makes interpretation of clinical trials difficult.

For relapsed patients, the standard treatment has been a regimen similar to the initial induction regimen (generally 7 + 3). More than 60% of relapsed patients achieve a complete remission that lasts a median of 8 months. In contrast, only 25% of patients with a brief initial remission respond to such reinduction, lasting a median of only 3 months. For refractory patients, the single most active agent in those who had relapses appears to be HiDAC, 2 to 3 g/m^2 intravenously every 12 hours for 4 to 6 days. Complete remission rates of up to 50% have been reported, lasting a median of 6 months, even in patients who failed to respond to conventional doses of cytarabine. It is not clear that when HiDAC is used in combination with an anthracycline or related drug, response rates are substantially increased.

Other agents with activity in relapsed and refractory patients include etoposide (VP-16), mitoxantrone, carboplatin, topotecan, diaziquone (AZQ). Each is associated with a 10% to 25% complete remission rate of brief duration.

Combinations of active agents studied to date generally do not enhance the complete remission rate or duration. The combination of high-dose etoposide (4.2 g/m^2) by continuous infusion over 26 to 69 hours, and cyclophosphamide 200 mg/kg on 3 or 4 consecutive days, has been reported to achieve complete remissions in more than 40% of refractory patients, lasting a median of 4 months.

Cells from patients with AML may acquire the multidrug-resistance (mdr-1) phenotype, and agents that have the potential to reverse this feature (*e.g.*, verapamil, R-verapamil, cyclosporine) are being evaluated to reverse clinical resistance.

DELAYED THERAPY

Patients with smoldering AML may not require therapy immediately at diagnosis but can wait until evidence of clinical deterioration. Delaying treatment for elderly patients with AML does not reduce the number of hospitalized days, and survival is inferior compared with that of patients who initially receive intensive remission induction chemotherapy.

The patient who does not want aggressive therapy, either as front-line therapy or in the case of refractory or relapsed disease, may respond to moderate doses of conventional agents (*e.g.*, prednisone, vincristine, methotrexate, 6-mercaptopurine [POMP]) administered on an outpatient basis. Hydroxyurea (2–20 g/day in divided doses, titrated against the WBC and platelet counts) can effectively control the WBC. Palliative therapy in the form of antibiotics, analgesics, and blood component therapy is another option.

Treatment for Disease-Related Complications

Treatment for disseminated intravascular coagulation and CNS relapse is discussed above. Treatment for infections is described in Chapter 59, and treatment for bleeding in Chapter 61.

LEUKOSTASIS

Patients with an exceptionally high WBC count (>100,000/μl) may develop a leukostasis syndrome from blasts aggregating in the capillaries. CNS and cardiopulmonary symptoms are most common and are associated with significant morbidity and mortality. This medical emergency requires rapid reduction of the WBC, including leukapheresis, chemotherapy (hydroxyurea, daunorubicin + cytarabine), and CNS or, rarely, pulmonary irradiation. Patients should be carefully observed for metabolic derangements from rapid lysis of tumor cells and should be treated appropriately (see Treatment of Adult Acute Lymphocytic Leukemias below, and Chap. 39).

TYPHLITIS

In a neutropenic patient who develops severe abdominal symptoms (most often only pain, less commonly bloody diarrhea, absent bowel sounds, rebound tenderness, and fever), the diagnosis of typhlitis (neutropenic enterocolitis) should be considered. Radiographs of the abdomen may suggest a soft-tissue mass in the right lower quadrant, a dilated colon, or pericecal edema. A mass in the cecum may also be suggested on barium enema.

The clinical picture may be indistinguishable from that of pseudomembranous colitis associated with antibiotic therapy, caused by *Clostridium difficile* and treated with vancomycin. The etiology of typhlitis is unclear but is likely related to Clostridium sp. (*e.g.*, *C. septicum*) or, possibly, other bacteria, including *Pseudomonas*, *Escherichia coli*, or *Klebsiella*. Stool cultures should be performed, and any pathogen treated appropriately.

The prognosis for patients with typhlitis is extremely poor. Medical management includes bed rest, maintenance of fluid and electrolyte balance, intravenous hydration, and no oral intake. Colonic resection may be warranted in some cases, although the risks must be considered in light of reports of survival with conservative management alone.

RENAL FAILURE

A number of etiologies exist for renal failure in patients with AML, including urate nephropathy, drug (*e.g.*, aminoglycoside) toxicity, sepsis, and renal infiltration by leukemia cells. The latter may be diagnosed by a careful examination of the urinary sediment after cytologic preparation. Renal infiltration may respond to systemic chemotherapy, but irradiation of the kidneys may also be required.

CHLOROMAS (MYELOBLASTOMAS, GRANULOCYTIC SARCOMAS)

These unusual tumors are composed of granulocytic precursor cells. "Chloroma" refers to their green color on cut surface, which is due to high levels of myeloperoxidase. Their appearance may antedate overt AML or chronic myelogenous leukemia in blast crisis by months to years, or they may appear during the course of the disease. They occur most commonly near neural structures, in bone and periosteum, and in soft tissue, lymph nodes (including mediastinum), skin, breasts, ovaries, and gastrointestinal tract.

Chloromas have responded to systemic chemotherapy given for active leukemia and also to radiation therapy, when disease is refractory to chemotherapy. Patients with a chloroma occurring as an isolated lesion in the absence of AML (documented by bone marrow examination) should receive local irradiation. Some investigators have recommended immediate treatment with combination chemotherapy, based on the observation that overt leukemia generally develops within 1 or 2 years. However, it is currently acceptable to follow such patients carefully, reserving systemic chemotherapy for overt leukemia. Marrow harvest and storage for future possible autologous bone marrow transplantation may also be considered.

TREATMENT OF ADULT ACUTE LYMPHOCYTIC LEUKEMIAS

Adult ALL accounts for 20% of acute leukemia in patients over the age of 15 years. Unfortunately, advances made in the treatment of childhood ALL have not been paralleled in adults. The reasons for this are unclear but may reflect, in part, an increasing frequency of the Philadelphia chromosome with age, which may be associated with greater drug resistance.

Classification

As with AML, the FAB classification is most widely used:

- L1 A relatively homogeneous population of lymphoblasts, of which 75% or more are small with scanty cytoplasm, a regular nuclear shape, finely dispersed chromatin, and inconspicuous nucleoli in most cells.
- L2 A heterogeneous population of lymphoblasts with regard to size, nuclear shape, and chromatin pattern. Prominent nucleoli are common.
- L3 A large and homogeneous population of lymphoblasts with regular nuclei and fine chromatin. The cytoplasm is abundant and basophilic with prominent vacuolization.

Common ALL is usually L1 or L2, as is T-cell ALL, whereas B-cell ALL more closely resembles Burkitt's cells and is characteristically L3.

A number of clinical and laboratory features have a negative prognostic impact: high WBC count (>15,000/μl) at presentation, presence of the Philadelphia (Ph^1) chromosome; t(4;11); age over 40 years; L3 morphology; null, T-cell, or especially B-cell phenotype (as opposed to cALLa-positive); expression of myeloid surface antigens; CNS disease; and prolonged induction phase to achieve a complete remission.

Preinduction Management

Although for the most part, the preinduction management of ALL is similar to AML, tumor lysis syndrome occurs more commonly than in AML, especially with L2 and L3 morphology. Major precipitating factors include large tumor burden, hyperuricemia, elevated lactic acid, and any impairment of renal function, including dehydration, obstructive uropathy, or renal involvement by tumor. Rapid destruction of tumor cells and release of cellular metabolic products lead to hyperuricemia, hyperkalemia, hyperphosphatemia, and hypocalcemia. The sequelae of such events can include cardiac arrhythmias and deposits of uric acid and calcium in the kidneys, with renal failure.

In patients at risk for acute tumor lysis syndrome, metabolic abnormalities should be corrected before treatment for leukemia is initiated. High doses of allopurinol (300–500 mg/m²/day either orally or intravenously) should be administered, and alkalinization of the urine (pH ≥ 7) is achieved by hydrating the patient with 3 liters/day or more of fluids including sodium bicarbonate (50 mEq/liter in intravenous solution). Patients who have developed tumor lysis syndrome and fail to respond rapidly may be candidates for dialysis (see Part VI of this text, Oncologic Emergencies).

Induction Therapy

As with AML, patients with ALL should be treated only by experienced physicians with access to adequate supportive care. The optimal regimen for ALL is a matter of controversy. The highest response rates and best long-term survival rate have been achieved with aggressive regimens, such as that of the German Multicenter Trial (Table 39-3). Intrathecal methotrexate and CNS irradiation are given during Phase II of this regimen. The reported complete remission rate is 74%, median remission duration is longer than 24 months, and there is a 39% probability of continuous complete remission at more than 5 years with a 49% 5-year survival for those with a complete remission.

Impressive results have also been reported with other aggressive, multiagent induction programs using intensive consolidation and maintenance. A regimen from the University of California, San Francisco, achieved an 88% complete remission rate with 42% projected to be alive and disease-free survival at 5 years. Such impressive results with intensive programs reinforce the need for aggressive postinduction therapy delivered over a prolonged (2- to 3-year) period.

Central Nervous System Therapy

PROPHYLAXIS

The importance of CNS prophylaxis for adult ALL is clearer than for AML. Over 40% of patients with ALL may develop leukemic involvement that can be prevented in the majority of cases. Optimal therapy is not defined; intrathecal methotrexate is probably adequate.

TREATMENT OF CNS LEUKEMIA

Of patients with ALL, 5% to 10% present with evidence of overt CNS leukemia. Treatment is similar to that for CNS AML: intrathecal methotrexate, generally in conjunction with cranial irradiation (24 cGy in 200-cGy daily fractions, 5 days/week). Craniospinal irradiation should be avoided, if possible, because it compromises the ability to administer further cytotoxic chemotherapy.

Postremission Therapy

MAINTENANCE

Earlier programs used a maintenance regimen patterned after childhood ALL, including methotrexate and 6-MP,

TABLE 39–3. GERMAN MULTICENTER REGIMEN FOR ADULT ALL

DRUG	DOSE (mg/m^2)	ROUTE	DAYS OF ADMINISTRATION
INDUCTION			
Phase I			
Prednisone	60	po	1–28 (then taper)
Vincristine*	1.5	iv	1, 8, 15, 22
Daunorubicin	25	iv	1, 8, 15, 22
L-asparaginase	5000 U/m^2	iv	1–14
Phase II			
Cyclophosphamide†	650	iv	29, 43, 57
Cytarabine	75	iv	31–34, 38–41, 45–48, 52–55
6-Mercaptopurine	60	po	29–57
Methotrexate‡	10	it	31, 38, 45, 52
REINDUCTION			
Phase I			
Dexamethasone	10	po	1–28
Vincristine	1.5	iv	1, 8, 15, 22
Doxorubicin	25	iv	1, 8, 15, 22
Phase II			
Cyclophosphamide	650	iv	29
Cytarabine	75	iv	31–34, 38–41
MAINTENANCE			
6-Mercaptopurine	60	po	daily—weeks 10–18, 29–130
Methotrexate	20	po/iv	weekly—weeks 10–18, 29–130

*Maximum single dose, 2 mg.
†Maximum single dose, 1000 mg.
‡Maximum single dose, 15 mg.
po = oral; iv = intravenous; it = intrathecal.

with or without intermittent pulses of vincristine and prednisone, resulting in a remission duration of 15 to 20 months and a 5-year disease-free survival of 25%.

Consolidation. Recently, more intensive consolidation programs (discussed previously) have increased the median duration of complete remission to more than 2 years, and the proportion of patients in continuous complete remission to 40% to 50% at 3 to 4 years. The optimal consolidation-intensification program has not been clearly defined.

Therapy at Relapse. As with AML, only bone marrow transplantation is associated with long-term remissions. A number of investigational regimens are being explored, and patients should be considered for these protocols.

MYELODYSPLASTIC SYNDROMES

Definition

Previously referred to as "smoldering leukemia," "oligoblastic leukemia," or "preleukemia," myelodysplastic syndromes (MDS) consist of a number of clonal disorders characterized by peripheral cytopenias with a cellular bone marrow, ineffective myelopoiesis, morphologic changes of dyserythropoiesis, and abnormal granulopoiesis and megakaryocytes. These disorders can occur *de novo* or following cytotoxic chemotherapy, frequently associated with abnormalities of chromosomes 5 and/or 7.

Classification

The FAB classification is most commonly used, and modifications have been suggested to better distinguish MDS, particularly refractory anemia with excess blasts in transformation (RAEB-T), from AML (Table 39-4), and M6 AML from MDS.

An additional related syndrome has been described in association with a deletion of part of the long arm of chromosome 5 (5q-), characterized by macrocytic anemia, generally with a relatively normal granulocyte count, with normal to increased platelets and morphologically abnormal megakaryocytes.

Treatment

WHEN TO TREAT

Patients with MDS may live for months or years with supportive measures alone, including transfusions and antibiotics. Nevertheless, the median survival is only 1 or 2 years, depending on the histologic subtype, and many patients suc-

TABLE 39–4. FRENCH-AMERICAN-BRITISH CLASSIFICATION FOR MYELODYSPLASTIC SYNDROMES

1. *Refractory anemia (RA)*: Anemia, reticulocytopenia, dyserythropoiesis, dysgranulopoiesis, with a normo- to hypocellular marrow with <5% blasts
2. *RA with ring sideroblasts* (acquired idiopathic sideroblastic anemia): Similar to above except for the presence of >15% of nucleated marrow cells being ringed sideroblasts
3. *RAEB*: Cytopenias of two or more marrow elements, with the peripheral blood revealing abnormalities of all three. Dysgranulopoiesis is common, as are circulating blasts, although usually <5%. The marrow is usually hypercellular with dyspoiesis of all three lines and, occasionally, ringed sideroblasts. Although there is evidence of granulocytic maturation, the percentage of marrow blasts is between 5% and 20%
4. *Chronic myelomonocytic leukemia (CMML)*: Characterized by an absolute monocytosis (>1 × 10^9/liter), often associated with an increase in mature granulocytes with or without dysgranulopoiesis. The marrow resembles RAEB except for the significant increase in monocyte precursors
5. *RAEB in transformation (RAEB-T)*: RAEB-T is characterized by cytopenias, with laboratory features that fit neither any of the above nor M1–6 AML. Generally exhibit >5% blasts in the peripheral blood with 20% to 30% blasts in the marrow, and Auer's rods in the granulocytic precursors

AML = acute myeloid leukemia.

cumb to infection and/or hemorrhage before the disease transforms into AML. Because patients with MDS tend to be elderly, any treatment for the disease, especially aggressive chemotherapy, is usually deferred until the disease progresses. Even when treatment is warranted, there is no "standard therapy," and participation in clinical trials is encouraged.

TREATMENT ALTERNATIVES

Supportive Care. Transfusions of red blood cells should be instituted in the presence of cardiopulmonary symptoms related to anemia; platelet transfusions should be reserved for significant bleeding episodes, and systemic antibiotics should be administered when appropriate.

Vitamin Therapy. Because the bone marrow in MDS is megaloblastoid, therapy with vitamin B_{12} or folic acid has been used empirically, but these are ineffective. Similarly, although pyridoxine may induce responses in some forms of sideroblastic anemia, it is not active in the MDS.

Hormonal Therapy

Glucocorticoids. Transient increases in blood counts have been reported in small series of patients treated with glucocorticoids. However, chronic use of steroids increases the risk of serious infection; therefore, this approach should be discouraged.

Androgens. Anecdotal responses have been reported, but the majority of clinical experience suggests that these agents are only minimally active. Danazol, a semisynthetic attenuated androgen, may be effective at a dosage of 600 mg daily in reversing immune-mediated thrombocytopenia and hemolysis that rarely accompany MDS, but not in the other cases.

Aggressive Chemotherapy. A number of case reports and small series suggest that antileukemic therapy (e.g., daunorubicin + cytarabine; HiDAC) can induce remissions in some patients with MDS. The reported frequency of complete remissions ranges from 15% to 50%, with an associated risk of treatment-related deaths of 25% to 40%. Other data suggest that aggressive chemotherapy may shorten the survival of these patients. It is likely that there are substantial differences among patient groups; younger patients (<50 years) and those with more aggressive histologies (e.g., RAEB, RAEB-T) whose behavior is more similar to that of AML patients should be considered candidates for intensive therapy in a clinical trials setting. However, these patients tend to have prolonged pancytopenia following treatment. Older patients tolerate multiagent therapy poorly, and this treatment cannot be recommended as a standard approach.

Bone Marrow Transplantation. Bone marrow transplantation using a variety of preparative regimens achieves prolonged disease-free survival in approximately half the reported cases; the results are better in younger patients, those with fewer bone marrow blasts, and those with less marrow fibrosis. Nevertheless, treatment-related deaths occur in 25% to 40% of cases. For patients with suitable donors, bone marrow transplantation remains the treatment of choice because it is currently the only curative therapy for MDS. The use of matched unrelated donors has been successful in select patients but with substantial treatment-related toxicities

Hematopoietic Growth Factors

Erythropoietin. Although patients with MDS are generally anemic, the response rate to erythropoietin, as determined by a reduction in transfusion requirements, is only about 20%. This limited effectiveness may reflect their tendency to have high endogenous erythropoietin levels.

Myeloid Growth Factors. G-CSF, GM-CSF, and IL-3 have been used to treat patients with MDS. Although each induces a granulocyte response in two thirds of cases, an increase in the platelet count is uncommon, and although there may be a reticulocytosis, there is no decrement in the transfusion requirement. An increase in the percentage of bone marrow blasts has been observed, and there is concern that these agents may accelerate the transformation to AML in some patients. They should not be considered "standard" therapy but may be useful as intermittent treatment for patients who develop an infection in the setting of neutropenia. The efficacy of combinations of growth factors is being evaluated. Chemical studies of the recently cloned thrombopoietin will be of interest.

Differentiating Agents. The observation that a number of drugs can induce differentiation of human leukemia cell lines and fresh leukemia cells in vitro has led to clinical evaluation of some of these agents. The drug most often used has been cytarabine at 5 to 25 mg/m2/day (10% to 20% of the conventional leukemia dose) for 14 to 21 days. Despite early encouraging results, complete remissions have been achieved in less than 20% of cases, and this approach was not demonstrated to be better than supportive care in a prospective randomized comparison.

Other potential differentiating agents are the retinoids. Trials in which patients were randomized to supportive care or placebo vs. 13-cis-retinoic acid failed to demonstrate a survival advantage for the treated patients. Recently published data have failed to demonstrate activity for ATRA in the MDS. The use of retinoids has also been associated with considerable toxicity, including fatigue, dry skin and cheilitis, hepatic dysfunction, bleeding, and pseudotumor cerebri.

Neither vitamin D analogs nor interferons alpha or gamma have been associated with meaningful responses in MDS patients. Other agents under investigation include 5-azacytidine and hexamethylene-bis-acetamide. Newer and more effective therapies are needed and should be evaluated in carefully designed clinical trials with correlative laboratory studies.

BIBLIOGRAPHY

Bennett JM, Catovsky D, Daniel M et al. Proposals for the classification of the acute leukaemias. Br J Haematol 33:451–458, 1976

Acute Myeloid Leukemia

Bennett JM, Catovsky D, Daniel M et al. Proposed revised criteria for the classification of acute myeloid leukemia. Ann Intern Med 103:626–629, 1985

Berman E, Heller G, Santorsa J et al. Results of a randomized trial comparing idarubicin and cytosine arabinoside with daunorubicin and cytosine arabinoside in adult patients with newly diagnosed acute myelogenous leukemia. Blood 77:1666–1674, 1991

Bishop JF, Lowenthal RM, Joshua D et al. Etoposide in acute nonlymphocytic leukemia. Blood 75:27–32, 1990

Brown RA, Herzig RH, Wolff SN et al. High-dose etoposide and cyclophosphamide without bone marrow transplantation for resistant hematologic malignancy. Blood 76:473–479, 1990

Cassileth PA, Lynch E, Hines JD et al. Varying intensity of postremission therapy in acute myeloid leukemia. Blood 79:1924–1930, 1992

Cheson BD, Cassileth PA, Head DR et al. Report of the National Cancer Institute sponsored workshop on definitions of diagnosis and response in acute myeloid leukemia. J Clin Oncol 8:813–819, 1990

Estey EH, Keating MJ, McCredie KB et al. Causes of initial remission induction failure in acute myelogenous leukemia. Blood 60:309–315, 1982

Estey E, Thall PF, Kantarjian H et al. Treatment of newly diagnosed acute myelogenous leukemia with granulocyte-macrophage colony-stimulating factor (GM-CSF) before and during continuous-infusion high-dose ara-C daunorubicin: Comparison to patients treated without GM-CSF. Blood 79:2246–2255, 1992

Frick J, Ritch PS, Hansen RM et al. Successful treatment of meningeal leukemia using systemic high-dose cytosine arabinoside. J Clin Oncol 2:365–368, 1984

Goldberg MA, Ginsburg D, Mayer RJ et al. Is heparin administration necessary during induction therapy for patients with acute promyelocytic leukemia? Blood 69:187–191, 1987

Herzig RH, Lazarus HM, Wolff SN et al. High-dose cytosine arabinoside with and without anthracycline antibiotics for remission reinduction of acute nonlymphocytic leukemia. J Clin Oncol 2:992–997, 1985

Kahn SB, Begg CB, Mazza JJ et al. Full dose versus attenuated dose daunorubicin, cytosine arabinoside, and 6-thioguanine in the treatment of acute nonlymphocytic leukemia in the elderly. J Clin Oncol 2:865–870, 1984

Kantarjian HM, Beran M, Ellis A et al. Phase I study of topotecan, a new topoisomerase I inhibitor, in patients with refractory or relapsed acute leukemia. Blood 81:1146–1151, 1993

List AF, Spier C, Greer J et al. Phase I/II trial of cyclosporine as a chemotherapy-resistance modifier in acute leukemia. J Clin Oncol 11:1652–1660, 1993

Löwenberg B, Zittoun R, Kerkhofs H et al. On the value of intensive remission-induction chemotherapy in elderly patients of 65+ years with acute myeloid leukemia: A randomized phase III study of the European Organization for Research and Treatment of Cancer Leukemia Group. J Clin Oncol 7:1268–1274, 1989

Mayer RJ, Davis RB, Schiffer CA et al. Comparative evaluation of intensive post-remission therapy with different dose schedules of ara-C in adults with acute myeloid leukemia (AML): Initial results of a CALGB phase III study (abstr 853). Proc ASCO 11:261, 1992

Rowe JM, Andersen J, Mazza JJ et al. Phase III randomized placebo-controlled study of granulocyte-macrophage colony stimulating factor (GM-CSF) in adult patients (55–70 years) with acute myelogenous leukemia (AML). A study of the Eastern Cooperative Oncology Group. Blood (in press)

Rubin EH, Andersen JW, Berg DT et al. Risk factors for high-dose cytarabine neurotoxicity: An analysis of a Cancer and Leukemia Group B trial in patients with acute myeloid leukemia. J Clin Oncol 10:948–953, 1992

Stone RM, Mayer RJ. The unique aspects of acute promyelocytic leukemia. J Clin Oncol 11:1913–1921, 1990

Warrell RP Jr, de Thé H, Wang Z-Y et al. Acute promyelocytic leukemia. N Engl J Med 329:177–189, 1993

Weick J, Kopecky K, Appelbaum F, et al. A randomized investigation of high-dose (HDAC) versus standard dose (SDAC) cytosine arabinoside with daunorubicin (DNR) in patients with acute myelogenous leukemia (abstr 856). Proc ASCO 11:261, 1992

Acute Lymphoblastic Leukemia

Clarkson B, Ellis S, Little C et al. Acute lymphoblastic leukemia in adults. Semin Oncol 12:160–179, 1985

Ellison RR, Mick R, Cuttner J et al. The effects of postinduction intensification treatment with cytarabine and daunorubicin in adult lymphocytic leukemia: A prospective randomized clinical trial by Cancer and Leukemia Group B. J Clin Oncol 9:2002–2015, 1991

Hoelzer D, Thiel E, Loffler H et al. Prognostic factors in a multicenter study for treatment of acute lymphoblastic leukemia in adults. Blood 71:123–131, 1988

Kantarjian HM, Walters RS, Keating MJ et al. Results of the vincristine, doxorubicin, and dexamethasone regimen in adults with standard- and high-risk acute lymphocytic leukemia. J Clin Oncol 8:994–1004, 1990

Kantarjian HM, Walters RS, Smith TL et al. Identification of risk groups for development of central nervous system leukemia in adults with acute lymphocytic leukemia. Blood 72:1784–1789, 1988

Linker CA. Treatment of acute leukemias in adults. Curr Opin Oncol 4:53–65, 1992

Linker CA, Levitt LJ, O'Donnell et al. Treatment of adult lymphoblastic leukemia with intensive cyclical chemotherapy: A follow-up report. Blood 78:2814–2822, 1991

Morra E, Lazzarino M, Inverardi D et al. Systemic high-dose ara-C for the treatment of meningeal leukemia and non-Hodgkin's lymphoma. J Clin Oncol 4:1207–1211,

Sobol RE, Mick R, Royston I et al. Clinical importance of myeloid antigen expression in adult acute lymphoblastic leukemia. N Engl J Med 316:1111–1117, 1987

Westbrook CA, Hooberman AL, Spino C et al. Clinical significance of the BCR-ABL fusion gene in adult acute lymphoblastic leukemia: A Cancer and Leukemia Group B study (8762). Blood 80:2983–2990, 1992

Myelodysplastic Syndromes

Andreef M, Stone M, Michaeli J et al. Hexamethylene bisacetamide in myelodysplastic syndrome and acute myelogenous leukemia: A phase II clinical trial with a differentiation-inducing agent. Blood 80:2604–2609, 1992

Cheson BD. The myelodysplastic syndromes: Current approaches to therapy. Ann Intern Med 112:932–941, 1990

Cheson BD. Chemotherapy and bone marrow transplantation for myelodysplastic syndromes. Semin Oncol 19:85–94, 1992

Cheson BD, Jasperse DM, Simon R et al. A critical appraisal of low dose cytosine arabinoside in patients with acute non-lymphocytic leukemia and myelodysplastic syndromes. J Clin Oncol 4:1857–1864, 1986

Foucar K, Langdon RM II, Armitage JO et al. Myelodysplastic syndromes: A clinical and pathologic analysis of 109 cases. Cancer 56:553–561, 1985

Goasguen JE, Bennett JM. Classification and morphologic features of the myelodysplastic syndromes. Semin Oncol 19:4–13, 1992

Greenberg PL. Treatment of myelodysplastic syndromes with hematopoietic growth factors. Semin Oncol 19:106–114, 1992

Matthew P, Tefferi A, Dewald GW et al. The 5q- syndrome: A single institution study of 43 consecutive patients. Blood 81:1040–1045, 1993

Negrin RS, Haeuber DH, Nagler A et al. Maintenance treatment of patients with myelodysplastic syndromes using recombinant human granulocyte colony-stimulating factor. Blood 76:36–43, 1990

Stein RS, Abels RI, Krantz SB. Pharmacologic doses of recombinant human erythropoietin in the treatment of myelodysplastic syndromes. Blood 78:1658–1663, 1991

John S. Macdonald, Daniel G. Haller, Robert J. Mayer, Eds. *Manual of Oncologic Therapeutics*, Third Edition.

40. CHRONIC LEUKEMIAS

Bruce D. Cheson

CHRONIC MYELOGENOUS (MYELOID, MYELOCYTIC) LEUKEMIA

Chronic myelogenous leukemia (CML) makes up 15% to 20% of adult leukemias. This neoplastic, clonal proliferation of pluripotent stem cells was the first recognized disorder with a characteristic chromosome abnormality, the Philadelphia chromosome (Ph^1), t(9;22)(q34;q11), which can be detected in more than 90% of patients. The Ph^1 involves the translocation of most of the ABL proto-oncogene from chromosome 9 to chromosome 22, where it is contiguous with the 5′ portion of the breakpoint cluster region (BCR) gene. The breakpoint in the BCR gene generally occurs in the major breakpoint region associated with Ph^1 CML, half the cases of Ph^1 acute lymphoblastic leukemia (ALL), and occasional cases of Ph^1 acute myeloid leukemia. This fusion results in the synthesis of the hybrid $p210^{bcr\text{-}abl}$ protein, which is presumed to be involved in the etiology of CML. The molecular lesion can be demonstrated even in most cases of Ph^1-negative CML.

The course of CML falls into three phases: the chronic phase (CML-CP) is the most common presentation and generally persists for about 4 to 5 years. The onset of fever, weight loss, and other constitutional symptoms along with laboratory evidence of increasing blasts in the bone marrow and peripheral blood, with or without the appearance of additional cytogenetic abnormalities, heralds the accelerated phase of the disease (CML-AP), which generally lasts from a few weeks to about 6 months. Over 80% of patients die during blast crisis (CML-BC), which is associated with the hematologic appearance of an aggressive acute leukemia, which is lymphoid in a third of cases, and myeloid in most of the remaining ones. CML-BC is particularly refractory to therapy and lasts only 2 to 6 months. Approximately 5% of patients with CML will present in CML-BC.

Prognostic factors associated with a more rapid transition to the more aggressive forms of CML include older age, large spleen, increased eosinophils and/or basophils, fever, additional cytogenetic abnormalities, skin infiltration, unexpected decrease or increase in platelet count, and lymphadenopathy.

TREATMENT FOR CML-CP

Conventional chemotherapy for CML neither delays transformation to CML-BC nor substantially prolongs survival. Therefore, therapy has traditionally been delivered to ameliorate symptoms or to manage anemia, thrombocytopenia, or thrombocytosis, not simply to lower the white blood cell (WBC) count below an arbitrary level (*e.g.*, 50,000/μl). Moreover, CML patients may experience periodic (*e.g.*, every 2 months) oscillations of blood counts. Therefore, a period of observation is often warranted before treatment is considered.

Single-Agent Chemotherapy

Whichever chemotherapy is planned, patients should be pretreated with allopurinol, 300 mg/day given orally, to prevent urate nephropathy.

HYDROXYUREA

Hydroxyurea is the current standard chemotherapy for CML-CP. This drug is generally given as 1 to 2 g/m^2/day orally in divided doses. Hematologic responses can be achieved in 60% to 80% of cases and are rapid (*i.e.*, occur within several days); however, cytogenetic responses are uncommon.

INTERFERON ALPHA

Recombinant interferon alpha (IFNα), 5×10^6 units/m^2/day given subcutaneously is active in controlling the WBC and platelet counts in CML. Between 50% and 80% of patients will achieve either a partial or a complete hematologic response, which may take several weeks to months to occur. In almost half of patients, partial suppression of the Ph^1 clone can be demonstrated, but complete disappearance is achieved in only 10% to 25%. In many patients with a complete cytogenetic response, the bcr-abl rearrangement is still detectable using polymerase chain reaction technology. Patients who achieve a complete cytogenetic response appear to have prolonged progression-free survival; however, whether that reflects drug effect or selection of patients who would have had a prolonged chronic phase is unclear. Randomized studies comparing IFNα with hydroxyurea demonstrate a response, time to progression, and survival advantage for the IFNα. Many clinicians would now consider IFNα to be the preferable initial therapy for CML.

Combinations of IFNα with other agents, such as low-dose cytarabine, have provided encouraging results that require confirmation in larger studies.

BUSULFAN

Busulfan appears to have a better response rate than other alkylators (*e.g.*, cyclophosphamide, chlorambucil) and is better at controlling blood counts and symptoms. Therapy is begun with 4 to 6 mg/m^2/day given orally. Loading doses provide no advantage and subject some particularly sensitive patients (10% to 20% of all patients) to excessive risk of prolonged myelosuppression. Because busulfan is eliminated slowly from the body, myelosuppression may persist for up to 6 to 8 weeks after discontinuation. Thus, to avoid neutropenia, therapy should be stopped when the WBC has been lowered to approximately 20,000/μl. Alternative schedules include pulses of 50 to 150 mg every 2 to 4 weeks, but the chronic administration at low doses is usually easier to manage. Over 75% of patients will respond to busulfan with a reduction in WBC, often accompanied by a decrease in platelet count in patients with thrombocytosis, and at least a partial resolution of splenomegaly. The development of resistance often heralds CML-AP or CML-BC.

A partial lack of cross-resistance between alkylators is demonstrated by the observation that over 30% of patients who are not responding to busulfan will respond to hydroxyurea. Like other alkylating agents, busulfan has an inherent risk of inducing acute myeloid leukemia (AML). Nevertheless, an accelerated rate of transformation has not been apparent. Randomized studies demonstrate that busulfan is inferior to hydroxyurea and IFNα. Moreover, busulfan therapy may compromise the outcome of subsequent bone marrow transplant. Therefore busulfan is no longer frequently used as clinical therapy.

HOMOHARRINGTONINE

Homoharringtonine is a cephalotaxine ester that has demonstrated activity in CML-AP and CML-CP. Attempts to combine this agent with IFNα are in development.

Combination Chemotherapy. Aggressive combination chemotherapy regimens result in transient disappearance of the clone in 30% of patients, but without an apparent impact on survival. Intensive chemotherapy programs increase morbidity and cannot be recommended as standard care.

Splenectomy. Splenectomy early in the course of CML has not resulted in a consistent survival advantage. However, the spleen has been described anecdotally as the initial site of blastic transformation. In practice, splenectomy should be reserved for patients who exhibit a hematologic response to chemotherapy but with persistent, symptomatic splenomegaly or for those who develop excessive thrombocytopenia with chemotherapy.

Splenic Irradiation. Brief responses have been observed, yet several reports suggest that this treatment may shorten survival.

Leukapheresis. Leukapheresis may induce not only a rapid decrease in the WBC count but a reduction in hepatosplenomegaly as well. These effects may last for several weeks. Such therapy may benefit patients who have hyperviscosity from sludging of circulating WBCs and may temporarily benefit pregnant women, until standard treatment can safely be delivered post partum.

Bone Marrow Transplantation. Allogeneic and syngeneic bone marrow transplantation (BMT) offer the only curative options for patients with CML. Candidates include patients who are younger than 55 years, with a histocompatible marrow donor. The probability of long-term survival for allogeneic BMT in the chronic phase is 60% to 70%, compared with 15% to 20% in the accelerated phase or blast crisis. Nevertheless, the relapse rate is 20%, and treatment-related deaths occur in 15% of cases.

The results appear to be better if BMT occurs within 1 year of diagnosis. Therefore, a potential candidate for BMT should be referred to a transplant center soon after diagnosis to obtain information about risks and potential benefits and to decide on an appropriate time for undergoing BMT.

In the absence of a human leukocyte antigen (HLA)-matched sibling, a one-antigen mismatch may provide comparable results; HLA-matched unrelated donors have been used with some success. There is an associated 50% prolonged disease-free survival, which varies considerably with a number of prognostic factors, including donor disparity, recipient age, disease status at transplant, and type of graft-versus-host-disease prophylaxis; the results are best for those in the first chronic phase and younger than 30 years of age. The 2-year disease-free survival for those undergoing transplantation in the first chronic phase is 30% to 35%; in the second or greater chronic phase or the accelerated phase of the disease, it is 20%; there are no long-term disease-free survivors in blast crisis. Patients who relapse after an allogenic bone marrow transplant may be reinduced into a durable hematologic remission following the administration of donor leukocytes.

Autografting for patients with CML is still investigational. The prolongation of survival suggested for patients with CML-CP may reflect patient selection. Those in CML-BC have a median survival of only 4 months. Autologous transplantation for patients who have achieved a complete cytogenetic remission following IFNα therapy is being evaluated. IFNα needs to be discontinued several weeks before transplantation to permit successful engraftment. The possibility of in vitro selection of normal progenitor cells is currently under study.

TREATMENT FOR CML-AP

No specific treatments are available for CML-AP. Patients usually experience only minor responses of brief duration to a succession of agents that are effective in CP. Transformation occurs within a few weeks to months.

TREATMENT FOR CML-BC

CML-BC remains one of the hematologic malignancies that is most refractory to treatment. A number of regimens induce complete hematologic remissions in up to 30% of patients, but median duration of survival is rarely longer than 6 or 7 months. Approximately 30% of cases of CML-BC undergo a lymphoblastic transformation, which appears to have a significantly higher rate of response to regimens that include vincristine and prednisone, although survival is only a few months. Tiazofurin, a nucleoside analog, may induce complete remissions in myeloid CML-BC; however, responses with current regimens are brief and current requirements for close pharmacokinetic monitoring make such therapy impractical.

CHRONIC LYMPHOCYTIC LEUKEMIAS

The chronic lymphocytic leukemias are a heterogeneous collection of B- and T-cell disorders characterized by a clonal accumulation of functionally deficient lymphocytes. Included are chronic lymphocytic leukemia (CLL), prolymphocytic leukemia, hairy cell leukemia, splenic lymphoma with villous lymphocytes, chronic T-cell lymphocytosis, Sézary syndrome, and adult T-cell leukemia/lymphoma (ATLL).

CLL is the most common of the B-cell lymphoproliferative disorders in Western countries, with 10,000 new cases diagnosed in the United States each year. Although generally considered a disease of the elderly, approximately 15% of patients who present are younger than age 50. The diagnosis is suspected with an unexplained, sustained increase (>5000/μl) of mature-appearing lymphocytes that have monoclonal light chain expression and low levels of surface immunoglobulins and that express pan–B-cell antigens (*e.g.*, CD19, CD20, CD23), and CD5. In practice, performing a node biopsy is rarely necessary to confirm the diagnosis. However, the bone marrow provides valuable information about prognosis, response to therapy, cytogenetic abnormalities, and molecular biology.

Staging

The Rai classification is the most widely used staging system in the United States, whereas the Binet system (Table 40-1) is often used in Europe. An attempt made by the International Workshop on CLL to integrate the two has not been widely adopted. The five-stage Rai system has been recently modified to three stages: low-risk (Stage 0), intermediate-risk (Stages I and II), and high-risk (Stages III and IV) (Table 40-2). Clinical stage is the strongest predictor of outcome in CLL. However, none of the currently staging systems accurately distinguishes patients who will experience a stable course from those who will soon progress; nor do they permit incorporation of newly identified prognostic factors.

Other clinical and laboratory features conferring a poor outcome include older age, male sex, diffuse pattern of bone marrow involvement, rapid lymphocyte doubling time (≤12

TABLE 40–1. THE BINET STAGING SYSTEM FOR CLL

STAGE	CLINICAL FEATURES	MEDIAL SURVIVAL (YEARS)
A	Fewer than three areas of clinical lymphadenopathy; no anemia or thrombocytopenia	>10
B	Three or more involved node areas; no anemia or thrombocytopenia	7
C	Hemoglobin ≤10 g/dl and/or platelets <100,000/μl	2

months), cytogenetic abnormalities, failure on prior therapy, elevated serum β_2-microglobulin. Such prognostic features, along with newer immunologic and biologic advances, may lead to even more useful staging systems.

Between 5% and 15% of CLL patients undergo an aggressive transformation. The most common is Richter's syndrome, an aggressive large cell lymphoma that occurs in 3% to 5% of cases and is associated with systemic symptoms, progressive lymphadenopathy, extranodal disease, an elevated lactate dehydrogenase (LDH) level, often with a monoclonal gammopathy. Other patients undergo a prolymphocytic transformation. Few durable responses are achieved; survival is brief once these terminal phases occur, and new treatments are needed.

Treatment

Most patients with CLL do not require immediate therapy; treatment neither cures nor prolongs survival of patients with early-stage disease. A number of factors should be considered in deciding when to treat. Whenever possible, patients should undergo a 3- to 6-month period of observation to assess the clinical course of their disease.

INDICATIONS FOR TREATMENT

Indications for therapy include evidence of "active" disease, such as the following:

1. Disease-related symptoms: These may include fevers and sweats without evidence of infection, weight loss, or fatigue.
2. Progressive bone marrow failure: Therapy should be considered for symptomatic anemia, especially with a requirement for repeated transfusions, or progressive thrombocytopenia (*e.g.*, platelet count < 100,000/μl or evidence of spontaneous bleeding other than cutaneous).
3. Autoimmune anemia and/or thrombocytopenia. Although laboratory evidence for autoimmune anemia or thrombocytopenia can be detected in 20% to 30% of

TABLE 40–2. THE MODIFIED RAI STAGING SYSTEM FOR CLL

RAI STAGE	THREE-STAGE SYSTEM	CLINICAL FEATURES	MEDIAL SURVIVAL (YEARS)
0	Low-risk	Lymphocytosis only in blood and marrow	>10
I	Intermediate-risk	Lymphocytosis + lymphadenopathy +	
II		splenomegaly ± hepatomegaly	7
III	High-risk	Lymphocytosis + anemia	1.5
IV		+ thrombocytopenia	

cases of CLL, these disease complications are clinically important in only 10%.

4. Massive and/or progressive lymphadenopathy.
5. Massive and/or progressive hepatosplenomegaly.
6. Recurrent infections: These include systemic or disseminated bacterial, viral, or fungal infections requiring systemic antimicrobial therapy, or localized infections (*e.g.*, abscesses) poorly responsive to conventional antimicrobial therapy.
7. Progressive lymphocytosis with a short (<6-month) doubling time or a 50% increase over 2 months.

Because Rai Stage 0 patients are usually asymptomatic and their disease may not progress for years to several decades of follow-up, they require no treatment. Treatment should even be discouraged for stable Stage I and Stage II patients, even for those with a psychological need for something to be done; all of the active agents have potentially serious side-effects, including a possible increase in secondary solid tumors. A high WBC count should not be the sole indication for therapy because hyperviscosity may not occur, even with a WBC over 500,000/μl.

ASSESSMENT OF RESPONSE TO TREATMENT

The widest used standardized criteria for response to therapy were published by the NCI-sponsored Working Group on CLL, and are presented in Table 40–3.

TREATMENT FOR CHRONIC LYMPHOCYTIC LEUKEMIA

Therapy for CLL should include allopurinol (300 mg/day given orally) for patients with a large tumor burden, particularly those who have not received prior therapy. Allopurinol can be discontinued at the same time as the antileukemic therapy.

Chemotherapy. Alkylating agents have been the mainstay of chemotherapeutic treatment. Nevertheless, they are merely palliative and do not substantially affect the natural history of the disease. Chlorambucil, the most active and

TABLE 40–3. DEFINITION OF CLINICAL RESPONSE FOR PATIENTS WITH B-CLL

	CR*	PR†	PD
Physical examination			
Nodes	None	≥50% decrease	≥50% increase, new nodes
Liver/spleen	Not palpable	≥50% decrease	≥50% increase, newly palpable
Symptoms	None	N/A	N/A
Peripheral blood			
PMN	≥1500/μl	≥1500/μl or >50% improvement from baseline	—‡
Platelets	>100,000/μl	>100,000/μl or >50% improvement from baseline	—‡
Hemoglobin (untransfused)	>11.0 g/dl	>11.0 g/dl or >50% improvement from baseline	—‡
Lymphocytes	≤4000/μl	≥50% decrease	≥50% increase
Bone marrow	<30% lymphocytes	N/A	N/A

*Complete remission (CR) requires fulfillment of *all* criteria for a duration of >2 months, at which time a bone marrow aspirate and biopsy are required to document response as complete.

†Partial remission (PR) requires fulfillment of the above-noted decrease in circulating lymphocytes, regression in either adenopathy and/or hepatosplenomegaly, and one other parameter listed above for a duration of >2 months.

‡In the absence of other indices of clinical progression, the presence of a ≥2 g/dl decrease in hemoglobin, or ≥50% decrease in platelet count and/or absolute granulocyte count, will not exclude a patient from continuing the study.

PMN = polymorphonucleotides; N/A = not applicable.

best tolerated, is administered at a dose of 6 to 14 mg/day given orally, with blood counts checked weekly, until the signs and symptoms that compelled therapy have diminished. The dose can then be reduced by 50% or even discontinued. No data support the use of maintenance programs. A suitable alternative is pulse administration of chlorambucil (20 to 30 mg/m^2 given orally every 2 to 4 weeks); these schedules have an efficacy similar to that of daily dosing, with less myelotoxicity and better patient compliance. With either schedule, responses can be expected in 30% to 50%, although complete remissions are uncommon (<10%).

Cyclophosphamide, 100 to 200 mg/day given orally, or 1 to 1.5 g given intravenously every 3 weeks is an acceptable alternative to chlorambucil and may have activity in some patients whose disease has failed to respond to chlorambucil, which suggests some degree of non–cross-resistance.

Other alkylators, such as busulfan and melphalan, appear to be less active.

Glucocorticoid Therapy. Transient partial responses can be achieved in 40% to 60% of CLL patients using prednisone, 30 to 60 mg/day given orally. Steroid therapy may be of particular value in patients with autoimmune hemolytic anemia or immune thrombocytopenia. Nevertheless, the associated toxicities (*e.g.*, diabetes, osteoporosis, infections) preclude long-term use.

Combination Therapy. Combinations of alkylators (*e.g.*, chlorambucil) and prednisone (40–60 mg/day for 5–7 days every month) have been used but are not clearly superior to alkylating agents alone yet have the increased risks associated with chronic steroid administration.

More intensive multiagent regimens, including the aggressive M-2 regimen (carmustine, melphalan, vincristine, prednisone, and cyclophosphamide) or doxorubicin-containing regimens, such as cyclophosphamide, doxorubicin, and prednisone (CAP), do not produce durable responses and have not demonstrated a survival advantage over less intensive programs. A report by the French Cooperative Group on CLL suggested a longer survival for patients with Binet Stage C disease treated with cyclophosphamide, doxorubicin, vincristine, and prednisone (CHOP) compared with cyclophosphamide, vincristine, and prednisone (COP); however, other groups have failed to reproduce these findings.

Newer Agents

Purine Analogs. Three purine analogs have demonstrated impressive activity in CLL: fludarabine (Fludara), 2-chlorodeoxyadenosine (CdA, cladribine, Leustatin), and 2′-deoxycoformycin (DCF, pentostatin, Nipent). The most active of these is fludarabine, which, at a dose of 25 mg/m^2/day for 5 days every month for 4 to 6 months, achieves complete remissions in 15% of refractory patients, with an overall response rate of 55%; the median duration of responses is approximately 16 months. In patients without prior therapy, complete remissions are achieved in 33%, with an overall response rate of over 80%. A large national trial comparing fludarabine, chlorambucil, and the combination of the two agents in previously untreated patients is nearly completed. When available, the results will redefine the initial approach to this disease. In a German study, response rates with fludarabine were superior to CAP (cyclophosphamide, doxorubicin, prednisone) in the previously treated and untreated patients.

CdA achieves responses in 50% of previously treated CLL patients, although few are complete remissions and the median duration of response is 4 to 5 months. Responses occur in 65% of untreated patients, but are not durable. Initial reports of CdA responses in fludarabine failures have not been confirmed, and such treatment has been associated with significant thrombocytopenia and infections. DCF has an overall response rate of 25% to 30% with few complete remissions.

These three agents share toxicities of myelosuppression with neutropenic fevers, immunosuppression and opportunistic infections, and, rarely, pulmonary or neurologic effects.

Biologic Therapy. IFNα has limited activity in either previously treated or untreated patients (15–20% response rate), with higher response rates in patients who have earlier-stage disease. The role of this agent remains undefined.

A number of new immunoconjugates, both immunotoxins and radioimmunoconjugates, are in the early stages of development and appear to have promise.

Radiation Therapy. Local disease control can be achieved with radiation therapy, including palliation of pain from lymphadenopathy or relief of an obstructed bronchus. Splenic radiation therapy results in partial responses in half of patients, although neutropenia, thrombocytopenia, and briefness of the responses limit the usefulness of this practice. Total-body irradiation is infrequently used because it is less effective at controlling disease than chlorambucil or fludarabine and induces more profound cytopenias.

Splenectomy. Indications include autoimmune anemia or thrombocytopenia refractory to systemic therapy, or persistent symptomatic splenomegaly in a patient who has otherwise responded to chemotherapy. Splenectomy has no influence on survival in CLL.

Bone Marrow Transplantation. Because about 15% of cases of CLL are diagnosed before age 50, and since complete remissions can be achieved with drugs such as fludarabine, allogeneic and even autologous bone marrow transplantation (ABMT) have been evaluated. There is no clear plateau on the disease-free survival curve following ABMT.

Results are more promising with allogenic bone marrow transplantation; however, whether patients are being cured with either approach remains to be determined. Moreover, treatment-related deaths occur in 25% to 40% of patients. These treatments should be conducted only on a clinical trial.

TREATMENT FOR DISEASE-RELATED COMPLICATIONS

Packed red blood cells or platelets may be administered for symptomatic anemia or thrombocytopenia, respectively, once an autoimmune cause has been excluded. Although high-dose intravenous immunoglobulin therapy is available for patients who are hypogammaglobulinemic, this therapy should be restricted to those with documented, recurrent bacterial infections.

Pneumococcal polysaccharide vaccines are probably not useful in CLL because patients are generally unable to respond adequately to an antigen challenge. Moreover, other immune defects, including impaired complement activation, may contribute to this increased susceptibility to infections. Purine analogs have dramatically altered the spectrum of infections in patients with CLL, from the encapsulated bacteria to a wide variety of opportunistic organisms.

Leukemic meningitis is rarely clinically apparent, although it is not an uncommon finding at autopsy. Responses have been reported with intrathecal methotrexate and cranial irradiation.

PROLYMPHOCYTIC LEUKEMIA

The B-cell variant of prolymphocytic leukemia (PLL) is more common than the T-cell variant (T-PLL). PLL is distinguished from CLL by the presence of 55% or more prolymphocytes in the peripheral blood and bone marrow. Clinical features include massive splenomegaly and lymphadenopathy, with skin infiltration in a substantial number of cases. The prognosis is worse for patients with PLL developing as a late event in the course of CLL rather than *de novo*.

Both fludarabine and DCF have demonstrated significant activity in PLL patients. CHOP chemotherapy has been used in patients younger than 60 years of age with adequate performance status, but with limited efficacy. Splenectomy, splenic irradiation, and leukapheresis have been used with minimal success.

HAIRY CELL LEUKEMIA

When to Treat

Hairy cell leukemia (HCL) is a rare chronic B-cell disorder. Bly-7 appears to be a diagnostic market for HCL cells. It may be associated with a very indolent course. Approximately 10% of patients may never require therapy. Therefore, treatment can be reserved for patients with active disease: those with a transfusion requirement, abnormal blood counts that are deteriorating or symptomatic, hemoglobin level less than 12 g/dl, granulocyte count less than 1000/μl, platelet count less than 100,000/μl, circulating hairy cell count more than 20,000/μl, recurrent infections requiring antibiotics, symptomatic splenomegaly, or vasculitis.

Treatment for Hairy Cell Leukemia

2-CHLORODEOXYADENOSINE

Following a single course at 1.0 mg/kg by continuous intravenous infusion or 2-hour infusion daily for 5 to 7 days, CdA achieves complete remissions in 65% to 85% of patients with HCL; most of the remainder achieve a partial response. These responses appear to be durable, although relapses are observed in 20% of patients, which raises the question of whether patients are being cured. Nevertheless, if therapy is needed, most recurrences respond to retreatment.

2-DEOXYCOFORMYCIN

The activity of DCF in HCL is comparable to CdA. Low doses of DCF (4 mg/m^2 given intravenously every other week for 4 to 6 months) achieve durable complete remissions in 60% to 80% of patients with HCL, with partial responses in most of the remaining patients. Late relapses have been observed, although few of these require re-treatment. A recently completed comparison of DCF vs. IFN demonstrated a clear advantage in complete remission, rate and duration of response in favor of the DCF.

Whether DCF or CdA is preferable for treatment is a matter of physician and patient preference based on convenience of schedule, cost, and toxicity profile. Responses to CdA have been reported in patients who failed to respond to or who could not tolerate DCF.

FLUDARABINE

Anecdotal reports suggest activity for fludarabine in HCL.

INTERFERON ALPHA

IFNα was the first major advance in systemic therapy for HCL. Recombinant IFNα 2b at doses of 2×10^6 units/m^2 three times weekly, or 3×10^6 units daily of alpha-2a, both subcutaneously, induce hematologic responses in 80% of patients, although complete remissions occur in only 10%. The recommended duration of therapy is 1 to 2 years, unless disease progression is observed. Therapy is reinstituted if relapse occurs more than 6 months after an initial response. Maintenance therapy appears to increase complications without an influence on survival. Both DCF and CdA successfully treat IFNα.

SPLENECTOMY

Splenomegaly is present in 80% to 90% of HCL patients and was the treatment of choice for HCL until the availability of the new effective systemic agents. A normal complete blood count is observed in 40%, although no pathologically complete remissions are achieved. Whether response translates into prolonged survival is controversial. Clinical features that appear to be associated with benefit from splenectomy include age less than 60 years, large spleen, and brief clinical history. DCF and CdA can effectively replace splenectomy as initial treatment in most patients.

SPLENIC IRRADIATION

Splenic irradiation may provide temporary symptomatic relief for patients unable to undergo splenectomy, but hematologic responses are uncommon.

CHRONIC T-CELL LYMPHOCYTOSIS

The chronic T-cell leukemias are a heterogeneous group of relatively rare disorders that differ significantly from B-cell leukemias with respect to their morphology, immunology, virology, biology, and response to therapy and should therefore be considered a distinct collection of diseases. The differential diagnosis includes large granular lymphocytic leukemia (LGL), T-PLL, Sézary syndrome, and adult T-cell leukemia/lymphoma (see discussion further on). LGL, the most common of these diseases, is a clonal disorder of unknown etiology that is often incidentally diagnosed in the setting of a lymphocytosis. The peripheral blood mononuclear cells exhibit characteristic azurophilic granulation. Proliferations of LGL may be either CD3+ (T-LGL) or CD3− (natural killer [NK]-LGL). Approximately 95% are CD4−, CD8+, although some cases may be CD4+, CD8−.

T-LGL presents at a median age of 57 years and is more common in women. Almost 40% experience recurrent infections. Most patients have neutropenia, which may be severe; there is bone marrow involvement in almost 90% of cases. Of interest is a 30% incidence of rheumatoid arthritis, occasionally with Felty's syndrome. Polyclonal hypergammaglobulinemia occurs in almost half of cases, and rheumatoid factor, antinuclear antibodies, and circulating immune complexes are commonly detected. NK cells are often decreased in numbers. Pure red-cell aplasia has been reported. Although LGL has seemed to be indolent, more than two thirds of patients eventually require therapy, primarily because of recurrent infections, which may be fatal in a third of cases. When indicated, alkylating agents with or without steroids have been effective. CdA, fludarabine, and DCF appear to have limited activity. Anecdotes suggest that cyclosporin A may induce responses. Splenectomy is generally not associated with long-term benefit.

The median age of patients with NK-LGL is 39 years, without a female predominance or an association with rheumatoid arthritis. Patients often present with fevers without obvious infection, and with other constitutional symptoms. Profound neutropenia is less common than with T-LGL, whereas massive splenomegaly is more frequent (>90%), and bone marrow infiltration is universal. The clinical course of NK-LGL tends to be rapid and aggressive, and the majority of patients succumb to their disease within a couple of months despite aggressive combination chemotherapy.

T-Prolymphocytic Leukemia

Patients with T-PLL generally present with massive splenomegaly; lymphadenopathy is seen in 40%, and skin infiltration in 20%. The presenting WBC count is often higher than 100,000/μl. The phenotype of the malignant cell is generally CD3+,CD4+,CD5+,CD7+,CD8−, CD25− although a third of cases are CD4+/CD8+ or CD4−/CD8+. There are no apparent clinical differences among these subsets. A consistent abnormality of chromosome 14 has been reported, with two breakpoints at 14q11 and 14q32.

The prognosis of T-PLL patients is poor, with a median survival of 7 months. The most active agent appears to be DCF, which has achieved complete remissions in up to 10% and partial remissions in a third of patients.

Adult T-Cell Leukemia/Lymphoma

Adult T-cell leukemia/lymphoma (ATLL) is most common in the Caribbean and southwestern islands of Japan. ATLL is usually associated with infection with the human T-cell leukemia virus 1 (HTLV-1) retrovirus. The immunophenotypic characteristics of the malignant cells include CD2+,CD3+,CD5+,CD4+,CD8−,CD25++,CD56/5−. The clinical spectrum of ATLL ranges from a preleukemic condition that progresses to symptomatic ATLL, then to, in 3% of patients, an indolent disease that may not require treatment for several years; finally it progresses to an extremely aggressive disease characterized by anemia, hypercalcemia, bone and skin lesions, splenomegaly, central nervous system involvement, opportunistic infections, circulating leukemia cells, and a very poor outcome. Factors reported to be associated with an unfavorable prognosis include a leukemic phase, high serum lactate dehydrogenase, poor performance status, and cytogenetic abnormalities. Activity has been suggested for DCF that is higher in previously untreated patients than in those with more advanced disease whose prognosis is poor (median survival of 6.5 months).

Sézary Syndrome

Approximately a third of patients with mycosis fungoides will have circulating malignant cerebriform cells at the time of diagnosis, which may be an independent negative prognostic factor. The frequency varies with the stage of the disease: 0% to 22% in patients with skin patches, 9% to 30% in those with plaques, 27% to 50% in those with skin tumors, and 90% to 96% in those with erythroderma. The treatment of mycosis fungoides is described elsewhere in this text.

BIBLIOGRAPHY

Binet JL, Auquier A, Dighiero G et al. A new prognostic classification of chronic lymphocytic leukemia derived from a multivariate survival analysis. Cancer 48:198–206, 1981

Cheson BD. New antimetabolites in the treatment of human malignancies. Semin Oncol 19:695–706, 1992

Cheson BD, Bennett JM, Rai KR et al. Guidelines for clinical protocols for chronic lymphocytic leukemia: Recommendations of the National Cancer Institute-sponsored Working Group. Am J Hematol 29:152–163, 1988

Döhner H, Ho AD, Thaler J et al. Pentostatin in prolymphocytic leukemia: Phase II trial of the European Organization for Research and Treatment of Cancer Leukemia Cooperative Study Group. J Natl Cancer Inst 85:658, 1993

Drobyski WR, Keever CA, Roth MS et al. Salvage immunotherapy using donor leukocyte infusions as treatment for relapsed chronic myelogenous leukemia after allogeneic bone marrow transplantation: Efficacy and toxicity of a defined T-cell dose. Blood 82:2310–2318, 1993

French Cooperative Group on Chronic Lymphocytic Leukemia. Long-term results of the CHOP regimen in stage C chronic lymphocytic leukaemia. Br J Haematol 73:334–340, 1989

French Cooperative Group on Chronic Lymphocytic Leukemia. Effects of chlorambucil and therapeutic decision in initial forms of chronic lymphocytic leukemia (stage A): Results of a randomized clinical trial on 612 patients. Blood 75:1414–1421, 1990

French Cooperative Group on Chronic Lymphocytic Leukemia. A randomized trial of chlorambucil versus COP in stage B chronic lymphocytic leukemia. Blood 75:1422–1425, 1990

Grossbard ML, Lambert JM, Goldmacher VS et al. Anti-B4-blocked ricin: A phase I trial of 7-day continuous infusion in patients with B-cell neoplasms. J Clin Oncol 11:726–737, 1993

Italian Cooperative Study Group on Chronic Myeloid Leukemia. A prospective study of interferon alpha-2A vs chemotherapy in chronic myeloid leukemia (CML): Karyotypic response and survival (abstr 980). Proc ASCO 12:300, 1993

Kantarjian HM, Deisseroth A, Kurzrock R et al. Chronic myelogenous leukemia: A concise update. Blood 82:691–703, 1993

Kantarjian HM, Keating MJ, Estey EH et al. Treatment of advanced stages of Philadelphia chromosome-positive chronic myelogenous leukemia with interferon-α and low-dose cytarabine. J Clin Oncol 10:772–778, 1992

Keating MJ, O'Brien S, Kantarjian H et al. Long-term follow-up of patients with chronic lymphocytic leukemia treated with fludarabine as a single agent. Blood 81:2878–2884, 1993

Marks DI, Cullis JO, Ward KN et al. Allogeneic bone marrow transplantation for chronic myeloid leukemia using sibling and volunteer unrelated donors. Ann Intern Med 119:207–214, 1993

O'Brien S, Kantarjian H, Beran M et al. Results of fludarabine and prednisone therapy in 264 patients with chronic lymphocytic leukemia with multivariate analysis-derived prognostic model for response to treatment. Blood 82:1695–1700, 1993

Ozer H, George SL, Schiffer CA et al. Prolonged subcutaneous administration of recombinant alpha-2b interferon in patients with previously untreated Philadelphia chromosome-positive chronic-phase chronic myelogenous leukemia: Effect on remission duration and survival. Cancer and Leukemia Group B study 8583. Blood (in press)

Piro LD, Saven A, Ellison D et al. Prolonged complete remissions following 2-chlorodeoxyadenosine (2-CdA) in hairy cell leukemia (HCL) (abstr 846). Proc ASCO 11:259, 1992

Rabinowe SN, Soiffer RJ, Gribben JG et al. Autologous and allogeneic bone marrow transplantation for poor prognosis patients with B-cell chronic lymphocytic leukemia. Blood 82:1366–1376, 1993

Raphael B, Andersen JW, Silber R et al. Comparison of chlorambucil and prednisone versus cyclophosphamide, vincristine, and prednisone as initial treatment for chronic lymphocytic leukemia: Long-term follow-up of an Eastern Cooperative Oncology Group randomized clinical trial. J Clin Oncol 9:770–776, 1991

Robertson LE, Pugh W, O'Brien S: Richter's syndrome: A report on 39 patients. J Clin Oncol 11:1985–1989

Saven A, Piro LD. Treatment of hairy cell leukemia. Blood 79:1111–1120, 1992

Saven A, Lemon RH, Piro LD. 2-Chlorodeoxyadenosine for patients with B-cell chronic lymphocytic leukemia resistant to fludarabine. N Engl J Med 328:812–813, 1993

Saven A, Carrera CJ, Carson DA et al. 2-Chlorodeoxyadenosine treatment of refractory chronic lymphocytic leukemia. Leuk Lymph 5:133, 1991

Talpaz M, Kantarjian H, Kurzrock R et al. Interferon-alpha produces sustained cytogenetic responses in chronic myelogenous leukemia. Philadelphia chromosome-positive patients. Ann Intern Med 114:532–537, 1991

John S. Macdonald, Daniel G. Haller, Robert J. Mayer, Eds. *Manual of Oncologic Therapeutics*, Third Edition.

41. HODGKIN'S DISEASE

George P. Canellos

Hodgkin's disease (HD) is one of the few malignancies whose natural history has been favorably altered by modern diagnosis and therapy. The mortality-to-incidence ratio was dramatically reduced between 1970 and 1980, when combination chemotherapy and linear accelerator radiation therapy achieved more widespread application. The success represents an achievement for diagnostic and therapeutic innovation in cancer management. The introduction of a universally accepted histopathologic and clinical staging system facilitated the communication between investigators and clinicians in community practice.

ETIOLOGY

Despite the progress in clinical staging and the success of therapeutic intervention, the cell of origin in HD remains an area of controversy. Some aspects of the epidemiology of HD suggest that transmission of an infectious agent may have an important etiologic role. The disease tends to occur primarily in children in the developing world, whereas it is concentrated in the 25 to 35 age group in Europe and North America. The Epstein-Barr virus (EBV), the etiologic agent in infectious mononucleosis, has been strongly associated with HD based on serology and the molecular *in situ* demonstration of EBV genome in Hodgkin's and Reed-Sternberg cells. With sensitive techniques, 50% to 90% of HD patients will have cellular molecular evidence of the EBV genome. Furthermore, the EBV genome is monoclonal. The presence of some surface antigens known to exist on normal, lymphoid cells — human leukocyte antigen-DR, CD30 (Ki antigen), and CD25 (interleukin-2 receptor) — suggests that the pathognomic Reed-Sternberg cell represents a transformed lymphoblastoid cell that, by and large, lacks the leukocyte common antigen (CD45) and specific markers of B- or T-cell origin. Rarely, in less than 10% to 20% of patients studied, there may be evidence of immunoglobulin or T-cell receptor gene rearrangement. Immunoperoxidase will detect CD15 (Leu-M-1) on the Reed-Sternberg cell in approximately 80% of patients. This is a granulocyte-monocyte marker. The current evidence suggests that lymphocyte-predominant HD, especially the nodular variant, is a low-grade B-lymphocytic proliferative disorder, because the Reed-Sternberg–like cell (L/H cell) and the lymphocytes demonstrate B-cell markers. It is controversial whether monotypic immunoglobulin light chains or immunoglobulin gene rearrangements are present in those B-lymphocytes.

PATHOLOGY

The pathologic classification has undergone few changes since the development of Lukes-Butler scheme, which classifies HD into four subgroups:

1. Lymphocyte-predominant HD (LPHD) (nodular and diffuse variant), which occurs in about 5% of cases and usually in young males. There is generally an indolent natural history with an excellent result from any therapeutic modality. Very late recurrences have been noted.
2. Nodular sclerosis HD (NSHD) occurs in about 80% of cases and is the common histology of young females. Some pathologists subclassify the cellular components surrounded by areas of fibrosis. A fixation artifact unique to NS results in retraction of tissue around the Reed-Sternberg cell, resulting in a "lacunar cell."
3. Mixed cellular HD (MCHD) occurs in 10% to 15% of series and is usually associated with a poorer prognosis and more advanced stage. It is the more common histology of patients over age 40.
4. Lymphocyte-depleted HD (LDHD) is a rare variant and is usually associated with advanced stage and an aggressive natural history. Some cases can be confused with large cell lymphoma.

The most important aspect of evaluating the patient suspected of having HD is the hematopathologic review. Other disorders have been confused with HD and should be differentiated by appropriate immunoperoxidase techniques designed to show the absence of LCA (CD45), and the presence of Leu-M-1 (CD15) and Ki (CD30). The latter has been seen in some cases of anaplastic (non-Hodgkin's) lymphoma, usually of T-cell phenotype. Patients with epithelioid (Lennert's) lymphoma, angioimmunoblastic lymphadenopathy, Castleman's angiofollicular lymphoid hyperplasia, and diffuse mixed (non-Hodgkin's) lymphomas have been confused with MCHD.

STAGING AND CLINICAL PRESENTATION

The majority of patients present with clinical manifestations above the diaphragm, such as supraclavicular or cervical adenopathy with radiographic evidence of an asymptomatic anterior mediastinal mass of varying size. Superior vena cava obstruction is rare despite the size of the mass. The majority, more than 50% to 60%, will not have the constitutional symptoms (B symptoms) characteristic of HD: fever, night sweats, and weight loss >10%. Rarely patients give a history of pruritus and alcohol-induced pain in nodal sites.

The assessment of dissemination to abdominal nodal (Stage III) and extranodal (Stage IV) sites requires an abdominal-pelvic computed tomographic (CT) scan and bone marrow biopsy. Dissemination to extranodal sites is more likely to occur with unfavorable histology (MCHD, LDHD). As opposed to non-Hodgkin's lymphoma, HD rarely involves the lymphoid tissue of Waldeyer's ring; epitrochlear, popliteal, and mesenteric nodes; or intestinal lymphoid tissue. Testicular, peripheral blood and central nervous system involvement is highly unusual.

Staging laparotomy is used to identify cryptic abdominal involvement, such as celiac, portahepatic, para-aortic, and splenic hilar nodes and the liver and spleen. This diagnostic procedure does not influence survival but rather the choice of therapy. It is still employed when radiation therapy is under consideration as the sole therapeutic modality. Abdominal involvement of any type, except perhaps minimal splenic involvement (one to four small nodules), usually suggests the need for systemic therapy. Patients who present with a mediastinal mass larger than one third of the diameter of the thorax or with four or more involved sites above the diaphragm will also require systemic therapy and should be spared a laparotomy. Conversely, young (<26 years) females who are asymptomatic with NSHD involving only one site above the diaphragm (Stage IA) do not require surgery because the yield is so low (<5%). Overall, 25% to 30% of patients with disease clinically confined above the diaphragm will have microscopic evidence of HD in the abdomen. The operation should be performed only if it will influence therapy.

Prognostic factors for detecting abdominal involvement (percentage with vs. percentage without) include male gender (29% > 18%), B symptoms (34% > 21%), and two or more sites (27% > 17%). About 40% of clinically suspected Stage III or IV patients will be downstaged. The hematologic and biochemical abnormalities associated with HD are rare and usually associated with more advanced stages. Anemia is usually microcytic and hypochromic with low serum iron and iron-binding capacity. Autoimmune disorders, such as autoimmune hemolytic anemia, thrombocytopenia, and nephrotic syndrome, are rare.

Leukocytosis, lymphopenia, eosinophilia, and an elevated sedimentation rate can occur in patients with more advanced stages. Undoubtedly many manifestations of HD are mediated by cytokines elaborated by the neoplastic cells.

A more recently introduced imaging technique is gallium scanning. The majority of HD patients will show positive avidity for the radionuclide, especially in sites above the diaphragm. It is not a substitute for CT scans or lymphangiography. The latter has a diminished role in staging, as it has been replaced by CT scans; the number of experienced radiographers is thus decreasing. The value of the gallium scan is in the interpretation of residual masses after therapy. A reversion to gallium negative has been defined as a positive sign for residual necrosis or fibrosis and would be negative on gallium scanning.

The Ann Arbor staging terminology was modified by the Cotswold Staging classification:

Stage I: single lymph node area involvement

Stage II: two or more lymph node sites on the same side of the diaphragm

Stage III: lymph node sites on both sides of the diaphragm

Stage III$_1$: splenic, celiac, portahepatic involvement

Stage III$_2$: para-aortic, iliac, mesenteric involvement

Stage IV: any of the above with involvement of an extranodal site

X: a mass >10 cm or a mediastinal mass larger than one third the thoracic diameter

E: involvement of a single extranodal site contiguous to a known nodal site

CS: clinical stage

PS: pathologic (postlaparotomy) stage

THERAPY FOR LOCALIZED DISEASE

The management of localized HD has changed considerably in the last 20 years. The addition of systemic therapy is known to decrease relapse, and that in turn obviates a staging laparotomy. Furthermore, there is a rising concern that the late appearance of solid tumors is related to radiation therapy directed at normal tissues. These include carcinomas and sarcomas and occur in 15% to 20% of patients at risk for 20 years of follow-up. Thus, the combined use of radiation therapy and chemotherapy may permit lower doses and smaller fields of radiation. This is under current investigation.

In general, patients in pathologic (postlaparotomy) Stage I/IIA treated with mantle, para-aortic fields to 35 to 45 cGy will have an 80% relapse-free survival with a higher overall survival because of the salvage value of systemic chemotherapy. Table 41–1 presents a scheme of options according to clinical presentation: radiation therapy only, combined modality therapy, and combination chemotherapy only.

SYSTEMIC THERAPY FOR ADVANCED DISEASE

The introduction of combination chemotherapy, especially the nitrogen mustard, Oncovin, procarbazine, and pred-

TABLE 41–1. THERAPEUTIC OPTIONS FOR LOCALIZED HODGKIN'S DISEASE

RADIATION THERAPY ONLY

1. Very favorable presentation (no laparotomy); asymptomatic young female, single site, favorable histology (LPHD, NSHD); asymptomatic young male with LPHD in a single site, no bulky disease
2. Pathologic I/IIA or B with limited disease above the diaphragm (after laparotomy)

COMBINED MODALITY THERAPY

1. Any but the favorable clinical presentations (above)
2. Mediastinal mass larger than one third the thoracic diameter, regardless of stage or histology
3. Advanced stage (III) with masses >10 cm (>7 cm in some series)

COMBINATION CHEMOTHERAPY ALONE

1. Theoretically any stage, except the favorable groups in which radiation therapy alone can be used
2. Stage IV with bone marrow, bone, hepatic, or extensive pulmonary disease

TABLE 41–2. COMMONLY USED REGIMENS IN TREATMENT FOR HODGKIN'S DISEASE

ALKYLATING AGENT REGIMENS	
MOPP	
Mustargen	6 mg/m² days 1, 8
Oncovin	1.4 mg/m² days 1, 8
Procarbazine	100 mg/m² days 1–14
Prednisone	40 mg/m² days 1–14
MVPP	
Mustargen	6 mg/m² days 1, 8
Vinblastine	10 mg/m² days 1, 8, 14
Procarbazine	100 mg/m² days 1–14
Prednisolone	40 mg days 1–14 q 42 d
ChlVPP	
Chlorambucil	6 mg/m² (not to exceed 10 mg) days 1–14
Vinblastine	6 mg/m² (not to exceed 10 mg) days 1, 8
Procarbazine	100 mg/m² days 1–14
Prednisolone	40 mg days 1–14 q 28 d
NONALKYLATING AGENT REGIMENS	
ABVD	
Doxorubicin†	25 mg/m² days 1, 15
Bleomycin	10 mg/m² days 1, 15
Vinblastine	6 mg/m² days 1, 15
Dacarbazine	375 mg/m² days 1, 15
EVA	
Etoposide	100 mg/m² days 1–3
Vinblastine	6 mg/m² day 1 q 28 d
Doxorubicin†	50 mg/m² day 1
MOPP/ABV ("hybrid")	
Nitrogen mustard	6 mg/m² day 1
Vincristine	1.4 mg/m² (max 2.0 mg) day 1
Procarbazine	100 mg/m² days 1–7
Prednisone	40 mg/m² days 1–14
Doxorubicin	35 mg/m² day 8
Bleomycin	10 mg/m² day 8
Vinblastine	6 mg/m² day 8

*Cycles 1,4 out of 6 q 28 d.

†Adriamycin.

nisone (MOPP) was a pivotal event in the management of HD presenting in a disseminated stage or as relapse from primary radiation therapy. This regimen and its analogs are still used, but a series of randomized trials have shown that MOPP alternating with doxorubicin (Adriamycin), bleomycin, vinblastine, and DTIC (ABVD) or a hybrid of MOPP-ABV was superior to MOPP in progression-free survival (Table 41-2). A number of randomized trials have shown no difference between the "hybrid" and MOPP alternating with ABVD. The choice of primary combination chemotherapy should be based on efficacy and toxicity. When ABVD (with or without radiation therapy) is compared with MOPP alone, there is a superiority in progression-free survival for the nonalkylating agent–containing regimen, ABVD. The absence of male and female sterilization and secondary myelodysplasia and acute myeloblastic leukemia, both known to occur with MOPP, has led to a wider use of ABVD with radiation therapy, especially in earlier-stage disease. It is unknown (and under investigation) whether the hybrid is superior to ABVD alone. Another factor that complicates the use of MOPP is the particularly toxic effect of this regimen on bone marrow stem cells, which limits the doses of drugs that can be given in subsequent cycles. At the present time, ABVD and the hybrid are the most commonly used regimens in North America. A number of variants for MOPP and ABVD attempt to reduce some of the acute toxicities. The British developed a regimen of chlorambucil, vinblastine, procarbazine, and prednisone (ChlVPP), which reduced the hair loss, neuropathy, and nausea and vomiting associated with MOPP with equal efficacy. Modifications of the ABVD regimen tend to omit the bleomycin to reduce pulmonary toxicity but have not been widely tested.

The expected benefits of chemotherapy are based on clinical prognostic factors. They include age, stage, number of extranodal sites, B symptoms in Stage IV, and performance status. Age is the most significant factor in most series. About 50% to 60% of patients in Stage III/IV will be cured of HD after receiving first-line therapy. For some other subgroups, such as those older than age 50 or those with Stage IV disease involving more than one extranodal site, the outcome is poorer (about 30%). Other series have used elevated serum alkaline phosphatase with elevated sedimentation rate to predict a poor outcome in Stage III/IV.

THERAPY FOLLOWING RELAPSE FROM COMBINATION CHEMOTHERAPY

Patients whose disease is refractory to first-line combination chemotherapy or who experience relapse from a complete remission within 12 months are in a particularly poor prognostic group. Second-line chemotherapy will result in a long-term salvage of only 10% to 20%. Patients who have late relapses (>12 months) with node-only sites and no symptoms have a very high salvage rate with second-line therapy, ranging from 50% to 75%. It is uncertain whether a "non–cross-resistant" regimen is required for those who have late relapses, since a repeat of the original regimen can achieve durable second-time remissions.

Patients who experience relapse early or whose disease is refractory to standard-dose therapy may be considered candidates for high-dose therapy with autologous stem cell in bone marrow support. This is a difficult modality to evaluate because of the lack of a true plateau in the survival curve. Regardless, poor-prognosis patients who demonstrate a chemotherapy-sensitive relapse are candidates for this form of dose intensification with a relatively small statistical chance of remaining free of disease at 3 years (~25%).

There are rare patients who have relapses late in a single nodal site without symptoms, and they may be salvaged with radiation therapy only. The vast majority, however, require systemic therapy. A number of third-line regimens have been used, consisting of etoposide, a nitrosourea, and methotrexate, if the patient has failed two more regimens. These are palliative treatments for patients with far-advanced disease.

BIBLIOGRAPHY

Canellos GP, Anderson JR, Propert KJ et al. Chemotherapy of advanced Hodgkin's disease with MOPP, ABVD, or MOPP alternating with ABVD. N Engl J Med 1992;327:1478–1484

DeVita VT Jr, Hubbard SM. Hodgkin's disease. N Engl J Med 1993;328:560–565

Longo DL, Young RC, Wesley M et al. Twenty years of MOPP therapy for Hodgkin's disease. J Clin Oncol 1986;4:1295–1306

Mauch P, Larson D, Osteen R et al. Prognostic factors for positive surgical staging in patients with Hodgkin's disease. J Clin Oncol 1990;8:257–265

Pinkus GS, Said JW. Hodgkin's disease, lymphocyte predominance type, nodular—further evidence for a B-cell derivation: L&H variants of Reed-Sternberg cells express L26, a pan B cell marker. Am J Pathol 1989;133:211–217

Selby P, Patel P, Milan S et al. ChlVPP combination chemotherapy for Hodgkin's disease: long-term results. Br J Cancer 1990;62:279–285

Urba WJ, Longo DL. Hodgkin's disease. N Engl J Med 1992;326:678–687

Viviani S, Santoro A, Negretti E et al. Results in patients relapsing more than twelve months after first complete remission. Ann Oncol 1990;1:123–127

John S. Macdonald, Daniel G. Haller, Robert J. Mayer, Eds. *Manual of Oncologic Therapeutics*, Third Edition.

42. NON-HODGKIN'S LYMPHOMA

Richard I. Fisher

Non-Hodgkin's lymphomas are malignancies of the lymphoid system. The number of cases is increasing dramatically. The most recent statistics from the American Cancer Society report that there were 43,000 new cases of non-Hodgkin's lymphomas in 1993. The increases are seen not only among immunosuppressed patients, such as those with acquired immunodeficiency syndrome (AIDS), but also in patients who are traditionally considered immunocompetent. The incidence of non-Hodgkin's lymphomas increases with age from childhood through age 80. Most non-Hodgkin's lymphomas are tumors of B cells or T cells.

The non-Hodgkin's lymphomas are not a single disease entity but rather a group of malignancies that arise from each stage of differentiation of B or T cells. Thus the normal cellular counterpart of each type of non-Hodgkin's lymphoma can be identified in the normal lymphatic system. It also follows that the non-Hodgkin's lymphomas can arise from any lymphatic organ. Although lymph nodes are usually involved, extranodal sites are much more commonly involved than in Hodgkin's disease. Finally, in contrast to Hodgkin's disease, which spreads in an orderly fashion from one lymphoid region to the next contiguous region, the non-Hodgkin's lymphomas have earlier blood-borne dissemination and may skip adjacent lymphatic regions.

Accurate identification of the various subtypes of the non-Hodgkin's lymphomas is necessary in order to predict the biologic behavior of a given tumor and to select appropriate therapy. Pathologic categorization is difficult, and a highly experienced hematopathologist is needed to establish an accurate diagnosis. Multiple pathologic classifications have been proposed. All provide relatively equivalent prognostic information. The Rappaport classification is the oldest and most commonly used in the United States. In 1982, an international study proposed a Working Formulation for Non-Hodgkin's Lymphomas that enables clinicians and pathologists to translate from one pathologic classification to another. Thus, investigators can report their results by using any pathologic system that they desire, but they must also include the Working Formulation. It is easy to translate from one system to the other as shown in Table 42–1.

The biologic behavior of the majority of the non-Hodgkin's lymphomas can be grouped into two categories: indolent and aggressive. The indolent, or favorable, lymphomas are not generally curable by current treatment methods. They do have a relatively long natural history. These patients frequently live with slow-growing disease for many years. The indolent lymphomas include diffuse well-differentiated lymphocytic, nodular poorly differentiated lymphocytic, and nodular mixed lymphoma. In contrast, the aggressive, or unfavorable, lymphomas are rapidly progressive and fatal in a short period of time if they are not successfully treated. However, recent improvements in therapy have resulted in long-term disease-free survival (*i.e.*, cure) for approximately 50% of these patients. The aggressive non-Hodgkin's lymphomas include nodular histiocytic, diffuse poorly differentiated lymphocytic, diffuse mixed, diffuse histiocytic, and diffuse undifferentiated lymphoma.

Lymphoblastic lymphoma is a unique subset of the non-Hodgkin's lymphomas that tends to behave like T-cell acute lymphocytic leukemia with early systemic dissemination and frequent metastases to the central nervous system. Treatment programs have therefore evolved to become highly similar to those used for poor-prognosis acute lymphocytic leukemia.

PRETREATMENT EVALUATION

The pretreatment evaluation is designed to establish the stage of the disease and to define sites of tumor involvement, so that the response to therapy can be assessed during and after treatment.

The complete pretreatment evaluation includes the following:

A. Detailed history and physical examination with careful measurements of all palpable lymph nodes, liver, spleen, Waldeyer's ring, subcutaneous nodules, thyroid, testes, *etc.*
B. Complete blood counts and chemistries
C. Chest radiography
D. Computed tomographic (CT) scans of chest and abdomen
E. Bilateral iliac crest bone marrow biopsies
F. Other staging studies based on patient complaints and institutional capabilities
   1. Bone scans
   2. Gallium scans
   3. Lymphangiograms
   4. Magnetic resonance imaging (MRI)
   5. Peritoneoscopy with liver biopsies
G. Staging laparotomy (rarely, if ever)

Usually the above tests will accurately define the patient's stage. However, other tests may occasionally be indicated. They include the following:

TABLE 42–1. TRANSLATION OF PATHOLOGIC CLASSIFICATIONS FOR NON-HODGKIN'S LYMPHOMA USING THE WORKING FORMULATION

WORKING FORMULATION	RAPPAPORT CLASSIFICATION
Low Grade	
A. Malignant lymphoma, small lymphocytic, consistent with chronic lymphocytic leukemia	Diffuse well-differentiated lymphocytic (DWDL)
B. Malignant lymphoma, follicular, predominantly small cleaved cell	Nodular poorly differentiated lymphocytic (NPDL)
C. Malignant lymphoma, follicular mixed, small cleaved and large cell	Nodular mixed lymphocytic-histiocytic (NM)
Intermediate Grade	
D. Malignant lymphoma, follicular, predominantly large cell	Nodular histiocytic (NH)
E. Malignant lymphoma, diffuse, small cleaved cell	Diffuse poorly differentiated lymphocytic (DPDL)
F. Malignant lymphoma, diffuse mixed, small and large cell	Diffuse mixed lymphocytic-histiocytic (DM)
G. Malignant lymphoma, diffuse large cell	Diffuse histiocytic (DH)
High Grade	
H. Malignant lymphoma, large cell, immunoblastic	Diffuse histiocytic (DH)
I. Malignant lymphoma, lymphoblastic	Diffuse lymphoblastic (LL)
J. Malignant lymphoma, small non-cleaved cell	Diffuse undifferentiated (DU)

A. Gastrointestinal x-ray series for patients with gastrointestinal complaints, guaiac-positive stools, and Waldeyer' s ring involvement
B. Lumbar puncture with cytology for patients with neurologic abnormalities, lymphoblastic lymphoma, or diffuse aggressive lymphomas with bone marrow involvement
C. Test of cardiac ejection scans and pulmonary function prior to therapy with Adriamycin and Bleomycin, respectively
D. Immunologic phenotyping of lymph node or bone marrow biopsies may separate reactive from monoclonal malignant infiltrates; similar studies can define involvement of peripheral blood; identification of tumors as being either T cell or B cell usually does not affect therapy

STAGING SYSTEM

The staging system used for the non-Hodgkin's lymphomas is the same as that originally proposed for Hodgkin's disease at the Ann Arbor conference in 1971 (Table 42–2).

In addition, patients are classified by the presence or absence of constitutional symptoms as follows:

A. Asymptomatic
B. Fever, night sweats, weight loss >10% of body weight

Extralymphatic sites of involvement are much more common in non-Hodgkin's lymphoma than in Hodgkin's disease. The indolent lymphomas present with Stage III or IV disease involving lymph nodes, bone marrow, or liver in 84% of cases. The aggressive lymphomas present as 10% Stage I,

TABLE 42–2. STAGING SYSTEM FOR NON-HODGKIN'S LYMPHOMA

Stage I	Involvement of a single lymph node region (I) or of a single extralymphatic organ or site (I_E)*
Stage II	Involvement of two or more lymph node regions on the same side of the diaphragm (II) or localized involvement of an extralymphatic organ or site and of one or more lymph node regions on the same side of the diaphragm (II_E)
Stage III	Involvement of lymph node regions on both sides of the diaphragm (III), which may also be accompanied by involvement of the spleen (III_S) or by localized involvement of an extralymphatic organ or site (III_E), or both (III_{SE})
Stage IV	Diffuse or disseminated involvement of one or more extralymphatic organs or tissues, with or without associated lymph node involvement

*The subscript E (e.g., I_E or II_E)is used to denote involvement of an extralymphatic site primarily or by direct extension, rather than hematogenous spread, as in the case of a mediastinal mass extending to involve the lung.

20% Stage II, and 70% Stage III or IV. Extranodal sites of involvement may include bone marrow, liver, gastrointestinal tract, spleen, bone, and less commonly, lung, thyroid, testes, and central nervous system.

TREATMENT

Stage I and II Indolent Lymphomas

Because fewer than 10% of all patients with indolent lymphomas present with Stage I or II disease, there are no large prospective series that define optimal therapy. However, several series suggest that a significant number of these patients have prolonged disease-free survival and may be cured following radiation therapy. Because these series were retrospectively reviewed, the fraction of all Stage I or II patients who were treated in this manner is unknown. Therefore, in the absence of prospective data, localized radiation therapy remains the standard treatment.

Stage III or IV Indolent Lymphoma

There are many acceptable ways to treat patients with advanced-stage indolent lymphoma. Many forms of therapy result in 60% to 75% complete remissions; however, these remissions are not durable, and none of the currently available treatments is curative. The median disease-free interval following completion of therapy is only 17 months. Patients who experience relapse can frequently be retreated with good results, but the complete remission rate and disease-free interval decrease with each retreatment. Thus, these patients frequently live with recurrent disease for a large part of their clinical course. Survival is good at 5 years (over 80%) but falls by 10 years (30% to 50%).

Alkylating agents have been used to treat these patients for many years. Chlorambucil at a daily oral dose of 0.1 to 0.2 mg/kg/day and cyclophosphamide at a daily oral dose of 1.5 to 2.5 mg/kg/day are commonly used. The dose of each is titrated to maintain a white blood cell count above 3000 and platelet count above 100,000. Responses occur slowly, and it may take several years to achieve complete remission. Acute toxicity is minimal, although long-term daily use of aklylating agents has been associated with an increased incidence of acute myelogenous leukemia in several other diseases.

Combination chemotherapy with three or four drugs is also used frequently. The CVP regimen consists of

Cyclophosphamide 400 mg/m^2 po qd × 5

Vincristine 1.4 mg/m^2 iv on day 1

Prednisone 100 mg/m^2 po qd × 5

Treatment is repeated every 21 days and continues for a minimum of six cycles or two cycles following achievement of a complete clinical response.

The C-MOPP regimen consists of

Cyclophosphamide 650 mg/m^2 iv on days 1 and 8

Vincristine 1.4 mg/m^2 iv on days 1 and 8

Procarbazine 100 mg/m^2 po days 1 to 14

Prednisone 60 mg/m^2 po days 1 to 14.

The cycle is repeated every 28 days. Although there are no universally accepted guidelines for selecting aklylating agents or combination chemotherapy, one must recall that antitumor responses are achieved much more slowly with the alkylating agents. Therefore, we prefer to use combination chemotherapy for any patient with high tumor burden, rapid tumor growth, or extensive marrow involvement. Conversely, alkylating agents may be utilized for patients with minimal tumor burdens who wish to avoid toxicity.

Total-body irradiation has also been used to treat these patients. Total doses of 150 to 300 rad given at a rate of 10 rad/day have been administered. Thrombocytopenia may result in some delays during treatment. Total nodal irradiation has been utilized, especially in Stage III patients.

The previously described therapies have all been shown to yield comparable results. Because these treatments are not curative and may not affect the natural history of the indolent lymphomas, Rosenberg, at Stanford University, has advocated no initial therapy for these patients. He demonstrated that asymptomatic patients may not need systemic treatment for several years after diagnosis. Large lymph nodes in one or two areas could be successfully palliated with local irradiation. Careful follow-up of these patients every 2 or 3 months is essential to this approach. Systemic therapy must be initiated before patients develop compression of visceral organs or bone marrow that is completely replaced by lymphoma.

Patients with nodular mixed lymphoma may represent a unique subset of the indolent lymphoma patients. Rosenberg showed that they require systemic therapy sooner than other indolent lymphoma patients. The National Cancer Institute reported a long disease-free survival in the majority of these patients who were initially treated with the previously described combination chemotherapy regimens. Long follow-up still has not clarified whether a percentage of these patients may be cured.

New approaches to the initial treatment of the other indolent lymphomas are desperately needed. The initial use of aggressive chemotherapy and biologic response modifiers is being evaluated. A few patients with low-volume indolent disease have undergone autologous bone marrow transplantation. Initial response rates are high, but follow-up is still much too short to know if any patients are cured. Some, but not all, studies of initial chemotherapy followed by maintenance therapy with interferon for 1 to 2 years suggested a prolongation of disease-free survival. Early analysis suggests that the benefit may be restricted to indolent lymphoma patients who have a high tumor burden and a more aggressive course.

As noted previously, most of the indolent lymphoma patients experience relapse after initial treatment. They can often be retreated with the same therapy, although the number and duration of responses will decrease, compared with the initial treatment results. Combination chemotherapy is the usual treatment modality selected for patients experiencing relapse. Several centers have begun to utilize autologous bone marrow transplantation in young patients with relapsed indolent lymphoma. Once again, responses are high but follow-up remains too short to determine whether any patients are cured.

Ultimately most indolent lymphoma patients become refractory to treatment. Approximately one third of cases will evolve into diffuse aggressive lymphoma. Therefore, rapidly growing tumor masses should be biopsied. Aggressive treatment of these patients with one of the new treatment programs for diffuse lymphomas (see below) may result in a complete remission.

Stage I or II Aggressive Lymphomas

Because patients with Stage I or II aggressive lymphoma frequently have microscopic dissemination of their disease to distant sites, combination chemotherapy is the standard treatment. Patients can be clinically staged, as previously outlined, and avoid a laparotomy. Miller and Jones have reported that 75% of these patients remained disease-free at 3 years. Most patients received eight cycles of CHOP chemotherapy on the following schedule:

Cyclophosphamide 750 mg/m^2 iv on day 1

Adriamycin 50 mg/m^2 iv on day 1

Vincristine 1.4 mg/m^2 iv on day 1

Prednisone 100 mg po qd $\times$ 5

Cycles were repeated every 21 days. Half of their patients also received involved-field radiation therapy after completing chemotherapy. The role of radiation therapy after chemotherapy remains indefinite. Toxicity was mild and manageable. Nausea, vomiting, hair loss, and moderate leukopenia without infectious complications were seen. Several other groups have obtained similar results with either chemotherapy alone or a three-cycle course of chemotherapy plus involved-field radiation therapy.

Stage III or IV Aggressive Lymphomas

Combination chemotherapy is the treatment of choice for all patients with Stage III or IV diffuse aggressive lymphomas. Several four- or five-drug combinations that were developed between 1965 and 1975 are capable of curing a subset of these patients. These regimens include CHOP; C-MOPP; bleomycin, Adriamycin, cyclophosphamide, vincristine, and prednisone (BACOP); and cyclophosphamide, vincristine, methotrexate with leucovorin rescue, and ara-C (COMLA).

Regardless of the chemotherapy regimen utilized, these patients represent complex problems. In addition to the complete blood count and chemistry tests required before each drug administration, a detailed history, physical examination, and tumor measurements are required at monthly intervals. Toxicity varies with each regimen, but the dose-limiting toxicity that is common to all regimens is almost always myelosuppression. Patients with fewer than 1000 granulocytes and fever must be hospitalized immediately, cultured, and empirically treated with broad-spectrum antibiotics. Platelet transfusion is performed if the platelet count falls to less than 20,000. Other common toxicities include nausea and vomiting, which can be lessened with antiemetics; reversible hair loss; and neurotoxicity.

These regimens produce complete remissions in 40% to 60% of all patients. Because partial remissions do not improve overall survival, it is essential to document "true" complete remission by a thorough re-evaluation of all previously involved sites of disease. This re-evaluation includes a careful physical examination, repetition of previously abnormal x-ray films or CT scans, biopsies of any residual abnormalities, and repeat biopsies of bone marrow or liver if they were the sites of initial tumor involvement. For most of these regimens, 50% to 80% of the complete responders will remain disease-free.

Most relapses occur in the first 2 years following treatment, but later relapses are not uncommon. Therefore, patients who achieve a complete remission should be examined monthly for 1 year, every other month in the second year, every third month in the third year, and then every 6 months. X-ray films and CT scans of previously involved tumor sites should be repeated every 6 months during the first 2 years. Overall, 30% to 40% of patients are therefore cured. This prolonged disease-free survival of the complete responders, and resultant cure, is in marked contrast to the behavior of the indolent lymphomas managed with these same regimens.

Retrospective analysis reveals that certain clinical factors are associated with a poor prognosis. An International Non-Hodgkin's Lymphoma Prognostic Factors Project presented a predictive model for survival of patients with aggressive lymphomas. Five factors were independently associated with poor survival. They included age over 60 years, Stage III or IV disease, two or more extranodal sites, poor performance status, and an abnormal serum lactate dehydrogenase level. Patients were grouped into low, low-intermediate, high-intermediate, and high-risk categories, on the basis of their presenting number of poor-risk factors. Patients with no or one risk factor were found to be low-risk, patients with two risk factors were low-intermediate risk, patients with three risk factors were high-intermediate risk, and patients with four or five risk factors were high-risk. Differences in the distribution of these prognostic factors from one study to another can cause major differences in therapeutic outcome.

More intensive regimens using six or seven drugs have been developed in the late 1970s and early 1980s in an attempt to increase the complete remission rate and subsequent cure rate. These regimens include prednisone, methotrexate, Adriamycin, cyclophosphamide, and etoposide, alternating with nitrogen mustard, vincristine, procarbazine, and prednisone (ProMACE-MOPP); prednisone, doxorubicin, cyclophosphamide, and etoposide followed by cytarabine, bleomycin, vincristine, and methotrexate with leucovorin rescue ProMACE-CytaBOM); methotrexate with leucovorin rescue, bleomycin, Adriamycin, cyclophosphamide, vincristine, and decadron (m-BACOD); and methotrexate with leucovorin rescue, doxorubicin, cyclophosphamide, vincristine, prednisone, and bleomycin (MACOP-B). In general these programs produce 70% to 75% complete remissions and 50% long-term survival. However, toxicity — especially bone marrow suppression and mucositis — are much more severe than in earlier regimens. The cost of these regimens is also significantly greater.

The Southwest Oncology Group and the Eastern Cooperative Oncology Group recently conducted a prospective, randomized Phase III comparison of CHOP vs. m-BACOD vs. ProMACE-CytaBOM vs. MACOP-B. Their goal was to make a valid comparison between the results obtained by treating patients with advanced stages of intermediate- or high-grade non-Hodgkin's lymphoma with first- and third-generation chemotherapy regimens. There were 1138 patients registered on the study. Known prognostic factors were equally distributed. There were no significant differences in either the partial or complete response rates between treatment arms.

At 3 years, 44% of all patients were estimated to be alive without disease (41% for CHOP and MACOP-B, and 46% for m-BACOD and ProMACE-CytaBOM; $p = .35$). Overall survival of all patients at 3 years was 52% (50% for both ProMACE-CytaBOM and MACOP-B, 52% for m-BACOD, 54% for CHOP; $p = .90$). No subset of patients was found to have significantly improved survival with the third-generation regimens. The received dose-intensity data were comparable to the data previously published for these regimens. Fatal toxicity was 1% for CHOP, 3% for ProMACE-CytaBOM, 5% for m-BACOD, and 6% for MACOP-B.

Based on similar failure-free and overall survivals with lower cost and lower incidence of severe toxicity, CHOP remains the best currently available treatment for patients with advanced-stage, intermediate- or high-grade non-Hodgkin's lymphoma.

Relapsed Aggressive Lymphomas

Based on the results of the intergroup study discussed earlier, approximately 55% to 65% of patients with advanced-stage intermediate- or high-grade non-Hodgkin's lymphoma either will be refractory to or will experience relapse after initial chemotherapy. These refractory or relapsed patients should be considered for bone marrow transplantation (usually autologous: ABMT), which offers an overall prolonged disease-free survival of 20% to 25%.

Although there is considerable variability in selection criteria among studies employing ABMT as salvage therapy, there have been several consistent findings across studies. Patients who are likely to achieve a complete response and possible cure are those who had a good response to initial therapy and who entered ABMT with no or minimal residual disease, having responded to salvage chemotherapy. Such patients are said to have a "sensitive" relapse. Patients with disease progression on salvage therapy before ABMT are unlikely to benefit; the same is true for patients who did not respond to initial therapy. A variety of preparative regimens have been used and shown to be effective. A commonly used regimen includes high-dose cytoxan and total-body irradiation.

Many patients will not be candidates for bone marrow transplantation because of age, bone marrow involvement, poor performance status, or poor medical condition. These patients are usually treated with conventional-dose salvage chemotherapy. Many of the reported salvage chemotherapy studies involve small numbers of patients, are retrospective, and are restricted to single institutions. In addition, it is extremely difficult to compare studies because of marked variation in the proportion of patients with poor risk factors, *e.g.*, disease resistant to initial therapy, older age, bulky disease at relapse, high lactate dehydrogenase level. To date, no randomized prospective studies have compared different salvage regimens in aggressive non-Hodgkin's lymphoma.

Despite these limitations, based on presently available data, one can draw tentative conclusions. The regimen of dexamethasone, high-dose ara-C, and cisplatin (DHAP) has been reported as salvage therapy in aggressive non-Hodgkin's lymphoma in almost 300 patients and has consistently produced response rates greater than 50% and complete response rates between 15% and 30%. DHAP is commonly used before ABMT to "debulk" the lymphoma, and the response to this regimen is frequently used to identify patients with sensitive vs. resistant relapse. This has important prognostic implications, as noted above. Whether or not anyone with resistant or relapsed NHL can be cured with conventional salvage combination chemotherapy is not clear. However, conventional salvage chemotherapy can produce prolonged disease-free survival, albeit in a minority of patients.

Phase II studies of new drugs or biologics are certainly indicated at this stage of the disease.

REFERENCES

Anderson T, Bender RA, Fisher RI et al. Combination chemotherapy in non-Hodgkin's lymphoma: Results of long term followup. Cancer Treat Res 61:1057–1066, 1977

Armitage JO. Bone marrow transplantation in the treatment of patients with lymphoma. Blood 73:1749–1758, 1989

Carbone PP, Kaplan HS, Musshoff K et al. Report of the Committee on Hodgkin's Disease Staging Classification. Cancer Res 31:1860–1861, 1971

Fisher RI, Gaynor ER, Dahlberg S et al. Comparison of a standard regimen (CHOP) with three intensive chemotherapy regimens for advanced non-Hodgkin's lymphoma. N Engl J Med 328:1002–1006, 1993

Jones SE, Miller TP, Connors JM. Long term follow-up and analysis for prognostic factors for patients with limited-stage diffuse large-cell lymphoma treated with initial chemotherapy with or without adjuvant radiotherapy. J Clin Oncol 7:1186–1191, 1989

The International Non-Hodgkin's Lymphoma Prognostic Factors Project. A predictive model for aggressive non-Hodgkin's lymphoma. N Engl J Med 329:987–994, 1993

Miller TP, Jones SE. Initial chemotherapy for clinically localized lymphomas of unfavorable histology. Blood 62: 413–418, 1983

The Non-Hodgkin's Lymphoma Pathologic Classification Project. National Cancer Institute sponsored study of classifications of non-Hodgkin's lymphomas. Summary and description of a working formulation for clinical usage. Cancer 49:2112–2135, 1982

Velasquez WS, Cabanillas F, Salvador P et al. Effective salvage therapy for lymphoma with cisplatin in combination with high-dose ara-C and dexamethasone (DHAP). Blood 71:117–122, 1988

John S. Macdonald, Daniel G. Haller, Robert J. Mayer, Eds. *Manual of Oncologic Therapeutics*, Third Edition.

43. PLASMA CELL DYSCRASIAS

Michael V. Seiden
Kenneth C. Anderson

Plasma cell dyscrasias are a heterogenous collection of clinical disorders characterized by increased numbers of plasma cells in the bone marrow or tissue. The natural history of these disorders is remarkably diverse. For example, patients with monoclonal gammopathies of unknown significance are often asymptomatic for life, whereas patients with plasma cell leukemias usually survive for only weeks or months.

EVALUATION OF THE PATIENT WITH ELEVATED GLOBULINS

With the availability of automated serum analyzers, it has become common to identify persons with elevated gamma globulin levels. In some cases, the rise of gamma globulins may result from recognized medical problems, whereas in others the finding is serendipitous and unexplained. Elevations in gamma globulins can be either polyclonal or monoclonal.

Polyclonal gammopathies are the result of the expansion of several different B-cell clones, each producing a different immunoglobulin. Polyclonal gammopathies are usually seen in chronic inflammatory conditions, such as chronic infections (tuberculosis, chronic hepatitis, osteomyelitis, bacterial endocarditis), or autoimmune disorders, such as inflammatory arthritides, vasculitides, or other rheumatologic disorders. Serum electrophoresis demonstrates a diffuse increase of gamma globulins (immunoglobulins) without evidence of a clonotypic or monoclonal paraprotein. Treatment in these cases is directed toward the primary disease.

Monoclonal gammopathies represent the expansion of a single B-cell clone. Each neoplastic cell secretes the identical immunoglobulin. Once a clone expands to a level of 10^8 to 10^9 cells, the clonotypic immunoglobulin product can be detected by serum immunoelectrophoresis. Except in cases of very advanced age or life-threatening comorbid disease, an attempt should be made to characterize further all monoclonal gammopathies. Over half the cases of monoclonal gammopathy represent an indolent, usually asymptomatic, disorder known as monoclonal gammopathy of unknown significance (MGUS). Approximately one third of the persons with monoclonal gammopathy have myeloma on initial evaluation, with most of the remaining patients having a lymphoid malignancy. Finally, there is a large collection of inflammatory disorders, infectious diseases, and dermatologic and idiopathic disorders that are occasionally associated with a monoclonal gammopathy. In some of these disorders the antibody can be demonstrated to bind an antigen associated with the underlying disease (*e.g.*, p24 in persons with acquired immunodeficiency syndrome [AIDS]).

In most cases, the monoclonal gammopathy causes no relevant clinical sequelae. In rare cases, the antibody has specificity for a biologically important molecule (*e.g.*, von Willebrand's factor, Factor VIII, myelin), and in these cases, plasmapheresis and/or chemotherapy may be required. Table 43–1 reviews the disorders associated with monoclonal gammopathies.

Patients presenting with monoclonal gammopathies should have a complete history and physical examination. In particular, patients should be questioned about a history of fevers, night sweats, bone pain, weight loss, fatigue, and malaise. Physical examination should confirm or exclude purpura, adenopathy, areas of bone tenderness, splenomegaly, hepatomegaly, and masses on the cranium. For all patients, laboratory tests should include a complete blood count (CBC). Most patients should have a bone marrow biopsy and aspirate as part of their initial evaluation. Asymptomatic patients with normal physical findings, normal CBC, a modest elevation in monoclonal protein (immunoglobulin G [IgG] <3.0 g/dl, immunoglobulin M [IgM] <500 mg/dl, and immunoglobulin A [IgA] <1 g/dl), and no hypogammaglobulinemia are likely to have MGUS, and a bone marrow examination can be omitted if follow-up is ensured. Likewise, radiologic evaluation in these patients is of low yield and is not recommended.

A small proportion of patients with monoclonal gammopathies will present with striking lymphocytosis, sometimes with lymphadenopathy, raising the suspicion of chronic lymphocytic leukemia. Other patients will have prominent lymphadenopathy, often with B symptoms, consistent with non-Hodgkin's lymphoma. Examination of the peripheral blood smear, a bone marrow biopsy, or a lymph node biopsy may be necessary for diagnosis. These disorders are associated with modest levels of IgM paraprotein, usually less than 1 g/dl.

Patients with a history of recurrent sinopulmonary infections, bone pain, fatigue, polyuria, polydipsia and/or hypercalcemia, or anemia are likely to have myeloma. A history of bruising, bleeding, confusion, and increasing somnolence in the setting of hepatosplenomegaly and an IgM monoclonal protein suggests Waldenström's macroglobulinemia. The evaluation of these disorders is discussed later in this chapter.

TABLE 43–1. DISORDERS ASSOCIATED WITH MONOCLONAL GAMMOPATHIES

MOST COMMON DISORDERS
Monoclonal gammopathy of unknown significance
Multiple myeloma
Chronic lymphocytic leukemia
Non-Hodgkin's lymphoma
UNCOMMON DISORDERS
PLASMA CELL DISORDERS
Waldenström's macroglobulinemia
Solitary osseous plasmacytoma
Extramedullary plasmacytoma
Amyloidosis
Heavy chain disease
INFLAMMATORY DISORDERS
Mixed cryoglobulinemia
Sjögren's syndrome
Cold agglutinin disease
OTHER DISORDERS (RARE)
Systemic lupus erythematosus
Lichen myxedematosus
Pyoderma gangrenosum
Sézary syndrome
Erythema elevatum diutinum
Diffuse plane xanthomatosis
Acquired immunodeficiency syndrome (AIDS)
Renal transplant recipients
Bone marrow transplant recipients
Idiopathic pulmonary fibrosis
Pulmonary alveolar proteinosis
Hashimoto's thyroiditis
Schönlein-Henoch purpura

TABLE 43–2. CRITERIA FOR MULTIPLE MYELOMA AND MONOCLONAL GAMMOPATHY OF UNKNOWN SIGNIFICANCE

MONOCLONAL GAMMOPATHY OF UNKNOWN SIGNIFICANCE
I. Monoclonal gammopathy
II. M component
IgG < 3.5 g/dl
IgA < 1.0 g/dl
III. Bone marrow plasma cells < 10%
IV. No lytic bone lesions
V. No symptoms consistent with myeloma
MULTIPLE MYELOMA
MAJOR CRITERIA
I. Plasmacytoma on tissue biopsy
II. Bone marrow plasma cells > 30%
III. Monoclonal gammopathy
IgG > 3.5 g/dl
IgA > 2.0 g/dl
Bence-Jones > 1.0 g/24-hour urine collection
MINOR CRITERIA
I. Bone marrow plasma cells 10–30%
II. Monoclonal gammopathy, but less than major criteria levels
III. Lytic bone lesions
IV. Hypogammaglobulinemia
IgM < 50 mg/dl
IgA < 100 mg/dl
IgG < 600 mg/dl
Diagnosis is confirmed when at least one major and one minor criteria are present or, alternatively, three minor criteria, including I and II.

IgA = immunoglobulin A; IgG = immunoglobulin G; IgM = immunoglobulin M.

MONOCLONAL GAMMOPATHY OF UNKNOWN SIGNIFICANCE

In general, persons with monoclonal gammopathy of unknown significance are asymptomatic, or at least have no symptoms directly related to their plasma cell dyscrasia. This entity is seen with the same frequency in both men and women. The incidence of MGUS is age-dependent and rises rapidly after the fifth decade of life. By definition, there is no evidence of hypercalcemia, lytic bone lesions, renal failure, anemia, or hypogammaglobulinemia. Levels of monoclonal protein are usually lower than those seen in myeloma (Table 43–2). Bone marrow biopsy results are usually normal and in all cases reveal fewer than 10% plasma cells.

Although this entity was previously referred to as "benign monoclonal gammopathy," this is clearly a misnomer. Long-term follow-up studies demonstrate that approximately 30% to 40% of patients will develop a hematologic malignancy within 30 years of their MGUS diagnosis. Patients with MGUS are at highest risk of developing multiple myeloma, although Waldenström's macroglobulinemia, amyloidosis, chronic lymphocytic leukemia (CLL), and non-Hodgkin's lymphoma are also seen. Patients with MGUS should be followed by history, physical examination, and quantitative gamma globulins as well as a CBC twice a year for the first few years. Patients with stable monoclonal immunoglobulin levels can be followed yearly. Serial bone marrow examinations and radiologic studies are unnecessary unless there are signs and symptoms suggestive of a hematologic malignancy, anemia, or rising gamma globulin level. Patients with rising monoclonal immunoglobulin levels (>0.5 mg/dl/year) should be re-evaluated for myeloma.

Patients with IgM monoclonal gammopathies have a 15% to 20% risk of developing Waldenström's macroglobulinemia over 20 years. In addition, another 15% of this population will develop CLL, lymphoma, or amyloidosis during the same period. Currently no therapy is known to be effective in preventing the progression of MGUS. Long-term exposure to alkylating therapy is leukemogenic and is contraindicated in this population.

MYELOMA

Presentation and Evaluation

Although myeloma can present in persons of almost any age, ranging from adolescents to the elderly, the mean age is approximately 60 and disease before the age of 40 is uncommon. The disease is relatively common. Mortality rates are age-, sex-, and race-dependent, with approximately 20 deaths per 100,000 persons at age 70. Men have a higher incidence of disease than women. Blacks have a two to three times higher incidence than whites. The incidence of the disease is increasing for unclear reasons, making it one of the most common hematologic malignancies. Currently, it is the second most common such malignancy in whites, and the most common hematologic malignancy in blacks.

Patients can present with a large range of symptoms due to the complications related to the anemia, hypogammaglobulinemia, lytic bone lesions, renal dysfunction, and/or hypercalcemia. Occasionally patients present with medical emergencies, including epidural spinal cord compression, hyperviscosity, life-threatening hypercalcemia, or congestive heart failure due to amyloidosis. Other patients may fortuitously be diagnosed while asymptomatic through the detection of either an elevated serum or urine protein or the discovery of a mild anemia.

Currently there are several therapies for myeloma. Each, however, is associated with its own morbidity, and it is useful to fully evaluate patients before initiating therapy. Evaluation should focus on a history of fevers or recurrent sinopulmonary infections. Pain is often present and should be documented. In particular, back pain and pain in the hips, thighs, and knees should not be ignored because they may be the site of future pathologic fracture. Bone pain can be referred. Radicular pain or herpes zoster should raise the suspicion of a dorsal root compression and, possibly, impending spinal cord compression. Knee or thigh pain may be referred from the hip or pelvis.

Physical examination should include palpation of the skull, which may reveal cranial plasmacytomas, and spine percussion may demonstrate areas of point tenderness secondary to involvement of the vertebral body with myeloma. Lymphadenopathy, hepatomegaly, and splenomegaly are usually not present and should raise the suspicion of an alternate or additional diagnosis. Finally, signs and symptoms including edema, dyspnea, orthopnea, dizziness, orthostatic hypotension, purpura, and hepatosplenomegaly may be present and suggest the possibility of amyloidosis.

Laboratory evaluation should include a CBC, blood urea nitrogen (BUN), creatinine, lactate dehydrogenase (LDH), calcium, C-reactive protein (CRP) and β_2-microglobulin. Serum and urine electrophoresis and a serum quantitative immunoglobulin should be performed. If Bence-Jones protein is present in the urine or there is an abnormality in renal function tests, a 24-hour urine specimen should be collected for calculation of creatinine clearance and total urinary protein. Nephrotic range proteinuria with little or no Bence-Jones proteinuria suggests amyloidosis.

Radiologic examination should be performed of all areas of bone pain or tenderness that are weight-bearing. Particular attention should be paid to patients with a principal complaint of back pain, since epidural cord compression is common and associated with potentially catastrophic complications in this population.

Median survival for patients with newly diagnosed myeloma is approximately 30 months. Currently, there are several different staging systems for myeloma, which divide patients into groups with more or less favorable survival times. The Durie-Salmon remains the one most extensively used staging systems for dividing patients into good, fair, and poor prognostic groups. This system uses lytic bone lesions, anemia, and hypercalcemia as surrogate markers for tumor burden and predicted survival (Table 43-3). Median survivals

TABLE 43–3. DURIE-SALMON STAGING SYSTEM

STAGE I
All of the following:
- Hemoglobin value > 10 g/dl
- Calcium value normal (<12 mg/dl)
- Radiologic evaluation reveals normal bone structure or solitary plasmacytoma
- Low M component
  - IgG value < 5 g/dl
  - IgA value < 3 g/dl
  - Bence-Jones < 4 g/24-hr urine collection

STAGE II
One or more values more abnormal than Stage I; no values as defined for Stage III

STAGE III
One or more of the following:
- Hemoglobin value < 8.5 g/dl
- Serum calcium value >12 mg/dl
- Advanced lytic bone lesions
- High M component
  - IgG value > 7 g/dl
  - IgA value > 5 g/dl
  - Bence-Jones > 12 g/dl

SUBCLASSIFICATIONS
A = relatively normal renal function with serum creatinine <2.0 mg/dl
B = abnormal renal function with serum creatinine >2.0 mg/dl

are longer than 60 months, 41 months, and 23 months for patients in Stages I, II, and III, respectively.

Recently, several new prognostic variables have been identified, including LDH, β_2-microglobulin, CRP, tumor labeling index, thymidine kinase, and serum interleukin 6 levels. The combination of CRP and β_2-microglobulin seems to be a powerful and simple prognostic staging system for myeloma. In a recent study, patients with CRP above 6 mg/liter and β_2-microglobulin above 6 mg/liter have a median survival of 6 months. Good-prognosis patients with a CRP less than 6 mg/liter and β_2-microglobulin above 6 mg/liter had median survivals of 54 months, with 25% of patients estimated to be alive at 8 years. Patients with only one elevated value had an intermediate prognosis.

Primary Treatment

Multiple myeloma is both radiosensitive and chemosensitive, and median survival of patients with this disease is approximately 2 to 3 years. As mentioned above, the median survival is somewhat misleading because many patients die within the first year of diagnosis despite aggressive therapy, whereas others survive for a decade with minimal therapy.

The first decision is whether the patient with newly diagnosed myeloma requires treatment. Any patients with hypercalcemia, myeloma-induced renal dysfunction, severe anemia, or recurrent infections in the setting of hypogammaglobulinemia should be treated with chemotherapy. Patients with multiple bone lesions should receive systemic therapy before radiation therapy. Patients with asymptomatic myeloma or in whom the diagnosis of myeloma vs. MGUS is unclear should be watched with careful follow-up. Solitary lesions may be successfully treated with radiation therapy and are discussed below.

Clinical responses in myeloma are often accompanied by improvement in bone pain, anemia, and hypercalcemia. Monoclonal protein levels usually drop, although this drop may be slow and may lag several months behind therapy because of the long half-life of some immunoglobulin subclasses. Complete responses are defined as less than 5% plasma cells found on bone marrow biopsy and absence of a monoclonal immunoglobulin on immunoelectrophoresis. Conventional-dose chemotherapy seldom produces a complete response. Partial responses have been defined as a 50% (Chronic Leukemia-Myeloma Task Force) or 75% (Southwestern Oncology Group) reduction in monoclonal protein. Patients with stable or responsive disease do better than the subset of patients with progressive disease. Curiously, patients with stable disease do as well as persons with partial responses.

In the last several years, there has been increasing interest in high-dose chemotherapy with either autologous or allogeneic stem cell rescue. To date there have been no randomized trials comparing these therapies to conventional therapy; therefore, the guidelines are not definitive. Nevertheless, several general conclusions can be made about the efficacy and toxicity associated with this therapy. Allogeneic bone marrow transplantation is associated with significant toxicity and a high complete response rate. Some of these complete responses have been associated with prolonged disease-free survival. Initial studies have been hampered by toxic deaths and deaths associated with graft-versus-host disease. Allogeneic transplantation performed with T cell–purged donor marrow is safer, although the efficacy of this approach is still under investigation. Despite the risks associated with this therapy, the young myeloma patient with a human leukocyte antigen–matched sibling should be considered for a clinical trial exploring the potential efficacy of this approach.

The role of autologous bone marrow transplantation is less clear. Published studies are contradictory: Some demonstrate little efficacy, whereas others appear promising. Despite several unanswered questions, it is clear that autologous transplantation can be performed with an acceptable peritransplant mortality rate (<5%) and high complete response rates in otherwise healthy patients with chemosensitive disease. A large, multigroup randomized trial examining the role of high-dose therapy with autologous bone marrow support is currently scheduled to begin accruing patients in 1994. Physicians caring for younger patients with myeloma should consider referring patients to one of the numerous centers participating in this trial.

For patients who are ineligible or inappropriate for high-dose chemotherapy trials, conventional chemotherapy offers effective palliation from many of the complications associated with myeloma. Active chemotherapy agents against myeloma include melphalan, cyclophosphamide, steroids, vincristine, doxorubicin (Adriamycin), and 1,3-bis(2-chloroethyl)-1-nitrosourea (BCNU). Melphalan plus prednisone remains the gold standard of safe and effective chemotherapy to which all newer regimens must be compared. Recent meta-analysis of randomized studies comparing combination chemotherapy regimens with melphalan plus prednisone revealed no survival advantage for combination chemotherapy regimens. Response rates for either melphalan plus prednisone or combination chemotherapy are approximately 50%. Hence oral melphalan plus prednisone seems to be a suitable first regimen for the majority of patients receiving chemotherapy for palliation of the symptoms associated with their myeloma.

Patients presenting with extremely high tumor burdens or life-threatening hypercalcemia may benefit from combination chemotherapy regimens such as vincristine, Adriamycin, dexamethasone (VAD), since responses may occur more rapidly with multidrug chemotherapy regimens. Single-agent high-dose dexamethasone is also a reasonable alternative in the patient presenting with pancytopenia or hypercalcemia. Table 43–4 reviews a few of the chemotherapy regimens used to treat patients with myeloma. Extensive treatment with alkylating agents (*i.e.*, melphalan) or with

TABLE 43–4. COMMON CHEMOTHERAPY REGIMENS FOR MULTIPLE MYELOMA

MELPHALAN AND PREDNISONE			
Melphalan	8–10 mg/m^2	po	days 1–4
Prednisone	1 mg/kg	po	days 1–4
Adjust melphalan for leukocyte nadir of 2000/cc^3; repeat every 21–28 days			
VAD			
Vincristine	0.4 mg/m^2	civ	days 1–4
Adriamycin	9 mg/m^2	civ	days 1–4
Dexamethasone	40 mg	po	days 1–4, 9–12, 17–20
Cycles repeated every 28 days			
HIGH-DOSE DEXAMETHASONE			
Dexamethasone	20 mg/m^2	po	days 1–4, 9–12, 17–20
Cycles repeated every 28 days			
M2			
Vincristine	0.03 mg/kg	iv	day 1
Melphalan	0.25 mg/kg	po	days 1–7
Cyclophosphamide	10 mg/kg	iv	day 1
BCNU	1 mg/kg	iv	day 1
Prednisone	1 mg/kg	po	days 1–7
Repeat every five weeks			

po = oral; civ = continuous intravenous; iv = bolus intravenous; BCNU = carmustine.

BCNU has deleterious stem cell effects and should be avoided in patients who might be future candidates for autologous bone marrow transplantation.

Currently, there are several different melphalan plus prednisone schedules, with no regimen demonstrating clear superiority. Absorption of oral melphalan is variable; some patients show significant myelosuppression with 45 to 50 mg/m^2 divided over 3 or 4 days, whereas other patients tolerate more than 100 mg/m^2 with relatively little myelosuppression. Melphalan doses should be tailored to the individual patient, with the initial cycle starting at 45 to 55 mg/m^2 total dose of melphalan divided over 4 days. Patients should be treated to best response. In most patients, monoclonal protein levels plateau at a lower level within 5 to 12 months of starting therapy. Typically, patients enjoy effective palliation with improvement in bone pain, resolution of hypercalcemia, and improvement in anemia. Renal function and hypogammaglobulinemia may also improve. Complete responses are rare. Prolonged chemotherapy, past the best response, is not recommended because prolonged exposure to alkylating agents may increase the risk of leukemia in these patients.

Recent evidence has suggested a potential role for interferon α_2b in the maintenance of the best response in patients with myeloma. Patients achieving significant cytoreduction with chemotherapy may have a prolonged response with interferon given subcutaneously three times per week. Initial studies have demonstrated an increase in progression-free survival but have failed to prove that overall survival is significantly enhanced with this therapy. It is possible that patients with Bence-Jones proteinuria or IgA myeloma may benefit more from maintenance interferon than those with the more common IgG myeloma.

New therapies targeting the multidrug resistance protein pump are currently under investigation. Finally, there is growing interest in the role of interleukin 6 in the growth of myeloma cells and its role in the bone resorption and anemia seen in patients with myeloma. Several therapies targeting interleukin 6 or the interleukin 6 receptor are currently under investigation.

Complications

LYTIC BONE LESIONS

Cytokine-mediated bone destruction represents the most striking type of morbidity associated with myeloma. Interleukin 1, interleukin 6, and other cytokines stimulate osteoclasts to increase bone absorption with resulting osteolytic bone lesions. Pathologic fracture is common. Unfortunately, the axial skeleton — in particular the spine — is particularly prone to destruction. Pain in a weight-bearing bone (spine, humerus, hip, leg) should prompt a thorough radiologic evaluation. Large, lytic lesions or lesions eroding the bone cortex may require orthopedic stabilization before radiation therapy. Painful lesions that are not associated with threatened fracture can usually be effectively palliated with chemotherapy in the chemotherapy-naive patient. Patients with known chemotherapy resistance usually require radiation therapy for effective palliation.

Epidural spinal cord compression is common in myeloma and should be treated with high-dose dexamethasone and radiation therapy. Surgery is reserved for three special situations: spine instability secondary to bone destruction, recurrent plasmacytoma in a region that has received maximal radiation therapy, and solitary undiagnosed spinal lesions.

Recent evidence suggests that "prophylactic" therapy with bisphosphonates (inhibitors of osteoclast-mediated bone absorption) may reduce the risk of future fractures and hypercalcemia.

ANEMIA

For many patients with myeloma, the clinically symptomatic anemia associated with this disease negatively affects their quality of life. The etiology of the anemia is multifactorial and includes factors such as marrow replacement, previous chemotherapy, and previous radiation therapy. In addition, cytokines produced by the myeloma cells and the surrounding marrow stromal cells may inhibit erythropoiesis. Systemic chemotherapy is often effective in improving the hematocrit in the early stages of the disease, when tumor cells are still drug-sensitive. Subsequent stages of disease are often associated with acquired chemoresistance and refractory anemia. Some of these patients will benefit from erythropoietin therapy. Patients not eligible for this therapy are usually treated with red cell transfusion therapy.

HYPERCALCEMIA

Hypercalcemia is a cytokine-mediated complication due to increased osteoclast-mediated bone resorption and subsequent calcium release. Therapy is principally directed to cytoreducing the systemic burden of plasma cells, which in turn reduces the rate of bone resorption. High-dose steroids, along with aggressive hydration, is an effective initial therapy. Bisphosphonates are also effective for temporarily controlling the hypercalcemia of multiple myeloma.

RENAL FAILURE

There are multiple causes of renal dysfunction in myeloma. Myeloma kidney is one of the most common forms of myeloma-related renal dysfunction due to a toxic effect of the clonotypic immunoglobulin light chain on the renal tubule. Curiously, some light chains are very toxic, whereas other clonotypes are essentially harmless to the renal tubule. Treatment is virtually futile unless the disease can be effectively controlled, usually through systemic chemotherapy. In addition to light chain disease, several other renal insults have been described, including hypercalcemia, hyperuricemia, pyelonephritis, and occasionally papillary necrosis in association with hyperviscosity. Fortunately, careful follow-up of the myeloma patient can avoid most of these problems. Finally, high-grade albuminuria with renal deterioration may be a sign of myeloma-associated glomerulopathy, but more likely is due to amyloidosis. Cytoreduction of the myeloma may temporarily stabilize the problem.

INFECTION

Multiple myeloma is associated with hypogammaglobulinemia and increased risks of infection. In particular, patients with myeloma are at increased risks of sinopulmonary infection and to a lesser extent urinary tract infection. Indeed, infection accounts for 20% to 50% of the deaths in multiple myeloma. Streptococcal pneumonia is the most commonly identified pathogen. Attempts to protect myeloma patients through pneumococcal vaccine have been disappointing, probably because of the poor humoral response to the vaccine. Prophylactic gamma globulin infusion has been investigated and is currently not recommended in all myeloma patients. Nevertheless, it may have some efficacy in the severely hypogammaglobulinemic patient with recurrent infections. The use of prophylactic antibiotics has not been extensively studied in this disease and is currently not recommended.

HYPERVISCOSITY

The hyperviscosity syndrome occurs when the viscosity of serum increases to a level that negatively affects the flow of blood through small vessels. Typically patients present with bleeding and a wide constellation of neurologic symptoms, including focal neurologic deficits, seizures, altered mental status, nystagmus, and vertigo. Diagnosis is made with the demonstration of an elevated blood or serum viscosity in the appropriate clinical context. Hyperviscosity is much more common in patients with IgM myeloma or Waldenström's macroglobulinemia, compared with patients with IgG or IgA myeloma. Clinical symptoms generally appear when serum viscosity exceeds 4 to 6 centipoises, although some patients do not experience symptoms at this level of viscosity. Therapy with plasmapheresis lowers viscosity and improves the bleeding diathesis and neurologic symptoms.

RELAPSED/REFRACTORY DISEASE

Unfortunately, most patients eventually develop progressive disease after an initial response to chemotherapy. In addition, approximately 25% of patients will present with primary refractory disease. VAD is considered one of the most effective palliative regimens available, but second responses tend to be of short duration. Several other alternatives, including high-dose dexamethasone alone; BCNU, etoposide, dexamethasone, cytosine arabinoside, *cis*-platinum (EDAP); or high-dose cyclophosphamide may be considered. Consolidation with dose-intensive melphalan or cyclophosphamide with total-body irradiation may offer long-term palliation in a subset of carefully selected patients responding to salvage chemotherapy.

SOLITARY PLASMACYTOMA

A small subset of patients present with a solitary mass that on biopsy proves to be a plasmacytoma. These masses may present in bone (solitary osseous plasmacytoma) or along the aerodigestive tract (extraosseous plasmacytoma).

Solitary osseous plasmacytoma can present essentially in any bone; however, the large majority of patients present with a lesion in the axial skeleton, in particular, the spine, skull, humerus, or femur. Evaluation should include serum electrophoresis, bilateral bone marrow biopsies, and a complete skeletal survey. Patients with no other evidence of disease should receive primary radiation therapy that provides rapid and effective local control. Although the majority of these patients do well in the short term, most develop multiple myeloma within 8 years of presentation. Patients with elevated serum β_2-microglobulin at diagnosis seem to be at increased risk for early relapse. There currently is no evidence to suggest that adjuvant chemotherapy after radiation therapy prolongs disease-free survival or overall survival in this uncommon disease. Patients with additional lytic lesions or excessive (>30%) plasma cells in their bone marrow should be treated with systemic chemotherapy. Radiation therapy and possibly surgery should be considered in patients with impending pathologic fracture and/or epidural spinal cord compression.

Some patients present with extraosseous lesions in the sinus cavities, mesentery, or other areas of the aerodigestive tract. Occasionally, patients present with multiple lesions. Evaluation is the same as with osseous plasmacytoma. Treatment for solitary lesions is radiation therapy, sometimes following surgical resection. These patients seem to enjoy a better prognosis than do patients with osseous plasmacytoma, but they are at risk for the subsequent development of multiple myeloma. Disease-free intervals can be remarkably long, sometimes spanning decades. There is no evidence that adjuvant chemotherapy is beneficial in patients with solitary extraosseous myeloma. Patients with multiple extraosseous plasmacytomas have a worse prognosis and should be treated with systemic chemotherapy.

WALDENSTRÖM'S MACROGLOBULINEMIA

In a large Mayo Clinic study, 56% of persons with monoclonal IgM protein had MGUS. Thirty-one percent of persons with monoclonal IgM proteins had Waldenström's macroglobulinemia. These patients have more than 1500 mg/dl of IgM protein and a mean age 60 years. Interestingly, IgM paraprotein in these patients often demonstrates reactivity to autoantigens, including IgG and myelin. Patients often present with neurologic symptoms, severe fatigue, and bleeding. Physical findings often include lymphadenopathy and hepatosplenomegaly. Lytic bone lesions and renal dysfunction are usually not seen. The clinical course of the disease is variable and often indolent. Eventually, the disease is complicated by pancytopenia and hyperviscosity. Hyperviscosity results from the aggregation of pentameric IgM that affects the rheologic properties of blood flow. Interestingly, this aggregation is highly dependent on the variable region of the IgM immunoglobulin; hence, blood viscosity is not directly related to the IgM paraprotein level. Symptoms of hyperviscosity include strokelike syndromes, confusion, headaches, somnolence, and bleeding from mucosal surfaces. Signs include venous engorgement (sausage retinal vessels), diminished mental status, purpura, and eventually coma. In symptomatic cases of mental deterioration and/or bleeding, plasmapheresis should be performed to lower IgM concentrations rapidly.

Treatment for Waldenström's macroglobulinemia is similar to that for low-grade non-Hodgkin's lymphomas. Generally, the aim of therapy is palliation. Asymptomatic patients are usually observed off therapy. Patients with hyperviscosity may be treated with plasmapheresis or chemotherapy. Persons with progressive hepatosplenomegaly, lymphadenopathy, profound fatigue, or pancytopenia should receive chemotherapy. Oral alkylating agents, such as chlorambucil, melphalan, or cyclophosphamide, are often effective. Combination therapy may be more effective than single-agent therapy, but controlled comparative studies are currently not available. Chemotherapy should be withheld until clear indications exist for its initiation. Once therapy is initiated, attempts should be made to minimize exposure to alkylating agents, since this therapy is associated with an increased risk of acute myelogenous leukemia. Patients with disease that is resistant to alkylating agents may benefit from therapy with 2-chloro-deoxyadenosine. Median survival is 5 years. Male patients, patients older than 60 years at diagnosis, and patients with a leukocyte count of under 4000/cc^3 have a worse prognosis.

BIBLIOGRAPHY

Alexanian R, Barlogie B, Dixon D. High-dose glucocorticoid treatment of resistant myeloma. Ann Intern Med 105:8, 1986

Alexanian R, Barlogie B, Dixon D. Renal failure in multiple myeloma. Pathogenesis and prognostic implications. Arch Intern Med 150:1693, 1990

Anderson KC. Plasma cell neoplasms. In Holland JF, Frei E III, Bast RC et al (eds). Cancer Medicine. Philadelphia, Lea & Febiger, 1993:2075

Barlogie B, Alexanian R, Jagannath S. Plasma cell dyscrasias. JAMA 268:2946, 1992

Bataille R, Boccadoro M, Klein B et al. C-reactive protein and beta-2 microglobulin produce a simple and powerful myeloma staging system. Blood 80:733, 1992

Berkman SA, Lee ML, Gale RP. Clinical uses of intravenous immunoglobulins. Ann Intern Med 112:278, 1990

Bloch KJ, Maki DG. Hyperviscosity syndromes associated with immunoglobulin abnormalities. Semin Hematol 10:113, 1973

Buzaid A, Durie B. Management of refractory myeloma: A review. J Clin Oncol 6:889, 1988

Chak LY, Cox RS, Bostwick DG et al. Solitary plasmacytoma of bone; treatment, progression, and survival. J Clin Oncol 5:1811, 1987

Crawford J, Cox EB, Cohen HJ. Evaluation of hyperviscosity in monoclonal gammopathies. Am J Med 79:13, 1985

Crawford J, Eye MK, Cohen JH. Evaluation of monoclonal gammopathies in the "well" elderly. Am J Med 82:39, 1987

Durie BG, Salmon SE. A clinical staging system for multiple myeloma. Cancer 36:842, 1975

Facon T, Brouillard M, Duhamel A et al. Prognostic factors in Waldenström's macroglobulinemia: A report of 167 cases. J Clin Oncol 11:1553, 1993

Gahrton G, Tura S, Flesh M et al. Allogeneic bone marrow transplantation in multiple myeloma. N Engl J Med 325:1267, 1991

Gasman, Pralle H, Haferlach T et al. Staging systems for multiple myeloma: A comparison. Br J Haematol 59:703, 1985

Gregory WM, Richards MA, Malpas JS. Combination chemotherapy versus melphalan and prednisone in the treatment of multiple myeloma: An overview of published trials. J Clin Oncol 10:334, 1992

Greipp PR, Lust JA, O'Fallon M et al. Plasma cell labeling index and β_2-microglobulin predict survival independent of thymidine kinase and C-reactive protein in multiple myeloma. Blood 81:3382, 1993

Hjorth M, Hellquist L, Holmberg E et al. Initial versus deferred melphalan-prednisone therapy for asymptomatic multiple myeloma stage I — a randomized study. Myeloma Group of Western Sweden. Eur J Haematol 50:95, 1993

Jacobson DR, Zolla-Pazner S. Immunosuppression and infection in multiple myeloma. Semin Oncol 13:282, 1986

Jagannath S, Barlogie B. Autologous bone marrow transplantation for multiple myeloma. Hematol Oncol Clin North Am 6:437, 1992

Kyle RA. Diagnostic criteria of multiple myeloma. Hematol Oncol Clin North Am 6:347, 1992

Kyle RA, Farton JP. The spectrum of IgM monoclonal gammopathy in 430 cases. Mayo Clin Proc 62:719, 1987

Kyle RA, Lust JA. Monoclonal gammopathies of undetermined significance. Semin Hematol 26:176, 1989

Lahtinen R, Laakso M, Palva I et al. Randomised, placebo-controlled multicentre trial of clodronate in multiple myeloma. Lancet 340:1049, 1992

MacKenzie MR. Macroglobulinemia. In Wiernik PH, Canellos GP, Kyle RA, Schiffer CA (eds). Neoplastic diseases of the blood, 2nd ed. New York, Churchill Livingstone, 1991:501

Mandelli F, Avvisati G, Amadori S et al. Maintenance treatment with recombinant interferon alfa-2b in patients with multiple myeloma responding to conventional induction chemotherapy. N Engl J Med 32:1430, 1990

Mohrbacher A, Anderson KC. Bone marrow transplantation in multiple myeloma. In Kyle RA (ed). Multiple Myeloma. Oxford, England, Oxford University Press (in press)

Mohrbacher A, Anderson KC. Plasmacytoma. In Williams CJ, Krikorian JC, Green MR, Raghavan D (eds). Textbook of Uncommon Cancer. Sussex, J Wiley & Sons, Ltd (in press)

Moore DF, Migliore PJ, Shullenberger CC et al. Monoclonal macroglobulinemia in malignant lymphoma. Ann Intern Med 72:43, 1970

Osterborg A, Bjorkholm M, Bjoreman B et al. Natural interferon-α in combination with melphalan/prednisone versus melphalan/prednisone in the treatment of multiple myeloma stages II and III: A randomized trial from Myeloma Group of Central Sweden. Blood 81:1428, 1993

Seiden MV, Anderson KC. Multiple myeloma. In Schiffer CA (ed). Current Opinion in Oncology. Philadelphia, Current Science (in press)

John S. Macdonald, Daniel G. Haller, Robert J. Mayer, Eds. *Manual of Oncologic Therapeutics*, Third Edition.

44. CANCERS OF UNKNOWN PRIMARY ORIGIN

Martin N. Raber

The term unknown primary carcinoma (UPC) refers to the presence of metastatic cancer in the absence of a demonstrable primary tumor. It has been reported in between 2% and 10% of all patients presenting with cancer.[1] Its frequency is variably reported because the criteria for diagnosis depend on the thoroughness of the search for a potential primary tumor. However one defines the entity, the literature suggests that these patients have a very poor prognosis, with most studies reporting median survival in the range of 4 to 6 months.[2] In fact, patients with UPC form a heterogeneous group in which the prognosis and treatment must be individualized.

EVALUATION

There remains some controversy over the evaluation of patients with UPC. Given the poor prognosis of the group as a whole, some authors favor a highly limited evaluation to rule out the treatable malignancies (*e.g.*, breast, ovarian, germ cell, and prostate cancer).[3] Others favor an in-depth search to establish the primary tumor at almost any cost. Given the realities of health care today, and the desire of the patient and physician to develop the optimal therapy and the most accurate prognosis, the specific evaluation of each patient should be based on the studies most likely to add meaningful information about primary source and extent of disease.

The most important first step, after obtaining a complete history and performing a physical examination, is a review of the pathologic material by an experienced pathologist. The most common pathologic subtype is adenocarcinoma (about 60%), followed by undifferentiated (or poorly differentiated) carcinomas (30%) and squamous carcinomas (6%). Although rare, neuroendocrine carcinomas (2%) form an important subset because of their unique natural history. (Where not otherwise referenced, data are based on an analysis of 927 patients referred to the M. D. Anderson Cancer Center with a diagnosis of UPC between 1987 and 1993).

In the group of patients with adenocarcinoma and squamous carcinoma, the focus is on elucidating the primary tumor, whereas in the patients with undifferentiated tumors, the focus is on immunohistochemistry and electron microscopy in an attempt to determine more accurately the histologic subtype. Thus a percentage of these patients will be found to have markers for sarcomas, lymphomas, melanomas, neuroendocrine tumors, and germ cell tumors.[4] In our own series, these histologies represent 6% of patients referred with a diagnosis of UPC and 18% of the primary tumors found.[5] Histochemical studies may also diagnose prostate cancer. Recently, molecular genetic studies have also proved helpful in determining the germ cell origin of undifferentiated tumors,[6] and these techniques will no doubt become more important in the future.

A directed approach for the evaluation of patients referred with UPC is outlined in Table 44–1. All patients should have a complete medical history and physical examination, including breast and gynecologic evaluation in women, and prostate and testicular examination in men. All patients should undergo chest radiography and computed tomographic (CT) scans of the abdomen and pelvis. A number of studies have demonstrated the usefulness of abdominal and pelvic CT scanning in diagnosing primary tumors and establishing the extent of disease.[7]

All women should undergo mammography. In the case of axillary nodes with a negative mammogram, breast ultrasonography should be considered. Patients with an abnormal chest x-ray film should be evaluated with chest CT, sputum cytology, and, where appropriate, bronchoscopy. Gastrointestinal imaging studies should be limited to patients with abdominal presentations or complaints. Patients with cervical nodes should be evaluated with a thorough head and neck examination, CT scan of the head and neck, and in the case of papillary adenocarcinoma, thyroid studies.

Although tumor marker studies may be helpful in suggesting a primary tumor, the adenocarcinoma markers (carcinoembryonic antigen [CEA], CA-125, CA15-3, CA19-9) have significant overlap and are rarely diagnostic, with the exception of prostate-specific antigen elevation in the blood and immunohistochemical confirmation of the pathologic material. Human chorionic gonadotropin-beta subunit in germ cell tumors and choriocarcinoma, and alpha fetoprotein in germ cell tumors and hepatomas may be helpful in establishing a diagnosis.

When these approaches are taken, about 25% of patients referred with a diagnosis of UPC will have a primary tumor discovered or will be found to have a specific diagnostic histology. In a recent series, the most commonly found primary tumor was lung cancer (30%), followed by cancer of the pancreas (10%) and breast (7.5%).[5] The survival of patients with identified primary tumors is comparable to the natural history of other patients who present with that specific tumor.

TABLE 44–1. EVALUATION OF PATIENTS PRESENTING WITH UNKNOWN PRIMARY CARCINOMAS

All patients	Complete history and physical examination Hematologic and biochemical screening studies Chest x-ray film CT scan: abdomen and pelvis
Men	PSA, CEA, hCG-β, αFP
Women	Gynecologic evaluation, mammography CEA, CA-125, CA15-3 hCG-β, αFP
Selected patients	
Cervical adenopathy	Head and neck examination CT scan Thyroid evaluation
Abnormal chest x-ray finding	Sputum and bronchoscopy
Abdominal presentation or guaiac-positive	Gastrointestinal imaging

CT = computed tomographic; PSA = prostate-specific antigen; CEA = carcinoembryonic antigen; hCG-β = human chorionic gonadotropin-beta subunit; αFP = alpha-fetoprotein.

NATURAL HISTORY AND THERAPY

Overall survival for UPC patients with this diagnosis is poor. The median survival of patients with adenocarcinomas (6 months) is worse than those with carcinomas (11 months). Nevertheless the clinical course of specific clinical presentations may be quite varied. About 40% of patients present with a single site (single organ) of disease. Common presentations include lymph nodes, lung, liver, bone, and pleural effusions. Less common sites of presentation include brain, peritoneum, adrenal gland, and skin. Patients who present with single-site disease appear to have a better prognosis, as might be expected.

A number of favorable clinical subsets have been identified. In these cases there is considerable agreement on the therapy of choice.

DISTINCT PATHOLOGIC SUBSETS

Patients identified as having lymphoma, melanoma, sarcoma, germ cell tumors, and prostate cancer should be treated by following established guidelines for these diseases. Their prognosis does not appear to be influenced by their presentation.[8] A distinct group of patients has been identified who have neuroendocrine carcinomas. These patients have a favorable prognosis compared with other patients with UPC (median survival 27 months). Like patients with neuroendocrine carcinomas from known sites, these patients may have slow-growing disease. When disease is confined to the liver, patients may benefit from long periods of observation and local therapy such as hepatic infarction; when disseminated, they should be treated with chemotherapy. The most often recommended regimen is etoposide plus cisplatin.[9] Similarly, a group of patients with small cell carcinomas presenting as UPC has been identified and should receive similar chemotherapy.[10]

DISTINCT CLINICAL SUBSETS

Lymph Node–Only Disease

Historically, patients presenting with lymph node–only disease have a better prognosis than those presenting with visceral disease (median survival 35 months vs. 9 months). For patients with nodal disease, the value of regional therapy should be considered. Patients with local or regional nodal disease often benefit from local therapy (surgery or radiation therapy). Two presentations merit specific discussion.

Patients presenting with squamous carcinoma in cervical lymph nodes have a unique natural history. They require intense evaluation for an occult head and neck primary tumor. If none is found, they should be treated with radiation therapy (in some cases, surgery) and may have a 5-year survival above 50%. This is true also of patients with undifferentiated histology.[11] Unfortunately, patients with affected supraclavicular lymph nodes and those with adenocarcinoma in any cervical location do not enjoy such good results.

Another favorable subset of patients are women with adenocarcinoma in axillary lymph nodes. These patients should be evaluated with mammography; if results are negative, they should undergo breast ultrasonography. They should be presumed to have breast cancer and should be treated accordingly, with axillary surgery, adjuvant chemotherapy, and control (either by surgery or by radiation therapy) of the ipsilateral breast. Their natural history is similar to that of Stage II breast cancer.[12]

Peritoneal Carcinomatosis

Although the literature has long suggested that UPC presenting as ascites carries a poor prognosis, recent studies suggest that there is a distinct subset of women with peritoneal carcinomatosis who in fact have a better prognosis. Often these women have papillary adenocarcinomas associated with elevated levels of the ovarian marker CA-125. However, even on close histologic review, their ovaries show no evidence of malignancy. Some investigators consider these tumors as arising from the peritoneum itself, whereas others think their origin is remnant müllerian tissue.

Whatever its origin, peritoneal carcinomatosis follows a natural history similar to that of ovarian cancer and should be managed accordingly. Its responsiveness to platinum-containing regimens is well established.[13] Its response to paclitaxel (Taxol) regimens is under investigation. Unfortunately, men with peritoneal carcinomatosis, and women with classic signet-ring mucinous adenocarcinomas do not have a similar favorable prognosis.

Germ Cell Equivalents

Previous studies have identified a subset of patients with UPC who appear to be highly responsive to chemotherapy and have the potential for prolonged survival. Earlier studies were limited to young male patients with midline undifferentiated tumors and positive germ cell markers; more recent studies suggest that this group includes patients of either sex who have undifferentiated or poorly differentiated carcinomas and some of the following characteristics: young age at presentation (<50), midline tumor, and rapid tumor growth. They usually do not have germ cell tumor markers. When treated with aggressive, platinum-containing chemotherapy regimens, these patients have high response rates: Up to 50% respond, and up to 30% achieve complete remission.[14] In this latter group, median survival is long (>5 years).[15] Unfortunately, this group probably represents only about 15% of patients who present with UPC. Similar approaches have been taken with patients presenting with poorly differentiated adenocarcinomas, although the results are not as promising.[14]

The majority of patients with UPC present with adenocarcinomas that do not fall into the above-mentioned groups. For this group of patients, UPC remains a devastating disease (median survival about 6 months). Although many chemotherapeutic regimens have been tried, none can really be considered satisfactory. Reported combinations include anthracycline-based regimens, such as (5-fluorouracil (5-FU), doxorubicin and mitomycin C (FAM) or platinum-based regimens, including etoposide and cisplatin and, more recently, 5-FU, leucovorin, and cisplatin.[2]

In unselected series of UPC, response rates of about 30% are reported with about 10% complete responders, but on closer examination the responders are usually accounted for by patients in the "favorable" groups listed above. For most patients there is no satisfactory therapy. Given this reality, patients should be encouraged to enter clinical trials, and aggressive chemotherapy should be used judiciously.

Patients with single-site disease should be considered for local or regional therapy. Isolated bone metastases should be irradiated. Pleural effusions should be drained and pleurodesis performed. Single-node or cutaneous sites should be considered for surgical removal, where feasible, or radiation therapy. Disease limited to the brain should be biopsied and similarly treated with surgery or radiation therapy. Patients with progressive disease requiring chemotherapy, if they are not on a clinical trial, may be treated as noted above. Given the results of treatment in patients with "germ cell–equivalent tumors," patients with disseminated undifferentiated or poorly differentiated carcinomas should be given a trial of a cisplatin-containing regimen.

CONCLUSION

UPC is a not-uncommon presentation in medical oncology. Although the overall prognosis is poor, a directed evaluation for a primary tumor should be undertaken. A number of important subsets of patients with more favorable outcomes have been identified, and on this basis, therapy should be individualized.

REFERENCES

1. Ultmann JE, Phillips TL. Cancer of unknown primary site. In DeVita VT Jr, Hellman S, Rosenberg SA (eds). Cancer Principles and Practice of Oncology. Philadelphia, JB Lippincott, 1985:1843–1853
2. Sporn JR, Greenberg BR. Empirical chemotherapy in patients with carcinoma of unknown primary. Am J Med 88:49, 1990
3. Stewart JF, Tattersall MHN, Woods RL et al. Unknown primary adenocarcinoma: Incidence of over investigation and natural history. Br Med J 1:1530–1533, 1979
4. Mackay B, Ordonez NG. Pathological evaluation of neoplasms with unknown primary tumor site. Semin Oncol 20:206–229, 1993
5. Lenzi R, Abbruzzese M, Abbruzzese JL et al. Diagnostic evaluation of patients (pts) with metastatic tumors of unknown primary (UPT). Proc Am Assoc Clin Oncol 11: 354, 1992
6. Ilson DH, Motzer RS, Rodriguez ES et al. Genetic analysis in the diagnosis of neoplasm of unknown primary tumor site. Semin Oncol 20:229–237, 1993
7. Karsell PR, Sheedy PF II, O'Connell MJ. Computed tomography in search of cancer of unknown origin. JAMA 248:340–343, 1982
8. Horning SJ, Carrier EK, Rouse RV et al. Lymphomas presenting as histologically unclassified neoplasms: Characteristics and response to treatment. J Clin Oncol 7:1281–1287, 1989
9. Moertel CG, Kvols LK, O'Connell MJ et al. Treatment of neuroendocrine carcinomas with combined etoposide and cisplatin: Evidence of major therapeutic activity in the anaplastic variants of these neoplasms. Cancer 68:227–232, 1991
10. Van Der Gaast, Verwey J, Prins E et al. Chemotherapy as treatment of choice in extrapulmonary undifferentiated small cell carcinomas. Cancer 65:422–424, 1990
11. Marcial-Vega VA, Cardenes H, Perez CA et al: Cervical metastases from unknown primaries: Radiotherapeutic man-

agement and appearance of subsequent primaries. J Radiat Oncol Biol Physiol 19:919–928, 1990

12. Ellerbroek N, Holmes F, Singletary E et al. Treatment of patients with isolated axillary nodal metastases from an occult primary carcinoma consistent with breast origin. Cancer 66:1461–1467, 1990
13. Strnad CM, Grosh WW, Baxter J et al. Peritoneal carcinomatosis of unknown primary site in women: A distinct subset of adenocarcinoma. Ann Intern Med 111:213–217, 1989
14. Hainsworth JD, Johnson DH, Greco FA. Cisplatin based combination chemotherapy in the treatment of poorly differentiated carcinoma and poorly differentiated adenocarcinoma of unknown primary site. J Clin Oncol 10:912–922, 1992
15. Hainsworth JD, Dial TW, Greco FA. Curative combination chemotherapy for patients with advanced poorly differentiated carcinoma of unknown primary site. Am J Clin Oncol 11:138–145, 1988

John S. Macdonald, Daniel G. Haller, Robert J. Mayer, Eds. *Manual of Oncologic Therapeutics*, Third Edition.

45. CANCERS IN CHILDREN

Marc E. Horowitz
Malcolm Smith
Ian T. Magrath
C. Philip Steuber
Lee Helman
Angela Ogden
ZoAnn E. Dreyer
Donald H. Mahoney, Jr.
Richard S.Ungerleider
Philip A. Pizzo
David G. Poplack

Although childhood cancers constitute less than 3% of all malignancies, they represent an important success story in oncology. Pediatric oncology has contributed significantly to our overall understanding of cancer, having elucidated that certain malignancies (*e.g.*, retinoblastoma) are genetically transmissible; that congenital immunodeficiency disorders (*e.g.*, Wiskott-Aldrich syndrome) can predispose one to lymphoreticular malignancies; and that clinical and laboratory features (ranging from age and sex to immunologic phenotyping and molecular analysis) can be used to classify common childhood cancers, assign a prognosis, and guide the intensity and duration of treatment. Most importantly, because many childhood cancers have been responsive to currently available therapies, they have served to delineate the principles of treatment now being applied to adult tumors. These include the value of adjuvant chemotherapy for patients with localized tumors, the use of intensive chemotherapy regimens and bone marrow transplantation for high-risk patients, the use of neoadjuvant chemotherapy and limb-sparing procedures, the importance of central nervous system (CNS) prophylaxis and maintenance therapy in acute leukemia and non-Hodgkin's lymphoma, and the importance of following patients for the long-term sequelae of cancer and its treatment.

In this chapter, the more common childhood malignancies are used to illustrate the principles of evaluation and therapy. We have not attempted to provide facile prescriptions for treatment but have chosen to discuss the overall approach to management. Approximately 80% of children with cancer nationwide are treated on a clinical research protocol. Collaborative group and single-institution protocols are available for the majority of clinical situations. It is imperative that a child be treated on a study whenever feasible. The benefit to the child is a treatment plan that reflects the state of the art designed by experts in the field. Additionally, we will continue to make progress toward every pediatric cancer specialist's goal — a cure for all. Information about available protocols can be obtained from the *PDQ*, the National Cancer Institute's on-line information service.

ACUTE LYMPHOBLASTIC LEUKEMIA OF CHILDHOOD

Acute leukemia is the most common childhood malignancy, with 2000 cases reported each year in the United States. Of these, approximately three quarters are diagnosed as acute lymphoblastic leukemia (ALL). The peak incidence of ALL in childhood is between 2 and 6 years of age; the disease is seen more commonly in boys than in girls. The record of therapeutic success in childhood ALL has been dramatic. Thirty years ago, ALL was uniformly fatal, whereas today more than half of the children who present with ALL are alive 5 years after initial diagnosis, with a majority of these patients being considered cured. In recent years, molecular, cytogenetic, and immunologic studies have demonstrated that there is marked heterogeneity of this disease. As a result, it is no longer appropriate to treat all patients with childhood ALL in an identical manner. Thus, the therapeutic approach to the patient with ALL has become increasingly complex.

The child with ALL can present with a variety of signs and symptoms that reflect both infiltration of the bone marrow with leukemic lymphoblasts and extramedullary spread of the disease. Reduction in the number of normal hematopoietic precursors produces anemia, thrombocytopenia, and neutropenia resulting in fatigue, pallor, anorexia, petechiae, purpura, bleeding, and infection. Extramedullary leukemic spread results in lymphadenopathy, including mediastinal enlargement, hepatomegaly, and splenomegaly. Overt CNS leukemia or testicular infiltration is relatively rare at diagnosis but is a not-infrequent site of relapse. Infiltration of the periosteum and bone is common, and patients frequently present with bone and joint pain. Other malignancies affecting the pediatric age group (*e.g.*, non-Hodgkin's lymphoma, retinoblastoma, neuroblastoma, and rhabdomyosarcoma) may also involve the bone marrow and must be included in the differential diagnosis.

Pretreatment Evaluation

A diagnosis of ALL is made when more than 25% of cells on a bone marrow aspirate are lymphoblasts. Morphologic assessment alone is inadequate. Bone marrow aspirates must be subjected to special cytochemical stains (*e.g.*, myeloperoxidase, periodic acid–Schiff), immunophenotyping, biochemical study (*e.g.*, terminal deoxynucleotidyl transferase [TdT] assay), and deoxyribonucleic acid (DNA) index and cytogenetic analysis. In addition to a careful physical examination, which permits assessment of the degree of extramedullary spread (*e.g.*, lymphadenopathy, hepatomegaly, splenomegaly), a chest film (to assess mediastinal involvement) and a lumbar puncture (to rule out CNS disease) should be obtained. Radiographic examination may reveal changes resulting from leukemic infiltration of the periosteum and bone, even in an asymptomatic patient.

In addition to an abnormal blood count, a child with ALL may manifest other abnormal laboratory findings. Hyperuricemia and its attendant threat of uric acid nephropathy and renal failure require adequate hydration, alkalinization, and allopurinol. Abnormalities in serum calcium, potassium, phosphate, and lactic acid dehydrogenase may be observed, especially in patients with large tumor burdens. Because the initial evaluation of the child with ALL requires relatively sophisticated laboratory techniques to perform the necessary immunologic, biochemical, and cytogenetic assays, and because the results of these studies are important in defining the most appropriate forms of therapy, the pretreatment evaluation of children with ALL should be performed in the setting of a pediatric cancer center.

Classification and Staging

Unlike the solid tumors or lymphomas, there is no formal staging system *per se* for childhood ALL. However, it is now common practice to categorize patients with ALL prognostically, on the basis of certain biologic features of their leukemic lymphoblasts and on certain clinical features of their disease evident at the time of its presentation. However, prognosis is intimately associated with treatment; 30 years ago *all* patients had a poor prognosis, regardless of their biologic or "prognostic" characteristics.

MORPHOLOGIC CLASSIFICATION

The French-American-British (FAB) cooperative working group has established a universally accepted system for morphologic classification of the lymphoblastic leukemias. Three morphologically distinct categories are recognized (see Chap. 39). The L1 subtype is seen in approximately 85% of children with ALL. Slightly less than 15% have L2 morphology, a type more frequently seen in adults; approximately 1% to 2% of children have L3 morphology. The FAB classification system appears to have prognostic value; patients with the L1 subtype have the best prognosis, whereas patients with blast cells of L3 morphology (cytomorphologically identical to Burkitt's lymphoma cells) have the worst prognosis. The L2 phenotype also carries a relatively poor prognosis. There is some suggestion that the FAB classification appears to function as an independent prognostic variable.

IMMUNOLOGIC CHARACTERIZATION

Until recently, standard techniques for cell surface marker characterization identified three major immunologic subsets of ALL. Approximately 15% to 20% of patients were classified as having T-cell ALL and approximately 1% to 2% as having B-cell ALL; the majority of children with ALL (70–80%) were believed to have non-T, non–B-cell lymphoblasts. It has now been shown that approximately 80% of patients with so-called non-T, non–B-cell disease have lymphoblasts that display a common ALL antigen. More recent studies have confirmed that the majority of patients formerly considered to have non-T, non–B-cell lymphoblasts actually have disease of early B-cell lineage. Those patients have been variously designated as having B-precursor or B-progenitor ALL.

Furthermore, approximately one fifth of these B-precursor cases show leukemic cells, which demonstrate the presence of cytoplasmic immunoglobulin and have been subclassified as pre-B ALL. These cells are frequently capable of differentiating *in vitro* cells with more mature B-cell markers. Molecular biologic studies have confirmed the early B lineage of these cells by demonstrating evidence of immunoglobin gene rearrangement. Study of the pattern of immunoglobulin gene rearrangement and the coordinate expression of a variety of B-cell lineage-specific monoclonal antibodies has made it possible to subclassify early B-lineage ALL into various stages of differentiation. For example, infants with ALL, a subgroup with a uniquely poor prognosis, have lymphoblasts that appear to have arisen from a relatively less differentiated B-cell precursor.

Recent information from studies of the molecular biology of T-cell leukemic lymphoblasts indicates that there is also heterogeneity among patients with T-cell disease in the rearrangement and expression of various T-cell receptor genes. The pattern of rearrangement correlates with the stage of T-cell differentiation.

CYTOGENETICS

At least two thirds of children with ALL have recognizable chromosomal abnormalities in their leukemic cells. There is a significant correlation between chromosome number and prognosis. Hyperdiploidy and a modal number greater than 50 appear to be associated with a relatively good prognosis, whereas pseudodiploidy and aneuploidy are associated with a poor prognosis. Using flow cytometry to estimate the leukemia cell chromosome number provides a rapid and useful measurement of ploidy and allows calculation of the DNA index (ratio of the DNA content of the leukemic cells to that of normal diploid cells). A DNA index above 1.16 strongly correlates with favorable outcome. In addition, specific translocations have been identified that place the patient at exceptionally high risk of relapse. These include the

Philadelphia chromosome and the t(1;19), t(4;11), and t(11;14) translocation abnormalities. Ongoing analyses suggest that there are some specific numeric abnormalities, such as the combined trisomies of chromosomes 4 and 10, which are indicative of a favorable outcome.

BIOCHEMISTRY

A variety of enzymatic assays can provide information useful for both the diagnosis and classification of ALL. TdT is not present in mature normal lymphocytes but is found in the lymphoblasts of all but true B-cell ALL, in which its expression varies. TdT expression may help differentiate ALL from acute nonlymphoblastic leukemia (ANLL), where it is rarely detected. The activity of various other enzymes may correlate with cell type and thus prognosis. For example, T-cell lymphoblasts have greater amounts of adenosine deaminase activity and lower 5′-nucleotidase and purine nucleoside phosphorylase activity. It has been suggested that the number of glucocorticoid receptors also has prognostic importance, although it is not clear whether determination of glucocorticoid receptors provides information different from that provided by more conventional prognostic factors.

CLINICAL PROGNOSTIC FACTORS

A variety of clinical features, determined at diagnosis, have prognostic value. The two most important are the white blood cell (WBC) count at diagnosis and the patient's age. Patients with high WBCs at diagnosis (*e.g.*, >50,000/mm^3) have a poor prognosis. Similarly, patients who are either very young (<2 years and particularly <1 year) at diagnosis or older than 10 years of age have a relatively poor prognosis compared with children between 2 and 9 years of age. Other clinical prognostic factors include cytogenetics, sex, race, degree of organomegaly and lymphadenopathy, presence of mediastinal mass, initial hemoglobin, platelet count, FAB classification, immunologic subtype, immunoglobulin levels at diagnosis, the presence or absence of CNS leukemia at diagnosis, and human leukocyte antigen (HLA) type. Many of these variables, however, are dependent rather than independent prognostic factors.

In most centers, patients with poor prognostic features are treated with more aggressive, intensive treatment approaches, whereas patients in the more favorable-risk categories receive therapy designed to be effective but associated with less toxicity. Unfortunately, however, because no single method of risk-group stratification is universally accepted, comparison of treatment results among different centers is difficult. For example, the Children's Cancer Study Group has used an algorithm based on the initial WBC, age at diagnosis, sex, FAB classification, degree of bulk disease, and immunophenotype to assign patients to one of five currently recognized risk groups. In addition to the good, average (intermediate), and high-risk groups (predominantly defined on the basis of initial WBC, age at diagnosis, and FAB morphology), they recognize two additional high-risk groups: those who present with lymphomatous features (the "lymphoma syndrome," characterized by the presence of bulky extramedullary disease), and infants younger than 12 months of age. The latter group of patients has the worst overall prognosis.

The Pediatric Oncology Group primarily uses the leukemic cell immunophenotype to stratify therapy and, within the B-precursor ALL subset, uses age, initial WBC, DNA index, presence or absence of CNS leukemia, and selected translocations to assign risk group. A recent collaborative ALL workshop sponsored by the National Cancer Institute (NCI) promises a standardization of risk hazard assignment parameters among groups and institutions in order to allow comparative analyses.

Treatment

The complexity of the initial workup, the need for appropriate risk-group assignment, and the degree of sophistication and the complexity of the current therapeutic strategies aimed at the various patient risk groups emphasize the importance of having children with ALL treated by a multidisciplinary team of pediatric cancer specialists. Although combination chemotherapy, with or without cranial radiotherapy, remains the primary therapeutic modality, the heterogeneity of ALL makes it inappropriate to define a single "standard" ALL treatment regimen. The basic goals of treatment are to control bone marrow and systemic disease successfully and to prevent relapse in sanctuary sites (*e.g.*, CNS). Treatment is divided into four phases: remission induction, CNS preventive therapy, consolidation, and maintenance therapy.

INDUCTION THERAPY

Using the three-drug regimen of vincristine, prednisone, and L-asparaginase, remission induction can be achieved in over 90% of patients. The addition of a fourth drug, daunorubicin, and even a fifth agent, cyclophosphamide, has been advocated for patients in higher risk groups. Although it is not possible to demonstrate that the addition of these agents increases the percentage of patients achieving remission, there is some indication that the four-drug combination produces longer remission durations.

The rapidity with which patients achieve a complete remission has prognostic significance. Patients who do not achieve a complete remission at the end of the usual 4-week induction period have a poor prognosis: M1 marrow by day 14 is associated with good prognosis.

CENTRAL NERVOUS SYSTEM PREVENTIVE THERAPY

Prior to the use of specific CNS-directed therapy, the meninges were the most common site of initial disease recurrence. Current therapeutic strategies administer specific treatment to the CNS that is designed to prevent CNS leukemia while minimizing toxicity. Identification of factors that place the patient at high or low risk of CNS relapse has led to the concept of tailoring CNS preventive therapy accordingly, using less intensive CNS treatment whenever possible. For example, patients with a good prognosis can be successfully treated without cranial radiotherapy; intrathecal chemotherapy (either methotrexate alone or methotrexate plus cytarabine and hydrocortisone) provides adequate prophylaxis. In contrast, for patients with a high risk of CNS relapse, cranial radiotherapy plus intrathecal methotrexate is commonly used.

The optimal form of CNS preventive therapy for patients in the intermediate-risk (average-risk) group is under study. Despite evidence that 1800 cGy of cranial radiation appears to be as effective as 2400 cGy, concern over the potential long-term toxicity of radiotherapy has prompted a number of studies examining whether cranial radiotherapy can be eliminated from the CNS preventive therapy regimens used to treat this group of patients. Other forms of CNS preventive therapy that may be equally effective include intrathecal chemotherapy alone, intermediate-dose systemic methotrexate with leucovorin rescue plus intrathecal chemotherapy, or high-dose intravenous methotrexate with leucovorin rescue alone.

MAINTENANCE AND CONSOLIDATION THERAPY

Once a complete remission is obtained, additional treatment is required to prevent recurrence. Therapy is usually continued for 2.5 to 3 years, although the optimal length of treatment has not been determined. The drugs typically used for maintenance therapy in good-risk ALL patients include weekly or biweekly methotrexate and daily oral 6-mercaptopurine (6-MP). The addition of intermittent pulses of vincristine and prednisone are also frequently employed. For patients in the higher-risk categories, other drug combinations and schedules have been used during maintenance in addition to 6-MP and methotrexate. Many centers add periodic drug pulses, which include vincristine, corticosteroids, anthracyclines, L-asparaginase, epipodophyllotoxins, cyclophosphamide, cytosine arabinoside, and/or intravenous intermediate- or high-dose methotrexate, in these high-risk patients.

The concept of an “intensive remission consolidation” or “postinduction intensification” has gained popularity and appears to have improved the outcome for higher-risk patients. This approach involves the use of high-dose therapy shortly after remission induction with agents that are unlikely to be cross-resistant with the initial induction regimen. An example of this approach is the West German BFM Study Group, which has obtained prolonged disease-free survival in more than 70% of children, including poor-prognosis patients.

Drug dosage and the route of administration are also important factors in maintenance therapy. Recent pharmacologic studies have shown that bioavailability of orally–administered 6-MP and methotrexate may vary from patient to patient, raising questions about whether maintenance chemotherapy is being optimally delivered with regimens that rely on the oral route. Lack of compliance in taking oral medications may further jeopardize the outcome in older children. In addition to variation in compliance and in bioavailability, there are increasing data to suggest that differences in the leukemic cell metabolism of therapeutic agents correlate with response. Clearly, these issues must be considered in patients who experience relapse on maintenance therapy.

SUPPORTIVE CARE AND MONITORING OF PATIENTS UNDERGOING TREATMENT

A comprehensive system of psychosocial support is essential for both the patient and the family. The need for hospitalization for patients is dictated to a great degree by the intensity of therapy they are receiving. Whereas good-risk patients may be managed largely in an outpatient setting, high-risk patients may require intensive support, including intermittent hospitalization.

Until recently, patients undergoing treatment were followed with periodic bone marrow aspirates to monitor the success of their therapy. This practice has been questioned, and many now restrict bone marrow examination to the time of diagnosis; the time of completion of induction therapy (to document complete remission), when clinically indicated during maintenance; and at the time of completion of chemotherapy. Surveillance for the possibility of CNS relapse, however, requires routine periodic lumbar punctures with cytospin examination, usually on an every 3-month basis.

SUCCESSFUL COMPLETION OF THERAPY

For patients who complete the full 2.5 to 3 years of maintenance chemotherapy without relapse, the overall prognosis is good. With modern therapies, approximately 80% of all children with ALL will fall into this category and 80% of those completing therapy will remain disease-free. The greatest risk of relapse occurs within the first year after therapy has been stopped. In subsequent years, the risk of relapse per year is rapidly reduced, so that 4 years from the time of cessation of chemotherapy, recurrence of disease is extremely unusual. Patients who have successfully completed treatment must, however, be followed periodically. The possibility of adverse late effects, such as CNS dysfunction, abnormal growth and/or reproductive capacity, second malignancies, and other sequelae of chemotherapy and radiotherapy, exists. Although most children who have undergone ALL therapy do not experience problems, the physician caring for these children must be sensitive to the possibility of late effects and should carefully monitor patients accordingly.

TREATMENT FAILURE

Bone Marrow Relapse

Bone marrow relapse is the principal form of treatment failure. The prognosis for the child who suffers a marrow recurrence is related to the timing of relapse. If it occurs either while the patient is receiving chemotherapy or within a year of discontinuation of treatment, the prognosis for long-term survival is exceedingly poor. In contrast, patients who experience a relapse more than 1 year following the discontinuation of initial therapy may be cured when aggressively retreated.

In those patients who suffer a bone marrow recurrence during or shortly after completing therapy and who have an HLA-identical sibling, bone marrow transplantation should be strongly considered. Traditionally, transplantation from an HLA-matched sibling donor has been the most successful approach. Recently, attempts have been made to circumvent the "HLA barrier." A variety of approaches, including matched, unrelated donors (identified through various bone marrow donor registries), partial mismatched related donors, and autologous bone marrow transplantation, using the patient's own marrow "purified" *in vitro* of leukemia cells by drug or monoclonal antibody treatment, are being studied. Some investigators believe that selected high-risk patients, particularly those with chromosomal translocations, might also benefit from bone marrow transplantation during first remission.

Testicular Relapse

The testes are a major site of extramedullary relapse in boys with ALL, and testicular relapse is a frequent cause of late treatment failure. Relapse in the testes frequently heralds bone marrow relapse. Until recently, many centers adopted the policy of performing testicular biopsies either routinely or in high-risk patients (those with a high initial WBC, T-cell disease, prominent lymphadenopathy and splenomegaly, or significant thrombocytopenia), either during or on completion of an apparently successful course of chemotherapy. The value of routine testicular biopsy, however, has been questioned because of its low yield and relatively high incidence of false-negative results.

Confirmation of a testicular relapse requires an aggressive treatment approach. Following bilateral wedge biopsies, patients should receive a minimum of 2400 cGy to both testes. Because of the subsequent increased risk of systemic (*i.e.*, bone marrow) relapse, intensified systemic therapy should also be instituted. This strategy has dramatically improved the prognosis for patients with testicular recurrence.

Central Nervous System Relapse

CNS relapse occurs in approximately 5% to 10% of children with ALL. The choice of treatment for CNS relapse must be guided by the type of CNS preventive therapy the patient received previously. For example, patients who had received CNS prophylaxis without cranial radiotherapy have achieved encouraging results when craniospinal radiotherapy is administered following successful reinduction of a CNS remission with intrathecal chemotherapy. However, for patients who have already received cranial radiotherapy, other approaches have been used, including intrathecal chemotherapy; intraventricular chemotherapy, administered via a surgically implanted Ommaya reservoir; and intraventricular chemotherapy with low-dose craniospinal radiotherapy. As in the case of testicular relapse, the frequent occurrence of bone marrow relapse following the development of overt CNS disease requires intensification of the systemic chemotherapy.

ACUTE MYELOID LEUKEMIA

Acute myeloid leukemia (AML) represents approximately 25% of cases of acute leukemia in childhood. As in ALL, the signs and symptoms present at diagnosis reflect a decrease in normal hematopoietic precursors and/or infiltration of other organs by leukemic cells. Anemia, thrombocytopenia, neutropenia, and infection are frequently seen at presentation. Hepatosplenomegaly is present in approximately half of the patients; lymphadenopathy is less common. Chloromas (localized soft-tissue leukemic masses) may be present, although they rarely develop as the first sign of leukemia. When present, they may involve the orbit, skin, spinal cord, or other tissues. CNS leukemia at presentation occurs with a frequency of 5% to 20%. CNS disease is more common in patients with M4 or M5 subtypes of AML. Coagulation abnormalities, which occur not infrequently in AML, are most common in patients with acute promyelocytic leukemia (the M3 subtype of AML).

Pretreatment Evaluation

It is not possible to distinguish between AML and ALL on clinical grounds alone. Examination of the bone marrow by using special stains (*e.g.*, myeloperoxidase) and enzyme studies (*e.g.*, TdT) as well as myeloid-specific monoclonal antibodies will help confirm the diagnosis. Cytogenetics should be performed. Abnormal karyotypes have been seen in over three quarters of the cases of children with AML, and with improving techniques, it is likely that virtually all patients with AML will be shown to have some karyotypic abnormality. Certain karyotypic abnormalities are associated with particular subtypes of AML. For example, the t(15;17) abnormality is more common in acute promyelocytic leukemia, and the t(8;21) is associated with M2 disease (acute myelogenous leukemia with differentiation). The −5, 5q−, and −7 abnormalities are seen more frequently in adults than in children and suggest a pre-existing myelodysplastic syndrome. In contrast, t(11q) and +19 are seen more frequently in children.

Following confirmation of the diagnosis, patients should begin therapy as soon as their clinical condition is stabilized. As in childhood ALL, appropriate hydration, alkalinization, and administration of allopurinol is indicated. The presence of severe anemia or bleeding requires appropriate transfusion support. The presence of disseminated intravascular coagulation (DIC) at presentation in a patient with acute promyelocytic leukemia may be an indication for administration of heparin.

In addition to hydration, leukapheresis or exchange transfusion may be required in patients with very high WBC counts (*i.e.*, >200,000/mm^3) to prevent the metabolic or hemorrhagic complications of hyperleukocytosis. Once therapy is initiated, careful attention must be paid to the possibility of the tumor lysis syndrome and its attendant metabolic complications.

Classification

Approximately 50% to 70% of children with AML are classified as having acute myelocytic leukemia; approximately 30% have acute monocytic leukemia. The FAB system has classified AML into seven subtypes, as outlined in Table 45–1.

The M5 subtype is particularly common in children less than 2 years of age. Both M5a (acute monoblastic leukemia) and M5b (acute monocytic leukemia) subcategories have a less favorable prognosis. Among other FAB subtypes, the responses to treatment appear to be similar. Not surprisingly, serum and urine levels of muramidase are highest in patients with the M4 and M5 subtypes. Patients with M6 disease may have extremely high levels of fetal hemoglobin.

TABLE 45–1. FAB SYSTEM OF CLASSIFYING ACUTE MYELOID LEUKEMIA

FAB CLASS	COMMON NAME
M1	Acute myelocytic leukemia without differentiation
M2	Acute myelocytic leukemia with differentiation
M3	Acute promyelocytic leukemia
M4	Acute myelomonocytic leukemia
M5	Acute monocytic leukemia
M6	Erythroleukemia
M7	Megakaryoblastic leukemia

FAB = French-American-British

Prognosis

Information regarding the influence of factors such as age, sex, and WBC on prognosis has been conflicting. Children less than 1 year of age at the time of diagnosis and those with a high WBC (>20,000/mm^3) are in a distinctly unfavorable prognostic group for the attainment of complete remission. The initial WBC, age at diagnosis, and FAB classification all have some prognostic value in terms of remission duration. Children between the ages of 3 to 10 years have the best prognosis; those with high WBCs (particularly >100,000/mm^3) are in a highly unfavorable prognostic group. The very poor prognosis observed in patients less than 2 years of age may be due to the fact that the M4 and M5 FAB categories are observed more frequently in these children. Unlike acute lymphocytic leukemia, the presence of CNS leukemia at diagnosis does not adversely affect prognosis. The chromosomal abnormalities (t8;21) and inv(16) confer a favorable prognosis. In contrast, deletions of chromosomes 5 and 7 are associated with poorer prognosis.

Treatment (Induction Therapy)

Children with AML have a better prognosis than adults. The progress in childhood AML, however, has not matched that in childhood ALL. The most effective regimens for remission induction include cytarabine together with an anthracycline (usually daunorubicin) either in a two-drug combination or together with additional drugs, including prednisone, vincristine, 6-thioguanine, or 5-azacytidine. Drug doses must be sufficiently high to induce profound marrow aplasia. As a consequence, the risk of morbidity and mortality following the initiation of therapy is not insignificant. With the most frequently used induction regimen, a 7-day continuous infusion of cytarabine plus 3 days of an anthracycline, approximately 70% to 85% of children with AML achieve a complete remission.

Central Nervous System Preventive Therapy

It has been suggested that the rate of occurrence of CNS leukemia in AML is similar to that in children with ALL. However, the actual incidence of CNS disease is lower, perhaps as a result of the shorter survival time of children with AML. Several studies have indicated that CNS preventive therapy is effective, and many centers use some form of CNS preventive therapy, including intrathecal chemotherapy with methotrexate or cytarabine, or cranial radiotherapy plus intrathecal chemotherapy.

Maintenance Therapy

Traditionally, consolidation and maintenance therapy is routinely used in childhood AML. A variety of strategies have been applied; the duration of treatment in most studies is approximately 2 years. One particularly effective regimen, from the Dana Farber Cancer Institute uses repetitive intensive pulses of therapy with combinations of several agents (including doxorubicin, cytosine arabinoside, 5-azacytidine, vincristine, methylprednisolone, 6-MP, and methotrexate). This monitoring approach has been associated with an improved (greater than 50%) predicted 3-year continuous complete remission rate.

Despite these results, however, conclusive data on the necessity for maintenance therapy in childhood AML do not exist. Recent results suggest that, as in the case of adult AML, if an intensive consolidation treatment is administered after initial remission is induced, further maintenance therapy may be unnecessary. This has recently been demonstrated by using intensive consolidation therapy with short courses of high-dose cytosine arabinoside.

Bone Marrow Transplantation During First Remission

Many centers recommend bone marrow transplantation for patients with AML who have achieved an initial complete remission and have an appropriate histocompatible sibling donor. Approximately 55% to 60% of children over 2 years of age who have received bone marrow transplants during first remission are surviving free of leukemia. The results of a recent randomized trial performed to test the value of bone marrow transplantation compared with conventional AML maintenance chemotherapy indicate some benefit for patients who received an allogeneic matched transplant. Although these results are encouraging, only approximately one third of patients have eligible histocompatible siblings. Another approach is autologous transplantation of remission bone marrow purged *in vitro* with chemotherapy (4-hydroperoxycyclophosphamide) or monoclonal antibodies. Recent studies suggest that survival after autologous transplantation in a first complete remission approximates the survival after allogeneic transplantation.

NON-HODGKIN'S LYMPHOMA

Optimal therapy for children with non-Hodgkin's lymphoma (NHL) requires knowledge of the cell type and extent of disease. For treatment purposes, NHL in children is often divided into lymphoblastic lymphomas and nonlymphoblastic lymphomas. In children, the non-Hodgkin's lymphomas are best considered a systemic disease, even when the clinical assessment reveals only localized involvement.

Patients with lymphoblastic lymphomas most commonly present with a mediastinal mass and often pleural effusions. If lymphadenopathy is present, it is likely to be located above the diaphragm — in the neck, the supraclavicular regions, or the axillae. These tumors, unlike nonlymphoblastic lymphomas, express TdT and most often have a T-cell phenotype corresponding to intermediate (CD7, CD5, CD2, CD1, CD4, and CD8) or late thymic compartments (CD7, CD2, CD3, and either CD4 or CD8). Only rare lymphoblastic lymphomas express the phenotype of pre-B cells as seen in acute lymphoblastic leukemia (*i.e.*, CD19, usually with common ALL antigen but without surface immunoglobulin).

Patients with nonlymphoblastic lymphomas almost always present with abdominal tumor. Lymphadenopathy is uncommon but if present, is likely to be inguinal or iliac in distribution. Nonlymphoblastic lymphomas are almost always of B-cell phenotype and express surface immunoglobulin, CD19, CD20, and HLA-DR, but are TdT-negative.

The distinction between lymphoblastic and nonlymphoblastic lymphomas can be made histologically in most cases, but phenotypic markers provide useful confirmation.

Pretreatment Evaluation

Adequate material is essential to establish the diagnosis. Wherever possible, tissue examination should include histology, immunophenotyping, and cytogenetics. It is important to determine the status of the patient's renal function promptly, because with extensive tumor burdens, uric acid nephropathy is frequently present and may require correction before chemotherapy is initiated. Allopurinol should be given to all patients. Imaging studies should include a chest film and computed tomographic (CT) scans and/or ultrasonography of the abdomen and chest. The gallium scan is a useful screening test for nonlymphoblastic lymphomas but is less helpful in lymphoblastic lymphomas. Bone scans rarely demonstrate tumor that is not detected by gallium scans. The bone marrow and cerebrospinal fluid (CSF) should also be examined. Other studies are indicated according to the patient's presenting signs and symptoms (*e.g.*, head magnetic resonance imaging [MRI] for cranial nerve abnormalities, or MRI or myelography for those with back pain or motor loss).

Staging Systems

Staging systems in childhood NHL predominantly reflect the tumor volume. There are several systems in use: the most widely used is the St. Jude staging system (Table 45–2). This system is applicable to all histologic types of childhood lymphoma and separates patients with limited-stage disease (one or two masses on one side of the diaphragm) from those with extensive intrathoracic or intra-abdominal disease. Patients with bone marrow involvement or CNS disease are separated into the worst prognostic group. Recently, it has been shown that as prognostic determinants, biochemical markers, such as lactate dehydrogenase (LDH) and interleukin-2 receptors, are as good as or better than clinical stage in patients with nonlymphoblastic lymphomas, probably because they more accurately reflect tumor burden.

Treatment

Patients with limited disease (Stage I or II by the St. Jude staging system; see Table 45–2) do not need treatment of the same intensity as those with intra-abdominal or intrathoracic disease and in most protocols achieve a long-term survival in excess of 90%. Results from the Children's Cancer Study Group (CCSG) do not show a clear advantage of the LSA_2-L_2 program vs. cyclophosphamide, vincristine (Oncovin), methotrexate, and prednisone (COMP) in limited-stage patients, although the COMP regimen may be less effective for lymphoblastic lymphoma. In nonlymphoblastic lymphomas, a high proportion of patients with limited disease are patients in whom all tumor has been removed surgically (Stage AR [intra-abdominal tumor with >90% of tumor surgically resected] in the NCI staging system, Stage II in the St. Jude system). Such patients are currently treated with as few as two cycles of therapy.

The most widely used chemotherapy regimens for patients with extensive lymphoblastic lymphomas are based on protocols designed for ALL, but not all such protocols are equally satisfactory. Anthracyclines are contained in the most successful drug combinations, including the German Cooperative Group protocol, the Memorial Sloan-Kettering LSA_2-L_2 protocol, and the Dana Farber's doxorubicin (Adriamycin), prednisone, vincristine (APO) regimen. The LSA_2-L_2 protocol as used by the CCSG gives a long-term survival rate of approximately 60% to 65% for patients with extensive disease. A recent report in which this protocol was supplemented with 10 administrations of high-dose methotrexate produced an event-free survival rate of 80%. Highly similar results have been reported for the German BFM protocol. The NCI regimen of alternating cycles of cyclophosphamide, doxorubicin [Adriamycin], vincristine, and prednisone (CHOP) and 42-hour methotrexate infusions, although not based on ALL therapy, has also been successful for patients with extensive lymphoblastic lymphoma, except for those in whom the bone marrow is involved. The APO protocol is also much less effective in patients with bone marrow involvement.

"Leukemia-like" regimens are generally suboptimal for the treatment of nonlymphoblastic lymphomas. Several protocols using cyclic cyclophosphamide-containing combinations have been shown to be highly effective in such patients. In several recent clinical trials, event-free survival rates of between 80% and 90% have been obtained, even for patients with the more extensive diseases, including the "B-cell ALL (L3)."

Regimens for both lymphoblastic and nonlymphoblastic lymphomas should include prophylactic treatment against CNS involvement with intrathecal cytarabine and methotrexate. There is no evidence that cranial irradiation is necessary in addition to intrathecal chemotherapy in nonlymphoblastic lymphomas.

TABLE 45–2. STAGING SCHEME OF ST. JUDE CHILDREN'S RESEARCH HOSPITAL FOR NON-HODGKIN'S LYMPHOMA

Stage I	A single tumor (extranodal) or single anatomical area (nodal), with the exclusion of mediastinum or abdomen
Stage II	A single tumor (extranodal) with regional node involvement Two or more nodal areas on the same side of the diaphragm Two single (extranodal) tumors with or without regional node involvement on the same side of the diaphragm A primary gastrointestinal tract tumor, usually in the ileocecal area, with or without involvement of associated mesenteric nodes only, grossly completely resected
Stage III	Two single tumors (extranodal) on opposite sides of the diaphragm Two or more nodal areas above and below the diaphragm All of the primary intrathoracic tumors (mediastinal, pleural, thymic) All extensive primary intra-abdominal disease All paraspinal or epidural tumors, regardless of other tumor sites
Stage IV	Any of the above with initial CNS or bone marrow involvement (<25%)

Monitoring of Response and Toxicity

During therapy, tumor response should be monitored by using the same imaging studies that were used to establish the extent of disease at presentation. These should be repeated monthly until complete remission is established. Toxicity is monitored by twice-weekly blood counts and weekly liver and renal function tests. Patients with nonlymphoblastic lymphomas are at risk of relapse in the first year from diagnosis (predominantly in the first 6 months), unlike those with lymphoblastic lymphomas who are at greatest risk in the first 24 to 30 months after diagnosis.

HODGKIN'S DISEASE

Treatment considerations for Hodgkin's disease are quite different from those for NHL. In the child, the toxicity of radiotherapy is much greater than in the adult, largely because of the effect of radiation on growing tissues, whether soft tissue or bone. Possible toxicities include short stature, hypoplasia of breasts and clavicles, hypothyroidism and thyroid neoplasia, pericardial fibrosis, radiation pneumonitis, azoospermia, and second malignancies. Accordingly, there has been a much greater effort to limit irradiation of children, and, as a consequence, to emphasize chemotherapy (although the latter is not without long-term effects, particularly azoospermia).

The use of chemotherapy means that exhaustive staging procedures are unwarranted. For example, the role of a staging laparotomy with splenectomy is of questionable value when the patient is going to receive chemotherapy, regardless of the result. Although there is a greater acceptance of combined-modality therapy in children than in adults, some still advocate surgical staging and radiotherapy in Stages I to IIIA in adolescents, accepting the higher relapse rate encountered with this approach on the grounds that salvage with chemotherapy is effective. This approach certainly exposes fewer patients to combined-modality treatment, but there is evidence that less than half of all patients who experience relapse achieve cure, so that this may ultimately prove to be an unacceptable approach. An increasingly explored alternative is the use of chemotherapy alone, because it remains to be shown that irradiation of bulk disease adds to the therapeutic efficacy of chemotherapy.

Pretreatment Evaluation

Physical examination of the patient is paramount in determining the extent of peripheral lymph node involvement, the presence of hepatosplenomegaly, and the involvement of the skin. A chest film to determine the presence of mediastinal involvement (a chest CT scan will provide more precision but is not mandatory), lymphangiography, and a CT scan of the abdomen to detect intra-abdominal disease—particularly para-aortic node involvement—should be performed. Bilateral bone marrow aspiration and biopsy should also be done. Liver biopsy is often done, although it is not mandatory. Further staging procedures depend on the treatment approach to be used. If radiotherapy alone is being considered, a staging laparotomy is performed. In patients with high cervical lesions, particularly on the right, the incidence of cryptic abdominal disease is so uncommon that laparotomy may be unnecessary, even if radiotherapy alone is to be used.

Staging System

The same staging system is used in adults and children (see Chap. 41). All stages are subdivided into A or B, according to the presence of systemic features of fever, night sweats, or weight loss of more than 10%.

Treatment

Combined-modality therapy (with nitrogen Mustard, vincristine [Oncovin], Procarbazine, and Prednisone [MOPP], doxorubicin [Adriamycin], bleomycin, vinblastine, and dacarbazine [ABVD], or alternating MOPP-ABVD) is recommended for children with Hodgkin's disease, although the results of involved-field radiotherapy alone in patients with localized upper neck disease are so good that this subgroup of patients is usually treated without chemotherapy. When chemotherapy is the primary treatment modality, radiotherapy can be much more limited and confined to only the site(s) of known disease (involved-field radiotherapy). Treatment according to stage of disease at diagnosis is described in the following sections.

EARLY STAGE (IA TO IIB)

In recent trials in which children were clinically staged with lymphangiography but without initial laparotomy, actuarial disease-free survival at 5 to 12 years in Stages IA to IIB was 88% to 91% after three to six cycles of MOPP chemotherapy and radiotherapy that ranged from a limited field to total nodal. Similar results were obtained in patients receiving chlorambucil, vinblastine, procarbazine, and prednisone combination with irradiation of initial bulk disease. No advantage was demonstrated for patients with early-stage disease who received six vs. three cycles of MOPP or who had limited, compared with more extensive, fields of radiation. Thus, laparotomy can clearly be omitted from staging without affecting long-term treatment outcome; when combined modality therapy is used in early stage disease. It is recommended that radiation be confined to the involved field.

Equally good survival has been reported for surgically staged patients treated with extended-field radiotherapy, but a higher relapse rate and the requirement for "salvage" chemotherapy in as many as 25% of patients must be expected. Radiotherapy alone would normally be used for Stages IA to IB only in patients who have achieved full growth. Only two trials have been reported in which chemotherapy has been used alone, but an overall survival of between 75% and 90% in early-stage disease has been observed.

Patients with massive mediastinal involvement occupying more than one third of the largest diameter of the chest) are treated with radiotherapy to the mediastinum after chemotherapy with an appropriate combination drug regimen. Half (*e.g.*, three cycles) or all of the chemotherapy may be given before radiotherapy.

STAGE IIIA

Patients with clinical Stage IIIA Hodgkin's disease have a significantly improved disease-free survival if treated with combined-modality therapy. This applies particularly to patients with extensive abdominal involvement (in surgically staged patients, involvement beyond the upper para-aortic nodes and spleen, including the iliac nodes [Stage IIIA2]). Recently, randomized trials comparing chemotherapy alone to chemotherapy plus radiotherapy in adults have not shown an advantage to the addition of radiotherapy. Similar data are not available in children.

STAGES IIIB AND IV

The primary treatment modality for Stages IIIB and IV is chemotherapy, although some investigators have included subsequent irradiation to sites of bulk disease. There is no clear evidence that local irradiation is of benefit, and no chemotherapy regimens have been shown to be definitely more effective than MOPP, although MOPP-ABVD or ABVD alone may be less toxic. Newer regimens that include an epipodophyllotoxin show promise, but the risk of secondary leukemia with such regimens needs to be assessed before they can be recommended. The dose intensity of the drugs delivered appears to be critical to the success of treatment. Survival rates in the range of 60% to 90% have been observed.

Toxicity

It is clear that excellent results can be achieved in childhood Hodgkin's disease. Because of this, much attention has been paid to the long-term effects of therapy. Combined-modality therapy increases the incidence of infections, both bacterial and fungal, and herpes zoster occurs in a high proportion (over 50%) of children. Azoospermia and the risk for developing a second malignancy are also worrisome complications. Thyroid neoplasia may occur in as many as 5% of patients 11 years following treatment. Secondary AML occurs at a rate of approximately 1% per year in patients who have received combined-modality therapy, and secondary NHL is only slightly lower in frequency. Splenectomy has recently been shown to increase the risk of secondary leukemia, an additional reason to avoid staging laparotomy when possible. These complications have prompted the evaluation of alternative chemotherapy programs (*e.g.*, ABVD).

WILMS' TUMOR

Wilms' tumor (nephroblastoma) is the most frequent renal malignancy in children, with approximately 500 new cases diagnosed yearly in the United States. It is a disease of early childhood, being infrequently seen beyond 7 years of age: the median age is 3.5 years. With integrated interdisciplinary treatment, Wilms' tumor has the best prognosis of the common childhood malignancies. The multidisciplinary approach to the successful therapy of this illness, as employed by investigators of the National Wilms' Tumor Study (NWTS) group, has resulted in a major success story in oncology.

Wilms' tumor generally presents as an upper abdominal mass, which may be accompanied by pain, micro- or macroscopic hematuria, hypertension, or fever, or may be asymptomatic. Additional abnormalities occasionally seen in these children include genitourinary anomalies, aniridia, and/or hemihypertrophy. The flank mass is typically firm and smooth, may extend across the midline, and may be bilateral. Metastases are noted at diagnosis in approximately 10% to 15% of patients and are most frequently pulmonary, although hepatic metastases also occur. Metastases to other sites are uncommon for Wilms' tumor but do occur for other childhood renal tumors, *e.g.*, bone and brain metastases in clear cell sarcoma of the kidney, and brain metastases in rhabdoid tumor of the kidney.

Pretreatment Evaluation

The major goals of the pretreatment evaluation are to confirm the diagnosis, to gather information that will assist the surgeon in planning the operative procedure, to elucidate the degree of systemic spread, and to obtain pertinent baseline values. The initial history should document the occurrence of cancer, especially Wilms' tumor, and congenital anomalies in family members. Duration of abdominal swelling and/or pain and the presence of hematuria should be ascertained. Bone or joint pain may indicate metastatic spread to bone.

Physical examination should include the patient's blood pressure, abdominal girth, whether the abdominal mass is unilateral or bilateral, liver and spleen size, and whether there is evidence of congenital anomalies (*e.g.*, aniridia, hemihypertrophy, genitourinary malfunctions). Routine laboratory studies include a complete blood count, blood urea nitrogen, creatinine, alanine aminotransferase, alkaline phosphatase, prothrombin time and partial thromboplastin time, and fibrinogen. Hypercalcemia may be observed in infants with rhabdoid tumor of the kidney or with mesoblastic nephroma. Urinalysis (noting the presence or absence of protein and white or red blood cells), urine vanillylmandelic acid/homovanillic acid (VMA/HVA) evaluation, and electrocardiography and echocardiography (if doxorubicin administration is anticipated) should be done.

Radiographic evaluation should include a plain film of the abdomen, abdominal CT, abdominal ultrasonography (to detect tumor foci in the contralateral kidney and tumor thrombi in the inferior vena cava or right atrium), and plain films of the chest. CT scans of the chest may detect small pulmonary metastases not recognized on plain films, but the prognostic significance of these small lesions is not clear. Excretory urograms may be requested at some institutions to assist the treating radiotherapist in defining treatment portals. Patients found at surgery to have clear cell sarcoma of the kidney should have a skeletal survey and CT (or MRI) of the brain. Patients found to have malignant rhabdoid tumor should have CT (or MRI) of the brain.

Staging

The most widely used method of staging is that developed by the NWTS group. Assignment of stage is based on the surgically determined extent of disease and the presence or absence of unfavorable (anaplastic or sarcomatous) histologic features (*e.g.*, Stage I, favorable histology or Stage III, unfavorable histology) (Table 45–3)

Treatment

Children with Wilms' tumor must be evaluated and treated by a multidisciplinary team of surgeons, pediatric oncologists, radiotherapists, radiologists, and pathologists because outcome may be compromised when treatment is attempted by caregivers who have limited experience with the tumor. Because of the relative rarity of this illness, every effort should be made to enter patients into organized clinical trials.

Ordinarily, treatment begins with an exploratory laparotomy using a transabdominal, transperitoneal approach for adequate exposure. The contralateral kidney is mobilized, palpated, and visualized, and the abdominal cavity is explored for metastases. Suspicious lymph nodes are excised, but routine nodal dissection is not recommended. The liver is inspected, and suspicious areas are biopsied. Radical nephrectomy is performed while avoiding rupture of the tumor capsule, with removal of the tumor, uninvolved kidney, hilum, a long section of ureter, and structures adherent due to tumor invasion. However, extraordinary attempts to remove all traces of tumor are not recommended. Unresected tumor is biopsied, and the margins of dissection and residual disease are marked with titanium clips.

Postsurgical therapy is determined by clinicopathologic stage and by histology. The therapies outlined in the paragraphs below are the "standard" arms of NWTS-4. Infants younger than 12 months of age should receive one half of the recommended dose of all chemotherapy agents, since excessive toxicity is observed when full doses are used. Also, diffuse anaplasia, clear cell sarcoma of the kidney, and rhabdoid tumor of the kidney are associated with poorer prognosis (with the exception of Stage I tumors with diffuse anaplasia). Patients with diffuse anaplasia Stages II to V should receive a four-drug regimen that includes cyclophosphamide in addition to vincristine, dactinomycin, and doxorubicin. Patients with clear cell sarcoma of the kidney benefit from a three-drug regimen that includes doxorubicin. Satisfactory treatment of rhabdoid tumor of the kidney has not been defined.

TABLE 45–3. STAGING OF WILMS' TUMOR

Stage I	Tumor is limited to the kidney and is completely excised; the surface of the renal capsule is intact; tumor is not ruptured before or during removal; there is no residual tumor apparent beyond the margins of resection
Stage II	The tumor extends beyond the kidney but is completely excised; there is regional extension of the tumor (*i.e.*, penetration through the outer surface of the renal capsule into perirenal soft tissues); vessels outside the kidney are infiltrated or contain tumor thrombus; the tumor may have been biopsied, or there has been local spillage of tumor confined to the flank; there is no residual tumor apparent at or beyond the margins of excision
Stage III	There is residual nonhematogenous tumor confined to the abdomen; any one or more of the following may occur: 1. The lymph nodes are found to be involved in the hilus, the para-aortic chains, or beyond 2. There has been diffuse peritoneal contamination by tumor such as by spillage of tumor beyond the flank before or during the surgery or by tumor growth that has penetrated through the peritoneal surface 3. Implants are found on the peritoneal surfaces 4. Gross or microscopic tumor remains postoperatively (*e.g.*, tumor cells are found at the surgical margin on microscopy of the specimen) 5. The tumor is not completely resectable because of local infiltration into vital structures
Stage IV	There are hematogenous metastases (*e.g.*, lung, liver, bone, or brain)
Stage V	There is bilateral renal involvement at diagnosis

STAGE I—FAVORABLE HISTOLOGY

Dactinomycin and vincristine are begun postoperatively and continued for 24 weeks. Radiotherapy is not given to Stage I patients.

STAGE II—FAVORABLE HISTOLOGY

Dactinomycin and vincristine are begun postoperatively and are administered over a 65-week period. Radiotherapy is not administered.

STAGE III—FAVORABLE HISTOLOGY

In addition to dactinomycin and vincristine, Stage III patients also receive doxorubicin (Adriamycin). Cycles of chemotherapy should continue over a 15-month period. Stage III patients should also receive radiotherapy, beginning no later than the ninth postoperative day, to the tumor bed with boosts to areas of residual disease that measure 3 cm or more in maximum diameter. The initial field is extended across the midline to include the relevant vertebral bodies (avoiding the contralateral kidney) to minimize the likelihood of scoliosis. Total abdominal radiotherapy is used when there has been preoperative tumor rupture, intraoperative tumor spillage, or diffuse peritoneal involvement.

STAGE IV—FAVORABLE HISTOLOGY; STAGES I TO IV, CLEAR CELL SARCOMA

The chemotherapy for these patients is similar to that for Stage III patients with favorable histology. Radiotherapy of the abdomen is given to all clear cell sarcoma patients, regardless of stage, and is given to Stage IV favorable histology patients if their primary tumor has Stage III characteristics. Radiotherapy is omitted for favorable-histology patients if the primary tumor has Stage I or II characteristics. Metastases are irradiated according to organ tolerance. Whole-lung radiotherapy should be accompanied by prophylactic trimethoprim-sulfamethoxazole for a total of 150 days.

STAGE V

The patient with bilateral tumor should be approached with curative intent. Resection of tumors is attempted only when sufficient uninvolved renal parenchyma will remain. Typically, bilateral biopsies are obtained, and postoperative chemotherapy with dactinomycin and vincristine is employed to reduce tumor bulk with the goal of making renal parenchyma-sparing surgery possible. If there is insufficient tumor shrinkage in response to two-drug therapy, then doxorubicin may be added. Second-look laparotomy is performed when renal parenchyma-sparing surgery appears feasible. Postlaparotomy chemotherapy depends on the tumor's response to the initial vincristine and dactinomycin treatment. Patients with good response to these two drugs continue to receive these agents, whereas patients with less satisfactory response also receive doxorubicin.

PATIENTS WITH INOPERABLE TUMORS

Wilms' tumors deemed unresectable by the surgeon can usually be removed following chemotherapy designed to reduce the bulk of the tumor. Such patients can be treated with chemotherapy as per Stage III patients and then re-evaluated for tumor shrinkage. Radiotherapy with weekly vincristine may be given if no tumor shrinkage occurs in response to initial chemotherapy. Excision should be undertaken once sufficient shrinkage has been documented (often within 6 weeks of diagnosis). Because of the significant error rate in the preoperative diagnosis of renal masses after roentgenographic assessment alone, biopsy should be obtained before preoperative chemotherapy is instituted. Postexcisional chemotherapy and radiotherapy should be similar to those for Stage III favorable-histology patients.

OBSERVATIONS DURING AND FOLLOWING THERAPY

Complete blood counts and liver and renal function tests should be performed regularly during therapy. Hematologic toxicity should be closely monitored during radiotherapy and for 2 to 3 weeks following actinomycin D or doxorubicin therapy. Severe hepatotoxicity in the early weeks of therapy when patients are receiving actinomycin D and weekly vincristine has occurred in 3% to 4% of patients treated on the NWTS-4 protocol, which emphasizes the need for careful monitoring of hepatic function. For patients without lung metastases at diagnosis, chest radiographs should initially be performed every 3 months and subsequently tapered to annual studies. Patients with lung metastases at diagnosis initially have more frequent chest radiographs to document complete response of metastatic disease. Abdominal imaging is annually performed for evaluation of the remaining kidney. Patients with metastatic disease at other sites (*e.g.*, bone, liver, brain) should have regular imaging of these areas. X-ray films of bones included in the radiation fields are appropriate yearly until full growth is attained, and then every 5 years indefinitely (because of the risk of malignant second tumors).

NEUROBLASTOMA

Neuroblastoma is the most frequently occurring solid tumor outside of the CNS in infants and children. It occurs primarily in the first decade of life. The majority of children, particularly those older than 2 years of age, have disseminated disease at diagnosis. Caucasian children are affected more often than African-American children.

Neuroblastoma originates from the neural crest and therefore can be found at any site of sympathetic nervous tissue. The most frequent sites of primary tumor involvement are the abdomen (the adrenal gland in particular) and the chest (*i.e.*, the posterior mediastinum). Metastatic involvement usually includes spread to regional lymph nodes and distant spread to bone marrow, bone, liver, and skin.

Among the most common presenting symptoms are general malaise, fatigue, weight loss, abdominal enlargement, difficulty in ambulation, diarrhea, and/or malabsorption syndrome. Physical examination may reveal an abdominal mass or symptoms associated with extension of paraspinous lesions (paresis, paralysis). Cervicothoracic primary tumors may be seen with Horner's syndrome, heterochromia iridis, and periorbital ecchymosis with or without proptosis.

Pretreatment Evaluation

The initial workup should include a careful history and thorough physical examination with specific attention to neurologic parameters. A complete blood count and bone marrow examination are necessary. Essential radiographic studies include a chest film, abdominal film, bone scan, and chest and abdominal CT scans to determine the extent of disease. A meta-idobenzylguanidine (MIBG) scan is often helpful. If neurologic symptoms or findings are present, plain films of the spine, MRI of the spine or myelography, and a CT scan of the head are obtained. Elevation of VMA and HVA in a 24-hour or spot urine collection is helpful in establishing the diagnosis and can be used to follow tumor regression or recurrence. However, normal levels of urinary catechols do not rule out the diagnosis of neuroblastoma. Elevations of serum ferritin and serum neuron-specific enolase suggest a poor prognosis, as does multiple N-myc copy number within tumor cells.

Biopsy of the primary lesion or an involved lymph node is warranted to establish the diagnosis when total resection of the primary lesion is not possible. It is imperative to obtain adequate tissue to allow appropriate tumor biological examinations to be performed. Determinations of N-myc gene copy number and tumor cell DNA content or ploidy are prognostic variables that are essential for defining appropriate therapeutic interventions.

Staging System

Several staging systems for neuroblastoma are currently in use. The Children's Cancer Study Group, St. Jude's, and Pediatric Oncology Group staging systems are based on clinical or surgical findings. Based on a retrospective analysis, Shimada and coworkers have recently introduced a staging system that is based on a pathologic classification in which the histologic pattern is correlated with survival.[1]

A new International Neuroblastoma Staging System has been proposed as an international standard. This system, which categorizes patients based on radiographic, surgical, and bone marrow findings, is outlined in Table 45–4.

TABLE 45–4. INTERNATIONAL NEUROBLASTOMA STAGING SYSTEM

Stage I	Localized tumor with complete gross excision, with or without microscopic residual disease; representative ipsilateral lymph nodes negative for tumor microscopically (nodes attached to and removed with the primary tumor may be positive)
Stage IIA	Localized tumor with incomplete gross excision; representative ipsilateral nonadherent lymph nodes negative for tumor microscopically
Stage IIB	Localized tumor with or without complete gross excision, with ipsilateral nonadherent lymph nodes positive for tumor; enlarged contralateral lymph nodes must be negative microscopically
Stage III	Unresectable unilateral tumor infiltrating across the midline with or without regional lymph node involvement; or localized unilateral tumor with contralateral regional lymph node involvement; or midline tumor with bilateral extension by infiltration (unresectable) or by lymph node involvement
Stage IV	Any primary tumor with dissemination of tumor to distant lymph nodes, bone, bone marrow, liver, skin, and/or other organs (except as defined for Stage IVS)
Stage IVS	Localized primary tumor (as defined for Stage I, IIA, or IIB), with dissemination limited to skin, liver, and/or bone marrow (<10% tumor cells, and MIBG scan negative in the marrow); limited to infants <1 year of age.

MIBG = metaiodobenzylguanidine.

Treatment

The treatment of children with neuroblastoma involves a multimodality approach that depends on prognostic variables such as age, stage of disease, N-myc gene copy number, and tumor cell ploidy. Because neuroblastoma is rare, all newly diagnosed patients must be enrolled in organized clinical trials if an impact is to be made on treatment outcome.

Therapy for Stage I patients is surgery only. Stages II and III patients should receive chemotherapy when the tumor is only partially resected. The current role of radiotherapy is under study. Treatment for Stage IV patients involves aggressive chemotherapy (usually with a combination of cyclophosphamide, doxorubicin, cisplatin, and etoposide [VP-16]) along with surgery where appropriate. Investigational treatment protocols involve intensive combination chemotherapy with various agents and high-dose chemotherapy and radiotherapy with bone marrow transplant rescue.

The overall prognosis for survival depends on the prognostic variables mentioned previously. Children under the age of 12 months have an excellent prognosis for survival. However, older children with advanced-stage disease have a very poor prognosis.

BRAIN TUMORS

Brain tumors are the most common solid tumors of childhood, with an annual incidence of approximately 25 new cases per million in the United States (see also Chap. 38). However, childhood brain tumors are quite diverse, and the incidence of individual histologic subtypes is relatively low.

The clinical presentation can vary widely and depends on the location of the tumor as well as on the histologic type and age of the patient. In contrast to brain tumors in adults, 50% to 60% of childhood brain tumors arise in the posterior fossa. Increased intracranial pressure resulting from an enlarging tumor mass or obstruction to the flow of CSF results in generalized symptoms including headache, vomiting, lethargy, and irritability. Other common presenting complaints include ataxia, gait disturbances, behavioral changes, diplopia, vertigo, hemiparesis, seizures, and head tilt.

Although the disease outcome varies with the histologic type and location, overall the prognosis is poor. In most cases, both morbidity and mortality are the result of local progression of the disease. On the other hand, medulloblastoma and, to a lesser extent, ependymoma and glioblastoma can metastasize within the neuraxis, with spinal and subarachnoid seeding of tumor. Extraneural spread is less common, although children account for 40% of reported cases. Medulloblastoma, for example, can metastasize to bone (producing blastic or lytic lesions) and bone marrow. Spread of tumor via ventricular shunts can occur. Permanent shunting should be avoided when possible.

Pretreatment Evaluation

The CT and MRI scans are sensitive and accurate techniques for demonstrating the presence of a brain tumor and defining its anatomical location. MRI is more sensitive for tumors of the posterior fossa and brain stem.

CT myelography or spinal MRI with contrast, and CSF cytology (when safe to obtain) are indicated to rule out seeding of the tumor along the spinal axis in children with medulloblastoma, ependymoma, germ cell tumor, and malignant glioma. Spread within the neuraxis is estimated to occur in 40% of children with malignant brain tumors. Bone marrow examination and a bone scan are useful for the detection of extraneural metastases in medulloblastoma and other primitive neuroectodermal tumors (PNET).

Follow-up studies for children with brain tumors should include repeated neurologic examinations, CT or MRI scans, and CSF cytology and spinal cord imaging for tumors capable of subarachnoid metastasis. Imaging of the primary tumor should be done postoperatively, before other therapy is instituted.

Staging System

There are currently no generally accepted staging systems for the various childhood brain tumors. Current protocols define risk groups based on the extent of disease and surgical resection.

Treatment

Surgical resection is the initial therapy for most childhood brain tumors. Complete resection is difficult to attain, because wide excisions may permanently impair neurologic function. However, gross total tumor removal appears to improve survival. Radiotherapy is used as an adjunct to surgery in patients with malignant, incompletely resected, or inoperable tumors. It is also useful for the treatment or prevention of tumor spread within the neuraxis. The role of chemotherapy in the treatment of childhood brain tumors is growing. Studies evaluating the efficacy of chemotherapy are being conducted in most types of tumors. All patients deserve to be considered for treatment on protocols available through the pediatric cooperative groups (*e.g.* Children's Cancer Study Group, Pediatric Oncology Group) or single centers. Specific therapies and outcomes for the more common types of childhood brain tumors are discussed below.

MEDULLOBLASTOMA

The goals of surgery for medulloblastoma are relief of obstruction to the flow of CSF and gross total resection of the tumor if possible. All patients should also receive craniospinal radiotherapy. Radiation doses of 3500 cGy to the whole brain, 5500 cGy to the posterior fossa, and 3500 cGy to the spinal axis are standard. The 5-year survival rate with this therapy is approximately 50%.

Patients with disease confined to the posterior fossa have a better prognosis. Most patients who experience recurrence do so within the first 2 years. Recurrence at the site of the primary tumor accounts for 70% of failures. Subarachnoid spread occurs in 20% of patients, and extraneural spread occurs in 5% to 10%.

The role of chemotherapy in the treatment of medulloblastoma is being studied. A number of agents have produced responses in patients with recurrent disease, including the nitrosoureas, procarbazine, vincristine, cyclophosphamide, cisplatin, methotrexate, aziridinyl benzoquinone, and dibromodulcitol. The use of adjuvant chemotherapy with lomustine (CCNU) and vincristine with or without prednisone following standard surgery and radiotherapy yielded an overall increase in disease-free survival in higher-risk patients. Patients with more extensive local tumor (subtotal resection or biopsy) may benefit most from chemotherapy. Studies within the cooperative groups are currently evaluating more aggressive therapy for high-risk patients and the optimal sequencing of chemotherapy and radiotherapy. Whenever possible, newly diagnosed patients should be referred to a center participating in these studies.

CEREBELLAR ASTROCYTOMAS

Astrocytomas of the cerebellum are usually low grade and are cystic in nature, presenting as a mural nodule. Surgical removal is the primary treatment, and the prognosis following resection is excellent (90–95%). The survival rate with complete excision is reported to be virtually 100%, and with partial resection, 79%. Histologic features of these lesions have prognostic significance. The more common juvenile type has an excellent prognosis (94%), compared with the diffuse type (38%). Recurrences usually occur within 2 to 5 years of surgery in patients with incompletely resected tumors or with the diffuse histologic subtype. Radiotherapy is usually reserved for the patient with progressive, unresectable disease. Chemotherapy has no role in the adjuvant setting, and experience in treating recurrent disease is extremely limited.

SUPRATENTORIAL ASTROCYTOMAS

Both low-grade (Stages I and II) and high-grade (Stages III and IV) astrocytomas occur supratentorially. The prognosis appears to be inversely related to the grade. Surgical resection is the primary mode of therapy for low-grade astrocytomas. As with cerebellar astrocytomas, the prognosis is relatively good, with 80% of patients (ages 0 to 19 years) surviving 5 years. Radiotherapy is generally deferred in patients with completely resected lesions. Local radiation has been recommended in patients with incompletely resected tumors. The recurrences are almost all local and can occur many years after the initial treatment.

The conventional treatment for high-grade astrocytomas (malignant astrocytoma and glioblastoma multiforme) has been the maximal surgical resection that is technically feasible, followed by high doses of radiation (5500 cGy). Randomized trials in adults have also shown a benefit from whole-brain irradiation. However, the outcome with this therapy has been poor, with a 5-year survival of less than 20%.

Chemotherapy has been studied in patients with high-grade lesions. Few agents, however, have demonstrated activity, and chemotherapy has been palliative at best. The alkylating agents appear to be the most active of the agents studied. In children, a clinical trial of adjuvant chemotherapy with CCNU, vincristine, and prednisone in high-grade lesions (Stages III and IV) yielded disease-free survival (in patients treated with chemotherapy) of approximately 45%, compared with 11% for those receiving radiotherapy alone. No other studies support that degree of benefit from chemotherapy. Clinical trials of new chemotherapeutic agents are under way.

BRAIN STEM GLIOMAS

The majority of brain stem tumors are high-grade astrocytomas, and they tend to be infiltrating lesions. The diagnosis is usually based on clinical and radiologic features. MRI is the most useful diagnostic test. Surgery has been reserved for exophytic or cystic lesions. A benefit of surgery in patients with cervicomedullary lesions has been recently suggested. Conventional therapy includes local high-dose radiotherapy (5000–6000 cGy). The prognosis is poor, with less than a 20% survival rate. Delivery of higher-dose hyperfractionated radiotherapy may be of benefit. A number of studies are addressing the role of chemotherapy in this disease, but it has not yet been shown to be of benefit.

EPENDYMOMAS

Althoug these tumors occur anywhere along the neuraxis, they are most commonly seen in the posterior fossa. Subarachnoid seeding occurs in approximately 10% of patients. Surgery is the initial mode of treatment, followed by radiotherapy. A gross total surgical resection may result in a significantly improved likelihood of survival. There is controversy as to the volume of CNS to irradiate because of the tendency of this tumor to seed CSF pathways. Local radiotherapy is generally used for low-grade supratentorial lesions, and craniospinal radiotherapy for the higher-grade posterior fossa lesions. Studies are under way to determine the need for craniospinal radiotherapy in low-grade posterior fossa lesions and high-grade supratentorial lesions. Adjuvant chemotherapy has not been adequately tested. Drugs that have demonstrated activity in patients with recurrent disease include nitrosoureas, cyclophosphamide, and cisplatin. This tumor tends to progress slowly, and the long-term prognosis is poor, with 5- and 10-year survivals of 45% and 35%, respectively. Clinical trials are exploring the roles of chemotherapy and hyperfractionated radiotherapy.

CRANIOPHARYNGIOMA

There is controversy over the relative merits of primary surgery or radiotherapy. Subtotal excision and local radiotherapy are advocated by some. Five-year survival of 80% can be achieved with combination therapy. Half of the patients treated with surgery alone experience recurrence and require radiotherapy. Endocrinopathies resulting from tumor growth or treatment may require hormone replacement therapy.

BRAIN TUMORS IN THE VERY YOUNG CHILD

Historically children less than 3 to 4 years old who develop brain tumors do poorly with conventional therapy. The developing CNS is highly susceptible to damage by radiotherapy. Recent studies have demonstrated the feasibility of primary chemotherapy to delay or avoid CNS irradiation. Overall progression-free survival at 2 years with chemotherapy alone is approximately 40%. Ongoing collaborative group studies are investigating new chemotherapy regimens to delay or avoid radiotherapy.

LATE SIDE-EFFECTS OF TREATMENT

Of major concern is the long-term effect of high doses of radiation on brain function in children. Intellectual deterioration as measured by lowered IQ and learning disabilities is not uncommon. Leukoencephalopathy may also occur. In addition, the incidence of endocrine abnormalities may be high. Chemotherapy may lead to hearing loss, second malignancies, and sterility. Methotrexate can increase the neurotoxicity of radiation.

OSTEOSARCOMA

Bone tumors account for approximately 5% of the tumors that occur in children (see also Chap. 33). Osteosarcoma is the most common of the pediatric bone tumors, arising most often in the femur, humerus, and tibia. The lung is the most frequent site of metastatic spread, although bones, lymph nodes, and CNS may also be involved. If the tumor arises in the bones of the extremity, the primary tumor can usually be removed surgically. However, if surgery is the only modality employed, at least 80% of patients can be expected to develop subsequent metastatic disease. Therefore, adjuvant chemotherapy is indicated.

Pretreatment Evaluation

Prior to starting therapy, evaluation of the lungs (by chest radiograph and CT scan) and the bones (by radionuclide scan) is necessary to determine the presence of metastatic disease. Evaluation of the primary site of involvement might include a CT scan, MRI, and arteriography, particularly if a limb-sparing procedure is contemplated.

Staging

There is no universally accepted staging system for osteosarcoma, and patients are considered as having either local disease (albeit with probably micrometastatic spread) or overt metastatic involvement. For treatment planning, most investigators also distinguish between patients whose primary site of tumor can be surgically removed and those whose tumor cannot. Serum LDH and alkaline phosphatase levels have prognostic significance.

Treatment

Standard treatment of patients without overt evidence of metastatic osteosarcoma includes both surgical extirpation of the primary tumor and adjuvant chemotherapy. The two most commonly used surgical approaches are amputation and resection of the tumor while sparing the limb. Limb-sparing surgery is performed whenever possible. If the primary disease is unresectable, radiotherapy in combination with chemotherapy may be used to control the primary lesion. This most commonly applies to patients with pelvic primary tumors.

Three approaches have been used for systemic therapy of patients with osteosarcoma: (1) postsurgical adjuvant chemotherapy, (2) presurgical chemotherapy (or "neoadjuvant") followed by surgery and then postsurgical adjuvant chemotherapy, and (3) presurgical neoadjuvant chemotherapy followed by an assessment of the response of the primary tumor both clinically *and* pathologically to the preoperative chemotherapy. The response to the neoadjuvant therapy (including a pathologic grading of the response) is then used to tailor the subsequent *postoperative* therapy. In addition to these three approaches, intra-arterial chemotherapy with cisplatin to achieve local tumor control has been investigated in pilot studies.

The chemotherapy regimens most commonly used include high-dose methotrexate (12 g/m^2 over 4 hours), and doxorubicin and cisplatin (given either together or separately). More than 80% of patients not receiving adjuvant chemotherapy eventually develop metastasis, compared with approximately 40% of patients who received chemotherapy. The long-term outcome of most trials that have used systemic chemotherapy have demonstrated a long-term disease-free survival of more than 60%. Recently, ifosfamide was demonstrated to be active in osteosarcoma. Its role is being studied in the next generation of adjuvant chemotherapy protocols.

The primary toxicities of these regimens are the acute toxicities of myelosupression, nephrotoxicity, and hearing loss. Late effects of therapy must always be considered in relation to pediatric cancers and their treatment.

The optimal management of metastatic disease in the lungs either at the time of initial diagnosis or subsequently requires surgery, usually with the addition of a systemic chemotherapy regimen. However, long-term surgical control is limited to patients with a limited number of pulmonary nodules (generally fewer than six). Multiple surgical procedures may be necessary to control pulmonary disease. Patients have been cured after as many as six procedures.

EWING'S SARCOMA/PERIPHERAL PRIMITIVE NEUROECTODERMAL TUMOR

Ewing's sarcoma, the second most common bone tumor in children and young adults, most often arises in the bones of the pelvis, femur, humerus, and ribs, although other sites may be involved as well. Ewing's sarcoma is of neural (parasympathetic) origin. Closer examination of these tumors with newer techniques has led to the diagnosis of peripheral neuroepithelioma being made more frequently. These tumors are considered related to Ewing's sarcoma and generally are treated as such. The most common sites of metastatic spread are the lungs, bones, and bone marrow; rarely, the CNS may be involved. Lymph nodes are usually not involved. If systemic therapy is not employed, more than 90% of patients can be expected eventually to develop metastases.

The location and extent of disease at diagnosis are the most important prognostic features in Ewing's sarcoma. Patients who have central axis or pelvic primary tumors or who present with evidence of metastases have a poorer prognosis than patients with tumor limited to an extremity. Histologic features are not generally of prognostic significance.

Pretreatment Evaluation

The extent of the primary tumor should be determined by CT and/or MRI. Serum LDH should be measured before therapy. In addition, sites of possible metastatic spread should be evaluated by chest radiograph and CT scan, radionuclide bone scan, and bone marrow aspirate and biopsy.

Staging

There is no universally accepted system of staging Ewing's sarcoma beyond division of patients into those with metastatic disease at diagnosis and those without it. However, patients can also be stratified into low- and high-risk groups according to the site of the primary disease (pelvic and proximal lesions faring worse and considered to be high-risk) and size of the primary tumor.

Treatment

Standard treatment of patients with nonmetastatic Ewing's sarcoma includes both eradication of the primary tumor and adjuvant chemotherapy. The most common approach to the primary tumor is with radiotherapy, usually more than 5000 to 6000 cGy over a 6-week period with 180- to 200-cGy fractions, using a shrinking-field technique. Surgical extirpation may be considered when the primary tumor involves an expendable bone (*e.g.*, fibula), especially in younger patients, and may replace or limit radiotherapy.

The adjuvant therapy of patients with Ewing's sarcoma usually consists of combination chemotherapy with vincristine, cyclophosphamide, and doxorubicin in two- or three-drug combinations. Dactinomycin is included in some protocols as continuation therapy. Ifosfamide and etoposide with sodium 2-mercaptoethase sulfonate (MESNA) uroprotection are being evaluated in treatment protocols. Complete remission can be achieved in up to 90% of patients with Ewing's sarcoma, but the duration of remission is related to whether the patient has low- or high-risk prognostic features. Accordingly, the intensity and length of therapy have varied according to the patient's prognostic factors. With multimodal therapy, the outcome for low-risk patients has improved so that more than 60% will be free of disease 5 years after completion of therapy.

The treatment of patients who have evidence of metastatic disease is generally similar to that of patients without metastatic disease. Patients who have evidence of metastases at the time of diagnosis have fared more poorly on both standard chemotherapy regimens and on very intensive regimens that have included high-dose chemotherapy, total-body irradiation, and autologous bone marrow reconstitution. Even with such an approach, less than 20% of those with metastatic disease can be expected to be disease-free at long-term follow-up. The need for radiotherapy to manage metastatic lesions is unknown.

The major toxicities encountered with these therapies are myelosuppression and the potential for long-term organ toxicity (*e.g.*, nephrotoxicity and cardiotoxicity). The incidence of long-term complications referable to the primary tumor site is also notable, either because of destruction of bone by tumor or because surgical biopsy or radiotherapy has violated the integrity of the bone. Pathologic fractures, abnormal extremity function, and secondary tumors occur frequently enough that future protocols will need to address ways to reduce these complications.

SOFT-TISSUE SARCOMAS

Rhabdomyosarcoma, the most common soft-tissue sarcoma in childhood, occurs most often in the head and neck region but may arise in virtually any site in the body (see also Chap. 33). The two main histologic subtypes are embryonal and alveolar, the alveolar histologic usually carrying a worse prognosis. The most common site of metastatic spread is the lung, although bones, lymph nodes, and bone marrow are also commonly involved.

Cytogenetic studies have provided biological confirmation of the clinicopathologic distinction between alveolar and embryonal subtypes of this tumor. A specific chromosomal translocation has been identified in alveolar rhabdomyosarcoma between band q 35 on chromosome 2 and band q 14 on chromosome 13 t(2;13) (q 35; q 14). The breakpoint has now been molecularly cloned, and PCR can be used for the identification of this specific translocation. Embryonal rhabdomyosarcomas have been shown to have loss of heterozygosity at 11p15, a compelling finding when coupled with the genetic linkage of 11p15 to Beckwith-Wiedemann syndrome that is known to lead to an increased risk of rhabdomyosarcoma.

Pretreatment Evaluation

Before initiation of therapy, a search for systemic spread is essential, because treatment is based on the stage, site, and histology of the tumor. The lungs are evaluated by chest radiograph and CT scan, the bones by radionuclide scan, the bone marrow by iliac crest aspiration and biopsy, and the lymph nodes by lymphangiography, CT scan, or biopsy, depending on primary tumor site and histology.

Staging

The staging system for rhabdomyosarcoma is currently evolving. Traditionally staging relied on a postsurgical grouping of patients: Group I refers to patients whose tumors have been completely resected; Group II refers to patients whose tumors have been grossly resected but with microscopic residual disease; Group III refers to patients whose tumors have gross residual disease after surgery; and Group IV refers to patients whose tumors may be of any size, but metastatic disease is present. The problem with this staging system is the reliance on a surgeon's expertise rather than intrinsic biological properties of the tumor. A presurgical staging system is being evaluated by the current Intergroup Rhabdomyosarcoma Study (IRS) study; it uses a modified TNM staging system and emphasizes the importance of site in the overall prognosis of patients.

Previous recommendations included whole-brain resolution as CNS prophylaxis in patients with tumors adjacent to the meninges. However, recent data suggest that with careful CT-guided radiotherapy, CNS prophylaxis is not necessary.

Treatment

Standard management of rhabdomyosarcoma includes therapy directed toward the primary tumor with surgery and/or radiotherapy and systemic chemotherapy. The choice of which modality to use to treat the primary tumor depends on a variety of factors, including the site and extent of the disease and the age of the child. When radiotherapy is required, standard fractionation is usually used. Hyperfractionation and brachytherapy are under investigation. Dose and volume are also related to a number of factors, but in general, 5000 to 6000 cGy is necessary for effective control.

Surgical extirpation of small tumors is usually preferred in order to avoid or limit the amount of radiation administered to a child. On the other hand, surgical resection of large tumors, or tumors in sites that require loss of function, has been replaced in many instances by radiotherapy.

The systemic therapy of patients with rhabdomyosarcoma is related to stage and postsurgical grouping, site of disease, and histology. The most commonly used agents are vincristine, usually on an initial weekly schedule; dactinomycin, on either a 1- or a 5-day schedule; and cyclophosphamide. Other agents that have activity in rhabdomyosarcoma and are being studied in the treatment of higher stages of disease are doxorubicin, etoposide, melphalan, and ifosfamide.

Local therapy is related to the extent of residual tumor after resection. If there is no evidence of microscopic residual disease following surgery, local radiotherapy is not necessary. In those with residual tumor, radiotherapy should be administered.

In addition to designating therapy according to the stage of disease, the site of tumor primary represents an additional consideration, as described in the following discussions.

HEAD AND NECK RHABDOMYOSARCOMA

The orbit and parameningeal sites (nasopharynx, sinuses, middle ear, pterygopalatine, and infratemporal fossae) are the most common. These lesions are usually inaccessible to surgical resection, and radiotherapy is the primary modality for local tumor control. Because patients with parameningeal primary tumors are at risk for contiguous tumor extension into the CNS, extended-field radiotherapy has been recommended, which, for some patients, includes CNS prophylaxis.

Patients with orbital tumors, on the other hand, have an excellent prognosis, and local radiotherapy together with two-drug (vincristine and actinomycin) adjuvant therapy results in a more than 90% disease-free state at 3 years.

EXTREMITY RHABDOMYOSARCOMA

These tumors occur predominantly in adolescents and are more likely to have alveolar histology. Amputation is not advocated. Patients with resectable disease should receive postoperative therapy unless they have been rendered clinical Stage (Group) I by surgery. Adjuvant chemotherapy should be administered to all patients.

GENITOURINARY RHABDOMYOSARCOMA

Nearly 20% of pediatric rhabdomyosarcomas arise in the genitourinary tract; the major sites are the prostate, bladder, vagina, and paratesticular regions. Aggressive surgical resection is not advocated, and chemotherapy has been used to reduce bulk disease as an alternative to surgery. Radiotherapy should be administered, and all patients should receive adjuvant treatment. For patients with paratesticular primary tumors, the para-aortic lymph nodes should be included in the radiation field unless lymphangiogram and node biopsy results are negative.

The major toxicities of this treatment are related to the myelosuppression caused by the chemotherapy. The presently ongoing protocols are attempting to reduce the morbidity of surgery (*i.e.*, avoidance of pelvic exenteration) while maintaining a high cure rate.

NONRHABDOMYOSARCOMATOUS SOFT-TISSUE SARCOMAS

Treatment of nonrhabdomyosarcomatous soft-tissue sarcoma (*e.g.*, synovial cell sarcoma, mesenchymal sarcoma, hemangiopericytomas) is usually related to histology, site, age of patient, and extent of disease. The most common sites of metastatic disease are the lung and lymph node, but other sites may be involved. The primary management is usually surgical, and the extent of surgery is again related to many clinical factors. Of prime importance is complete resection of the lesions. Radiotherapy may be required if complete surgical extirpation is not ensured; however, this is again related to histology and patient age.

The role of chemotherapy, usually a doxorubicin- and cyclophosphamide-based regimen, has not yet clearly been established. Some adult trials have suggested a benefit from adjuvant chemotherapy for extremity soft-tissue sarcomas; however, whether this information can be correctly applied to all children and adolescents with all subtypes of soft-tissue sarcomas in all sites is not yet clear.

The prognosis carried by most localized and resectable tumors is very good. The prognosis carried by most unresectable or metastatic tumors is poor.

REFERENCE

1. Shimada H et al. Histopathologic prognostic factors in neuroblastic tumors: definition of subtypes of ganglioneuroblastoma and an age-linked classification of neuroblastomas. J Natl Cancer Inst. 73:405, 1984

John S. Macdonald, Daniel G. Haller, Robert J. Mayer, Eds. *Manual of Oncologic Therapeutics*, Third Edition.

V. REGIONAL THERAPY FOR METASTATIC DISEASE

46. CARCINOMATOUS MENINGITIS

David R. Macdonald

Diffuse infiltration of the leptomeninges (leptomeningeal metastases, carcinomatous meningitis) is a well-known problem in acute leukemias and non-Hodgkin's lymphomas and is an increasingly common complication of solid tumors, especially carcinomas of the lung and breast and melanoma. Untreated, carcinomatous meningitis is, with rare exception, a rapidly progressive, fatal neurologic illness. Mild headache, subtle mental and behavioral change, and minor low back or extremity pain are followed within weeks by stupor, multiple asymmetric cranial neuropathies, flaccid areflexic quadraparesis, and incontinence. Early diagnosis is essential if major disability is to be averted. This requires a high index of suspicion and a willingness to investigate thoroughly any seemingly minor neurologic symptoms in cancer patients. Early diagnosis is emphasized because of the limited ability of the nervous system to recover from, or compensate for, significant injury. Following a normal enhanced computed tomographic (CT) scan, the spinal fluid should be examined for malignant cells in any cancer patient with unexplained behavioral or cognitive change, persistent headache, cranial neuropathy, radicular pain in the extremities, persistent low back pain, sphincter disturbance, or unexplained loss of deep tendon reflexes, particularly if asymmetric.

DIAGNOSIS

Carcinomatous meningitis is clinically suspected when neurologic symptoms and signs point to involvement of more than one level of the neuraxis. A careful, detailed neurologic history and examination are important in cancer patients with new neurologic symptoms because the clinical features and findings of early carcinomatous meningitis may be subtle. Neuroradiologic investigations, such as contrast-enhanced CT brain scan, gadolinium-enhanced magnetic resonance imaging (MRI) of the brain, gadolinium-enhanced MRI of the spine, or myelography may strongly suggest the diagnosis of carcinomatous meningitis. Radiologic findings strongly suspicious for carcinomatous meningitis include hydrocephalus, contrast enhancement of the basal cisterns, cortical sulci, or tentorium, obliteration of the basal cisterns or cortical sulci, multiple small, enhancing cortical nodules, diffuse or focal thickening or enhancement of spinal nerve roots, especially the cauda equina, and multiple small, enhancing subarachnoid spinal nodules. Irregular filling of the subarachnoid space due to thickening and nodularity of nerve roots, sometimes causing a spinal subarachnoid block, are the typical myelographic features of carcinomatous meningitis. Gadolinium-enhanced MRI is probably more sensitive than CT or myelography in demonstrating leptomeningeal metastases. Carcinomatous meningitis may also be present in patients with brain or spinal metastases. A CT scan or MRI of the brain should be done in any patient with cancer and neurologic symptoms possibly referable to the brain, before a lumbar puncture is performed, to exclude intracranial mass lesions, or obstructive hydrocephalus that would make a lumbar puncture hazardous. In addition, thrombocytopenia or a coagulopathy should be excluded before a lumbar puncture is performed, particularly in patients who have recently received chemotherapy.

The single most important diagnostic test is careful examination of the cerebrospinal fluid (CSF). In patients with neoplastic meningitis the CSF is virtually always abnormal in some respect; typical CSF findings include some or all of the following: elevated pressure, lymphocytic pleocytosis, increased protein, and decreased glucose. These changes are nonspecific; it is the presence of malignant cells in the spinal fluid that establishes the diagnosis. False-positive cytologic findings are rare. Reactive lymphocytes are occasionally mistaken for malignant cells. False-negative results are common even when the clinical picture is highly characteristic of carcinomatous meningitis. At times, repeated examinations of the CSF fail to reveal malignant cells, even when leptomeningeal tumor is ultimately identified at autopsy. The initial CSF examination reveals malignant cells in only 50% to 60% of patients with carcinomatous meningitis, and in many patients multiple samples must be analyzed to establish the diagnosis. Carcinomatous meningitis is unlikely if the CSF is totally normal, but it is not excluded by a single negative cytology result. Some false-negative cytology results are undoubtedly the result of improper handling of CSF specimens. Whenever possible, the spinal fluid should be promptly delivered to a forewarned cytology laboratory. At night and on weekends the CSF should be "fixed" by adding an equal volume of 50% alcohol before sending the specimen to the laboratory. Provided the lumbar CSF is examined on multiple occasions and large volumes of fluid are sent for analysis, there is little advantage in routinely sampling the cisternal fluid; however, cisternal CSF is sometimes abnormal when the lumbar CSF is negative for malignant cells. Patients with Ommaya reservoirs or ventriculoperitoneal shunts may have no malignant cells in the ventricular fluid but may have positive cytology results in the lumbar CSF, or sometimes vice versa.

Because carcinomatous meningitis is usually rapidly progressive, it may be unwise to delay treatment for an extended period while awaiting the unequivocal identification of malignant cells in the spinal fluid. If the clinical findings strongly suggest leptomeningeal metastases, then relatively nonspecific spinal fluid abnormalities, such as an elevated protein or depressed glucose, should lead one to make the diagnosis and institute treatment. If the clinical features are not diagnostic, then the physician should demand other supportive evidence of carcinomatous meningitis before beginning treatment — ideally, a positive CSF cytology result. If the CSF cytology results are repeatedly negative, circumstantial evidence of neoplastic meningitis may be provided by CT scan, MRI, myelography, or analysis of CSF markers. Elevated levels of beta-glucuronidase, carcinoembryonic antigen, lactate dehydrogenase isoenzymes, beta$_2$-microglobulin, beta-human chorionic gonadotropin, and alpha-fetoprotein may be of diagnostic value in selected cases. Flow cytometry of CSF may be useful in leukemic or lymphomatous meningitis in evaluating a monoclonal lymphocytic infiltrate.

TREATMENT

Early diagnosis is vitally important because stabilization is a more realistic expectation of treatment than is a dramatic neurologic improvement. Current treatment is usually not curative and is considerably more effective for leukemia, lymphoma, and carcinoma of the breast than for other tumor types. Adrenocorticosteroid hormones, radiation therapy, and intrathecal or intraventricular chemotherapy, in varying combinations, may be highly effective in some patients.

Steroids (*e.g.*, dexamethasone, 4 mg four times daily) may promptly relieve headaches, vomiting, drowsiness, and back pain, but they rarely reverse cranial neuropathies or paraparesis. Steroids may also help minimize acute side-effects due to cranial radiation therapy and intraventricular chemotherapy. There is no evidence that steroids significantly alter the disease process or prolong survival. For patients with malignant meningitis, radiation therapy may be the single most effective treatment modality. It is recommended for symptomatic areas (*i.e.*, brain, basal meninges, cauda equina) and areas of bulky disease. In patients for whom there is no effective systemic chemotherapy, a strong case can be made for whole-neuraxis radiation therapy as the sole treatment. However, neuraxis radiation therapy is not considered standard because it may produce severe bone marrow depression in heavily pretreated patients and may substantially limit future systemic chemotherapy in those for whom this is an option.

Lumbar intrathecal or intraventricular instillation of chemotherapeutic agents is required to deliver adequate concentrations of medication to the CSF. Only a few cytotoxic drugs can be used safely. Methotrexate is considered by many to be the drug of choice, it is usually given in a dose of 7 mg/m^2 to children, or a fixed dose of 10 to 15 mg in adults. Headache, nausea, vomiting, fever, meningeal signs, and confusion have been reported following intraventricular or intrathecal administration of methotrexate, and are probably due to a chemical meningitis. Transient and permanent paraplegia and acute fatal meningoencephalopathy are rare complications of treatment. Repeated administration of methotrexate may be associated with a delayed leukoencephalopathy. The risk of leukoencephalopathy is substantially increased in patients who have had previous cranial radiation therapy or high-dose systemic methotrexate, or in those who have had an intraventricular injection in the presence of obstructive hydrocephalus.

Methotrexate may occasionally escape into the systemic circulation, causing severe mucositis and profound myelosuppression. To guard against systemic toxicities, oral folinic acid (*e.g.*, 10 mg orally twice a day for 3 days, beginning 12 hours after treatment) should be given. Complete blood counts should be checked periodically in patients receiving intrathecal or intraventricular methotrexate, and treatment should be withheld or delayed if the peripheral white blood cell count is less than 3000/mm^3 (absolute neutrophil count <1000/mm^3) or the platelet count is less than 100,000/mm^3.

Cytarabine (cytosine arabinoside, ara-C) has a narrower spectrum of antitumor activity (usually effective only against leukemia or lymphoma) and is not recommended as initial treatment for most patients with carcinomatous meningitis. The usual dose for intraventricular or intrathecal use is 30 to 50 mg/m^2 (or a fixed dose of 50 to 100 mg). Myelosuppression and acute or delayed neurotoxicity have been reported. Thiotepa has been demonstrated to have activity against meningeal leukemia, lymphoma, and solid tumors; the usual dose is 10 to 15 mg. Myelosuppression and neurotoxicity may occur. Methotrexate, cytarabine, and thiotepa have been used in varying combinations. Combination therapy is more toxic, and there is no evidence that it is substantially more effective than single-agent therapy. High-dose systemic chemotherapy with methotrexate, cytarabine, or thiotepa is occasionally useful in patients with leukemic or lymphomatous meningitis.

Several new, experimental chemotherapeutic agents are under development for intrathecal use in carcinomatous meningitis: nimustine, a water-soluble nitrosourea (ACNU), DTC 101 (an extended-release form of cytarabine encapsulated in DepoFoam, microscopic spherical particles containing numerous nonconcentric aqueous chambers bounded by a single bilayer lipid membrane), diaziquone, 4-hydroperoxycyclophosphamide (mafosfamide, a pre-activated cyclophosphamide derivative), and radiolabeled monoclonal antibodies. These experimental agents show promise in animal and human trials, but their efficacy and toxicity must be determined by more extensive testing. New agents are required because existing chemotherapeutic agents for intrathecal use have limited effectiveness in many patients.

Treatments are given twice weekly until neurologic symptoms and signs stabilize or diminish, and malignant cells begin to be cleared from the CSF. Following initial improvement, treatments are given weekly on an outpatient basis. If improvement is maintained, the treatment interval may be lengthened to biweekly or monthly. (The frequency of treatments in patients who respond is somewhat arbitrary; there are no firm guidelines.) Response is determined by stabilization or abatement of clinical signs and symptoms, reduction of number or elimination of malignant cells from the CSF, normalization of CSF protein or glucose levels, or reduction of previously elevated levels of CSF markers. Progressive symptoms or signs and lack of improvement in CSF parameters within 1 month of starting intrathecal treatment usually implies failure (or development of a complication, such as hydrocephalus). Continued treatment with the same agent is seldom beneficial, and a new treatment approach should be considered. If clinical improvement and improvement in CSF parameters are observed — even if the CSF cytology results remain positive for malignant cells — treatment should continue, provided there are no unacceptable complications. Quantitative CSF cytopathology analysis may show a reduction in the number of malignant cells as a sign of response.

Chemotherapeutic agents for intrathecal use must be *preservative-free* and must be diluted in preservative-free solutions. Many of the transient and irreversible complications of intrathecal chemotherapy have been linked to preservatives in bacteriostatic diluents. Many chemotherapeutic agents (such as vincristine or doxorubicin) are lethal when injected into the CSF. The physician must be extraordinarily careful in mixing medications, and there must be adequate supervision of junior and inexperienced staff when intraventricular and intrathecal chemotherapeutic agents are given.

Until arrangements can be made for placement of an Ommaya reservoir, chemotherapy is given by the lumbar intrathecal route (by lumbar puncture). Intraventricular instillation is the preferred means of drug delivery because chemotherapy injected by the lumbar route may be inadvertently delivered to the subdural or epidural space, repeated lumbar punctures are often uncomfortable for the patient and technically difficult for the physician, and intraventricular instillation provides more uniform distribution of drug in the subarachnoid space. Scanning of the neuraxis following the injection of a radioisotope into the Ommaya reservoir is a simple means of ascertaining that the catheter tip is properly positioned in the lateral ventricle, that there is no obstruction to CSF outflow from the ventricular system, that CSF flows over the cerebral hemispheres, and that isotope is delivered to the entire spinal subarachnoid space. A substantial number of patients with carcinomatous meningitis have CSF flow disturbances, a knowledge of which may be important in treatment planning.

Hydrocephalus in patients with carcinomatous meningitis poses special problems. Management must be individualized and is influenced by a variety of factors, including the type of hydrocephalus (communicating vs. noncommunicating) and the need for ventricular drainage or shunting. Radiation therapy may relieve ventricular obstruction, thereby normalizing CSF flow, but frequently it does not. If a ventriculoperitoneal shunt is required, an on-off valve and reservoir should be included in the system. Chemotherapy planning (*i.e.*, route, dose, frequency) may be facilitated by visualizing CSF flow patterns after both lumbar and intraventricular injections of radionuclide. Spinal subarachnoid blockage to CSF flow may be relieved by focal irradiation. As a general rule, chemotherapeutic agents should not be injected into the ventricular system when there is evidence of outflow obstruction (*i.e.*, noncommunicating or obstructive hydrocephalus).

The treatment of carcinomatous meningitis is difficult and often ineffective. Up to 75% of patients with meningeal leukemia or lymphoma and 60% of patients with carcinomatous meningitis from breast cancer or small cell carcinoma of the lung will stabilize or improve with treatment. However, responses are often short-lived, especially for solid tumors, and many solid tumors fail to respond at all. Safe, effective central nervous system prophylaxis, improved methods for early diagnosis, and more effective chemotherapeutic agents are needed. The incidence of carcinomatous meningitis can be expected to increase as the effectiveness of treatment for systemic cancer improves and as patients survive longer, only to develop late complications of metastatic disease.

BIBLIOGRAPHY

Berg SL, Balis FM, Zimm S et al. Phase I/II trial and pharmacokinetics of intrathecal diaziquone in refractory meningeal malignancies. J Clin Oncol 10:143–148,1992

Chamberlain MC, Corey-Bloom J. Leptomeningeal metastases: ^{111}Indium-DTPA CSF flow studies. Neurology 41:1765–1769, 1991

Chamberlain MC, Sandy AD, Press GA. Leptomeningeal metastasis: A comparison of gadolinium-enhanced MR and contrast-enhanced CT of the brain. Neurology 40:435–438, 1990

Giannone L, Greco FA, Hainsworth JD. Combination intraventricular chemotherapy for meningeal neoplasia. J Clin Oncol 4:68–73, 1986

Grossman SA, Finkelstein DM, Ruckdeschel JC et al. Randomized prospective comparison of intraventricular methotrexate and thiotepa in patients with previously untreated neoplastic meningitis. J Clin Oncol 11:561–569, 1993

Grossman SA, Trump DL, Chen DCP et al. Cerebrospinal fluid flow abnormalities in patients with neoplastic meningitis. Am J Med 73:641–647, 1982

Jaeckle KA, Krol G, Posner JB. Evolution of computed tomographic abnormalities in leptomeningeal metastases. Ann Neurol 17:85–89, 1985

Kim S, Chatelut E, Kim JC et al. Extended CSF cytarabine exposure following intrathecal administration of DTC101. J Clin Oncol11:2186–2193, 1993

Kochi M, Kuratsu J, Mihara Y, et al. Ventriculolumbar perfusion of 3-[(4-amino-2-methyl-5-pyrimidinyl) methyl]-1-(2-chloroethyl)-1-nitrosourea hydrochloride. Neurosurgery 33: 817–823, 1993

Olson ME, Chernik NL, Posner JB. Infiltration of the leptomeninges by systemic cancer: A clinical and pathologic study. Arch Neurol 30: 122–137, 1974

Phillips PC, Than TT, Cork LC et al. Intrathecal 4-hydroperoxycyclophosphamide: Neurotoxicity, cerebrospinal fluid pharmacokinetics, and antitumor activity in a rabbit model of VX2 leptomeningeal carcinomatosis. Cancer Res 52: 6168–6174, 1992

Rogers LR, Duchesneau PM, Nunez C et al. Comparison of cisternal and lumbar CSF examination in leptomeningeal metastasis. Neurology 42: 1239–1241, 1992

Russak V, Kim S, Chamberlain MC. Quantitative cerebrospinal fluid cytology in patients receiving intracavitary chemotherapy. Ann Neurol 34: 108–112, 1993

Sze G, Abramson A, Krol G et al. Gadolinium-DTPA in the evaluation of intradural extramedullary spinal disease. Am J Radiol 150: 911–921, 1988

Wasserstrom WR, Glass JP, Posner JB. Diagnosis and treatment of leptomeningeal metastases from solid tumors: Experience with 90 patients. Cancer 49: 759–772, 1982

John S. Macdonald, Daniel G. Haller, Robert J. Mayer, Eds. *Manual of Oncologic Therapeutics*, Third Edition.

47. SURGICAL TREATMENT OF ISOLATED METASTASES OF LIVER, LUNGS, AND BRAIN

M. Margaret Kemeny

LIVER METASTASES

The use of surgery to remove metastatic deposits from the liver has become the standard of practice only in the last decade. The mortality associated with elective surgery on the liver was prohibitive until well into the second half of the twentieth century. A better understanding of liver anatomy, new surgical tools, and improved perioperative care have enabled the surgical oncologist to include hepatic resection in the armamentarium of antimetastatic weapons. The resection of liver metastases is almost always done for colorectal primary tumors. The other tumor types that occasionally have isolated metastases to the liver and are resected include soft-tissue sarcomas, breast cancer, germ cell tumors, and Wilms' tumors.

Techniques used for liver resections have become more sophisticated over the last decade. The use of intraoperative ultrasonography to detect small nonpalpable liver metastases is now standard procedure at many centers. Hepatic lobectomies are generally being abandoned for smaller resections, such as segmentectomies or metastasectomies, in which only the tumor and a rim of normal tissue are removed. The total vascular exclusion technique, borrowed from experience in liver transplantation, allows for more hemostatic removal of large tumors that are close to the vena cava or hepatic veins. Dissection of the liver parenchyma can be facilitated by the ultrasonic dissector (Cavitron) or the laser dissector. Some surgeons think that fibrin glue can help stop oozing from the raw liver surface. Mortality for major liver resections done at large centers is now usually less than 5%.

The resection of metastases to the liver had primarily been limited to solitary lesions from colorectal primary tumors. Numerous studies from the early 1970s showed that resection of solitary metastases resulted in a 26% to 45% 5-year survival rate for these patients (Table 47-1). More recent work extended the resectability criteria from solitary lesions to three lesions, with an expected 5-year survival of at least 25%. Currently, numerous centers disagree about the upper limits of metastatic nodules that can be removed with acceptable results in 5-year survival, but there is general agreement that three or fewer metastases should be resected with an expected survival benefit (see Table 47-1).

The one reliable criterion for excluding a patient from resection of hepatic metastases is the presence of extrahepatic intra-abdominal disease. Other factors are prognostic indicators but should not be used to exclude patients from resections. These include the presence of mesenteric lymph node involvement with the primary colorectal lesion (5-year survival with no lymph node involvement, Dukes B is 32% to 52% vs. lymph node involvement, Dukes C, which is 24% to 11%) and the disease-free interval between the colorectal resection and appearance of the liver lesions (synchronous — 5-year survival is 27%; metachronous within the first 12 months after colorectal resection — 5-year survival is 31%; or 12 months or more after the colorectal resection — 5-year survival is 42%) (see Table 47-1).[1]

Postoperative chemotherapy, including continuous hepatic artery infusions, are being studied in randomized settings to see if there is a benefit to survival and decreased hepatic recurrence.

Excision of liver metastases resulting from gastrointestinal primary cancers other than colon cancer is rare because most gastrointestinal malignancies with spread to the liver are rapidly fatal, such as gastric and pancreatic cancer.

Resection of hepatic metastases from primary tumors that are not gastrointestinal represents a different logical paradigm. Because all of the gastrointestinal organs drain into the portal vein, the liver is the first capillary bed through which these metastatic cells pass. As a result, an isolated metastasis to the liver may well represent the only spread of these tumors. Removal of this metastatic disease, even though it is done at significant risk of mortality (≤5%), can be condoned because of the real prospect of cure (25%).

In contrast, any blood-borne metastatic cells from an extra-abdominal organ must pass through the pulmonary capillary bed to get to the liver. The hypothesis that the liver could be the only site of metastatic disease seems less likely, and the concept of doing a hepatic resection in the setting of extrahepatic disease is not considered justifiable. Nonetheless, there are scattered reports of liver resections for metastatic breast cancers, generally of solitary hepatic lesions in patients with no other evidence of metastatic disease. In one of the larger reported studies of a group of 18 patients with isolated liver metastases from breast cancer, only 66% had resectable hepatic metastatic disease. Only two patients had no evidence of disease at 17 and 29 months after resection. The authors concluded that hepatic resection was not a successful treatment modality for the few patients who had isolated hepatic metastases from breast cancer.[2]

TABLE 47–1. RESECTION OF HEPATIC METASTASES FROM COLORECTAL CANCERS

PROGNOSTIC FACTORS	5-YEAR SURVIVAL (%)
Number of lesions	
Solitary	26–45
2–3	10–37
>3	0–40*
Synchronous	27
Metachronous	
1–12 months	31
>12 months	42*
Dukes B (no mesenteric lymph node involvement)	32–52
Dukes C (mesenteric lymph node involvement)	11–32*

*Statistically significant.

In summary, hepatic resection for metastatic disease to the liver from colorectal primary tumors can be resected with an expected 25% 5-year survival if the disease is contained in the liver and there are three or fewer metastatic deposits.

PULMONARY METASTASES

The history of pulmonary resections for metastases from sarcomas or carcinomas (resection of lymphomas and germ cell tumors are not discussed) goes back to the first half of the twentieth century. Since the lungs are overwhelmingly the most common site of metastases from sarcomas, both soft-tissue and osteogenic forms, there has been a great deal of interest in the resection of these metastases to prolong survival. Multiple resection of tumors from osteogenic sarcomas has been practiced throughout the United States for over 20 years, mostly in children. In adults, in whom soft-tissue sarcomas metastases are more common, a number of studies have investigated survival after pulmonary resection of metastases.[3,4]

Most studies agree that a number of important prognostic variables affect survival and help with the selection of patients for resection (Table 47-2). The disease-free interval between the appearance of lung metastases and the primary sarcoma is one of the most important of these variables. Patients with a disease-free interval of less than 12 months had a less than 5% 4-year survival, whereas patients with a disease-free interval of longer than 12 months had a 30% to 40% 4-year survival. The number of metastatic nodules was also important. Patients with four or fewer lesions survived for a median of 23 months, whereas those with four or more nodules had a median survival of 6 months. In contrast, bilaterality of the tumors and the tissue type of sarcoma were not important predictors of survival.

For patients with resectable pulmonary metastases from carcinoma, the most common sites of primary were the colon, breast, and skin (melanoma). Other less common primary sites included kidney, head and neck, and gynecologic organs.

For patients with melanoma, the most important prognostic indicators for survival after pulmonary resection are (1) the number of pulmonary nodules (patients with solitary lesions do better than patients with multiple lesions, and many surgeons think that more than two nodules should not be resected) and (2) the disease-free interval from the time of diagnosis to the time of the occurrence of pulmonary metastases (especially if the pulmonary metastases appear more than 5 years after the primary lesion). Resections of metastatic disease should be reserved for patients in whom the disease is confined to the lung. Most studies have shown a 5-year survival rate of 20% for patients who underwent resection of isolated pulmonary metastases from melanoma.[5]

In patients with breast cancer, the lung is often a site of metastatic disease, but generally the disease is not isolated to the lung. A study from M.D. Anderson suggested that 21% of patients who die from metastatic breast cancer have isolated metastases to the lung that are potentially resectable some time during the course of their disease. The most important prognostic variable for patients undergoing pulmonary resection from metastatic breast cancer was a disease-free interval after primary resection of longer than 12 months (an interval of 12 months or longer carried a median survival of 82 months and a 5-year survival of 57% vs. an interval of 12

TABLE 47–2. PULMONARY METASTASES PROGNOSTIC FACTORS FOR PULMONARY RESECTION DEPENDENT ON PRIMARY CANCER TYPE

SOFT-TISSUE SARCOMA	BREAST	COLON	MELANOMA
DFI > 12 months	DFI > 12 months	Solitary lesion	Solitary lesion
Four or fewer nodules	ER + tumors	CEA < 5	DFI > 12 months
	One or two nodules	DFI not critical	No extrapulmonary disease

DFI = disease-free interval; ER = estrogen receptor; CEA = carcinoembryonic antigen.

months or less, which carried a median survival of 15 months and 5-year survival of 0%). Patients who were estrogen receptor–positive had improved survival over patients who were estrogen receptor–negative (81 months median survival vs. 23 months). Most patients receiving resection had a solitary nodule, but there was no significant survival difference between the patients with two or more nodules and those with solitary pulmonary nodules.[6]

One of the most common carcinomas to metastasize to the lung is colorectal cancer. It is estimated that approximately 1000 patients per year will develop resectable pulmonary metastases from colorectal cancer. The majority of these patients will have solitary lesions. A large study from the Mayo clinic found that the disease-free interval for patients with colorectal cancer was not a significant prognostic indicator for survival after pulmonary resection (27% 5-year survival with a disease-free interval of less than 2 years vs. a 31.8% 5-year survival with a disease-free interval of greater than 2 years). Patients with colon cancer who had resectable extrapulmonary disease and had it resected did not have a significantly poorer survival than did those without extrapulmonary disease.

For patients with colon cancer the number of pulmonary metastases seemed important to survival. Patients with solitary metastases had a 36.9% 5-year survival vs. 19.3% for patients with two metastases and 7.7% for those with more than two metastases. Another significant variable for patients with colon cancer was the carcinoembryonic antigen (CEA) level. Patients with a CEA level of more than 5 did significantly worse than patients who had a CEA level of less than 5 at the time of pulmonary resection. Most of the resections done for metastatic disease were wedge resections. No data suggested that extended resections increased survival. The use of chemotherapy before or after resections was variable for the different diseases.[7]

In summary, the role of resection of pulmonary nodules seems to be different for different primary tumors. There does seem to be a place, however, for resection of solitary and even multiple pulmonary nodules in various tumor types, including sarcomas, colon cancer, melanoma, and breast cancer. The overall rule for these resections includes the ability to control disease outside of the lungs and a low number of metastatic lesions. There are differences in the other variables that guide the surgeon's decision to operate, depending on the cell of origin for the metastasis.

Disease-free interval is the major criterion for resection of a metastatic sarcoma but seems to be a less important factor for metastases from colorectal cancer. The limitation to one or at most two metastases is critical for melanoma, but for sarcoma the number of resectable lesions can be up to four, and for osteogenic sarcoma there seems to be almost no limit. Because of these and other differences, the thoracic surgeon must know about the tendencies of the specific pulmonary metastases before attempting a resection.

BRAIN METASTASES

Brain metastases occur with variable frequency according to the primary cancer type, but overall they occur in from 10% to 30% of cancer patients, with the majority from lung primary tumors. At least one third of these metastases are solitary. Radiation therapy has been the standard treatment for brain metastases, but the increasing frequency of reports of success with surgical resection has influenced physicians to consider this modality as well. In a randomized study from 1990 reported in the *New England Journal of Medicine*, surgery and radiation therapy were superior to radiation therapy alone for patients with solitary brain metastases from cancers outside of the central nervous system.[8] The group of patients who received the combined modalities had a lower recurrence rate (28% vs. 52% $p < .02$), longer survival (40 vs. 15 weeks, $p < .01$), and were functionally independent for a longer period of time (38 vs. 8 weeks, $p < .005$).

Brain metastases, in contrast to liver and pulmonary lesions, need to be solitary and accessible to be potentially resectable. Control of the primary disease is the single most important survival factor in most studies. Lung cancer is the most common carcinoma to metastasize to the brain. In a study from Memorial Sloan-Kettering Cancer Center, the 5-year survival was 13% for the 185 patients with resection of brain metastases from non–small cell lung cancer. They reported no survival difference in patients with synchronous lesions, compared to those with metachronous lesions. The stage of the primary tumor also had no influence on survival; however, if the primary lung cancer could not be completely resected, patients did worse.[9]

In a retrospective review at the Mayo Clinic of over 200 cerebral resections, 37% were metastases from lung, 12% from breast, and 11% from melanoma. The tissue of origin was not important to survival in these patients. The most significant variable for survival was whether the primary disease was controlled. For patients in whom there was systemic disease at the time of craniotomy, the median survival ranged from 5 to 7 months and 3-year survival was 6%. No patient in this group lived past 3.6 years. These patients did not seem to have improved survival over patients receiving radiation therapy alone. For these reasons, craniotomy does not seem to be justified for patients whose primary disease is not under control.[10]

In contrast, patients with no systemic disease who underwent resection of their solitary brain metastases had a median survival of 11.7 months and a 10% 5-year survival. These patients did better than those treated with radiation therapy alone (historical control).

In summary, craniotomy can be considered a reasonable treatment option for patients who have a solitary brain metastasis from an extracranial primary and whose primary disease is under control. Craniotomy will improve disease-free survival, functionally independent survival (*i.e.*, quality of life), and may even offer a small chance of cure for selected patients.

REFERENCES

1. Kemeny N, Kemeny M, Lawrence T. Liver metastases. In Abeloff, Armitage, Lichter et al (eds). Clinical Oncology. Churchill Livingstone (in press)
2. Elias D, Lasser P, Spielmann M et al. Surgical and chemotherapeutic treatment of hepatic metastases from carcinoma of the breast. Surg Gynecol Obstet 172:461–464, 1991
3. Roth JA, Putnam JB, Wesley MN et al. Differing determinants of prognosis following resection of pulmonary metastases from osteogenic and soft tissue sarcoma patients. Cancer 55:1361–1366, 1985
4. McCormack PM, Martini N. The changing role of surgery for pulmonary metastases. Ann Thorac Surg 28(2): 139–145, 1979.
5. Harpole DH, Johnson CM, Wolfe W et al. Analysis of 945 cases of pulmonary metastatic melanoma. Thorac Cardiovasc Surg 4: 743–750, 1992
6. Lanza LA, Natarajan G, Roth JA et al. Long-term survival after resection of pulmonary metastases from carcinoma of the breast. Ann Thorac Surg 54:244–248, 1992
7. McAfee MK, Allen MS, Trastek VF et al. Colorectal lung metastases: Results of surgical excision. Ann Thorac Surg 53:780–786, 1992
8. Patchell RA, Tibbs PA, Walsh JW et al. A randomized trial of surgery in the treatment of single metastases to the brain. N Engl J Med 322:494–500, 1990
9. Burt M, Wronski M, Arbit E et al. Resection of brain metastases from non-small cell lung carcinoma. Results of therapy, Memorial Sloan-Kettering Cancer Center Thoracic Surgical Staff. J Thorac Cardiovasc Surg 103:339–410, 1992
10. Smalley SR, Laws EF, O'Fallon JR et al. Resection for solitary brain metastasis: Role of adjuvant radiation and prognostic variables in 229 patients. J Neurosurg 77:531–540, 1992

John S. Macdonald, Daniel G. Haller, Robert J. Mayer, Eds. *Manual of Oncologic Therapeutics*, Third Edition.

48. REGIONAL CHEMOTHERAPY

Maurie Markman

In an effort to improve the efficacy of cytotoxic chemotherapy for tumors principally confined to particular regions of the body, investigators have infused antineoplastic agents directly into arteries (intra-arterial therapy) feeding the organ, or into cavities (intracavitary therapy) where the cancer is localized. The goal of such therapy is to increase local drug concentrations in contact with tumor while at the same time decreasing systemic exposure to the agent. It is hoped this will lead to greater cell kill (if the cytotoxic effect of the drug against the tumor is concentration dependent) and reduced toxicity. Over the last decade multiple trials of regional chemotherapy involving several areas of the body have been reported, with varying degrees of success (Table 48–1).

REGIONAL THERAPY FOR THE LIVER

Since the liver is responsible for metabolizing a number of chemotherapeutic agents, regional therapy for tumors principally confined to the liver (primary and metastatic) has been actively investigated. Drugs that are rapidly and extensively metabolized during their first passage through the liver would be predicted to demonstrate the most favorable pharmacokinetic advantage following either portal vein infusion (PVI) or hepatic artery infusion (HAI). Indeed, a two- to three-log difference in exposure of the liver to several such drugs (*e.g.*, 5-fluorouracil [5-FU] or floxuridine [5-FUdR]) has been demonstrated. Conversely, if the liver is not a major site of metabolism (*e.g.*, cisplatin), or if the liver is unable to metabolize a large portion of the agent during its first passage through the liver (*e.g.*, caffeine), direct liver perfusion will yield at most only a modest increase in exposure of the liver compared with that of the systemic circulation.

While a similar pharmacokinetic advantage will result from either PVI or HAI, the latter is preferable for treating hepatic tumor masses. In several experimental systems about 95% of the blood supply to established macroscopic tumors comes from the hepatic artery, while for microscopic tumors the delivery of nutrients by the two vascular systems is essentially equal (suggesting a possible role for PVIs for adjuvant therapy of tumors with a high likelihood of subclinical hepatic metastasis).

The availability of totally implantable catheter-delivery systems and long-term infusion devices has made it possible to treat patients with continuous HAI on an ambulatory basis. The most commonly employed drugs in clinical trials have been 5-FU and 5-FUdR. Most reported response rates using these two drugs by HAI are in the 40% to 50% range for patients with colon carcinoma metastatic to the liver. Patients failing to respond to systemically delivered 5-FU may respond to the same drug delivered by HAI.

Several randomized controlled trials have compared HAI with standard intravenous drug administration. In one of the largest studies reported to date, Kemeny and coworkers have found a significantly higher response rate in patients treated with 5-FUdR by HAI compared with patients receiving 5-FUdR by continuous intravenous infusion. In this trial there was no statistically significant difference in survival between the two treatment groups. These data are similar to that reported by other investigators. Unfortunately, a number of the trials examining HAI compared to systemic treatment of metastatic colon cancer to the liver have permitted crossover to regional therapy following failure of intravenous treatment, including the study of Kemeny noted above. This trial design has made it difficult to interpret the impact of HAI on survival in this clinical setting.

For physicians considering HAI, the regimen reported by Kemeny is associated with a reasonable response rate and toxicity profile. In this study patients received 5-FUdR delivered as a continuous infusion for 14 days via an Infusaid pump at a starting dose of 0.3 mg/kg/day. Following a 2-week break, the therapy is repeated. Dose reductions were common in this study, so that by the completion of the third cycle the median dose was 0.2 mg/kg/day.

The toxicity of HAI is not insignificant. In addition to the risks associated with catheter placement, toxicity includes gastrointestinal disturbances (gastritis and/or ulcers in up to 50% of patients), hepatitis, and sclerosing cholangitis.

A summary of the currently available data concerning HAI with 5-FU or 5-FUdR for metastatic colon carcinoma suggests the following:

1. Overall, there is a higher response rate in the liver than that achieved with systemic administration.
2. A survival advantage for HAI compared with bolus systemic drug administration has yet to be demonstrated.
3. Responses in the liver can be observed in patients who fail to respond to systemically delivered drug.
4. Relapses frequently appear systemically while the response continues in the liver.
5. HAI can offer important palliation for patients with disease confined principally to the liver.

Other drugs that have been delivered via HAI include mitomycin, cisplatin, and doxorubicin, or a combination of agents. Recent data suggest the combination of 5-FUdR and leucovorin administered by the hepatic arterial route may re-

TABLE 48–1. THE ROLE OF REGIONAL THERAPY IN THE TREATMENT OF CANCER

DEFINITE CLINICAL UTILITY:
Intrathecal therapy of meningeal leukemia
Intravesical therapy of bladder tumors
Intrahepatic artery therapy of established metastatic tumor in the liver from colon carcinoma
Intra-arterial therapy of locally recurrent or unresectable extremity malignant melanoma

PROBABLE CLINICAL UTILITY:
Intraperitoneal therapy (cisplatin-based) of persistent ovarian carcinoma (minimal residual disease) in patients who have previously responded to systemic cisplatin or carboplatin
Intra-arterial therapy of extremity soft-tissue and skeletal sarcomas (with doxorubicin and radiation therapy)

POSSIBLE CLINICAL UTILITY:
Intraperitoneal therapy of malignant mesothelioma (cisplatin or doxorubicin)
Adjuvant portal vein infusion or intraperitoneal therapy for colorectal cancer
Intra-arterial therapy of tumors other than those involving the liver or sarcomas of the extremity
Intraperitoneal therapy of ovarian carcinoma following systemic chemotherapy in those individuals achieving a surgically defined complete remission
Intraperitoneal therapy as part of the initial chemotherapy program in patients with advanced ovarian carcinoma

sult in a higher objective response rate compared to 5-FUdR alone. Unfortunately, the combination appears to be associated with increased hepatic toxicity. Further evaluation of this strategy seems indicated.

OTHER INTRA-ARTERIAL APPROACHES

The intracarotid administration of carmustine (BCNU) and cisplatin can result in higher concentrations of drug in tumor cells in the brain, cerebrospinal fluid, and normal brain tissue than that achieved with systemic administration. In addition, objective response rates to such therapy have been the highest reported to cytotoxic chemotherapy for brain tumors and may be higher than intravenous drug administration. However, a survival advantage for this technique of drug administration has not been demonstrated. In addition, toxicity can be substantial. Specifically, intra-arterial high-dose cisplatin can produce blindness, paresis, eye pain, and encephalopathic coma. Patients receiving BCNU have developed seizures, ipsilateral blindness, abnormal mental status, and eye pain. This therapy should be given only by those highly trained in the technique of administration and familiar with the serious side effects of such therapy. For the present, intracarotid drug delivery for brain tumors should be considered investigational.

Intracarotid therapy for head and neck cancers has also been attempted with some success. Unfortunately, as noted above, there is a limited pharmacokinetic rationale for this form of therapy and the technique has yet to demonstrate superiority to standard systemic drug administration in randomized clinical trials. Alternative approaches to treating head and neck cancers, including neoadjuvant chemotherapy, have greater appeal both from the theoretical and safety points of view.

Intra-arterial therapy for extremity tumors has been investigated by several groups. Eilber and coworkers have administered intra-arterial doxorubicin with and without local radiation for soft tissue and skeletal sarcomas. Toxicity has included arterial thrombosis, wound slough, lymphedema, and fracture. This technique is appealing because it often allows limb-sparing surgery. The incidence of local tumor recurrence following such surgery and intra-arterial chemotherapy (plus radiotherapy) is an important end point of treatment to examine. In a treatment program that employed intra-arterial doxorubicin and local radiation to 1750 cGy, limb salvage was possible in 93% of patients with skeletal sarcomas (2 of 103 consecutive patients requiring amputation) and in 97% of patients with soft tissue sarcoma (5 of 190 consecutive patients requiring amputation). In a control population (nonrandomized) of patients treated at the same time with either limb-sparing surgery alone or surgery plus postoperative radiotherapy, 34 of 60 (56%) patients with skeletal sarcomas and 19 of 74 (30%) patients with soft-tissue sarcomas required amputation. While these results are quite impressive, the series was not randomized and it remains unclear whether the intravenous administration of doxorubicin would produce comparable results with a lower incidence of side effects. Intra-arterial therapy is time consuming, requires hospitalization and angiography, and is associated with significant local toxicity. This therapeutic approach should only be attempted by individuals and in institutions with the appropriate technology and required skills.

Intra-arterial therapy has also been employed for recurrent tumors in the pelvis (cervical, colorectal) and chest wall (breast), with and without local radiation therapy. Complications have included systemic side effects of the administered drugs (mitomycin, cisplatin, doxorubicin) and significant local toxicity (deep necrotic ulcers, pain, erythema, blisters, impaired wound healing, arterial thrombosis, necrotic cellulitis). Significant palliation of pain and tumor regression have been noted in several trials, but the impact on survival or the relative efficacy of such an approach compared with standard therapy (*e.g.*, local radiation alone) is unknown at present. In view of the potential for serious toxicity associated with this therapeutic approach and the limited information available about appropriate drugs, dosing, and schedules, for the present this treatment strategy must remain a research technique.

Finally, intra-arterial therapy employing isolation-perfusion techniques has been used in patients with unresectable, recurrent, or locally advanced metastatic melanomas confined to an extremity. This approach, with the use of several chemotherapeutic agents including melphalan, cisplatin, and nitrogen mustard, is effective in palliating symptoms and producing long-term disease-free survival in a subset of patients. The technique has also been employed in the adjuvant setting in patients with a high risk for the development of recurrent disease. Unfortunately, despite encouraging reports in nonrandomized trials, unequivocal clinical benefit has yet to be demonstrated, and the use of regional isolation perfusion as an adjuvant to surgery remains investigational.

INTRACAVITARY CHEMOTHERAPY

Intracavitary drug administration for cancer principally confined to body cavities (including the pleura, peritoneum, and pericardium) was attempted in the earliest days of the modern chemotherapeutic era. Unfortunately, with the drugs available at that time local toxicity was excessive and objective antitumor responses were rare. However, significant palliation from the problems associated with recurrent fluid was noted (due to the sclerosing effect of the agents), and this form of therapy is commonly used in clinical practice to control malignant fluid reaccumulation. Bleomycin is probably the most commonly used antineoplastic agent at present for the treatment of malignant pleural effusions. A dose of 60 units delivered intrapleurally appears to be as effective in preventing fluid reaccumulation as higher dose regimens. The intraperitoneal administration of bleomycin to treat malignant ascites is less effective than intrapleural drug delivery.

Interest in intracavitary (principally intraperitoneal) administration of chemotherapeutic agents for their cytotoxic rather than sclerosing properties was renewed after mathematical modeling studies suggested a sound theoretical rationale for this approach. A major pharmacokinetic advantage for peritoneal cavity exposure compared with systemic exposure was postulated for certain drugs, particularly those metabolized in the liver, since a major route of exit from the cavity is by way of the portal circulation. This model has been shown to be remarkably accurate in clinical trials conducted with a number of antineoplastic agents, including 5-FU, doxorubicin, cisplatin, mitoxantrone, carboplatin, methotrexate, and taxol.

The importance of using large treatment volumes (≥ 2 liters) to achieve adequate drug distribution when employing this technique in the peritoneal cavity has been shown both in an animal model and in the clinical setting. Patients only able to receive a limited treatment volume because of adhesion formation or tumor masses should not be treated by this technique, because it is highly unlikely that tumor in the cavity will come in contact with the drug-containing fluid. One or two liters of fluid with radiolabeled albumin can be administered intraperitoneally prior to the initiation of therapy to determine if there will be any difficulty with drug distribution.

A second important consideration is adequate access to the peritoneal (or pleural) cavity. While patients can be treated by percutaneous placement of peritoneal dialysis or thoracentesis catheters when fluid is present, there is considerable risk with blind percutaneous catheter placement in patients who have undergone one or more operations with resultant adhesion formation. Most investigators prefer surgical placement of Tenckhoff catheter-type delivery systems for patients who are to be treated with multiple courses of intraperitoneal chemotherapy. These catheters can be attached to subcutaneous ports (*e.g.*, Port-a-cath) to improve patient acceptance of the device and to reduce the risk of infection. Such catheters can also be used to drain malignant fluid or to assess cytologies during and following treatment. Unfortunately, 40% to 60% of these catheters become "one-way" valves, allowing one to deliver treatment but not to withdraw fluid. This seems to be due to the formation of tight fibrous bands around the catheter that do not prevent fluid exit from the catheter openings but do prevent fluid entry into it. Fortunately, it is not necessary to drain fluid from the cavity following the completion of treatment to prevent excessive toxicity for most of the agents that have been clinically evaluated, including cisplatin, carboplatin, and 5-FU.

A major theoretical concern with the use of intracavitary chemotherapy is the question of the depth of penetration of the drugs into tumor nodules. Experimental evidence suggests that agents can penetrate to a maximum depth of 1–3 mm. Thus, the patients who might benefit most from intracavitary drug administration are those with *minimal residual* intraperitoneal disease either following surgery or initial systemic chemotherapy.

Patients with bulky intra-abdominal disease are unlikely to demonstrate major clinical benefit from the direct uptake of drug into the tumor nodules, but the combination of this effect plus that achieved by drug entering the systemic circulation and reaching tumor by capillary flow may still be more effective treatment than that achieved by systemic therapy alone. Thus, when considering a single-drug or combination regimen for intraperitoneal therapy, it is important to recognize the benefit of agents that do escape from the peritoneal cavity in significant concentrations to achieve this "dual" delivery to tumor cells. If the dose-limiting toxicity of a particular drug is *not* local toxicity, then it should be possible (at least in theory) to escalate the dose delivered to the point where as much is leaking into the plasma (and therefore delivered to the tumor by capillary flow) as would be present if the drug were administered by the systemic route. Drugs such as cisplatin and melphalan fall into this category, while agents such as doxorubicin, mitomycin, and mitoxantrone which exhibit significant local toxicity that severely limits the total dose of drug, will not achieve significant systemic levels following intraperitoneal delivery.

Toxicity of intracavitary chemotherapy includes the expected systemic effects of specific cytotoxic agents (emesis, nephrotoxicity, neurotoxicity), and local toxic effects (pain, fever, ileus, adhesion formation leading to bowel obstruction, infection).

There is currently sufficient experience with the use of cisplatin-based intraperitoneal chemotherapy in the treatment of persistent ovarian carcinoma following front-line systemic chemotherapy to define a patient population most likely to benefit from this therapeutic approach. While between 30% and 50% of patients whose largest tumor mass is ≤ 1 cm in diameter (including microscopic disease) will respond to treatment, fewer than 10% of individuals with any tumor > 1 cm in diameter at the initiation of intracavitary therapy will demonstrate evidence of a major antitumor effect. Twenty to 30% of patients with very small tumor bulk at treatment initiation can be anticipated to achieve a surgically defined complete remission. Complete responses are very rarely observed in patients with tumor masses > 1 cm in diameter. In addition, patients who have previously *failed* to exhibit a response to systemically administered cisplatin *rarely* respond to intraperitoneal cisplatin, despite having very small volume disease at the initiation of salvage treatment. Thus, in general, patients with clinically defined platinum-refractory ovarian cancer should *not* be considered candidates for regional therapy with a cisplatin or carboplatin-based regimen.

Several different cisplatin treatment regimens have been examined in patients with refractory ovarian carcinoma, and, at this time, it is unclear whether any one program is superior to another. Table 48–2 lists a number of cisplatin-based regimens reported to demonstrate both safety and efficacy in the treatment of persistent small volume residual ovarian carcinoma following front-line systemic chemotherapy.

It is important to note that it is unknown at present if the responses observed in the salvage setting will be translated into a survival advantage. Also, it remains to be shown that this therapeutic approach is superior to other forms of second-line therapy. However, based on the currently available data, it is reasonable to suggest that for patients with minimal residual ovarian carcinoma following cisplatin-based chemotherapy who have demonstrated a response to initial systemic therapy, intraperitoneal cisplatin (using one of the programs outlined in Table 48–2) would be a rational therapeutic option.

Intracavitary therapy for other tumors, including mesothelioma (cisplatin, doxorubicin) and colon carcinoma (5-FU, mitomycin), has been reported to produce objective tumor remissions and palliation of symptoms (principally ascites formation). What role, if any, such therapy will play in the standard practice of treating these malignancies remains to be defined. Similarly, while responses to intrapleural and intrapericardial drug administration have been reported (reduction in malignant fluid reaccumulation), it is unknown at present whether the toxic or financial costs justify the routine use of such treatment when alternative approaches are available (standard sclerosing therapy). Clinical trials currently in progress and planned for the future will possibly answer these important questions.

TABLE 48–2. CISPLATIN-BASED INTRAPERITONEAL CHEMOTHERAPY OF PERSISTENT OVARIAN CARCINOMA IN PATIENTS PREVIOUSLY EXHIBITING A RESPONSE TO SYSTEMIC CISPLATIN OR CARBOPLATIN

REGIMENS	DOSAGES (IN 2 LITERS)	FREQUENCY
Cisplatin	50 mg/m^2	q 3 week × 6
Cisplatin	60–150 mg/m^2	q 2–3 week × 6–10
(plus IV sodium thiosulfate for any renal toxicity)		
Cisplatin	200 mg/m^2	q 4 week × 4–6
(plus IV sodium thiosulfate in all patients)		
Cisplatin	90 mg/m^2	
5-FU	1000 mg	q 3–4 week × 8
Cisplatin	200 mg/m^2	
Etoposide	350 mg/m^2	q 4 week × 6
(plus IV sodium thiosulfate in all patients)		
Cisplatin	100 mg/m^2	
Etoposide	200 mg/m^2	q 4 week × 6

Intravenous sodium thiosulfate is administered to protect against cisplatin-induced renal insufficiency. A typical schedule is as follows: 4 g/m^2 bolus (over 10 minutes) in 250 ml sterile water (with initiation of cisplatin intraperitoneal instillation), plus 12 g/m^2 infusion (over 6 hours) in 1 liter sterile water. Use of sodium thiosulfate is limited to investigational settings.

BIBLIOGRAPHY

1. Collins JM. Pharmacokinetic rationale for regional drug delivery. J Clin Oncol 2:498–504, 1984
2. Cumberlin R et al. Isolation perfusion for malignant melanoma of the extremity: A review. J Clin Oncol 3:1022–1031, 1985
3. Hohn DC et al. A randomized trial of continuous intravenous versus hepatic intra-arterial floxuridine in patients with colorectal cancer metastatic to the liver: The Northern California Oncology Group trial. J Clin Oncol 7:1646–1654, 1989
4. Kemeny N et al. Intrahepatic or systemic infusion of fluorodeoxyuridine in patients with liver metastases from colorectal carcinoma: A randomized trial. Ann Intern Med 107:459–465, 1987
5. Kemeny N et al. Randomized trial of hepatic arterial floxuridine, mitomycin, and carmustine versus floxuridine alone in previously treated patients with liver metastases from colorectal cancer. J Clin Oncol 11:330–335, 1993
6. Markman M. Intraperitoneal chemotherapy. Semin Oncol 18(3):248–254, 1991
7. Markman M et al. Responses to second-line cisplatin-based intraperitoneal therapy in ovarian cancer: influence of a prior response to intravenous cisplatin. J Clin Oncol 9:1801–1805, 1991
8. Markman M et al. Impact on survival of surgically defined favorable responses to salvage intraperitoneal chemotherapy in small-volume residual ovarian cancer. J Clin Oncol 10:1479–1484, 1992

John S. Macdonald, Daniel G. Haller, Robert J. Mayer, Eds. *Manual of Oncologolic Therapeutics*, Third Edition.

49. RADIATION THERAPY FOR METASTATIC DISEASE

Thomas F. DeLaney
Timothy J. Kinsella

INTRODUCTION

Radiation therapy (RT) plays a major role in the sometimes curative, but more commonly palliative, treatment of metastatic disease in children and adults. RT may be used as a single modality or may be integrated with surgery and/or chemotherapy in a combined modality approach to metastases. The choice of optimal palliative therapy for metastatic disease can vary depending on the site of metastasis, the severity of physiological or functional compromise associated with the metastasis, the overall functional status of the patient, the presence of other metastatic disease, and, of course, the prior history of cancer treatment. Clearly, a decision on effective palliative treatment can be complex, often requiring input from surgical, medical, and radiation oncologists. In this chapter, the clinical management of bone metastases, brain metastases, and liver metastases will be discussed briefly with particular emphasis on treatment with radiation therapy. The clinical management of superior vena cava syndrome and spinal cord compression will be covered elsewhere.

BONE METASTASES

Up to 50% of patients with breast, lung, and prostate cancer will develop bone metastases, and these three cancers constitute more than 80% of all patients with bone metastases. Localized pain is the most common symptom associated with cortical bone destruction and periosteal expansion. Radicular pain may occur with metastases to the sacrum or vertebrae. Vertebral metastases may also be associated with an extradural soft-tissue growth and possible cord compression. In patients with back pain and even subtle neurologic signs, a more comprehensive workup, including an MRI scan, vertebral CT scan and/or myelogram, is indicated.

Bone metastases require treatment to relieve pain, to prevent development or progression of neurologic signs, and to prevent fracture, in particular in weight-bearing bones. The vast majority of patients will have multiple sites of bone involvement, making radical surgical approaches unrealistic. Pathologic fractures in weight-bearing bones or subluxation of a vertebral body require internal fixation, often followed by RT.

The major goal of treatment is to keep patients ambulatory with little or no pain. Most patients (>75%) will respond to localized RT, sometimes with prompt (within 2 to 3 days) and dramatic relief of pain. Patients with metastatic breast and prostate cancer are more likely to achieve complete pain relief than patients with lung and other primary tumors.[1] Several studies suggest that low–dose, short-course irradiation (500–2000 cGy in one to five fractions) is as effective as a longer radiation course (3000–4000 cGy over 2 to 4 weeks).[1,2] In practical terms, the radiation fractionation schedule depends on the field size, the volume and type of normal tissue (*e.g.* bowel) within the radiation field, and the patient's performance status. For example, focal rib metastases may be treated with a single fraction of 800 cGy, whereas a lytic lesion eroding the cortex of the femur is often treated to 3000 cGy in 10 fractions over 2 weeks. A solitary bone metastasis, particularly in the cervical or thoracic spine, in a patient with good performance status might be treated to 4000 cGy in 3 to 4 weeks since long-term control is desired. The total dose and fractionation schedule as outlined above allows for consideration of retreatment with RT in patients with recurrent symptoms.

Hemibody irradiation has been used in selected patients with widespread symptomatic bone metastases. In one series of metastatic breast cancer patients treated with 600 cGy to 800 cGy half-body irradiation, 12 of 21 patients experienced excellent pain relief within 2 days of treatment.[3] While these treatment results are impressive, hemibody irradiation must be reserved for patients without a history of excessive systemic treatment. Bone marrow suppression, especially thrombocytopenia, results and recovery can require several weeks to months. Additionally, moderate nausea, vomiting, and diarrhea may result acutely from upper hemibody irradiation. Hemibody irradiation usually cannot be repeated, and the resulting prolonged myelosuppression often precludes the use of subsequent systemic therapy.

More recently, there has been renewed interest in the use of systemically administered radionuclides with the approval of Strontium-89 (^{89}Sr), a bone-seeking nuclide with a low energy beta emission, for the treatment of patients with blastic bony metastases. Another radionuclide, Phosphorus-32 (^{32}P)had been shown to be an effective agent in palliating bony pain in approximately 70% of patients, but was associated with a 25% frequency of severe hematological toxicity because of its marrow incorporation. Because strontium-89 is handled physiologically as a calcium analogue, it is not incorporated into marrow or leukocytes, resulting in less common and less severe hematological toxicity. A recent study in patients in which patients with metastatic prostate cancer receiving local field radiotherapy were randomized to also receive ^{89}Sr or placebo indicates that ^{89}Sr is an effective adjuvant to local field radiotherapy.[4] It reduces the number of subsequent painful bony sites with resultant improvement in quality of life, reduction in analgesic requirement, and reduced need for subsequent local field radiotherapy.

BRAIN METASTASES

Brain metastasis is a frequent problem confronting the oncologist, particularly in dealing with patients with lung and breast cancer and melanoma. The cerebrum is the most common site of metastases, with cerebellar metastases being less frequent and brain stem metastases the least frequent. Approximately two-thirds of patients with brain metastases will present with multiple metastases.

Patients with brain metastases present most commonly with headaches, seizure activity, loss of motor function, and cerebellar signs. Early diagnosis is of major importance in an attempt to minimize the physical and psychological consequences of brain metastases. Immediate computed tomographic (CT) scanning is indicated even in the presence of very subtle neurologic symptoms and signs. Once the diagnosis is established, mildly symptomatic patients are started on oral corticosteroids, usually dexamethasone, 8 mg to 16 mg daily. Patients with marked papilledema, severe neurologic signs, and a midline shift on CT scan require more vigorous medical management with intravenous corticosteroids and/or dehydrating agents such as mannitol or urea. Anticonvulsants, usually phenytoin, are necessary in patients presenting with seizures.

RT is usually the treatment of choice. An occasional patient with good performance status and a surgically accessible, isolated metastasis in a "silent" area of the brain may be considered for resection. These solitary metastases are most commonly associated with melanoma, renal cell carcinoma, or osteosarcoma. In such patients, a randomized trial has demonstrated that resection followed by whole-brain radiotherapy increases median survival and intracranial tumor control compared to whole-brain radiotherapy alone.[5] Stereotactic radiosurgery, a non-invasive focal radiation procedure, in combination with whole brain external beam RT appears to provide comparable results to resection and whole brain RT.[6] Whole-brain irradiation is recommended for the typical patient with multiple metastases documented by CT or MRI scanning. The Radiation Therapy Oncology Group has evaluated several different radiation fractionation schemes ranging from 2000 cGy in 1 week to 4000 cGy in 4 weeks in patients with symptomatic brain metastases.[7] Most patients (>75%) improved at least one functional category. Patients receiving the larger fractions and shorter courses demonstrated a more prompt response. No fractionation scheme was superior in terms of the frequency of response, extent of neurologic improvement, or duration of response. The median survival varied between 15 to 18 weeks, with progression of brain metastases as a cause of death in less than 50% of patients. The radiation schedule recommended for most patients is 3000 cGy in 2 weeks to the whole brain. However, in ambulatory patients with brain metastases as the only site of disease, a higher total dose of 4500 cGy to 5000 cGy is recommended with 1500 cGy to 2000 cGy being given as a boost to localized metastatic sites in the brain. Retreatment of brain metastases is possible, particularly in patients demonstrating a response to previous irradiation and who received a dose of less than 4000 cGy over 3 to 4 weeks.[8]

LIVER METASTASES

Typically, the patient referred for RT has bilobar involvement, which can be associated with significant pain, right upper quadrant tenderness, and jaundice. Since the entire liver is necessarily included within the radiation portal, the radiation tolerance of normal liver limits the dose of conventional external-beam irradiation to 2000 cGy to 3000 cGy fractions over 2 to 3 weeks, often using simple anteroposterior-posteroanterior fields.[9] The major clinical experience with liver irradiation involves patients with symptomatic metastatic colorectal carcinoma, usually with a performance status of one to three using Eastern Cooperative Oncology Group (ECOG) criteria or a Karnofsky performance level of >40. A majority of patients (>75%) will experience significant pain relief, and some (up to 40%) may have an objective response to treatment. Patients with liver metastases from colorectal cancer respond more frequently than those with liver metastases from other primary sites.[10] Pain relief is prompt, occurring within a median of 1.7 weeks, with a median duration of relief of 3 months. Survival is generally short, in the range of 4 months in several series.

Recently, there has been some enthusiasm for combining liver irradiation with hepatic arterial infusion chemotherapy, most commonly using the fluoropyrimidine (5-FU, FUdR). Using a similar radiation treatment schedule, the objective response rates for this combined-modality approach are in the range of 50% to 70%, which compares favorably with studies using intra-arterial chemotherapy alone (50%). Patient selection, the type and duration of infusional chemotherapy, and the timing of radiation and infusion have varied considerably in these studies, which makes a direct comparison of treatment results difficult.

Recent advances in radiation treatment planning using computer-assisted three-dimensional treatment planning have permitted escalation in administered radiation doses to focal lesions in the liver.[11] Lesions have been given boost radiation doses up to 4500–6000 cGy without evidence of radiation hepatitis or other normal tissue injury. Focal radiation has also been given to patients with interstitial brachytherapy catheters using afterloaded Iridium-192.[12] The latter has been done in selected patients found to be unresectable at the time of attempted resection of liver metastases. Because of their technical complexity, both of these radiation techniques should be reserved for patients with good performance status.

The major toxicity of whole-liver irradiation is the development of radiation "hepatitis," which consists of the rather acute onset of jaundice, ascites, and tender hepatomegaly usually 4 to 6 weeks following treatment. The major differential diagnosis is progressive tumor. Histologically, sinusoidal congestion and partial to complete occlusion of the small central veins are found. While radiation hepatitis is uncommon (<10%) following a whole-liver dose of 2500 cGy to 3000 cGy, it can progress to hepatic coma and death. Medical treatment of radiation hepatitis with protein restriction and judicious use of diuretics for ascites is recommended. The role of corticosteroids is not established. More aggressive measures such as a LeVeen shunt have not been used routinely in these patients. Retreatment of previously irradiated liver metastases is not recommended.

REFERENCES

1. Hendrickson FR, Shehata WM, Kirchner AR. Radiation therapy for osseous metastasis. Int J Radiat Oncol Biol Phys 1:275, 1976
2. Price P, Hoskin PJ, Easton D, et al. Prospective randomized trial of single and multifracation radiotherapy schedules in the treatment of painful bony metastases. Radiother Oncol 6:247, 1986
3. Bartelink H, Battermann J, Hart G. Half body radiotherapy. Int J Radiat Oncol Biol Phys 6:87, 1980
4. Porter AT, McEwan AJB, Powe JE, et al. Results of a randomized phase-III trial to evaluate the efficacy of strontium-89 adjuvant to local field external beam irradiation in the management of endocrine resistant metastatic prostate cancer. Int J Radiat Oncol Biol Phys 25:805, 1993
5. Patchell RA, Tibbs PA, Walsh JW et al. A randomized trial of surgery in the treatment of single metastases to the brain. N Engl J Med 322:494, 1990
6. Metha MP, Rozenthal JM, Levin AM et al. Defining the role of radiotherapy in the management of brain metastases. Int J Radiat Oncol Biol Phys 24:619, 1992
7. Borgelt B, Gelber R, Kramer S, et al. The palliation of brain metastases: Final results of the first two studies by the Radiation Therapy Oncology Group. Int J Radiat Oncol Biol Phys 6:1, 1980
8. Cooper JS, Steinfeld R, Lerch IA. Cerebral metastases: Value of re-irradiation in selected patients. Radiology 174:883, 1990
9. Kinsella TJ. The role of radiation therapy alone and combined with infusional chemotherapy for treating liver metastases. Semin Oncol 10:215, 1983
10. Leibel SA, Pajak TF, Massullo V et al.: A comparison of misonidazole sensitized radiation therapy to radiation therapy alone for the palliation of hepatic metastases: Results of a Radiation Therpy Oncology Group randomized prospective trial. Int J Radiat Oncol Biol Phys 139:1057, 1987
11. Lawrence TS, Tesser RJ, Ten Haken RK. An application of dose volume histograms to the treatment of intrahepatic malignancies with radiation therapy. Int J Radiat Oncol Biol Phys 19:1041, 1990
12. Dritschilo A, Harter KW, Thomas D et al. Intraoperative radiation therapy of hepatic metastases: Technical aspects and report of a pilot study. Int J Radiat Oncol Biol Phys 14:1007, 1988

John S. Macdonald, Daniel G. Haller, Robert J. Mayer, Eds. *Manual of Oncologolic Therapeutics*, Third Edition.

VI. ONCOLOGIC EMERGENCIES

50. CENTRAL NERVOUS SYSTEM EMERGENCIES

Kevin R. Fox

Neurological manifestations of malignancies will often require urgent or emergency treatment in order to preserve quality of life and neurological function while maintaining patient comfort and well-being. The management of four conditions: spinal cord compression, brain metastases, seizures, and carcinomatous meningitis will be considered in this section.

SPINAL CORD COMPRESSION

Although metastasis to the epidural space with resulting spinal cord compression and injury is not the most common neurological complication of cancer, it must be considered the most emergent, and the most capable of producing harm if not recognized and treated with great speed.

Tumors gain access to the epidural space by a variety of means: most commonly, involvement of the anterior elements of the vertebral body (and far less commonly the posterior elements, or neural arch) by metastatic tumor to bone will result in extrinsic compression of the spinal cord. Less commonly, direct extension of tumor via the neural foramina will produce a similar result; rarely, seeding of the dura and subdural spaces by carcinomatous meningitis will be severe enough to cause frank spinal cord compression.

Breast and lung cancer alone will probably account for over one fourth of all spinal cord compressions, and for over one half in many series. Lymphoma, melanoma, prostate cancer, and tumors of "unknown primary" will account for a substantial portion of the remainder. The likely site of cord compression, thoracic, cervical, or lumbosacral, is proportional to the size and number of vertebral bodies in a given segment of the spine, and thus over two-thirds of cord compressions will involve the thoracic spine.

The clinical hallmark of spinal cord compression is back pain, which is present in more than 90% of all patients, often for many weeks or months prior to diagnosis. Frank weakness or loss of sensory function, or both, may follow. Frank paraplegia and bladder dysfunction are late and ominous findings. The pain with which patients present may be radicular rather than central, and may be exacerbated rather than relieved by recumbency, and exacerbated by sneezing, coughing, or the Valsalva maneuver.

The diagnostic evaluation of the patient depends upon the clinical presentation. The patient with pain and any evidence of neurologic impairment, whether subjective or objective, deserves emergent evaluation. The magnetic resonance imaging scan (MRI) has essentially replaced myelography as the diagnostic procedure of choice, and views of the entire spine should be obtained, as multiple levels of compression or threatened compression may be present. The patient with unrelenting pain but without neurologic symptoms and signs should be considered for plain radiographic evaluation: an abnormal X-ray is a strong predictor of cord compression; a normal X-ray, however, does not guarantee against epidural compression. Unrelenting pain alone is justification for MRI scanning, although the emergent nature of this situation is unknown.

The treatment of spinal cord compression begins with the administration of corticosteroids. Dexamethasone at a dose of 10 mg intravenously (some physicians recommend 100 mg) followed by 4 mg every 6 hours (some recommend higher doses) should begin when clinical suspicion is present. Consultations with the radiotherapist, neurologist, and neurosurgeon should be obtained as quickly as possible.

The outcome of therapy depends upon the patient's neurological status at the time the treatment is initiated. Ambulatory patients have a high expectation for remaining ambulatory (greater than 60%) while paraplegic patients have limited chances of regaining ambulatory function (less than 10%). A minimally impaired patient may progress to paraplegia during the diagnostic period within hours. The need for prompt action is thus underscored.

Radiation therapy remains the mainstay of treatment in the opinions of most experts, with a dose of 3000 cGy in approximately ten fractions delivered to the site of cord compression, and one to two vertebral bodies cephalad and caudad to this area. Radiation therapy should be initiated immediately in any patient with neurological symptoms or signs with radiographic evidence of spinal cord compression.

The role of neurosurgery in the treatment of spinal cord compression is evolving. Neurosurgery, either alone or in combination with radiotherapy, may have some role in selected patients with spinal cord compression. Circumstances demanding neurosurgical intervention are listed in Table 50–1.

BRAIN METASTASES

Brain metastases remain the most common neurological complication of cancer; most patients present with nonemergent symptoms and signs, including headache, disturbances of cognitive function, disturbances of mood, and weakness. However, the development of seizures, or an acute neurological deficit, or a progressive neurologic deficit may herald a true emergent consequence of brain metastasis, and must be dealt with accordingly.

Brain metastases produce these emergent complications by a variety of mechanisms. Rapid tumor growth *per se* may produce seizures or neurologic deficits. Cerebral hemorrhage, hydrocephalus, or progressive cerebral edema may produce herniation syndromes which constitute the greatest of CNS emergencies. These same herniation syndromes may, of course, be caused by nonmalignant events to which the cancer patient may be predisposed, including stroke, subdural hematoma, hemorrhage, or abscess formation.

In general, herniation syndromes will be tonsilar (posterior), uncal (temporal), or central, depending upon the predominant site of tumor involvement. Herniation syndromes are characterized generally by their progressive nature, and the development of stupor/coma, pupillary abnormalities, gaze abnormalities, posturing, and ventilatory and hemodynamic changes.

The fundamental approach to the treatment of suspected cerebral metastases includes the prompt administration of corticosteroids (loading dose of dexamethasone, 10 mg to 100 mg intravenously, followed by maintenance doses of 4 mg to 24 mg every 6 hours) coupled with a prompt diagnostic procedure, either a computed tomographic (CT) scan or MRI scan, each done preferably with appropriate contrast agents.

Patients with suspected herniation syndromes, or patients who have rapidly become stuporous or comatose, or who are deteriorating rapidly will require acute intervention that exceeds mere steroid therapy. General guidelines for management of such patients are included in Table 50–2. All measures are directed toward a reduction of intracranial pressure, and will afford stabilization while the appropriate diagnostic scan is performed. Prompt neurosurgical consultation should be obtained for all such patients, as many causes of acute deterioration, including hemorrhage, herniation, edema, or hydrocephalus may be remedied by decompression. Stabilization may require intubation with hyperventilation, osmotic therapy with mannitol, and steroid therapy. Although the optimum dose of dexamethasone has never been established, there is little value in deliberating this issue in the acutely ill patient, and higher doses are recommended.

In the absence of the need for emergent neurosurgical decompression, radiation therapy remains the mainstay of definitive therapy for brain metastases, and should be commenced electively, but promptly upon stabilization. Typical

TABLE 50–1. INDICATIONS FOR NEUROSURGICAL INTERVENTION IN PATIENTS WITH SPINAL CORD COMPRESSION

Need for tissue diagnosis
Neurologic progression despite radiotherapy
Cord compression in a previously radiated area
Spinal instability
Invasion of the spinal cord or epidural space by bone or bone fragments

TABLE 50–2. INTERVENTIONS IN MANAGEMENT OF ACUTE CENTRAL NERVOUS SYSTEM DETERIORATION

Hyperventilation—intubation with pCO_2 maintained at 25–30 mmHg
Osmotic therapy—mannitol 50 g to 100 g bolus dose, repeated as necessary, or
Glycerol 1 g/kg bolus dose, repeated as necessary
Steroid therapy
Dexamethasone 100 mg loading and 24 mg q6h
Neurosurgical consultation

TABLE 50–3. CONDITIONS FOR ELECTIVE SURGICAL RESECTION OF BRAIN METASTASES

DIAGNOSTIC UNCERTAINTY
NO KNOWN PRIMARY TUMOR
POSSIBLE NONMALIGNANT ETIOLOGY (MENINGIOMA, BENIGN DISEASE, INFECTION)
SOLITARY METASTASIS
AMBULATORY PERFORMANCE STATUS
SURGICALLY ACCESSIBLE LESION IN NONCRITICAL LOCATION
PRIMARY DISEASE AND OTHER METASTATIC DISEASE WELL-CONTROLLED

doses of 3000 cGy over two weeks will bring about symptomatic improvement in the majority of patients. Elective surgical resection of brain metastases is usually not necessary, but may be beneficial if the metastasis is solitary and other conditions are met (Table 50–3); or in cases of diagnostic uncertainty.

SEIZURES

Although seizures are not the most common presenting manifestation of cerebral metastases, they are the most common acute manifestation, occurring as the presenting manifestation in 15% of patients with brain metastases. Conversely, brain metastases are the most common cause of seizures in cancer patients. Seizures may result from a variety of conditions in the absence of frank cerebral metastases, including carcinomatous meningitis and the nonmalignant causes listed in Table 50–4.

Every patient with a new onset of seizures should be approached emergently. Repeated seizures (status epilepticus) should be managed with benzodiazepines (diazepam or lorazepam, intravenously) for stabilization and intravenous diphenylhydantoin (approximately 15 mg/kg. loading at a rate not to exceed 50 mg/minute and a maintenance dose of 5 mg/kg/day) for prophylaxis. Single seizures or suspected seizures may be treated with oral loading of diphenylhydantoin 1 gram over approximately 24 hours, with similar maintenance doses as above. The same treatment philosophy should be used for both focal and generalized seizures, although the former may be more difficult to control.

TABLE 50–4. NONMALIGNANT CAUSES OF SEIZURES IN CANCER PATIENTS

Hyperglycemia	Narcotic withdrawal
Hypoglycemia	Cerebrovascular accident
Uremia	Cerebral hemorrhage
Hyponatremia	Subdural hematoma
Hypernatremia	Disseminated intravascular coagulation
Hypomagnesemia	Marantic endocarditis
Hypocalcemia	Infectious meningitis
Hepatic failure	Brain abscess
Hypoxia	Sinus thrombosis

Such pharmacologic stabilization may proceed while diagnostic evaluation begins. Routine assessment of electrolytes, tests of liver and kidney function, blood gases, blood counts, and coagulation studies should be obtained as the history and neurological examination proceed. CT or MRI imaging of the brain (contrast-enhanced) should be performed in virtually every patient with a known primary malignancy and new onset seizures, even when a frank metabolic abnormality is noted and corrected. The role of diagnostic lumbar puncture is less clearly defined, but generally should follow imaging studies unless clinical suspicion for infectious meningitis is high, and should be avoided if clinical or radiographic evidence of herniation or increased intracranial pressure are present.

Anticonvulsant therapy is generally not recommended for prophylaxis against seizures in patients with known brain metastases who have never had seizures. Correction of metabolic deficits that cause seizures obviates the need for ongoing anticonvulsant therapy, providing that brain metastases or carcinomatous meningitis are absent. For patients intolerant of diphenylhydantoin, phenobarbitol remains the drug of second choice.

The role of electroencephalography (EEG) in the evaluation of seizures in the cancer patient is less well defined. This study is of little value in patients with demonstrable metastases, and is probably best reserved for patients without an obvious structural or infectious cause, and for patients who continue to seize despite anticonvulsant therapy and correction of obvious electrolyte abnormalities.

CARCINOMATOUS MENINGITIS

Carcinomatous meningitis is an uncommon but well-recognized consequence of metastatic carcinoma, particularly lung and breast carcinoma. Infiltration of the leptomeninges is also a well-known phenomenon in the lymphoid malignancies (non-Hodgkin's lymphoma) and the acute leukemias. The pathological process begins when the leptomeningeal membranes become infiltrated by malignant cells. This process can occur at any point or points along the neuraxis; the array of potential presenting signs and symptoms is broad and varied.

In general, most reviews pinpoint headache, mental status change, diplopia, hearing loss, visual disturbances, weakness, paresthesias, and back pain as the more common presenting symptoms. True "meningitic" signs, such as neck rigidity and pain on leg-raising are absent in most patients. The clinical diagnosis of carcinomatous meningitis thus requires a high index of suspicion in any cancer patient who presents with neurological complaints of recent onset, particularly if those complaints or the attendant physical findings involve more than one level of the neuraxis.

Whether or not carcinomatous meningitis constitutes a true neurological emergency is not a valid issue; although the natural history of this condition is quite variable, this phenomenon can cause acute and permanent neurological injury by a variety of mechanisms. First, the association of seizures with carcinomatous meningitis is well known; they may be the presenting symptom in up to 10% of patients. Second, brain metastases will co-exist with carcinomatous meningitis in up to one fourth of patients; such patients will presumably be predisposed to all of the potential for acute deterioration that exists in a patient with brain metastases alone. Third, the co-existence of epidural metastases in more than one fourth of carcinomatous meningitis patients has been described, raising the potential for acute epidural cord compression. Finally, a rapidly progressing, high-growth fraction tumor may produce rapidly progressive neurological symptoms by virtue of its growth rate alone.

The diagnostic evaluation of patients with suspected carcinomatous meningitis should proceed swiftly. Comatose or seizing patients, although uncommon in this setting, should be offered the same emergent care as described in the above sections. The lumbar puncture remains the diagnostic mainstay of carcinomatous meningitis. It is prudent, however, first to obtain emergent MRI scanning of the brain in any patient who develops progressive mental status changes or signs of increasing intracranial pressure. Patients with back pain and neurological signs or symptoms should be presumed to have epidural metastases until proven otherwise, and whole-spine MRI scanning should precede the lumbar puncture.

The diagnosis of carcinomatous meningitis rests upon the demonstration of malignant cells in the cerebrospinal fluid. A single lumbar puncture is successful in demonstrating these malignant cells in only about half of patients, although virtually all patients will have some abnormality in CSF glucose, protein, cell count, or opening pressure. An abnormality of any of these parameters with normal cytology mandates repeated lumbar punctures; sometimes as many as six spinal taps are required to establish the diagnosis. If a positive cytology cannot be obtained promptly in a severely symptomatic or deteriorating patient, gadolinium-enhanced MRI scanning of the neuraxis may provide radiographic clues (Table 50–5) that justify commencement of therapy in the absence of positive cytology.

Treatment of carcinomatous meningitis is directed at symptom relief and stabilization of neurological deficits. The treatment consists usually of some combination of steroids, radiation therapy, and chemotherapy. Dexamethasone in doses similar to those used in the treatment of brain metastases or epidural spinal cord compression will relieve headache, nausea, and pain. Radiation therapy is recommended for all patients with site-specific symptoms. Cranial radiation therapy in doses of approximately 3000 cGy over two weeks may relieve headache, nausea, and mental status changes. Base of skull radiotherapy may reverse some cranial nerve deficits. Radiation therapy should be given to sites of back and radicular pain and should be given, of course, to any site of epidural cord compression or bulky epidural disease.

TABLE 50–5. RADIOGRAPHIC (MRI OR MYELOGRAPHIC) SIGNS OF CARCINOMATOUS MENINGITIS

Meningeal enhancement
Tentorial enhancement
Nerve root enhancement
Cisternal enhancement
Enhancement of sulci
Thickening or nodularity of nerve roots
Multiple dural nodules
Hydrocephalus

The institution of intrathecal chemotherapy is recommended for patients with meningitis of leukemic or lymphoid origin, for most breast cancer and small-cell lung cancer patients, and for other patients who cannot be successfully palliated by other means. Chemotherapy may be required emergently in severe cases of leukemic or lymphomatous meningitis, and if so, methotrexate in doses of 7 mg/m^2, maximum dose 15 mg, should be administered via the lumbar route, and should be co-administered with oral calcium leuzovorin. A leucovorin dose of 10 mg orally or intravenously every 6 hours for 4 to 6 doses should begin approximately 24 hours following methotrexate administration. Cytosine arabinoside or thiotepa serve as alternatives for patients intolerant of methotrexate. There is no indication for combination therapy (see Table 50–6).

Patients who do not require emergent intrathecal chemotherapy are best treated via the intraventricular route, using an implantable (Ommaya) reservoir.

In general, intrathecal chemotherapy by whatever route is continued twice weekly until clinical stabilization and cytologic normalization are achieved. The frequency of treatment is then decreased arbitrarily but gradually after maximum response is achieved, and may ultimately be discontinued.

TABLE 50–6. INTRATHECAL CHEMOTHERAPEUTIC DOSING OPTIONS IN THE TREATMENT OF CARCINOMATOUS MENINGITIS

Methotrexate 7 mg/m^2 (10–15 mg) with leucovorin 10 mg (po or iv) q 6 h for 4–6 doses 24 hr post methotrexate
Cytosine arabinoside 30–100 mg
Thiotepa 10–15 mg

REFERENCES

DeLorenzo R. Status epilepticus. In Johnson RT (ed): Current Therapy in Neurologic Disease Part 3. Philadelphia, Decker, 1990:47

Gilbert RW, Kim J, Posner JB. Epidural spinal cord compression from metastatic cancer: Diagnosis and treatment. Ann Neurol 8:361, 1980

Glover DJ, Grabelsky S, and Glick JH. Oncological emergencies and special complications. In Calabresi P, Schein P. Medical Oncology (2nd ed.). New York, McGraw-Hill, 1993:1021

Haller DG, Fox KR, Schuchter LM. Special complications of metastatic disease. In Fowble B, Goodman RL, Glick JH, Rosato EF. Breast Cancer Treatment: A Comprehensive Guide to Management. St. Louis, Mosby, 1991:420

Patchell RA, Tibbs PA, Walsh JW. A randomized trial of surgery in the treatment of solitary metastases to the brain. N Engl J Med 322:494, 1990

Sarpel S, Sarpel G, Yu E. Early diagnosis of spinal epidural metastasis by magnetic resonance imaging. Cancer 59:1112, 1987

Wasserstrom WR, Glass JP, Posner JB. Diagnosis and treatment of leptomeningeal metastases from solid tumors. Cancer 49:759, 1982

John S. Macdonald, Daniel G. Haller, Robert J. Mayer, Eds. *Manual of Oncologic Therapeutics*, Third Edition.

51. METABOLIC EMERGENCIES

Donna Glover

HYPERCALCEMIA

The most frequent metabolic emergency in oncology is hypercalcemia, which develops when the rate of calcium mobilization from bone exceeds the renal threshold for calcium excretion. Neoplastic disease is the leading cause of hypercalcemia among inpatients.[1–3] The tumors most commonly associated with hypercalcemia are carcinomas of the breast and lung, hypernephroma, multiple myeloma, squamous cell carcinoma of the head and neck, and esophageal and thyroid cancer.[2] Parathyroid carcinoma is a rare malignancy associated with intractable hypercalcemia due to elevated parathyroid hormone (PTH) levels.

Although over 80% of patients with hypercalcemia have osseous metastases, the extent of bony disease does not correlate with the level of hypercalcemia.[2] During the course of their disease, from 40% to 50% of patients with breast carcinoma metastatic to the bone will develop hypercalcemia. In most settings, hypercalcemia suggests progression of disease. However, patients with metastatic breast cancer involving bone may develop hypercalcemia when they are placed on hormonal therapy. Estrogen and anti-estrogens stimulate breast cancer cells to produce osteolytic substances that increase bone resorption.[4] Within several days of initiating hormonal therapy for metastatic breast cancer, the calcium level may rise and the bone pain may increase. This tumor flare in response to hormonal therapy usually implies that the patient will subsequently have an excellent antitumor response to hormonal treatment. However, the hormonal therapy may have to be temporarily delayed and the hypercalcemia corrected before the hormone is reinstituted.

In the majority of patients with bone metastases, bone resorption occurs when malignant cells metastatic to bone produce humoral substances which stimulate osteoclast activity and cause hypercalcemia. However, 20% of solid tumors associated with hypercalcemia show no evidence of osseous spread. In these situations, investigators have demonstrated humoral substances, such as parathyroid hormone-like substances and cytokines, which are secreted by tumor cells. In multiple myeloma, hypercalcemia occurs because of production of cytokines such as interleukin-I by the abnormal plasma cells.[2]

Bone metastases or the indirect effects of ectopic humoral substances directly stimulate osteoclast activity and proliferation. Although osseous metastases are frequently surrounded by a zone of osteoclasts, it is not clear whether hypercalcemia results from direct neoplastic bony destruction or from release of osteolytic substances from the malignant cells. *In vitro* studies have shown that some cancer cell lines are capable of resorbing bone without increasing osteoclast activity.[2–4]

Patients with squamous cell carcinoma of the head and neck, lung, and esophagus may develop a clinical syndrome that suggests hyperparathyroidism due to ectopic secretion of a parathyroid hormone peptide, which is structurally similar to PTH. In association with hypercalcemia, patients develop hypophosphatemia, increased urinary cyclic adenosine monophosphate, and elevations in bone alkaline phosphatase.[2] Although it is clear that parathyroid carcinoma cells produce excessive parathyroid hormones, in other tumor types recent data suggest that ectopic parathyroid hormone production is a rarer cause of hypercalcemia than previously reported. Except in parathyroid carcinoma, extractable PTH is rarely present in neoplastic tissues. Most cases of hypercalcemia that were presumed to be secondary to ectopic PTH production are now felt to be due to ectopic secretion of PTH-like substances that bind to PTH receptors. In contrast to hypercalcemia due to hyperparathyroidism, these patients have impaired production of 1,25-dihydroxy vitamin D and no evidence of renal bicarbonate wasting.[4]

Osteolytic prostaglandins have been detected in hypercalcemic patients with carcinomas of the lung, kidney, and ovary.[5–8]

Lymphokines and cytokines are the "Osteoclast Activating Factors" (OAF), potent osteolytic peptides which cause bone resorption and secondary hypercalcemia in multiple myeloma and lymphoma. However, despite the potent osteolytic activity of OAF *in vitro*, patients with elevated levels of OAF do not always develop hypercalcemia unless there is renal dysfunction.[4] Patients with lymphoma due to the human T-cell lymphotrophic virus present with severe hypercalcemia due to ectopic production of several osteotrophic factors (OAF, colony-stimulating factor, gamma-interferon, and an active vitamin D metabolite).[4]

Clinical Presentation and Diagnostic Evaluation

Hypercalcemia is rarely a presenting sign of malignancy, except in patients with parathyroid carcinoma, HTLV-1 T-cell lymphomas, or multiple myeloma. Most hypercalcemic patients present with nonspecific symptoms of fatigue, anorexia, nausea, polyuria, polydipsia, and constipation. Neurologic symptoms from hypercalcemia begin with vague muscle weakness, lethargy, apathy, and hyporeflexia. Without treatment, symptoms progress to profound alterations in mental status, psychotic behavior, seizures, coma, and death. Patients with prolonged hypercalcemia eventually develop permanent renal tubular abnormalities with renal tubular acidosis, glucosuria, aminoaciduria, and hyperphosphaturia.[3] Sudden death from cardiac arrhythmias may occur when the serum calcium rises acutely.[1-2] Except in parathyroid cancer, hypercalcemic cancer patients rarely live long enough to develop signs of chronic hypercalcemia.

All hypercalcemic patients should have serial serum calcium measurements and measurements of phosphate, alkaline phosphatase, electrolytes, blood urea nitrogen (BUN), and creatinine levels. In malnourished patients with low albumin levels, the ionized calcium value may be helpful in deciding on therapy, since hypercalcemic symptoms correlate with elevation in ionized rather than protein-bound calcium. Patients with multiple myeloma may have elevated serum calcium levels secondary to abnormal calcium binding to paraproteins without an elevation in ionized calcium, while malnourished patients with hypoalbuminemia may have symptoms of hypercalcemia with normal serum calcium levels. The electrocardiogram often reveals shortening of the QT interval, widening of the T wave, bradycardia, and PR prolongation.[2]

Therapy

The cause of hypercalcemia, the severity of associated clinical signs, and the chances of response to effective antitumor therapy determine the most appropriate hypocalcemic therapy. Mild hypercalcemia is frequently corrected with intravenous hydration alone. If effective antitumor therapy is available, the serum calcium will gradually decline as the tumor regresses. However, most hypercalcemic cancer patients require additional hypocalcemic therapy until an antitumor response is obtained. Calcium balance can be corrected by directly decreasing bone resorption, promoting urinary calcium excretion, and decreasing oral calcium intake. Patients should be mobilized to avoid osteolysis. Constipation should be corrected. Medications such as thiazide diuretics or vitamins A and D, which may elevate calcium levels, should never be used.[2]

All hypercalcemic patients are dehydrated because of polyuria from renal tubular dysfunction. Intravenous hydration with normal saline will increase urinary calcium excretion since the urinary clearance rates for calcium excretion parallel sodium excretion.[2] When hypercalcemia is life-threatening, aggressive hydration (*e.g.*, 250–300 ml/hour) and intravenous furosemide should be employed to decrease calcium resorption. However, hypercalcemia will not be corrected unless a potent osteoclast inhibitor or inhibitor of bone resorption is given.

Corticosteroids are effective hypocalcemic agents in multiple myeloma, lymphoma, breast cancer, and leukemia. Corticosteroids block bone resorption caused by cytokines and lymphokines. High-dose steroids may also have hypocalcemic effects by increasing urinary calcium excretion, inhibiting vitamin D metabolism, decreasing calcium absorption, and, after long-term use, by producing negative calcium balance in bone.[2-4] High doses of corticosteroids are generally required for several days before an effective hypocalcemic response is seen. Most patients require up to 100 mg. of prednisone daily.[2-9]

Hypercalcemia can be easily treated with intravenous biphosphonates (*e.g.* etidronate, disodium pamidronate). These drugs have rapid hypocalcemic effects; they act by inhibiting osteoclast activity. Etidronate was the first diphosphonate to be marketed in the United States. Intravenously, this drug produces normal calcium levels in 75% to 100% of patients with malignancy associated with hypercalcemia. In addition to its inhibition of bone resorption, etidronate may also decrease new bone formation. Etidronate should be infused over two hours, since high bolus doses in animals have caused renal damage. Because of limited experience in patients with renal failure, caution should be used when the drug is administered to patients with elevated creatinines. Oral etidronate is generally well tolerated and may be useful for prolonging the duration of normocalcemia in patients initially treated with the IV form. The dose of etidronate disodium is 7.5 mg/kg IV per day, infused over 2 hours to reduce renal toxicity. The drug is less effective orally than intravenously; it is not an optimal choice for initial or sole treatment of hypercalcemia.

Newer drugs of the bisphosphonate series, such as disodium pamidronate, are able to inhibit bone resorption at doses that have little effect on bone mineralization. Hypocalcemic effects are observed within one day, and the calcium usually normalizes within one week. This drug has a safety and efficacy profile for oral administration that makes it a promising outpatient regimen for hypercalcemia. Disodium pamidronate is a more potent hypocalcemic agent than etidronate. In randomized studies the magnitude and duration of the hypocalcemic effects were greater following pamidronate compared to etidronate.

In vitro, gallium nitrate produces a dose-dependent reduction in the osteolytic response to PTH and certain lymphokines and cytokines that cause hypercalcemia. In initial studies, gallium nitrate was infused intravenously at doses ranging from 100 to 200 mg/m^2 daily for 5 consecutive days to control hypercalcemia associated with malignant conditions. In 86% of patients the serum calcium concentration normalized with 200 mg/m^2 dose compared to 60% of patients who received 100 mg/m^2. The hypocalcemic response was usually seen within 2 days and was maintained for 4 to 14 days after the drug was discontinued. The main treatment-associated side effect was transient serum creatinine elevation of 2 mg/dl or less. A controlled trial compared gallium nitrate at 200 mg/m^2 to salmon calcitonin 8 I.U./kg every 6 hours for 5 days. Seventy-five percent of patients treated with gallium nitrate became normocalcemic compared to 31% treated with calcitonin. Gallium nitrate is contraindicated in patients with renal insufficiency, while the hypocalcemic effects of the other agents seem to be due to another mechanism.

Ten years ago, many hypercalcemic patients required treatment with mithramycin, a chemotherapeutic agent that decreased bone resorption by reducing osteoclast number and activity. Mithramycin is effective in patients with hypercalcemia from either bone metastases or ectopic humoral substances.[11] Mithramycin is a sclerosing agent and must be given as a bolus through a freshly started intravenous line. If extravasation occurs, patients will develop ulceration and ultimately fibrosis of the underlying tissues. Hypercalcemic patients will often require one or two injections of mithramycin (15 μg–20 μg/kg) per week, unless effective antitumor therapy is initiated. The serum calcium level will begin to fall within 6 to 48 hours. If no response occurs within the first 2 days, a second dose should be administered.[2,9,11,12] Since only low doses of mithramycin are necessary to control hypercalcemia, the majority of patients do not develop the side-effects generally seen with high doses of the drug (*e.g.*, thrombocytopenia, coagulopathy, hypertension, liver function abnormalities, or nephrotoxicity).[11–12] Now mithramycin is used rarely, due to less toxic alternative therapies.

When hypercalcemia occurs following therapy for metastatic breast cancer, patients should be treated with hydration, steroids, and, if necessary, bisphosphonates. When severe hypercalcemia occurs after hormonal therapy for breast cancer, the hormone should be discontinued immediately. Once the calcium level normalizes, the hormone can be restarted in lower doses and gradually increased. When mild hypercalcemia is precipitated by hormonal therapy, the hormone frequently can be continued without undue risk while the patient is managed with hydration alone.[2]

Calcitonin promptly inhibits bone resorption, causing a fall in serum calcium within hours of administration.[2,13] Although a prompt hypocalcemic response is obtained, tachyphylaxis develops unless glucocorticoid therapy is given with calcitonin. If the serum calcium begins to rise with calcitonin, the drug may be temporarily discontinued and then reinstituted; occasionally for unclear reasons a secondary response will occur within 48 hours. Calcitonin is given in daily doses of 3 to 6 Medical Research Council (MRC) units/kg intravenously or twice daily by intramuscular or subcutaneous injection (100–400 MRC units).[2,14]

Although initial clinical trials suggested that inhibitors of prostaglandin synthesis (*e.g.*, indomethacin or aspirin) were hypocalcemic agents, subsequent trials have failed to confirm the initial reports.[1,2,9]

The majority of patients are effectively managed with hydration, mobilization, effective antitumor therapy, and gradually tapering doses of bisphosphonates or, in steroid responsive malignancies, corticosteroids. If effective antitumor therapy is not available, patients must be maintained on hypocalcemic therapy indefinitely. Serum calciums should be monitored at least twice weekly. If corticosteroids are used, the dose can be gradually tapered to the lowest effective therapeutic dose. If mithramycin is used chronically, one can generally lengthen the interval between injections. Similarly, if hypercalcemia is controlled with calcitonin, the injections can be gradually increased from 12 to 24 hours.[2]

URIC ACID NEPHROPATHY

Uric acid nephropathy is usually associated with malignancies that have an increased rate of cell turnover. Although this can occur spontaneously, uric acid deposition in the urinary tract most frequently is reported as a complication of cytotoxic therapy that produces a rapid antitumor response. With rapid cell death, increased uric acid production results in hyperuricemia and uric acid crystal deposition in the urinary tract.[15–17] Hyperuricemia and associated renal uric deposition occur most commonly with the tumor lysis syndrome, which is often associated with Burkitt's lymphoma. Although most episodes of uric acid nephropathy are associated with effective cytotoxic chemotherapy or radiotherapy in hematologic malignancies, spontaneous hyperuricemic nephropathy has been occasionally reported in patients with aggressive lymphoma and leukemia.[16] Untreated leukemics have increased uric acid excretion. The degree and incidence of hyperuricemia correlate with the cytologic type of leukemia, rather than with the degree of white count elevation. For example, uric acid excretion is typically higher in "aleukemic" acute myelocytic leukemia than in chronic lymphocytic leukemia.[2,15]

Uric acid stones are seen in less than 10% of hyperuricemic cancer patients in recent series. Uric acid calculi occur most often in patients with chronic hyperuricemia (*e.g.*, those with chronic myeloproliferative syndromes).[2,16]

The incidence and severity of hyperuricemic nephropathy have decreased with prophylactic allopurinol, vigorous hydration, and akalinization of the urine. In previous studies, mortality rates from hyperuricemic nephropathy ranged from 47% to 100%. However, with aggressive medical therapy, now the majority of patients regain normal renal function within a few days of treatment after the serum uric acid level falls below 10 mg/dl.[16]

The tumors most commonly associated with hyperuricemia are leukemia and lymphoma, but case reports of uric acid nephropathy have been reported among patients with chronic myeloproliferative syndromes, multiple myeloma, and squamous cell carcinomas of the head and neck.[2,16]

Clinical Presentation and Diagnostic Evaluation

Since patients rarely develop ureteral obstruction, flank pain and gross hematuria are uncommon.[16] The majority of patients present with signs of uremia, including nausea, vomiting, lethargy, and oliguria.[2,16,17] With early treatment, there is an excellent chance of rapidly reversing renal dysfunction.[2,16,17] Often, it is difficult to differentiate acute uric acid nephropathy from other causes of renal failure with secondary hyperuricemia. In acute uric acid nephropathy, the mean serum uric acid level at presentation is 20.1 mg/dl (ranging from 9.2 to 92 mg/dl).[16] Since hyperuricemia increases the incidence of dye-induced renal dysfunction, intravenous contrast should be avoided. In the tumor lysis syndrome, hyperphosphatemia and hypocalcemia often occur disproportionately with the degree of renal insufficiency.[16] Serial blood studies for electrolytes, blood urea nitrogen, creatinine, calcium, phosphorus, and uric acid must be obtained. The urinalysis will be helpful if uric acid crystals are seen, but their absence does not exclude the diagnosis since crystalluria and hematuria occur only in the acute phase.[16,17] Kelton has demonstrated that a urinary uric acid to creatinine ratio greater than one is relatively specific for hyperuricemia nephropathy.[2]

Therapy

The primary goal of therapy should be the prevention of hyperuricemia. Patients at high risk should be treated with allopurinol, vigorous hydration, and urinary alkalinization for at least 48 hours prior to cytotoxic therapy. Drugs that block tubular reabsorption of uric acid (*e.g.*, aspirin, radiographic contrast, probenecid, and thiazide diuretics) should be avoided.[17] Prior to chemotherapy, the serum uric acid level should be normal, the urine pH above 7, and the urine volume greater than 3 liters per day.[2,15,16,18] To alkalinize the urine, intravenous sodium bicarbonate 100 mEq/m^2 daily should be given. When the urinary pH is above 7.5, uric acid solubility is maximal. Therefore, it is not necessary to produce significant metabolic alkalosis, which may complicate the clinical situation.[16–18] Serum potassium and magnesium levels should be followed closely. Allopurinol should be administered in doses ranging from 300 mg to 800 mg daily. Allopurinol decreases uric acid production by competitively inhibiting xanthine oxidase.[15,16,18] Although high xanthine levels might precipitate xanthine stones, this has not been reported in patients treated for hyperuricemic nephropathy.[2,17] Prophylactic colchicine is not required when allopurinol is administered, since patients rarely develop acute gouty arthritis.

If oliguria or anuria develops, ureteral obstruction must be excluded by renal ultrasound or antegrade or retrograde pyelography. Nephrotoxic contrast must be avoided. Once ureteral obstruction is excluded, mannitol or high-dose furosemide should be given in an attempt to restore urine flow. A Foley catheter should be inserted to measure urine output accurately. If prompt diuresis does not occur within a few hours, emergency hemodialysis will be necessary to reverse uric acid obstruction of the renal tubules.[16]

A hollow-fiber kidney apparatus will decrease serum uric acid levels more rapidly than either peritoneal or coil hemodialysis.[2,15] With hemodialysis, all patients in Kjellstrand's series had rapid normalization of renal function and a prompt diuresis when the serum uric acid level fell below 10 mg to 20 mg/dl. Within 6 hours of hemodialysis, uric acid levels generally fall by 50%. Most patients will require 6 days of dialysis before hyperuricemia resolves and renal function returns to baseline normal values.[16]

In patients undergoing dialysis, a low-calcium dialysate should be used to prevent calcium phosphate precipitation, which theoretically would increase nephrotoxicity. Aluminum hydroxide antacids may also help to decrease gastrointestinal phosphate absorption.[16] If hemodialysis cannot be employed, uric acid clearance can be improved by adding albumin to the peritoneal dialysis. Albumin will increase uric acid protein binding and removal.[17] Alkalinizing the dialysate to a neutral pH with sodium bicarbonate will also enhance uric acid clearance.[19] Fortunately, with aggressive measures for prevention and treatment, acute uric acid nephropathy now has an extremely low morbidity rate and mortality rate.[2,16]

HYPONATREMIA

Only 1% to 2% of patients with malignancy develop the syndrome of inappropriate antidiuretic hormone secretion (SIADH). Despite a low plasma osmality, the urine is inappropriately concentrated with a high sodium concentration. Since this situation can also occur in renal disease, hypothyroidism, and adrenal insufficiency, these disorders must be excluded to confirm the diagnosis of SIADH.[20–22] The majority of patients are asymptomatic unless the serum sodium concentration falls abruptly.[2]

Ectopic antidiuretic hormone secretion has only been confirmed in patients with bronchogenic carcinoma. Small cell anaplastic carcinoma of the lung is the most common malignancy associated with SIADH.[2] At presentation, over 50% of patients with small cell lung cancer may develop hyponatremia following a water load, but less than 15% of patients will develop clinically significant hyponatremia.[2,23] SIADH has also been reported with cancers of the prostate, adrenal cortex, esophagus, pancreas, colon, head and neck, carcinoid, thymoma, lymphoma, and mesothelioma.[2,22]

Since ectopic antidiuretic hormone production is rarely seen except in patients with small cell carcinoma, SIADH is more frequently associated with pulmonary or central nervous system metastases. Inappropriate antidiuretic hormone secretion can also occur with medications such as morphine, vincristine, and cyclophosphamide.[20,21] With advanced malignancy, patients may also develop hyponatremia due to a "reset osmostat." In this situation, the serum sodium is usually mildly depressed and with effective antitumor therapy may return to normal levels. Kerns and co-workers reported that SIADH secretion can occur with pituitary prolactinomas.[24] These tumors may produce SIADH without detectable arginine vasopressin levels. In this setting, bromocriptine induces both tumor regression and correction of hyponatremia.

Adrenal insufficiency due to withdrawal of corticosteroids or metastases to the adrenal or pituitary glands may cause mild hyponatremia. In the setting of severe liver disease, heart failure, or acute renal insufficiency, patients may develop dilutional hyponatremia.[20,21] Vomiting, diarrhea, ascites, or diuretics may precipitate hyponatremia.[21] Patients with plasma cell dyscrasias may have artifactual hyponatremia. Electrolytes should be followed when the patients are treated with high-dose cisplatin and mannitol diuresis.[25]

Pathophysiology

With increased antidiuretic hormone (ADH) secretion, excessive water is reabsorbed in the collecting ducts. This leads to increased distal sodium delivery by producing a mild increase in intravascular volume. Volume expansion also increases renal perfusion, decreases proximal tubular reabsorption of sodium, and decreases aldosterone effect.[5] Ectopic ADH secretion has been measured in patients with small cell lung carcinoma.[25] In other conditions associated with increased ADH secretion, there is excessive production of ADH by the posterior pituitary.[2]

Dilutional hyponatremia occurs in volume-overloaded states secondary to cardiac, hepatic, or renal dysfunction. Although the total body sodium and water content are increased, the circulating plasma volume is reduced. With impaired renal perfusion, there is greater absorption of water in the collecting ducts and increased ADH secretion, resulting in a dilutional hyponatremic state.[20] With dehydration, total body salt and water content are generally decreased. This results in decreased renal perfusion and increased ADH secretion. Diuretics, interstitial renal disease, and mineralocorticoid deficiency are also associated with excessive renal sodium losses. Pseudohyponatremia is associated with excessive renal sodium losses. Pseudohyponatremia is associated with elevated paraprotein levels in patients with plasma cell dyscrasias. Since the plasma sodium concentration is measured as the sodium concentration per unit of plasma, with elevated paraprotein levels the percentage of water in plasma is decreased.[20] With mannitol infusion or hyperglycemia, an osmotic gradient produces increased water movement into the extravascular spaces, resulting in hyponatremia.[2]

Clinical Presentation

With mild hyponatremia, patients may complain of anorexia, nausea, myalgias, and subtle neurologic symptoms. When hyponatremia develops rapidly or the sodium falls below 115 mg/dl, patients frequently have alterations in mental status ranging from lethargy to confusion and coma. Seizures and psychotic behavior have also been reported.[21,22] With profound hyponatremia, alterations of mental status, pathologic reflexes, papilledema, and (rarely) focal neurologic signs may be found on physical examination.[21,22] The cause of hyponatremia must be determined before appropriate therapy can be initiated. If pseudohyponatremia due to hyperproteinemia, hyperlipidemia, or hyperglycemia is suspected, serum protein electrophoresis, lipids, and glucose levels should be checked. Medication records should be reviewed since chemotherapeutic agents (*e.g.*, vincristine or cyclophosphamide), mannitol, morphine, diuretics, and abrupt steroid withdrawal may contribute to hyponatremia.[2]

A careful history and physical examination and review of patient's intake and output will help to determine whether the patient is volume-expanded, dehydrated, or euvolemic. Serum and urine electrolytes, osmolality, and creatinine should be measured. With SIADH, there is inappropriate sodium concentration in the urine for the level of hyponatremia. The urine osmolality is greater than plasma osmolality but is never maximally dilute. With SIADH, the BUN is usually low from volume expansion. Hypouricemia and hypophosphatemia may result from decreased proximal tubular reabsorption of these ions.[2,20,21] Thyroid and adrenal dysfunction should be ruled out if laboratory studies suggest SIADH. Chest films and CT scans of the brain may reveal pulmonary or neurologic disorders that may cause ADH production.

Therapy

Ideally, treatment should be directed at the cause of the hyponatremia. SIADH resolves when the underlying cause of excessive antidiuretic hormone production is removed. Following effective combination chemotherapy for small cell lung cancer, the sodium will rise to normal levels. Corticosteroids and radiotherapy may alleviate SIADH due to brain metastasis. If drug-induced SIADH occurs, the serum sodium will return to normal once the offending agent is discontinued.[2] If the etiology of excessive ADH secretion cannot be corrected, the initial therapy is water restriction. If free water intake is restricted to 500 ml to 1000 ml per day, the negative free water balance will correct the hyponatremia within 7 to 10 days.[2,20–22,26] If the serum sodium does not correct with water restriction, demeclocycline may correct hyponatremia by decreasing the ADH stimulus for water reabsorption in the collecting ducts.[20,21,27,28] Demeclocycline produces a dose-dependent reversible nephrogenic diabetes insipidus.[20,27,29]

With demeclocycline, despite liberal fluid intake, the average pretreatment serum sodium (121 mEq/liter) rose above 130 mEq/liter within 3 to 4 days of initiating treatment.[22] The only side effect of demeclocycline is reversible nephrotoxicity.[2, 22] Renal dysfunction develops in less than half of patients and is generally mild. The majority of patients who experienced nephrotoxicity were either receiving other nephrotoxic drugs or received higher doses of demeclocycline. Since demeclocycline is excreted in the urine and bile, patients with renal or hepatic dysfunction should either avoid this drug or receive reduced doses.[2,22,27] The initial daily demeclocycline dose is 600 mg; however, lower doses should be used in patients with liver or renal disease or when other nephrotoxic drugs are administered.[26] Doses may be increased up to 200 mg daily if hyponatremia persists. The total daily dose should be divided into two or three doses per day.[2]

Patients with coma or seizures from SIADH should receive 3% hypertonic saline or isotonic saline with intravenous furosemide, 1 mg/kg.[2] In volume-expanded patients, hyponatremia will resolve if the associated cardiac, renal, or liver dysfunction can be corrected. Dehydrated hyponatremic patients are managed with intravenous isotonic saline solutions.[20,21]

HYPOGLYCEMIA

Fasting hypoglycemia occurs with insulinomas and, rarely, other islet cell tumors of the pancreas. Most of the other associated tumors are large bulky mesenchymal malignancies, including fibrosarcomas, mesotheliomas, and spindle cell sarcomas.[2,30–32]

Normally, glucose homeostasis is maintained by appropriate hormonal regulation of gluconeogenesis and glycogenolysis in patients with adequate caloric intake.[2] Tumor-induced hypoglycemia may be caused by secretion of insulin or an insulin-like substance, increased glucose utilization by the tumor, or alternations in the regulatory mechanisms for glucose homeostasis. Although insulin levels are elevated in patients with hypoglycemia from islet cell cancers, increased insulin secretion has not been observed with other neoplasms.[2,31] Using bioassays, increased levels of substances with insulin-like activity have been measured in serum samples from patients with hypoglycemia and non-islet cell malignancies. These substances are now referred to as nonsuppressible insulin-like activity (NSILA). Only 5% to 10% of their insulin-like activity can be neutralized with anti-insulin antibodies. NSILA appears to be a combination of somatomedins A and C, high-molecular-weight glycoproteins, and low-molecular-weight growth factors. These substances have both the growth-promoting and metabolic effects of insulin. However, the growth-promoting effects of the low-molecular-weight substances are about 50% greater than insulin's effects, while their metabolic effects are only 1% to 2% as potent. The high-molecular-weight substances have minimal growth-promoting capabilities but maintain their metabolic effects.[2]

Elevated levels of the low-molecular-weight NSILA have been demonstrated in patients with non-islet cell tumors, causing hypoglycemia. Elevated levels of these substances have been observed in patients with hemangiopericytomas, hepatomas, pheochromocytomas, adrenocortical carcinomas, and large mesenchymal tumors. Low to normal levels of NSILA have been measured in patients with hypoglycemia in association with leukemia, lymphoma, or gastrointestinal primaries.[2,31] The majority of hypoglycemic patients with fibrosarcomas will have elevated high-molecular-weight NSILA levels.[2] When there is a rapid reduction in glucose levels in the normal patient, counter-regulatory mechanisms should increase secretion of adrenocorticotropic hormone (ACTH), glucocorticoids, growth hormone, and glucagon. However, in patients with tumor-induced hypoglycemia, the fall in glucose is usually not rapid enough to produce an increase in these hormone levels.[31]

Cancer patients have reduced rate of hepatic gluconogenesis, reduced glycogen breakdown following epinephrine or glucagon, and decreased hepatic glycogen stores.[2,33] Data suggest that impaired glucose homeostasis may contribute to tumor-induced hypoglycemia. In the past, increased glucose utilization by the tumor was thought to be one of the causes of hypoglycemia. However, in this situation, increased glycogen breakdown and gluconeogenesis should compensate for increased glycolysis. Before assuming that the metabolic abnormality is due to the malignancy, one should exclude the more common causes of hypoglycemia (*i.e.*, exogenous insulin use, oral diabetic agents, adrenal failure, pituitary insufficiency, ethanol abuse, or malnutrition).[2]

Most patients will complain of excessive fatigue, weakness, dizziness, and confusion. Patients will rarely have symptoms that suggest reactive hypoglycemia. Hypoglycemic symptoms tend to occur after fasting in the early morning or late afternoon. If the blood sugar remains depressed below 40 mg/dl, seizures may result.

Fasting and late afternoon glucose levels are most helpful in making the diagnosis. Patients with insulinomas will have increased insulin levels with fasting glucose levels below 50 mg/dl, while patients with non-islet cell tumors will have normal to low insulin levels during the period of hypoglycemia.[2,31] Leukemic patients with high leukocyte counts may have artifactual hypoglycemia when blood remains in collection tubes for prolonged periods.[2]

Insulinomas produce large amounts of proinsulin and have elevated proinsulin: insulin ratios. Higher proinsulin levels are seen with malignant insulinomas. If technically feasible, insulin-like plasma factors should be measured by bioassays or radioreceptor techniques.[2]

Hypoglycemia is corrected rapidly with intravenous injections of 50% dextrose. This should be followed by a continuous infusion of 10% dextrose. Insulinomas are frequently cured by surgery. The rare patient with an inoperable insulinoma can be managed with chemotherapy or diazoxide.[2]

If effective antitumor therapy is available for non-islet cell tumors associated with hypoglycemia, the metabolic abnormalities should resolve with tumor regression. Following surgical resection of fibrosarcomas, hypoglycemia will resolve. Effective chemotherapy regimens for mesotheliomas have also corrected hypoglycemia.[31] To prevent nocturnal hypoglycemia, patient should be awakened from sleep for meals and should have frequent between-meal and bedtime snacks. In an occasional patient, corticosteroids may provide temporary relief. Patients have also benefited from intermittent subcutaneous or long-acting intramuscular glucagon injections.[2]

LACTIC ACIDOSIS

Most malignant cell lines have increased rates of glycolysis, which result in increased lactate production. However, even patients with rapidly growing tumors rarely have significant lactate accumulation because of effective hepatic clearance. Lactic acidosis occurs most often with a rapidly growing neoplasm and associated liver dysfunction. The tumors that most commonly cause lactic acidosis are acute lymphocytic leukemia, acute myelogenous leukemia, Hodgkin's disease, and high-grade lymphomas. Isolated cases of lactic acidosis have also been described in association with cancers of the lung, breast, colon, and osteosarcoma.[34–36] If effective systemic chemotherapy is available lactic acidosis will resolve as the tumor regresses.[37] Mild lactic acidosis may also occur as a reversible complication of hypertonic dextrose solutions, which are used for parenteral hyperalimentation.[36–38]

Increased lactate accumulation produces hyperpnea, fatigue, anorexia, and alterations in mental status. The diagnosis is suspected when an increased anion gap is noted in a patient with normal renal function. The diagnosis may be confirmed if the lactate level is over 2 mmol/liter.[36–39] The majority of cancer patients develop lactic acidosis because of circulatory insufficiency, cardiopulmonary complications, or sepsis. These disorders must be excluded before one assumes that lactic acidosis is related to altered tumor metabolism.[36,39]

If lactic acidosis is related to the patient's underlying malignancy, effective antineoplastic therapy should be initiated promptly. Patients may be maintained on oral or intravenous bicarbonate to control the acidosis. However, unless a significant antitumor response is obtained, the prognosis is very poor.

TUMOR LYSIS SYNDROME

The tumor lysis syndrome can occur after effective systemic chemotherapy for rapidly growing, bulky, chemosensitive tumors. Rapid tumor lysis results in release of intracellular uric acid, phosphate, and potassium, which causes hyperuricemia, hypocalcemia, hyperkalemia, and hyperphosphatemia. In the presence of elevated serum phosphate levels, hypocalcemia develops as a result of calcium and phosphate precipitation. Without effective treatment, renal failure occurs rapidly from both uric acid nephropathy and calcium-phosphate deposition in the renal tubules. Since the kidney is the main source for excreting uric acid, potassium, and phosphate, metabolic abnormalities are more likely to occur in patients with preexisting renal dysfunction.[36,40,41]

The tumors most commonly associated with tumor lysis are acute lymphoblastic lymphoma, acute lymphocytic leukemia, Burkitt's lymphoma, and rapidly growing, diffuse, undifferentiated lymphomas.[35,36,41] The syndrome has been described rarely with other non-Hodgkin's lymphomas, myeloproliferative disorders, and chronic myelocytic leukemia in blast crisis.[36,40] Since rapid tumor regression is uncommon in solid tumors, tumor lysis is an infrequent complication of therapy, but it has been found following effective chemotherapy for small cell lung cancer.[36,42] Risk factors for the development of tumor lysis syndrome include a sensitive tumor type, increased tumor bulk, elevated lactate dehydrogenase levels, rapid growth rate, decreased renal function, and high uric acid levels prior to treatment. Tumor lysis occurs within 1 to 5 days of initiating effective chemotherapy.

Treatment should be preventive. Chemotherapy should be delayed until metabolic disturbances are corrected. Ideally, patients should be pretreated with allopurinol, 300 mg twice a day, to normalize uric acid levels prior to chemotherapy. All patients at risk should be prehydrated at a rate of 200 ml to 300 ml per hour for at least 1 day prior to chemotherapy and for 3 to 5 days thereafter. To enhance uric acid excretion, the urine should be alkalinized prior to chemotherapy. However, if alkalinization is continued when phosphate levels rise, this may lead to calcium phosphate precipitation. In patients at high risk for developing the tumor lysis syndrome, blood studies should be obtained twice daily to measure serum electrolytes, calcium, phosphorus, creatinine, and uric acid. Input and output must be carefully recorded.[36]

Hemodialysis is necessary if potassium increases above 6 mEq/liter; uric acid above 10 mEq/dl; creatinine above 10 mg/dl; or phosphorus above 10 mg/dl. Other indications for hemodialysis include volume-overloaded states in association with renal insufficiency and symptomatic hypocalcemia. When methotrexate is employed, serial methotrexate levels should be obtained to determine the need for prolonged leucovorin rescue.[35,36,41]

REFERENCES

1. Besarb A, Caro JF. Mechanisms of hypercalcemia in malignancy. Cancer 41:2276–2285, 1978
2. Glover DJ, Glick JH. Oncologic emergencies and special complications. In Calabresi P, Schein PJ, Rosenberg SA (eds): Medical Oncology: Basic Principles and Clinical Management of Cancer. New York, Macmillan, 1985:1261–1326
3. Mazzaferri EL, O'Dorisio TM, LoBuglio AF. Treatment of hypercalcemia associated with malignancy. Semin Oncol 5:141–153, 1978
4. Mundy GR. Pathogenesis of hypercalcemia of malignancy. Clin Endocrinol 23:705–714, 1985
5. Brereton HD, Halushka PV, Alexander RW et al. Indomethacin-responsive hypercalcemia in a patient with renal cell adenocarcinoma. N Engl J Med 291:83–85, 1974
6. Josse RG, Wilson DR, Heersche JNM et al. Hypercalcemia with ovarian carcinoma: Evidence of a pathogenetic role for prostaglandins. Cancer 48:1233–1241, 1981
7. Shane E, Bilezikian JP. Parathyroid cancer: A review of 62 patients. Endor Rev 3:218–226, 1982
8. Tashjian AH. Prostaglandins, hypercalcemia, and cancer. N Engl J Med 293:1317–1318, 1975
9. Bockman RS. Hypercalcemia in malignancy. Clin Endocrinol Metab 9:157–333, 1980
10. Mundy GR, Raisz LG, Cooper RA et al. Evidence for the secretion of an osteoclast stimulating factor in myeloma. N Engl J Med 291:1041–1046, 1974
11. Elias EG, Evans JT. Hypercalcemic crisis in neoplastic diseases: Management with mithramycin. Surgery 71:615–635, 1972
12. Perlia CP, Gubisch NJ, Wolter J et al. Mithramycin treatment of hypercalcemia. Cancer 25:389-394, 1970
13. Binstock MO, Mundy GR. Effect of calcitonin and glucocorticoids in combination on the hypercalcemia of malignancy. Ann Intern Med 93:269–272, 1980
14. Body JJ. Cancer hypercalcemia: Recent advances in understanding and treatment. Eur J Cancer Clin Oncol 20:865–869, 1984
15. Garnick MB, Mayer RJ. Acute renal failure associated with neoplastic disease and its treatment. Semin Oncol 5:156–165, 1978
16. Kjellstrand CM, Campbell DC II, Von Hartizsch B, Buselmeier TJ. Hyperuricemic acute renal failure. Arch Intern Med 133:349–359, 1974
17. Klinenberg JR, Kippen I, Bluestone R. Hyperuricemic nephropathy: Pathologic features and factors influencing urate deposition. Nephron 14:99–115, 1975
18. Seyberth HW, Sewgre GV, Moran JL et al. Prostaglandins as mediators of hypercalcemia associated with certain types of cancer. N Engl J Med 293:1278–1283, 1975
19. Knochel JP, Mason AD. Effect of alkalinization on peritoneal diffusion of uric acid. Am J Physiol 210:1160, 1966
20. DeFronzo RA, Thier SO. Pathophysiologic approach to hyponatremia. Arch Intern Med 140:897–902, 1980
21. Goldberg M. Hyponatremia. Med Clin North Am 65:251–269, 1981
22. Trump DL: Serious hyponatremia in patients with cancer. Cancer 47:2098–2912, 1981
23. Lockton JA, Thatcher N. A retrospective study of 32 patients with small cell bronchogenic carcinoma and inappropriate secretion of antidiuretic hormone. Clin Radiol 37:47–50, 1986
24. Kerne PA, Robbins RJ, Bichet D et al. Syndrome of inappropriate antidiuretics in the absence of arginine vasopressin. J Clin Endocrinol Metab 62:148–152, 1986
25. Spencer HW, Yarger WE, Robinson RE. Alterations of renal function during dietary-induced hyperuricemia in the rat. Kidney Int. 9:489–500, 1976.
26. Thomas TH, Morgan DB, Swaminathan R. Severe hyponatremia: A study of 17 patients. Lancet 1:621–624, 1978
27. Geheb M, Cox M: Renal effects of demeclocycline. JAMA 243:2519–2520, 1980
28. Skrabanek P, Powell D. Ectopic insulin and Occam's razor. Reappraisal of the riddle of tumor hypoglycemia. Clin Endocrinol 9:141–154, 1978
29. Forrest JN Jr., Cox M, Hong C et al. Superiority of demeclocycline over lithium in the treatment of chronic syndrome of inappropriate secretion of antidiuretic hormone. N Engl J Med 298:173–177, 1978
30. Anderson N, Lokich JJ. Mesenchymal tumors associated with hypoglycemia: Case report and review of the literature. Cancer 44:785–790, 1979
31. Kahn CR. The riddle of tumor hypoglycemia revisited. Clin Endocrinol Metab 9: 335–360, 1980
32. Smitz S, Legros J, Franchimont P, LaMaire M. High molecular weight vasopressin: Detection of a large amount in the plasma of a patient. Clin Endocrinol 23:379–384, 1985
33. Chandalia HB, Boshell BR. Hypoglycemia associated with extrapancreatic tumors. Arch Intern Med 129:447–456, 1985
34. Block JB. Lactic acidosis in malignancy and observations on its possible pathogenesis. Ann NY Acad Sci 230:94–102, 1974
35. Cohen LF, Balow JE, Magrath IT et al. Acute tumor lysis syndrome: A review of 37 patients with Burkitt's lymphoma. Am J Med 64:486–491, 1980
36. Fields ALA, Josse RG, Bergsagel DE. Metabolic emergencies. In DeVita VT, Hellman S, Rosenberg SA (eds). Cancer: Principles & Practice of Oncology. Philadelphia, JB Lippincott, 1985:1874–1876
37. Field M, Block JB, Levin R et al. Significance of blood lactate elevations among patients with acute leukemia and other neoplastic proliferative disorders. Am J Med 40:528–547, 1966
38. Goodgame JT, Pizzo P, Brennan MF. Iatrogenic lactic acidosis in association with hypertonic glucose administration in a patient with cancer. Cancer 42:800–803, 1978
39. Roth GJ, Porte D. Chronic lactic acidosis and acute leukemia. Arch Intern Med 125:317–321, 1970
40. Schlisky RL. Renal and metabolic toxicities of cancer chemotherapy. Semin Oncol 9:75–83, 1982
41. Tsokos GC, Balow JE, Spiegel RJ et al. Renal and metabolic complications of undifferentiated and lymphoblastic lymphomas. Medicine 60:218–229, 1981
42. Vogelzang NU, Nelimark RA, Nath KA. Tumor lysis syndrome after induction chemotherapy of small cell bronchogenic carcinoma. JAMA 249:513–514, 1983

BIBILIOGRAPHY

Dudley FJ, Blackburn CRB. Extraskeletal calcification complicating oral neural-phosphate therapy. Lancet 2:628–630, 1970

Epstein FM. Calcium and the Kidney. Am J Med 45:700–714, 1968

Gordon P, Hendricks CM, Kahn CR et al. Hypoglycemia associated with non-islet cell tumor and insulin-like growth factors. N Engl J Med 305:1452–1455, 1981

Gutman AB, Yu TF. Uric acid nephrolithiasis. Am J Med 45:756–779, 1978

McLellan G, Baird CW, Melick R. Hypercalcemia in an Australian hospital adult population. Med J Aust 2:354–356, 1968

Mundy GR, Ibbotson KJ, D'Souza SM et al. The hypercalcemia of cancer. Clinical implications and pathogenic mechanisms. N Engl J Med 150:1718–1727, 1984

Singer I, Robenberg D. Demeclocycline-induced nephrogenic diabetes insipidus. Ann Intern Med 79:679–683, 1973

John S. Macdonald, Daniel G. Haller, Robert J. Mayer, Eds. *Manual of Oncologic Therapeutics*, Third Edition.

52. SUPERIOR VENA CAVA SYNDROME

Rita Axelrod

The superior vena cava syndrome (SVCS) is a well-defined symptom complex traditionally designated an oncologic emergency. While still recognized as urgent, it only rarely justifies treatment in the absence of a diagnosis.

SVCS is caused by obstruction of blood flow in the superior vena cava, limiting return of blood from the head, neck and upper trunk to the right heart. This results in symptoms of face, neck, chest wall, and arm swelling; prominence of neck veins and plethora; observation of the development of collateral channels, sometimes including a dilated venous pattern over the anterior chest wall; less frequently, elevated CNS pressure and symptoms; dysphagia; and (rarely) stridor with tracheal compression.

PATHOPHYSIOLOGY

The superior vena cava, a delicate, thin-walled conduit suited to a low-pressure system, is situated in a relatively noncompliant compartment, the superior mediastinum. The superior mediastinum is limited by bones in the front and back (sternum and vertebral column). The SVC is surrounded by lymph nodes, including the paratracheal[1,2] and the right anterior superior mediastinal lymph nodes. These nodes drain all of the structures of the right thoracic cavity and lower left thorax. The SVC is in direct contact with the ascending aorta, the right pulmonary artery, left atrium (fixed at one portion to the pericardium), right pulmonary veins, and right main stem bronchus.

Collateral circulation between the SVC and the inferior vena cava (IVC) is abundant and has been described as four main systems.[1] These are 1: internal mammary veins, including the internal mammary, intercostal and superficial veins of the thorax; 2: vertebral veins, including the innominate and dural sinuses of the intercostal lumbar and sacral veins; 3: the azygous route, which connects the SVC and IVC and receives part of the blood from internal mammary and vertebral channels; and 4: the lateral thoracic veins, including the paraesophageal and thoracoepigastric lateral thoracic veins, intercostal and periumbilical veins. When a SVC obstruction occurs above the azygous vein, blood drains from the right and left neck through external jugular veins to superficial veins of the anterior chest wall and other intercostal veins, and through the left accessory hemizygous veins into the right atrium. This has been demonstrated in animal models and is the most common type of obstruction seen clinically.[3] When the obstruction occurs distal to the azygous arch, venous blood returns to the heart through the IVC via collaterals: the veins of the abdominal wall, femoral, and iliac veins.[2] In animal models this type of obstruction carries a higher mortality when created acutely. Retrograde blood flow in the azygous and esophageal veins forms a connection between the portal and systemic venous shunts. This explains the occurrence of varices of upper esophagus in acute SVCS or in the whole esophagus in chronic SVCS.[2,4]

ETIOLOGY

The first English language account of SVCS was published in 1757 by John Hunter[5], who described a case of obstruction of the SVC by aortic aneurysm proven by postmortem findings. Others have summarized cases from the literature since, notably McIntire and Sykes,[1] who summarized published series through 1946 and added 2 cases of their own, and Parish,[6] who published 86 cases from 20 years of the Mayo Clinic record. The etiologic distribution of SVC obstruction has changed since Hunter's original description,[5] with a shift towards malignancy and away from complications of infection and aortic aneurysm.

Benign causes of SVC syndrome include syphilitic aortic aneurysm, tuberculous mediastinitis, other mediastinitis and fibrosis, including histoplasmosis.[6] McIntire and Sykes[1] noted a drop in SVCS caused by syphilitic mediastinitis from 28.6 to 0.9% from 1904 to 1946, although approximately one third of the SVCS they reported was attributable to aneurysm, presumably syphilitic. Other less frequent benign causes include thymoma,[1] substernal goiter,[7] and congenital malformations including aneurysm and fistula between SVC and other structures.[8] Primary thoracic tumor and syphilis (*i.e.*, aneurysm) each accounted for approximately one third of the cases of SVCS in 1948.[1]

Iatrogenic SVC may be related to indwelling catheters or pacemaker wires. These may act as a nidus around which clot can form, may cause intimal proliferation, or the infusion of drugs themselves (*e.g.*, fluorouracil) may be thrombogenic. The catheters may be placed for either malignant or benign disease (*e.g.*, chronic renal disease, hyperalimentation). In this situation the development of the SVC obstruction may be sudden and dramatic, related to the formation of a thrombus. Intervention varies with life expectancy and can include surgery, angioplasty, or thrombolytic therapy.[6,9,10]

Malignant tumors are now the most common cause of SVC syndrome, most frequently bronchogenic carcinoma. Right-sided lesions predominate, as would be expected given the proximity of the right main stem bronchus to the

SVC.[2,11] The most commonly histologic type is small cell carcinoma,[12,13,14] followed by squamous cell carcinoma of the lung. Other causes include lymphoma (a more common cause in children) including Hodgkin's disease, metastatic disease including breast cancer and melanoma, stomach cancer, and embryonal rhabdomyosarcoma.[15]

CLINICAL PRESENTATION AND DIAGNOSIS

Acute symptoms of SVCS are manifested by sudden onset of obstructive symptoms, including a sense of dizziness or shortness of breath, sudden swelling of the face and neck, and obtundation due to cerebral edema. When accompanied by stridor due to tracheal obstruction, it represents a true emergency, and immediate intervention to maintain airway is needed. Hypoxia may occur due to bronchial compression or edema as well. This is more likely to occur in children or as a result of the underlying tumor which caused the SVC obstruction. Chronic SVC syndrome is characterized by the more insidious onset of the symptom complex. It may persist for months or years without threatening life.

When the history and physical examination suggest SVCS, diagnostic procedures usually include a chest film and contrast-enhanced CT scan.

The chest film may show mediastinal widening (most common), pleural effusion, right hilar mass, right upper lobe collapse, anterior mediastinal mass, or rib notching. Occasionally the chest film is normal, but this does not exclude the presence of the syndrome when a clinical diagnosis is entertained.[3,6]

The contrast-enhanced CT scan is the single most useful diagnostic test. Decreased opacification of the innominate or SVC below the obstruction may be observed, or collateral patterns of venous drainage may be opacified. CT diagnosis of SVC obstruction requires intraluminal filling defects (which may be unreliable due to dilution of contrast or laminar flow of contrast) and external compression of the mediastinal venous channels with collateral vessel opacification. The presence of collateral vessels alone on CT scans is considered by some to be a highly sensitive and specific sign of SVCS.[16] In addition to helping to establish the diagnosis of SVCS, the CT scan can identify primary and metastatic mediastinal masses. This helps to plan the radiotherapy field, shows the entire mediastinum, and allows evaluation of the liver and adrenal glands for presence of metastases. It may also afford the opportunity for CT-guided needle biopsy for sampling.[3,4]

Phlebography of the SVC, an earlier standard for diagnosis, shows the collateral circulation well. It may be useful in planning venous bypass, which will not likely be entertained in the patient with malignant disease. Scintigraphy with technetium may demonstrate SVCS, but is generally not as useful as CT scanning.[17] MRI can be helpful in defining vascular structures in the mediastinum, will help to distinguish hilar vessels from nodes, and may be helpful in distinguishing late radiation fibrosis from recurrent tumor.[18]

TREATMENT

There has been much discussion about the urgency of treatment, especially when SVCS occurs in patients as the first evidence of malignancy.[12] Biopsy of an accessible superficial lymph node or bronchoscopy with biopsy, sputum cytology, and mediastinoscopy may each be used to achieve a tissue diagnosis. Radiation before diagnosis is rarely justified, and is likely to distort tissue subsequently sampled, making firm diagnosis difficult or impossible. Because the initial treatment plan is crucial in the ultimate outcome of lymphoma and small cell lung carcinoma, tissue diagnosis is imperative. It has not been established that sampling of structures under increased venous pressure leads to life-threatening complications. Further, regression of symptoms is not necessarily a response to therapy, but may be due to the spontaneous opening of collateral channels. Obstruction of the SVC superior to the azygous vein in dogs[12] resulted in cyanotic listless animals, with resolution of the symptoms within one week due to collateral blood flow. Schechter and Ziskind's series[19] describes ten patients with no improvement after therapy who were followed for 3 months. All but one of the patients at autopsy had obstruction due to infiltration of the vessel wall; of two early deaths in this series (before therapy began), one resulted from aspiration of blood from massive epistaxis and another from tracheal compression by mediastinal nodes, with the SVC block the accompanying rather than the primary finding.

Once a diagnosis has been established, the mainstay of treatment for SVCS is radiation therapy, usually delivered with high dose fractionation of 400 rads daily for the first three or four days and then followed by treatment with 150 rads per day, with the total dose varying with histology of tumor and condition of the patient.[20] Rate of resolution is best when relatively large fractions are used to initiate therapy (300–400 rads per day). Field size varies with histology. The entire mantle may be irradiated in Hodgkin's disease, but only contiguous structures may be irradiated with solid tumors.[11,13,20,21,22,23,24]

Chemotherapy was introduced early as an adjunct to radiation therapy. Karnofsky described the use of nitrogen mustard combined with radiation in the treatment of bronchogenic carcinoma.[25] SVCS resulting from small cell lung cancer may be treated as effectively with chemotherapy alone as with combination radiation and chemotherapy. In Maddox's series at MD Anderson, 100% of the patients treated with chemotherapy alone responded with prompt resolution vs. 64% of those treated with radiotherapy alone, with no influence of the initial treatment on survival.[14] Initial chemotherapy may shrink the tumor size of a chemosensitive mass, decreasing the volume of lung that must be irradiated. SVCS due to non-Hodgkin's lymphoma is another example in which initial treatment with chemotherapy alone or with the combination of radiation and chemotherapy for SVCS are without difference in response.[26]

SVCS due to complications of vascular access catheters calls for removal of the catheter and consideration of anticoagulants and fibrinolytic therapy. New techniques include angioplasty; for those with long life expectancy, surgical repair could be considered.[27]

Palliative measures to relieve SVCS include elevation of the head of bed and supplemental oxygen. Diuretics and phlebotomy can help to reduce blood volume and give some relief, but hemoconcentration may also facilitate further thrombosis. Steroids may relieve edema around nerves and vessels and allow shrinkage of lymphoma, but is not advised unless there is a known diagnosis, since it can distort histology.

SUMMARY

In summary, SVCS is a long-recognized clinical syndrome resulting from obstruction of the SVC and the expansion of its collateral channels. By itself it is rarely immediately life-threatening. Rather, the prognosis depends on underlying illness, with benign causes consistent with survival for many years. The syndrome is now usually caused by malignancy, most frequently bronchogenic carcinoma. There is also an emerging group of iatrogenic SVCS in patients with indwelling venous access devices. The appearance of the syndrome is a signal for prompt assessment of true risk of immediate consequence due to airway compromise or cerebral edema; measures to establish the extent of disease in the chest, usually including chest film and CT scan; establishment of a pathologic diagnosis (if unknown prior to SVCS) by sputum cytology, biopsy of an accessible node or other involved tissue, CT-guided needle biopsy, bronchoscopy with biopsy, or, if necessary, thoracotomy; and institution of diagnosis-appropriate therapy with high fraction radiation and sometimes chemotherapy.

REFERENCES

1. McIntire FT, Sykes Jr. EM. Obstruction of the superior vena cava: A review of the literature and report of two personal cases. Ann Intern Med 30:925–60, 1949
2. Roswit B, Kaplan G, Jacobson HG. The superior vena cava obstruction syndrome in bronchogenic carcinoma. Radiology 61:722–37, 1953
3. Yedlicka JW, Schultz K, Moncada R, Fisak M. CT findings in superior vena cava obstruction. Seminars in Roentgenology 24(2):84–90, 1989
4. Dudiak CM, Olson MC, Posniak HV. Abnormalities of the azygos system: CT evaluation. Seminars in Roentgenology 24(1):47–55, 1989
5. Hunter W. The history of an aneurysm of the aorta with some remarks on aneurysms in general. Med Obs Inq (London) 1:323–357, 1757
6. Parish JM, Marschke Jr. RF, Dines DE, Lee RE. Etiologic considerations in superior vena cava syndrome. Mayo Clinic Proceedings 56:407–13, 1981
7. Silverstein GE, Burke G, Goldberg D, Halko A. Superior vena caval system obstruction caused by benign endothoracic goiter. Dis Chest 56(6):519–23, 1969
8. Madani MA, Loughran EH, Cooke Jr. JA. Congenital venous aneurysm of superior mediastinum. New York State Journal of Medicine 73:289–90, 1973
9. Puel V, Caudry M, LeMetayer P et al. Superior vena cava thrombosis related to catheter malposition in cancer chemotherapy given through implanted ports. Cancer 72(7):2248–52, 1993
10. Woodyard TC, Mellinger JD, Vann KG, Nisenbaum J. Acute superior vena cava syndrome after central venous catheter placement. Cancer 71(8):2621–3, 1993
11. Lokich JJ, Goodman R. Superior vena cava syndrome. JAMA 231(1):58–61, 1975
12. Ahmann FR. A reassessment of the clinical implications of the superior vena caval syndrome. Journal of Clinical Oncology 2(8)961–69 1984
13. Perez CA, Presant CA, Van Amburg III AL. Management of superior vena cava syndrome. Seminars in Oncology 5(2)123–134 1978
14. Maddox AM, Valdivieso M, Lukeman J et al. Superior vena cava obstruction in small cell bronchogenic carcinoma. Cancer 52(11):2165–72, 1983
15. Ghosh BC, Cliffton EE. Malignant tumors with superior vena cava obstruction. New York State Journal of Medicine 73:283–88, 1973
16. Kim HJ, Kim HS, Chung SH. CT diagnosis of superior vena cava syndrome: Importance of collateral vessels. American J of Roentgenology 161:539–42, 1993
17. Scarantino C, Salazar OM, Rubin P et al. The optimum radiation schedule in treatment of superior vena caval obstruction: Importance of ^{99m}Tc scintiangiograms. Int J Radiation Oncology Biol Phys 5(11&12)87–95, 1979
18. Bragg DG. Imaging in primary-lung cancer: The roles of detection, staging, and follow-up. Seminars in Ultrasound, CT, and MR 10(6):453–466, 1989
19. Schechter MM and Ziskind MM. The superior vena cava syndrome. American Journal of Medicine 18:561–66, 1955
20. Davenport D, Ferree C, Blake D, Raben M. Response of superior vena cava syndrome to radiation therapy. Cancer 38:1577–80, 1976
21. Davenport D, Ferree C, Blake D, Raben M. Radiation therapy in the treatment of superior vena caval obstruction. Cancer 42:2600–03, 1978
22. Rubin P, Green J, Holzwasser G, Gerle R. Superior vena caval syndrome. Radiology 81:388–401, 1963
23. Fisherman WH, Bradfield JS. Superior vena caval syndrome:

Response with initially high daily dose irradiation. Southern Medical Journal 66(6):677–80, 1973

24. Avasthi RB, Moghissi K. Malignant obstruction of the superior vena cava and its palliation. J of Thoracic and Cardiovascular Surgery 74(2):244–48, 1977
25. Karnofsky DA, Abelmann WH, Craver LF, and Burchenal JH. The use of the nitrogen mustards in the palliative treatment of carcinoma. Cancer 1:634–56, 1948
26. Perez-Soler R, McLaughlin P, Velasquez WS et al. Clinical features and results of management of superior vena cava syndrome secondary to lymphoma. J Clin Oncol 2:260, 1984
27. Wisselink W, Money SR, Becker MO et al. Comparison of operative reconstruction and percutaneous balloon dilatation for central venous obstruction. American J of Surgery 166(2):200–4, 1993

John S. Macdonald, Daniel G. Haller, Robert J. Mayer, Eds. *Manual of Oncologic Therapeutics*, Third Edition.

53. THE ACUTE ABDOMEN IN THE CANCER PATIENT

John H. Raaf
Raphael S. Chung

CAUSES OF ACUTE ABDOMEN IN THE CANCER PATIENT

Management of the acute abdomen in cancer patients requires both art and science. These patients can develop abdominal pain due to the "benign" causes seen in individuals without cancer, but the problem becomes more complex because the pain may be tumor related or even treatment related. Abdominal pain in these patients can present a major diagnostic and therapeutic challenge.

Intra-abdominal inflammation, obstruction, perforation, or hemorrhage may be due to benign processes such as appendicitis, pancreatitis, diverticulitis, duodenal ulcer, or incarcerated hernia. Alternatively, the problem may be tumor related, such as from obstruction of the bowel lumen by primary or metastatic tumor, or pressure on or invasion of an adjacent organ by the tumor. Intussusception resulting in abdominal pain and bowel obstruction may result from a primary (*e.g.*, polypoid hamartoma) or metastatic (*e.g.*, melanoma) tumor in the wall of the small bowel.

Peritonitis due to tumor-related bowel perforation may give rise to an acute abdomen. Infected bile associated with cholangitis can result from duct blockage due to carcinoma of the pancreas or common bile duct. Malignant biliary obstruction does not generally result in cholangitis without externally introduced organisms, but the patient may become frankly septic following instrumentation. Pyelonephritis related to obstruction of a ureter may also complicate tumor growth and may develop behind an obstructed ureter after retrograde studies.

Inflammation of the cecum ("typhlitis") typically occurs in a leukemic patient with neutropenia and is difficult to distinguish clinically from acute appendicitis.

Retroperitoneal tumors may cause back pain by nerve compression. Pancreatic or gastric carcinoma can infiltrate the celiac plexus, while pelvic sarcoma or rectal carcinoma can compress the lumbosacral nerve roots. Tumor invasion of the psoas muscle may cause psoas spasm with radiation of pain in the distribution of the genitofemoral nerve or the lateral cutaneous nerve of the thigh.

Hemorrhage due to a solid tumor may be intraperitoneal, retroperitoneal, or into the tumor itself, the abdominal wall, or the lumen of the gastrointestinal tract. Tumors such as melanoma commonly undergo central necrosis, which can lead to bleeding within the tumor. This type of hemorrhage may cause sudden, painful enlargement of a tumor mass. Liquefaction of the center of the tumor is seen on computed tomography (CT). The bleeding may be sufficient to cause a change in the hematocrit, and a tender mass may become palpable on physical examination.

Hemoperitoneum as a result of bleeding from an intra-abdominal tumor (classically a hepatoma) into the free abdominal cavity causes sudden pain, fluid in the abdomen, pallor, and hypovolemia. If bleeding occurs into a retroperitoneal tumor, cutaneous discoloration may be evident when blood seeps into the subcutaneous space (Grey Turner's sign).

Tense ascites may be painful, particularly when the accumulation has been rapid. Hemorrhage into the ascitic fluid or secondary infection further aggravates the pain. Ascitic fluid due to tumor may be gelatinous, as in the case of ovarian carcinoma or pseudomyxoma peritonei. Serosanguinous ascitic fluid is found for several other tumor types and may be palliated by placement of a peritoneovenous (LeVeen) shunt in patients who have failed management with diuretics and repeated paracentesis. Such shunts will function longer if the ascitic fluid is cytologically negative for malignant cells. An infected LeVeen shunt can cause abdominal pain.

Splenic enlargement in patients with lymphoma or leukemia may result in hypersplenism (decreased white blood count and platelet count), pain due to stretching of the splenic capsule, splenic infarcts, anorexia secondary to pressure on the stomach, or even frank rupture of the splenic capsule leading to shock. The benefit of elective splenectomy in these patients is controversial.

An acute abdomen may be treatment related. Adhesions due to radiation therapy may cause bowel obstruction. Neutropenia from bone marrow toxicity of chemotherapeutic drugs can result in infection or abscess formation. Effective cancer treatment may result in tumor necrosis, perforation, or rupture. Massive tumor necrosis following a good response to chemotherapy may lead to sudden perforation of an involved viscus. Necrosis of tumor involving the gut can also lead to fistula formation or gastrointestinal bleeding. The same complication may follow irradiation, although less frequently. Treatment with chemotherapeutic agents, particularly of lymphoma, can cause rapid lysis of tumor with consequent pain, fever, and the picture of sepsis. Occasionally, a solid tumor mass may rupture into the peritoneal cavity.

Large bulky tumors on pedicles (*e.g.*, ovarian carcinoma) may undergo axial torsion and detorsion, giving rise to the characteristic syndrome of rapid onset and rapid relief, without much pain between episodes. Multilevel obstruction of the intestine by metastatic tumor leads to closed-loop obstruction, perhaps followed by intestinal perforation, despite nasogastric drainage.

Necrosis of tumors may be difficult to differentiate from abscess formation; fever, pain, and leukocytosis are common to both. The distinction is more than academic since a liver abscess should be managed by open drainage while a necrotic liver tumor should not.

Drug toxicity from chemotherapeutic agents such as the vinca alkaloids can cause neuropathy that manifests as abdominal pain. Such pain following the administration of vincristine should be carefully evaluated, but conservative, nonsurgical treatment is usually indicated. Steroids, on the other hand, may mask symptoms related to bowel perforation, so in steroid-treated patients the surgeon may need to be aggressive even when signs and symptoms are mild. Steroid treatment can lead to gastric ulceration or perforation, which may be preceded by upper gastrointestinal bleeding. Acute pancreatitis may follow steroid administration.

Complications of cancer surgery may result in acute abdomen. Intraoperative injury to intestine, ureter, or bile ducts can result in intra-abdominal suppuration and fistula formation. Necrosis from devascularization following extensive nodal dissection may also lead to sepsis. Internal herniation or adhesion formation can result in intestinal obstruction.

Certain acute abdominal conditions are encountered in patients subjected to stress and cachexia. Acute perforation of peptic ulcers and acalculous cholecystitis are two examples. Fecal impaction and stercoral ulceration may occur in any debilitated patient.

DIAGNOSTIC EVALUATION

As in the patient without cancer, a careful history and physical examination are the essential starting points. The medical background is vital: a detailed knowledge of tumor histology and stage, drug history, courses of chemotherapy and irradiation, and the nature of previous surgery.

A careful analysis of the symptom of pain is valuable. The rapidity of onset, the nature and variation in intensity, and the localization of the point of maximum tenderness all give important clues. Peritoneal irritation is indicated by cough tenderness; pelvic irritation is indicated by tenesmus and frequency of urination. Typical referral pain patterns should be noted.

When there is much vomiting, this should be compared with the degree of abdominal distention. High intestinal obstruction is characterized by copious vomiting with little abdominal distention, while low small bowel obstruction gives rise to the most distention of all. Left colonic obstruction can give rise to a "peripheral" type of abdominal distention due to the competent ileocecal valve, which spares the small bowel from being distended. Failure to pass gas must be distinguished from simple constipation.

In the examination of the abdomen, the presence of muscle guarding indicates peritonitis; but the degree of guarding varies greatly with the age and strength of the subject. In the frail and debilitated patient, frank peritonitis may not be accompanied by muscular guarding. An obstructive pattern of high-pitched bowel sounds, particularly when synchronized with pain, is strong evidence of early obstruction, while a silent and distended abdomen is suggestive of ileus. Rectovaginal examination (feeling for a "rectal shelf" of tumor, or pelvic "drop metastases") with guaiac testing of stool provides essential information.

Depending on the differential diagnosis, further evaluation is carried out using appropriate biochemical and hematologic laboratory studies, contrast x-ray studies, gastrointestinal endoscopy, or CT scan. Complete blood count, liver function tests, and serum amylase are routinely determined.

Plain films of the chest and abdomen, including an upright view, may show free air, indicating perforation of a viscus. Multiple fluid levels are suggestive of obstruction, while abnormal gas-fluid collections provide evidence of suppuration. Ultrasonography or CT scan can further define the location and extent of an intra-abdominal mass felt on examination. When the mass is identified to be a fluid collection, guided needle aspiration may furnish more diagnostic information or may even be therapeutic. Diagnostic tapping of ascites should be performed, with cytologic examination for malignant cells and bacterial culture.

When urine output can be maintained only with increasing amounts of fluid infusion ("third-spacing"), peritonitis and ileus should be suspected as sources of fluid sequestration. The diagnosis of peritonitis is strengthened if acute abdominal pain is accompanied by signs of toxicity, such as fever, leukocytosis, and dehydration.

Diagnostic laparoscopy for the acute abdomen has recently been resurrected after long years of neglect, due to current enthusiasm for elective laparoscopic surgery. In the critically ill patient who may not tolerate an open exploratory laparotomy, a negative laparotomy may worsen the outcome. In such a patient, laparoscopy is a valuable option. The procedure may be performed under local anesthesia with conscious sedation or under general anesthesia, followed by a definitive surgical procedure once the diagnosis is made. With the modern video endoscope the entire abdomen can be systematically examined, including the general and pelvic peritoneal cavity and the viscera therein. The subphrenic spaces can be inspected better laparoscopically than at open operation.

Using appropriate retractors and holders inserted via accessory ports, the small bowel can be traced and its mesentery inspected. Findings of peritonitis (fibrinous exudate, adhesions, pus, and edema) with or without evidence of perforation (intestinal fluid or contents) mandate laparotomy, while edema alone without purulence suggests conservative measures. Hemorrhagic ascites may be found in association with gangrenous bowel or pancreatitis, the latter also suggested by fat saponification in the omentum. Bloody ascites alone without associated lesions is a grey area; our limited experience supports placing a drain and subsequent careful clinical observation.

A few simple therapeutic procedures, such as suturing a small perforation, removal of the appendix, drainage of an intra-abdominal abscess, directed biopsy of omental metastasis or of the liver, and placement of an enterostomy tube for decompression or for feeding, can be accomplished laparoscopically. Sound judgment is most important; the surgeon must resist the temptation to expediency at the expense of safety. As stated by Schwartz, magnified visualization through the video endoscope cannot always replace tactile sensation and two-point discrimination by the surgeon's hand. Open exploration is still the best approach for definitive diagnosis and staging of most abdominal cancers.

TREATMENT

If there are signs of frank peritonitis, no time should be wasted on unnecessary investigations. Instead, the patient should be rapidly prepared for surgical exploration. Initial therapy consists of nasogastric suction, analgesics, intravenous fluids to correct dehydration and electrolyte imbalance, and parenteral broad-spectrum antibiotics that cover *Enterobacteriaceae*, *Pseudomonas aeruginosa*, and anaerobes. Coagulopathies should be treated pre- or intraoperatively with fresh frozen plasma and/or platelet transfusion.

Aggressiveness of treatment depends on the status of the patient, the expected responsiveness of the tumor to therapy, and the wishes of the patient and family. Multiple sequential examination of the patient's abdomen (*e.g.*, hourly) is an effective way to determine whether the patient is improving or getting worse. The potential for doing harm is often great in a patient with cancer, so unnecessary exploratory laparotomy should be avoided if at all possible.

If a leukemic patient has a white blood count less than $1000/mm^3$ and develops right lower quadrant pain, one may first treat with broad-spectrum antibiotics and conservative measures rather than proceed immediately to exploratory laparotomy. Exploration of the abdomen under these circumstances is likely to reveal only an inflamed cecum and surrounding phlegmon (perityphlitis) that will resolve in most cases if the white blood count recovers. Other areas in the gastrointestinal tract in such a patient may also be inflamed (neutropenic enterocolitis), due perhaps to invasion of enteric bacteria through mucosal breaks and to decreased host resistance.

Patients with widespread intraperitoneal tumor may have intermittent episodes of bowel obstruction that can be palliated by nasogastric suction using a long tube passed into the small bowel using a mercury-weighted tip. In an abdomen that is "frozen" due to malignancy, this is often the preferred initial treatment, in contrast to bowel obstruction in a patient who appears in an emergency room and likely has a benign cause. The latter type of patient with, for example, a strangulated hernia, is in danger of developing necrotic bowel, whereas tissue necrosis with perforation is less likely if obstruction is due to partial blockage by tumor. An upper gastrointestinal series with small bowel follow-through using Gastrografin may help to determine whether the blockage is only partial and will possibly improve without surgical intervention. Surgical resection of the tumor or bypass of the obstructed loop may be required.

On the other hand, one should be quite aggressive in managing most cancer patients with bowel perforation or gastrointestinal bleeding (see Chap. 55), although judgment as to whether to undertake surgery in a poor-risk individual should always be tempered by a realistic assessment of the long-term prognosis. The morbidity and mortality of patients receiving active chemotherapy treatment who undergo an emergency operation to correct a life-threatening problem are substantial despite modern intensive care unit support.

Previous treatment may increase surgical risk in such patients by contributing to renal toxicity (cisplatin), cardiomyopathy (doxorubicin), pulmonary fibrosis (bleomycin or radiation therapy), or neutropenia and thrombocytopenia (many myelosuppressive drugs). Malnutrition, steroid treatment, and previous radiation can substantially delay wound healing. To optimize the surgical outcome in such cases, the surgeon must use meticulous surgical technique, careful skin preparation, perioperative antibiotic coverage, and supplementary enteral or parenteral nutrition in patients who are malnourished.

BIBLIOGRAPHY

Baker AR. Surgical emergencies. In DeVita Jr VT, Hellman S, Rosenberg SA (eds): Cancer: Principles & Practice of Oncology, 4th ed. Philadelphia, JB Lippincott, 1993: 2141–2158.

Berci G, Sackier JM, Paz-Parlow M. Emergency laparoscopy. Am J Surg 151:332–335, 1991

Cheung DK, Raaf JH. Selection of patients with malignant ascites for a peritoneovenous shunt. Cancer 50:1204–1209, 1982

Ferrara JJ, Martin EW, Carey LC. Morbidity of emergency operations in patients with metastatic cancer receiving chemotherapy. Surgery 92:605–609, 1982

Katz JA, Wagner ML, Gresik MV et al. Typhlitis, an 18-year experience and postmortem review. Cancer 65:1041–1047, 1990

Mitchell EP, Schein PS. Gastrointestinal toxicity of chemotherapeutic agents. Semin Oncol 9:52–64, 1982

Raaf JH. Techniques for avoiding surgical complications in

chemotherapy-treated cancer patients. Recent Results in Cancer Research 98:46–52, 1985

Schwartz SI. The sensate surgeon. Contemp Surg 44:264, 1994

Shamberger RC, Weinstein HJ, Delorey MJ, Levey RH. The medical and surgical management of typhlitis in children with acute nonlymphocytic (myelogenous) leukemia. Cancer 57:603–609, 1986

Skibber JM, Matter GJ, Pizzo PA, Lotze MT. Right lower quadrant pain in young patients with leukemia: A surgical perspective. Ann Surg 206:711–716, 1987

Starnes HF, Moore Jr FD, Mentzer S et al. Abdominal pain in neutropenic cancer patients. Cancer 57:616–621, 1986

Torosian MH, Turnbull ADM. Emergency laparotomy for spontaneous intestinal and colonic perforations in cancer patients receiving corticosteroids and chemotherapy. J Clin Oncol 6:291–296, 1988

Turnbull AD. The surgical oncologist's role in the intensive care unit. In Howland WS, Carlon GC (eds): Critical Care of the Cancer Patient. Chicago, Year Book Medical Publishers, 1985:318–338

Warshaw AL, Fernandez-del Castillo C. Laparoscopy in preoperative diagnosis and staging for gastrointestinal cancers. In Zucker KA (ed): Surgical Laparoscopy. St. Louis, Quality Medical Publishing, 1991:101–114

John S. Macdonald, Daniel G. Haller, Robert J. Mayer, Eds. *Manual of Oncologic Therapeutics*, Third Edition.

54. GASTROINTESTINAL BLEEDING IN THE CANCER PATIENT

Raphael S. Chung
John H. Raaf

ASSESSMENT

The first consideration in the management of gastrointestinal bleeding in any patient is evaluation of the magnitude of blood loss, the stability of the circulation, and the activity of the bleeding. Treatment of hypovolemic shock, regardless of the bleeding source, must take immediate priority.

Orthostatic hypotension occurs after a rapid loss of at least 20% of blood volume. Tachycardia, restlessness, and peripheral vasoconstriction are signs of shock and indicate that supportive measures must be instituted immediately. Signs of continued bleeding include frequent bloody bowel movements, hematemesis, continued gastric fullness and nausea, and hyperactive bowel sounds. In patients with poor liver function, active bleeding may precipitate encephalopathy. Acute changes in hematocrit often underestimate the magnitude of bleeding, because time is required for equilibration.

Emergency Intervention

Volume repletion must be monitored. In the patient with good cardiac reserve, parameters as simple as vital signs, urine output, or the color and warmth of the extremities may be adequate, but in frail subjects measurement of the right atrial pressure or pulmonary wedge pressure is often required for adequate monitoring. Intravenous lactated Ringer's solution may be safely given as a preliminary measure in all patients with hypovolemic shock while awaiting blood replacement.

Platelet transfusion and therapy with other blood components are indicated for specific defects identified by coagulation studies. Platelet transfusion usually is utilized in patients with decreased production such as that induced by antineoplastic agents, or when antiplatelet agents such as aspirin have been used. Fresh frozen plasma and other colloids may be used to maintain peripheral circulation before blood is available. When packed cells are transfused, one should remember that there is little to be gained by raising the hematocrit above 30% in a patient with adequate volume.

Sources of Bleeding

Common benign bleeding conditions such as esophagitis, peptic ulcer, or diverticulitis may occur in cancer patients. In addition, the cancer patient can bleed from tumors arising from or invading the gut, or from complications of chemotherapy or radiotherapy. Coagulation abnormalities, particularly platelet depletion, must be ruled out in all cases. Side-effects of chemotherapeutic agents such as thrombocytopenia and mucosal ulceration should be suspected. Primary squamous or adenocarcinoma of the esophagus, stomach, and colon as well as lymphomas and leiomyosarcomas of the gut are noted for their tendency to hemorrhage. Metastatic tumor in the bowel wall such as melanoma or breast carcinoma, as well as directly invasive pancreatic cancer, can bleed profusely. Infectious lesions of the gut associated with immunosuppression are potential bleeding sources (*e.g.*, herpes ulcers of the esophagus, esophageal moniliasis, and cecal ulcerations). Diffuse ulcerations of the colon or even of the entire gut are characteristic of graft-versus-host reaction.

Gastric erosions associated with salicylates, steroids, cytotoxic drug administration, sepsis, and stress are common in the cancer patient population. During the last decade, the widespread prophylactic use of intensive antacid titration of the gastric *p*H to neutrality and the administration of H_2 blockers such as cimetidine and ranitidine in critically ill patients have drastically reduced the incidence of massive bleeding from gastric erosions. Orally administered sucralfate also appears to protect the upper gastrointestinal mucosa, perhaps by forming a barrier to diffusion of hydrogen ions rather than by neutralization of gastric acid.

HISTORY AND PHYSICAL EXAMINATION

Hematemesis strongly suggests a source of bleeding in the upper gastrointestinal tract. By contrast, passage of blood mixed with recognizable stool indicates a bleeding source in the part of the alimentary tract where the contents are no longer semifluid, which generally means distal to the right colon. Maroon-colored bloody movements are suggestive of right colonic or lower small bowel origin, but massive bleeding in the upper tract is still one of the most common causes of rectal bleeding. The rate of bleeding is not of much diagnostic value by itself. However, a rapid rate may indicate bleeding from a single sizable vessel, which stands a better chance of being demonstrated (and even treated) radiologically. Intermittent slow blood loss occurs in granulation beds, such as those associated with radiation enteritis or necrotic tumors. Active bowel sounds usually accompany active bleeding, but when heard in the presence of abdominal distention, intestinal obstruction must be considered. A tender abdomen may indicate a concomitant perforation, as in bleeding-perforating ulcers of the stomach or cecum.

DIAGNOSTIC INVESTIGATION

Nasogastric tube aspiration is simple to perform and gives useful information: when positive, the bleeding source is proximal to the ligament of Treitz; when negative (if the patient is still actively bleeding), a source proximal to the pylorus can be confidently excluded. Sigmoidoscopy is helpful in ruling out bleeding lesions in the rectum and anus and may even identify the source if it is in the sigmoid. With few exceptions, these two simple maneuvers should be the first steps in the investigation of gastrointestinal bleeding.

The most useful and accurate investigation of gastrointestinal hemorrhage is fiberoptic endoscopy, particularly for bleeding in the upper tract. A major advantage of endoscopy is that various therapeutic modalities may be used at the same time, as soon as the diagnosis has been made. This procedure can be readily performed with little or no patient sedation, and extensive lavage is required only in exceptional cases. The esophagus is easily traversed endoscopically and can be readily inspected. A stomach containing blood can be visualized completely if the endoscopist turns the patient from one side to the other to expose areas previously submerged in blood. Unless a bleeder occurs behind a stenotic pylorus, most bleeding duodenal lesions are accessible to the endoscope, including ampullary lesions. Colonoscopy is highly accurate in patients with active bleeding in the lower tract because blood acts as a cathartic. However, when the bleeding has stopped, the blood-filled colon requires tedious preparation since water absorption renders the content viscous and tenacious. One practical benefit of sigmoidoscopy is that if blood is seen continuously entering the sigmoid, colonoscopy should be performed immediately and should have a good yield. Endoscopic biopsy of all undiagnosed bleeding lesions, in either the upper or lower gastrointestinal tract, is mandatory (see Chaps. 5 and 6).

A technetium-99m-sulfur colloid scan may show the bleeding location, but in practice often serves only to confirm that the patient is actively bleeding from the gastrointestinal tract and is of use mainly as a screening test to increase the yield of angiography. Technetium-99m labelled red cell scan, however, may increase the yield if the patient is scanned sequentially at appropriately close intervals, since the test material stays in the circulation for up to 48 hours. Angiography is diagnostic when the rate is sufficiently rapid (> 0.5 ml/min), but nonvisualization of extravasation is not helpful. Angiography is most useful when the suspected location is out of reach of conventional endoscopes, such as in hemobilia or small bowel bleeding. Contrast studies, once all-important, are much less frequently used nowadays because the tests do not indicate active bleeding, nor do they distinguish bleeding from nonbleeding lesions when multiple lesions are demonstrated.

Occasionally the small intestine may harbor an obscure source of chronic bleeding, in the so-called "no man's land" beyond the reach of the conventional upper gastrointestinal endoscope and the colonoscope. Such a patient presents with chronic blood loss over time, requiring multiple blood transfusions, and repeated conventional endoscopy has been negative. In this circumstance enteroscopy is indicated and may help to localize such lesions. These include leiomyoma, lymphoma, angiosarcoma, adenocarcinoma, metastatic cancer (*e.g.*, breast carcinoma, melanoma), and A-V malformation (angioectasia).

"Push" enteroscopy allows examination of 60–120 cm of jejunum beyond the ligament of Treitz. The push enteroscope is simply a long (160 cm) conventional endoscope. An alternative technique is Sonde enteroscopy. The Sonde enteroscope is a very small diameter but very long endoscope (the same diameter as a nasogastric tube, but 5 meters long). It is passed passively, relying on peristalsis of the small bowel to carry the Sonde enteroscope to the terminal ileum, which takes 4–6 hours. The enteroscope is then withdrawn, and examination of the bowel is performed during this withdrawal phase. Unfortunately this enteroscope, being thin and long, has no biopsy channel, and tip deflection is limited. With this instrument it may be difficult to ascertain the exact location of any lesion discovered.

A third technique is operative enteroscopy, which is total examination of the intestinal lumen at open laparotomy by passing a long endoscope either per oram, per anum, or both. The surgeon helps the endoscopist when there is an obstacle to progress. This technique is appealing because it offers the opportunity to render definitive surgical treatment upon diagnosis.

TREATMENT

When GI bleeding is other than a terminal event in a patient with an extremely poor prognosis, volume repletion should be expeditious. Diffuse bleeding associated with abnormal coagulation is usually treated by correction of the coagulation abnormality. Platelet dysfunction and platelet depletion from decreased production ($<20{,}000/mm^3$) are corrected by platelet transfusion. Fresh frozen plasma is a shotgun method of treating coagulation defects and is quite practical. Vasopressin infusion (up to a dose of 0.4 unit/min) has been used for diffuse bleeding, but the side effects can be serious; systemic acidosis, hypertension, bradycardia, and coronary or visceral ischemia are dangerous sequelae.

Bleeding from a single, discrete source often stops spontaneously. However, the patient with no reserve can ill afford the luxury of "expectant" treatment, probably the most common judgmental error in the management of such patients. Since many cancer patients are poor surgical risks, therapeutic endoscopy or radiology should be an early consideration. When the lesion is accessible to the endoscope, a variety of modalities may be employed depending on the nature of the bleeding lesion. For example, varices and bleeding arteries may be injected with sclerosants. Bleeders other than varices may be treated by many options, including bipolar or monopolar electrocoagulation, laser photocoagulation (Argon or Nd:YAG), or heat coagulation with the heater probe. Some modalities require great expertise since the safety margin is relatively small, but others, such as the heater probe and sclerosant injection, are reasonably safe and are readily available. Although survival is often not substantially changed by therapeutic endoscopy, emergency surgery may be avoided by the successful use of these techniques. Sclerotherapy for acute bleeding from esophageal varices is a good example.

A particularly useful therapeutic endoscopic modality, proven to be effective in randomized, controlled trials, is injection of the bleeding vessel with 1 : 10,000 epinephrine, using relatively large volumes (10 ml/site, up to 50 ml). Epinephrine causes local vasoconstriction without tissue damage, unlike other agents such as dehydrated ethanol, which causes further ulceration. The hemostatic effect of epinephrine, while temporary, is usually sufficient to bring about thrombosis and arrest bleeding from a localized site. The efficacy of various methods to achieve endoscopic hemostasis has been evaluated at a Consensus Conference of the National Institutes of Health.

The newer endoscopic modalities are particularly helpful when bleeding is from a nonresectable tumor. Bleeding from an advanced gastric carcinoma, for example, is appropriately treated symptomatically with Nd:YAG photocoagulation of the offending bleeder or bleeding surface.

Upper gastrointestinal tract bleeders may be suitable for selective radiologic embolization, particularly when first demonstrated during angiography. Arteries such as the gastroduodenal may require superselective catheterization and embolization of a tertiary branch, often from both ends of the collateral flow. Gelfoam and steel coils are popular, but detachable miniature balloons can also be used; the latter are retrievable if misplaced in an inappropriate vessel. Colonic vascular lesions are generally not suitable for embolization since infarction may occur, leading to perforation. A load of contrast material can precipitate renal failure in a hypovolemic patient, so adequate renal function is a prerequisite to angiography.

Surgery is indicated for failure of hemostasis after exhaustion of nonoperative treatment, when a discrete source has been demonstrated. The surgeon should not overlook common benign surgical conditions simply because the patient has cancer. The decision to operate, however, should be a logical one rather than one made in desperation. "Blind" gastrectomy or "blind" subtotal colectomy should rarely be performed; unfortunate situations can be avoided if a logical sequence of investigation is followed. The best surgical results are obtained when surgery is used with precision, both in timing and in scope. There is no better illustration of the importance of integration of multispecialty care than in the treatment of gastrointestinal hemorrhage in the cancer patient.

BIBLIOGRAPHY

Chung RS. Management of upper gastrointestinal bleeding: The role of diagnostic and therapeutic endoscopy. In Chung RS: Therapeutic Endoscopy in Gastrointestinal Surgery. New York, Churchill Livingstone, 1987:5–37

Fath RB Jr, Kurtz RC. Gastrointestinal problems in the critically ill cancer patient. In Howland WS, Carlon GC (eds): Critical Care of the Cancer Patient. Chicago, Year Book Medical Publishers, 1985:86–113

Hunt PS, Korman MG, Hansky J et al. Bleeding duodenal ulcer: Reduction of mortality with a planned approach. Brit J Surg 66:633–640, 1979

Proceedings of the Consensus Conference on Therapeutic Endoscopy in Bleeding Ulcers. Gastrointest Endosc 36(5 Suppl):S1–S65, 1990

Sherlock P, Winawer SJ. Differential diagnosis of upper gastrointestinal bleeding and cancer. Cancer 28:7–16, 1978

Technology Assessment Committee of ASGE. Status Evaluation: Enteroscopy. Gastrointest Endosc 37:673–677, 1991

John S. Macdonald, Daniel G. Haller, Robert J. Mayer, Eds. *Manual of Oncologic Therapeutics*, Third Edition.

55. UROLOGIC EMERGENCIES

Nicholas J. Vogelzang
Glenn E. Gerber
Robert L. Vogelzang

The purpose of this chapter is to focus on those urologic events in cancer patients which are true medical emergencies and to distinguish such events from those which necessitate urgent, but not emergent, intervention. This chapter will deal with the following topics:

1. Ureteral obstruction, either unilateral or bilateral.
2. Gross hematuria, including hemorrhagic cystitis.
3. Acute renal failure.
4. Bladder outlet obstruction leading to acute urinary retention.

URETERAL OBSTRUCTION

Ureteral obstruction is frequently seen in patients with advanced cancer arising from a variety of sites. The most common malignancy causing ureteral obstruction is invasive transitional cell carcinoma of the bladder. This is usually secondary to tumor arising at or near the ureteral orifice blocking the flow of urine within the intramural ureter. As tumor commonly originates in the urothelium at the ureteral-vesical orifice, unilateral hydronephrosis secondary to obstruction is commonly a presenting sign or symptom of bladder cancer. The symptoms of acute hydronephrosis include flank pain, nausea, backache, and occasionally hematuria. Since obstructive uropathy caused by bladder cancer can be insidious and slow to develop, it may be completely asymptomatic. In many cases the symptoms of unilateral or bilateral hydronephrosis are extremely subtle and only a minor change in the serum creatinine heralds the onset of the syndrome. In those patients immediate renal ultrasound should be performed to confirm the presence of collecting system dilatation. Retrograde pyelograms are almost never necessary for diagnosis. Care should be taken not to obtain computerized tomography (CT) scans with iodinated contrast media, as contrast toxicity can be synergistic with obstructive uropathy injury. Hydronephrosis can also occur following a transurethral resection of a bladder cancer since the transurethral resection itself may cause fibrosis in the area of the ureteral orifice leading to unilateral obstruction. Similarly, transitional cell carcinomas can, on rare occasions, occur primarily in the ureter or renal pelvis and cause unilateral ureteral obstruction.

The next most common malignancy causing ureteral obstruction is cervical cancer. This usually results from direct invasion into the base of the bladder with resultant blockage of the distal ureter(s). A similar mechanism of obstruction occurs in men with locally advanced prostate cancer. In this case, the tumor grows into the bladder base and trigone, leading to urinary obstruction. Alternatively, the ureters may be compromised more proximally in their course within the retroperitoneum or pelvis secondary to lymphadenopathy. As cervical cancer is treated with extensive pelvic surgery, inadvertent surgical ligation of the ureters has been one of the dreaded complications of treatment of this cancer. The incidence of this complication has declined dramatically with careful attention and with routine pre- and post-operative urinary tract visualization studies. Finally, less common causes of obstruction in cervical cancer include radiation fibrosis, which leads to stricturing of the ureter, perhaps secondary to compromised ureteral blood flow and inadvertent clipping of the ureter during pelvic laparoscopy. As might be expected, it is not uncommon for patients with advanced cervical cancer and bulky local disease to die of uremia.

Less common causes of malignant ureteral obstruction include metastatic cancers originating from the breast, lung, and GI tract. Even less common causes are sarcomas, tumors of the testicle, and lymphomas which may cause ureteral obstruction due to massive retroperitoneal disease. Testicular tumors and lymphomas are, of course, effectively treated with combination chemotherapy while the other tumors are generally refractory to chemotherapy. Thus, stents need to be in place only until the exquisite sensitivity of lymphomas and testicular tumors to chemotherapy has been defined, while in the other malignancies stents probably will be permanent.

Although the cause of obstructive uropathy varies with the cancer type, the clinical/physiologic outcome is similar in all cases. The pathophysiology of obstructive uropathy has been recently reviewed;[1,2] outcome depends largely on the degree of obstruction and the length of time that it has been present. Short-term ureteral blockage of 3 to 7 days duration will not lead to long-term renal damage. However, a significant amount of renal function can be permanently lost when obstruction persists for weeks to months, even if there is only partial obstruction. The amount of renal function lost can be anatomically estimated by assessing the degree of renal cortical atrophy present on the ultrasound or pyelogram. Extensive atrophy suggests irretrievable loss of renal function. On rare occasions obstruction may lead to rupture of a renal calyceal fornix and extravasation of urine into the renal sinus and retroperitoneum. Therefore, the finding of

TABLE 55–1. RETROGRADE CYSTOSCOPIC URETERAL DECOMPRESSION VERSUS ANTEGRADE PERCUTANEOUS URETERAL DECOMPRESSION

RETROGRADE URETERAL DECOMPRESSION		PERCUTANEOUS ANTEGRADE URETERAL DECOMPRESSION	
ADVANTAGES	DISADVANTAGES	ADVANTAGES	DISADVANTAGES
No need for external drainage bag Requires no special care by patient or nurse	Cytoscopy and general anaesthesia necessary for insertion or replacement of stent May cause lower urinary tract pain or irritation Frequently associated with stent occlusion or migration and recurrent ureteral obstruction; need regular stent changes	Reliable drainage of kidney achieved Large 10 French ureteral stents can be placed No need for general anesthesia	External drainage bag sometimes needed Systemic anticoagulation or coagulopathy is relative contraindication Local care of external tube sometimes necessary

unilateral hydronephrosis should lead to the prompt institution of corrective measures but does not require emergency intervention unless there is sepsis or severe pain secondary to the obstruction. Bilateral obstruction requires more emergent therapy.

Treatment of obstructive uropathy can be rapidly accomplished with antegrade percutaneous nephrostomy tubes placed under ultrasound guidance by an interventional radiologist or by the cystoscopic placement of a ureteral stent by a urologist. Both of these methods have advantages and disadvantages (Table 55–1).

Initial percutaneous decompression of malignant ureteral obstruction could be followed by an attempt to cross the distal ureteral obstruction and place ureteral stents. The latter maneuver can be accomplished in *at least* 90% of cases; in patients in whom the obstructing tumor resists passage, ureteral drainage *can* continue via the existing catheter(s).

When percutaneous nephrostomy tubes cannot be placed or are unsuccessful, placement of the stent via cystoscopy or via an endoscopic placement of a stent by an endourologist is then necessary. In most circumstances, relief of ureteral obstruction can be accomplished. There is a 40% to 50% failure rate when stents are placed cystoscopically in the presence of extrinsic ureteral obstruction.[3] Therefore, percutaneous drainage is a more reliable means of decompressing a hydronephrotic kidney and should be used in most urgent situations where prompt upper urinary tract decompression is needed. Due to the expense and high initial failure rate of cystocopically placed stents, percutaneous nephrostomies are the preferred method of management.[4]

Complications of ureteral stents, whether placed from an antegrade or retrograde approach, can occur. The "double J" stents may cause bladder spasm and hematuria as well as proteinuria. In selected patients the bladder spasms can be difficult to manage and may require removal of the stent and maintenance of percutaneous nephrostomy tubes for the remainder of the patient's life. Infection of the nephrostomy tubes or stents should not be ignored since bacterial biofilm ("slime") develops rapidly in stents exposed to cutaneous gram-positive organisms.[5] Bacterial biofilm build-up and encrustation necessitates stent changes every 3 to 4 months, although larger diameter stents may allow longer intervals between changes. Since patients with indwelling stents often have chronic pyuria or hematuria, signs of urinary tract infections maybe obscured. Thus, a patient with a stent who experiences foul-smelling urine should be immediately started on antibiotic therapy and stent change considered. Chronic suppressive antibiotic therapy is not indicated as it allows overgrowth of drug-resistant bacteria and *Candida*.

In conclusion, ureteral obstruction, either unilateral or bilateral, is a common accompaniment of advanced pelvic malignancies. In patients who are candidates for further hormone or chemotherapy, every attempt should be made to relieve the hydronephrosis immediately. An elevated serum creatinine will cause such patients to be ineligible for standard or investigational therapies which usually require a serum creatinine of less than or equal to 1.5 mg/dl. Because the complication rate of stenting is low and the quality of life is high, the usual clinical practice is to stent or to drain percutaneously all patients who present with or develop obstructive uropathy. Only the very rare patient is allowed to experience unilateral renal loss or bilateral renal failure and death secondary to obstructive uropathy.

GROSS HEMATURIA

Gross hematuria can occur secondary to a number of causes in patients with malignancies. While it is rare for patients to have life-threatening hematuria, the presence of bloody urine frequently alarms patients, nurses, and physicians, leading to urgent evaluation. The causes of gross hematuria in cancer patients are listed in Table 55–2.

The most common presenting symptom of a variety of primary urinary tract tumors is gross or microscopic hematuria. These include renal cell carcinoma, transitional cell carcinoma of the kidney, ureter or bladder and urethral cancer. Other tumors, such as adenocarcinoma of the prostate or benign prostatic hyperplasia, may also present with hematuria. Gross hematuria may also be seen in patients with nonurinary tract malignancies that either metastasize or invade locally into the genitourinary system. While this may potentially occur with a wide variety of tumors, it is most commonly encountered in patients with cervical or lower gastrointestinal malignancies.

Hematuria may also be frequently caused by factors not directly related to tumor invasion. Many patients who are immunosuppressed secondary to advanced malignancy or chemotherapy will be prone to upper or lower urinary tract infections. The risk of such infection is significantly increased by the presence of a nephrostomy tube or stent. Although most patients will have other symptoms, it is not uncommon for significant hematuria to occur secondary to infection alone.

Another common cause of hematuria is hemorrhagic cystitis secondary to oxazaphosphorine agents, cyclophosphamide and isophosphamide.[6] Urologic side effects are a significant source of morbidity in the use of these agents and in many cases, are very difficult to treat effectively. The cause of the urotoxicity is acrolein, a hepatic metabolite of the oxazaphosphorine agents, which damages the bladder wall by direct contact. The risk of hemorrhagic cystitis can be reduced by the use of hydration and N-acetyl cysteine (Mesna), which binds acrolein in the urine. Unfortunately, some patients still develop hemorrhagic cystitis despite these measures. Hemorrhagic cystitis may also be caused by radiation injury to the bladder. Urgency, frequency, and dysuria are usually seen in addition to gross hematuria. External beam radiation in patients with cervical or prostate cancer is the most common cause and it is estimated that as many as 5%–10% of patients receiving full dose pelvic radiation therapy will develop bleeding. Finally, patients with rapid cell death and turnover secondary to chemotherapy may develop uric acid stones. The most common symptom in such cases is flank pain, but patients may occasionally experience hematuria.

TABLE 55–2. CAUSES OF HEMATURIA IN CANCER PATIENTS

Benign and malignant urinary tract neoplasms
Invasion of urinary tract by other malignant tumors
Infection
Medications and chemical toxins
Kidney stones
Radiation injury to the urinary tract
Urinary tract irritation from indwelling catheters

As mentioned earlier, hematuria is rarely life-threatening. Initially, if patients are able to void and are not passing blood clots, no immediate intervention is generally needed. Patients should be instructed to increase their fluid intake or the rate of intravenous fluid infusion should be increased. When bleeding is severe with passage of large blood clots, it is usually best to insert a large urethral catheter (20–24 F) and irrigate manually with saline to remove the blood clots from the bladder. It is often helpful to use a catheter with multiple drainage holes to facilitate clot evacuation. If bleeding continues to be severe, a "three-way" catheter should be inserted, which allows for continuous bladder irrigation.[4] This continuous irrigation does not improve hemostasis but merely prevents occlusion of the catheter and accumulation of clots.

Evaluation of the source of hematuria is based on the degree of bleeding and the clinical situation. If an upper urinary tract source is suspected, radiologic evaluation is necessary. This can be performed using ultrasonography, excretory or retrograde urography, or computerized tomography. The choice of radiologic procedure must be individualized. In most cases, however, the lower urinary tract will be the site of bleeding. Cystoscopy is generally the procedure of choice to evaluate the urethra and bladder and may also allow for control of hemorrhage by tumor resection, fulguration of bleeding sites, or introduction of hemostatic agents. In some cases, mere endoscopic evacuation of blood clots will lead to prompt cessation of bleeding.

Hemorrhagic cystitis secondary to radiation or chemotherapeutic agents is very difficult to treat. Initially, continuous irrigation and correction of anemia, thrombocytopenia, and elevated clotting parameters should be attempted and will often be successful. However, many patients will continue to have severe bleeding and under such circumstances, a variety of intravesical agents have been used with moderate success, including alum, silver nitrate, and prostaglandins. When hemorrhage remains significant despite these measures, cystoscopy is necessary. The bladder usually will show evidence of bleeding from the entire surface, making it impossible to achieve hemostasis successfully by fulguration. Intravesical formalin can then be instilled and in most cases will control bleeding. However, this must be performed under general anesthesia, and a preoperative cystogram is necessary to rule out vesicoureteral reflux. If present, balloon occlusion catheters may be inserted in each ureter to prevent upper tract damage from the formalin. Patients may develop severe irritative symptoms secondary to formalin and occasionally bladder contracture will occur. Therefore, this treatment should only be given when severe hemorrhage cannot be controlled by any other means. Finally, urinary diversion by the placement of percutaneous nephrostomy tubes or hyperbaric oxygen treatments may also allow for hemostasis.

ACUTE RENAL FAILURE

The causes of acute renal failure in the cancer patient are multiple and are shown on Table 55–3.

Although acute renal failure from any cause is a urologic emergency, we will deal only with renal failure secondary to chemotherapy, tumor lysis syndrome, or antibiotics. Acute renal therapy can be secondary to a number of drugs but the most common drug causing renal failure is cisplatin. The usual reported incidence of acute renal failure is 1%–3% of patients. In selected circumstances such as patients with severe diarrhea, dehydration, or pre-existing renal dysfunction, the incidence of acute renal failure secondary to cisplatin may approach 25%. During phase I and early phase II trials in unhydrated patients, acute renal failure occurred in upwards of 75% of patients who received cisplatin doses over 50 mg/m^2. These early clinical trials led to the widespread use of forced diuresis in the prevention of cisplatin nephrotoxicity. Aggressive fluid management, with 2 to 3 liters of fluid and urine output of greater than 100 cc per hour prior to a cisplatin dose of over 50 mg/m^2 as a single dose, has dramatically lowered the rate of cisplatin nephrotoxicity. For doses between 20 and 50 mg/m^2 many physicians use only 1 to 2 liters of fluid hydration and do not insist upon 100 cc per hour of urinary output. For patients receiving 100 mg/m^2 and greater doses the risk of acute renal failure significantly increases. These patients should be hydrated for a minimum of 6 hours prior to chemotherapy. Furosemide induced diuresis may be necessary. Patients should have urine outputs of at least 100 cc per hour prior to and following the cisplatin dose. Many clinicians routinely infuse cisplatin over 6 hours so as to avoid high peak levels of unbound or free cisplatin. The high peak levels of unbound cisplatin have been shown to be the proximate cause for acute renal failure. Although no randomized controlled studies have compared hydration schemes or schedules of cisplatin using the endpoint of renal function, there has been ample clinical experience to suggest that brief high doses of platinum are not only associated with abnormal serum creatinine levels but also with a higher incidence of renal tubular abnormalities such as magnesium wasting, potassium wasting, and hypophosphatemia.

TABLE 55–3. CAUSES OF ACUTE RENAL FAILURE IN CANCER PATIENTS

Nephrotoxic chemotherapeutic agents
Tumor lysis syndrome with calcium, phosphorus and uric acid deposition in the kidneys
Radiographic contrast media-induced renal failure
Drug-induced renal failure secondary to antibiotics especially aminoglycoside therapy
Bilateral invasion of the kidneys by lymphoma or leukemia
Membranous glomerulo-nephritis or immune complex nephritis
Dehydration and acute tubular necrosis secondary to hypovolemia induced by diarrhea, nausea, vomiting, or other fluid losses
Hypotension induced by immunotherapeutic agents such as tumor necrosis factor or interleukin-2
Septic shock
Adult respiratory distress syndrome
Acute bilateral hydronephrosis

Even after a single dose of cisplatin there is biochemical and cytological evidence of tubular damage. The rate of recovery of the renal function following a single dose of platinum is usually 2 to 3 weeks. Thus, regardless of how careful oncologic professionals are, cisplatin, at any dose, causes kidney damage. The degree to which the kidney recovers from cisplatin nephrotoxicity is highly variable, with the majority of patients experiencing full recovery and normal serum creatinine levels for many years after therapy. The longest follow-up experience with cisplatin has come in patients with testicular cancer. Follow-up studies of patients treated with cisplatin 10 or more years ago document a small decrease in the creatinine clearance and an increase in the serum creatinine, though the values typically lie within the upper normal range of the laboratory tests. Such patients also apparently experience mildly increased rates of hypertension. Bosl et al. have documented that these patients have alterations of the renin-angiotensin system, possibly mediated by magnesium losses induced by cisplatin tubular damage. Patients who are to receive cisplatin should be warned of its toxicity and should be treated cautiously with hydration, careful attention to urinary output, and cessation of cisplatin in the face of diminished renal function.

Newer methods of prevention of cisplatin nephropathy have included circadian dosing of cisplatin. Hrushesky et al. have shown that administration of cisplatin at 6:00 P.M. is less nephrotoxic than cisplatin administered at 6:00 A.M. This time of administration is obviously not practical for most outpatient facilities. Nonetheless administration of cisplatin in the afternoon may have some advantage over morning cisplatin.

Several new drugs can ameliorate cisplatin nephrotoxicity. These include WR2721, antabuse, and a variety of other drugs.

The most common nephrotoxic antibiotics are those of the aminoglycoside family. Although they are highly effective, in most clinical situations third generation cephalosporins or quinolones are easily substituted for aminoglycosides. Nonetheless aminoglycosides remain an important weapon in the treatment of patients with life-threatening gram negative sepsis, especially those with severe neutropenia. When patients are on aminoglycoside therapy, careful pharmacodynamic monitoring should occur, with serum levels of aminoglycosides being monitored by an in-hospital dosing service. Usually this service is provided to the physicians and oncologic professionals by the pharmacy staff. The development of a non-nephrotoxic aminoglycoside therapy has been unsuccessful.

Another toxin which can cause acute renal failure is uric acid. The syndrome of acute tumor lysis has been well-documented in medical literature. This syndrome occurs through the rapid death, perhaps by programmed cell death (apoptosis), of fast-growing tumors such as lymphomas, leukemias, small cell lung cancer, and breast cancer, when treated with chemotherapy. The medical literature documents acute tumor lysis syndrome following therapy for virtually all types of malignancies. The pathogenesis of tumor lysis syndrome induced acute nephrotoxicity is apparently mechanical deposition of calcium, phosphorus, and uric acid crystals within the renal tubule. The deposition of insoluble material leads to acute tubular necrosis. In most cases, with conservative management, including dialysis, renal function will recover fully. The degree of permanent renal damage is a function of the duration of anuria. Prevention of this syndrome should be the responsibility of all oncologic professionals who administer chemotherapy. Patients who are at risk for this syndrome, particularly those with acute leukemia and Burkitt's lymphoma, should be pretreated with allopurinol, alkalinization of the urine with oral bicarbonate, and forced diuresis. Monitoring of serum calcium, phosphorus, uric acid, and lactate dehydrogenase (LDH) should be performed at 12-hour intervals during the first 3 to 4 days of chemotherapy. It should be noted that occasional patients have had tumor lysis syndrome following a single dose of intrathecal methotrexate for leukemia or a single oral dose of hydrocortisone for treatment of nausea prior to systemic therapy of a lymphoma. Thus all patients with these rapidly proliferating tumors should be considered to be at risk for this rare but clinically spectacular syndrome.

URETHRAL OBSTRUCTION

The cause of urethral obstruction in the cancer patient is usually due to prostate cancer, although less common malignancies such as primary urethral transitional cell carcinomas, sarcomas of the prostate, primary malignancies of the penis, and primary malignancies of the vaginal introitus can occasionally cause acute urethral obstruction. Benign causes of bladder outlet obstruction include radiation fibrosis, urethral stricture, or blood clots. The management of acute urinary retention secondary to these conditions involves emergent urologic consultation. Placement of a Foley catheter is usually easily accomplished in females. Occasionally, the urethral meatus has retracted to a position in the anterior vagina making catheter insertion slightly more difficult. In contrast, prostatic enlargement, radiation changes, or urethral strictures frequently prevent passage of a urethral catheter in males. In the presence of significant hyperplasia of the prostate, the use of a coude tipped catheter, which has a slight upward angulation at the distal tip, may allow catheter placement with little risk of urethral injury. However, urethral strictures require dilation which can be accomplished using a variety of techniques. These are best reserved for those experienced with these methods. The most direct means of draining the bladder when passage of a catheter is difficult is with a percutaneously placed suprapubic tube. In the presence of a distended bladder this is usually straightforward. However, if pelvic or lower abdominal surgery has been previously performed it is best to place the suprapubic tube using sonographic guidance to avoid inadvertent puncture of the large or small intestine, which may be adherent between the anterior bladder surface and the abdominal wall.

Both prostate cancer and benign prostatic hypertrophy (BPH) are extremely common, and can be difficult to distinguish clinically. A considerable number of patients are presumed to be obstructed secondary to BPH, but in fact are found to have prostatic malignancy. Since placement of a Foley catheter and the attendant trauma and local inflammation may cause release of PSA (prostate specific antigen) into the serum, the clinical picture can be quite confusing. In no case is it a urologic emergency. Patients with an indwelling Foley catheter secondary to BPH and an elevated PSA may be considered for biopsy if medical management of the BPH is insufficient. Medical management of BPH usually includes finastride (Proscar) 5 mg/day or terazosin (Hytrin).

The symptom of urethral obstruction, namely complete anuria with suprapubic/abdominal pain, is clinically striking and emergent care is required. Patients can develop neurogenic bladders, may not experience symptoms of urinary obstruction, and will have overflow continence. In those situations, placement of Foley catheter and chronic drainage for up to several months may be required for some return of bladder tone. Ultimately patients who require chronic indwelling Foley catheters require careful management by the urologists. In many patients the technique of chronic self-catheterization is preferred over chronic indwelling catheters.

REFERENCES

1. Jones DA, George NJ. Interactive obstructive uropathy in man. Br J Urol 69:337–345, 1992
2. Abramson AF, Mitty HA. Update on interventional treatment of urinary obstruction. Urol Radiol 14:234–236, 1992
3. Docimo SG, DeWolf WC. High failure rate of indwelling

ureteral stents in patients with extrinsic obstruction: Experience at 2 institutions. J Urol 142:277–279, 198
4. Russo P. Urologic emergencies. In DeVita VT, Hellman S, Rosenberg SA, (eds). Cancer: Principles & Practice of Oncology, 4th ed. Philadelphia, JB Lippincott, 1993:2159
5. Christensen GD. The sticky problem of staphylococcus epidermidis sepsis. Hosp Practice, 27–38, September 30, 1993
6. Levine LA, Richie JP. Urological complications of cyclophosphamide. J Urol 141:1063–69, 1989
7. Zagoria RJ, Hodge RG, Dyer RB, Routh WD. Percutaneous nephrostomy for treatment of intractable hemorrhagic cystitis. J Urol 149:1449–51, 1993
8. Vogelzang NJ. Nephrotoxicity from chemotherapy: Prevention and management. Oncology Williston Park, 5:97–103, 1991
9. Vogelzang NJ, Nelimark RA, Nath KA. Tumor lysis syndrome following induction chemotherapy of small cell bronchogenic carcinoma. JAMA, 249:513–514, 1983

John S. Macdonald, Daniel G. Haller, Robert J. Mayer, Eds. *Manual of Oncologolic Therapeutics*, Third Edition.

VII. SUPPORTIVE CARE AND REHABILITATION

56. PAIN

Beth Popp
Russell K. Portenoy

INTRODUCTION

Chronic pain is experienced by more than 70% of cancer patients during their illness.[1,2] *Pain* is an inherently subjective phenomenon, which has been defined as "an unpleasant sensory and emotional experience associated with actual or potential tissue damage, or described in terms of such damage."[3] Although acute pain may be associated with objective behavioral (*e.g.*, grimacing, guarding, or limping) or autonomic (*e.g.*, tachycardia, hypertension, or diaphoresis) signs, chronic pain typically occurs without these indicators. In the absence of an objective test for pain, it is best if the physician simply accepts the patient's report.

Acute pain has a well-defined onset and a temporal course characterized by transience. Opioid or non-opioid analgesics are usually required and diagnosis of the underlying cause is a critical aspect of the assessment. Numerous acute cancer-related pain syndromes have been described (Table 56–1) and treatment approaches have been recently reviewed in the Clinical Practice Guidelines for Acute Pain Management developed in conjunction with the Agency for Health Care Policy and Research.[4]

Chronic pain has a prolonged course or is associated with a lesion that is not expected to resolve. Most chronic pain fluctuates and is associated with discrete episodes of *breakthrough pain* (known as *incident pain* when precipitated by a voluntary action such as walking). The chronic pain syndromes associated with cancer can be classified based on underlying pathophysiology or etiology (Table 56–2). This classification and other issues related to the assessment of chronic cancer pain have been extensively reviewed in recent publications.[5,6]

COMPREHENSIVE ASSESSMENT

Comprehensive assessment of pain is critical to effective management. Pain should be explicitly queried during the initial consultation and at every follow-up encounter. The history should elicit the pain locations, severity, quality, exacerbating or relieving factors, onset, course, and associated circumstances. The effect of the pain on functional status, including activities of daily living, work, and social interactions, should be determined, and both the extent of the cancer and other medical diseases should be clarified. This information can be used to understand the characteristics, etiology, and pathophysiology of the pain and categorize the specific pain syndrome. Each of multiple pain complaints should be considered in the same systematic fashion.

An important element in this assessment is the elucidation of the presumed pathophysiology of the pain. The term *nociceptive pain* is applied to a pain syndrome that can be attributed to the activation of specific sensory receptors in somatic or visceral organs. *Somatic nociceptive pain* is usually well localized and often has an aching, throbbing, or sharp quality. *Visceral nociceptive pain* is often poorly localized, may be referred to remote cutaneous sites (such as shoulder pain from diaphragmatic irritation), and frequently has a deep aching, cramping, or gnawing quality. The term *neuropathic pain* is applied to a pain syndrome that can be attributed to aberrant somatosensory processing in the peripheral or central nervous system. Neuropathic pain may be de-

TABLE 56–1. ACUTE CANCER-RELATED PAIN SYNDROMES

ACUTE PAIN ASSOCIATED WITH DIAGNOSTIC AND THERAPEUTIC INTERVENTIONS	ACUTE PAIN ASSOCIATED WITH ANTI-CANCER THERAPIES	ACUTE PAIN ASSOCIATED WITH INFECTION
Acute pain associated with diagnostic interventions	Acute pain associated with chemotherapy infusion techniques	Acute hepatic neuralgia
Bone marrow biopsy	Intravenous infusion pain	Oropharyngeal candidiasis
Lumbar puncture	Intraperitoneal chemotherapy pain	
Colonoscopy	Acute pain associated with chemotherapy toxicity	
Percutaneous biopsy	Mucositis	
Thoracentesis	Steroid pseudorheumatism	
Acute postoperative pain	Painful peripheral neuropathy	
Acute pain caused by therapeutic interventions	Acute pain associated with hormonal therapy	
Pleurodesis	Hormone-induced pain flare in breast cancer	
Percutaneous nephrostomy	Gynecomastia	
Acute pain associated with analgesic techniques	Acute pain associated with immunotherapy	
Injection pain	Diffuse bone pain due to colony stimulating factors	
Epidural injection pain	Interferon-induced acute pain	
Opioid headache	Acute pain associated with radiation therapy	
	Incident pain associated with positioning	
	Oropharyngeal mucositis	
	Acute radiation enteritis and proctitis	

TABLE 56–2. CHRONIC CANCER-RELATED PAIN SYNDROMES

TUMOR-RELATED CHRONIC PAIN SYNDROMES	CHRONIC PAIN SYNDROMES ASSOCIATED WITH CANCER THERAPY
Bone pain	Post-chemotherapy pain syndromes
Multiple bony metastases	Chronic painful peripheral neuropathy
Marrow expansion	Postherpetic neuralgia
Back pain and epidural compression	Chronic post-surgical pain syndromes
Headache and facial pain	Postmastectomy pain syndrome
Intracerebral tumor	Post-thoracotomy pain
Leptomeningeal metastases	Phantom pain syndromes
Base of skull metastases	Phantom breast pain
Tumor involvement of the peripheral nervous system	Phantom limb pain
Tumor-related radiculopathy	Postsurgical pelvic floor myalgia
Cervical plexopathy	Chronic post-radiation pain syndromes
Brachial plexopathy	Radiation-induced brachial plexopathy
Malignant lumbosacral plexopathy	Radiation-induced lumbosacral plexopathy
Tumor-related mononeuropathy	Chronic radiation enteritis and proctitis
Pain syndromes of the viscera	Burning perineum syndrome
Hepatic distention syndrome	
Chronic intestinal obstruction	
Peritoneal carcinomatosis	
Miscellaneous tumor-related syndromes	
Malignant perineal pain	
Malignant pelvic floor myalgia	
Ureteric obstruction	
Paraneoplastic pain syndromes	
Tumor-related gynecomastia	

scribed as a dysesthesia, an "abnormal" pain often depicted as burning, tingling, or electrical. Because they are sustained by processes in the nervous system itself, neuropathic pain syndromes may persist after the underlying cause is eliminated.

Assessment of the psychosocial status of the patient is an essential part of the comprehensive pain assessment. The patient's current level of anxiety and depression, presence of suicidal ideation, and degree of functional incapacity should all be assessed. Information about psychiatric illnesses and the response to prior medical problems is also highly valuable, and may identify patients who are at high risk for psychological deterioration during the current illness.

The physical examination, which must include a complete neurologic examination, can clarify the pain syndrome and extent of disease, and indicate the need for imaging or laboratory procedures. Additional evaluation may be also warranted, however, in the absence of physical signs. Unless there is a clear understanding of the pain, further assessment should be directed by the patient's history, combined with knowledge of the natural history of the cancer and the pain syndromes with which it is associated.

Treatment of pain during the diagnostic evaluation will improve the patient's ability to participate in the necessary procedures, reduce the physical and psychological debilitation that may accompany unrelenting pain, and convey the message that the physician takes the complaint of pain seriously. Adequate pain control will not obscure the diagnosis.

The *goals of care* should be clarified during the pain assessment. Some patients, particularly those at the end of life, have comfort as the primary goal, and express less concern about the maintenance of function. Others value comfort and function equally. Therapeutic decision-making is profoundly affected by these goals. Decisions about the goals of therapy must be made jointly by the patient, medical care givers, and family or friends assisting in day-to-day care.

The onset or worsening of pain in a cancer patient commonly, but not invariably, indicates recurrence or progression of disease. Consequently, repeated pain assessment is needed whenever the pain changes, and each assessment requires a new definition of the extent of disease. In some cases, such as postmastectomy syndrome following surgical trauma to the intercostobrachial nerve, cancer will be excluded as the etiology, whereas in others, such as post-thoracotomy pain syndrome following resection of a lung tumor, recurrent cancer is typically found.

PRIMARY THERAPY

Primary therapy attempts to ameliorate the underlying cause of the pain. Primary therapies include radiation therapy, surgical resection of tumor, cytotoxic chemotherapy, immunotherapy, hormonal therapy, and antibiotics for infection. With the exception of radiotherapy, primary antineoplastic therapies are seldom administered for pain palliation alone. Other antineoplastic approaches may have analgesic consequences, however, and the presence of pain often influences treatment decisions. This highlights the importance of an up-to-date knowledge of analgesic therapy. Although the potential for pain relief should be considered when weighing the risks and benefits of primary therapy, the importance of this factor cannot be clarified without adequate information about traditional analgesic therapies.

Focal pain usually responds to external beam radiation therapy, particularly if the tumor is known to be radiosensitive. The use of radiotherapy for pain palliation should always be considered if the underlying lesion is focal and the response to analgesics is not satisfactory. Local toxicities (*e.g.*, mucositis or proctitis), the time and cost involved, and the occasionally significant loss of bone marrow reserve following irradiation of bony regions are the major disadvantages.

Cytotoxic chemotherapy can palliate pain in chemoresponsive disease, even when it does not prolong survival; poorly relieved pain is occasionally an appropriate indication for therapy. For example, back pain from retroperitoneal lymphadenopathy related to germ cell tumors, lymphomas, or chronic lymphocytic leukemia may respond well to chemotherapy and obviate the need for analgesics. The potential for pain relief from chemotherapy must be balanced against the time and cost of receiving the therapy and any negative effects on quality of life that may result from the side effects of the treatment.

In highly selected cases, cancer surgery is considered primarily for pain management. Relief of persistent bowel obstruction, some orthopedic procedures (*e.g.*, spine stabilization, joint replacement, and claviculectomy), and resection of recurrent abscesses may be effective in refractory pain. Surgery must be considered in the context of the expected survival of the patient and the severity of the pain syndrome.

In a study of patients referred to the pain service at Memorial Sloan-Kettering Cancer Center[7], 4% had undiagnosed infection as the etiology of the pain. Treatment of infection with antibiotics, and other measures such as abscess drainage, may produce dramatic relief of pain. Empiric antibiotic therapy is sometimes warranted for patients who develop escalating pain that may be due to occult infection, such as those who have been previously irradiated for head and neck cancer and have skin changes that could represent cellulitis, and those with an ill-defined deep pelvic soft tissue mass following radiotherapy for a pelvic tumor.

SYSTEMIC ANALGESIC PHARMACOTHERAPY

The WHO Analgesic Ladder

Guidelines based on the World Health Organization's (WHO) "analgesic ladder" approach[8] (Figure 56–1) are now widely accepted for the treatment of cancer pain.[6,9–11]

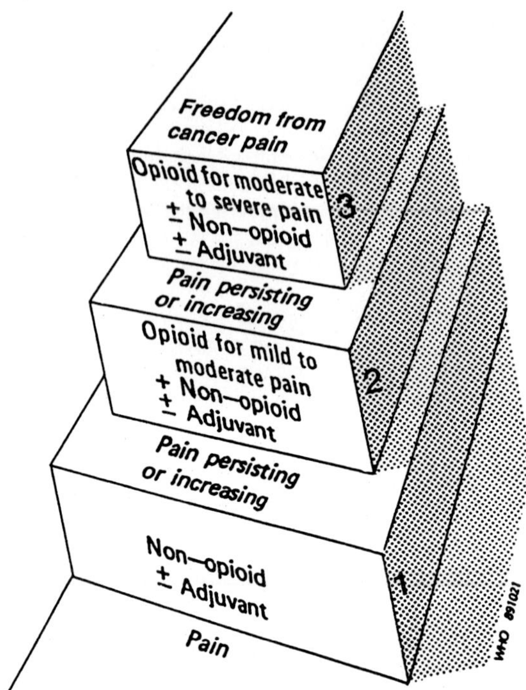

Figure 56–1. The World Health Organization "analgesic ladder"

Studies suggest that 70%–90% of patients with cancer pain can attain adequate relief using this approach.[12,13]

Analgesic drugs can be categorized into 1) non-opioid analgesics, including aspirin, acetaminophen, and the nonsteroidal anti-inflammatory drugs; 2) opioid analgesics, such as propoxyphene, codeine, oxycodone, morphine, hydromorphone, fentanyl, levorphanol, and methadone; and 3) the adjuvant analgesics, which are those drugs that have primary indications other than pain but are analgesic in certain settings. The analgesic ladder approach requires familiarity with a few drugs in each of these three categories.

The WHO approach matches the analgesic to the intensity of the pain. Non-opioids are first line therapy for the cancer patient with mild to moderate pain. The patient who fails to attain adequate relief with a non-opioid, or who presents with moderate to severe pain, should be treated with an opioid conventionally used for pain of this severity. This therapy is combined with adjuvant drugs (either treatments for opioid side effects or adjuvant analgesics), if specific indications exist. Patients who present with severe pain or who fail to respond to the opioid selected from the second "rung" of the analgesic ladder should be treated with an opioid conventionally selected for severe pain, combined with adjuvant drugs if needed.

NON-OPIOID ANALGESICS (TABLE 56–3)

All non-opioid analgesics have a "ceiling dose," above which there is no additional analgesic benefit from dose escalation. There is substantial variability in the dose-response relationships observed among patients given the same drug and in the overall response of a single patient given different drugs. The use of these drugs is not associated with tolerance or physical dependence.

Aspirin is the prototype for the analgesic, anti-inflammatory and antipyretic effects of the non-opioid analgesics. It is inexpensive, available for oral and rectal administration, and often combined in a fixed ratio with codeine, oxycodone, or propoxyphene in commercially available formulations. Its use in the cancer population is limited by gastrointestinal adverse effects, platelet inhibitory effects, and antipyretic effects. These effects may be especially problematic for patients who are receiving myelosuppressive chemotherapy.

Acetaminophen has analgesic and antipyretic activity comparable to aspirin, but is a weak anti-inflammatory agent. Like aspirin, it is inexpensive, available for oral or rectal administration, and is often combined in a fixed ratio with an opioid conventionally used on the second "rung" of the analgesic ladder (*e.g.*, codeine, oxycodone, or propoxyphene). It causes less gastrointestinal irritation and does not affect platelet function. The potential for hepatic toxicity limits the dose to 4–6 g/24 hr; doses should be limited further in those patients with significant liver disease or history of alcoholism.

Nonsteroidal anti-inflammatory drugs (NSAIDs) also have analgesic, antipyretic and anti-inflammatory activity comparable to aspirin. These drugs have diverse pharmacokinetic profiles and durations of analgesic action (Table 56–3). Nonacetylated salicylates, such as choline magnesium trisalicylate and salsalate, are effective analgesics, anti-inflammatory drugs and antipyretics that tend to cause less gastrointestinal distress and platelet dysfunction than aspirin. Ibuprofen and naproxen are available over-the-counter, and depending on dose, may be relatively convenient and inexpensive. Ketorolac is unique among NSAIDs available in the United States in having both oral and parenteral formulations. Experience with this drug is limited and long-term use cannot presently be recommended. Many other NSAIDs are available and the clinician should be familiar with several drugs for the purpose of sequential trials, if indicated.

The gastrointestinal toxicity of the NSAIDs may limit their usefulness in the treatment of chronic cancer-related pain. Nausea and upper abdominal pain are common. The risk of gastric ulcers increases fivefold and complications of ulcers increase threefold during NSAID therapy. These drugs are relatively contraindicated in patients with other risk factors for ulcers, such as concurrent treatment with steroids or a history of ulcer disease; older patients are at increased risk. Dyspepsia is a poor predictor of ulceration, and most patients are asymptomatic until the complication oc-

TABLE 56–3. EXAMPLES OF NON-OPIOID ANALGESICS

ANALGESIC	DOSE RANGE	DURATION OF ANALGESIC EFFECT	PHARMACOLOGIC $T_{1/2}$
aspirin	650 mg po q 6 hours	4–6 hours	varies with dose
acetaminophen	650–1000 mg po q 4–6 hours maximum 4000–6000 mg/day	4–6 hours	1–4 hours
ibuprofen	200–400 mg po q 6 hours maximum 2400 mg/day	4–6 hours	2 hours
naproxen	250–500 mg po q 6 hours	8–12 hours	14 hours
choline magnesium trisalicylate	500–750 mg po q 8–12 hours	8–12 hours	9–17 hours
diflunisal	500–1000 mg po q 12 hours	8–12 hours	8–12 hours
ketorolac (parenteral)	30–60 mg im or iv loading dose then 15–30 mg q 6 hours maximum daily dose 120 mg/day (150 mg/day on first day) Should not be used for more than 5 consecutive days	6–8 hours	4–6 hours

curs. Although many prophylactic therapies are used (*e.g.*, antacids, H_2 blockers, sucralfate, omeprazole, misoprostol), only misoprostol has been clearly shown to reduce the risk of gastric ulceration. This drug is recommended in patients with other potential risk factors for ulceration and those whose medical condition is too fragile to tolerate a new gastrointestinal complication.[14]

NSAID-induced renal toxicity, which varies in severity from mere volume expansion to renal failure due to interstitial nephritis or papillary necrosis, is more likely in the elderly and those with pre-existing renal or liver disease, dehydration, cardiac failure, or diabetes. Hepatotoxicity, manifest as hepatocellular damage, is rare with currently available NSAIDs.

OPIOID ANALGESICS

The opioid analgesics can be categorized into the pure agonists, mixed agonist-antagonists and partial agonists on the basis of receptor interactions. Only the agonists have a substantial role in the treatment of chronic pain related to cancer.

The mixed agonist-antagonist drugs (pentazocine, nalbuphine, and butorphanol) and the partial agonist drugs (buprenorphine and probably dezocine) are not preferred for the management of chronic pain because, unlike the pure agonists, they have a ceiling effect for analgesia, can precipitate a withdrawal syndrome in patients who are physically dependent on opioid agonists, and with the exception of pentazocine, have no oral formulations. Additionally, the mixed agonist-antagonists have dose-dependent psychotomimetic side effects that exceed those of the pure agonists.

Opioids conventionally used on the second "rung" of the analgesic ladder were previously labelled "weak" opioids, a misnomer that was not based on the known pharmacology of these drugs, but rather, on the customary way they are used. These drugs are often administered with aspirin or acetaminophen in a fixed dose combination product for oral administration. Dose escalation of these combination products is limited by the potential for aspirin or acetaminophen toxicity; hence these products are only useful for the management of moderate to severe pain in the relatively nontolerant patient. In clinical practice, these drugs are usually administered for convenience and the patient is switched to an alternative opioid on the third "rung" of the analgesic ladder when the maximum dose of the co-analgesic (*e.g.*, acetaminophen 4–6 g/day) is reached. The recent availability in the United States of oxycodone without a co-analgesic has underscored the fact that a drug traditionally viewed as a "weak" opioid can in fact be used much like oral morphine.[15]

Opioids for severe pain, the prototype of which is morphine, have previously been termed "strong" opioids. This appellation, too, is a misnomer. With these drugs, the development of adverse effects, such as confusion, sedation, nausea, and vomiting, imposes practical limits on dose escalation. A favorable balance between analgesia and side effects determines a favorable outcome, regardless of dose.[16] Some patients with severe pain attain this favorable balance and others do not (see below).

General Principles of Opioid Pharmacotherapy

SELECTING A DRUG

A trial of systemic opioid therapy is indicated for the treatment of moderate or severe cancer-related pain, regardless of its characteristics. Although morphine is the prototype opioid analgesic, there is a great deal of intra-individual variability in the response to different opioids and sequential trials of the various opioids may be needed to identify the one with the most favorable balance between analgesia and side effects. Patients with severe pain are usually offered morphine first, because it is available in a variety of tablet strengths and in both immediate and controlled-release preparations.

Like the agonist-antagonist opioids, meperidine (Demerol) has characteristics that make it less desirable for chronic use. It is metabolized to a relatively toxic compound, normeperidine. Compared to meperidine, this metabolite is twice as potent as a convulsant and half as potent as an analgesic. Normeperidine has a half-life 4–5 times that of meperidine and accumulates for a longer period after dosing begins or increases. Normeperidine toxicity can result in dysphoria, tremulousness, multifocal myoclonus, and, most importantly, seizures.[17] Naloxone will not reverse these seizures, and indeed, may precipitate them by selectively reversing the CNS-depressant effects of meperidine and leaving the convulsant effects of normeperidine unopposed.[18] These toxicities are most likely in the elderly and those with impaired renal function, but they have also been observed in younger patients with normal renal function.

A unique toxicity of meperidine can occur when it is administered to a patient receiving a monoamine oxidase (MAO) inhibitor antidepressant (*e.g.*, tranylcypromine [Parnate], and phenelzine [Nardil]). This combination can produce hyperpyrexia, muscle rigidity, seizures, and circulating collapse, the etiology of which is not understood. The reaction can be fatal, and administration of an MAO inhibitor within two weeks is considered an absolute contraindication to the use of meperidine.

During the course of their illness, cancer patients may be offered treatment with several opioids. To optimize drug selection, prior experience with these drugs should be assessed carefully. Many patients report an "allergy" to an opioid, notwithstanding the rarity of this phenomenon. A history of nausea or vomiting after postoperative administration of a parenteral opioid may be labelled an allergy by the patient, rather than a side effect. The clinician should recognize that such a history does not contraindicate the use of that drug. Similarly some commercial preparations of oral oxycodone contain sulfites which can trigger an allergic reaction in sensitized patients; these patients can tolerate oxycodone preparations without sulfites. Finally, many patients report that they were given an opioid in the past and "it didn't work." This should also be explored further to determine whether or not the dose was appropriately escalated to dose-limiting toxicity. If the dose was not increased to the point of dose-limiting toxicity, it should not be assumed that therapy would fail at appropriate doses. Reports of inadequate analgesia due to dose-limiting toxicity should be respected and lead to the choice of alternative opioids or routes of administration, unless intervening events provide reason to expect that the patient's analgesic needs or sensitivity to the adverse effects have changed.

SELECTING AN APPROPRIATE ROUTE

The routes of opioid administration can be classified based on invasiveness. The least invasive, safest route by which effective analgesia can be achieved should be chosen. As the patient's clinical situation changes, the route of administration may also require change. In one survey, the majority of patients with advanced cancer required at least two routes of administration, and 25% required at least three, prior to death.[19]

Non-invasive routes include oral, rectal, transdermal, intranasal, sublingual, and transmucosal. Oral administration is preferred in most cases, unless there is a clear indication for an alternative route, such as impaired swallowing, gastrointestinal dysfunction, patient preference, or the need for a large number of tablets to give an adequate dose.

Rectal suppositories are commercially available for oxycodone, hydromorphone, oxymorphone, and morphine. Commercially available controlled-release morphine can also be administered per rectum.[20] Compounded suppositories containing other drugs can be obtained from experienced pharmacists in occasional cases. The potency of opioids administered per rectum is believed to be equivalent to oral dosing.[21]

Fentanyl is the only opioid currently available for transdermal administration. The delivery system provides a constant rate of drug delivery over time. This route has been demonstrated to be effective in postoperative and cancer pain,[22,23] but it is not recommended for acute pain. Patches are available that deliver 25, 50, 75, and 100 μg/hr. Although patients who require doses in excess of 100 μg/hr may use more than one patch at a time, the application of more than 3 patches simultaneously is usually impractical. Patches must be changed every 48–72 hours, with the majority of patients using a 72-hour dosing interval. At the start of therapy and after the dose is increased, drug effects typically begin to evolve after a period of hours. At least 24 hours are required to approach a new steady state plasma level and evaluate the effect of the change. Provision for an alternative short-acting opioid (usually by the oral or subcutaneous route) is necessary to manage breakthrough pain in patients using transdermal fentanyl.

There are currently no pure agonist opioids available for intranasal administration. Butorphanol, a mixed agonist-antagonist drug, is available by this route, but is not recommended for chronic cancer-related pain.

Sublingual administration is of limited value due to a lack of sublingual formulations, poor absorption of most drugs,[24] and difficulty in delivering large doses. Favorable reports of sublingual morphine administration have appeared,[25] but this efficacy may relate, in large part, to swallowing part of the dose. Sublingual absorption is better for more lipophilic opioids, such as fentanyl and methadone.

The sublingual route is occasionally used for injectable opioid formulations in nontolerant patients who temporarily lose the ability to use the oral route.[26]

Oral transmucosal fentanyl has recently been approved, but its role in the treatment of pain has not yet been fully studied. This route may provide a convenient method for the treatment of breakthrough pain in patients without the ability to use the oral route.

Invasive routes of administration include intravenous (IV), subcutaneous (SC, SQ) and intramuscular (IM). Repeated boluses may be given intermittently by any of these routes. This approach may be limited by the occurrence of toxicity at peak plasma concentration and/or breakthrough pain at trough plasma concentration, commonly known as the *bolus effect*. Repeated IM injections are not recommended; they are painful, offer no pharmacokinetic advantage over the SQ or IV routes, and may produce erratic drug absorption in a cachectic patient with advanced cancer. If a patient does not experience prominent bolus effects, IV or SQ bolus injections can be used. In such cases, the number of skin punctures can be minimized by injecting via an indwelling infusion device. While IV devices are in common use (*i.e.*, heparin wells or saline locks), the analogous SQ device is not as well known outside of the palliative care setting. Such a device consists of a 27-gauge "butterfly" needle, which is inserted into the subcutaneous tissue, covered with an occlusive dressing and left *in situ* for up to 7 days.

Intravenous bolus administration has the most rapid onset of action (range 2–15 minutes, depending on the degree of lipophilicity of the opioid). A trial of this route is recommended for patients with pre-established venous access who are unable to tolerate oral medications (such as post-operative patients or those with bowel obstruction), those with severe breakthrough pain who have a need for especially rapid relief, and those with very severe pain who require rapid dose changes. When used to gain rapid control over very severe pain, the interval between IV bolus doses can be as brief as that required to reach peak effect after each dose. Close monitoring is necessary when doses are administered in rapid succession.

Continuous intravenous infusions (CIVI) or continuous subcutaneous infusions (CSCI) may be extremely useful for patients who cannot maintain a noninvasive route of opioid administration, including those who cannot swallow and do not have an enteral feeding tube, and those with poor enteral absorption.[27–30] CSCI and CIVI can be easily used in ambulatory or bedbound patients. Dosing for both routes is comparable.

Considerable experience exists with morphine and hydromorphone CSCI. Although the technique is feasible with most parenteral opioid formulations, experience suggests that methadone is relatively irritating to the skin, and this drug is not preferred for this reason.[31] An opioid CSCI is administered via a 27-gauge "butterfly" needle, as described previously. The infusion rate should not exceed 3–5 ml/hr to minimize discomfort at the infusion site. Patients can receive higher flow rates if hyaluronidase (used anecdotally in the range of 100–750 I.U. per liter) is added to the infusate. If hyaluronidase is added, the infusion rate can be high enough to provide hydration via CSCI,[32] which is termed *hypodermoclysis*. Medications for the treatment of nausea (metoclopramide, haloperidol, scopolamine, chlorpromazine, or methotrimeprazine), anxiety (one of the neuroleptics, hydroxyzine, or midazolam), or agitated delirium (haloperidol, methotrimeprazine, chlorpromazine, or midazolam) can be added to the opioid or hypodermoclysis solution for CSCI.[29,33,34]

For patients with previously placed intravenous access devices, there may be no advantage to the subcutaneous route. The IV route is preferred for patients receiving large doses of opioids that cannot be highly concentrated (such as fentanyl or oxymorphone) or are irritating by the SQ route (usually methadone). Placement of a central venous access device or a peripherally inserted central catheter (PICC) line facilitates this approach and minimizes crises due to interruption of intravenous access.

Pumps for CIVI and CSCI vary in terms of capacity, complexity, expense, and ability to administer patient-controlled supplementary doses in addition to the infusion. The option of *patient controlled analgesia* (PCA) eliminates the logistic delay entailed in administration of parenteral *"rescue" doses* (*i.e.*, supplemental "as needed" doses for breakthrough pain) by nurses or family members. It can also permit careful titration of the opioid dose in patients with rapidly changing pain, and relieve considerable anxiety in patients with rapid onset breakthrough pains. Patients with severe mucositis during bone marrow transplantation required less total analgesic and felt more satisfied with PCA than similar patients offered a nurse controlled dosing regimen.[35] The potential value of long-term PCA for the treatment of chronic cancer-related pain that cannot be adequately managed by less invasive means is now well established.[30,36]

RELATIVE POTENCY AND EQUIANALGESIC DOSES

Relative potency is the ratio of the dose of two analgesic drugs that produces equal analgesic effects. The standard comparison for reference is 10 mg of parenteral morphine.[37] The table of equianalgesic doses (Table 56–4) is based on relative potency data and provides the information necessary to change routes of administration or opioid drugs. The values in this table are guidelines for dosing and should not be construed as appropriate starting doses for a particular patient. Dose selection is also influenced by pain intensity, prior opioid exposure, age, metabolic disturbances, and other factors.

CHANGING ROUTES OF ADMINISTRATION

Changes in routes of administration are often necessary.[19] The conversion should be based on relative potency data (Table 56–4) and other clinical factors, as discussed above.

TABLE 56–4. OPIOID AGONIST DRUGS CONVENTIONALLY USED FOR SEVERE PAIN

OPIOID ANALGESIC	APPROXIMATE EQUIANALGESIC PARENTERAL DOSE	APPROXIMATE EQUIANALGESIC ORAL DOSE	APPROXIMATE EQUIANALGESIC DOSE BY ALTERNATE ROUTE*	DURATION OF ANALGESIC EFFECT (HOURS)	ELIMINATION $t_{1/2}$ (HOURS)
MORPHINE (MSIR, MS Contin, Oramorph, RMS)	10 mg	30–60 mg*	30–60 mg pr	2–4	2–3
HYDROMORPHONE (Dilaudid)	7.5 mg	1.5 mg	10 mg pr	2–4	2–3
OXYMORPHONE (Numorphan)	1 mg	N/A	10 mg pr	3–6	2–3
LEVORPHANOL (Levo-dromoran)	2 mg	4 mg	N/A	3–6	10–15
METHADONE (Dolophine)	10 mg	20 mg	N/A	4–8	15–200
MEPERIDINE[‡] (Demerol, pethidine)	75 mg	300 mg	N/A	2–4	2–3
OXYCODONE (alone as Roxicodone or combined with acetaminophen or aspirin as Tylox, Roxicet, Rowaprin, Percocet, Percodan)	N/A	30 mg	N/A	3–6	2–3
FENTANYL CITRATE (Sublimate)	100 μg bolus dose equivalent to morphine sulfate 10 mg bolus 50 μg/hr infusion is equivalent to morphine sulfate 1 mg/hr infusion			Variable[§]	3–15 (with chronic or continuous administration)
FENTANYL TTS (Duragesic)	Fentanyl TTS 50 patch (delivers 50 μg/hr) is equivalent to morphine sulfate 1 mg/hr infusion			48–72	13–24

*Equianalgesic dose of oral morphine varies with dosing schedule; 30 mg po is equivalent to 10 mg parenterally when administered on a chronic around-the-clock basis; 60 mg po is equivalent to 10 mg parenterally when it is administered as a single dose or intermittently.

[†]Equianalgesic conversions for rectal administration are more variable due to dual blood supply and resultant pharmacokinetic differences.

[‡]Due to accumulation of the metabolite normeperidine, meperidine administration should be limited to 800 mg/day and should not be used for more than 48 hours.

[§]Duration depends on clinical setting; during chronic administration by infusion or transdermal system, a bolus can provide analgesia for several hours, similar to rescue doses of other short-acting opioids.

For the IM, SQ, and IV routes, potencies are assumed to be essentially equivalent, as are the oral and rectal routes. Following a change in route, the need for subsequent dose titration should be anticipated. Stepwise conversion over several days (*e.g.*, when converting from parenteral to oral administration) can minimize the risk of over- or underdosing.

SCHEDULING OF OPIOID ADMINISTRATION

A key facet of the WHO approach for the treatment of chronic cancer-related pain is the administration of analgesics "around the clock." This technique is clearly preferable for patients with continuous or frequently recurrent pain. However, patients with no previous opioid exposure (particularly the elderly or medically frail) and those who are beginning treatment with a long half-life opioid (*i.e.*, methadone or levorphanol) may be at some increased risk of toxicity when this approach is used from the start. Appropriate monitoring is needed, and in some cases, temporary use of "as needed" dosing is prudent. Given the difficulty in initiating treatment with methadone, which has both a long and variable half-life, "as needed" dosing is strongly recommended when this drug is begun. Patients who undergo an anesthetic, neuroablative, or other definitive palliative therapy may have rapidly decreasing analgesic needs and may also be able to benefit from a modified "as needed" regimen, in which a minimum dose is maintained to prevent opioid withdrawal. Patients with intermittent pains may also be manageable with "as needed" dosing alone.

While an "around the clock" regimen may prevent recurrence of pain, it is important to provide a rescue dose for episodes of breakthrough pain. Rescue doses should be available no more often than the time to peak effect for the particular drug and route being used. Oral rescue doses are typically offered every 1–2 hours, while parenteral rescue doses can be offered every 15–60 minutes. Based on clinical experience, the dose should be 5%–15% of the 24–hour scheduled dose regimen.[38] Alternatively, 50% of the dose administered every 4 hours (orally or parenterally) or 50%–100% of the dose administered each hour as a CSCI or CIVI can be used as guidelines for the rescue dose.

The rescue dose should be required relatively infrequently (4 or fewer times per day), if the scheduled dose regimen is adequately titrated. The need for rescue doses can be used as a guide when adjusting the scheduled dose. The size of the rescue dose should be increased as the baseline dose is escalated during dose titration.

Controlled-release preparations of short-acting opioids can provide additional convenience for patients on around-the-clock dosing. Currently, two controlled-release morphine sulfate preparations are available (MS Contin [Purdue Frederick], and Oramorph SR [Roxane Laboratories]) in a variety of doses (15 mg, 30 mg, 60 mg, and 100 mg tablets). These drugs permit dosing every 8–12 hours, rather than every 3–4 hours for conventional oral morphine preparations. Controlled-release preparations of oxycodone and hydromorphone are currently in development. The transdermal fentanyl administration system may be viewed as a controlled-release formulation of a short-acting opioid.

The two currently available controlled-release morphine preparations have been shown to be both safe and effective in the treatment of chronic cancer-related pain.[39,40] These drugs can each be converted on a milligram-to-milligram basis from immediate release morphine, but they are not bioequivalent to each other. Each of these drugs reach peak plasma levels 3–5 hours after administration. Each change in dose requires 24–48 hours to approach a new steady state plasma level. As a consequence, controlled-release morphine is not optimal for the rapid titration of dose in patients with severe pain; a short-acting drug is usually preferred.

DOSE SELECTION AND TITRATION

Patients who have had limited exposure to opioids (*e.g.*, a combination product on the second "rung" of the WHO analgesic ladder) should generally begin use of an opioid for more severe pain equivalent to 5–10 mg of parenteral morphine sulfate every 4 hours. This dose must then be titrated to effect. When patients are starting a new opioid after previous treatment with another opioid from the third "rung" of the WHO ladder, the starting dose of the new drug should be reduced by 25%–50% of the calculated equianalgesic dose to account for incomplete cross-tolerance between opioids. The reduction should be relatively less if the patient has severe pain at the time of the switch, and relatively more if the patient has prominent opioid-related side effects or is medically frail. The exception to this general rule is conversion to methadone, which should be reduced by 50%–75% of the calculated equianalgesic dose based on clinical experience.

Gradual dose escalation should continue until either analgesia is adequate or dose-limiting side effects ensue. As discussed previously, there is no ceiling effect for analgesia, and hence no fixed maximum opioid dose. For each increment in dose, the scheduled dose should be increased by 30%–50%, or by the quantity of rescue doses required during the previous 24-hour period.

The rate of dose titration depends on the severity of the pain and the half-life of the drug. Patients who present with very severe pain, a *pain emergency*, require rapid dose titration. This can be accomplished using a short-acting opioid by repeated administration of parenteral boluses every 15–30 minutes until the pain begins to be relieved. The total parenteral loading dose can then be used to calculate the rate of a maintenance IV or SQ infusion using guidelines that were developed for the treatment of acute pain,[41] but which have been found to be clinically applicable to the treatment of a pain crisis in cancer patients. Specifically, the initial hourly maintenance infusion rate can be approximated as the total loading dose divided by twice the half-life of the drug.

Patients with inadequate analgesia who do not require

emergent treatment should have their opioid dose increased more slowly, usually at intervals that permit steady state plasma levels to be approached. The time to steady state is approximately 4–5 times the half-life of the drug, independent of the route of administration. As a result, the dose of short-acting opioids, such as morphine, hydromorphone, and oxycodone, can be adjusted every 12–24 hours. Controlled-release oral morphine and transdermal fentanyl can be adjusted every 24–48 hours.

Most patients can be maintained on a stable dose of opioid for long periods.[42,43] Inadequate analgesia after a stable period is usually indicative of progression of disease, an intercurrent complication such as infection, or increasing psychological distress.[44] True pharmacologic *tolerance* to analgesic effects, the phenomenon whereby exposure to the drug induces an attenuation of effect, appears to be rare in the clinical setting. In contrast, tolerance to the non-analgesic effects of opioids, such as respiratory depression, sedation, and nausea, occurs commonly and typically permits aggressive escalation of the opioid dose. Tolerance to these non-analgesic effects appears to develop at varying rates in each patient; tolerance to the constipating effects of the opioids develops most slowly.[44]

Fear of the development of tolerance is common among physicians, nurses, patients, and families. Concerns about tolerance should be allayed by the clinician and not impede the use of opioids early in the course of the illness. Worsening pain in a patient receiving stable doses of opioids should be investigated rather than ascribed to tolerance.

MANAGEMENT OF OPIOID ADVERSE EFFECTS

The successful management of chronic cancer-related pain is defined by a favorable balance between analgesia and adverse effects. Management of side effects, therefore, is a fundamental aspect of treatment, which increases the likelihood of a favorable outcome and contributes independently to patient comfort. Extensive experience suggests effective strategies for the management of common opioid side effects.

Respiratory Depression. Respiratory depression is the most serious potential toxicity of opioid therapy. Opioids can depress respiratory rate and tidal volume, and hence minute ventilation. When tidal volume is diminished, respiratory rate may transiently increase in an attempt at compensation. As a consequence, a "normal" respiratory rate can mask subclinical depressant effects of opioids on pulmonary function. This may explain the clinical observation that opioid-treated patients appear to be at increased risk for respiratory decompensation if a concurrent pulmonary insult, such as pneumonia, pulmonary edema, or pulmonary embolism occurs.

Clinically significant respiratory depression is always accompanied by signs of central nervous system depression, specifically somnolence and bradypnea. Respiratory insufficiency associated with tachypnea and anxiety is never due to primary opioid toxicity.

Tolerance to the respiratory depressant effects of opioids appears to develop rapidly, usually in a matter of hours to days. This permits the management of chronic cancer-related pain to proceed with little risk of significant respiratory depression. Pain and anxiety may also stimulate respiration and further reduce the risk. If pain is suddenly eliminated, such as after a neurolytic procedure, clinically important respiratory depression can occur if the opioid dose is not appropriately reduced.

Opioid-induced respiratory depression can be reversed by the opioid antagonist naloxone. Patients with multifactorial respiratory compromise may transiently improve if naloxone reverses the opioid-induced component. For this reason, improvement after administration of naloxone should not be taken as evidence that the opioid was the sole cause of the respiratory depression. Other potential contributing causes must always be investigated carefully.

Naloxone can precipitate a severe abstinence syndrome and recurrent pain if administered to patients who are physically dependent on an opioid drug. Consequently, naloxone is not a benign therapy and should not be used unless there is the potential for life-threatening respiratory depression. Patients who are easily arousable should not be given naloxone if enough time has passed since the last opioid dose to ensure that peak plasma opioid concentration has been observed. These patients should be carefully monitored with pulse oximetry and/or arterial blood gases. Cautious naloxone administration is appropriate if there is significant respiratory compromise and the peak effect of the opioid has not yet occurred, or the patient is not arousable. Endotracheal intubation should be considered for unarousable patients, or preparations made for possible emergent intubation to prevent aspiration after naloxone is administered. Due to the complexity of issues related to intubation in advanced cancer patients, each case must be considered individually, based on the goals of care for the particular patient at that point in the illness. When naloxone is given, a dilute solution (an ampule of 0.4 mg diluted in 10 ml of saline) should be administered in small aliquots (*i.e.*, 0.04 mg or 1 ml of the dilute solution), titrating to improvement in pulmonary function; full reversal of the opioid effect is neither necessary or desirable. A naloxone infusion may be a useful method for careful titration of the dose.[45]

Sedation. Tolerance to the sedating effect of opioids usually develops over days to weeks. Nonetheless, sedation may be a problem each time the dose is escalated significantly, and appropriate restrictions on potentially hazardous activities, such as driving, are prudent during these periods. Centrally-acting anxiolytics, antiemetics, and antidepressants can augment sedation due to opioid analgesics.

If sedation does not clear after a dose escalation, re-evaluation of the need for other centrally-acting medications should be undertaken. The presence of metabolic abnormalities that may cause sedation, such as hypercalcemia, should also be assessed and corrected if possible. If a primary cause cannot be identified and reversed, and analgesia is adequate, the opioid dose can be decreased by 25%. If analgesia is inadequate, barely adequate, or sedation persists despite dose reduction, the addition of a psychostimulant, such as methylphenidate, dextroamphetamine, or pemoline, should be considered. Experience with methylphenidate in the cancer population is most extensive.[46,47] Pemoline may also be a useful drug and its availability as a chewable tablet may be an advantage. When dextroamphetamine or methylphenidate is used, the starting dose is usually 2.5–5 mg by mouth administered either once daily in the morning, or twice daily in the morning and at midday. The starting dose for pemoline is 18.75–37.5 mg. Dose escalation is often needed. These drugs should be used with caution in patients with cardiac arrhythmias, agitated delirium, paranoid personality disorder, or a history of prior amphetamine abuse.

Other options can also be considered in the management of persistent sedation. Changing to an alternative opioid sometimes results in a better balance between analgesia and adverse effects. Selection of the new drug is by trial-and-error. It may also be appropriate to consider an anesthetic (*e.g.*, intraspinal opioid) or neuroablative (*e.g.*, nerve block or cordotomy) procedure, which may decrease the need for opioid analgesics and thereby reduce the magnitude of adverse effects.

Confusion and Delirium. Confusion and delirium, and the fear of these effects, can be serious barriers to optimal pain management for cancer patients.[48] Mild cognitive impairment is common during the days to weeks after initiation of therapy or significant dose escalation.[49] Tolerance usually develops during this period.

The management of confusion and delirium parallels the management of sedation. It should include elimination of non-essential centrally-acting medications, reversal (if possible) of contributing metabolic or infectious causes, and a trial of dose reduction if pain is controlled. When these maneuvers are unsuccessful, a trial of a psychostimulant (unless the patient is agitated) or a neuroleptic, such as haloperidol 0.5–1 mg PO or IV, should be considered. Changing to an alternative opioid may also result in a better balance between analgesia and adverse effects and should be considered. Finally, patients with confusion or delirium that persists despite these measures should be considered for anesthetic or neuroablative procedures.

Constipation. Constipation is the most common adverse effect of chronic opioid therapy. Although rarely life-threatening, it can cause significant impairment in the quality of life.[50] Prophylactic prescription of laxative medications is reasonable in the elderly and those who may be predisposed to constipation by the use of other drugs or disease-related factors. There are no controlled trials comparing various laxative regimens in cancer patients. One common approach combines a stool softener (*i.e.*, docusate 100–200 mg two or three times a day) and a cathartic (*i.e.*, senna 1–2 tablets two or three times a day). Doses may need to be increased, and a supplemental osmotic laxative, such as milk of magnesia, should be available if needed. Some patients prefer treatment with an osmotic laxative alone, such as milk of magnesia every 2 days or daily lactulose therapy. Occasionally, oral naloxone is administered for very refractory constipation. Oral naloxone, which has a very low bioavailability (about 3%), is thought to reverse constipation by selectively antagonizing the opioid receptors in the gastrointestinal tract. There is some chance of precipitating withdrawal symptoms as the dose is escalated; the initial dose should be 0.8–1.2 mg once or twice daily, with dose escalation to 3–12 mg if needed.[51,52]

Nausea And Vomiting. Opioids produce nausea and vomiting through three mechanisms: stimulation of the medullary chemoreceptor trigger zone, increased vestibular sensitivity, and decreased gastrointestinal motility.[53] In ambulatory patients, nausea and vomiting occur in 10%–40% at the start of opioid therapy.[54] Tolerance to the emetogenic effects of opioids usually develops over weeks. While routine prophylactic administration of antiemetics is not necessary, provision for antiemetics, if needed, is prudent. Metoclopramide or prochlorperazine is effective for the majority of patients. Anxiolytics (*e.g.*, lorazepam and hydroxyzine), steroids (*e.g.*, dexamethasone), and other neuroleptics (*e.g.*, haloperidol) have antiemetic effects, and may be helpful in some patients. Patients with vertigo or prominent movement-induced nausea appear to benefit from drugs used in the treatment of vertigo, including meclizine or scopolamine. Patients with nausea associated with symptoms of delayed gastric emptying, such as early satiety, bloating, or postprandial vomiting, may benefit most from metoclopramide therapy. The role of serotonin antagonists, such as ondansetron, remains ill-defined.

Myoclonus. Multifocal myoclonus is a dose-related adverse effect of opioid drugs. Occasional mild myoclonus is common and does not require specific therapy. More frequent or severe myoclonus can precipitate episodes of pain due to involuntary movement. When myoclonus requires intervention, benzodiazepines such as clonazepam have been helpful.[55] Severe myoclonus is an indication for trial of an alternative analgesic.

Urinary Retention. Opioid analgesics cause an increase in smooth muscle tone, which may produce bladder spasms or urinary retention. This adverse effect is uncommon and is often managed acutely with urecholine or catheterization. If it persists and contributing factors cannot be eliminated, a trial of an alternative opioid is appropriate.

Pulmonary Edema. Noncardiogenic pulmonary edema has been reported in patients with advanced cancer who received high, rapidly escalating doses of opioids.[56] The mechanism of this rare event is not understood.

DEPENDENCE AND ADDICTION

The fear of physical dependence and addiction is among the major barriers to the optimal treatment of cancer pain.[48,57] These phenomena are often misunderstood by medical professionals and the lay public alike.

Physical Dependence. *Physical dependence* is a pharmacologic property of opioid drugs defined by the development of an abstinence syndrome, or withdrawal. Physical dependence can be assumed to be present when patients have taken an opioid on a regular basis for a period of days to weeks. Physical dependence is only a problem if opioid antagonists are administered or treatment is abruptly discontinued. Physical dependence is entirely distinct from the phenomenon of addiction.

Addiction. *Addiction* is characterized by a loss of control over drug use, compulsive use, and continued use despite harm. Typically, there is evidence of craving for the drug to achieve a psychic effect and aberrant drug-related behaviors, such as compulsive drug-seeking in the setting of adequately controlled pain or unsanctioned dose escalation.

The appropriate medical use of opioids very rarely results in iatrogenic addiction.[58,59] Occasionally, patients with inadequate analgesia may exhibit drug craving and related behaviors that mimic addiction, but disappear entirely when pain is relieved. This has been termed *pseudoaddiction*.[60] These behaviors, including concern about opioid availability, unsanctioned dose escalation, and "clock-watching," often cause a great deal of anxiety among the professional staff, who fear they may have contributed to development of an addiction problem. It is critically important that the clinician carefully assess any aberrant drug-related behavior and determine the degree to which it is driven by uncontrolled pain or other factors, such as psychiatric disease apart from addiction. Incorrectly labeling the patient as an addict can compromise the relationship with the patient and exacerbate the undertreatment of pain.

Adjuvant Analgesics

Adjuvant analgesics have primary indications other than pain, but are analgesic in some conditions (Table 56–5). These drugs are in diverse pharmacological classes and are used extensively in the treatment of non-cancer-related pain. In the management of cancer pain, they usually supplement therapy with opioid or non-opioid analgesics on any of the three "rungs" of the WHO analgesic ladder.

Although data from controlled clinical studies is largely lacking, dose-dependent analgesic effects are presumed to occur with most adjuvant analgesics. Dose titration is usually attempted, unless adverse effects occur at the initial low dose. Interindividual variability in the response to the adjuvant analgesics is substantial and sequential trials are often useful. Unlike the opioids, the latency of analgesic effect can be weeks, often resulting in the need for prolonged trials.[61]

MULTIPURPOSE ADJUVANT ANALGESICS

Corticosteroids. Corticosteroids are among the most widely used adjuvant analgesics. They have beneficial effects in treating pain, anorexia, nausea, and lassitude. The mechanism of analgesia is probably multifactorial, determined in part by anti-inflammatory and anti-edema effects. Dexamethasone is the most commonly used agent, perhaps because of its low mineralocorticoid potency, but methylprednisolone, prednisolone and prednisone have all been used successfully.

Patients with severe bone pain or neuropathic pain that does not promptly respond to opioid therapy can often achieve dramatic relief from a short course of high dose steroids (*i.e.*, dexamethasone 100 mg as a single dose, followed by 24 mg every 6 hours). This treatment is tapered over weeks while other analgesic approaches, such as radiation or nerve blocks are instituted.[62] Patients with less severe pain, typically those with multiple symptoms related to advanced disease, are commonly offered a trial of a low dose steroid regimen (*e.g.*, 1–2 mg of dexamethasone twice daily). Side effects of this type of regimen are usually acceptable; they include oropharyngeal candidiasis, dyspepsia, weight gain, Cushingoid habitus, edema, echymoses, and neuropsychological effects.[63] Other more serious adverse ef-

TABLE 56–5. ADJUVANT ANALGESICS

CONTINUOUS NEUROPATHIC PAIN	LANCINATING NEUROPATHIC PAIN	BONE PAIN	VISCERAL PAIN
Antidepressants	Anticonvulsants	Corticosteroids	Glycopyrrolate
Corticosteroids	Baclofen	Calcitonin	Atropine
Local anesthetics	Clonazepam	Strontium-89	Scopolamine
Clonidine	Local anesthetics	Pamidronate	
Capsaicin	Antidepressants	NSAIDS	

fects (*e.g.*, osteoporosis and myopathy) are possible but rarely preclude therapy in this population.

Methotrimeprazine. Neuroleptics are used frequently to treat nausea and delirium. The use of these drugs as analgesics is limited. Methotrimeprazine is a phenothiazine with established analgesic efficacy, which may be useful in patients with both anxiety and pain, or those who are particularly sensitive to the gastrointestinal adverse effects of opioids. Because orthostatic hypotension and sedation are dose-limiting side effects, it is most useful in bedridden patients with advanced disease. There is extensive experience with subcutaneous[29] and intravenous administration in cancer patients. Treatment is usually begun with 5–10 mg every 6 hours, or 1–1.5 mg/hr by SQ or IV infusion, followed by titration to effect.

ADJUVANTS USED FOR NEUROPATHIC PAIN

Antidepressants. The tricyclic antidepressants, particularly the tertiary amine subgroup (amitriptyline, doxepin, and imipramine) may be effective in the treatment of cancer-related neuropathic pain that does not respond adequately to an optimal opioid regimen.[64–66] The secondary amine tricyclic drugs (desipramine and nortriptyline) have fewer side effects, but there is less compelling evidence for efficacy. Because the side effects of the tricyclic antidepressants (*e.g.*, sedation, constipation, urinary retention) overlap with those of the opioid analgesics, a low starting dose (*e.g.*, 10–25 mg of amitriptyline) and gradual dose titration (*e.g.*, an additional 10–25 mg every 3 days) is recommended. Dose escalation can proceed to a total dose of 50–150 mg in most patients. If relief is inadequate at these doses after 1–2 weeks, it may be useful to check plasma drug concentrations before deciding whether to increase the dose or proceed to a trial of another adjuvant agent. Concentration-dependent effects are likely, but there is no evidence that benefit is gained at concentrations above those associated with antidepressant effects.

There is less evidence to support analgesic efficacy of the "newer" antidepressants, such as maprotiline, trazodone, paroxetine, and fluoxetine. Of these agents, evidence is best that maprotiline and paroxetine have analgesic efficacy in neuropathic pain.[67,68] Monoamine oxidase inhibitors are rarely used in cancer patients, largely because of concern over the risk of toxicity, but there is some limited evidence that they may be helpful in some pain syndromes.

Systemic Local Anesthetics. Both continuous and lancinating neuropathic pain syndromes may be improved by systemic administration of local anesthetics: mexiletine, tocainide, flecainide, and subcutaneous lidocaine.[61,69–71] All of these drugs have the risk of inducing cardiac arrhythmias and are preferred in patients without any significant cardiac disease who have not had relief with less toxic agents. Mexiletine is believed to be the safest of these drugs, and should be started at a dose of 100–150 mg/day. The dose should be titrated upward until analgesia or therapeutic blood levels are reached, usually no more than 900 mg/day.

Clonidine. This a-2 adrenergic agonist is used primarily to treat hypertension, but has a well established role as an adjuvant analgesic. Although it is viewed as a multipurpose analgesic in the non-cancer setting, it is generally used for refractory neuropathic pain in the cancer population. One advantage is its availability in oral and transdermal formulations.

Anticonvulsants. Anticonvulsants are conventionally used to treat lancinating or paroxysmal neuropathic pains. Carbamazepine is the most commonly used, perhaps because of experience in the treatment of trigeminal neuralgia. Bone marrow toxicity manifested as leukopenia or thrombocytopenia may complicate its use in the cancer patient population, however. Phenytoin, valproate, and clonazepam are also used. All these drugs are administered for pain in a manner identical to their use for seizures.

Baclofen. Baclofen, a gamma aminobutyric acid (GABA)-agonist compound used primarily to treat spasticity, has been shown to be effective in the treatment of trigeminal neuralgia. Based on this experience, baclofen has been used successfully in the management of other paroxysmal neuropathic pains. The initial dose of 5 mg every 8–12 hours can be gradually increased to a total dose of 30–90 mg/day, or higher in some patients. Sedation and confusion may limit dose escalation.

ADJUVANTS FOR BONE PAIN

Bisphosphonates. Bisphosphonates are pyrophosphate analogues that inhibit osteoclast activity and reduce bone resorption. Their primary indication is hypercalcemia, but analgesic effects have been suggested in patients with diffuse bony metastases.[72]

Radiopharmaceuticals. Bone-seeking radiopharmaceuticals that are absorbed into areas of high bone turnover have been evaluated as therapy for metastatic bone pain. Historically, phosphorus-32 was found to be effective, but its use was limited by marrow toxicity. Recently strontium-89 and rhenium-186 have been shown to have significant clinical response with acceptable hematologic toxicity.[73] Strontium-89 was recently approved for the treatment of pain related to diffuse bony metastatic disease. The drug may reduce marrow reserve and should not be used in patients who remain candidates for myelosuppressive chemotherapy. Due to the risk of persistent thrombocytopenia, it should also be used very cautiously in patients with platelet counts below 100,000 cells/μL and is usually contraindicated if the platelet count is less than 60,000 cells/μL.

Calcitonin. Although the mechanism by which calcitonin produces analgesia is unknown, there is a favorable experience for diffuse pain due to bony metastases. Objective data are limited, however. The dose is often begun at 25 I.U. SC once or twice daily, then gradually increased to 100–200 I.U. SC once or twice daily.[74]

The Patient Refractory To Systemic Opioid Therapy

Clinical experience suggests that approximately 10% of cancer patients will fail to achieve a favorable balance between analgesia and side effects using the WHO approach. For these patients, trials of alternative approaches must be considered (Table 56–6).

Anesthetic approaches consist of trigger point injections, somatic and sympathetic nerve blocks, and intraspinal administration of opioids or other drugs.[75] Nerve blocks are generally used for localized pain caused by an identifiable structural lesion. A temporary block utilizing a local anesthetic may be followed in selected patients by a permanent block using absolute alcohol or phenol, both of which are neurolytic.

Intraspinal administration of opioids, with or without local anesthetics, may be implemented via an implanted epidural or subarachnoid catheter. These approaches deliver smaller doses of opioids nearer the presumed site of action, thereby minimizing the adverse effects of systemic administration.[76]

Neuroablative procedures have a long history in cancer pain management. Cordotomy is the most commonly used approach and is usually considered for patients with refractory unilateral pain, particularly pain below mid-chest. Cordotomy involves sectioning the anterolateral quadrant of the cervical or upper thoracic spinal cord to interrupt the lateral spinothalamic tract and other ascending pain pathways. This may be done as an open surgical procedure involving a laminectomy or percutaneously at the cervical level. Initial pain relief is excellent, often as high as 90%, but this figure drops to 60% at one year.[77] Phrenic nerve paralysis, leg paresis, and urinary retention are potential complications, which occur infrequently. Seven to ten percent of patients will develop pain on the side ipsilateral to the cordotomy, which is known as *mirror pain*.[78]

Neurostimulatory approaches provide analgesia by stimulating afferent pathways. These approaches include counterirritation, transcutaneous electrical nerve stimulation (TENS), and invasive techniques such as dorsal column stimulation. There are no controlled trials of these techniques in cancer patients. The non-invasive techniques are safe and simple, and therefore merit consideration in patients with localized pain who are unable to obtain relief from systemic analgesics without excessive side effects. TENS is contraindicated in patients with pacemakers.

Physiatric techniques, such as use of orthoses and prostheses, may provide some additional comfort and/or improve functional status, usually with little risk to the patient. Similarly, behavioral and cognitive approaches, such as biofeedback, hypnosis, distraction, and relaxation training, are widely used in the treatment of non-cancer pain and may provide benefit to the cancer patient as well. Because these methods offer the potential to minimize the amount of systemic medication and consequently diminish adverse effects in patients with a narrow therapeutic window, they should be used to supplement pharmacotherapy in motivated patients.

SEDATION AS PAIN THERAPY

Rare patients experience pain at the end of life that is poorly controlled despite aggressive analgesic therapies.[79] In addition to continued efforts to find effective analgesic strategies, the option of sedation may be desirable for some patients.

TABLE 56–6. MANAGEMENT OF DOSE-LIMITING TOXICITY FROM SYSTEMIC OPIOID THERAPY

NON-INVASIVE MEANS	INVASIVE MEANS	OTHER
Treat dose-limiting side-effects	Regional anesthetic techniques	Sedation
Reduce opioid needs	Neuroablative techniques	
Institute primary therapy	Invasive neurostimulatory approach	
Add a non-opioid analgesic		
Use a cognitive technique for pain management		
Use a physiatric technique for pain management		
Use a behavioral technique for pain management		
Orthotic		
TENS		

Sedation can be accomplished with systemic opioid infusions, benzodiazepine infusions (*e.g.*, lorazepam or midazolam), neuroleptics (*e.g.*, methotrimeprazine), or barbiturates.[80] Experience with all of these approaches is anecdotal.

Sedation as a medical strategy for the treatment of refractory symptoms is ethically sound and is based on the *principle of double effect* in the setting of informed consent. This principle distinguishes between the beneficient therapeutic intent (the relief of pain) and an unavoidable adverse consequence (the reduction of consciousness and possible shortening of the time remaining until death).[81] If the clinician acts to achieve the desirable effect after discussion with the patient and family, unavoidable negative consequences are acceptable. Such a choice requires careful consideration by the physician, patient, and family. Consultation with a religious counselor, social worker, or clinical ethicist may be helpful. It is critical that the patient, family, and all involved staff have a comprehensive understanding of this intervention.

CONCLUSION

Ongoing assessment and opioid pharmacotherapy are the mainstays of treatment for chronic cancer-related pain. Most patients achieve a favorable balance between analgesia and adverse effects. Although therapeutic strategies that have been developed to manage refractory symptoms may require the input of experienced practitioners, all clinicians can acquire the skills necessary to provide enhanced comfort and improved quality of life to a large majority of patients.

REFERENCES

1. Bonica JJ. Treatment of cancer pain: current status and future needs. In: Fields HL, Dubner R, Cervero F (eds): Proceedings of the Fourth World Congress on Pain. New York, Raven Press, 1989:589. (Advances in Pain Research and Therapy, vol 9)
2. Portenoy RK. Cancer pain: pathophysiology and syndromes. Lancet 339:1026, 1992
3. International Association for the Study of Pain: Subcommittee on taxonomy. Pain Terms: A list with definitions and notes on usage. Pain 8:249, 1980
4. Acute Pain Management Guideline Panel. Acute pain management: operative or medical procedures and trauma. Rockville, MD: Agency for Health Care Policy and Research, Public Health Service, US Department of Health and Human Services, 1992:145. (Clinical Practice Guideline; AHCPR Pub. No. 92–0032)
5. Cherny NI, Portenoy RK. Cancer pain: principles of assessment and syndromes. In: Wall PD, Melzack R (ed): Textbook of Pain, 3rd ed. London, Churchill Livingstone, 1994:787
6. Cherny NI, Portenoy RK. Cancer pain management: current strategy. Cancer (Supplement) 72(11):3393, 1993
7. Gonzales GR, Elliott KJ, Portenoy RK, Foley KM. The impact of a comprehensive evaluation in the management of cancer pain. Pain 47(2):141, 1991
8. World Health Organization. Cancer Pain Relief and Palliative Care. Geneva: World Health Organization, 1990:75
9. Jacox A, Carr DB, Payne R et al. Management of Cancer Pain. Clinical Practice Guideline No. 9. Rockville, MD: Agency for Health Care Policy and Research, U.S. Department of Health and Human Services, Public Health Service, 1994:257. (AHCPR Publication No. 94-0592; vol 1)
10. Cherny NI, Portenoy RK. Practical issues in the management of cancer pain. In: Wall PD, Melzack R (ed): Textbook of Pain, 3rd ed. London, Churchill Livingstone, 1994:1437
11. American Pain Society. Principles of analgesic use in the treatment of acute pain and cancer pain, 3rd ed. Skokie, Illinois: American Pain Society, 1992:41
12. Ventafridda V, Tamburini M, Caraceni A, De Conno F, Naldi F. A validation study of the WHO method for cancer pain relief. Cancer 59(4):850, 1987
13. Grond S, Zech D, Schug SA, Lynch J, Lehman KA. Validation of World Health Organization guidelines for cancer pain relief during the last days and hours of life. J Pain Symptom Manage 6(7):411, 1991
14. Ingham JM, Portenoy RK. Drugs in the treatment of pain: NSAIDs and opioids. Curr Opinion Anaesth 6:838, 1993
15. Glare PA, Walsh TD. Dose-ranging study of oxycodone for chronic pain in advanced cancer. J Clin Oncol 11(5):973, 1993
16. Portenoy RK, Foley KM, Inturrisi CE. The nature of opioid responsiveness and its implications for neuropathic pain: new hypotheses derived from studies of opioid infusions. Pain 43(3):273, 1990
17. Kaiko RF, Foley KM, Grabinski PY et al. Central nervous system excitatory effects of meperidine in cancer patients. Ann Neurol 13(2):180, 1983
18. Umans JG, Inturrisi CE. Antinociceptive activity and toxicity of meperidine and normeperidine in mice. J Pharmacol Exp Ther 223(1):203, 1982
19. Coyle N, Adelhardt J, Foley KM, Portenoy RK. Character of terminal illness in the advanced cancer patient: pain and other symptoms during the last four weeks of life. J Pain Symptom Manage 5(2):83, 1990
20. Kaiko RF, Cronin C, Healy N, Pav J, Thomas G, Goldenheim PD. Bioavailability of rectal and oral MS-Contin. Proceedings of the American Society of Clinical Oncology 8:abstract 1307, 1989
21. Beaver WT, Feise G. Comparison of the analgesic effect of oxymorphone by rectal suppository and intramuscular injection in patients with postoperative pain. J Clin Pharmacol 17:276, 1977
22. Miser AW, Narang PK, Dothage JA, Young RC, Sindelar W, Miser JS. Transdermal fentanyl for pain control in patients with cancer. Pain 37:15, 1989
23. Gourlay GK, Kowalski SR, Plummer JL, et al. The efficacy of transdermal fentanyl in the treatment of postoperative pain; a double blind comparison of fentanyl and placebo systems. Pain 40:21, 1990
24. Weinberg DS, Inturrisi CE, Reidenberg B, et al. Sublingual absorption of selected opioid analgesics. Clin. Pharm. Therap. 44:335, 1988

25. Hirsch JD. Sublingual morphine sulfate in chronic pain management. Clin. Pharmacy 3:585, 1984
26. Ripamonti C, Bruera E. Rectal, buccal, and sublingual narcotics for the management of cancer pain. J Palliat Care 7(1):30, 1991
27. Portenoy RK. Continuous intravenous infusion of opioid drugs. Med Clin North Am 71(2):233, 1987
28. Bruera E, Brenneis C, Michaud M et al. Use of the subcutaneous route for the administration of narcotics in patients with cancer pain. Cancer 62(2):407, 1988
29. Storey P, Hill HH Jr, St. Louis RH, Tarver EE. Subcutaneous infusions for control of cancer symptoms. J Pain Symptom Manage 5(1):33, 1990
30. Swanson G, Smith J, Bulich R, New P, Shiffman R. Patient-controlled analgesia for chronic cancer pain in the ambulatory setting: a report of 117 patients. J Clin Oncol 7(12):1903, 1989
31. Bruera E, Fainsinger R, Moore M, Thibault R, Spoldi E, Ventafridda V. Local toxicity with subcutaneous methadone. Experience of two centers. Pain 45(2):141, 1991
32. Bruera E, Legris MA, Kuehn N, Miller MJ. Hypodermoclysis for the administration of fluids and narcotic analgesics in patients with advanced cancer. J Pain Symptom Manage 5(4):218, 1990
33. Burke AL, Diamond PL, Hulbert J, Yeatman J, Farr EA. Terminal restlessness — its management and the role of midazolam. Med J Aust 155(7):485, 1991
34. Hutchinson HT, Leedham GD, Knight AM. Continuous subcutaneous analgesics and antiemetics in domiciliary terminal care (Letter). Lancet 2(8258):1279, 1981
35. Hill HF, Chapman CR, Kornell J, Sullivan K, Saeger L, Benedetti C. Self-administration of morphine in bone marrow transplant patients reduces drug requirement. Pain 40:121, 1990
36. Citron M, Johnston-Early A, Boyer M, Brasnow S, Hood M, Cohen M. Patient-controlled analgesia for severe cancer pain. Arch Intern Med 146:734, 1986
37. Houde RW, Wallenstein SL, Beaver WT. Evaluation of analgesics in patients with cancer pain. In: Lasagna L (ed): International Encyclopedia of Pharmacology and Therapeutics, vol. 1. New York, Pergamon Press, 1966:59
38. Portenoy RK, Hagen NA. Breakthrough pain: definition, prevalence and characteristics. Pain 41(3):273, 1990
39. Kaiko RF. Controlled-release oral morphine for cancer-related pain: European and North American Experiences. In Foley KM, Bonica JJ, Ventafridda V (eds): Second International Congress on Cancer Pain. New York, Raven Press, 1990:171. (Advances in Pain Research and Therapy, vol 16)
40. Walsh TD, MacDonald N, Bruera E, Shepard KV, Michaud M, Zanes R. A controlled study of sustained-release morphine sulfate tablets in chronic pain from advanced cancer. Am J Clin Oncol 15(3):268, 1992
41. Edwards WT, Breed RJ. Treatment of postoperative pain in the post-anesthesia care unit. Anesthesiology Clinics of North America 8:235, 1990
42. Kanner RM, Foley KM. Patterns of narcotic drug use in a cancer pain clinic. Ann NY Acad Sci 362:161, 1981
43. Brescia FJ, Portenoy RK, Ryan M, Krasnoff L, Gray G. Pain, opioid use, and survival in hospitalized patients with advanced cancer. J Clin Oncol 10(1):149, 1992
44. Foley KM. Clinical tolerance to opioids. In Basbaum AI, Besson JM (eds): Towards a new pharmacotherapy of pain. Chichester, John Wiley & Sons, 1991:181
45. Bradberry JC, Reabel MA. Continuous infusion of naloxone in the treatment of narcotic overdose. Drug Intelligence and Clinical Pharmacy 15:85, 1981
46. Bruera E, Brenneis C, Paterson AH, MacDonald RN. Use of methylphenidate as an adjuvant to narcotic analgesics in patients with advanced cancer. J Pain Symptom Manage 4(1):3, 1989
47. Bruera E, Chadwich S, Brenneis C, Hanson J, MacDonald RN. Methylphenidate associated with narcotics for the treatment of cancer pain. Cancer Treatment Report 71:67, 1987
48. Cleeland CS. Pain control: public and physicians' attitudes. In Hill CS, Fields WS (eds): Drug Treatment of Cancer Pain in a Drug-Oriented Society. New York, Raven Press, 1989:81 (Advances in Pain Research and Therapy, vol 11)
49. Bruera E, Macmillan K, Hanson J, MacDonald RN. The cognitive effects of the administration of narcotic analgesics in patients with cancer pain. Pain 39(1):13, 1989
50. Walsh TD. Prevention of opioid side effects. J Pain Symptom Manage 5(6):362, 1990
51. Sykes NP. Oral naloxone in opioid associated constipation. Lancet 337:1475, 1991
52. Culpepper-Morgan JA, Inturrisi CE, Portenoy RK et al. Treatment of opioid-induced constipation with oral naloxone: a pilot study. Clin Pharmacol Ther 52(1):90, 1992
53. Allen SG. Nausea and vomiting. In Doyle D, Hanks GW, MacDonald N (eds): Oxford Textbook of Palliative Medicine. Oxford, Oxford University Press, 1993:282.
54. Campora E, Merlini L, Pace M et al. The incidence of narcotic-induced emesis. J Pain Symptom Manage 6(7):428, 1991
55. Eisele JH, Grigsby EJ, Dea G. Clonazepam treatment of myoclonic contractions associated with high dose opioids: a case report. Pain 49(2):231, 1992
56. Bruera E. Narcotic-induced pulmonary edema. J Pain Symptom Manage 5(1):55, 1990
57. Foley KM. The decriminalization of cancer pain. In Hill CS, Field H (eds): Drug Treatment of Cancer Pain in a Drug-Oriented Society. New York, Raven Press, 1989:5 (Advances in Pain Research and Therapy, vol 11)
58. Chapman CR, Hill HF. Prolonged morphine self-administration and addiction liability. Cancer 63:1636, 1989
59. Schuster CR. Does treatment of cancer pain with narcotics produce junkies? In Hill CS, Fields WS (eds): Drug Treatment of Cancer Pain in a Drug-Oriented Society. New York, Raven Press, 1989:1 (Advances in Pain Research and Therapy, vol 11)
60. Weissman DE, Haddox JD. Opioid pseudoaddiction—an iatrogenic syndrome. Pain 36:363, 1989
61. Portenoy RK. Adjuvant analgesics in pain management. In Doyle D, Hanks GW, MacDonald N (eds): Oxford Textbook of Palliative Medicine. Oxford, Oxford University Press, 1993:187
62. Greenberg HS, Kim J, Posner JB. Epidural spinal cord compression from metastatic tumor: results with a new treatment protocol. Annals of Neurology 8:361, 1980
63. Hanks GW, Trueman T, Twycross RG. Corticosteroids in terminal cancer. Postgrad Med J 59:702, 1983
64. Magni G, Arsie D, DeLeo D. Antidepressants in the

treatment of cancer pain. A survey in Italy. Pain 29(3):347, 1987

65. Panerai AE, Bianchi M, Sacerdote P, Ripamonti C, Ventafridda V, De Conno F. Antidepressants in cancer pain. J Palliat Care 7(4):42, 1991
66. Walsh TD. Antidepressants in chronic pain. Clinical Neuropharmacology 6:271, 1983
67. Watson CPN, Chipman M, Reed K, Evans RJ, Birkett N. Amitriptyline versus maprotiline in postherpetic neuralgia: a randomized, double-blind, crossover trial. Pain 48:29, 1992
68. Sindrup SH, Gram LF, Brosen K, Eshoj O, Mogensen EF. The selective serotonin reuptake inhibitor paroxetine is effective in the treatment of diabetic neuropathy symptoms. Pain 42:135, 1990
69. Dejgard A, Petersen P, Kastrup J. Mexiletine for treatment of chronic painful diabetic neuropathy. Lancet 1:9, 1988
70. Lindstrom P, Lindblom U. The analgesic effect of tocainide in trigeminal neuralgia. Pain 28:45, 1987
71. Brose WG, Cousins MJ. Subcutaneous lidocaine for treatment of neuropathic cancer pain. Pain 45(2):145, 1991
72. Clarke NW, Holbrook IB, McClure J, George NJ. Osteoclast inhibition by pamidronate in metastatic prostate cancer: a preliminary study. Br J Cancer 63(3):420, 1991
73. Robinson RG, Preston DF, Spicer JA, Baxter KG. Radionuclide therapy of intractable bone pain: emphasis on strontium-89. Semin Nucl Med 22(1):28, 1992
74. Hindley AC, Hill AB, Leyland MJ, Wiles AE. A double-blind controlled trial of salmon calcitonin in pain due to malignancy. Cancer Chemotherapy Pharmacology 9:71, 1982
75. Cousins MJ, Bridenbough PO (ed): Neural blockade in clinical anesthesia and management of pain, 2nd ed. Philadelphia, Lippincott, 1988:1171
76. Cousins MJ, Plummer JL. Spinal opioids in acute and chronic pain. In Max MB, Portenoy RK, Laska EM (eds): The Design of Analgesic Clinical Trials. New York, Raven Press, 1991:457 (Advances in Pain Research and Therapy, vol 18)
77. Rosomoff HL, Papo I, Loeser JD, Bonica JJ. Neurosurgical operations on the spinal cord. In Bonica JJ (ed): The Management of Pain, 2nd ed. Philadelphia, Lea & Febiger, 1990:2067
78. Nagaro T, Amakawa K, Kimura S, Arai T. Reference of pain following percutaneous cervical cordotomy. Pain 53:205, 1993
79. Ventafridda V, Ripamonti C, De Conno F, Tamburini M, Cassileth BR. Symptom prevalence and control during cancer patients' last days of life. J Pall Care 6(3):7, 1990
80. Cherny NI, Portenoy RK. Sedation in the management of refractory symptoms: Guidelines for evaluation and treatment. J Pall Care 10(2): In press.
81. Latimer EJ. Ethical decision-making in the care of the dying and its applications to clinical practice. J Pain Symptom Manage 6:329, 1991

John S. Macdonald, Daniel G. Haller, Robert J. Mayer, Eds. *Manual of Oncologic Therapeutics*, Third Edition.

57. TREATMENT OF EMESIS

Richard J. Gralla
Rita Axelrod

TYPES OF EMESIS

Acute Chemotherapy-Induced Emesis

Differences in the potential for causing emesis and in the pattern of emesis exist, but certain common factors are of importance (Table 57–1). Typically, nausea and vomiting begin 90 minutes to 3 hours after the administration of chemotherapy for the majority of previously untreated patients. The period of maximum emesis often persists for 2 to 6 hours. Important exceptions to this pattern are seen with intravenous cyclophosphamide and carboplatin, where emesis more commonly begins 9 to 18 hours after the start of chemotherapy. Also, with many agents, the likelihood of emesis or its severity may be dose-related.

Delayed Emesis

This problem is frequently observed with highly emetogenic chemotherapy, especially with cisplatin given in high total doses (>100 mg/m^2). Emesis may be well controlled with appropriate antiemetics during the period in which the acute onset would occur, but nausea or vomiting may then become a problem 1 to 4 days later (the peak period of risk being 48 to 72 hours after high-dose cisplatin). While delayed emesis is not as severe as that seen acutely, it still interferes with comfort and proper nutrition.

Anticipatory Emesis

Emesis conditioned by prior poor emetic control reinforces the need to prevent this problem by using the optimal antiemetic regimens with each chemotherapy administration. This problem is more common after highly emetogenic chemotherapy, and its incidence is lessened by attention to control of acute emesis.

Emesis Not Induced by Chemotherapy

Commonly, all nausea or vomiting is attributed to chemotherapy. When the pattern of emesis is not typical of the chemotherapy administered, other causes should be considered. Frequently, other medications (opiates, bronchodilators, antibiotics), tumor-related problems (intestinal obstruction, brain metastases), or other problems such as gastritis may be the cause of the emesis and require a different approach.

PHYSIOLOGY OF EMESIS

The CTZ, or chemoreceptor trigger zone, has been identified in the area postrema of the medulla. It is postulated that stimulation of neurotransmitter receptors in this area can lead to emesis through further involvement of the medullary emetic center, which then initiates and coordinates the complex actions of emesis. Additionally, gut receptors may stimulate vomiting via afferents to the emetic center. It would appear that nausea, vomiting, and retching are all related through these pathways.

Since several different types of neuroreceptors are found in the CTZ, including dopamine, opiate, and serotonin receptors, blockade of one or more of these can lead to effective emetic control. The newest agents (ondansetron, granisetron) are selective for 5-HT3 (Type 3 serotonin) receptors. This selectivity improves or preserves the antiemetic effect of high-dose metoclopramide, which blocks both dopaminergic (D2) and 5-HT3 receptors while also eliminating the dystonic reactions that result from D2 blockade.

PATIENT CHARACTERISTICS

Chronic High Alcohol Intake

With appropriate antiemetics, it is easier to control chemotherapy-induced nausea and vomiting in patients with this history. It is not current alcohol intake that is of importance, but the chronic history. If emesis does occur, it is generally less severe in this group. It must be emphasized that full and appropriate doses of antiemetics are mandatory for these patients, but that the likelihood of excellent emetic control is enhanced.

Age

Age only indirectly affects the control of emesis. Younger patients are more likely to experience acute dystonic reactions with antiemetics that block dopamine receptors. Fractionating treatment over several consecutive days can also increase dystonic reactions. Studies to date in children and young adults suggest that 5-HT3 antagonists are effective and do not produce acute dystonia or akathisia.

Emesis with Prior Chemotherapy

These patients may already have some degree of anticipatory emesis, and control with antiemetics directed only at acute

TABLE 57–1. EMETOGENIC POTENTIAL OF COMMONLY USED CHEMOTHERAPEUTIC AGENTS OR CLASSES

HIGH	MODERATE	LOW
Cisplatin	Anthracyclines	5-Fluorouracil
Dacarbazine	Nitrosoureas	Bleomycin
Dactinomycin	Cytarabine	Vinca alkaloids
Mechlorethamine	Carboplatin	Chlorambucil
Cyclophosphamide*	Ifosfamide	Mitomycin C
		Methotrexate

*Associated with late onset of emesis.

emesis may not be sufficient. If a patient previously received a good antiemetic regimen but failed to have adequate control, he or she may be an individual with more resistent emesis for reasons that are not presently definable. In that instance, changing antiemetics may be worthwhile.

CHEMOTHERAPEUTIC AGENTS

The potential of individual agents for causing emesis is outlined in Table 57–1; the typical patterns and time courses of emesis with common agents are discussed in the previous section on acute chemotherapy-induced emesis.

When combinations of chemotherapeutic agents are given, the individual emetic properties of each agent in a combination must be considered. Thus, for a patient receiving cyclophosphamide plus doxorubicin plus vincristine, the early onset of emesis with doxorubicin must be addressed as well as the late onset with cyclophosphamide. Since vincristine rarely causes emesis, no provisions for this agent are generally needed. Clearly, treating only for cisplatin-induced emesis may be sufficient for a cisplatin plus vinca alkaloid regimen but not for chemotherapy that includes cisplatin plus cyclophosphamide.

ANTIEMETIC AGENTS

Doses, schedules, and recommended regimens are given in Table 57–2. Other details of frequently used agents are given below.

Selective Serotonin Antagonists

A growing experience with the selective serotonin antagonists indicates antiemetic properties equal to or greater than metoclopramide, without associated extrapyramidal side effects. Studies indicate utility in pediatrics and in younger adults receiving several days of cisplatin treatment, without dystonic reactions or increased toxicity. Side effects reported to date are generally mild, including occasional headache and transient minor elevation of SGOT.

Ondansetron is the first of this class to be widely available. The recommended dose is 0.15 mg/kg intravenously (or 6mg/m^2) in both adults and children. The initial dose is given over 15 minutes, beginning one-half hour prior to

TABLE 57–2. RECOMMENDED ANTIEMETIC REGIMENS

INDICATION: Cisplatin ≥ 75mg/m^2, high dose cyclophosphamide, or high dose dacarbazine

1. Ondansetron* 0.15 mg/kg prior to and at 4 and 8 hours after chemotherapy *plus* dexamethasone, 20 mg IV, given over 5 minutes with initial dose of ondansetron
2. Granisetron,* 10 μg/kg infused over 5 minutes, with dexamethasone, 20 mg IV over 5 minutes; may add lorazepam, 1 or 2 mg PO or IV

INDICATION: Cisplatin < 75mg/m^2 or cyclophosphamide or high doses of anthracyclines

1. Ondansetron* *or* granisetron* with dexamethasone as above
2. Metaclopramide* 2 mg/kg IV over 30 minutes, before cisplatin with diphenhydramine, 25 mg PO or IV, *plus* dexamethasone 10 to 20 mg IV; may add lorazepam 1 or 2 mg PO or IV; may repeat at 90 min post-cisplatin

INDICATION: Low to moderate dose anthracycline with cyclophosphamide; or ifosfamide 1g/m^2

1. Ondansetron* *or* granisetron* with dexamethasone as above
2. Prochlorperazine 10 mg IV, as a bolus or over 10 minutes with decadron, 20 mg IV; may add lorazepam 1 mg PO or IV.

Above given just prior to chemotherapy; may repeat all or part at 6 hours

CAVEAT: Children and adults, <age 30 avoid phenothiazines; use 5-HT3 receptor antagonist with or without steroids when possible. Use diphenhydramine 25 mg IV as an antidote to extrapyramidal (dystonic) reactions from phenothiazines; may repeat once.

CAVEAT: elderly patients: avoid intravenous benzodiazepines.

*Initial dose 20 to 30 minutes before chemotherapy.

chemotherapy. Studies have typically administered a total of three doses with the subsequent doses given every 2, 4, or 6 hours. Although the recommended schedule is every 4 hours, the every 2-hour regimen is as effective and may be more convenient in many settings.

More recent studies have used initial intravenous doses of 8 to 32 mg of ondansetron with comparable success. The drug also has been released in the United States in oral formulation in 4- and 8-mg tablets. The oral agent has good bioavailability and is useful after initial intravenous treatment when the patient is away from the clinic.

A second 5-HT-3 receptor antagonist, granisetron, has recently entered the United States market for intravenous use. The recommended dose is 10 µg/kg, given as a 5-minute infusion, 30 minutes prior to highly emetogenic agents. Recent studies show comparable results with granisetron and ondansetron in control of cisplatin-induced emesis. Dexamethasone, in doses of 12 to 20 mg given over 5 minutes in combination with granisetron or ondansetron, has been shown to improve antiemetic control of cisplatin-induced vomiting. Tropisetron, another agent of this class, has also been studied.

Dopamine-Blocking Agents

SUBSTITUTED BENZAMIDES

Metoclopramide is most effective when given in high intravenous doses. In comparison trials it is as active as or superior to all other agents except ondansetron. Side effects include mild sedation, dystonic reactions, restlessness (akathisia), and possibly diarrhea.

BUTYROPHENONES

Several studies using intravenous dosing of haloperidol and droperidol have shown favorable results. Side effects are similar to those reported for metoclopramide.

PHENOTHIAZINES

Oral and intramuscular regimens are inferior to other available routes and agents against the chemotherapeutic agents most likely to induce emesis. High intravenous doses appear to be more effective than the oral and intramuscular phenothiazines; however, orthostatic hypotension can be a potential toxicity. Other side effects are similar to those with butyrophenones and metoclopramide.

Other Agents

CORTICOSTEROIDS

Dexamethasone and methylprednisolone are active parenterally and orally and have shown activity in a variety of settings. Although the mechanism of action is not defined, it appears to be different from that of other antiemetics. Thus, steroids are easy to use in combination antiemetic regimens and enhance the activity of other active antiemetics. Side effects are generally mild and well described.

BENZODIAZEPINES

Lorazepam has only modest objective antiemetic effects, but together with its antianxiety and amnestic properties it has high subjective acceptance. It is also effective in reducing akathisia and appears useful in lessening dystonic reactions. The major side effect is sedation. Lorazepam is recommended as an addition to effective antiemetics and not as a single agent.

CANNABINOIDS

Nabilone and dronabinol are oral agents with activity similar to or greater than oral phenothiazines. Side effects appear greater than with phenothiazines and include moderate sedation, dizziness, ataxia, orthostatic hypotension, dry mouth, and dysphoria. In that cannabinoids have great popularity in the lay press, independent of their tested properties, every few years their use becomes an issue. With the availability of dronabinol (THC), the next controversy became the use of inhalant marijuana. One well-conducted (random assignment, double binded, crossover) study comparing oral THC with marijuana has been reported. Both agents had similar activity, with a trend toward patient preference for the THC among those who expressed a preference. Overall, neither agent was particularly good, with 75% of patients experiencing emesis.

TREATMENT OF SPECIFIC PROBLEMS

Acute Chemotherapy-Induced Emesis

Table 57–2 outlines suggested antiemetic regimens for chemotherapeutic agents by the severity of the emesis likely to be induced. There can be no substitute for careful consideration and for familiarity with both the antiemetic and chemotherapeutic agents. These regimens are intended as suggestions and not as "cookbook" recipes.

Delayed Emesis

Studies have shown that oral antiemetics after high-dose cisplatin are effective. For the vulnerable 4-day period beginning 12–24 hours after the administration of cisplatin (>100 mg/m^2), our current recommendations are given in Table 57–3. Starting the suggested regimen the morning after cisplatin (about 12–24 hours later) is a practical approach in that the mechanism causing this problem, and the exact time of onset, are not well defined.

Anticipatory Emesis

While prevention of this problem through the use of the most effective antiemetics with each course of chemotherapy remains the best approach, treatment once the problem has occurred can be helpful. Behavior therapy techniques

TABLE 57–3. RECOMMENDATIONS FOR PREVENTION OR TREATMENT OF DELAYED EMESIS

INDICATION: For patients who have received high doses of cisplatin (≥75 mg/m^2), in one dose or over several days

1. On day of chemotherapy, use an effective combination regimen from Table 57–2
2. Beginning the morning after cisplatin (12–24 hours after cisplatin), dexamethasone, 8 mg PO bid for 2 days, then 4 mg PO bid for 2 additional days, plus metoclopramide, 0.5 mg/kg PO qid for 2 days.

with desensitization have been shown to be useful. The utility of antianxiety agents has not been well studied.

BIBLIOGRAPHY

Dilly SG, Friedman C, Yocom K. Contribution of dexamethasone to antiemetic control with granisetron is greatest in patients at high risk of emesis. Proc ASCO vol B (abstract 1500), 1994

Gralla RJ, Tyson LB, Kris MG, Clark RA: The management of chemotherapy-induced nausea and vomiting. Med Clin No Amer 71:289–301, 1987.

Levitt M. Fairman C, Hawks R, et al: Randomized double-blind comparison of delta-9-tetrahydrocannabinol (THC) and marijuana as chemotherapy antiemetics. Proc Am Soc Clin Oncol 3:91, 1984.

Kris MG, Gralla RJ, Clark RA, et al: Phase II trials of the serotonin antagonist GR38032F for the control of vomiting caused by cisplatin. J Natl Cancer Inst 81:42–46, 1989.

Kris MG, Gralla RJ, Tyson LB et al: Controlling delayed vomiting: double-blind, randomized trial comparing placebo, dexamethasone alone, and metoclopramide plus dexamethasone in patients receiving cisplatin. J Clin Oncol 7:108–114, 1989.

Marty M, Pouillart P, Scholl S, et al: Comparison of the 5-hydroxytrypamine 3 (serotonin) antagonist ondansetron (GR38032F) with high dose metoclopramide in the control of cisplatin-induced emesis. N Engl J Med 322:816–821, 1990.

Morrow GR, Morrell C: Behavioral treatment for the anticipatory nausea and vomiting induced by cancer chemotherapy. N Engl J Med 307:1476–1480, 1982.

Roila F, Tonato M, Cognetti F, et al: Prevention of cisplatin-induced emesis: A double-blind multicenter randomized crossover study comparing ondansetron and ondansetron plus dexamethasone. J Clin Oncol 9:675–678, 1991.

Ruff P, Paska W, Goedhals L, et al. Ondansetron compared with granisetron in the prophylaxis of cisplatin-induced acute emesis. Oncology 51; 113–118, 1994.

John S. Macdonald, Daniel G. Haller, Robert J. Mayer, Eds. *Manual of Oncologic Therapeutics*, Third Edition.

58. NUTRITIONAL SUPPORT IN THE CANCER PATIENT

Linda S. Callans
John M. Daly

Malnutrition is a common finding in oncology patients. One third to three quarters of patients with cancer present with anorexia, and 50% to 80% have weight loss. Cancer cachexia is characterized by anorexia, marked weakness, tissue wasting, and organ dysfunction and does not necessarily correlate with stage or tumor burden. Many factors contribute to cancer cachexia, including reduced oral intake, local effects of the tumor, metabolic abnormalities, and treatment toxicities (Table 58–1). Oncology patients have poor nutrient intake due to anorexia, physiologic alterations in taste, and learned food aversions. Tumors of the gastrointestinal tract most commonly produce symptoms related to obstruction, but occasionally malabsorption syndromes occur. Oropharyngeal and esophageal cancers can cause odynophagia and dysphagia. Gastric cancers or large tumors of the upper abdomen can present with symptoms of early satiety or partial gastric outlet obstruction with nausea and vomiting. Small or large bowel cancers or metastatic disease with carcinomatosis can produce intestinal obstruction and, occasionally, blind loop syndrome with bacterial overgrowth and subsequent malabsorption. Pancreatic carcinoma can present with malabsorption due to exocrine insufficiency, but this occurs more commonly following surgical resection or radiation.

The metabolic alterations associated with cancer cachexia differ from the adaptive changes found in the setting of starvation (Table 58–2) and are thought to be mediated by cytokines such as tumor necrosis factor (TNFα), interleukin-1 (IL-1), IL-6, and interferon gamma (IFNA) produced by the tumor-bearing host or the tumor itself. In starvation, the basal metabolic rate is reduced, fat stores are used preferentially as a source of fuel with relative sparing of skeletal muscle, and whole body protein and glucose turnover are reduced. In cancer cachexia, the basal metabolic rate is unchanged or increased and fat, protein, and carbohydrate metabolism are altered. There is equal mobilization of fat and skeletal protein with increased lipolysis, proteolysis, and whole body protein turnover. Glucose production and utilization are increased, and insulin resistance can often be identified. Thus, the adaptive changes seen in the setting of starvation do not occur in cancer cachexia and tissue wasting is accelerated.

Antineoplastic therapies not only increase metabolic demands and exacerbate the preexisting metabolic abnormalities found in cancer patients but also produce their own toxicities that can further interfere with nutrient intake or absorption. Surgery can be complicated by prolonged ileus, infections, anastamotic stricture, and postgastrectomy syndromes. Chemotherapy can be associated with anorexia and altered taste, severe nausea and vomiting, mucositis, stomatitis, oral candadiasis, diarrhea, or obstipation. The complications due to radiation therapy correlate with the dose of radiation and the site and volume of tissue irradiated. Radiation can cause anorexia, nausea and vomiting, xerostomia, stomatitis, radiation enteritis and stricture.

The initial evaluation of cancer patients should include a complete nutritional assessment and consideration of the indications for nutritional support. Other factors compounding poor nutritional status should be addressed, and periodic reassessment of a patient's nutritional status should be performed during treatment.

INDICATIONS FOR NUTRITIONAL SUPPORT IN ONCOLOGY PATIENTS

The goals of nutritional support may vary from maintenance of adequate caloric intake to repletion of the severely malnourished patient. Clearly, terminally ill patients should not be offered nutritional support, while patients with normal nutritional status and tumors that respond rapidly to therapy may not require nutritional support. In general, attempts should be made to identify and correct nutritional deficits before or concomitant with cancer treatment. Intervention may include dietary counseling and antiemetics, oral supplementation, enteral tube feedings, or total parenteral nutrition (TPN) via a central venous catheter.

Malnutrition in the cancer patient is associated with significant morbidity and mortality. Weight loss is a significant prognostic variable predicting poorer survival following cancer treatment independent of performance status and tumor stage. In addition, malnourished patients have a higher incidence of complications associated with antineoplastic therapy. Perioperatively, malnourished patients have poor wound healing, prolonged ileus, increased wound infections and other septic complications related to the immunosuppression seen in severe malnutrition, and prolonged hospital stay. These patients are also more susceptible to septic episodes related to cytotoxic chemotherapy and neutropenia.

Cancer cachexia and the associated metabolic changes can be quite difficult to treat, and the indications for nutritional support in these patients remain somewhat controversial. Efforts to improve overall survival and decrease treatment-related morbidity by replenishing the malnourished

TABLE 58–1. FACTORS CONTRIBUTING TO CANCER CACHEXIA

REDUCED ORAL INTAKE
Anorexia
Nausea, vomiting
Altered taste and smell

LOCAL EFFECTS OF TUMOR
Odynophagia, dysphagia
Early satiety
Intestinal or gastric outlet obstruction
Malabsorption (blind loop syndrome)

ALTERED PROTEIN, GLUCOSE AND FAT METABOLISM

CYTOKINES (TNFα, IL-1, IL-6, INFγ)

EFFECTS OF CANCER TREATMENT
Postoperative
  Altered mastication, swallowing
  Postgastectomy syndromes
  Pancreatic insufficiency with malabsorption
  Anastomotic stricture
Chemotherapy-Induced
  Nausea, vomiting
  Altered taste and smell
  Stomatitis, mucositis
  Diarrhea
Radiation-Induced
  Anorexia, nausea, vomiting
  Altered taste and smell
  Xerostomia, stomatitis
  GI mucosal damage
  Late strictures
Psychosocial
  Depression, grief
  Anxiety
  Learned food aversions

cancer patient and reversing the metabolic abnormalities seen in cancer cachexia have been ineffective. There is little evidence that aggressive nutritional support improves the tolerance or efficacy of antineoplastic therapy, although many of the studies are flawed by small numbers, heterogeneous patient populations, and inadequate or varied nutrition regimens.

TPN is rarely indicated in the setting of chemotherapy except in the severely malnourished patient, patients undergoing bone marrow transplantation, or patients with severe toxicity such as neutropenic colitis that prohibits oral or enteral feeding. Similarly, no outcome benefit has been demonstrated in patients undergoing radiation therapy, and nutritional support should be considered only in the severely malnourished patient or in the setting of severe toxicity. Prospective randomized trials, however, have demonstrated decreased surgical morbidity and mortality in severely malnourished patients treated with TPN in the perioperative setting. To achieve this benefit, preoperative TPN should be administered for a minimum of 7 days prior to surgery.

TPN is currently indicated for cancer patients in the following categories:

1. Severely malnourished patients undergoing major surgery or cytotoxic drug therapy
2. Postoperative patients who have a prolonged paralytic ileus, infection, or fistula preventing enteral feeding;
3. Patients with complications of antineoplastic therapy prohibiting the use of the gastrointestinal tract; and
4. Bone marrow transplant patients.

Enteral feedings in the immediate postoperative period have also been shown to be beneficial, and the enteral route is preferred for nutritional support. Patients undergoing major abdominal surgery, particularly those with upper gastrointestinal cancers who are anticipated to undergo sequential multimodality therapy, should have a feeding jejunostomy placed at the time of their original surgery. Enteral feedings can then be instituted in the early postoperative period and continued as needed according to the patient's nutritional requirements.

NUTRITIONAL ASSESSMENT

The malnourished cancer patient usually has a combination of marasmus (simple starvation due to prolonged reduced intake of protein and calories) and kwashiorkor (protein deficiency in the setting of adequate caloric intake). Forty-five percent of hospitalized cancer patients have lost more than 10% of their usual body weight; as many as twenty-five percent have lost more than 20%. Although advanced cancer cachexia may be clinically obvious, many cancer patients have more subtle deficits, and a formal assessment of nutritional status should be included in the pretreatment evaluation with periodic reassessment during treatment. Nutritional status can be determined by history and physical examination, anthropomorphic measurements, and determination of serum protein levels and immunologic function (Table 58–3). On the basis of these parameters, a patient can be classified as normal or mildly, moderately, or severely malnourished in order to identify the high-risk patient who would benefit from aggressive nutritional support.

History and Physical Examination

Nutritional assessment begins with a complete history and physical examination. Patients should be questioned regarding weight loss, anorexia, and GI symptoms, including nausea, vomiting, dysphagia, early satiety, abdominal pain, and change in bowel habits. Prior gastric or intestinal resections may result in vitamin and mineral deficiencies and malabsorption syndromes; underlying chronic illnesses may also affect the nutritional status.

TABLE 58–2. METABOLIC CHANGES IN STARVATION AND CANCER CACHEXIA

	STARVATION	CANCER CACHEXIA
METABOLIC RATE		
Resting energy expenditure	Decreased	Normal/increased
Respiratory quotient	Decreased	Unchanged
O_2 consumption, CO_2 production	Decreased	Unchanged
Nitrogen balance	Negative	Negative
PROTEIN METABOLISM		
Whole body protein turnover	Decreased	Unchanged
Urinary nitrogen excretion	Decreased	Unchanged
Skeletal muscle catabolism	Decreased	Increased
Skeletal muscle anabolism	Decreased	Decreased
Hepatic protein synthesis		Increased
CARBOHYDRATE METABOLISM		
Whole body glucose turnover	Decreased	Increased
Hepatic gluconeogenesis	Increased	Increased
Glucose tolerance	Decreased	Decreased
Insulin sensitivity	Decreased	Decreased
Blood glucose	Decreased	Unchanged
Serum insulin	Decreased	Unchanged
Blood lactate	Unchanged	Increased
Cori cycle activity		Increased
FAT METABOLISM		
Lipolysis and fatty acid mobilization	Increased	Increased
Lipoprotein lipase activity	Unchanged	Decreased
Serum triglycerides		Increased

If possible, the patient's body weight should be documented at 2 months, 6 months, and 1 year before presentation. A recent weight loss of more than 10% of the usual body weight is indicative of significant malnutrition and an increased risk of morbidity and mortality. A 24-hour dietary recall should be elicited to estimate the patient's average daily caloric and protein intake. The dietary history should also inquire about food aversions as well as abnormalities in taste sensations that often include sour and salty foods.

TABLE 58–3. METHODS TO ASSESS NUTRITIONAL STATUS

History and physical examination
Laboratory studies
  Serum proteins
  Total lymphocyte counts
  Anergy testing
  Creatinine-height index (CHI) = actual Ucr/standard Ucr × 100
  Nitrogen balance
Anthropometric measurements
  MMC = Arm circumference (cm) − (0.134 × TSF(mm))
  TSF
Prognostic nutritional index (PNI)
  PNI (%) = 158 − 16.6 ×(ALB) − 0.78 (TSF) − 0.20 (TFN) − 5.8 (DH)

ALB, albumin (g/dl); DH, delayed hypersensitivity (0 = negative, 1 = <5 mm reactivity, 2 = ≥5 mm reactivity); MMC, midarm muscle circumference (cm); TFN, transferrin (mg/dl); TSF, triceps skinfold (mm); Ucr, 24-hour urinary creatinine (mg)

Physical examination may reveal findings suggestive of malnutrition such as pallor, atrophic skin, muscle wasting and decreased muscle strength, pitting edema, and skin lesions. Patients with marasmus may have decreased subcutaneous fat and lean muscle mass, while those with kwashiorkor may also have anasarca, ascites, hepatomegaly, alopecia, and psychomotor changes. Signs of vitamin and mineral deficiencies may be evident in malnourished patients (Table 58–4).

Anthropometrics

Anthropometric measurements are useful for estimating body fat and lean muscle composition based on a patient's body weight, height, skinfold thickness, and upper arm circumference. These measurements are compared to a standard based on age- and sex-matched population controls. However, unless a patient is significantly malnourished, anthropometrics may be helpful only after serial measurements to monitor change.

The triceps skinfold (TSF) thickness is an indirect measure of body fat. The TSF is generally measured using

TABLE 58–4. VITAMIN AND MINERAL DEFICIENCIES

SITE	SIGN OR SYMPTOM	DEFICIENCY
Hair	Dryness	Zinc
	Alopecia	Zinc
	Easy pluckability	Vitamins E and A
	Corkscrew hair	Vitamin C
	Color change	Biotin
Nails	Dystrophic	Iron
Skin	Hyperpigmentation	Niacin
	Erythema	Niacin
	Scrotal dermatitis	Niacin
	Follicular keratosis	Vitamin A
	Acneiform lesions	Vitamin A
	Xerosis	Vitamin A, linoleic acid
	Ecchymosis	Vitamins C and K
	Petechiae	Vitamins C and K
	Nasolabial seborrhea	Vitamin B_6
Eyes	Angular palpebritis	Vitamin B_2
	Bitot's spots	Vitamin A
	Conjunctival keratosis	Vitamin A
	Keratomalacia	Vitamin A
Mouth	Glossitis	Vitamin B_{12}, niacin, folate
	Angular stomatitis	Vitamin B_2
	Cheilosis	Vitamin B_2
	Magenta tongue	Vitamin B_2
	Scarlet, raw tongue	Niacin
	Atrophic papillae	Niacin
	Swollen, bleeding gums	Vitamin C
Neurologic	Peripheral neuropathy	Thiamine, niacin, B_6
	Wernicke's encephalopathy	Thiamine
	Encephalopathy (pellagra)	Niacin
	"Burning feet" syndrome	Pantothenic acid
	Loss of deep tendon reflexes	Thiamine, vitamin B_1, and B_{12}
Musculoskeletal	Osteomalacia	Vitamin D
	Joint pain	Vitamin C
	Tender muscles	Thiamine
Hematologic	Hemolytic anemia	Vitamin E
	Macrocytic anemia	Vitamin B_{12}, folate
	Microcytic anemia	Vitamin B_6, iron, copper
	Coagulopathy	Vitamin K
	Thrombocytopenia	Linoleic acid
Visceral	Congestive heart failure	Thiamine
	Diarrhea	Folate, zinc, niacin
	Goiter	Iodine
	Hepatosplenomegaly	Zinc

Adapted from Rombeau JL, Caldwell MD (eds): Enteral and Tube Feedings, p 129. Philadelphia, WB Saunders, 1984

calipers at a point midway between the acromial process and the olecranon of the nondominant arm. The arm should be relaxed and hanging freely at the patient's side or folded across the chest. A lengthwise fold of skin is pinched 1 cm above the midline and pulled away from the underlying muscle, and the thickness of the pinched skinfold is measured at a depth equal to the thickness of the fold.

Midarm muscle circumference (MMC) is an indirect assessment of lean muscle mass and is calculated from the arm circumference with an adjustment for the subcutaneous fat as measured by the TSF (see the MMC equation in Table 58–3). The arm circumference is measured in centimeters using a measuring tape placed midway between the acromial process and the olecranon of the nondominant arm without constricting the skin.

Laboratory Studies

Serum proteins such as albumin, transferrin, prealbumin, and retinol-binding protein reflect visceral protein status.

Because of their longer half-lives, albumin and transferrin levels are better indicators of nutritional status, whereas prealbumin and retinol-binding protein levels reflect recent dietary changes. Once nutritional support is instituted, significant increases in serum albumin and transferrin levels may be seen after 7 to 10 days and 4 days, respectively. However, factors other than nutritional status may affect serum protein levels and limit their reliability as nutritional indicators (Table 58–5).

Determinations of immune function such as total lymphocyte count and anergy to antigen skin testing may reflect nutritional status but are generally of limited value for this purpose. Total lymphocyte counts correlate with weight loss and other measures of visceral protein status but are also affected by chemotherapy, radiation therapy, infection, and immunosuppressive drugs. Skin testing for delayed cutaneous hypersensitivity (DCH) is performed by intradermal injection of a panel of antigens including purified protein derivative (PPD) of tuberculin, mumps, *Trichophyton*, and *Candida* followed by examination of the sites at 24 and 36 hours after injection. A positive test is scored with a minimum of 10 mm of induration. Anergy to skin testing, however, is not a sensitive or specific indicator of malnutrition. Substantial protein depletion is required before anergy due to malnutrition is evident, and many other factors such age, malignancy, sepsis, immunosuppressive medications, surgery, and radiation therapy can result in a negative anergy panel.

The creatinine–height index (CHI) uses 24-hour urinary creatinine excretion as a measure of skeletal muscle mass. The CHI is defined as the ratio of the patient's creatinine excretion to a standard creatinine excretion for a normal adult of the same sex and height. Assuming normal renal function, a CHI of less than 80% of the standard correlates with significant depletion of lean body mass and protein-calorie malnutrition.

The Prognostic Nutritional Index

Based on the above parameters, a patient can be classified as normally nourished or mildly, moderately, or severely malnourished (Table 58–6). The Prognostic Nutritional Index (PNI) is a scoring system based on the triceps skin fold (TSF), serum albumin and transferrin levels, and delayed cutaneous hypersensitivity (DCH) to recall antigen skin testing (see Table 58–3). The PNI has been correlated with morbidity and mortality. In a large retrospective study, surgical patients with a PNI less than 30% had a 12% complication rate with 2% mortality whereas those with a PNI greater than 60% had a complication rate of 81% with 59% mortality. In another study, cancer patients with a PNI over 40% had a significant decrease in postoperative morbidity and mortality when treated with TPN whereas those with a PNI less than 40% showed no difference. The PNI quantifies the degree of malnutrition, allowing more accurate serial assessments, and can guide decisions regarding nutritional intervention by identifying patients at high risk for complications associated with malnutrition.

TABLE 58–5. MEASURES USED TO ASSESS PROTEIN STATUS

SERUM PROTEIN	HALF-LIFE (DAYS)	AFFECTED BY
Albumin	20	Extracellular fluid changes; Liver or kidney disease
Transferrin	8	Iron deficiency
Prealbumin	2	Traumatic injuries, sepsis
Retinol-binding protein	0.5	Renal failure, stress

MANAGING THE MALNOURISHED CANCER PATIENT

Management of Cancer Cachexia

The metabolic changes associated with cancer cachexia are often resistant to nutritional therapy. However, many factors that contribute to cancer cachexia may be amenable to treatment, thereby lessening their impact on the patient's nutritional status (Table 58–7). Animal studies suggest that many aspects of cancer cachexia can be reversed by blocking the effects of TNFα using anti-TNF antibodies, but this not been tested in the clinical setting. Anti-IFNγ antibodies have been similarly implicated. Although it is considered experimental, hydrazine sulfate has been implicated in the treatment of cachexia by blocking excessive glucose production.

Anorexia is a prominent component of cancer cachexia, and several studies have demonstrated improved appetite and oral intake with megestrol acetate as well as other medications. The nausea and vomiting associated with chemotherapeutic agents or radiation therapy can be averted by premedication with antiemetics, some of which are listed in Table 58–7. The serotonin antagonist ondansetron is particularly effective in this setting. Analgesics can relieve pain from mucositis and stomatitis and enhance food intake. Limitations of nutrient intake related to local effects of the tumor or post-treatment complications such as stricture are often ameliorated by surgical resection or bypass. Dietary counseling may enable the patient to maintain a balanced diet, replace offensive foods with more palatable foods, and alter texture and consistency of foods to facilitate mastication and swallowing. Attention should also be given to the problems of xerostomia, dentition, gastrointestinal dysmotility, diarrhea, depression, and anxiety.

TABLE 58–6. ASSESSING DEGREE OF MALNUTRITION

	NORMAL	MILD	MODERATE	SEVERE
% Weight loss	0%	<5%	5–9%	>10%
Albumin (g/dl)	3.5–5.8	3.0–3.5	2.4–3.0	<2.4
Transferrin (mg/dl)	200–400	150–200	100–150	<100
Prealbumin (mg/dl)	16–43	10–15	5–10	<5
Total lymphocyte count	>2000	1200–2000	800–1200	<800
% Positive skin test	80	53		50
MMC	>40%	35–40%	30–34%	<30%
TSF	>40%	35–40%	30–34%	<30%
CHI	>90%	81–90%	61–80%	<60%
PNI		<40%	41–50%	>50%

CHI, creatinine–height index; MMC, midarm muscle circumference (cm); PNI, prognostic nutritional index; TSF, triceps skinfold (mm)

Nutritional Management of the Cancer Patient

Once clinical and laboratory assessment has determined the degree of malnutrition, the indications for nutrition therapy should be considered. The goal of therapy may be maintenance of nutritional status during sequential multimodality cancer treatment, repletion of deficits in a severely malnourished patient, or support during a period of gastrointestinal nonfunction in the perioperative period or due to complications of antineoplastic therapy. The daily nutrient requirements should be calculated, the patient's oral intake estimated based on dietary history and calorie counts, and the additional nutrients needed to meet the patient's daily requirements determined. Oral supplements or enteral feedings are preferred, although TPN may be indicated in selected circumstances.

TABLE 58–7. MANAGEMENT OF FACTOR PREDISPOSING TO MALNUTRITION IN CANCER PATIENTS

ANOREXIA
Metoclopramide (Reglan)
Megestrol acetate
Dexamethasone (Decadron)
Tetrahydrocannabinol (THC)

NAUSEA/VOMITING
Ondansetron (Zofran)
Metoclopramide (Reglan)
Prochlorperazine (Compazine)
Promethazine (Phenergan)
Droperidol (Inapsine)
Haloperidol (Haldol)
Corticosteroids (Decadron, Solumedrol)
Tetrahydrocannabinol (THC)

LOCAL TUMOR EFFECTS
Surgical resection or bypass
Radiation therapy

DIARRHEA/MALABSORPTION
Antidiarrheal agents
Pancreatic enzyme replacement
Antibiotics (blind loop syndrome)

ALTERED TASTE/FOOD AVERSIONS
Dietary counseling
Alter texture and consistency of foods

PSYCHOSOCIAL ASPECTS
Antidepressants
Anxiolytics
Analgesics

Daily Nutrient Requirements

The average protein requirement for maintenance in normal individuals is 0.8 g/kg per day for maintenance and 1.2 to 1.5 g/kg per day for anabolism. Hospitalized cancer patients have increased requirements and should be given 1.5 to 2.0 g/kg per day. Dietary nitrogen should be supplied with a calorie-to-nitrogen ratio ranging from 125 to 150 calories per gram of nitrogen (1 g of nitrogen = 6.25 g of protein). A 24-hour urine collection for urinary urea nitrogen can be performed to calculate the nitrogen balance and assess the adequacy of protein delivery in meeting the patient's needs.

The daily caloric requirement is calculated based on sex, age, weight, and height using the Harris-Benedict equation (Table 58–8). The basal energy expenditure is then adjusted by a correction factor based on activity level and clinical status to estimate a patient's caloric expenditure (Table 58–9). The correction factor ranges from 1.2 in an ambulatory, nonstressed patient to 1.8 in major sepsis. In general, a factor of 1.3 is used in hospitalized cancer patients for maintenance goals and 1.5 for repletion.

A more accurate measure of the resting energy expenditure (REE) is obtained by indirect calorimetry that measures gas exchange in a thermoneutral environment (see Table 58–8). Oxygen consumption and carbon dioxide production are determined at least 2 hours after eating after the patient has rested in the supine position for 30 minutes. When possible, periodic indirect calorimetry should be used to determine the patient's REE more precisely and guide nutritional support recommendations.

TABLE 58–8. DETERMINATION OF ENERGY REQUIREMENTS

HARRIS-BENEDICT EQUATION (BASAL ENERGY EXPENDITURE)
For women: BEE (kcal/d) = 655 + [9.6 × weight (kg)] + [1.7 × height (cm)] − [4.7 × age (years)]
For men: BEE (kcal/d) = 66 + [13.7 × weight (kg)] + [5.0 × height (cm)] − [6.8 × age (years)]
Resting energy expenditure (REE) = BEE × energy correction factor*

INDIRECT CALORIMETRY (RESTING ENERGY EXPENDITURE)
REE (kcal/d) = $((3.9 \times Vo_2) + (1.1 \times Vco_2)) \times 1440$ min/d

ENERGY CONVERSION BY NUTRIENT SOURCE
1 g glucose = 3.4 kcal
1 g fat = 9 kcal
1 g protein = 4 kcal

BEE, basal energy expenditure; REE, resting energy expenditure; Vo_2, O_2 consumption (l/min); Vco_2, CO_2 production (l/min)

*See Table 58-9 for energy correction factors.

Nonprotein calories are supplied as a combination of carbohydrates and fats. The maximal rate of glucose oxidation in the adult is 7 g/kg per day; additional caloric requirements should be met using lipids. To avoid essential fatty acid deficiency, a minimum of 1000 ml of a 10% lipid emulsion should be given each week.

Attention must also be given to the management of fluids and electrolytes (Table 58–10). Maintenance fluid requirements average 30 ml/kg per day. Depending on the patient's nutrient and fluid requirements and the particular enteral formula or TPN solution chosen, it may be necessary to supply additional free water or administer a diuretic. Ongoing urinary and gastrointestinal losses of fluid and electrolytes must be considered and specific electrolyte, vitamin, or mineral deficiencies identified and corrected. Required daily vitamins and minerals are included in most enteral formulas or can be provided as multivitamin and trace element preparations. Multivitamin preparations supply vitamins A, D, E, B_2, B_6, B_{12}, C, and folic acid, but vitamin K must be provided separately.

TABLE 58–9. ENERGY CORRECTION FACTORS AS DETERMINED BY CLINICAL STATUS

CONDITION	CORRECTION FACTOR
Activity	
Confined to bed	1.2
Ambulatory	1.3
Elective surgery	1.2
Fever	1.0 + 0.13 per °C
Peritonitis	1.2 − 1.5
Soft tissue trauma	1.2 − 1.37
Major sepsis	1.4 − 1.8
Starvation	0.7

TABLE 58–10. DAILY REQUIREMENTS FOR NUTRITIONAL SUPPORT

PROTEIN
1.5 to 2.0 g protein/kg/day

NONPROTEIN CALORIES
Harris-Benedict equation*
Indirect calorimetry*
35 to 45 kcal/kg/day

FLUIDS
30 ml/kg/day

MULTIVITAMINS
(Vitamin K must be administered separately)

ELECTROLYTES	
Sodium	60–120 mEq
Potassium	60–100 mEq
Chloride	60–120 mEq
Magnesium	8–10 mEq
Calcium	200–400 mg
Phosphorus	300–400 mg
TRACE METALS	
Zinc	2.5–4 mg
Copper	0.5–1.5 mg
Chromium	10–15 µg
Manganese	0.15–0.8 mg

*See Table 58-8.

Route of Feeding

Patient education, dietary counseling, and oral supplements may be all that is required to establish adequate intake in patients who can tolerate a regular diet. If nutritional support is indicated and the patient is unable to take adequate protein and calories by mouth, enteral feedings should be considered. Enteral nutrition is preferred if the gastrointestinal tract is functional because it is less expensive, easier to administer, and safer than TPN; further, intestinal structure and integrity are maintained and nutrient utilization is enhanced. GI tract function and aspiration risk should be evaluated before enteral feedings are instituted. Feedings into the stomach by nasogastric or gastrostomy tube are contraindicated in patients with gastric outlet obstruction, absent gag reflex, or mental obtundation, but these patients may be candidates for jejunostomy tube feedings. Contraindications to enteral feeding include intestinal obstruction, paralytic ileus, toxic megacolon and neutropenic colitis, fistulae, radiation enteritis, severe diarrhea, and malabsorption. When the enteral route is contraindicated, TPN should be considered.

ENTERAL FEEDING

The enteral route is preferred if the GI tract is functional. A variety of tubes are available, and tube selection and enteral access should be individualized to meet each patient's needs. For short-term support, a small-bore flexible nasogastric or nasoduodenal tube may be well tolerated. For longer periods, a surgically, endoscopically, or laparoscopically placed tube should be considered. Patients undergoing major intra-abdominal procedures should have a feeding jejunostomy tube placed for nutritional support in the postoperative period and during subsequent courses of adjuvant therapy.

The type and size of an enteral feeding tube are determined by the route of access and the method of infusion as well as the viscosity and osmolality of the formula selected. Larger tubes are required for blenderized formulas (#12 to 14 French), high caloric density formulas (#10 Fr), and bolus or gravity feedings (#10 to 12 Fr); smaller tubes (#8 Fr) are adequate for isotonic chemically defined formulas and pump infusions. The smallest bore tube that allows adequate flow without clogging should be selected.

Small-bore (#8 to 10 Fr) polyurethane or silicon elastomer tubes are fairly well tolerated for nasoenteral feedings. Shorter tubes (91 cm) are used for feeding into the stomach, and 109-cm tubes with weighted tips can be placed into the duodenum for postpyloric infusions in patients at risk for aspiration. Inner stylets are often included to facilitate positioning of the tubes; water injected into the tube before placing the stylet facilitates removal of the stylet once the tube is in the proper position. After testing the gag reflex, nasoenteric intubation is performed with the patient in the semi-Fowler's position leaning his head forward. The tip is lubricated and placed through the nostril along the floor of the nasal passageway. The patient can assist tube passage into the esophagus by swallowing a small amount of water. The stylet should be removed once the tube reaches the stomach (50-cm marking) and the position checked by aspirating gastric contents, insufflating air while listening with a stethoscope for air bubbling over the stomach, and obtaining a radiograph. For postpyloric placement of weighted tubes, the patient should be placed on the right side for several hours to allow gravity and peristalsis to advance the tube. Alternatively, the tube can be placed with fluoroscopic guidance.

If more than 4 to 6 weeks of enteral nutrition is anticipated, gastrostomy or jejunostomy tube placement should be considered. Gastric feedings are generally well tolerated due to the distensibility and dilutional function of the stomach as well as pyloric regulation of emptying into the duodenum. Gastrostomy tubes are easily cared for and bolus or intermittent gravity feeding of blenderized food is less expensive and potentially more convenient. However, patients with severe gastroesophageal reflux, absent gag reflex, or altered mental status are at significant risk for aspiration and are not candidates for gastric feedings. Endoscopic placement of gastrostomy tube (percutaneous endoscopic gastrostomy [PEG]) is easily accomplished with local anesthesia and intravenous sedation. Patients with obstructing head and neck or esophageal cancers require a surgical gastrostomy that can be performed laparoscopically under general anesthesia or using an open technique under local, regional, or general anesthesia.

Jejunostomy tubes are indicated in patients at high risk for aspiration and patients with upper gastrointestinal cancers involving the stomach, pylorus, or duodenum. Jejunostomy tubes can be placed into the proximal jejunum at the time of the original cancer surgery or at a separate sitting using a standard Witzel technique and tacking the bowel to the anterior abdominal wall. Alternatively, a laparoscopic approach can be employed.

Enteral Formulas

A wide variety of enteral preparations are available. These differ in nutrient source, caloric density, osmolality, viscosity, expense, and ease of preparation (Table 58–11). Enteral formulas fall into four general categories — blenderized formulas, nutritionally complete commercial formulas, chemically defined preparations, and modular formulas — and should be selected based on the patient's nutritional requirements, clinical situation, and tolerance.

Blenderized formulas are prepared by the patient from any food that can be blenderized. The long preparation time may be offset by the low cost and the convenience of intermittent bolus or gravity infusions. Blenderized preparations can be used only with a gastrostomy tube, and a large-bore tube (#14 Fr) is required due to viscosity. The caloric content of these preparations usually ranges from 0.6 to 1.3 kcal/ml. Various additives such as corn syrup, vegetable oils, or powdered milk can provide additional calories and protein.

Many nutritionally complete, sterile, ready-to-use formulas are commercially available for enteral feeding, some of which are flavored for use as oral supplements. These are polymeric formulas with intact proteins; most are lactose-free and some have added fiber to reduce diarrhea. Most are isotonic with a caloric density of 1.0 kcal/ml, but high-calorie and high-nitrogen, hyperosmolar formulas that provide 1.5 to 2.0 kcal/ml are available. Continuous pump infusions are recommended for delivery into the stomach or jejunum to avoid gastrointestinal complications.

Chemically defined formulas contain hydrolyzed proteins and crystalline amino acids and are more readily absorbed. These lactose-free, very-low-residue preparations provide 1.0 kcal/ ml and are usually hyperosmolar. Elemental diets are indicated in patients with severe radiation enteritis, intestinal fistulas, and malabsorption.

Modular formulas consist of core modules of protein or carbohydrate or fats. Modules of vitamins or minerals are also available. Modular formulas can be used as supplements

TABLE 58–11. SELECTED ENTERAL FORMULAS

	CALORIC DENSITY*	OSMOLALITY	FLAVORED?	COMMENT
BLENDERIZED DIET	0.6–1.3			
NUTRITIONALLY COMPLETE				
Sustacal (Mead Johnson)	1.06	I	Y	
Isocal (Mead Johnson)	1.06	I	N	
Isocal HCN (Mead Johnson)	2.0	H	N	
Ensure (Ross)	1.06	H	Y	
Ensure PLUS (Ross)	1.5	H	Y	
Osmolite (Ross)	1.06	I	N	
Jevity (Ross)	1.06	I	N	Added fiber
CHEMICALLY DEFINED				
Criticare HN (Mead Johnson)	1.06	H		
Vital HN (Ross)	1.0	H	Y	
Vivonex T.E.N. (Norwich Eaton)	1.0	H	N	Powder; flavor packets available
MODULAR	**TYPE**		**FORM**	
Propac (Sherwood)	Protein		Powder	
Moducal (Mead Johnson)	Carbohydrate		Powder	
Sumacal (Sherwood)	Carbohydrate		Powder	
Nutrisource (Sandox)	Carbohydrate		Liquid	
MCT oil (Mead Johnson)	Fat		Liquid	
Nutrisource (Sandoz)	Fat		Liquid	

*Caloric density = kcal/ml

H, hyperosmolar; I, isotonic; Y, Yes; N, No.

with other enteral formulas or combined in different ways to meet an individual's specific requirements. These may be indicated in patients with specific organ dysfunction such as hepatic or renal failure.

Except for blenderized formulas, all enteral feeding should be delivered by continuous gravity or pump infusion. After tube placement, infusion is begun with a 5% dextrose solution at 30 ml per hour for the first 12 to 24 hours. It is then switched to full strength formula at the same rate. The rate of infusion can then be increased by 20- to 30-ml increments every 12 to 24 hours as tolerated by the patient until the goal regimen is met. Tube feedings can then be gradually cycled, ultimately providing the required volume at a more rapid rate for 12 to 14 hours overnight. This is generally well tolerated and improves quality of life and patient acceptance.

Complications of Enteral Nutrition

Although enteral nutrition is considered safer than TPN, gastrointestinal, mechanical, metabolic, and infectious complications do occur (Table 58–12). Gastrointestinal complications include nausea, vomiting, cramping, bloating, and diarrhea, and are commonly related to hyperosmolar solutions and to the rate of infusion. Persistent diarrhea can be treated with loperamide (Imodium) orally or added directly to the enteral formula. Mechanical complications include erosions, tube malfunction or displacement, and intestinal obstruction. Metabolic abnormalities such as hyperglycemia, electrolyte imbalances, and overhydration or dehydration can occur. Infectious complications include aspiration pneumonia, bacterial overgrowth in the feeding tube, and occasionally abdominal wall cellulitis or abscess. In general, however, the complications associated with enteral feeding are less severe than those seen with TPN and many can be prevented with careful monitoring.

TOTAL PARENTERAL NUTRITION (TPN)

Parenteral nutrition may be indicated in severely malnourished cancer patients undergoing major surgery or aggressive cytotoxic chemotherapy, patients with gastrointestinal complications of surgery, radiation, or chemotherapy precluding oral or enteral feeding, and bone marrow transplant patients. Peripheral parenteral nutrition can be provided with amino acid solutions and lipids, but calorie delivery is limited by the osmolality and sclerosing properties of the concentrated glucose solutions. For full parenteral nutritional support, central venous access must be established, with special attention given to sterile technique. A double- or triple-lumen venous catheter placed into the subclavian vein using the

TABLE 58–12. COMPLICATIONS ASSOCIATED WITH ENTERAL FEEDING

COMPLICATIONS	DIAGNOSIS	THERAPY	PREVENTION
GASTROINTESTINAL			
Offensive smell	Smell, nausea, vomiting	Add flavorings	Use polymeric formulas
Gastric retention	Gastric residual > 100 ml 4 h after a bolus, or > 115% of volume/h, nausea and vomiting	Dilute formula	Dilute formula and gradually increase concentration
Rapid infusion	Nausea and vomiting	Decrease rate, advance 25 ml/h every 12 to 24 h	Start gastrointestinal feedings at 40 ml–50 ml/h, jej. & duo feedings @ 20–25 cc/h, advance 25 ml/h every 12 to 24 h
Lactose intolerance	Review of history, diarrhea, nausea, vomiting, lactose intolerance test	Switch to nonlactose formula	Use formulas with low lactose content
Excessive fat in diet	Review of history, nausea, vomiting	Switch to low-fat diet	Provide < 30%–40% of calories by fat
Fat malabsorption	Review of history, 72-h fecal fat assessment	Pancreatic enzyme supplements	Use low-fat formulas
Hyperosmolar solution	Osmolality > 300 mOsm, diarrhea, increased stool water content	Dilute to isotonicity, stop for 12 h, resume at slow rate, use Kaopectate, Lomotil	Use isotonic solutions, start at slow rate (40–50 ml/h), and increase in 12- to 24-h increments
Cold feedings	Tubing cold to touch, diarrhea	Discontinue feedings until formula is warm	Start recently refrigerated formulas at 40 ml/h
Protein malnutrition	Albumin < 3 g/dl, diarrhea	Dilute solutions to isotonicity, use antidiarrheal	Start at slow rate (20–25 ml/h) and increase in 12- to 24-h increments
Diarrhea	Diarrhea	Decrease flow rate to 25–50 ml/h or discontinue, use parenteral feeding	
Dehydration	Orthostatic hypotention, dry mucous membranes, constipation	Supplemental fluids	Monitor intake and output
Impaction	Rectal examination, constipation	Digital disimpaction	Monitor intake and output
Obstruction	Nausea, vomiting, constipation, obstructive series	Surgery	
MECHANICAL			
Nasopharyngeal discomfort	Mouth breathing, sore throat, hoarseness	Sugarless gum, gargling with warm water and mouthwash, anesthetic lozenges	Use soft small-bore tubes
Nasal erosions	Erosions of nasal ala	Tape tube without pressure on nasal ala	Use soft small-bore tubes
Abscess of nasal septum	Pain, fever, chills	Remove tube, drainage, antibiotics	Use soft small-bore tubes, proper taping
Acute sinusitis	Pain, nasal congestion, fever, malodorous breath	Remove tube, hot compresses, analgesics	Use soft small-bore tubes

continued

TABLE 58–12. COMPLICATIONS ASSOCIATED WITH ENTERAL FEEDING *(Continued)*

COMPLICATIONS	DIAGNOSIS	THERAPY	PREVENTION
Acute otitis media	Severe throbbing ear pain, fever, chill, dizziness	Change tube to other nostril, antibiotics	
Rupture of eosophageal varices	Hematemesis, melena, radiographic studies	Sedation, rest of esophagus	Use soft small-bore tubes
Esophagitis	Heartburn, substernal and epigastric burning	Remove tube	Keep head of bed at 45° angle
Esophageal ulceration	Dysphagia, radiologic studies	Remove tube, esophagoscopy, dilatation	Use soft small-bore tube; with persistent vomiting, consider a a jejunostomy tube
Tracheoesophageal fistula	Fistula present	Symptomatic	Use soft small-bore tube; use gastric or jejunostomy tube
Knotting tube	Unable to remove tube	Cut tube and allow to pass per rectum, use McGill forceps to bring tube out mouth to cut tube	None
METABOLIC			
Hypokalemia	Insulin administration, diarrhea, severe malnutrition	K^+ supplements	Check electrolytes
Hypophosphatemia	Insulin administration, severe malnutrition	Phosphate supplements	
Hyponatremia	Overhydration	Water restriction	
Hyperphosphatemia	Renal insufficiency	Switch to low phosphate feeding	
Hypomagnesemia	Decreased carrier protein, inadequate delivery	Magnesium supplements	
Hypocupremia (elevated transaminases)	Activation of hepatic enzymes		
Vitamin K deficiency	Inadequate delivery	Vitamin K replacement	
Essential fatty acid deficiency	Low linoleic acid	Parenteral fat 5 ml safflower oil daily	

Seldinger guide wire technique provides a designated TPN port with additional access for phlebotomy or medication infusion.

TPN Solutions

The protein and caloric requirements of the patient to receive TPN should be determined as described above (see also Tables 58–8 and 58–10). TPN solutions composed of amino acids, glucose, and lipids can then be formulated to meet the patient's requirements (Table 58–13). In general, 500 ml of an 8.5% amino acid solution is mixed with 500 ml of a 50% glucose solution ($D_{50}W$) to provide a liter of 4.25% amino acids and 25% glucose. Each liter of standard TPN contains 42.5 grams of protein and 850 kcal as glucose. Thus, 2 liters of a standard TPN solution and 500 ml of 10% intralipid would approximate the caloric and protein requirements for a 6-foot-tall (180 cm) 50-year-old man weighing 70 kg calculated using the Harris-Benedict equation and an energy correction factor of 1.3. Additional protein can be provided for the severely malnourished or catabolic patient.

Alternative amino acid solutions may be indicated in certain circumstances. Ten percent stock amino acid solutions and solutions high in branched-chain amino acids (BCAA) are available. High BCAA solutions may be indicated in the setting of hypermetabolism with persistent negative nitrogen balance, glucose intolerance, and hepatic failure. Patients with renal failure can receive their full protein and nutrient goals and undergo dialysis to eliminate the excess fluid and nitrogen waste produced. When dialysis is not possible, a low-protein (25 to 50 g per day) regimen should be instituted or a specific renal failure solution containing only essential amino acids initiated if the low protein formulation is not tolerated (BUN greater than 90 or uremic syndrome).

TABLE 58–13. SAMPLE STANDARD TPN REGIMEN

NUTRIENT SOURCE	AMOUNT PER LITER
$D_{50}W$	500 ml (850 kcal)
Amino acids (8.5%)	500 ml (42.5 g protein)
Electrolytes	
Sodium	42 mEq
Chloride	58 mEq
Potassium	30 mEq
Calcium	5 mEq
Phosphate (mM)	7 mM
Magnesium	8 mEq
Acetate	0
Multivitamins	5 ml
Trace metals	
Heparin	1000 units
Intralipid (10%)	500 ml daily (450 kcal)

Lipid emulsions are an additional source of nonprotein calories (450 kcal per 500 ml of 10% intralipid or 900 kcal per 500 ml of 20% intralipid) and can be used to provide up to 30% of a patient's caloric goal for efficient nutrient utilization. Further, patients with glucose intolerance requiring excessive insulin administration or CO_2 retention complicating high glucose regimens may benefit from replacing glucose nutrients with lipids. Lipids can be infused separately or mixed in the pharmacy with the amino acid and glucose nutrients in a 3-liter IV bag. Generally, adults can tolerate no more than 2 to 4 grams of fat per kilogram per day, and serum triglycerides should be monitored to confirm adequate fat metabolism. If lipids are not used as an integral part of the TPN regimen, a minimum of 1000 ml of 10% intralipid should be given each week to avoid essential fatty acid deficiency.

In addition to protein, carbohydrate, and lipids, the TPN solution should provide the daily requirements for electrolytes, trace minerals, and vitamins (Table 58–10). Electrolyte concentrations can be altered based on serum levels to correct deficiencies and account for ongoing losses. Acetate (sodium or potassium acetate) can be added to maintain acid–base status.

Daily fluid requirements must be provided intravenously in the patient with a nonfunctional GI tract. Some patients may require diuresis to avoid overhydration depending on the volume necessary to deliver the patient's recommended protein and caloric goals. Other patients may need supplemental IV fluids to replace ongoing GI and urinary losses. Clearly, each patient's regimen should be individualized and the fluid status monitored closely.

TPN solutions are generally administered by continuous infusion over a 24-hour period. Low-dose heparin (1000 units per liter) can be added to decrease the incidence of catheter or subclavian vein thrombosis. Some intravenous medications such as cimetidine are compatible with TPN solutions and can be added directly to the mixture.

Complications of Parenteral Nutrition

Complications of TPN are infectious, mechanical, and metabolic (Table 58–14). Catheter infections are most commonly caused by gram-positive organisms, although gram-negative bacteria and yeast can also be pathogens. Clinical presentation can range from unexpected fever to frank sepsis; patients usually respond to removal of the infected catheter, although a course of an appropriate antibiotic may be required. A central venous line should always be regarded with suspicion in patients with fever. In addition to a complete physical examination, blood should be withdrawn from the catheter for culture, the central line changed over a sterile guide wire, and the catheter tip cultured. When a patient is frankly septic or a positive culture is obtained, the central line should be removed and replaced at a different site. Mechanical complications occur primarily during catheter

TABLE 58–14. COMPLICATIONS ASSOCIATED WITH TOTAL PARENTERAL NUTRITION

COMPLICATIONS	DIAGNOSIS	THERAPY	PREVENTION
MECHANICAL			
Pneumothorax	Dyspnea, chest film	Tube thoracostomy, observation	Avoid emergency procedures; use Trendelenburg position
Hemothorax	Dyspnea, chest film	Remove catheter, observation	
Venous thrombosis	Inability to cannulate	Remove catheter, heparin therapy	Use silicon catheters; add heparin
Air embolism	Dyspnea, cyanosis, hypotension, tachycardia, precordial murmur	Trendelenburg, left lateral decubitus positions	Trendelenburg position, Valsalva maneuver; tape connections
Catheter embolism	Sheared catheter	Fluoroscopic retrieval	Never withdraw catheter through needle
Arrhythmias	Catheter tip in atrium		
Subclavian artery injury	Pulsatile red blood	Remove needle, apply pressure, chest film	Review anatomy
Catheter tip misplacement	Chest film	Redirect with a guidewire	Direct level of needle caudally
METABOLIC			
Hyperglycemic, hyperosmolar nonketotic coma	Dehydration with osmotic diuresis, disorientation, lethargy, stupor, convulsions, coma; glucose >1000 mg/dl; Osm >350 MOsm/liter	Discontinue TPN, administer 5% dextrose half-normal saline at 250 ml/h; insulin 10–20 units/h; bicarbonate; monitor glucose, potassium, pH	Monitor glucose
Hypoglycemia	Headache, sweating, thirst, convulsions, disorientation, paresthesias	$D_{50}W$ intravenously	Taper TPN by one half for 12 h; then 12 hr of D_5W at 100 ml/h
CO_2 retention	Ventilator dependence, high RQ	Taper glucose	Provide 30% to 40% of calories with fat
Azotemia	Dehydration, elevated blood urea nitrogen	Increase nonprotein calories	Monitor fluid balance
Hyperammonemia	Lethargy, malaise, coma, seizures	Discontinue amino acid infusions, infuse arginine	Avoid casein or fibrin hydrolysate
Essential fatty acid deficiency	Xerosis, hepatomegaly, impaired healing, bone changes	Fat administration	Provide >25–100 mg/kg/day of essential fatty acids
Hypophosphatemia	Lethargy, anorexia, weakness	Supplemental phosphate	Treat causative factors: alkalosis, gram-negative sepsis, vomiting, malabsorption; provide >20 mEq/1000 cal; provide balanced TPN solution
Abnormal liver enzymes	Fatty infiltrate in liver	Evaluate for other causes	Supply >0.35–0.45 mEq/kg/day
Hypomagnesemia	Weakness, nausea, vomiting, tremors, depression, hyporeflexia	Infuse 10% magnesium sulfate	Monitor serum levels
Hypermagnesemia	Drowsiness,nausea, vomiting, coma, arrhythmia	Dialysis, infuse calcium gluconate	

placement but may also include venous thrombosis related to an indwelling catheter.

Metabolic complications can generally be avoided by careful assessment of a patient's caloric and nitrogen requirements and serial monitoring of glucose, electrolytes, and fluid balance. Glucose intolerance is usually treated with insulin added to the TPN mixture to maintain normoglycemia although severe hyperglycemia may require discontinuation of the infusion or changing the formulation to provide more calories as lipids and less as glucose. Phosphorus, calcium, magnesium, and potassium are necessary for anabolic pathways and must be supplemented appropriately.

MONITORING PATIENTS ON NUTRITIONAL SUPPORT

Patients receiving enteral and parenteral nutrition should be closely monitored to prevent metabolic complications and to assess the adequacy of the therapy. Close monitoring of fluid status, glucose tolerance, and electrolytes on initiation of nutrition support is essential. In stable patients on a steady regimen, the monitoring interval can be extended; home nutritional support patients are generally followed on a monthly basis (Table 58–15).

Initially, I's and O's should be carefully documented as an assessment of the patient's fluid status. Weight changes on a daily basis reflect hydration, while weight gain measured over a more prolonged period indicates increasing lean body mass. High serum glucose and glucosuria are indicative of glucose intolerance, and insulin therapy should be instituted. Insulin requirements can be determined using a sliding scale system adjusting the amount of insulin administered based on the degree of hyperglycemia. For patients on TPN, the 24-hour insulin requirements can be added directly to the TPN solution once a steady dose has been achieved. Severe glucose intolerance may require replacing glucose calories with a lipid source. Serum electrolytes, calcium, phosphate and magnesium should be monitored and supplemented as necessary, and liver function studies should be checked periodically. Elevated blood urea nitrogen may reflect dehydration and prerenal azotemia or protein delivery, while serum triglyceride levels obtained 6 to 8 hours after lipid infusion confirm adequate fat metabolism. The prothrombin time should be checked intermittently to assess vitamin K supplementation.

In addition to monitoring for metabolic complications of nutritional support, the patient's nutritional status should be reassessed periodically to guide further treatment. Serum proteins including albumin, prealbumin and transferrin may be helpful, and serial anthropometric measurements provide an ongoing assessment of muscle mass and body fat. Particularly during the postoperative period, septic episodes, and aggressive adjuvant therapy, repeated indirect calorimetry (see Table 58–8), and nitrogen balance determinations should be used to assess changes in a patient's metabolic demands and protein requirements. Nitrogen balance can be estimated from measurements of 24-hour urinary urea nitrogen (UUN) using the following equation:

TABLE 58–15. MONITORING NUTRITIONAL SUPPORT PATIENTS

TEST	STARTING NUTRITIONAL SUPPORT	STABLE HOSPITALIZED PATIENT	HOME PATIENT
Body weight	Daily	Daily	Twice weekly
Intake	Every 8 h	Daily	Twice weekly
Output (urine, stool)	Every 8 h	Daily	Twice weekly
Urine glucose	Every 8 h	Every 8 hr	Twice weekly
Blood			
Glucose	Daily	Every other day	Weekly
Electrolytes	Daily	Every other day	Monthly
BUN/creatinine	Daily	Weekly	Monthly
Complete blood count	Weekly	Weekly	Monthly
Calcium, phosphorus	Weekly	Weekly	Monthly
Total protein, albumin	Weekly	Weekly	Monthly
Prealbumin, transferrin	Weekly	Weekly	Monthly
Liver function tests	Weekly	Weekly	Monthly
Prothrombin time	Weekly	Weekly	Monthly
Triglycerides	Weekly	Monthly	Monthly
Anthropometrics	Initial	Monthly	Monthly
Indirect calorimetry	Twice monthly	Twice monthly	As indicated
Nitrogen balance	Weekly	As indicated	As indicated

Nitrogen balance =

$$\frac{\text{protein (g) delivered}}{\text{6.25 g protein/g nitrogen}} - (\text{UUN(g)} + 4)$$

A negative nitrogen balance indicates a persistent catabolic state with ongoing depletion of visceral proteins and the need for additional protein supplementation. Indirect calorimetry and nitrogen balance calculations thus allow a more accurate definition of an individual's nutrient goals and optimization of the nutritional regimen.

SPECIALIZED FORMULAS

Although considered investigational, specific nutrients added to TPN or enteral solutions may play a protective role in decreasing morbidity and mortality associated with antineoplastic therapy and depressed immunity. L-Glutamine (1 to 2%) provided in TPN or added to polypeptide-based or elemental enteral formulas seems to have a protective effect on the intestinal tract and decrease chemotherapy-induced mucositis and enterocolitis. Other nutrients such as arginine, RNA, and omega-3 fatty acids may enhance immune function and affect morbidity and mortality in oncology patients. In addition to enhancing cellular immunity, arginine is a potent secretagogue inducing secretion of growth hormone, insulin, glucagon, and several GI hormones. RNA in the diet is essential for maturation of T cells in animal models. Omega-3 fatty acids in the diet alter prostaglandin synthesis and improve immune response to infectious challenges in animals. A recent clinical trial in postoperative patients with upper GI malignancies compared a standard enteral diet to a diet supplemented with arginine, RNA, and omega-3 fatty acids. Decreased wound complications, infections, and length of hospital stay were demonstrated in the supplemented group. Clearly, further clinical trials are indicated to confirm the potential benefits of these specialized regimens.

BIBLIOGRAPHY

Buzby GP. Perioperative total parenteral nutrition in surgical patients. The Veterans Affairs Total Parenteral Nutrition Cooperative Study Group. N Engl J Med 325:525–532, 1991

Buzby GP. Overview of randomized clinical trials of total parenteral nutrition for malnourished surgical patients. World J Surg 17:173–177, 1993

Daly JM, Lieberman MD, Goldfine J, et al. Enteral nutrition with supplemental arginine, RNA, and omega-3 fatty acids in patients after operation: immunologic, metabolic, and clinical outcome. Surgery 112:56–67, 1992

Daly JM, Redmond HP, Hallagher H. Perioperative nutrition in cancer patients. JPEN 16:100S–105S, 1992

De Cicco M, Panarllo G, Fantin D, et al. Parenteral nutrition in cancer patients receiving chemotherapy: Effects on toxicity and nutritional status. JPEN 17:513–518, 1993

DeWys D, Begg C, Lavin PT, et al. Prognostic effect of weight loss prior to chemotherapy in cancer patients. Am J Med 69:491–497, 1980

Guidelines for the use of parenteral and enteral nutrition in adult and pediatric patients. JPEN 17:1SA–26SA, 1993

Heber DB, Lauri O, Tchekmedyian NS. Hormonal and metabolic abnormalities in the malnourished cancer patient: Effects on host–tumor interaction. JPEN 16:60S–64S, 1992

Lipman TO. Clinical trials of nutritional support in cancer. Hematol/Oncol Clin North Am 5:91–102, 1991

Moldawer LL, Rogy MA, Lowry SF. The role of cytokines in cancer cachexia. JPEN 16:43S–49S, 1992

Nelson DA, Walsh D, Sheehan FA. The cancer anorexia–cachexia syndrome. J Clin Oncol 12:213–225, 1994

Rombeau JL, Caldwell MD. Clinical nutrition: Enteral and tube feeding. 2nd ed. Philadelphia: WB Saunders, 1990

Rombeau JL, Caldwell MD. Clinical nutrition: Parenteral nutrition. 2nd ed. Philadelphia: WB Saunders, 1993

Tchekmedyian NS, Halpert C, Ashley J, Heber D. Nutrition in advanced cancer: Anorexia as an outcome variable and target of therapy. JPEN 16:88S–92S, 1992

Weisdorf SA, Lysne J, Wind D, et al. Positive effect of prophylactic total parenteral nutrition on long term outcome of bone marrow transplantation. Transplantation 43: 833–838, 1987

Windsor JA. Underweight patients and the risks of major surgery. World J Surg 17:165–172, 1993

John S. Macdonald, Daniel G. Haller, Robert J. Mayer, Eds. *Manual of Oncologic Therapeutics*, Third Edition.

59. INFECTION IN THE PATIENT WITH NEOPLASTIC DISEASE

Robert W. Finberg

INTRODUCTION

Infections are the major cause of death in a variety of malignancies. Autopsy studies reveal infection as the cause of death in 75% of patients with acute leukemia, 50% of patients with lymphoma, and many patients with metastatic carcinoma. In addition approximately 80% of patients with acute leukemia and the majority of patients with a variety of other cancers (including chronic leukemias and multiple myeloma) develop infections, often multiple infections, during the course of their therapy for cancer[1,2].

With the advent of platelet transfusions to prevent bleeding complications and the use of more intensive chemotherapy, the number of patients who have infections complicating their course has increased. The number of infectious disease emergencies has increased as the number of emergencies related to bleeding has diminished.

This review will focus on defining the manner in which tumors predispose to infection, as well as the presentation and therapy of infections which present acutely or more subacutely in relation to an underlying diagnosis of malignancy. Therapy of each infectious complication will be addressed along with the underlying disease. Finally guidelines for the prevention of infections which complicate treatment of cancer will be considered.

WHY ARE PATIENTS WITH CANCER PREDISPOSED TO INFECTIONS?

Non-immune Predispositions

Patients with cancer are predisposed to develop infections for many completely different reasons (Table 59–1). Any break in the skin or mucous membrane layer which serves as the body's initial defense against the external environment may lead to bacterial invasion. The skin protects the host against infection in different ways: the intact skin provides a barrier which bacteria cannot penetrate, and the skin provides a dry surface which is not optimal for growth of most bacteria and fungi. For this reason skin tumors or any tumor which lead to breaks in the skin may create a new space for bacteria or fungi to invade the host. The use of occlusive dressings leads to an environment much more conducive to the growth of both fungi and bacteria. The outbreak of *Rhizopus*[3] associated with occlusive dressings or the association between *Aspergillus*[4] and catheters are examples of alterations in the skin leading to serious infections. The placement of an intravenous catheter provides a superhighway for bacteria to travel from the skin directly into the bloodstream.

Any tumor which occludes a tube or prevents the host from removing waste will lead to pooling of secretions and infection. An excellent example of this problem is the high incidence of pyelonephritis in patients who, as a result of either primary renal cancer or metastasis, occlude the ureters. Although pyelonephritis is most often an ascending disease found in women (because of the short urethra), in the setting of ureteral occlusion it may be seen in men and can occur with a very small bacterial inoculum (because the normal clearance mechanism of urine is compromised). For this reason a cancer-related mechanical occlusion will lead to an infection as a direct result of impairment of a normal clearance mechanism. Another example of this phenomenon is the case of a patient with lung cancer who occludes a bronchus and has a series of pneumonias. In this case the failure of the normal clearance mechanism leads to pooling of bacteria in the alveolar spaces with consequent pneumonia.

Both of these examples emphasize the need for the oncologist treating a patient with cancer to be aware of the risks of infection in patients with normal immune function but with cancer-associated mechanical compromise. The solution to such problems lies in finding some method of opening the closed tube (either radiation to remove compression in the case of the lung cancer patient, or conduits to open up ureters). In the case of a break in the skin, the best we can do is utilize our knowledge of bacterial and fungal growth requirements to minimize the opportunity for these pathogens to flourish.

Immune Predispositions

Aside from simple mechanical issues, host defense can be compromised in a large number of ways, all of which lead to infectious complications (Table 59–1). In addition to the cancer itself, chemotherapy compromises the body's response to microorganisms (Table 59–2). Treatment of cancer, especially in patients with hematologic malignancies who receive cytotoxic chemotherapy, is often complicated by the development of neutropenia. An absolute neutrophil level below 1000 cells/cc is correlated with an increased risk of developing infection[5,6]. This risk rises even further when the granulocyte level falls to less than 500. A falling granulo-

TABLE 59–1. HOW TUMORS PREDISPOSE PATIENTS WITH CANCER TO INFECTION

PREDISPOSING FACTOR	TYPE OF CANCER
BREAKS IN INTEGUMENT	Skin or epithelial Other tumors which penetrate skin or mucosal surfaces
OCCLUSION OF ORIFICES	Head and neck tumors, lung tumors, renal tumors, colon or rectum tumors which metastasize to abdominal and pelvic organs
LACK OF GRANULOCYTES	Leukemias, tumors metastating to the bone marrow
LACK OF ANTIBODIES	B cell malignancies, catabolic states or severe protein loss (through GI tract or third spacing)
IMPAIRED T-CELL IMMUNITY	Hodgkins disease, lymphomas, hairy cell leukemia

cyte level or a patient in relapse is even more predictive of infection[5,6].

Based on these data most clinicians use a figure of less than 500 granulocytes as a marker for a high risk of infection. A patient with less than 500 granulocytes has a much higher likelihood of having a bacterial or fungal infection, and having a serious or fatal infection. The setting also has prognostic implications. Patients whose granulocyte counts are increasing are much less likely to have fatal infections than those whose cell counts are falling[5,6]. In general the initial infections associated with neutropenia are likely to be bacterial. However, after a prolonged period of neutropenia (particularly following the use of anti-bacterial antibiotics), fungal infection becomes likely[7].

TABLE 59–2. MECHANISMS BY WHICH CHEMOTHERAPY PREDISPOSES TO INFECTION

Alkylating agents and DNA damaging drugs lead to a failure of wound healing and to breaks in the skin and mucosal surfaces.
A variety of chemotherapeutic agents lead to decreases in granulocytes and lymphopenia (especially alkylating agents).
Other drugs may specifically suppress lymphocyte function (*e.g.*, fludarabine).

INFECTIOUS DISEASE EMERGENCIES IN ONCOLOGY

Infections in cancer patients can be viewed as either acute or chronic. The infectious disease problems described below are unique because they demand an immediate response by the oncologist caring for the patient.

Overwhelming Infection Following Splenectomy

Patients with cancer are often splenectomized either for diagnostic reasons (*e.g.*, as part of staging for Hodgkin's disease) or for therapeutic reasons (*e.g.*, in hairy cell leukemia where the procedure is often utilized to avoid infections related to neutropenia). Even entirely normal hosts are put at risk by the loss of a spleen. The rate of overwhelming sepsis in patients with traumatic splenectomy has been estimated to be 0.18 cases per 100 person years with an estimate of serious infection at 7.16 infections per 100 years[8]. Although the immunologic consequences of splenectomy are often overrated (splenectomized patients will respond to antigenic challenge in a close to normal manner), the role of the spleen as a filter is often underrated by clinicians. The initial response to infection by *S. pneumonia*, *N. meningitis* or *H. influenza* involves a containment process by the spleen prior to antibody production. Without this splenic filter an otherwise minor infection may be lethal. Thus all patients who are splenectomized should be vaccinated against encapsulated organisms. In addition it is wise to counsel splenectomized patients to seek medical attention with any sign of infection and some clinicians give their patients antibiotics to take in case of infection; this is one of the rare infections in medicine in which a delay in treatment by a few hours can result in a fatal outcome. Treatment of the splenectomized patient with an undiagnosed infection should always include antibiotics with efficacy against *S. pneumonia*, *H. influenza*, and *N. meningitidis*.

Meningitis in Immunocompromised Patients

Although the most common causes of meningitis in normal hosts are *S. pneumonia* and *N. meningitidis*, and adults with meningitis are often treated with penicillin or third generation cephalosporins, a patient receiving cancer chemotherapy may be much more likely to have disease caused by *Listeria monocytogenes* or *Pseudomonas aeruginosa*[9]. Thus treatment with ampicillin (for *Listeria*) and antibiotics effective against aerobic gram-negative rods (usually a third generation cephalosporin — see below), especially if there has been associated bacteremia, is indicated in the absence of a diagnosis. *Cryptococcus neoformans* should be high in the list of differential diagnoses in any patients with Hodgkin's disease, other lymphomas, or in any patients post-transplantation or receiving steroid chemotherapy.

Similarly, although brain abscess in normal hosts is likely to be caused by a mixture of anaerobic and aerobic bacteria, in cancer patients, fungal abscess is probably more likely. Neutropenic patients are prone to the development of brain abscesses with *Candida*, *Nocardia*, and *Aspergillus* as a result of hematogenous infection. As in patients with AIDS, *Toxoplasmosis* is a common cause of both brain abscess and meningitis in immunocompromised cancer patients[9]

Other Infectious Disease Emergencies in Cancer Patients

In addition to CNS presentations, other infectious disease emergencies in this patient population include situations in which the tumor (or its therapy) result in the blockage of a natural drainage pathway for organisms (see Table 59–1). In situations such as occluded ureters it is imperative to deal quickly with the situation in order to avoid permanent renal damage. Similarly occlusion of the GI tract or lung may result in a situation which requires urgent intervention. A series of malignancies are associated with defects which predispose to specific infections (Table 59–3). Granulocytopenia (neutropenia) is a common result of chemotherapy for several cancers (see below).

An Approach to Febrile Patients Who Are Neutropenic

One of the most common infectious disease emergencies seen in cancer patients occurs in the setting of neutropenia. As noted above, patients with neutropenia not only have a higher incidence of infection but also a higher incidence of fatalities when they are infected. The recognition that it was necessary to treat patients with fever and neutropenia with antibiotics prior to documentation of the specific infection has led to a great improvement in the outcomes in treatment of patients with fever and neutropenia. Initial studies using narrow spectrum antimicrobial agents in this setting resulted in the appearance of organisms not covered by the antibiotics used. Much of the literature which deals with patients in this clinical setting (and the literature is voluminous) is based on studies with patients with hematological malignancies (particularly AML)[10]. Since these tumors do not usually present with fever as a sign of the tumor it is a reasonable assumption in this setting that the presence of fever means there is an infection. In the case of many solid tumors (especially renal cell carcinoma and metastatic tumors of the liver) the presence of fever may be attributed to the tumor alone. Thus the patient's underlying disease as well as the history of previous infectious problems is critical in approaching diagnosis and treatment of the febrile cancer patient.

TABLE 59–3. INFECTIOUS DISEASE EMERGENCIES

LIFE-THREATENING	UNDERLYING PREDISPOSING FACTOR
Overwhelming bacterial infection	Splenectomy
Overwhelming bacterial infection	Granulocytopenia
Overwhelming bacterial infection	Antibody deficiency
Overwhelming viral infection	T-cell deficiency
Overwhelming parasitic infection	T-cell/B-cell deficiency

In the 1970s most infections in patients with leukemia were caused by gram-negative aerobic rods (especially *Pseudomonas aeruginosa*). These organisms are frequently normal gut organisms although they may be nasopharyngeal organisms which have colonized patients entering the hospital. In recent years bacteremias in most cancer hospitals have been caused by gram-positive organisms. *Staphylococcus aureus*, *S. epidermidis*, and *Streptococcus viridans* have been the most common organisms isolated from neutropenic patients at the Dana-Farber Cancer Institute (DFCI) in the last 3 years (R. Finberg, M. Lew, unpublished). However, because of the possibility of infection with gram-negative rods it is still necessary to provide treatment for a broad spectrum of organisms. The following is a general approach to the diagnosis and treatment of infection in cancer patients with fever and neutropenia.

1. *Physical examination with careful attention to sites likely to be infected in this patient population is indicated.*
   Of note is the fact that many diseases which present with characteristic physical findings in patients with adequate white cells, have different physical findings in neutropenic patients (*e.g.*, pneumonia often presents without consolidation and even without X-ray changes). Cellulitis may present with minimal erythema. The perirectal area is more likely to be a problem in monocytic leukemias but may be a site of infection in AML or ALL as well[11]. Those infections are associated with bacteremias with Enterobacteriaceae, and coverage for Bacteroides fragilis is not necessary. In fact, although perirectal problems are common, most clinical experience indicates that ticarcillin and an aminoglycoside provides excellent coverage[11,12,13]. In the last decade, with the increased use of long-term indwelling iv access devices, these devices have become a major portal of infection and now account for many (if not most) of our infections in neutropenic patients[14].
2. *Laboratory studies to be obtained in the initial evaluation of a patient with fever in the setting of neutropenia.*
   A reasonable series of microbiological studies to obtain on a febrile, neutropenic patient are outlined in Table 59–4. Obviously the history is important in determining whether other studies may be important. A history of exposure to TB as well as a travel history and history of exposures to parasites is important in the initial approach to the host. Table 59–4 lists a series of cultures which should be obtained.

TABLE 59–4. INITIAL MICROBIOLOGICAL STUDIES IN PATIENTS WITH FEVER AND NEUTROPENIA

At least 2 blood cultures
Urine (including gram stain), as cells may be absent in the face of infection
Throat and stool cultures to look for a predominant pathogen
Sputum (if possible)
Fluid samples: pleural or peritoneal fluid if indicated, aspiration of vesicles
Skin biopsy of suspicious lesions
CSF—only with CNS symptoms (look for organisms in the absence of cells in these patients)

X-ray studies are also likely to be useful in the initial evaluation, as well as in following the progression of neutropenia. Chest X-rays are mandatory (since physical exam is likely to be negative). Neutropenic patients are likely to have findings on X-ray but lack physical exam findings[15,16]. CAT scans with sinus cuts or MRI studies should be obtained if nasal lesions, facial cellulitis, or tenderness suggest disease.

3. *Initial antibiotic regimens for treatment of patients with fever and neutropenia.*
The approach to the febrile neutropenic patient should be determined not only by the patient's past history but also by the antibiotic resistant pattern of the hospital or community in which the patient has been living. Possible initial antibiotic treatment approaches are discussed below and some dosage guidelines follow:
   a. Use of a penicillin/aminoglycoside combination. A combination of a semi-synthetic penicillin with activity against *Pseudomonas aeruginosa* (*e.g.*, mezlocillin) in combination with an aminoglycoside is still a good initial therapy for patients with fever and neutropenia in hospitals without many resistant organisms[10,13].
   b. A cephalosporin (or cephamycin or carbapenem) with anti-*Pseudomonas* activity (see p. 420 for several possibilities) alone may be substituted for patients with serious renal dysfunction or pre-existing auditory or vestibular problems, in whom *Pseudomonas* is not suspected. In some trials single antibiotics (third generation cephalosporins) have been associated with the development of resistance to these antibiotics (especially by *Pseudomonas*)[17]. A large study predominated by patients with leukemia indicates that ceftazidime is useful as a single agent with the same caveats as above[18]. The advantage of ceftazidime lies in its coverage of *Pseudomonas* and the theoretical possibility that its poor anaerobic activity leads to less disruption of the bowel flora. Imipenem is also efficacious in this setting. However imipenem, which has much better anaerobic coverage, may lead to C. *difficile* diarrhea. The same argument probably applies to Timentin (ticarcillin and clavulinic acid) and Zosyn (piperacillin and tazabactam). A series of papers document the fact that double β-lactam combinations are similarly efficacious, but they are not demonstrably better. Cases of antagonism have been documented, and bone marrow depression may occur as a result of the use of β-lactam antibiotics[19,20,21].
   c. For patients with a history of severe reactions to penicillins (urticaria and anaphylaxis) a variety of alternatives have been shown to be acceptable: clindamycin has been used with gentamicin, and trimethoprim/sulfamethoxazole can also be used together with an aminoglycoside in this setting[22]. Ciprofloxacin, although it has a broad spectrum of activity, should not be given as a single agent in this setting because of its poor gram-positive activity[23]. The combination of vancomycin and aztreonam has a broad spectrum of activity (but would be a poor choice if anaerobic infection was a possibility).
   d. In the setting of *Pseudomonas* bacteremia (and possibly other gram negatives), one should always use a β-lactam/aminoglycoside combination for a prolonged course of therapy[24]. Tobramycin is more effective in the treatment of *Pseudomonas* than gentamicin.
   e. Guidelines for antibiotic dosing and administration.
      i. Aminoglycoside dosing
      Gentamicin (and tobramycin) are usually dosed at 1–2 mg/kg iv every 8 hours. In young people with normal renal function dosing should probably begin at 2 mg/kg. Amikacin is dosed at 7.5 mg/kg every 12 hours. Serum levels should be checked within 24–48 hours and monitored at least weekly. Therapeutic peak gentamicin levels are between 4 and 12 μg/ml. We usually aim for a peak of 6–10 μg/ml. The peak level is routinely measured $\frac{1}{2}$ hour after a $\frac{1}{2}$ hour infusion of the drug has ended. The trough levels are measured immediately prior to the next dose. Trough levels >2 and peak levels >12 correlate with toxicity. High trough levels are the most reliable predictors of toxicity. Therapeutic amikacin levels are between 20 and 30 mg/ml and toxic levels >60.
      Patients who are young, lean and febrile may require very large doses of aminoglycosides. Although single dosing of aminoglycosides has not been extensively tested in this patient group there is no evidence that more frequent dosing (more than 3 times per day) is indicated. Conversely, aminoglycosides should be given with care in the elderly and in patients with renal failure. Audiograms should be performed on patients who will receive long-term aminoglycoside therapy.
      ii. Because of the problem with gram-positive organisms (particularly S. *epidermidis*) many

patients are treated with vancomycin at some time during the course of their neutropenic episode. It is not clear that the vancomycin needs to be added prior to isolation of *S. epidermidis*, however[25]. Some guidelines about vancomycin follow:

(a) Vancomycin is not an antipyretic. It will not make neutropenic patients become afebrile. The concept of "planned progressive" antibiotic dosing (the practice of adding more and more antibiotics to patients who remain febrile) is not of proven efficacy, and may lead to more side effects rather than more efficacy.

(b) Vancomycin should be given iv over at least 30 minutes. Rapid infusion leads to histamine release and the "red-man" or "red-neck" syndrome. It may also be associated with hypotension and the "pain and spasm syndrome." The incidence of occurrence of these symptoms ranges from 3%–47% depending on the series[26,27]. These symptoms may be overcome by giving 500 mg over 1 hr or 1 gm over 2 hr, although it has been our experience that some patients have trouble tolerating the drug despite slow infusion as well as prophylactic antihistamines.

(c) Vancomycin can be given at a dose of 500 mg q 6 h or 1 gm q 12 h. It is more convenient to give it q 12 h.

(d) Vancomycin is not nephrotoxic in patients who have normal renal function. It may be a problem when given with an aminoglycoside (particularly if not carefully monitored)[28].

(e) In patients who have improved, renal function levels should be measured (troughs less than ten are reasonable) and dosage can be calculated on the basis of the nomogram of Matzke et al.[29].

f. What are the indications for coverage of anaerobic organisms in patients with fever and neutropenia? Bacteremias from most perirectal lesions in the febrile neutropenic patient are associated with aerobic gram negatives. If *Bacteroides fragilis* is documented or strongly suspected as a pathogen (bowel perforation or abscesses), clindamycin or metronidazole (Flagyl) could be used. In general, metronidazole is preferred. However, this is a rare cause of morbidity in this patient population. In fact patients with rectal lesions (which are common with acute leukemia — particularly monocytic leukemias) most commonly have infections with gram-negative aerobic rods, and these respond well to penicillins and aminoglycosides[11,12]. It is usually not necessary to add metronidazole.

g. What is the role for additional antibiotics in this setting?

i. Aminoglycosides

(a) **Tobramycin:** more active against *Pseudomonas* than gentamicin but less active against some *E. coli* and *Serratia*. Tobramycin should be employed if there is reason to suspect *P. aeruginosa* infection.

(b) **Amikacin:** likely to be active against gentamicin (and tobramycin) resistant gram-negative rods; should be employed if there is reason to suspect resistant organisms.

ii. Penicillins

(a) **Ticarcillin:** This drug has better anti-*Pseudomonas* activity than carbenicillin (and at half the dosage of carbenicillin and therefore less salt, less platelet dysfunction). Ticarcillin has replaced carbenicillin but has the same broad spectrum of activity, including good anaerobic activity[29].

(b) **Azlocillin:** more active than ticarcillin against *Pseudomonas* (2–4 fold) but less active against other gram negatives

(c) **Piperacillin:** has more activity against *Klebsiella* than azlocillin. See below for piperacillin and tazobactam

(d) **Mezlocillin:** has approximately the same activity as ticarcillin against *Pseudomonas*, but like azlocillin more activity against *Klebsiella* and *Serratia*, and less salt[29].

(e) **Timentin:** This is a combination of ticarcillin with clavulinic acid (a β-lactamase inhibitor), and expands the activity of ticarcillin to include oxacillin sensitive *S. aureus*. It is not active against oxacillin resistant *S. aureus* or resistant *S. epidermidis*. Therefore, we have not seen any reason to use it routinely. It has the disadvantage of being effective against *B. fungilis* and therefore is likely to wipe out the anaerobic flora, eliminate "colonization resistance," and predispose to *C. difficile* diarrhea.

(f) **Unasyn:** ampicillin and sulbactam — similar to timentin (above) in that it is a semi-synthetic with a β-lactamase inhibitor, but the half-life of sulbactam is longer and parallels the half-life of the ampicillin, making it a better combination. It is used in children to treat *H. influenzae* as well as gram positives.

(g) **Zosyn** (the brand name for piperacillin/tazobactam combination): This combination of piperacillin and a β-lactam inhibitor has a wide spectrum of activity (including *B. fragilis*), but does not have any more activity against *Pseudomonas aeruginosa* than piperacillin alone. The recommended adult dose is 3 grams piperacillin/375 mg tazobactam every 6 hours. The efficacy of this drug in the neutropenic population is not yet established, and it should not be used for serious *Pseudomonas* infections.

iii. Cephalosporins and related drugs

(a) **Cefazolin (Kefzol. Anef):** This drug has a spectrum similar to cephalothin, can be given im, and is not advised for *Staph endocarditis*, since failures have been noted in this setting.

(b) **Cefamandole (Mandol):** The spectrum of this agent includes *H. influenzae*, certain cephalothin-resistant Enterobacteriaceae, including resistant *E. coli*, Enterobacter, and indole positive proteus. Both cefamandole and cefoxitin (see below) are potent inducers of β-lactamases and both *in vitro* and *in vivo*[19] resistance has been reported to develop with treatment. Resistance usually develops in the extended spectrum organisms (cephalothin-resistant *E. coli*, Enterobacter). For this reason it is contraindicated to give either cefamandole or cefoxitin with another penicillin or cephalosporin. It is not to be used for *Pseudomonas* infections.

(c) **Cefoxitin (Mefoxitin):** Extends spectrum of cephalothin to include *Bacteroides fragilis* as well as some of resistant *E. coli, proteus, serratia. Cefoxitin and cefamandole are potent inducers of β lactamases and should not be given with other β lactam antibiotics (see above). This may apply to the drugs listed below, but has not been established.*

(d) **Cefotaxime (Claforan):** Cefotaxime has good gram-positive activity and can be used for treatment of susceptible meningitis. It is a first line drug for meningitis due to susceptible organisms, but it is not effective against *Listeria*.

(e) **Ceftazidime (Fortaz):** Ceftazidime has good activity against *Pseudomonas*, relatively poor staph activity, and is a poor anaerobic agent. This drug can be used as a first-line agent in febrile neutropenic patients in whom no culture data are available[18]. The maximum dose is 2 grams q 8 h.

(f) **Ceftriaxone (Rocephin):** This long-acting broad spectrum agent can be given on a daily or twice a day basis. It has a good gram-negative (although activity against *Pseudomonas* is not as good as ceftazidime) and gram-positive spectrum. It is given at doses of 1–2 g every 12–24 hours. The chief advantages are (1) it crosses into cerebrospinal fluid (CSF) well and (2) it can be given daily.

(g) **Cefoperazone (Cefobid):** Cefoperazone is a third generation cephalosporin which is associated with disulfiram-like reactions after alcohol ingestion. It has a broad gram-negative (although it does not have good activity against acinetobacter) and gram-positive activity.

(h) **Ceftizoxime (Ceftizox):** Ceftizoxime is a third generation cephalosporin with activity against *Pseudomonas* and some activity against anaerobes. The recommended dose is 1–4 g q 8 h.

(i) **Cefsulodin (Cefomonil):** Poor gram-positive coverage; useful only against *Pseudomonas*; may be used in *Pseudomonas* infections.

iv. Other antibiotics and combinations

(a) **Imipenem: thienamycin/cilastatin (Primaxin):** This is a drug combination consisting of carbapenem (thienamycin — a modified β-lactam drug compound) which is given with another drug (cilastatin) to prevent degradation and assure urine levels. Imipenem has a good gram-negative and gram-positive spectrum (includes *S. fecalis* but not *S. fecium*) with good activity against *Listeria* and nocardia and good anaerobic coverage (including *B. fragilis*). It may been given in a dose of 1 g q 6 h and has utility against *enterococcus* and resistant *Pseudomonas*[31]. Its exact place in the therapeutic armamentarium has not been defined. *Because of its association with seizures (particularly in patients with renal failure) it may not be good therapy for patients with seizure disorders and dosing should be adjusted for renal failure.*

(b) **Aztreonam (Azactam):** A monobactam (these have increased stability to β-lactamases), is active against most gram-negative organisms (but not acinetobacter, *P. maltophila* or *P. cepacia*)[32]. It is not active against staph, streptococci, anaerobes. The dose is 1–2 g q 6–8 h. *It is not a substitute for an aminoglycoside and should not be used this way.*

(c) **Norfloxacin (Noroxin):** Norfloxacin is a nalidixic acid derivative which has efficacy as a prophylactic agent equal to trimethoprim/sulfa. It is a good urinary tract drug but does not assure high serum levels. This agent has been used in antibiotic prophylaxis studies.

(d) **Ciprofloxacin(Cipro):** Ciprofloxacin is a nalidixic acid derivative with a very broad spectrum of activity which includes *Pseudomonas aeruginosa*. It is well absorbed po but can be given iv. A prophylactic study in bone marrow transplants at DFCI demonstrates efficacy[33].

(e) **Metronidazole (Flagyl):**Metronidazole is an excellent anaerobic drug. It is a good agent for use in the treatment of bowel perforation. It has little activity against aerobes (so it is usually given in combination with other agents in this setting. This drug is the drug of choice for fusobacterium and *Bacteroides fragilis* infections. The dose is 7.5 mg/kg (usually approximately 500 mg with a maximum dose not to exceed 4 g/day).

v. What about synergistic antibiotic combinations?

When the newer penicillins are combined with cefoxitin and (to a lesser extent cefamandole) there may be antagonism between the two drugs. Therefore it is contraindicated to give them together[19]. The possibility of antagonism with third generation cephalosporins (*e.g.*, cefotaxime, ceftazidime) has not been defined. In our hospital we usually discourage double β-lactam combinations in neutropenic patients because antibiotic resistance is not a problem; they may be marrow toxic[20,21], and they lead to more rashes. There is very little data that double β-lactam combinations are superior to single drugs, and since the toxicity and allergic reactions are multiplied by using two, we don't usually recommend their use. The issue is not settled, however, and may vary depending on the resistance pattern of a given hospital[10].

4. *Management after 48 to 72 hours (when cultures are back)*

a. Microbiologically documented infections

If an organism is documented as the causative agent of the infection in this setting, the antibiotics should be adjusted to the organisms found without sacrificing spectrum. In the case of gram-negative bacteremia it is best to treat with both a penicillin (or cephalosporin) plus an aminoglycoside to which the organism is sensitive[24]. However the spectrum should not be sacrificed, because this may lead to infection with organisms which are not covered by the antibiotics used. We can consider the following possibilities in the case of episodes in which we have isolated an organism:

i. Patient becomes *afebrile, neutrophils increase*

(a) If no focus of infection has been demonstrated (and the organism isolated is presumed to have come from the bowel as a consequence of chemotherapy) we usually favor a very short course of therapy.

(b) If a focus of infection is found (pneumonia, abscess, pyelonephritis, sinusitis) a full course of therapy (7–14 days) is indicated.

ii. Patient remains *febrile, neutrophils increase*:

If the patient remains febrile despite a rise in the granulocyte count to a "safe level" (greater than 500 neutrophils) the clinician should consider a hidden site of infection, drug fever, or an abscess. If the patient does not respond after a course of therapy but cultures are negative, antibiotics should usually be stopped. In this case either drug fever or an occult focus of infection (which is not being treated by the current regimen) should be high on the list of differential diagnoses.

iii. Patient becomes *afebrile* but *neutrophils* remain *low;* most clinicians will continue the antibiotics until neutrophils increase (see below).

iv. Patient stays *febrile* and *neutrophils* remain *low*

In this setting most clinicians will consider early empiric amphotericin. The presence of a culture for a bacterial pathogen does not rule out fungal infection and the longer the patient is neutropenic and on antibacterials, the higher the possibility of fungal infection[7, 34, 35].

b. Fever and neutropenia without documented infection

If there is no organism isolated we still presume that the patient is infected as long as he/she is febrile and neutropenic. The following are the clinical possibilities for this situation with guidelines as to management.

i. Afebrile, neutrophils > 500 — stop antibiotics

If the patient defervesces and the granulocytes rise most clinicians will stop antibiotics immediately.

ii. Febrile, neutrophils > 500 — stop antibiotics

If the patient remains febrile but the granulocytes rise the patient is no longer at high risk for a fatal infection, and under most circumstances the antibiotics can be stopped in this situation unless there is evidence of infection.

iii. Afebrile, neutrophils down — continue antibiotics. Pizzo et al. found an increased incidence of fatal complications in those patients who stopped antibiotics after 7 days at a time when they were afebrile[36]. Because the patient is still at high risk for fatal infections most clinicians will continue to treat neutropenic patients with antibiotics in this setting.

iv. *Febrile*, neutrophils low, what do you do?

Pizzo et al. randomized a small group of patients in this category[35]. Those who stopped antibiotics (to prevent superinfection) had a much higher risk of bacterial death than those who were continued on anti-bacterial agents. Those who did not receive amphotericin-B had a much higher incidence of fungal infection[35].

It is our practice to add amphotericin-B if there is a high clinical suspicion of fungal disease. We do not *automatically* treat with amphotericin-B because of the high morbidity of treatment in adults (especially elderly patients). A cooperative group study does demonstrate a difference in incidence of deep seated fungal disease in patients treated with amphotericin B beginning on day 4 of antibiotic treatment[34]. A number of studies suggest that empiric addition of amphotericin-B is a logical maneuver.

Because of the problem with fungal infections many groups have looked at alternative treatment protocols. Whether fluconazole, which clearly has activity in prophylaxis of *Candida* infection (see below), will be as effective in this patient population has yet to be thoroughly studied. Similarly, whether itraconzole (which has a wider spectrum of activity and is a better *aspergillus* drug) would be a better agent, or whether one of the new imidazoles (*e.g.*, saperconazole) will have activity is not yet settled.

5. *Subsequent management 72 hours+*
If no organism is isolated after the initial evaluation, consider the following clinical situations:
   a. If the patient continues to be febrile, repeated physical exams and chest X-rays are indicated[37]. Blood cultures are the single most reliable tool for documenting infections in this setting.
   b. What if the patient develops "breakthrough" bacteremia?
   If sensitivities are not known and the patient is desperately ill, it might be reasonable to switch to another antibiotic on the presumption that the offending organism is resistant (*e.g.*, vancomycin in the case of gram-positive cocci and amikacin in the case of gram-negative rods). However, the frequency with which this maneuver is employed depends on the resistance pattern of the hospital (as well as prior exposure of the patient to antibiotics) . Some "breakthrough" bacteremias are with sensitive organisms. Optimization of antibiotic therapy is certainly indicated (with high peak levels and frequent aminoglycoside doses). In general we use two drugs to which the organism is sensitive for initial therapy of gram-negative rods in neutropenic patients[24]. There are no data which mandate the use of two drugs for gram-positive organisms (except enterococcus). *In general switching antibiotics is not indicated for fever alone, as this only leads to drug toxicity and confusion.*
6. *When do you take out the line?*
In general, patients with acute leukemia tolerate Hickman lines well, and we treat many infected lines with antibiotics without removal (particularly if the infecting organism is *S. epidermidis*[14]. However, subcutaneous tunnel infections are an indication for removal and a local cellulitis may lead to extensive skin necrosis in a neutropenic patient. It is a difficult issue to decide when to pull the line. All authorities agree that most of the time it is not necessary, and there are circumstances when pulling the line will either save the patient's life or prevent major reconstructive surgery in the future. Treatment of lines infected with *Candida* is especially likely to fail. Line infections with *S. aureus* infection can be problematic[38]. Passing a new catheter over a guide wire is probably not a good idea[14].
7. *When do you give granulocyte transfusions?*
Early reports indicated that therapeutic administration of granulocytes were helpful in cases of documented gram-negative bacteremia[39,40]. The data are most convincing in the case of *Pseudomonas* bacteremia. Recent reports have emphasized the lack of success in many instances (particularly when only small numbers of cells are administered[41]) and the side effects of therapy (cytomegalovirus transmission and unexplained pulmonary infiltrates, particularly when patients are receiving amphotericin-B) have made investigators chary about the use of granulocytes even in the presence of gram-negative bacteremia. Investigators are currently giving donors cytokines (*e.g.*, G-CSF) to increase their yields with the hope that they may be able to utilize this modality more effectively.

ORGAN SYSTEM SPECIFIC INFECTIOUS COMPLICATIONS OF CHEMOTHERAPY

In approaching the cancer patient with an infection the clinician should note that certain characteristic findings may allow a specific diagnosis to be made. We have grouped these signs by organ system and their therapeutic implications are briefly described

Skin

Careful attention to examination of the skin may be very informative. Ecthyma can present in an amazingly innocent manner and can be a warning to begin, increase antibiotic doses, or switch antibiotics. Disseminated candidiasis may present as a macular-papular rash and biopsy (with histology) may be more sensitive than blood cultures for making a diagnosis.

CNS

Approximately 20% of patients with disseminated *Candida* infection have retinal lesions, making a careful ophthalmological exam mandatory. However in most cases the lesions are not seen until the granulocytes increase, so a "false negative" result may be obtained if you look during the period of neutropenia.

As noted above, meningitis in cancer patients may be caused by an entirely different group of organisms than is seen in normal hosts[9]. In addition to conventional pathogens toxoplasmosis must be considered as a cause of space-occupying lesions in the brain.

GI

Oral lesions are common in patients receiving chemotherapy and may be a portal of entry for bacteria or fungi. Acute necrotizing ulcerative gingivitis (ANUG) is an opportunistic spirochetal infection sometimes reported in young people. It may be a forerunner of NOMA (also referred to as *Cancrum oris* or gangrenous mucositis). Although originally described in children with poor oral hygiene it is more common in patients on chemotherapy[42,43]. Fusospirochetes, nonfragilis bacteroides and gram-negative aerobes (including *Pseudomonas*) have been implicated in NOMA. *Clostridium difficile* may cause toxin-related diarrhea or pseudomembranous colitis. Although *C. difficile*-induced diarrhea usually responds to stopping antibiotics, if the drugs are to be continued, treatment is often warranted. Vancomycin 125 mg q 6 h po is acceptable therapy[44].

Typhlitis is defined as a necrotizing colitis which specifically affects the cecum. It is seen in the setting of granulocytopenia and presents with severe abdominal pain (sometimes localized to the right lower quadrant (RLQ) so that it mimics appendicitis), and fever. The disease appears to be more common in children and is said to be responsible for 50% of surgical abdomens in children with leukemia[45,46].

Pathologically the disease process is confined to the cecum and there are few polys present. *Pseudomonas* is the most commonly isolated organism. It may be present with or without an associated vasculitis[45,46].

The most common radiologic finding is a mass effect in the right lower quadrant. Bowel edema may result in "thumb printing" in some cases, or thickening of the bowel wall[47].

Therapeutically, the early cases reported were made at autopsy and no intervention was recommended; however, later reports have demonstrated that the patients can successfully withstand surgery and some have recommended cecectomies [46].

Rectal infection is common in acute leukemia (and as noted previously is usually associated with aerobic gram-negative rods). In general we do not drain infectious sites unless there is an accumulation of pus, but in the case of necrotic lesions or expanding fasciitis, there may be a role for surgery[48], and drainage of a local accumulation may be indicated in the face of persistent bacteremia.

Veno-occlusive disease (VOD) is characterized by fever, right upper quadrant (RUQ) tenderness and abnormal liver function tests, and is seen in approximately 10% of bone marrow transplants. It is attributed to the effects of chemotherapy on the endothelial surface. Pathologically there is obliteration of the small venules without fibrin. The differential diagnosis of this complex of symptoms includes CMV infection, GVH (in allogeneic transplant patients), and obstructive biliary disease. Liver-spleen scan (said to demonstrate a characteristic shift in the blood flow to the lungs) and ultrasound (to rule out Budd-Chiari syndrome) may be helpful in sorting out the diagnosis. Clinically this syndrome usually presents with ascites and a bilirubin which is raised out of proportion to the other LFTs.

Lung Infections in Cancer Patients

Pulmonary infiltrates are one of the most difficult problems to deal with in immunocompromised patients. As a general rule, if culture from the histological examination of bronchial lavage fluid (especially in the case of *P. carinii* pneumonia) is not diagnostic, a biopsy will be necessary to make a definitive diagnosis[49]. However, transbronchial biopsies are often impossible in this group of patients, because of thrombocytopenia. If the patient has an X-ray picture compatible with *Pneumocystis carinii* in a disease where this organism is likely, it is wise to treat initially with trimethoprim and sulfa. In patients who have received irradiation, radiation- or drug-induced pneumonitis should be considered, and may respond dramatically to steroids. It is worth remembering that diffuse interstitial infiltrates are unlikely to be caused by bacterial processes, and if a therapeutic decision is to be made on the basis of a biopsy, it is better to do it *earlier in the course rather* than after it is already too late.

Diffuse infiltrates are compatible with viral illnesses which may be much more severe in immunocompromised hosts. Measles virus may cause severe disease[50]. Other respiratory viruses have been reported to cause persistent or fatal infections. Both respiratory syncytial virus (RSV) and parainfluenza have produced severe disease in bone marrow transplant recipients[51,52].

CHRONIC INFECTIONS IN ONCOLOGY PATIENTS

The herpes group viruses (HSV, VZV, CMV, EBV, HHu6), by virtue of their prevalence in the population and their ability to reactivate during periods of immunosuppression, are a major cause of morbidity and mortality in cancer patients (Table 59–5). In situations in which intensive chemotherapy is used (*e.g.*, bone marrow transplantation), 80% of patients excrete herpes simplex[53]. Herpes simplex is a cause of a variety of infections in patients with hematological malignancy and can cause fatal pneumonia in some individuals[53].

The majority of viral infections in children or adults on chemotherapy are uneventful. However, the family of herpes

TABLE 59–5. CHRONIC INFECTIONS ASSOCIATED WITH MALIGNANCY

Tuberculosis
Varicella zoster virus
Cytomegalovirus
Herpes simplex
Human herpes virus 6
Epstein-Barr virus
BK, JC viruses
HTLV-1
HIV-1

viruses (herpes simplex viruses, types 1 and 2; cytomegalovirus, varicella-zoster virus, and Epstein-Barr virus) cause potentially life-threatening disease in some immunosuppressed children. Herpes virus 6 (HHV6) has also been reported to cause disease in immunocompromised patients (Table 59–5).

In addition to the herpes group viruses, several other persistent viruses have been associated with disease in cancer patients. Progessive multifocal leukoencephalopathy (PML) is a neurological disorder presenting with dementia, seizures, and a variety of focal neurologic defects. The disease is seen in immunocompromised patients. It has been associated with the papovavirus JC which, like the BK virus, can be cultured from the urine of immunocompromised patients[55]. Treatment of PML with interferon and cytarabine has been reported[56], but the disease is usually fatal.

HIV infection should be considered in patients who have been transfused or have other risk factors.

Because of the frequency and severity of the herpes group virus infections in cancer patients we will discuss each and its consequences and therapy.

Herpes Simplex

Both HSV-1 and HSV-2 can cause severe disease in patients receiving chemotherapy. Chronic progressive mucocutaneous lesions are seen in both the oral and genital area. Acyclovir has been demonstrated to be very efficacious in treatment of these infections[56]. In addition acyclovir prophylaxis is effective in the prevention of HSV reactivations in these patients[53,57]. In bone marrow transplant recipients reactivation occurs in 80% of patients and is associated with severe mucositis. Prophylaxis with acyclovir is effective in preventing virus replication and in ameliorating mucositis[53].

Varicella Zoster

Chickenpox is the expression of primary VZV infection in the nonimmune person. The reported mortality of chickenpox in children with ALL or lymphomas is 5%–10%, and 30% will have disseminated disease. The clinical features of the disease include an incubation period of 10–21 days with new vesicle formation occuring longer than in normal patients (1–5 days). New vesicle formation beyond 7 days predicts a severe course.

Visceral involvement, including pneumonia (with an X-ray picture of nodular densities superimposed on perihilar infiltration and patchy consolidation) is the most frequent cause of death, and there is a high rate of associated bacterial sepsis (50%). Other complications, including a mild hepatitis, pancreatic disease, and small bowel obstruction have been reported. Susceptibility to chickenpox is determined by history and/or presence of serum antibody to VZV. Patients with history of chickenpox are not at risk of varicella (except possibly bone marrow transplant recipients), but they may develop zoster.

Unexposed patients with negative history of chickenpox may be candidates for VZV vaccine if it becomes licensed. An investigational live attenuated VZV vaccine was shown to be efficacious when given to children with ALL in remission for at least one year. If an immunocompromised patient with negative history is exposed to chickenpox, serology for VZV should be obtained immediately. If the VZV antibody titer is negative or unknown, Varicella Zoster immune globulin (VZIG) should be administered within 4 days of exposure, but preferably as early as possible. The dose is 1 vial per 10 kg im to a maximum of 5 vials.

Patients with lesions compatible with Varicella should have the base of the lesion scraped and applied to a slide for immunofluorescence antibody staining to confirm the diagnosis. After diagnosis they should immediately begin treatment with iv Acyclovir 500 mg/m^2 or 10 mg/kg every 8 hours for 7 days (or until the lesions have crusted). Note that this is more than twice the dose recommended for Herpes Simplex (5 mg/kg q 8 h) or 250 mg/m^2).

The patients should be isolated in negative pressure rooms and VZIG (Varicella Zoster immune globulin) may begiven to susceptible clinic or hospital contacts.

Herpes Zoster (shingles) occurs in persons who have previously had chickenpox. In normal people, the incidence of zoster is 0.1% in the first decade of life, and rises to approximately 10% by the seventh decade. The clinical episode begins with pain in the involved dermatome. Fever occurs within days, accompanied by a localized vesicular eruption, which may persist for up to three weeks. Severe post-herpetic neuralgia is a serious problem in older patients, but is infrequent in children. Zoster is roughly ten times more common in patients on chemotherapy. A St. Jude's study found the incidence of zoster to be 22% in childhood Hodgkin's, 9% in ALL, 5% in children with solid tumors, and 0.72% in childhood AML. Zoster is less worrisome than chickenpox in this population (bone marrow transplants are an exception). In the St. Jude's study, 50% had spread beyond the dermatome (cutaneous dissemination), but only 12% had visceral complications (pneumonia, encephalitis, hepatitis, iritis, pancreatitis), and only 3% died[58].

The standard treatment for immunocompromised patients is iv Acyclovir (500 mg/m^2 or 10 mg/kg every 8 hours for 5 to 7 days). Since administration of this regimen requires iv therapy and/or hospitalization, it should be reserved for patients who are likely to have severe disease (marrow transplants, marked immunosuppression) or who show rapid early progression (early and extensive cutaneous dissemination or any evidence of visceral dissemination). Oral acyclovir has been used for suppression of HSV. Its efficacy for prophylaxis of VZV when given orally seems assured, but its therapeutic efficacy may depend on the clinical situation. In recent studies it has shown efficacy in the non-immunocompromised population when given orally for either varicella or zoster. BV-araU is an investigation agent with 1000 times more activity against VZV *in vitro*. It looks promising *in vivo*.

Cytomegalovirus (CMV)

This agent causes severe morbidity and mortality in both renal transplant and bone marrow transplant patients. The urine is usually the easiest place to culture for CMV. Conventional culture methods may take a week or more for a positive result. However, using the "shell vial" technique, a result can be obtained in 24–48 hours. Patients with demonstrated CMV infection (this is tricky, because isolation of CMV from the urine alone does not imply disseminated disease) can be treated with ganciclovir. In the setting of intersitial pneumonitis in bone marrow transplants, ganciclovir alone is not efficacious, and patients respond better to a combination of ganciclovir and intravenous gamma globulin.[58]

Epstein-Barr Virus (EBV)

EBV induces polyclonal B cell transformation. With immunosuppression, EBV may be activated and appear in the oropharynx. Proliferation of multiple B cells can lead to a lymphoma-like disease in immunocompromised hosts. Although the overall incidence of EBV lymphoproliferative disease in patients being treated for cancer is low[59], there have been cases documented after bone marrow transplant[60]. In a few cases the virus appears to have been transmitted to an immune incompetent host with resulting fatal EBV disease. In other cases it has been related to T-cell depletion or the use of cyclosporine. A combination of IFN-α and immune globulin has been used in a series of such patients[60].

PROBLEMS UNIQUE TO BONE MARROW TRANSPLANT RECIPIENTS

The infectious problems of bone marrow transplant patients are usually divided into three groups based on the time post-transplant.

Early Infections (<30 days after transplant)

The infections seen in the first days post bone marrow transplantation are similar to infections seen in granulocytopenic leukemia patients (*i.e.*, predominantly bacterial and fungal infections). However, approximately 85% of HSV-1 seropositive patients will have culturable HSV in the pharynx at this time[53]. EBV can also be found in the pharynx at this time.

Early studies indicated a role for laminar air flow rooms and non-absorbable antibiotics in the prevention of infections in bone marrow transplant patients. We have demonstrated (in a double-blind placebo-controlled trial) that ciprofloxacin at a dose of 750 mg po bid prevents bacteremias and decreases the number of febrile days[33]. The question of whether antibiotics affect GVHD incidence is still debated.

Middle Infections (30–100 days)

During this period, 1–3 months post-transplantation, the patients' granulocytes begin to come back and in the allogeneic setting the patients become subject to graft-versus-host disease. Veno-occlusive disease is most often seen at this time (though it may be found earlier). Aside from being subject to fungal disease (and other intracellular parasites, *e.g.*, toxoplasmosis, TB, *M. avian intracellulare*), CMV is the major pathogen. This illness may be the result of new infection in a seronegative individual (it may be acquired by transfusion) or reactivation in a seropositive patient.

Typically CMV presents as pneumonia or hepatitis in this setting. As a cause of pneumonitis it is fairly non-specific in its X-ray appearance (may be unilateral or bilateral, nodular or diffuse), but usually presents as an interstitial infiltrate. The differential diagnosis in this setting thus includes both infectious causes of pneumonia (fungus, pneumocystis as well as drug-induced pneumonitis — associated with either radiation or chemotherapy) and GVH-associated pneumonitis (if this is a real entity). Pneumonitis (as well as fever and skin rash) has been reported to occur as a result of human herpes virus 6 post bone marrow transplantation[61].

Hepatitic abnormalities during this time period are even more difficult to define. Both CMV and GVH are associated with hepatitis (which leads to more obstructive findings than evidence of hepaticellular destruction). Veno-occlusive disease also presents a similar picture at this time. All involve fever, elevated alkaline phosphatase, and hepatomegaly. Since this is a classic picture for *Candida* hepatitis, this is a very tricky problem in differential diagnosis and treatment. The treatment for CMV and *Candida* involves the administration of a toxic drug (ganciclovir or amphotericin) and stopping steroids, while treatment of GVH may involve increasing steroid dose.

Whether it is possible to obtain a liver or lung biopsy at this time will depend on the patient's bleeding parameters and a variety of secondary issues. Looking for skin evidence of GVH (a skin biopsy is much more benign than a liver biopsy) or *Candida*, or cryptococcal serology may be helpful in making a diagnosis in this setting. In general, a liver biopsy showing CMV will be of questionable significance anyway, so that we do not usually recommend liver biopsies in this setting.

Several studies suggest that administration of IVIG may decrease the incidence of CMV[62] and high doses of acyclovir may reduce the incidence of CMV-induced disease[63]. Ganciclovir alone given prophylactically after engraftment will prevent CMV disease, but its administration is complicated by neutropenia[64].

TABLE 59–6. USE OF PROPHYLACTIC ANTIBIOTICS IN PATIENTS WITH CANCER

UNDERLYING DISEASE	INFECTIOUS PROBLEM	PROPHYLACTIC ANTIBIOTICS
Acute hematologic malignancies	Infection with extracellular bacteria	Broad spectrum (*e.g.*, TMP sulfa or quinolones)
Solid tumors, especially lung cancer	Tuberculosis	Isoniazid
Multiple myeloma or CLL	Infection with encapsulated organisms	Agents active against *S. pneumonia, H. influenza*
ALL, patients with lymphoma receiving immunosuppressive agents	*P. carinii* infection	TMP/sulfa (pentamidine and dapsone are alternatives)

Late Infections (>6 months)

The majority of allogeneic bone marrow transplants (and perhaps almost as many syngeneic transplants) will develop herpes zoster infection at some point between 6 months and 2 years post-transplant[53]. It is our practice to give acyclovir prophylactically in this setting. In addition, we give trimethoprim/sulfamethoxazole prophylaxis (1 tab daily) for at least 1 year following bone marrow transplantation as prophylaxis for *P. carinii* and *T. gondii*. This therapy is effective against pneumococcus and *H. influenzae* bacteremias. Late pneumococcal bacteremias have been reported after bone marrow transplantation, and we are currently assessing the efficacy of vaccination at various times post-transplantation.

PROPHYLAXIS AGAINST INFECTION IN ONCOLOGY PATIENTS

Antibiotic Prophylaxis

As a general rule it is relatively easy to prevent infection with a single organism using antibiotic prophylaxis over an ex-

TABLE 59–7. VACCINATION OF PATIENTS RECEIVING CHEMOTHERAPY FOR CANCER

VACCINE	PATIENTS RECEIVING CHEMOTHERAPY	BONE MARROW TRANSPLANT RECIPIENTS
Tetanus Diphtheria	As for other patients, boost when not receiving chemotherapy	Reimmunize after transplant
Poliomyelitis Seasonal influenza	Inactivated vaccines preferred Vaccine should not be given with chemotherapy; either given when not in chemo Rx or mid-cycle	Use only inactive vaccine Indicated—no contraindication
Pneumococcus *H. influenza* Meningococcus	Especially important in splenectomized patients	Protein conjugate vaccines have efficacy after immune reconstitution Pure polysaccharide vaccines should be given at 12 and 24 months post transplant
Measles, mumps, rubella		Appears safe in most patients 24 months post transplant

tended period. On the other hand, it is only possible to prevent infection with a large number of organisms over a short period. This is because over a long period of antibiotic pressure resistant organisms will tend to be selected and may become predominant.

Prevention of infection by *Pneumocystis carinii* is effective (even if given 3x/week) over a long period[65]. We recommend trimethoprim/sulfamethoxazole prophylaxis against *P. carinii* in all bone marrow transplant recipients (for the first year post-transplantation), as well as in cancer patients receiving high dose steroids or drugs (such as fludarabine) which impair T-cell responses.

Prophylaxis against bacterial and fungal infections is more problematic and there is not uniform agreement on its use. The disadvantage to prophylaxis against a large number of organisms is that it is easy to select for resistance in this way. Therefore we restrict this form of prophylaxis to patients with a very high risk of bacteremia, and give it for the shortest possible time. In the setting of bone marrow transplantation we have found that prophylaxis with ciprofloxacin decreases the number of gram-negative bacteremias during the neutropenic period[33]. Recent studies have demonstrated that fluconazole prophylaxis will decrease *Candida* infections in this setting. The disadvantage to either of these approaches is the risk of the development of resistance to the agents used, both in the patient and the hospital. For this reason these decisions have to be made carefully and may be different for different institutions. An outline of strategies by disease is presented in Table 59–6.

IVIG

The administration of intravenous globulin has been demonstrated to be life-saving for patients with agammaglobulinemia. Since a high percentage of patients with myeloma, CLL, and other cancers (and those recovering from bone marrow transplantation) have low immunoglobulin levels, the prophylactic administration of IV globulin has been proposed as a means of preventing infections. Although this agent may have some efficacy, its expense and difficulty of administration merit careful consideration in terms of the extent of its use[66].

Vaccination

A good general rule for the use of vaccines in immunoincompetent patients (*e.g.*, patients on high dose steroids or immediately after bone marrow transplantation) is to avoid live vaccines. However the measles, mumps, rubella vaccine has been shown to be safe when given to bone marrow transplant recipients without graft-versus-host disease 2 years following transplantation[67]. The major problems in giving purified protein or polysaccharide vaccines relate to the fact that these vaccines are not very immunogenic under the best of circumstances, and in patients receiving chemotherapy they are unlikely to elicit any response. For this reason the optimum time to give vaccines is when the patient is not receiving chemotherapy. If the patient is on a multicycle protocol and needs a vaccination for influenza, then it should be done mid-cycle (possibly during the period of neutropenia) in order to ensure the best possible response. Multiple doses of vaccines are being investigated by some centers. A basic approach to vaccines is outlined in Table 59–7.

The importance of immunizing splenectomized patients cannot be overstated, especially with the development of new pneumococcal vaccines which are likely to be much more effective than currently available vaccines. Physicians caring for splenectomized patients should instruct these people to seek medical attention with any febrile illness, and they should be given pills to carry with them for treatment of *S. pneumonia*, *H. influenza*, and *N. meningitidis*, since infections with these organisms are rapidly fatal in splenectomized hosts.

REFERENCES

1. Casazza AR, Duvall CP, Carbone PP. Infection in lymphoma–histology, treatment, and duration in relation to incidence and survival. JAMA 197:710, 1966
2. Hersh EM, Bodey GP, Nies BA, Freireich EJ. Causes of death in acute leukemia. A ten-year study of 414 patients from 1954–1963. JAMA 105, 1965
3. Keys T, Haldorson A, Rhodes K et al. Nosocomial outbreak of *Rhizopus* infections associated with Elastoplast wound dressings — Minnesota. MMWR 27:33, 1978
4. Grossman ME, Fithian EC, Behrens C et al. Primary cutaneous aspergillosis in six leukemic children. J Am Acad Dermatol 12:313–318, 1985
5. Bodey GP et al. Quantitative relationships between circulating leukocytes and infection in patients with acute leukemia. Ann Int Med 64:328, 1966
6. Gill FA et al. The relationship of fever, granulocytopenia, and antimicrobial therapy to bacteremia in cancer patients. Cancer 39:1074, 1977
7. Meunier AU et al. Fungemia in the immunocompromised host. Changing patterns, antigenemia, high mortality. Am J Med 71:363, 1981
8. Schwartz PE, Sterioff S, Mucha P et al. Postsplenectomy sepsis and mortality in adults. JAMA 248:2279, 1982
9. Armstrong D, Polsky B. Central nervous system infections in the compromised host. In: Rubin RH, Young LS (eds): Clinical Approach to Infection in the Compromised Host, 2nd ed. New York, Plenum Publishing, 1988:165
10. Hughes WT et al. Guidelines for the use of antimicrobial agents in neutropenic patients with unexplained fever. J Infect Dis 161:381–396, 1990
11. Shimpff SC et al. Rectal abscesses in cancer patients. The Lancet 2:844, 1972
12. Barnes SG et al. Perirectal infections in acute leukemia. Annal Int Med 100:515, 1984
13. EORTC International Antimicrobial Group: Three antibi-

otic regimens in the treatment of infection in febrile granulocytopenia patients with cancer. J Infect Dis 137:14, 1978
14. Raad II, Bodey GP: Infectious complications of indwelling vascular catheters. Clin Infect Dis 15:197, 1992
15. Sickles EA, Yong VM, Greene WH. Pneumonia in acute leukemia. Ann Intern Med 79:528, 1973
16. Sickles EA, Greene WH, Wiernik PH. Clinical presentation of infection in granulocytopenic patients. Arch Intern Med 135:715, 1975
17. Bolivar R, Fainstein V, Elting L, Bodey GP. Cefoperazone for the treatment of infections in patients with cancer. Rev Infect Dis 5[suppl]:S181-187, 1983
18. Pizzo PA et al. A randomized trial comparing ceftazadime alone with combination therapy in cancer patients with fever and neutropenia. N Engl J Med 315:552, 1986
19. Saunders CC, et al. Resistance to cefamondole: A collaborative study of emerging clinical problems. J Inf Dis 145:118, 1982
20. Neftel KA et al. Inhibition of granulopoiesis *in vivo* and *in vitro* by β-lactam antibiotics. J Infect Dis 152:90, 1985
21. Charak BS, Louie R, Malloy B, Twomey P, Mazumder A. The effect of amphotericin B, aztreonam, imipenem, and cephalosporins on the bone marrow progenitor cell activity. J Antimicrob Chemother 27:95, 1991
22. Bodey GP, Grose WE, Keating MJ. Use of trimethoprim-sulfamethoxazole for treatment of infections in patients with cancer. Rev Infect Dis 4:579, 1982
23. Meunier F, Zinner SH, Gaya H et al. Prospective randomized evaluation of ciprofloxacin versus piperacillin plus amikacin for empiric antibiotic therapy of febrile granulocytopenic cancer patients with lymphomas and solid tumors. Antimicrob Agents Chemo 35:873, 1991
24. EORTC International Antimicrobial Therapy Cooperative Group. Ceftazidime combined with a short or long course of amikacin for empirical therapy of gram-negative bacteremia in cancer patients with granulocytopenia. N Engl J Med 317:1692, 1987
25. Rubin M et al. Gram-positive infections and the use of vancomycin in 550 episodes of fever and neutropenia. Ann Int Med 108:30, 1988
26. Wallace MR, Oldfield EC III. Prospective evaluation of "red man" syndrome [letter]. J Infect Dis 169:700, 1994
27. O'Sullivan TL, Ruffing MJ, Lamp KC et al. Prospective evaluation of "red man" syndrome in patients receiving vancomycin. J Infect Dis 168:773, 1993
28. Farber CF, Moellerng RC Jr. Retrospective study of the toxicity of preparations of vancomycin from 1974 to 1981. Antimicrob Agents Chemo 23:138, 1983
29. Matzke GR et al. Pharmacokinetics of vancomycin in patients with various degrees of renal function. Antimicrob Agents Chemo 25:433, 1984
30. Drusono GL et al. The acylampicillins: mezlocillin, piperacillin, and azlocillin. RID 6:13, 1984
31. Barza M. Imipenem: first of a new class of β-lactam antibiotics. Ann Int Med 503:552, 1985
32. Jones PG et al. Aztreonam therapy in neutropenic patients with cancer. Am J Med 81:243, 1986
33. Lew MA Kehoe K, Ritz J, et al. Prophylaxis of bacterial infections with ciprofloxacin in patients undergoing bone marrow transplantation. Transplantation 51:630, 1991
34. EORTC International Antimicrobial Therapy Cooperative Group. Empiric antifungal therapy in febrile granulocytopenia patients. Am J Med 86:668, 1989
35. Pizzo PA et al. Empiric antibiotic and antifungal therapy for cancer patients with prolonged fever and granulocytopenia. Am J Med 72:101, 1982
36. Pizzo PA et al. Duration of empiric antibiotic therapy in granulocytopenic patients with cancer. Am J Med 67:1894, 1979
37. Donowitz GR, Harman C, Pop T, Stewart M. The role of the chest roentgenogram in febrile neutropenic patients. Arch Intern Med 151:701, 1991
38. Dugdale DC, Ramsey PG. Staphylococcus aureus bacteremia in patients with Hickman catheters. Am J Med 89(2):137, 1990
39. Higby DJ et al. Filtration leukapheresis for granulocyte transfusion therapy: Clinical and laboratory studies. N Engl J Med 292:761, 1975
40. Herzig RH et al. Successful granulocyte transfusion therapy for gram-negative septicemia: A prospectively randomized controlled study. N Engl J Med 296:701, 1977
41. Winston DJ et al. Therapeutic granulocyte transfusions for documented infections: A controlled trial in ninety-five infectious granulocytopenic episodes. Ann Intern Med 97:509, 1982
42. Ghosal SP et al. Noma neonatorum: Its etiopathogenesis. Lancet II:289, 1978
43. Limongelli WA et al. Nomalike lesion in a patient with chronic lymphocytic leukemia. Oral Surg 41:40, 1976
44. Fekety R, Silva J, Kauffman C, Buggy B, Deery HG. Treatment of antibiotic-associated *Clostridium difficile* colitis with oral vancomycin: comparison of two dosage regimens. Amer J Med 86:15, 1989
45. Sherman NJ et al. The ileocecal syndrome in acute childhood leukemia. Arch Surg 107:39, 1973
46. Varki AP et al. Typhilitis in acute leukemia. Cancer 43:695, 1979
47. Alexander JE, Williamson SL, Seibert JJ et al. The ultrasonographic diagnosis of typhilitis (neutropenic colitis). Pediatr Radiol 18:200, 1988
48. Huber P Jr et al. Necrotizing soft-tissue infection from rectal abscess. Am Soc Colon and Rectal Surg 26:507, 1983
49. Graeve, AH et al. Role of different methods of lung biopsy in the diagnosis of lung lesions. Am J Surg 140:742, 1980
50. Breitfeld V, Hashida Y, Sherman FE et al. Fatal measles infection in children with leukemia. Lab Invest 28:279, 1973
51. Wendt CH, Weisdorf DJ, Jordan MC, Balfour HH, Hertz MI. Parainfluenza virus respiratory infection after bone marrow transplantation. N Engl J Med 326:921, 1992
52. Harrington RD, Hooton TM, Hackman RC, Storch GA et al. An outbreak of respiratory syncytial virus in a bone marrow transplant center. J Inf Dis 165:987, 1992
53. Meyers JD, Thomas ED. Infection complicating bone marrow transplantation. In: Rubin RH, Young LS (eds): Clinical Approach to Infection in the Compromised Host, 2nd ed. New York. Plenum Publishing, 1988:525.
54. Shepp DH, Newton BA, Dandliker PS et al. Oral acyclovir therapy for mucocutaneous herpes simplex virus infections in immunocompromised marrow transplant recipients. Ann Int Med 102:783, 1985

55. Iida T, Kitamura T, Guo J et al. Origin of JC polyomavirus variants associated with progressive multifocal leukoencephalopathy. Proc Natl Acad Sci USA 90:5062, 1993
56. Steiger MJ, Tarnesby G, Gabe S et al. Successful outcome of progressive multifocal leukoencephalopathy with cytarabine and interferon. Annals of Neurology 33:407, 1993
57. Saral R, Burns WH, Laskin OL. Acyclovir prophylaxis of herpes simplex infection. N Engl J Med 305:63, 1981
58. Feldman S, Lott L. Varicella in children with cancer: impact of antiviral therapy and prophylaxis. Pediatrics 80:465, 1987
58. Reed EC, Bowden RA, Dandliker PS et al. Treatment of cytomegalovirus pneumonia with ganciclovir and intravenous cytomegalovirus immunoglobulin in patients with bone marrow transplants. Ann Int Med 109:783, 1988
59. Zutter MM, Martin PJ, Sale GE et al. Epstein-Barr virus lymphoproliferation after bone marrow transplantation. Blood 72:520, 1988
60. Shapiro RS, McClain K, Frizzera G et al. Epstein-Barr virus-associated B cell lymphoproliferative disorders following bone marrow transplantation. Blood 71:1234, 1988
61. Yoshikawa T, Suga S, Asano Y et al. Human herpes virus-6 infection in bone marrow transplantation. Blood 78:1381, 1991
62. Winston DJ et al. Intravenous immune globulin for prevention of cytomegalovirus infection and interstitial pneumonia after bone marrow transplantation. Ann Intern Med 106:12, 1987
63. Meyers JD, Reed EC, Shepp DH et al. Acyclovir for prevention of cytomegalovirus infection and disease after allogeneic marrow transplantation. N Engl J Med 318:70, 1988
64. Winston DJ, Ho WG, Bartoni K et al. Ganciclovir prophylaxis of cytomegalovirus infection and disease in allogeneic bone marrow transplant recipients. Results of a placebo-controlled, double-blind trial. Ann Int Med 118:179, 1993
65. Hughes WT et al. Successful intermittent chemoprophylaxis for Pneumocystis carinii pneumonitis. N Engl Med 26:1627, 1987
66. Weeks JC, Tierney MR, Weinstein MC. Cost effectiveness of prophylactic intravenous immune globulin in chronic lymphocytic leukemia. N Engl J Med 325:81, 1991
67. Ljungman P, Fridell E, Lonngvist B et al. Efficacy and safety of vaccination of marrow transplant recipients with a live attenuated measles, mumps, and rubella vaccine. J Inf Dis 159:610, 1989

John S. Macdonald, Daniel G. Haller, Robert J. Mayer, Eds. *Manual of Oncologic Therapeutics*, Third Edition.

60. COMMON PSYCHIATRIC SYNDROMES IN THE CANCER PATIENT

Carol L. Alter

INTRODUCTION

The diagnosis of cancer often brings with it a series of emotional responses which can be considered both within, and extending beyond, the normal range. Such responses and reactions are often related to the stage of illness or treatment and vary for each individual. However, when levels of distress become excessive and interfere with a patient's routine functioning or ability to receive treatment adequately, then psychiatric intervention is often both useful and necessary. The following chapter will discuss normal responses to cancer, and the most common psychiatric disorders (*e.g.*, depression, anxiety and delirium) that occur as complications of cancer and the psychological consequences of pain for the cancer patient. While evidence of pre-morbid psychiatric disorders may complicate patients' emotional response to cancer, these topics will not be covered in detail in this chapter. However, it is important to note that in these particular cases, early psychiatric consultation may be helpful.

NORMAL RESPONSES TO THE STRESS OF CANCER

For each phase of the diagnostic and treatment experience, there are normal emotional and psychological responses that a patient may exhibit. When a patient is initially diagnosed, there is often a sense of shock and disbelief, which may be followed by symptoms including sleeplessness, anxiety, decreased appetite, irritability, decreased concentration, and a diminished ability to function in normal daily activities. Thoughts about the diagnosis may intrude and patients may have concerns and fears about what is to come. There may be fears that the diagnosis is a death sentence and patients may be highly distressed. However, these symptoms tend to dissipate within 1 to 2 weeks. While these symptoms are often common at diagnosis, they may also occur at the time of relapse or treatment failure and may even be worse under those circumstances.

Following this initial response, many patients develop ongoing feelings of depression, poor sleep, and poor concentration that may persist for a few weeks but then resolve on their own. Ideally, patients will then reach a level of adaptation where they can begin to adjust to the new information, think about the disease in a less panic-stricken or anxiety-laden way, and begin to resume normal activities. This often occurs after about 2 weeks, and more often than not corresponds with the initiation of treatment and entering the chronic phase of illness and treatment. In many cases, these responses may be modulated by use of the patient's existing support systems such as family and friends. The patient's physician, nurses, and social workers within the treatment area may also offer reassurance to the patient.

While these responses are considered normal and should resolve, for those patients complaining of excessive distress use of mild anxiolytics such as alprazolam 0.25 mg to 0.5 mg 3 times a day or a sedative-hypnotic, *e.g.*, temazepam 15 mg at bedtime may be useful in decreasing these symptoms and allowing the patient some opportunity for rest and an ability to continue functioning. If it appears that symptoms have not resolved within 2 weeks a psychiatric consultation may be indicated. The consulting psychiatrist can not only offer emotional support, but will also attempt to evaluate the presence of more significant psychiatric disturbance that may require more intensive intervention.

PREVALENCE OF PSYCHIATRIC DISORDERS

A question that has often been raised in the oncologic setting is whether or not patients experiencing cancer diagnosis and treatment have a higher rate of psychiatric disorders than that noted in the general population. Studies that have examined this issue in cancer patients have revealed that while there may be a higher rate overall of psychiatric disorders, the rate of major psychiatric disorders such as anxiety or depression is actually comparable to that seen in the general population. A large multi-site study was undertaken by the Psychosocial Collaborative Oncology Group, which found that 47% of patients studied (n = 219) met some Diagnostic & Statistical Manual of Mental Disorders, third edition (DSM III) psychiatric diagnosis. Of those diagnoses, 68% represented adjustment disorders, that is levels of depression, anxiety, or mixed depression and anxiety that were elevated yet related almost wholly to the stress of illness and without evidence of serious neurovegetative signs. Thirteen percent of those (6% of the total number studied) met criteria for major depressive disorder. This number is comparable to the number found in large epidemiologic studies of well patients. Eight percent of those patients meeting criteria were diagnosed with organic mental disorders, the majority of which were defined as delirium. Four percent of these patients met criteria for an anxiety disorder. Eleven percent of patients studied had prior psychiatric problems, indicating that most psychological disorders in cancer patients arise from the stress of illness and its treatment.

DEPRESSION IN CANCER PATIENTS

While only 6% of all cancer patients studied met formal criteria for major depressive disorder, 12% of patients also met criteria for an adjustment disorder with depressed mood. These figures indicate that close to 20% of all patients with cancer will report depression as a symptom that may be disruptive for them to some degree. The diagnosis of depression is based on the presence of several symptoms, including depressed or dysphoric mood, hopelessness and helplessness, loss of interest or pleasure in usual activities, feelings of worthlessness and/or guilt, and decreased ability to concentrate, as well as the presence of suicidal ideation. In addition, a patient must have neurovegetative signs of depression, including diminished appetite, weight loss, insomnia, fatigue, decreased libido, or psychomotor retardation. Difficulties arise in the cancer patient in that many of the somatic symptoms associated with cancer treatment or illness are also those required for meeting criteria for a major depressive disorder. Therefore, it is often of little value to include the somatic signs of depression as criteria for formal diagnosis.

There are numerous aspects of the cancer illness and treatment which may also cause depression in the cancer patient. Metabolic abnormalities such as an increase in calcium need to be evaluated. Nutritional decompensation may also contribute to an impression of depressed mood or psychomotor retardation. Endocrine abnormalities have also been associated with depression, and certainly neurologic involvement may also lead to signs of depression. Several chemotherapeutic agents have also been associated with depression, including the vinca alkaloids, procarbazine, and interferon. Other medications associated with depression have been cimetidine, benzodiazepines, propranolol, and estrogens. In addition, steroids (both high dose and tapering of steroids) can lead to a depressive syndrome as well. Whole brain radiation and central nervous system metastases can also present as depression. A thorough evaluation of such organic causes must be undertaken to rule out etiologic factors that should be considered in understanding the source of the disorder.

Treatment of Depression

When evaluating a patient, it is important for the psychiatrist to understand the meaning of the cancer diagnosis and treatment and how the patient sees this in his or her life. Often such considerations may be helpful in providing emotional support to the patient and putting the illness in perspective. Secondly, although there is a distinction between major depressive disorder and a milder adjustment disorder with depressed mood, various treatment modalities may be considered based on the level of disruption in the patient's life and also an understanding of where the patient may be in terms of treatment. For the patient who may have some mild symptoms of emotional distress, hopelessness, and helplessness, it may be possible to reassure and offer support. In addition, for many patients there are prevailing medical reasons why an antidepressant may not be helpful, and psychological therapies may be indicated. It has been found that both psychopharmacologic and psychologic treatment modalities are equally effective in the treatment of depression. For those patients with persistent symptoms who do not respond to supportive intervention and who clearly are experiencing disruption in their lives, then consideration of a psychopharmacologic agent is indicated.

Pharmacologic Approaches

Once a diagnosis of depression is made, organic causes for depression have been ruled out, and a decision is made to consider psychopharmacologic treatment, then the treatment approach to depression in the cancer patient is much like that utilized in the non-medically ill patient. The first-line approach to the treatment of depression has traditionally been use of a tricyclic antidepressant. Such medications work by increasing levels of neurotransmitters such as norepinephrine and serotonin in the central nervous system. The choice of antidepressant is based on the symptoms the patient presents with, such as insomnia or anxiety, as well as the medical problems present, such as presence of stomatitis or constipation and the side effect profile of the particular tricyclic antidepressant.

Tricyclic antidepressants have a host of side effects which may be particularly troubling to patients who have concurrent medical illness. They all have a component of anticholinergic effects which may cause dry mouth, constipation, and urinary hesitancy. They all may lead to a greater or lesser degree of orthostatic hypotension and palpitations and may be contraindicated in patients with certain cardiac conduction abnormalities. Some patients may develop skin rashes and allergies; and, due to the drug's activity in the central nervous system, there may be evidence of sedation, delirium, or excessive stimulation. In addition, it has been noted that many of the tricyclic antidepressants can lead to weight gain and impotence in some patients. Because of such side effects, choose a tricyclic antidepressant which will have the least number of side effects, but will provide good antidepressant efficacy as well as sedation as needed for those patients complaining of insomnia. The two medications with the least number of side effects are desipramine or nortriptyline, often the drugs of choice for patients receiving a tricyclic antidepressant. Tricyclics should be started at a low dose, *e.g.*, 10 mg to 25 mg a day, and increased slowly by

25 mg every 1 to 2 days. It has been found that patients with cancer require therapeutic levels of antidepressant in order to receive therapeutic benefit and while doses of 300 mg of desipramine are often recommended in the psychiatric patient in order to reach therapeutic blood levels, such levels may be reached at between 150 mg and 200 mg of desipramine in cancer patients (see Table 60–1).

Recently there has been release of several new agents which have selective activity on the serotonin neurotransmitter system. The selective serotonin reuptake inhibitors (SSRIs) are of particular interest in the oncologic setting when compared to tricyclics because they have relatively fewer side effects, are known to be significantly less cardiotoxic, and may be better tolerated in patients with concomitant medical illness. Medications such as fluoxetine, paroxetine, and sertraline are now available and have been shown to be equally if not more efficacious in the depressed cancer patient. Side effects of the SSRIs may include transient nausea, anxiety, and mild complaints of dry mouth. In addition, these medications are not associated with weight gain. While these medications are by and large less sedating than the tricyclic antidepressants, their ability to assist in treating a patient's depression-related insomnia is excellent once therapeutic levels have been achieved. Doses vary for the particular agent chosen, but again standard doses are recommended.

The course of treatment and length of treatment in cancer patients again parallel that which is recommended in the healthy patient. It often may take anywhere between 2 and 3 weeks of therapeutic levels of antidepressant medication for a patient to begin to see signs of improvement. It is important during this 2-week period that doses are raised to a level at which side effects occur, to ensure that therapeutic levels are reached. In addition, tricyclic antidepressants can be monitored through blood levels if clinical indicators are not present. For those patients experiencing significant insomnia that is not relieved with the initiation of antidepressant medication, the antidepressant dosage is often sup-

TABLE 60–1. ANTIDEPRESSANT MEDICATIONS USED IN CANCER PATIENTS

DRUG NAME	STARTING DAILY DOSAGE (mg/po)	THERAPEUTIC DAILY DOSAGE (mg/po)
TRICYCLIC ANTIDEPRESSANTS		
Amitriptyline	25	75–100
Doxepin	25	75–100
Imipramine	25	75–100
Desipramine	25	75–100
Nortriptyline	25	75–100
SELECTIVE SEROTONIN REUPTAKE INHIBITORS		
Fluoxetine	20	20–60
Sertraline	20	20–60
Paroxetine	25	25–100
SECOND-GENERATION ANTIDEPRESSANTS		
Bupropoin	15	200–450
Trazodone	50	150–200
HETEROCYCLIC ANTIDEPRESSANTS		
Maprotiline	25	50–75
Amoxapine	25	100–150
MONOAMINE OXIDASE INHIBITORS		
Isocarboxazid	10	20–40
Phenelzine	15	30–60
Tranylcypromine	10	20–40
LITHIUM CARBONATE	300	600–1200
PSYCHOSTIMULANTS		
Dextromethamphetamine	2.5 at 8:00 am and noon	5–30
Methylphenidate	2.5 at 8:00 am and noon	5–30
Pemoline	18.75 in am and noon	37.5–150
BENZODIAZEPINES		
Alprazolam	0.25–1	0.75–6.0

plemented with a low dose of benzodiazapine. Alprazolam has been found efficacious in relieving both anxiety and depression and is often used in combination with antidepressant medication to augment the antidepressant response.

For those patients who have a prior history of depressive disorder, or who may come to cancer treatment already on an antidepressant, it is suggested that treatment begin with the medication found to be most effective in the past for that particular patient. While currently use of the second generation antidepressants such as trazodone, bupropion, maprotiline, and amoxapine are not considered first-line approaches to depression, some patients may have been taking these medications in the past. In most cases, these medications can be continued without incident. Caution should be exercised in the use of amoxapine, because of its strong dopamine blocking activity; thus with patients who are taking other dopamine blockers such as anti-emetics there may be an increased risk of developing extrapyramidal symptoms and movement disorders.

Psychostimulants

The psychostimulants, dextroamphetamine, methylphenidate, and pemoline, have been found to be effective in some patients with medical illness and depressive symptoms. They have been found to be most effective in patients with significant psychomotor slowing and cognitive deficits thought to be secondary to depression. They all have a very rapid onset of action which can be noted within hours to a day of initiating treatment, and have few side effects compared to the other antidepressants mentioned. The difficulty with these medications is that there may be agitation associated with their use, and they may not be as long-lasting as the traditional antidepressants. For those patients who appear to require long-term antidepressant dosing, it may be useful to initiate treatment with a psychostimulant (a starting dose of 2.5 to 5 mg of methylphenidate given in the morning and noon or 18.75 mg of pemoline) followed by the addition of a traditional antidepressant after several days.

Psychostimulants may also be used alone, especially for patients in the end stages of disease, who have significant pain, or who have too much physical debility to be able to tolerate a course of antidepressant medication. In low doses, psychostimulants can promote a sense of well being, may increase appetite, and also relieve feelings of weakness or fatigue. In addition, these medications are often very helpful in the pain patient, in that they can counteract the daytime sedation and sleepiness found with narcotic use. Occasionally, they can produce nightmares and/or insomnia, or even psychosis. Given the short half life of all these agents, if side effects are noted, doses can be either lowered or the drug can be stopped with reversibility of side effects.

Other Treatments for Depression

Other treatments for depression which have been used in healthy individuals may be utilized in cancer patients but often require significant thought and caution. Monoamine oxidase inhibitors (MAOIs) are used routinely in healthy individuals and are very effective in the treatment of depression; however, the strict dietary restrictions required for use of MAOIs (*e.g.*, tyramine restricted diet) is often thought to be contraindicated in patients who are having difficulty with appetite and maintaining weight. Secondly, most MAOIs have significant presence of orthostatic hypotension and autonomic instability, which may be contraindicated in cancer patients. For those patients who have been successfully treated with such medications in the past, attempts should be made to continue treatment, but with cautious review and oversight.

Lithium

Lithium carbonate can be used in the oncologic setting; however, several cautions apply. Lithium toxicity may be precipitated in the patient experiencing dehydration secondary to chemotherapy and thus lithium should be withheld the day before and the day of treatment. There is no risk of toxicity with radiation treatment. However, it is recommended that lithium be discontinued during cranial radiation as the risks of seizures may be increased with lithium use.

Electroconvulsive Therapy (ECT)

ECT is occasionally used for the depressed cancer patient who has life-threatening depression with psychotic features or significant psychomotor retardation, in whom emergency psychiatric treatment or intervention is required. ECT is rapidly effective; increased intercranial pressure is the only absolute contraindication to its use.

Anxiety

The experience of anxiety is a normal and common complaint of patients throughout the diagnostic and treatment aspects of illness. It is most commonly seen while patients are waiting to hear the diagnosis, before procedures are performed (*e.g.*, bone marrow aspiration, start of chemotherapy, irradiation, dressing changes), and commonly while awaiting test results. The usual and normal levels of anxiety often will dissipate once the stressful event has passed and is very amenable to reassurance by the physician and other members of the medical team. Although such non-invasive interventions are useful for many patients, use of anxiolytics on the night before the surgery or procedure may also help the patient be more comfortable. In those cases where the anxiety appears to be interfering with the patient's functioning or ability to understand or cooperate in a procedure, or if the patient has other signs of anxiety besides the objective sensation of nervousness or tension, such as complaints of tachycardia, tremors, or sweating, then a daytime anxiolytic (alprazolam, oxazepam, or lorazepam) can be prescribed.

Anxiety Symptoms Related to Medical Problems

As with the assessment of depression or other psychiatric problems in the medically ill, one needs to evaluate for organic etiologies of anxiety. There are numerous medical problems that can mimic anxiety in the cancer patient. These include: poorly controlled pain, abnormal metabolic states such as hypoxia or sepsis, or often the use of anxiety-producing drugs, specifically steroids. In many cases treatment of the medical source of anxiety will lead to diminution of symptoms. Steroid-related anxiety will dissipate with the discontinuation of steroids, but in many cases this is not possible because the steroids are required to maintain treatment. Under those circumstances concurrent use of anxiolytic agents can diminish patient discomfort and allow the medical regimen to continue. Another common presentation of anxiety is related to the use of various anti-emetic regimens, especially those utilizing dopamine agonists such as prochloroperazine or metochlopromide. Patients may often complain of restlessness, anxiety, or tremors which are similar to symptoms experienced by patients receiving neuroleptics for psychiatric conditions. This akathisia is remedied with the discontinuation of the anti-emetic and it is recommended in those patients that a more highly potent neuroleptic such as haloperidol with combination of lorazepam be utilized, or that patients be considered for a trial of odansetron to treat their nausea and vomiting.

Another important cause of anxiety that may often be overlooked is withdrawal from alcohol or other addictive substances (narcotics and benzodiazepines). It is always important to take a thorough history of alcohol use as well as a thorough history of detoxification or withdrawal syndromes which may alert the physician to potential problems. Secondarily, it is important to note what medications the patient has been using to treat nausea and vomiting, given the fact that many patients receive lorazepam for treatment of nausea and may not acknowledge the fact that they are taking such drugs when asked if they are taking any drugs for pain or for nerves.

Treatment for alcohol withdrawal is necessary because untreated delirium tremens has a mortality of 15%. Commonly, detoxification can be accomplished with chlordiazepoxide, starting at a dose of 50 mg orally every 6 hours with extra doses of 25 mg as needed. This dose can then be tapered at 10% per day. More rapid detoxification can occur if the patient is stable. If parenteral medication is required, lorazepam can be used, but it should be noted that lorazepam in the parenteral form has an active half life of between 1 and 2 hours and therefore needs to be dosed more frequently than chlordiazepoxide. Patients who are thought to be dependent on other substances such as benzodiazepines or narcotics should, similarly, be placed on doses to cover their tolerance.

Phobias and Panic

Phobia, which is an acute, distressing fear of a situation, and panic rarely occur for the first time during treatment for cancer. More commonly, patients with a history of either phobia or panic may experience such symptoms during the stressful periods of treatment. When this does occur, it can complicate treatment and significantly impair a patient's ability to complete the treatment regimen suggested. In cases where such symptoms interfere with treatment (for instance, a patient develops a needle phobia or becomes claustrophobic in the setting of the laminar air flow room of a bone marrow transplant), psychiatric consultation may help to devise a treatment plan which can address the patient's symptoms. For those patients undergoing a long-term treatment plan such as weekly chemotherapy, distraction and relaxation techniques may help them learn to cope with the distress of the needle stick or the procedure. For those patients in a more acute setting requiring response immediately, use of benzodiazepines are recommended and is very successful. In addition, in most cases, emotional support and reassurance can also help the patient. Combinations of both drug and behavioral treatments can also be successful for most patients.

Pharmacological Treatment of Anxiety Disorders

The most commonly used medications for the treatment of anxiety include the benzodiazepines; however, for some patients other treatments may also be utilized, including antihistamines, antipsychotics, beta blockers, and antidepressants. While barbiturates have been used in the past to treat anxiety, they are no longer recommended because of their severe addictive potential and their significant impact on respiratory function.

Benzodiazepines

For medically ill patients, recommended use of benzodiazepines includes those agents which are most short-acting, including alprazolam, lorazepam, and oxazepam (Table 60-2). Oxazepam also is the drug of choice for those patients who have hepatic impairment. Benzodiazepines can be used both on an as-needed basis and also in regular doses depend-

TABLE 60–2. COMMONLY PRESCRIBED BENZODIAZEPINES IN CANCER PATIENTS

DRUG	APPROXIMATE DOSE EQUIVALENT	INITIAL DOSAGE (mg/po)	ELIMINATION HALF-LIFE DRUG METABOLITES (HOUR)	ACTIVE METABOLITES
SHORT ACTING				
Alprazolam	0.5	0.25–0.5 (3 times daily)	10–15	Yes
Oxazepam	10	10–15g (3 times daily)	5–15	No
Lorazepam	1	0.5–2 (3 times daily)	10–20	No
MODERATELY LONG ACTING				
Chlordiazepoxide	10	10–25 (3 times daily)	10–40	Yes
Clonazepam	0.5	0.5–1 (2 times daily)	18–50	No
LONG ACTING				
Diazepam	5	5–10 (2 times daily)	10–100	Yes
Clorazepate	7.5	7.5–15 (2 times daily	30–200	Yes

ing on patient presentation. For those patients whose anxiety is limited to procedures or situational concerns, an as-needed dose may be very effective. For example, alprazolam can be dosed at 0.25 to 0.5 mg by mouth, 3 to 4 times daily with good effect. For those patients who are experiencing more significant anxiety that appears to last throughout the day and is not related to specific events, then fixed dosing is more effective and will diminish the cycle of anxiety and distress that may occur as a result of as-needed dosing. Similarly, for those patients who have had a history of anxiety, are enduring chronic distressing events, and whose anxiety impairs their ability to receive treatment, one can choose a longer-acting agent such as clonazepam which can be dosed on a twice daily basis and may be very effective in treating such distress.

It is also important to note that not all benzodiazepines have the same efficacy. While lorazepam may be very effective for agitation and for nausea, it may not be as adequate an anti-anxiety agent as alprazolam. Similarly, the anti-anxiety agents may not be as effective for sedation and insomnia as the medications that are considered to be sedative-hypnotics, such as temazepam, triazolam, and estazolam. In addition, there is some evidence that some benzodiazepines may be effective in treating depression and augmenting pain relief (alprazolam and clonazepam).

The most common side effects with use of benzodiazepines include drowsiness, sedation, and confusion. If such symptoms occur, the initial response is to lower the dose until the side effects are no longer present. Commonly, elderly patients who have been taking sedative-hypnotics on a regular basis may also develop delirium.

Acute panic is best treated with alprazolam, although antidepressants have also been shown to be effective in this population. In addition, the beta blocker propranolol has also been shown to be effective and can be utilized if there is concern about using benzodiazepines. Other approaches to anxiety include the use of antihistamines and antidepressants. Antidepressants with sedating properties such as imipramine can be very effective as anti-anxiety and antipanic medications. Antihistamines are excellent at diminishing short term anxiety in some patients and may serve as a hypnotic in others without leading to the confusion and drowsiness that some patients experience with benzodiazepine use.

ORGANIC MENTAL DISORDERS: DELIRIUM

The second most common psychiatric diagnosis seen in cancer patients is delirium. Delirium is defined as an acute confusional state thought to be secondary to some change in the central nervous system (CNS) and is reversible if those changes can be corrected. The specific causes of delirium in the cancer patient may be any single one or combination of the following: direct effect of the tumor on the central nervous system, the indirect effects on the central nervous system of complications of the disease and treatment (medications, electrolyte imbalance), a vital organ or systemic infection, vascular complications, or any pre-existing cognitive impairment or dementia.

Early signs of delirium include changes in sleep patterns, with restlessness and transient periods of disorientation often occurring in the evening, increased irritability, anger or temper outburst, withdrawal and refusal to talk to staff or relatives, and forgetfulness. Later and more severe changes secondary to delirium include overt signs of anger, including swearing, shouting, behavioral complications such as demanding behaviors, pacing the corridor, becoming lost, changes in perceptual abilities including hallucinations and delusions, and also misidentifying family members and staff.

In any patient showing such changes in mental status, a diagnosis of delirium must be entertained and an evaluation should be initiated to determine the cause of the change in mental status.

A major contributing factor to the onset of delirium in addition to presence of disease in the central nervous system is (either singly or in combination) the medications used both to treat cancer and medications to support the patient. There are numerous chemotherapeutic agents which are known to cause delirium, including fluorouracil, methotrexate, the vinca alkaloids, ifosfamide, and cisplatin. In addition, steroids are frequently implicated in the onset of mental status changes. Narcotic analgesics such as morphine sulfate and meperidine often cause confusional states which may be worse in patients with other compromise, such as the elderly, those who are terminally ill, and those who may also have other causes for central nervous system compromise.

Management of Delirium

The most important treatment for delirium is to arrive at an understanding of the cause of delirium and begin to initiate changes to reverse that cause. This includes a thorough review of the patient's current medical status, including laboratory findings and medications. Once that has been undertaken, and corrections have been made, there are several other ways of approaching such patients. First and foremost is to provide frequent reassurance to the patient and explanations to the family about the transient nature of delirium, and help to reassure the patient that the staff understands the confusion. Although many patients may appear severely confused and disoriented, they are often very frightened as a result of this and will respond to reassurance and support from staff and family alike.

Pharmacologic intervention is often most effective in helping to treat agitation, provide sedation, and diminish any perceptual difficulties that may occur. Low dose haloperidol is most effective in this setting. In addition, it is available in multiple forms including oral, intravenous, and intramuscular preparations. The dose can be repeated frequently in the intravenous setting and can be given in doses of 0.25 mg to 0.5 mg iv, every 30 minutes until symptom control is received. Oral doses usually can be started at 0.5 mg and can be titrated to anywhere between 2.5 and 5 mg daily. While haloperidol has few side effects, there may be an increased rate of movement disorders, including acute dystonia, and extrapyramidal side effects which can be controlled with the use of anti-Parkinsonian agents such as diphenhydramine and trihexyphenidyl. While lorazepam is often recommended for use in agitated patients, there can be a syndrome of disinhibition in the patient with delirium; thus, haloperidol is the first-line drug of choice, and if agitation persists, lorazepam can be added.

CANCER PATIENTS WITH PAIN

A large percentage of cancer patients experience significant pain at some point during their illness and treatment. While not all pain syndromes are accompanied by psychological distress, it is not uncommon for anxiety and depressive symptoms to accompany the presence of a pain diagnosis in patients. For this reason, it is important to diagnose and control pain aggressively as well as respond to whatever symptoms of acute anxiety, depression, and despair may occur along with the pain. Pain in and of itself may also present not only with subjective somatic complaints, but may present solely as an acute onset of anxiety, depression, agitation, irritability, uncooperativeness, insomnia, or even suicidal ideation. These symptoms are not labeled as a psychiatric disorder unless they persist after the pain is adequately controlled.

Specific treatments for pain management include nonnarcotic analgesics and narcotic analgesics, but these may also may be augmented with various psychopharmacologic agents. Antidepressants may be used in the cancer pain patient to augment narcotic analgesic effectiveness and may have specific efficacy in the area of bone pain. Certain benzodiazepines such as clonazepam and other antiseizure medications such as carbamazepine and phenytoin may also be effective in the treatment of nerve pain. Cognitive and behavioral interventions, such as relaxation, imagery, and systemic desensitization may also be very useful for some cancer patients with pain. While most patients can be effectively treated for pain with standard pharmacologic treatment, other patients who have persisting psychological distress can achieve optimal benefit with a combination of psychological support, medications, and behavioral techniques.

SUICIDE AND THE CANCER PATIENT

Suicidal ideation, that is, thoughts about ending one's own life, are common in cancer patients; however, it does not necessarily indicate suicidal intent or plan. However, there are several vulnerability factors which may increase the rate of suicidal ideation in patients with cancer. Advanced illness and poor prognosis, the presence of depression and/or pain, delirium, fatigue, and loss of control clearly raise the level at which one might be concerned about suicidal ideation. In addition, patients with either preexisting psychopathology, that is, a prior history of depressive disorder or a prior suicide history either in themselves or in their family may also indicate a higher risk for suicidal ideation. When a patient voices suicidal ideation it is imperative that a psychiatric evaluation be conducted to rule out serious intent and determine whether or not there is evidence of any other coexisting psychiatric disorder that can be treated and thus diminish the suicidal potential. If a depressive disorder or delirium is present, it can then be treated with diminution of suicidal risk.

BIBLIOGRAPHY

Bidder TC. Electroconvulsive therapy in the medically ill patient. Psychiatric Clinics of North America 4:391–405, 1981

Breitbart W. Suicide in cancer patients. Oncology 1:49–53, 1987

Breitbart W, Holland JC. Psychiatric Aspects of Symptom Management in Cancer Patients. Washington, DC, American Psychiatric Press, 1993

Bukberg J, Penman D, Holland JC. Depression in hospitalized cancer patients. Psychosomatic Medicine 66:199–212, 1984

Cohen-Cole SA, Kaufman KG. Major depression in physical illness: diagnosis, prevalence, and antidepressant treatment (A ten year review: 1982–1992) Depression 1:181–204, 1993

Derogatis LR, Morrow GR, Fetting J et al. The prevalence of psychiatric disorders among cancer patients. JAMA 249:751–757, 1983

Foley KM. The treatment of cancer pain. NEJM 313:84–95, 1985

Fordyce WE. Behavioral Methods for Chronic Pain and Illness. St. Louis, CV Mosby, 1976

Greenberg DB, Younger J, Kaufman SD. Management of lithium in patients with cancer. Psychosomatics 34(5):388–394, 1993

Hall RCW, Popkin MK, Stickey SK et al. Presentation of the steroid psychosis. Journal of Nervous and Mental Disease, 167:229–236, 1979

Lipowski Z. Delirium: Acute Confusional States. New York, Oxford University Press, 1990

Massie MJ, Lesko LM. Psychopharmacological management. In Holland JC, Rowland JR (eds): Handbook of Psychooncology: Psychological Care of the Patient with Cancer, 440–70, 1989

Massie MJ, Holland JC, Glass E. Delirium in terminally ill cancer patients. American Journal of Psychiatry 140:1048–50, 1983

Massie MJ. Depression. In Holland JC, Rowland JR (eds): Handbook of Psychooncology: Psychological Care of the Patient with Cancer, 283–290, 1989

Woods SW, Tesar GE, Murray GB et al. Psychostimulant treatment of depressive disorders secondary to medical illness. Journal of Clinical Psychiatry, 47:12–15, 1986

John S. Macdonald, Daniel G. Haller, Robert J. Mayer, Eds. *Manual of Oncologic Therapeutics*, Third Edition.

61. TRANSFUSION SUPPORTIVE CARE

Edward J. Lee
Charles A. Schiffer

The prognosis for patients with cancer responsive to intensive chemotherapy has improved considerably over the past 10 to 15 years. This can be attributed partly to improvements in chemotherapy and also to the improvement in the treatment and control of infection and hemorrhage that are the limiting toxicities of the treatment. This chapter reviews current approaches for the use of red blood cell, platelet, and granulocyte transfusions for patients with cancer.

RED BLOOD CELL TRANSFUSION THERAPY

Most patients with cancer require red blood cell (RBC) transfusions during the course of their disease. Excessive blood drawing and disruption of mucosal barriers due to the disease or its treatment contribute to blood loss, while chemotherapy, radiation therapy, and malignant disease may impair bone marrow function. Thus, many patients slowly develop anemia, which requires transfusion.

RBC for transfusions are obtained from healthy adult donors. One unit of packed RBCs is prepared from a 450-ml donation and usually has a final volume of 200 ± 20 ml of RBCs with 75 ml to 100 ml of plasma. The remainder of the whole blood donation is used for the preparation of other products such as platelet concentrate, fresh frozen plasma (FFP), and cryoprecipitate. Once packed RBCs are prepared, storage is possible for 6 weeks at 4°C depending on the specific additive used to maintain RBC metabolic processes. In most active hospital blood banks, however, RBCs are transfused within 1 week of procurement.

Whole blood is rarely, if ever, indicated. Even patients with massive hemorrhage can initially receive packed RBCs with FFP or albumin solutions given as further colloid replacement. If replacement of clotting factors is needed, FFP is usually the best product, although patients who are deficient primarily in fibrinogen can receive cryoprecipitate. Platelet concentrate is the appropriate product if thrombocytopenia is present. The platelets and white blood cells contained in stored whole blood function poorly and are not present in useful quantities.

Patients who experience minor nonhemolytic transfusion reactions should receive acetaminophen and diphenhydramine prior to all future transfusions. Should transfusion reactions persist, a leukocyte-depleted RBC product should be given. Inverted centrifugation of packed cells with removal of the buffy coat, saline washing, or processing by passage through a variety of commercially available filters is effective in reducing the number of white blood cells (WBC). Because of its relative ease, filtration is now used most commonly as the initial maneuver. Once packed RBCs have been modified by any of the methods listed, the product must be used within 24 hours. If transfusion reactions persist, frozen deglycerolized RBCs represent the RBC product with the greatest depletion of WBCs. With any modification of the initial packed RBC product, 15% to 20% of the RBCs may be lost, and the subsequent rise in hematocrit may be somewhat less than with standard RBCs. Saline washing to eliminate donor plasma is indicated for the occasional patient with immunoglobulin A deficiency. The use of modified RBC products increases both the preparation time and expense. Such products are indicated only in patients who are at risk for transfusion reactions, such as those with a history of reactions or those who have serologic evidence of alloimmunization (see Platelet Transfusion Therapy). The complications of RBC transfusions are similar to those of transfusion of any blood component and will be discussed in a separate section.

PLATELET TRANSFUSION THERAPY

Collection and Storage

Platelets for transfusion may be given in the form of pooled platelet concentrates (PC) prepared from multiple donors. A single unit of PC is prepared at the time of whole-blood donation. The PC from such a donation generally contains 0.7 to 0.9×10^{11} platelets, representing approximately 80% of the platelets contained in the original unit of whole blood. These PC units may be stored for up to 5 days with nearly normal post-transfusion recovery, survival, and hemostatic effectiveness.

Platelets for transfusion can also be collected by plateletpheresis of a single donor using any of a variety of cytopheresis machines, which yield from 4 to 12 units of functionally normal platelets in $1\frac{1}{2}$ to 3 hours. Such single-donor (SD) platelets can be stored for as many as 5 days if collected using a closed system. In the past, most SD collections have been used to provide histocompatible platelets from selected donors to alloimmunized patients. Because of the increased time and expense required to obtain SD platelets, this product should not be routinely used in the place of random-donor PC. However, SD platelets are used often as the product of choice to limit exposure to large numbers of donors. This choice may be appropriate if donor exposures are likely to be limited, but is not cost-effective if multiple transfusions are anticipated.

Dose and Distribution

The number of units given varies with the size of the patient. Adults will usually be given six to eight units of PC with an expected post-transfusion increase in the platelet count of 10,000 platelets/μl for each unit transfused. It is unnecessary to attempt to elevate the platelet count to normal levels because adequate hemostasis can usually be achieved with platelet counts of 50,000 to 70,000/μl. Although no data are available to provide guidelines for patients needing surgical procedures, certain recommendations can be made based on clinical experience. Minimally invasive procedures that allow direct compression of the puncture site are feasible even at very low (less than 20,000/μl) platelet counts. These include bone marrow aspiration or biopsy, radial artery puncture, and needle aspirations of soft-tissue masses. If platelet transfusion is planned in any event, however, it is advisable to do the procedure after the transfusion. Lumbar punctures should be performed only if platelet counts are above 30,000 whenever possible, because of the very slight risk of epidural hematoma, but they may be done at lower counts if necessary. Tooth extractions and more invasive procedures such as the placement of indwelling central venous access devices or bronchoscopy can lead to significant bleeding. Optimal patient safety requires a platelet count in excess of 40,000/μl and the absence of coagulopathy. Patients who can be maintained at such levels and who do not have concomitant coagulopathy can also undergo major surgery if necessary. It is preferable, however, to delay elective surgery until bone marrow function returns and platelet transfusion is unnecessary.

Studies with radiolabeled platelets have shown that transfused platelets are distributed to two pools. The circulating platelet pool is measured by the blood platelet count and contains approximately two thirds of the total body platelet mass in normal individuals. The remaining platelets are distributed to the splenic pool, which is in dynamic equilibrium with the blood pool. After transfusion, equilibration between the two pools occurs within 15 minutes. When the spleen is enlarged, the proportion of platelets in the (non-circulating) splenic pool increases substantially. Thus, patients with enlarged spleens often have significantly poorer responses to platelet transfusions when measured by post-transfusion platelet counts, but a great deal of variability exists. Platelets should not be withheld from patients with splenomegaly if they are otherwise indicated.

Indications for Platelet Transfusion

The need for platelet transfusion is dictated by either the risk or the presence of hemorrhage in a thrombocytopenic patient. This risk is related to the platelet count, the functional capacity of the circulating platelets, the etiology of the thrombocytopenia, and the presence of concomitant coagulopathy, infection, or mucosal-barrier disruption. Therefore, platelet transfusion should not be ordered for all patients with platelet counts below a certain number (20,000/μl is frequently cited) but rather only after a careful assessment of the clinical course and condition of each patient with thrombocytopenia. Patients with thrombocytopenia due to autoimmune processes or to drug- or infection-related peripheral destruction, who have normal bone marrow function, should receive platelet transfusions only in the presence of severe hemorrhage. Transfusing such patients when they are clinically stable is inappropriate because the transfused platelets generally suffer the same rapid destruction as endogenous platelets. Platelet transfusion is primarily reserved, therefore, for patients with thrombocytopenia due to decreased marrow production.

Platelets are frequently administered prophylactically to nonbleeding patients with acute leukemia who have undergone intensive chemotherapy at platelet counts between 10,000 and 20,000/μl to prevent spontaneous bleeding that may occur at platelet counts of less than 10,000/μl. The most catastrophic spontaneous bleeding is central nervous system hemorrhage, which occurs rarely as a consequence of thrombocytopenia alone, but may occur in patients with other ongoing clinical problems such as coagulopathy, infection, hyperleukocytosis (WBC count > 100,000/μl), and protracted emesis. More common manifestations of thrombocytopenic bleeding are microscopic hematuria, epistaxis, and the presence of occult blood in the stool. When bleeding from mucosal sites is minimal, platelet transfusions should be given only if further decrease in the platelet count is anticipated, or if other complicating factors such as infection or coagulopathy are present. Prophylactic transfusions are needed less often in patients with solid tumors because the chemotherapy given is usually associated with shorter and less profound periods of marrow aplasia. Patients with aplastic anemia should not receive prophylactic platelet transfusions unless severe infection or coagulopathy is present because of the indefinite duration of the thrombocytopenia and the higher risk of alloimmunization.

The presence of factors associated with an increased risk of bleeding mandates transfusion of platelets at a higher platelet count. Patients receiving heparin for disseminated intravascular coagulation (DIC) associated with acute progranulocytic leukemia, patients with leukemia with very high blast counts, and patients with significant ongoing bleeding should all be maintained above 40,000 platelets/μl until these associated problems are resolved. It may be necessary to transfuse patients more frequently, even multiple times per day in such settings. The presence of coagulopathy, infection, bleeding, or hepatic or renal disease requires at least daily reevaluation of the need for platelet transfusion to each thrombocytopenic patient.

Complications of platelet transfusion occur frequently and are discussed below. Alloimmunization to histocompatibility antigens is the most significant long-term complication of platelet transfusions and merits a detailed discussion.

Alloimmunization

In alloimmunized patients, transfused platelets are destroyed rapidly by recipient antibody directed at antigens on the platelet surface, primarily HLA-A and B antigens. This complication occurs in 30% to 50% of patients with acute leukemia treated with intensive chemotherapy. Patients with aplastic anemia who require transfusion support have a higher frequency of alloimmunization, probably related to the absence of immunosuppressive chemotherapy at the time when exposure to sensitizing antigens is initiated. Most patients with acute leukemia develop alloimmunization within 4 to 8 weeks of their initial transfusion. Data from the University of Maryland Cancer Center has shown that relatively few patients become alloimmunized after 8 weeks despite multiple further transfusions and that the development of alloimmunization is independent of the number of platelet transfusions received. Thus, platelet transfusions given for an appropriate indication should not be withheld in an attempt to delay the onset or to reduce the incidence of alloimmunization.

The diagnosis of alloimmunization should be suspected when clinically stable patients do not achieve adequate post-transfusion platelet count elevation. The effectiveness of any given platelet transfusion is best assessed by obtaining a post-transfusion platelet count 10 minutes after completion of the transfusion. Traditionally, a 1-hour post-transfusion count has been used, but the 10-minute count provides equivalent information and is more convenient.

The post-transfusion platelet count increment, or corrected count increment (CCI) is calculated as follows:

$$\text{CCI} = \frac{\text{BSA}(\text{m}^2) \times (\text{post-pre-platelet count})}{\text{No. of platelets administered } (\times 10^{11})}$$

The CCI is useful in distinguishing alloimmunization from other causes of poor platelet survival. Bleeding, infection, fever, or DIC reduce platelet survival, but platelet recovery, as measured by the 10-minute post-transfusion CCI, is usually adequate. However, patients with marked splenomegaly or sepsis may also have very poor platelet recovery. It may be impractical to obtain 10-minute post-transfusion platelet counts after all transfusions. Patients who demonstrate poor platelet survival and require transfusion daily or every other day should clearly have a 10-minute post transfusion platelet count done and the CCI calculated. Occasionally, patients exhibit adequate platelet recovery (10-minute post-transfusion CCI) and impaired platelet survival (18–24 hour post transfusion CCI) during the early phase of the development of alloimmunization. Thus, serial 10-minute post-transfusion platelet counts are often appropriate in selected patients.

The diagnosis of alloimmunization may be confirmed by the presence in recipient serum of antibody directed against HLA antigens. This antibody can be detected by standard microlymphocytotoxicity assays, and the presence of significant activity correlates with a poor CCI 10 minutes after transfusion.

The management of the alloimmunized patient is a major challenge in the supportive care of patients with acute leukemia. The cornerstone of management has been the use of HLA-matched single-donor platelets. HLA-A and HLA-B antigens can be detected on the platelet surface and are the most critical in terms of donor selection and matching. All patients with acute leukemia should have their lymphocytes typed prior to undergoing chemotherapy anticipating that HLA-matched platelets may be needed. In many blood centers large numbers of HLA donors who are available for pheresis are listed in computers. Extreme polymorphism occurs at the HLA loci and more than 70 HLA-A and HLA-B antigens have been identified to date, appearing with substantial variation in frequency. Large numbers of donors are therefore required to provide the best chance of obtaining a suitable match for a patient with relatively uncommon HLA antigens. When a complete match is not available, it is sometimes possible to selectively mismatch for certain antigens in some patients. These antigens may be "cross reactive" with patient antigens and therefore may not be recognized as foreign by the recipient antibody, or they may be expressed to a lesser extent on platelets compared with lymphocytes and thereby allow improved survival of transfused platelets. Alternatively, platelets from different donors can be crossmatched with serum from a refractory patient in a variety of antiplatelet antibody assays. This approach can provide effective platelet transfusions for alloimmunized patients whose HLA type is unknown. However, these strategies are not uniformly successful. Indeed, the transfusion of perfectly HLA-matched platelets is ineffective in approximately 20% of transfusions for reasons that are obscure. Possibilities include: (1) antibody directed against platelet-specific (non-HLA) antigens; (2) drug-related antiplatelet antibody, with cephalosporins, trimethoprim-sulfamethoxazole, and the penicillins as the most likely candidates in leukemia patients; (3) circulating immune complexes; (4) mismatching at the BW4/BW6 system, which is a biallelic HLA system associated with the HLA-B locus; (5) ABO (blood group) incompatibility. Any of these possibilities may be the explanation in a given patient, but probably none contributes in a high percentage of patients.

Management is difficult when no donors are available whose platelets produce effective transfusions. Under such circumstances, alloimmunized patients should not receive routine prophylactic transfusions. Hemorrhagic complications are best managed by the infusion of large numbers of random-donor PC in the hope that some of the units may be compatible or that transient absorption of recipient antibody may occur. The use of unmatched single-donor platelets is not recommended. Maneuvers that are successful in autoimmune thrombocytopenia, such as corticosteroid therapy, splenectomy, or high-dose intravenous gamma globulin, are not effective in restoring responsiveness to random-donor PC in alloimmunized patients.

Alloimmunized patients may also be supported with autologous PC. Briefly, patients who achieve remission undergo intensive plateletpheresis. Platelets can then be frozen using dimethylsulfoxide as a cryoprotectant and stored at liquid nitrogen temperature for years with preservation of the capacity to circulate and function hemostatically after transfusion. This technology, although not technically demanding, is presently available in only a few centers across the country.

In as many as 30% of all patients with alloimmunization, the activity of the lymphocytotoxic antibody present in recipient blood may diminish or disappear. This decrease is associated with an improved response to random-donor PC and may be sustained for weeks to months. Thus, patients with leukemia who continue to receive chemotherapy should have serial measurements of lymphocytotoxic antibody to plan optimal transfusion management.

As the problems posed by platelet alloimmunization are costly to manage, affect decisions about further treatment for malignant disease, and can result in life-threatening hemorrhage, prevention of platelet alloimmunization is the subject of considerable study. Three methods have been proposed: the use of single-donor platelets, irradiation of platelet products with ultraviolet B (UVB) light, and leukocyte depletion. Little data are available except regarding the use of leukocyte depleted platelet products.

Several published trials purport to show an advantage for leukocyte depletion. Many of these trials include patients with a variety of diagnoses other than acute myelo leukemia (AML). The incidence of alloimmunization has not been carefully studied in patients with malignancies other than AML or in patients undergoing bone marrow transplantation. Some trials did not include concurrent controls, all are small, and the methods of producing leukocyte depletion vary considerably. Nonetheless, no trial shows leukocyte depletion to be associated with a higher frequency of alloimmunization. However, filtration of platelets to prevent alloimmunization will also mandate filtration of red cell products, and is an expensive proposition. Furthermore, filters are not uniformly effective and are also associated with removal of approximately 20% of the platelets as well. Therefore, there is no clear-cut solution to the problem of how best to prevent alloimmunization. For this reason, the National Heart Lung and Blood Institute (at NIH) has funded a multi-center trial comparing random-donor platelet concentrates, UVB irradiated random-donor PC, filtered random-donor PC, and filtered single donor platelets. Accrual is expected to be complete in 1995.

GRANULOCYTE TRANSFUSION THERAPY

Despite the continued development of newer and more effective antibiotics, patients with cancer still die of infection. Patients with acute leukemia who have prolonged periods of bone marrow aplasia are particularly subject to this complication. In selected circumstances, granulocyte transfusion can be a useful modality that complements antibiotic therapy. The transfusion of granulocytes should be reserved for infected patients with severe (less than 100–200/μl) granulocytopenia in whom bone marrow recovery is not anticipated within a week. Indications for granulocyte transfusion include progressive infection in the face of optimal antibiotic therapy, infection with antibiotic-resistant organisms, and gram-negative bacteremia with pneumonia. Although granulocyte transfusions have been given and should be considered in patients with progressive fungal infections (both *Candida* and *Aspergillus*), the benefits of such transfusions have not been documented.

Dose and duration of granulocyte transfusion are important issues. If normal donors are used, the donor should be premedicated with corticosteroids in order to increase the granulocyte yield to the range of 20 to 50×10^9 leukocytes obtainable using continuous-flow methods of leukopheresis. Transfusions should be given daily for at least 4 to 5 days in order to determine whether any benefit can be seen and can be continued in continuously granulocytopenic patients who benefit from and tolerate the transfusions. Patients with chronic-phase chronic myelocytic leukemia may also be used as donors. Large doses of leukocytes in the range of 100 to 300×10^9 may be obtained from a single procedure without corticosteroid premedication if the white count is elevated. These leukocytes appear to function normally in the recipient, and continued division by immature myeloid precursors can often occur, providing continued quantities of leukocytes without the need for further transfusion. Granulocyte yields from normal donors may be considerably enhanced by administration of a cytokine such as G-CSF 12–16 hours prior to leukopheresis, but experience with this is limited.

Alloimmunization may also affect the results of granulocyte transfusion. In patients who are not alloimmunized, granulocytes from unmatched donors can rapidly migrate to sites of infection. Thus, random donors can be utilized for such patients. In contrast, in alloimmunized patients, migration does not occur if random donors are used, and pulmonary sequestration of labeled leukocytes has been documented. Thus, the transfusion of unmatched granulocytes is not likely to be of benefit to alloimmunized patients because granulocytes do not reach the site of infection. In addition, the incidence of transfusion reactions is markedly increased in alloimmunized patients. Patients who experience severe transfusion reactions should not be rechallenged with random-donor granulocytes, although some alloimmunized patients may benefit from granulocytes from histocompatible family members or HLA-matched donors.

COMPLICATIONS OF BLOOD COMPONENT THERAPY

Complications of transfusion occur frequently. Many can be ameliorated or prevented by various means, as described below.

Transfusion Reactions

Transfusion reactions are the most common complication of transfusion. Symptoms and signs vary from hives and pruritus to fever with shaking chills and, rarely, respiratory decompensation and hypotension. Transfusion reactions may result from sensitization to transfused cellular antigens or plasma proteins. In some patients with febrile reactions to platelet transfusions and adequate post-transfusion elevation of the platelet count, it may be possible to reduce the frequency of such reactions by leukocyte depletion. Patients who experience reactions to RBC transfusions should receive RBC products modified to reduce leukocyte content as well.

Hypervolemia

Hypervolemia can be the result of transfusing 350 ml to 500 ml (6–8 units) of PC or other blood products to either small children or to older patients with compromised cardiac function. Although pooled PC can be concentrated by centrifugation followed by resuspension of the platelet pellet in a smaller volume of plasma, this is not routinely recommended because platelet viability is reduced by storage at high platelet concentrations. If necessary, the concentrated pooled PC should be administered immediately after preparation.

Infection

A variety of infections can occur following transfusions. All components now released by transfusion centers in the United States have been screened for the presence of the human immunodeficiency virus (HIV). Because of the sensitivity of the assay, directed donations by an individual for a specific recipient have been discouraged. Viral hepatitis is the most frequent significant problem in blood transfusion recipients. Because of routine screening for hepatitis B, most transfusion-related viral hepatitis is due to hepatitis C. Recent institution of testing to detect exposure to the hepatitis C virus in donors should decrease the incidence of this problem in the future. Bacterial infection may be transmitted by the transfusion of stored PC, although the frequency with which this occurs is very low. Presumably, bacteria contaminate the PC due to inadequate aseptic technique at the time of collection and proliferate during storage at room temperature. If a severe reaction characterized by fever and chills occurs shortly after initiation of a transfusion of stored platelets, then the transfusion should be discontinued and appropriate cultures taken from the platelet bag and patient. Rarely, other infections such as malaria, toxoplasmosis, or salmonella may be transmitted by transfusion to normal recipients. Severely immunocompromised hosts who have no prior exposure to cytomegalovirus (CMV), especially those who have undergone bone marrow transplantation, should receive blood products obtained from donors who are serologically negative for CMV exposure because of the extremely poor prognosis of CMV infection in this setting.

Graft-Versus-Host Disease

Transfusion associated graft-versus-host (TGVH) disease is due to the incidental transfusion of viable lymphocytes contained in blood products. The true incidence of TGVH is unknown but an increasing number of cases are being reported. Patients who have undergone allogeneic or autologous bone marrow transplantation, patients with Hodgkin's disease, and, to a somewhat lesser extent, other lymphoproliferative malignancies are at greater risk of this complication. Such patients should receive gamma-irradiated blood products whenever possible. The recommended dose is 2500 centigray. As TGVH has been described in patients who are not immunocompromised, some centers have taken the approach that all blood products should be irradiated. While this seems excessive, data about incidence of TGVH are not available to provide guidelines, and this somewhat conservative approach at least solves the problems of tracking appropriate patients.

Hemolysis

Hemolysis of recipient red cells is an uncommon complication of transfusing plasma from ABO-mismatched platelet donors. Although a positive direct Coombs' test may occur following transfusion, recipient hemolysis is rare because multiple donors are used, few of whom are likely to have high-titer antibodies.

BIBLIOGRAPHY

Anderson K. Transfusion associated graft-versus-host disease (editorial). J Clin Oncol 9:727–730, 1991

Bowden RA, Cays M, Schoch G et al. Comparison of filtered blood (FB) to seronegative blood products (SB) for prevention of cytomegalovirus (CMV) infection after marrow transplant. Blood 82:204a, 1993

Daly PA, Schiffer CA, Aisner J, Wiernik PH. One-hour post-transfusion increments are valuable in predicting the need for HLA-matched preparations. JAMA 243:435–438, 1980

Duquesnoy RJ, Filip DJ, Rodey GE et al. Successful transfusion of platelets "mismatched" for HLA antigens to alloimmunized thrombocytopenic patients. Am J Hematol 2:219–226, 1977

Dutcher JP, Schiffer CA, Aisner J, Wiernik PH. Long-term follow-up of patients with leukemia receiving platelet transfusions: Identification of a large group of patients who do not become alloimmunized. Blood 58:1007–1011, 1981

Gmur J, Burger J, Schanz U et al. Safety of stringent prophylactic platelet transfusion policy for patients with acute leukemia. Lancet 338:1223–1226, 1991

Hussein MA, Lee EJ, Schiffer CA. Platelet transfusions administered to patients with splenomegaly. Transfusion 30:508–510, 1990

Lee EJ. Indications for platelet transfusion therapy. In Kurtz SR, Brubaker DB (eds): Clinical Decisions in Platelet Therapy, American Association of Blood Banks, Bethesda, MD, 31–43, 1992

O'Connell B, Lee EJ, Schiffer CA. The value of 10-minute post-transfusion platelet counts. Transfusion 28(1):66–67, 1988

O'Connell BA, Schiffer CA. Donor selection for alloimmunized patients by platelet crossmatching of random donor platelet concentrates. Transfusion 30:314–17, 1990

Petz LD. Red blood cell transfusion. Clin Oncol 2:505–527, 1983

Schiffer CA. Granulocyte transfusions: an overlooked therapeutic modality. Transfusion Medicine Reviews, 4:2–7, 1990

John S. Macdonald, Daniel G. Haller, Robert J. Mayer, Eds. *Manual of Oncologic Therapeutics*, Third Edition.

62. BOWEL DYSFUNCTION IN THE CANCER PATIENT

Michael L. Kochman
Peter G. Traber

Bowel dysfunction and abdominal complaints are common in patients with cancer. The high prevalence of these disorders can lead to multiple physician visits and hospitalizations. Knowledge of the common abnormalities that manifest themselves as a result of the primary malignancy or as a result of treatment can lead to an improvement in the diagnostic and treatment plans for these complicated patients.

DISTURBANCES OF NORMAL BOWEL FUNCTION

Constipation

Constipation is the source of multiple patient complaints and is the most commonly encountered bowel dysfunction syndrome, affecting over 4,000,000 people per year.[1] Constipation affects women 3 times as often as men and is increased in incidence over the age of 65.[2] Oncology patients, who are often seen frequently by physicians, are likely to complain of symptoms of constipation during treatment. A common definition of constipation is a frequency of defecation of less than two times per week. An abdominal X-ray may demonstrate feces throughout the colon and an abnormal small bowel air pattern in severe cases. Multiple factors are implicated in the pathogenesis including medications, lack of exercise, and alteration of diet. Narcotic analgesics and anticholinergics are the medications most often responsible; decreasing the dosage of these medications is often beneficial.

A multi-faceted approach should be taken to the management of constipation, dependent upon the degree and symptomology. Ambulation of the patient can be of benefit, though this may be a difficult goal due to the overall patient status. Enemas may be needed to clear the colon. We recommend the use of tap-water enemas; avoid phosphate-based enemas if there is any renal or cardiac impairment. After the colon is cleared, a regimen of fiber and laxatives is instituted. Psyllium can be introduced at the dose of 1 tablespoon in 8 ounces of water once per day and increased to twice per day. The patient should drink an additional glass of liquid after the psyllium is ingested and maintain good hydration. If this regimen is not satisfactory milk of magnesia, 30 cc po qhs, can be added. In refractory patients we occasionally use lactulose or a balanced electrolyte cathartic (such as Colyte). We try to avoid the use of anthraquinone cathartics due to the potential risk of inducing an atonic neuropathic bowel, although this may not be an issue in a patient with a limited life expectancy.

Paraneoplastic Pseudo-obstruction

The destruction of the myenteric plexus by an immune mediated process is a well-established sequela of small-cell carcinoma of the lung.[3] These patients present with the radiographic findings of small bowel obstruction or with intractable diarrhea due to bacterial overgrowth. They often have been operated on for a presumed small bowel obstruction and no surgically correctable lesion was found. Almost all reported cases have occurred in patients who have, or are subsequently diagnosed with, small cell carcinoma of the lung. Diagnosis of the syndrome can be made by the demonstration of a lymphocytic infiltration in the myenteric plexus and by the finding of a diagnostic serum titer for the IgG anti-enteric neuronal antibodies.

Broad-spectrum oral antibiotics are useful for the treatment of bacterial overgrowth in the palliation of the diarrhea and abdominal pain that are a consequence of the intestinal stasis. Typically the antibiotics used include tetracycline, metronidazole, and ciprofloxacin. The antibiotics may be cycled and alternated every few weeks to help avoid resistance. Promotility agents such as metoclopramide and cisapride may be tried, but usually are not efficacious in this disorder. In some cases of antibiotic failure octreotide has been used as a palliative treatment. It may be administered subcutaneously at a dose of 50 μcg t.i.d. increasing to a typical maximum of 200 mcg t.i.d. Long-term palliative support may occasionally require the use of gastrostomy or jejunostomy feeding tubes.

Acute Colonic Pseudo-obstruction

In this syndrome, sometimes called Ogilvie's Syndrome, the colon becomes acutely and/or severely dilated within the context of a serious medical illness and may mimic an intestinal obstruction with similar symptoms, signs, and X-ray findings. This term is now also used to refer to post-operative ileus or ileus arising in patients who have received chemotherapeutic agents.[4] Dilation of the cecum leads to increased cecal wall tension and decreased blood perfusion, potentially leading to transmural ischemia and subsequent perforation.

A plain abdominal X-ray is the most useful test to confirm the diagnosis and will demonstrate cecal dilatation with air in the rectum and relatively few air/fluid levels in the small intestine. Importantly, the patients tend not to have peritoneal signs or evidence of intraperitoneal free air. The setting may vary, but the diagnosis must include the acute onset of abdominal distention and radiographic confirmation of colonic dilation to greater than 10 cm without evidence for mechanical obstruction or an infectious etiology such as toxic megacolon. Occasionally a rectal contrast study may be indicated if concern exists about a distal mechanical obstruction. Complications of this syndrome are inability to feed the patient and colonic perforation.

Stepwise treatment may avert the need for invasive measures. Surgical decompression was the treatment in the recent past, but attendant with this was a high morbidity and mortality rate. Now the mortality rate is roughly 15% for patients treated conservatively and 30% for those treated with surgery, in comparison to 40% for those with perforated or ischemic colon. Treatment should include correction of metabolic abnormalities and sepsis, coupled with the discontinuation of any potential anti-motility agents including anticholinergics and narcotics. Placement of a nasogastric tube may help make the patient more comfortable. Enemas may be tried, but they must not be phosphate-containing preparations, as these may lead to lethal electrolyte abnormalities. The placement of a rectal decompression tube may be of benefit. Currently the treatment of choice for failure of a medical regimen or dilatation of the cecum to greater than 12 cm includes decompressive colonoscopy with or without the placement of a colonic decompression tube.[5] Colonoscopy is carefully performed due to the distention of the bowel wall and the potential for perforation of the dilated cecum. The placement of a decompression tube by colonoscopy is not mandatory, but may aid in the short-term prevention of recurrent severe dilatation. Motility agents, such as cisapride, may be of value in selected cases. Occasionally a decompressive cecostomy, for a cecal diameter greater than 12 cm, may be needed if colonoscopic therapy is unsuccessful or if colonic ischemia or perforation is felt to have occurred.

Diarrhea

The term diarrhea merits definition, as the patient and the physician may not always agree.[6] More than 200 g of stool per day indicates a diarrheal state in most adults, though frequent low-volume watery bowel movements may qualify with less total volume. Some patients have frequent bowel movements but do not have more than 200 g per day of stool, which may indicate proctitis or another anorectal disorder. Incontinence may be exacerbated by loose liquid stools. Factitious diarrhea and medication-induced causes of diarrhea, such as enteral feedings or the administration of magnesium-containing antacids, must always be considered. Most diarrheal states can be simply classified as either osmotic or secretory, though diarrhea that results from enterocyte damage, as seen with radiation therapy and chemotherapy, has a mixed picture. The onset of diarrhea concurrent with the institution of radiation treatment or chemotherapy is not unexpected, occurring in upwards of 90% of patients receiving certain treatment regimens. 50 Gy to the gastrointestinal tract will cause symptoms in about 5% of patients, while 75 Gy may cause symptoms in 50% of patients. Most patients receiving 5-FU will experience some diarrhea, though this is self-limited in most cases.

Non-specific therapy may be instituted for diarrhea simultaneously with evaluation for specific etiologies of diarrhea such as antibiotic associated colitis or radiation proctitis. The administration of stool binders, including aluminum-containing antacids, fiber products, and antimotility agents may serve to decrease the patient's diarrhea to a tolerable level, while intravenous hydration will volume replete the patient. Typical starting doses for aluminum antacids are 30 cc t.i.d., for psyllium 1 tablespoon b.i.d., and loperamide may be started at 2 mg q.i.d. In refractory cases octreotide may be instituted starting at 50 μcg t.i.d.

INFECTIOUS

Infectious diarrhea is typically of acute onset and of less than 2 weeks duration and may be difficult to differentiate from the initial presentation of inflammatory bowel disease or treatment-induced diarrhea. Infectious diarrhea may be due to all of the common etiologies implicated in non-hospitalized patients including bacterial, viral, and parasitic etiologies. Most often *E. coli*, *Salmonella*, *Campylobacter*, and *Shigella* will be encountered, but as a much lower total percentage of the overall number of cases. In contrast, *Clostridia difficile* will be encountered more frequently.

The diagnostic algorithm in an ambulatory or recently hospitalized patient should first include a determination of the severity of the diarrhea. If the patient has not had a prolonged course and bloody diarrhea, systemic signs, and dehydration are not present, symptomatic therapy may be sufficient treatment. If the patient requires hospitalization as a result of the diarrhea, or manifests any systemic signs, then thorough investigation is warranted. Intravenous or oral rehydration should be instituted with empiric antibiotic therapy of intravenous antibiotics covering for gram negative flora.

For all non-hospitalized patients routine stool cultures for enteric flora and aerobes, including *Campylobacter*, *Shigella*, and *Salmonella* should be obtained. A stool toxin assay for *C. difficile* should be sent along with stool samples for ova and parasites. Upper endoscopy with aspiration to evaluate for the presence of *Giardia* and *Strongyloides* may be needed as hyperinfection may occur in the immunocompromised patient. If the patient is hospitalized and subsequently develops acute diarrhea the differential diagnosis is markedly different. *C. difficile* accounts for well over 50% of the cases of nosocomial infectious diarrhea. Stool evaluation for *Salmonella*, *Shigella*, *Campylobacter* and for ova and parasites is usually not rewarding and cannot be obtained in many hospitals if ordered after greater than a 72–hour hospitalization. Viral etiologies increase in relative importance in hospitalized oncology patients, particularly for patients who have received bone marrow transplants. Significant morbidity and mortality have been associated with adenoviral, rotaviral, and *Coxsackie* infections in these patients.[7] Once the specific etiology of the diarrhea is found antimicrobial therapy may be instituted. Specific antibiotic recommendations are beyond the scope of this manual and may be found in most gastroenterology and infectious disease reference books.

ANTIBIOTIC ASSOCIATED COLITIS

Many oncology patients are treated with antibiotics at some point. Some patients develop self-limited diarrhea as a direct result of the administration of antibiotics, such as ampicillin, while others may develop severe diarrhea or systemic complaints.[8] Antibiotic associated colitis is classically associated with clindamycin, ampicillin, and the broad spectrum antibiotics. In oncology patients the administration of chemotherapy increases the incidence of antibiotic associated colitis. Selection of *Clostridium difficile* with its subsequent production of toxin A is responsible for the symptoms. An awareness of the disease is necessary as the symptoms are not markedly different from many chemotherapy and radiation related abdominal complaints. Typically the patient will have loose watery diarrhea and may manifest a fever or leukocytosis. Abdominal pain may not be present in mild cases, but is usually present if the patient is febrile or has a leukocytosis. *C. difficile* induced diarrhea may progress to pseudomembranous colitis. In pseudomembranous colitis systemic toxicity is observed and toxic megacolon may develop in 10% of cases and lead to subsequent perforation. Diagnosis is easy with the ready availability of assays for the *C. difficile* toxin. Culture for *C. difficile* is not accurate as over 40% of hospitalized patients may be colonized yet toxin negative. Sigmoidoscopy is a relatively simple and quick method of establishing the diagnosis and may be performed concurrently with the toxin assay. In 10% of cases *C. difficile* colitis may present with only right colonic involvement and require colonoscopy for diagnosis. Once the toxin is found the patient should be placed on enteric precautions as nosocomial transmission occurs.

Treatment consists of discontinuation of antibiotics, if possible, and the institution of specific antibiotic treatment for *Clostridium*. Oral vancomycin, 125 mg po q.i.d., or metronidazole, 250 mg po q.i.d., for ten days are usually adequate for treatment. Metronidazole iv may be administered in patients who are nil per mouth. Relapse may occur in up to 20% of cases and retreatment with the same antibiotic regimen is usually sufficient. Recurrent infection may warrant the use of cholestyramine or adjunctive administration of *Lacto-bacillus* to aid in the reconstitution of normal enteric flora.

Fecal Incontinence

Fecal incontinence can be incapacitating because of the social stigma attached. Patients may soil themselves not due to an inability to sense a defecatory urge, but due to inability to mobilize themselves or to communicate the need to defecate to others. Patients with intact sphincters may also experience fecal incontinence in the setting of diarrhea, often as the result of fecal impaction. It is necessary to eliminate pseudo-incontinence, which is not due to a diarrheal state, as the treatment will differ. Pseudo-incontinence may be due to inflammatory bowel disease, sexually transmitted disease, or hemorrhoids.

Continence is a complex interplay of cognition, stool quality, colonic reserve, and anorectal function. Neurologic loss due to either the malignancy, metastases, or surgery may result in loss of sensation or defecatory control.[9] The anorectal function is a result of internal and external anal sphincters and the puborectalis muscle. Disruption of any of the sympathetic or parasympathetic neural pathways will potentially lead to incontinence. The cause of incontinence often can be easily discerned. Occasionally a barium enema, sigmoidoscopy, or anorectal manometry may be indicated in the evaluation, though in most cases these tests will confirm the clinical diagnosis.

Treatment of incontinence is multifaceted. Fecal impaction is the leading cause in the elderly and should be treated aggressively. Manual disimpaction may be needed and institution of an aggressive bowel program necessary. Other causes of incontinence usually respond to simple measures. The institution of a high-fiber diet along with bulking agents, such as psyllium (1 to 2 tablespoons per day), will decrease symptoms in a majority of patients. If this is insufficient the addition of an antimotility agent such as loperamide, starting at 2 mg q.i.d., or a narcotic agent such as paregoric, starting at 1 teaspoon q.i.d., will be useful. Occasionally biofeedback training or surgical correction of documented sphincter defects will be needed. In severe cases, the placement of an appliance bag over the anus may aid in skin care and allow the patient some measure of freedom.

THERAPY-RELATED CAUSES OF BOWEL DYSFUNCTION

Narcotic-induced

Narcotics have been reported to cause both constipation and diarrhea. The finding of chronic abdominal pain, vomiting, weight loss, and chronic intestinal pseudo-obstruction in the setting of prolonged (>2 weeks) use of narcotics should suggest the possibility of this entity. Other causes need to be systematically ruled out so that serious disorders are not overlooked. The abdominal X-ray may reveal an ileus or large amount of feces. These patients are often seen in the emergency room and given narcotics, which will relieve the pain.

These patients need institution of an aggressive bowel regimen and may require treatment with psyllium and cathartics.

The narcotic bowel syndrome is felt to be due to the effects of narcotic withdrawal on the gut.[10] Withdrawal symptoms may include diarrhea, myalgia, and pilo-erection. The syndrome will respond to an alteration in the dosing regimen to alleviate withdrawal symptoms during narcotic nadirs. In instances where narcotic withdrawal is possible or necessary, the dose of the narcotic is reduced or eliminated completely and clonidine .1 mg po every 6 to 12 hours may be administered. This regimen may be continued for 7 days on an inpatient basis and over 90% of patients will successfully be weaned off the narcotics without severe withdrawal symptoms.

Radiation Enterocolitis

Radiation-induced bowel injury may present any time after the institution of high-dose radiation treatment. Despite efforts to minimize incidental injury to the bowel by shielding and multiple ports, radiation injury is still commonly seen. Prior intra-abdominal adhesions, abdominal surgery, and vascular insufficiency are associated with an increased incidence of symptomatic injury. Chemotherapy combined with radiation therapy increases the incidence when compared with radiation therapy alone.

Treatment of acute radiation induced enterocolitis includes a change in the radiation port, reduction in dosage, and/or cessation of the radiation therapy. Symptomatic treatment is given as needed with the liberal use of anti-emetics and antimotility and anticholinergic agents. The use of either hyoscamine or loperamide in escalating doses can be effective in helping to decrease the tenesmus and frequency associated with radiation. Chronic radiation-induced damage presents more difficult management issues. Chronic strictures related to radiation injury can be recalcitrant to endoscopic management due to the intense fibrosis that occurs, and surgical correction is often required. Before surgical correction it is necessary to make an effort with small bowel radiologic studies and barium enema exam to define the most likely physiologically significant strictures, as this differentiation is difficult to make during laparotomy.

Chronic blood loss and anemia may result after radiotherapy for pelvic malignancies. Chronic intestinal blood loss is due to the formation of telangiectasia and often can be managed medically. Colonoscopy should be performed to rule out a mass lesion and to obtain biopsies from the mucosa to rule out inflammatory bowel disease and to look for vascular ectasia and fibrosis. Symptomatic treatment of the patient may be undertaken with additional therapy dependent upon the severity. In some instances institution of fiber therapy will reduce rectal symptoms, decrease the bleeding, and alleviate the anemia when coupled with iron supplements. More severe cases may require the use of endoscopic laser therapy to eliminate the telangiectasia. Anecdotal reports have claimed the utility of per rectum estrogen creams in decreasing the frequency of blood transfusions.

Typhlitis

Typhlitis (neutropenic colitis) is an acute bacterial infection of the wall of the cecum and ascending colon. Most often *Clostridium septicum* is associated with the syndrome though gram-negative bacteria, including *Pseudomonas aeruginosa*, may be found.[11] Other intra-abdominal events, including free perforation and appendicitis, should be included in the differential diagnosis.

The usual setting is a patient with neutropenia as the result of chemotherapy. The patients often present with fever and peritoneal signs localizing to the right lower quadrant which may become non-focal with time. CT scan may show thickening of the right colon and cecum with no evidence for free air or a perforation. Aggressive medical therapy is warranted as the recent literature contains numerous reports of high morbidity associated with surgical intervention for this entity, in contrast to early literature that suggested nonsurgical therapy was unsuccessful. Patients should be kept NPO, closely followed with serial abdominal exams, and started on broad-spectrum antibiotics. Most patients improve within 48 to 72 hours. Deterioration should prompt consideration of laparoscopy or open surgery to rule out other intra-abdominal processes. The use of granulocyte-macrophage colony-stimulating factors has been discussed in case reports and holds theoretical hope as a viable treatment modality.

Mucositis

Inflammatory response to cytotoxicity from chemotherapy or radiation may occur throughout the gastrointestinal tract. The symptoms and complaints may vary from an oral ulcer to severe abdominal pain that might require differentiation from an acute surgical emergency.

Oral mucositis is most often seen after chemotherapy-induced leukopenia. Secondary infection may lead to systemic complications in a neutropenic patient. The finding of poor oral hygiene before chemotherapy should prompt institution of measures to improve dentition. Following chemotherapy a variety of infectious agents may infect the oral mucosa, including cytomegalovirus and herpes virus. Oral cultures and mucosal biopsies may need to be obtained to institute specific therapy for these infections.

Esophagitis should be considered when the patient complains of odynophagia or dysphagia. This is seen in the setting of radiotherapy with a port which encompasses the mediastinum or after chemotherapy. The symptoms may be due to radiation injury, fungal infections, viral infections, and rarely, bacterial causes. Occasionally esophagitis may be seen as a result of peptic reflux disease, especially in patients who have had prolonged nasogastric tube intubation or are bedridden. *Candida, Herpes simplex,* and *Cytomegalovirus* esophagitis are the most often encountered infections in the neutropenic patient. Systemic treatment with broad-spectrum antibiotics also predisposes to *Candida* esophagitis.

The evaluation of esophagitis is dependent upon the severity of the patient's symptomology. Therapy is often aimed at the most likely etiology, *Candida*. Upper endoscopy with biopsy and cytology are used for those who are refractory to antifungal therapy or who do not have evidence for oral thrush. Patients felt to have *Candida* esophagitis may be empirically treated with Nystatin swish and swallow, 400,000 units q.i.d. Patients who do not respond to this therapy will most likely require endoscopy to ascertain the exact etiology. If *Candida* is found ketoconazole (100 mg b.i.d.) or fluconazole (200 mg per day) may be instituted. If the patient is found to have invasive *Candidiasis* intravenous amphotericin B will be required. Patients found to have *Herpes* esophagitis may be treated with acyclovir, 750 mg/m^2/day split into 3 doses per day, for 7 days. A swish and swallow of lidocaine gel may provide significant symptomatic relief for many patients.

Stercoral/Neutropenic Ulcers in Rectum

Fecal impaction proximal to a narrowing of the colon increases the likelihood of a stercoral or ischemic ulcer. This entity should be considered in oncology patients since they are at increased risk for constipation and have a decreased ability to mount a mucosal inflammatory response. Stercoral ulcers may progress to colonic perforation and require surgical intervention. Concomitant use of nonsteroidal agents may increase the likelihood of perforation.[12] Treatment includes the alleviation of constipation and the avoidance of nonsteroidal agents.

Perirectal Cellulitis and Abscess

Proctitis may be related to radiation or chemotherapy and may be the initial symptom of a perirectal abscess. Most often perirectal infections occur in patients with prolonged neutropenia, though the incidence appears to be decreasing due to the widespread use of antibiotics for febrile neutropenia. If the patient is neutropenic the local signs may only include pain and relatively mild erythema that may mask a deep abscess or cellulitis. Digital and sigmoidoscopic exams under sedation may be required to adequately evaluate for an abscess. Endoscopy with endorectal ultrasound examination may yield the most rewarding information.[13] Therapy should include aggressive antibiotic therapy and surgical drainage, if the patient manifests systemic signs, or does not respond quickly to antibiotics.

Ascites

Fluid collections in the abdomen of a cancer patient may occur as a direct result of the malignancy, occult liver disease, poor nutritional status, or as a result of lymphatic disruption. The diagnosis of the specific etiology is made by paracentesis. Ascitic fluid should be analyzed for cell count with differential, albumin, triglyceride, bacterial culture, and cytology. If malignant ascites is suspected then a large volume paracentesis may be required. Determination of the serum-ascites albumin gradient is useful for determining the contribution of intrinsic liver disease to the ascites.[14] An albumin gradient (serum-ascitic) of less than 1.1 g/dl suggests a malignant etiology for the ascites.

The etiology of the ascites will determine the optimal manner in which to manage the fluid. If the ascites is the result of intrinsic liver disease treatment should include a low-salt (2 g Na) diet and diuretics such as spironolactone, starting at 50 mg b.i.d. Additional treatment recommendations are beyond the scope of this manual and may be found in any hepatology text. The investigation of ascites will occasionally lead to the finding of obstruction of the vena cava, Budd-Chiari syndrome, or unsuspected peritoneal carcinomatosis.

Chylous Ascites

Chylous ascites is most often seen as a postsurgical complication of retroperitoneal lymph node dissection or thoracic duct disruption, though lymphatic obstruction from tumor may also be seen.[15] The onset is typically within the first 6 weeks after surgery and may be initially subtle, though occasionally a rapid presentation with signs of peritoneal inflammation may be seen. The definitive diagnosis of chylous ascites is made by diagnostic paracentesis. Lymphangiography may help to localize the site of leakage. The fluid appears milky with high triglyceride and protein levels and fat globules upon staining with Sudan black.

If direct extension of tumor is responsible for chylous ascites, attempts to treat the malignancy are warranted. Surgical disruption responds better to treatment. Dietary manipulation is the primary therapy for either etiology; repeat paracentesis and diuretic therapy should be discouraged. Dietary limitation of long-chain triglycerides, which are the main form transported by the thoracic duct, and supplementation with medium-chain fatty triglycerides will decrease lymphatic flow from over 200 cc/minute to 1 cc/minute. If this is unsuccessful in patients in whom malignant obstruction is not present, total parenteral alimentation coupled with bowel rest should be tried. In some refractory cases surgical correction of the leak is necessary when conservative maneuvers have failed.

MALIGNANT ASCITES

Malignant ascites presents a difficult management problem.[16] Typically the patient suffers from massive hepatic metastasis or peritoneal carcinomatosis. Malignant ascites caused by carcinomatosis tends to be resistant to diuretic therapy while ascites caused by hepatic metastasis responds to diuretic therapy. If peritoneal carcinomatosis is present diuretic therapy should not be used. Large-volume paracentesis on a weekly or biweekly basis may benefit symptomatic patients. Patients with hepatic metastasis appear to respond to diuretics in a fashion similar to cirrhotic patients, if the serum-ascites albumin gradient is greater than 1.1 g/dl. These patients should be placed on a low-salt diet and diuretic therapy instituted with spironolactone at 50 mg b.i.d. and increased to achieve a diuresis of 0.5 kg/day.

REFERENCES

1. Shafik A. Constipation: pathogenesis and management. Drugs 45(4):528–40, 1993
2. Mezwa DG, Feczko PJ, Bosanko C. Radiologic evaluation of constipation and anorectal disorders. Radio Clin NA. 31(6):1375–93, 1993
3. Lennon VA, Sas DF, Busk MF et al. Enteric neuronal auto-antibodies in pseudo-obstruction with small cell lung carcinoma. Gastro 100:137–42, 1991
4. Dorudi S, Berry AR, Kettlewell MGW. Acute colonic pseudo-obstruction. Br J Surg 79:99–103, 1992
5. Nano D, Prindiville T, Pauly M et al. Colonoscopic therapy of acute pseudo-obstruction of the colon. Amer J Gastro. 82(2):145–8, 1987
6. Park SI, Giannella RA. Approach to the adult patient with acute diarrhea. Gastro Clin NA 22(3):483–97, 1993
7. Yolken RH, Bishop CA, Townsend RT et al. Infectious gastroenteritis in bone marrow transplant recipients. N Engl J Med 306 (17):1010–2, 1982
8. Pothoulakis C, LaMont JT. *Clostridium difficile* colitis and diarrhea. Gastro Clin NA 22(3):623–37, 1993
9. Madoff RD, Williams JG, Caushaj PF. Fecal incontinence. NEJM 326(15):1002–7, 1992
10. Sandgren JE, McPhee MS, Greenberger NJ. Narcotic bowel syndrome treated with clonidine. Ann Int Med 101:331–4, 1984
11. Hiruki T, Fernandes B, Ramsay J et al. Acute typhlitis in an immunocompromised host. Dig Dis Sci 37(8):1292–6, 1992
12. Hollingworth J, Alexander-Williams J. Non-steroidal anti-inflammatory drugs and stercoral perforation of the colon. Ann Royal Col Surg 73:337–40, 1991
13. Cataldo PA, Senagore A, Luchtefeld MA. Intrarectal ultrasound in the evaluation of perirectal abscesses. Dis Colon Rectum 36(6):554–8, 1993
14. Kajani MA, Yoo YK, Alexander JA et al. Serum-ascites albumin gradients in nonalcoholic liver disease. Dig Dis Sci. 35(1):33–7, 1990
15. Browse NL, Wilson NM, Russo F et al. Aetiology and treatment of chylous ascites. Br J Surg. 79:1145–50,1992
16. Pockros PJ, Esrason KT, Nguyen C, et al. Mobilization of malignant ascites with diuretics is dependent on ascitic fluid characteristics. Gastro. 103:1302–6,1992

John S. Macdonald, Daniel G. Haller, Robert J. Mayer, Eds. *Manual of Oncologic Therapeutics*, Third Edition.

63. URINARY DYSFUNCTION

Michael M. Lieber

SUPPORTIVE CARE AND REHABILITATION

Ill patients often require the use of an indwelling urethral catheter to provide bladder drainage. While insertion of a small-caliber latex or silicone Foley urethral catheter is usually straightforward, providing bladder drainage in a cancer patient can occasionally require a fair amount of urologic skill and wisdom. Basic guiding principles should be never to force a urethral catheter and always to use plenty of lubrication.

Urethral catheterization in a female is rarely difficult unless the patient has had extensive vulvar or vaginal surgery. In the male, however, an enlarged prostate gland, bladder neck contracture after previous prostate surgery, changes in the prostatic urethra caused by prostate carcinoma and radiation therapy, and urethral stricture can make urethral catheterization difficult or even impossible. If the catheter advances through the anterior urethra and appears to hang up at the level of the prostate or bladder neck, then one should attempt to pass a small Coude catheter of about 12- to 14-French diameter. Very often the bend in the Coude catheter tip will permit passage of the catheter over a prominent middle lobe of the prostate or through a tight bladder neck contracture, when a standard straight urethral catheter will not pass into the bladder.

For the male patient with obvious stricture in the penile urethra, dilatation of the stricture after passage of filiforms is usually the best course to follow. Use of filiforms and followers should be done by a urologist. Gentle passage of lubricated, very fine, straight or dogleg filiform catheters will often allow urethral catheterization through a tight stricture. With the filiform passing through the stricture and into the bladder, gentle dilation of the stricture can then be carried out using woven followers that screw on to the external end of the filiform catheter. In an emergency a woven hollow follower catheter passed into the bladder can be taped in place to the penis and serve as a temporary urethral drainage device. Unfortunately, such a catheter is usually not long-lasting, and replacement with a more permanent device that has an inflatable balloon to position it in the bladder is usually necessary. If the urethral strictures can be dilated enough, usually to 18-French or greater, a special Council-tip urethral catheter can be passed over a metal mandarin having at its end a male-threaded tip, which screws into the female external end of the filiform and permits safe guided passage of the catheter into the bladder.

Too much emphasis should not be given to blind tactile attempts to pass urethral catheters retrograde. In many cases, if this is not done by an experienced and gentle catheterizer, profound damage to the urethra results and retrograde catheterization becomes impossible after false passages are generated. Urethral bleeding can also be severe, and permanent scarring and stricture often result. It is much better to consult a urologist early on. With modern cystoscopic instruments, such as a cold knife urethrotome, urethral strictures can be visualized endoscopically, a urethral catheter or guidewire can be passed retrograde through the stricture, and then the stricture can be incised using the cold knife instrument. Subsequently, using a split-sheath attachment to the urethrotome, an 18- or 20-French urethral catheter can be positioned in the bladder under direct vision. Use of this newer type of urethral instrumentation accomplished under direct vision is preferred when the patient's general condition permits a trip to the cystoscopic examining room and a brief anesthetic.

For patients in whom a urethral catheter cannot be passed retrograde and a distended bladder fundus is palpable above the symphysis pubis, insertion of a percutaneous transabdominal cystostomy tube is highly recommended. Numerous commercial kits contain all of the necessary instruments and tubes, including a cystostomy tube ranging from 8- to 14-French diameter, which is passed on or through a stylet introduced 4 cm to 5 cm above the symphysis pubis under local anesthesia. Prospecting for the urine-filled bladder using an 18-gauge spinal needle is recommended before using the much larger diameter metal trocar provided with the cystotomy kit. One must be sure that a urine-filled bladder is available for puncture. In particular, after previous pelvic surgery such as anteroposterior resection of the rectum, the intrapelvic anatomy can be quite abnormal. The bladder can be far from the anterior abdominal wall, and blindly prospecting for the bladder with a large trocar is not recommended. On the other hand, a large, readily palpable bladder fundus in a thin patient provides a straightforward target for the suprapubic cystostomy tube.

URETHRAL CATHETERS AND INFECTION

With sterile insertion techniques, application of povidone-iodine (Betadine) salve to the urethral meatus, and closed urinary drainage devices, the lower urinary tract and the catheter can be maintained sterile for a number of days. Unfortunately, however, many cancer patients require prolonged drainage. After a period of days, whether the patient is on prophylactic antibiotics or not, the urine will become infected because the catheter is a foreign body communicating with the outside world. Unless the patient is clinically septic, treatment of a urinary tract infection (UTI) with a urethral catheter or suprapubic catheter in place is usually not advisable. Although the initial infecting organism is commonly treatable, its replacement by resistant superinfecting bacteria is virtually inevitable. Thus, an *Escherichia coli* UTI is commonly converted to a pseudomonas or yeast infection. Attempts to eradicate organisms such as *Pseudomonas* or *Serratia* with aminoglycoside antibiotics are ill-advised because the antibiotics may result in nephron injury and decreased renal function in an otherwise asymptomatic UTI. Unless the patient is septic, catheter-associated UTI should be simply ignored.

Many patients with a chronic indwelling urethral catheter, in addition to the inevitable UTI, develop purulent urethritis and occasionally severe pyogenic epididymitis. The development of such acute suppurating epididymitis should be suspected in any septic cancer patient who has an indwelling urethral catheter. Infected urine freely draining from the catheter is rarely a source of sepsis, but infected secretions traveling down the vas deferens and causing purulent epididymitis are a common source of infection in the debilitated male patient. Combination antimicrobial chemotherapy and often emergency orchiectomy are necessary for the patient with pyogenic epididymitis. In contrast, acute bacterial prostatitis or prostatic abscess is extremely rare in the patient with a chronic indwelling urethral catheter and not a likely source of sepsis in cancer patients.

NEPHROSTOMY TUBES

Supravesical urinary obstruction, usually bilateral tumor obstruction of the distal ureters, sometimes requires long-term or permanent nephrostomy drainage in patients with many types of intra-abdominal malignancy. At present, such nephrostomy tubes are usually placed percutaneously by the uroradiologist using fluoroscopic and angiographic techniques, as opposed to the open surgical insertion commonly used a decade ago. The dilated renal pelvis identified by excretory urography or ultrasound represents a fairly easy target for the experienced uroradiologist; puncture of the renal pelvis and passage of a guidewire into the pelvis or down the ureter generally is possible. Commonly, a 7- to 8-French angiographic catheter with a "J" or ring-curved tip can then be positioned in the renal pelvis to provide adequate drainage.

This type of percutaneous nephrostomy tube provides the most common supravesical diversion for cancer patients at the present time. Often, when bleeding from the initial percutaneous nephrostomy tube placement has subsided, the nephrostomy tract can be enlarged with passage of dilators over a guidewire and a larger, more permanent nephrostomy tube, less likely to occlude with clot or debris, can be placed before the patient is discharged from the hospital. In many cases, a 14- to 16-French silastic Foley catheter with the balloon inflated in the renal pelvis is a more desirable nephrostomy tube than an angiographic catheter positioned in the renal pelvis, which is easier to dislodge or occlude. Like urethral catheters, nephrostomy tubes commonly infect the urinary tract after several days of external drainage. Once again, the presence of an asymptomatic UTI from an indwelling nephrostomy tube is not a reason for treatment with antibiotics; doing so simply selects for resistant organisms. Nephrostomy tubes generally need to be exchanged every 3 to 4 months to prevent obstruction by debris. Significant leakage of urine around the nephrostomy tube is an indication to exchange the tube. The changing of nephrostomy tubes under fluoroscopic guidance as necessary can avoid many technical problems. After nephrostomy access to the renal pelvis has been achieved by the uroradiologist, it often is possible to pass an angiographic guidewire antegrade down the ureter into the bladder and then subsequently to pass a permanent indwelling double-J ureteral stent over the guidewire from the renal pelvis into the bladder. Use of such antegrade-inserted double-J ureteral stents is now common treatment for patients with ureteral obstruction due to retroperitoneal malignancy. In such patients, the nephrostomy tube placed for access can be plugged or withdrawn, and urine will be expelled from the bladder and urethra in the usual manner. Such internal urethral stent drainage is preferred over nephrostomy tube drainage, with its necessity for external collection bags, frequent catheter changes, and the local pain or discomfort associated with permanent external nephrostomy tube drainage.

For patients who require supravesical urinary diversion and who have a moderately indolent tumor, a life expectancy measured in months to years, and no contraindications to surgery, creation of an ileal conduit (or bilateral cutaneous ureterostomies, if the ureters are dilated from distal obstruction) may be a better long-term solution. Preservation of renal function and prevention of recurrent UTI are easier in the absence of foreign bodies in the urinary tract.

The existence of sophisticated techniques for ensuring urinary drainage does not exempt the physician from exercising judgment as to when drainage procedures may or may not be appropriate. In the presence of a malignancy for which all meaningful anticancer therapy has been exhausted, progressive uremia may be the most humane exodus available. Placement of percutaneous nephrostomy tubes in a patient with an advanced malignancy should not, therefore, become a reflex decision made by an inexperienced physician.

John S. Macdonald, Daniel G. Haller, Robert J. Mayer, Eds. *Manual of Oncologic Therapeutics*, Third Edition.

64. THE SWOLLEN EXTREMITY

Deborah M. Axelrod
Michael P. Osborne

ETIOLOGY

The major causes of unilateral leg edema are venous or lymphatic obstruction. In patients with a malignancy, direct invasion or compression by tumor or by fibrosis secondary to radiation or surgery can result in venous occlusion. Exacerbation of previous venous disease may be due to extrinsic compression in association with the hypercoagulable state that occurs in some patients with malignancy. Obstructive lymphedema may result from lymphadenectomy; irradiation, fibrosis, and inflammation of subcutaneous tissues; or tumor invasion of lymphatics and regional lymph nodes. In postoperative cancer patients who develop a swollen limb years after surgery, tumor metastases must be a primary consideration.

Unilateral upper extremity swelling may also be venous or lymphatic in origin. Venous etiologies include Pancoast tumor or invasion of the superior vena cava and axillary vein thrombosis. The most frequent cause of upper limb lymphedema is axillary dissection associated with breast cancer treatment (radical or modified radical mastectomy). Postmastectomy lymphedema ranges in incidence from 6.7% to 52.5% after radical mastectomy; the incidence is increased with preoperative or postoperative radiation therapy and gross nodal involvement. At Memorial Hospital the incidence of arm edema was 4.7% in patients having undergone limited resection, axillary dissection, and breast radiation therapy, compared with 12.5% in patients following modified radical mastectomy.

Although upper extremity lymphedema can occur in the immediate postoperative period from adventitial dissection of the axillary vein during surgery, often associated with flap necrosis, hematoma, or infection, it more commonly occurs months to years later. Early edema is usually mild and occurs before compensatory lymphatic channels or lymphovenous communications develop following surgery. Late edema is debilitating and is almost always the result of a low-grade infection in the extremity. The subsequent fibrosis increases the accumulation of interstitial fluid.

CLINICAL FEATURES

Patients may present with the clear-cut clinical signs of venous or lymphatic disease. In other cases, a complex presentation occurs, and the diagnosis must be established to allow appropriate treatment.

Dark and brawny firm edema, brownish discoloration, dermatitis, and skin ulceration usually result from impaired capillary perfusion in venous insufficiency. Venous disease rarely involves the toes, while in lymphatic disease the edema often begins most distally. Patients with deep venous thrombosis may have a history of recurrent thrombophlebitis. These patients present with tenderness, warmth, erythema, and edema localized to the site of involvement, or the entire leg may be involved as in ileofemoral venous thrombosis. Pain and cyanosis may be present (phlegmasia cerulea dolens). Thirty percent of patients who present with ileofemoral thrombosis have an occult malignancy.

In contrast to the edema of venous disease, lymphedema is usually painless in the absence of lymphangitis and cellulitis. The swelling is symmetrical and in long-standing lymphedema may be accompanied by fatigue, functional impairment of the limb, and cosmetic deformity. Unlike venous disease, ulceration is rare. Small blisters containing edema fluid with high protein content or hyperkeratosis of the skin may occur ("pigskin"). In mediastinal disease or axillary vein thrombosis, marked cutaneous collaterals may be evident over the upper extremity.

DIAGNOSTIC TESTS

Although physical examination constitutes the initial step in the diagnosis of the swollen extremity, noninvasive tests such as Doppler studies, ultrasound, impedance plethysmography, and B-mode ultrasonography can demonstrate the patency of the venous system. Invasive tests should be avoided if at all possible because the edematous limb is extremely susceptible to infection.

Computed tomography (CT) and ultrasonography may pick up pelvic neoplasms. In addition, CT may also demonstrate the characteristic "honeycomb" pattern of the subcutaneous compartment in lymphedema. Ultrasonography may differentiate lymphedema and phlebitis. Radionuclide scanning may be used to measure protein tissue clearance. Clearance of the isotope (usually radioiodinated human serum albumin) depends on the extracellular fluid volume and lymphatic drainage; because diffusion is increased in the lymphedematous limb, clearance measurements may be normal and so serial scans need to be performed.

In most cases, mild edema will respond to exercise, compression, and elevation, and no further investigative workup need be pursued; *when edema occurs late or with sudden onset*, however, recurrent neoplasm must be ruled out. Phlebography or less invasive techniques such as color

Doppler vascular mapping may define venous abnormalities such as thrombosis. This procedure is safer than conventional lymphangiography, a study obtained by forceful injection of oily contrast media directly into a cannulated lymphatic channel. This can cause lymphangitis, cellulitis, or phlebitis. On rare occasions, pulmonary oil embolism may result if a vein is injected erroneously or if a lymphovenous fistula exists. Currently, radioisotope lymphoscintigraphy has supplanted lymphangiography. This procedure requires a single subcutaneous injection (using technetium-99m–antimony trisulfide colloid) into the involved extremity.

COMPLICATIONS

The sequelae of venous stasis includes dermatitis, ulceration, and infection. Acute venous occlusion may be segmental or may progress to involve the entire leg, if there is ileofemoral thrombosis. In rare circumstances, rapid progression of phlegmasia cerulea dolens can lead to subsequent venous gangrene. Pulmonary embolism is a major complication of venous thrombosis.

Long-standing or severe lymphedema is characterized by fibrosis and lymph stasis, which predisposes the patient to recurrent lymphangitis and cellulitis, the major complications of lymphedema. Lymphangitis, in turn, accelerates the fibrosis, which causes more fluid to accumulate, hence more complications. Repeated bouts of infection may produce skin breakdown. Protein-rich edema fluid provides an ideal culture medium for bacteria; the beta-hemolytic streptococcus is most often implicated in lymphangitis/cellulitis.

Lymphangiosarcoma is a rare complication associated with chronic postmastectomy lymphedema (Stewart-Treves syndrome). This tumor generally appears 10 years or more after the onset of lymphedema in 0.5% to 10% of patients. Hematogenous metastases (particularly to the lung) appear early in the course of the disease and the prognosis is very poor. Amputation is reserved for cases without evident metastases.

TREATMENT

Medical Management

The goals of therapy include mobilization of fluid, prevention of infection, and maintenance of an edema-free state. Most patients respond to simple measures and rarely require surgery.

Before initiating treatment, baseline limb girth measurements should be obtained using a tape measure. Circumference changes of the lower limb should be measured at fixed points from the floor for reproducibility. A significant reduction in symptoms may be accompanied by only a modest decrease of edema. Early institution of compression is undertaken to control edema and prevent its progression to tissue fibrosis. Circumferential limb measurements may not accurately reflect volume measurements. Newer studies (*i.e.*, multiple frequency bioelectric impedance analysis) may more accurately monitor extracellular fluid changes before and after treatment and therefore effectiveness of treatment.

Elevation and compression are the mainstays of treatment. The edematous limb should be elevated above the level of the heart. Stockings with graded elastic compression should be worn continuously. Custom-fitted stockings generate pressures of 30 mmHg to 50 mmHg at the ankle level; for "off-the-shelf" stockings, pressures are approximately 24 mmHg. These stockings, made of Spandex, are relatively inexpensive and conform to a variety of different-shaped limbs. In patients with mild lymphedema or venous stasis, "off-the-shelf" stockings are effective in decreasing volume, circumference, and symptoms. In more severe cases custom-fitted stockings may be necessary. Patients who have undergone deep dissection of the iliac or obturator nodes are advised to avoid prolonged standing and to wear an elastic stocking to prevent lymphedema. Patients should be carefully instructed in how to wear these. Compliance has improved over the years because stockings are more fashionable and elastic arm sleeves lighter in weight.

In addition to continuous compression, various inflatable compression devices are now on the market for continued ambulatory treatment. These should be used in conjunction with elastic stockings, which provide continuous support. Sequential pneumatic compression, which produces a "milking" type of action, is effective in the treatment of lymphedema. One example is the *Lymphapress*, a multicompartmental, high-pressure pneumatic compression device. Most other pneumatic equipment, until recently, had only one inflatable chamber and did not exert a pressure gradient which seems to be more effective in controlling lymphedema. Repeated treatments with pneumatic compression devices are more effective in the improvement of limb lymphedema. Intermittent compression is effective in the treatment of edema caused by venous disease. The use of these inflatable devices is contraindicated in the presence of lymphangitis, cellulitis, phlebitis, and decompensated cardiac failure. Another drawback is the additional cost. Improvement in edema due to pneumatic compression devices is greatest at the distal sites compared with proximal sites.

Massage therapy has become a popular technique in the United States in the relief of lymphedema following axillary lymphadenectomy. It is not a new concept, having been introduced in the 1930s by Dr. Emil Vodder from Denmark. The Vodder method is a massage technique (manual lymphatic drainage) which should be practiced only by licensed massage therapists trained in this technique. Four basic movements are applied: stationary circles, rotary, pumping, and scooping movements, to ensure adequate drainage of the extremity. The goal (as seen with pneumatic compression devices) is actively to shunt extracellular fluid to those areas where lymphatic vessels are intact.

Massage therapy is also included in another technique, complex physical therapy. This combines massage therapy with skin care, compression bandaging, and (later) garments and exercises. Introduced in Australia, there have been several reports indicating high success rate with significant reduction in edema with initial therapy and further significant reductions with repeated courses of treatment.

Meticulous hygiene is crucial to the prevention of infection. Cracks and fissures in the thickened skin can serve as a potential portal of infection, and blisters may predispose to cellulitis. The skin should be cleansed with a mild antiseptic soap; use of a body lotion will suffice to keep the skin soft and to prevent it from cracking. Extra care must be taken to avoid cuts and burns. After mastectomy and axillary dissection, patients are cautioned against nail biting and cutting cuticles. Injections into and blood drawing from the dissected arm should be strongly discouraged and the contralateral arm should be used. Topical antifungal agents should be applied between the toes and on the soles of the feet in patients with fissures and cracks in the skin. Miconazole (Mica Tin) 2% cream, clotrimazole (Lotrimin) 1% cream, haloprogin (Halotex) 1% cream, or tolnaftate (Tinactin) 1% cream are effective antifungal agents.

The patient should be alerted to the early symptoms and signs of infection, including pain, tenderness, redness, streaking, and fever. Lymphangitis and cellulitis must be promptly treated with bedrest, leg elevation, and systemic antibiotics. Patients with a history of recurrent infection should be treated prophylactically with phenoxymethyl penicillin, 250 mg four times a day for 10 days periodically, or erythromycin for patients allergic to penicillin.

In the patient presenting with an acutely edematous leg, deep venous thrombosis should be investigated promptly and treated appropriately with anticoagulation.

Diuretics may help to reduce temporarily limb size. However, the risks may outweigh the benefits. Schirger recommends the intermittent use of thiazide diuretics such as hydrochlorthiazide (25 mg) in combination with a potassium-sparing agent, triamterene (50 mg), given every other day or three to four times per week, to aid in the maintenance of an edema-free state.

Mobilization of fluid removes only the water content and not the protein from the interstitial compartment. Drugs such as benzopyrones, which induce proteolysis, have been used in continental Europe and in Australia but are not approved for use in the United States and Great Britain.

SURGICAL MANAGEMENT

When conservative methods are unsuccessful in managing the lymphedematous extremity and there is functional impairment of the limb or recurrent lymphangitis and cellulitis, surgical treatment may be indicated. Cosmesis is a controversial indication because in the majority of cases the affected limb can never be expected to achieve a relatively normal physical appearance.

The sequential pneumatic compression device has been used to facilitate surgery for lymphedema of the limbs. It has been used before surgery to reduce lymphedema, during surgery to enlarge lymphatic vessels and facilitate creation of anastomoses, and after surgery to avoid early occlusion of the anastomosis.

Surgical approaches include physiological procedures and excisional methods; these may be combined. The goal of physiological operations is to increase drainage of lymphatic fluid. Creation of a lymphatic pedicle (preferably small bowel) to drain the affected limb is an example. However, the level of obstruction must be sufficiently proximal to bypass and avoid tension on the pedicle. O'Brien proposed microlymphaticovenous anastomosis with anastomosis of lymphatic channels into adjacent superficial veins. Degni reported a 75% reduction of edema in the lower extremity, having studied 77 patients with a follow-up period ranging from 1.5 months to 11 years.

Excisional methods involve removal of skin, subcutaneous tissue, and deep fascia. Charles originally described this procedure for elephantiasis of the scrotum, and it has been applied to both the lower and upper extremity. Split-thickness skin grafts are applied to the exposed muscle (and perineum). Advocates of the Charles procedure claim the most consistent postoperative improvement with the lowest associated risk. Liposuction has been reported to be used in conjunction with other surgical methods or alone in the treatment of primary and secondary lymphedema. Other reports suggest an exacerbation of lymphedema with liposuction.

In general, the results of surgery have been disappointing. Nevertheless, some patients do experience functional improvement. Complex procedures for patients with malignancy must be weighed against prognosis of the cancer, and surgery is contraindicated when recurrent disease is present.

BIBLIOGRAPHY

Britton RC, Nelson PA. Causes and treatment of post-mastectomy lymphedema of arm: Report of 114 cases. JAMA 180:95–102, 1962

Casley-Smith JR, Morgan RC, Piller NB. Treatment of lymphedema of the arms and legs with 5,6-benzopyrone. NEJM 329:1158–1163, 1993

Casley-Smith JR. Modern treatment of lymphedema I. Complex physical therapy: the first 200 Australian limbs. Australasian Journal of Dermatology 33(2):61–68, 1992

Degni M. Surgical management of selected patients with lymphedema of the extremities. J Cardiovasc Surg 25:481–488, 1984

Foldi E, Foldi M, Clodius I. The lymphedema chaos: a lancet. Ann Plast Surg 22:505–515, 1989

Golueke PJ, Montgomery RA, Petronis JD et al. Lymphoscintigraphy to confirm the clinical diagnosis of lymphedema. J Vasc Surg 10:306–312, 1989

Hadjis NS, Carr DH, Banks L, Pflug JJ. The role of CT in the diagnosis of primary lymphedema of the lower limb. Am J Radiol 144:361–364, 1985

Handley WS. The surgery of the lymphatic system. Br Med J 1:853, 1910

Johnson G Jr. Graded compression stockings: Custom versus noncustom. Arch Surg 117:69–72, 1982

Kinmonth JB, Taylor CW, Harper RK. Lymphangiography: A technique for its clinical use in the lower limb. Br Med J 1:940, 1955

Krylor V, Milanor N, Ab Almasor K. Microlymphatic surgery of secondary lymphoedema of the upper limb. Ann Chir Gynaecol 71:77–79, 1982

Latham A, English TC (eds). Elephantiasis Scroti: A System of Treatment, Vol 3, p 416. London, J & A Churchill, 1912

McCormick B. The incidence of arm edema following modified mastectomy, versus limited resection, axillary dissection and breast radiation therapy. Presented at meeting of Curie Society, Paris, April 1986

O'Brien B McC. Microlymphaticovenous and resectional surgery in obstructive lymphedema. World J Surg 3:3, 1979

Richmand DM, O'Donnell TF Jr, Zelikovksi A. Sequential pneumatic compression for lymphedema. Arch Surg 120:1116–1119, 1985

Schirger A. DDX and management of leg edema in the elderly. Geriatrics 37:26–32, 1982

Thompson N. Surgical treatment of chronic lymphedema of the lower limb. Br Med J 2:26–32, 1962

Yeh HC, Rabinowitz JG. Ultrasonography of the extremities and pelvic girdle and correlation with computed tomography. Radiology 143:519–525, 1982

Zelikovski A, Deutsch A, Reiss R. The sequential pneumatic compression device in surgery for lymphedema of the limbs. J Cardiovasc Surg 24(2):122–126, 1983

John S. Macdonald, Daniel G. Haller, Robert J. Mayer, Eds. *Manual of Oncologic Therapeutics,* Third Edition.

65. ORAL CARE OF THE CANCER PATIENT

Ted P. Raybould
Gerald A. Ferretti

INTRODUCTION

More than one million Americans develop cancer annually. Management of malignancies require procedures such as local or radical surgical excision, radiation therapy, chemotherapy, and transplantation. Unfortunately, many cancer treatments affect both normal and cancerous cells and tissues. As treatments for cancer have evolved, they have become therapeutically more successful but are usually more intensive. The side effects on normal cells and tissue integrity have also increased. The oral cavity is a frequent site of such side effects. Each year, as many as 400,000 patients undergoing cancer therapy may develop oral complications (direct or indirect) (Table 65–1), that are either acute or chronic in nature. Acute oral complications associated with cancer therapy are a frequent and potentially serious problem. The frequency for these problems can range from 12% of patients receiving adjunctive chemotherapy to essentially 100% of patients receiving radiation to their oral cavity when doses exceed a total of 5000 cGy. The most common complications include mucosal inflammation, ulceration, infection, hemorrhage, and salivary gland dysfunction. These complications are often painful and difficult to treat. Patients can become discouraged, depressed, anorexic, and physically weakened due to weight loss and inadequate sleep. All of these can further complicate the course of care and jeopardize the success of therapy. Research has also demonstrated that the oral cavity may serve as a portal of entry for acute, life-threatening, or fatal systemic infection.

The long-term consideration of the effects of cancer treatments cannot be ignored. Chronic conditions include osteoradionecrosis, salivary gland dysfunction, secondary malignancies, growth and development abnormalities of hard and soft tissues of the head and neck, and taste dysfunction.

As various cancer therapies become more intensive and survival rates increase, treatment side effects take on even greater significance. It is important that the management of the cancer patient is performed by an interdisciplinary care team approach. Optimal care for the cancer patient often includes a team consisting of the physician, dentist, nurse, social worker, and dietician. This concept of care has evolved because of an increasing emphasis on preventing or minimizing complications. Pre- and intra-therapy support care interventions can have a significant impact on the incidence and the severity of certain oral side effects.

A primary function of the oral mucosa is to serve as a protective barrier for underlying tissues and organs. The oral mucosa consists of a stratified, squamous epithelium that is capable of variable rates of cellular differentiation and maturation in order to meet the functional demands placed on it. Even in normal function, the mucosa of the oral cavity is subjected to a wide variety of traumatic insults and is challenged by the endogenous microflora. The basal cells in the deep germitive layers of the oral epithelium divide, mature, and migrate to the surface and finally desquamate at the surface as a result of the challenges to the surface epithelium. The time from basal replication to desquamation is less than that of the gut epithelium, but greater than that of skin. Also, the epithelial renewal rate is different for selected anatomical areas of the mouth. The nonkeratinized mucosa of the ventral surface of the tongue, labial mucosa, and soft palate have rates that have been estimated to be 1.5 to 5 times greater than masticatory mucosa of the attached gingiva and hard palate. The average epithelial turnover rate in the oral cavity varies between 4 and 14 days.

The intent of cancer chemotherapy is to maximize the destruction of tumor cells with minimal harm to normal cells. However, antitumor drugs do not fully distinguish between malignant cells and normal cells, and are thus potentially damaging to both. Many anticancer drugs have a narrow margin of safety between the tumoricidal and toxic doses. Virtually all chemotherapeutic agents can cause some degree of stomatitis. They can damage dividing cells in a variety of manners based on the type of agent used. For instance, alkalating agents damage nucleic acids, causing a breakdown of DNA. Antimetabolites interfere with metabolic pathways critical for DNA synthesis and cell function. Antibiotics and plant alkaloids are antimeiotic agents that disrupt cellular structures that are necessary for complete cell division. Other agents include asparaginase, procarbazine, and hormonal agents such as estrogen and corticosteroids. The potential for oral mucositis varies greatly among these agents. Among those most often associated with mucositis are methotrexate, adriamycin, 5-fluorouracil, bleomycin, and cisplatinum. In addition to the specific drug, the frequency and severity of oral complication is related to such factors as the dose and schedule of drug administration, single or combined usage, age, oral health, and the presence of existing mucosal irritation and trauma. Mucositis and other oral complications in chemotherapy patients are more predictable by diagnosis and corresponding aggressiveness of chemotherapy protocol. For example, the range of oral complications is as low as 12% for breast cancer, 33% for non-Hodgkin's lymphoma, and over 70% for certain types of leukemias. Younger patients (under the age of 20 years old) tend to have oral mucositis more frequently. Patients with impaired renal and/or hepatic function are at increased risk

TABLE 65–1. ORAL COMPLICATIONS OF CANCER THERAPY

DIRECT COMPLICATIONS	INDIRECT COMPLICATIONS	CHEMOTHERAPY COMPLICATIONS
MUCOSITIS	INFECTIONS	ORAL MUCOSITIS/STOMATITIS
Epithelial atrophy	Bacterial	
Pseudomembranous fibrin clots	Fungal	
	Viral	
Erythema/inflammation	HEMORRHAGE	
Edema		
SALIVARY GLAND DYSFUNCTION		
NEUROTOXICITIES		
TASTE DYSFUNCTION		

for mucositis due to reduced metabolism and/or secretion of administered drugs. Persistent blood and tissue levels of cytotoxic agents delay re-epithelialization. Also, the combination of head and neck radiation with chemotherapy (as seen with primary head and neck tumors and bone marrow transplantation) may dramatically increase the degree of mucositis. Mucositis resulting from depressed cell replication and maturation of the oral epithelium is considered a direct effect of the chemotherapy. Oral mucositis may also result from indirect effects of the chemotherapy by causing myelosuppression and immune suppression. These indirect effects are expressed by oral infection and hemorrhage.

Chemotherapy may also affect salivary gland function by acting initially to stimulate salivation, resulting in drooling and sialorrhea. Subsequently, this is followed by the shutdown of the acinar cells, causing xerostomia. Saliva serves a broad spectrum of physiologic needs relative to oral health and function, including lubrication of oral tissues, hydration of mucosa, and modulation and control of microbial colonization. Consequently, salivary gland dysfunction may not only result in xerostomia, but will also increase the risk of trauma and irritation to oral tissues increasing the potential incidence and severity of mucositis and oral infection. Oral mucositis can be generalized or localized. Severity can range from barely perceptible mucosal erythema and atrophy to severe mucosal inflammation and ulceration, often resulting in tremendous discomfort. Severe oral mucositis can prevent all oral nutritional intake and verbalization. In many instances, such as during bone marrow transplantation (BMT) or head and neck radiation, oral pain can be severe enough to require high dose systemic narcotic analgesics to control it. Many patients require an alternative means of receiving nutritional intake. In rare occasions the patient may require intubation in order to maintain an adequate airway. Also, mucositis can be so severe that it is necessary to suspend or reduce treatment doses to allow the oral tissues to recover. An often overlooked, yet significant consequence of oral mucositis is the potential for orally induced systemic infection with resultant increased morbidity and, potentially, mortality.

Mucositis from direct toxicity will usually occur within 7–10 days following initiation of chemotherapy and will heal after the end of treatment. Indirect mucositis resulting from mucosa secondarily infected by bacterial, fungal, and viral organisms occurs most frequently 12–16 days after initiation of chemotherapy and will heal as the neutrophil count returns to normal.

MANAGEMENT OF ORAL MUCOSITIS

The direct stomatotoxic effects of radiation and chemotherapy remain basically unpreventable. Therefore, the strategies to minimize or treat oral mucositis have only met with moderate success. The elimination of pre-existing dental disease as sources of mucosa irritation and trauma prior to cancer treatment can reduce the frequency and severity of many oral complications, including stomatitis. Even with the standard of care set forth by the 1990 NIH consensus conference on "Oral Complications of Cancer Therapy" recommending oral evaluation and care before and during cancer therapy, few oncology centers utilize dentists as part of the cancer treatment team. The direct stomatotoxic effects of chemotherapy remain basically unpreventable. There have been advances made in the management of oral mucositis, but they remain, to a large extent, palliative. There is evidence, however, that the use of antimicrobial mouth rinses may play a role in the reduction of oral complications of cancer chemotherapy. Chlorhexidine has been shown to decrease the incidence and severity of oral mucositis in patients receiving cancer chemotherapy. This drug appears to exert its effect by reducing the load of oral bacteria, thus reducing the secondary impact of oral bacteria on oral mucositis. Chlorhexidine has also been shown to have antifungal properties, including effectiveness against *Candida albicans*. Concerns regarding the high alcohol content of the available chlorhexidine rinse, Peridex, have been addressed by simply diluting the rinse 50% with sterile water and doubling the time of the rinse, when it causes discomfort.

The management of oral mucositis pain is directed in

two stages. The first is to use planned rinses, for example, Chlorhexidine, saline and sodium bicarbonate solutions, or antacid rinses, and topical anesthetics, including lidocaine, benzocaine, dyclonine, and diphenhydramine. Cellulose film-forming preparations have recently shown a great deal of promise in the management of mild to moderate mucositis pain. A number of other agents are being investigated. Benzydamine has consistently reduced the severity of stomatitis, but it is not currently available in the United States. Sucralfate suspension has shown some potential for reducing mucositis. Additionally, research with granulocyte colony stimulating factors have shown reduction of stomatitis as an unexpected side effect. None of these agents, however, have shown sufficient relief from the pain of severe mucositis. In these cases, where mucositis pain cannot be relieved with topical measures, pain management focuses primarily on the systemic use of narcotic analgesics. Since hemorrhage is a concern, platelet toxic analgesics, such as those containing aspirin, should be avoided. The non-steroidal prostaglandin inhibitors, such as ibuprofen, which causes a reversible decrease of platelet aggregation for only several hours, may be tried sparingly before advancing to the narcotic analgesics which may include such side effects as nausea and vomiting.

ORAL INFECTIONS

Odontogenic and Periodontal Infections

The oral cavity is under constant challenge by endogenous and opportunistic microorganisms. Microorganisms in supragingival plaque include *streptococcus, actinomyces, rothia, lactobacillus, veillonella, fusobacterium,* and *bacteroides*. Microorganisms are commonly found in subgingival plaque, including *bacteroides, actinobacillus, capnocytophaga,* and *treponema*. Dental plaque contains approximately 2×10^{11} microbes per gram, or the microbial density of a centrifuge pellet. Without sufficient accumulation of oral microbes, bacterial products cannot initiate and sustain damage to oral host tissues. Dental plaque is in a continuous state of dynamic fluctuation, succession, and change. Bacterial composition of plaque may vary from tooth surface to tooth surface as well as tooth to tooth. Even in an otherwise healthy individual, microbially induced oral disease can bring about significant morbid side effects and even, in rare cases, be life-threatening. Certainly in the immunosuppressed individual. underlying oral disease can become exacerbated and present significant complications to the individual's health and well being.

Pericoronitis, an infection originating around an erupting tooth, or one that has a flap of tissue covering the occlusal surface, may easily be overlooked. Food and debris collect between the tooth and the tissue flap and are decomposed by oral flora. In an immunosuppressed individual fever and trismus may occur in the absence of pain and discomfort. On clinical exam, the tissue flap may exhibit tenderness to palpation, even if it is not obviously inflamed. A *lateral periodontal abscess* is a very similar type of infection. Clinical findings include deep gingival pocketing associated with fever and painful irritated gingiva; subduration and necrosis may also be present. It differs from *pericoronitis* by affecting periodontically diseased gingiva rather than a residual tissue flap.

Another closely related condition is *acute necrotizing ulcerative gingivitis* (ANUG) also known as Vincent's stomatitis. *Fusiform* bacillus is commonly the causative organism, along with an oral spirochete, *Borrelia vincenti*. ANUG classically presents as an acute liquidification necrosis of the interdental papillary gingiva. The gingival papillae appear eroded or destroyed and may display pseudomembrane formation. Patients may complain of spontaneous bleeding, a fetid breath, and metallic taste. Neutropenic patients may not show the typical suppuration, nor have the classic fetid breath.

Periapical dental abscess, easily recognized in the general population, may present as an occult infection in immunosuppressed patients. It is caused by an infected or necrotic pulp. Diagnosis may be difficult and requires a detailed clinical and radiographic evaluation for dental caries, tooth fracture, subtle discoloration, and hyperocclusion. Various testing might be done, including sensitivity to percussion, palpation, and thermal and electric pulpal stimulation, as well as careful evaluation of dental radiographs. Periapical radiographs are preferred over panoramic radiographs for their clarity and detail. Chronic, occult, or dormant periapical abscesses may exacerbate acutely in the immune suppressed patient. In patients having any of the periodontal or odontogenic bacterial infections mentioned, transfusion with functional granulocytes may result in migration of white cells to the infected tissue, precipitating acute tissue reactions within minutes of the infusion. Pale and normal appearing gingiva may enlarge and undergo liquidification necrosis. In cases of pericoronitis and lateral periodontal abscesses, rapid onset swelling and necrosis have been seen.

Oral Mucosal Infections

Oral mucosal infections may occur by mucosal seeding of odontogenic or periodontal bacterial infection. Noma or gangrenous stomatitis is a complication of ANUG which involves the spread of infection from the gingiva, producing necrotizing or ulcerative lesions in the labial and buccal mucosa. Eventually, penetration in the outer skin surface may occur, with eventual systemic bacteremia that can be life-threatening.

Oral infection can also be superimposed with drug- or radiation-induced mucositis. The patient's general malaise and mouth pain impair oral hygiene and permit bacterial multiplication. Ulceration allows normal flora to invade underlying soft tissues and sometimes bone. Systemic bacteremias may occur. Prolonged antimicrobial therapy may permit an overgrowth of opportunistic organisms. Gram negative enteric bacteria and fungi usually predominate, with resistant strains emerging as antimicrobial therapy continues. Immunosuppressive and myelosuppressive effects of chemotherapy therefore make an oral infection potentially life-threatening.

FUNGAL INFECTIONS

One of the most frequent causes of infection in patients undergoing immunosuppressive therapy is from opportunistic overgrowth of fungal organisms. The most common fungal pathogens are the *Candida*, *Aspergillus*, and *Mucor* species. *Candida* represents over 90% of the fungal infections. The greater the degree and duration of the neutropenia or lymphocytopenia, the greater the risk of infection. Patients with a granulocyte or lymphocyte count of less than 100/mm^3 have a greater than 50% chance of developing an infection in some part of the body. If this level of granulocytopenia persists for 3 weeks or more, the risk increases to 100%. The most common sites of oral candidiasis are the ventral and dorsum of the tongue, the buccal, gingival, and palatal mucosa, and the commissures of the lips. Four distinct types of oral mucosal lesions are caused by overgrowth and infection by *Candida* species. These are pseudomembranous candidiasis (removable white plaques), erythematous candidiasis (patching or diffuse mucosal erythema), hyperplastic candidiasis (leukoplakia-like plaques that do not rub off), and angular cheilitis (sores radiating from angles of lips). Fungal cultures, potassium hydroxide (KOH) smears, and gram stain smears are helpful diagnostic tools. The white removable plaques of the pseudomembranous form of candidiasis are the most obvious to the examiner, and may have a tendency to coalesce and blanket large areas of the lining of the oral cavity. Forcible removal of the growth exposes the painful, raw, erythematous, often superficially ulcerated and bleeding mucosal surface. These organisms may infect other sites in the gastrointestinal tract and cause esophagitis and/or diarrhea. In neutropenic patients, mucosal infections with *Candida* spp. may lead to systemic infection and be life-threatening.

Mucormycosis, which classically occurs in uncontrolled diabetics, and aspergillosis have been noted to have significant incidence in patients receiving cancer chemotherapy. These infect the oral cavity, nares, and paranasal sinuses, and initially present as vague sinonasal or dental symptoms, but can rapidly progress by local extension along blood vessels and infarct large areas of bone and soft tissue. These can be fatal without early diagnosis and aggressive medical, and possibly surgical, intervention.

BACTERIAL INFECTIONS

Most of the oral bacterial infections that develop during treatment with antineoplastic drugs are caused by aerobic gram-negative bacilli, specifically *Pseudomonas*, *Klebsiella*, *Serratia*, *Enterobacter*, *Proteus*, and *Escherichia* spp. Lesions produced by *Pseudomonous* spp. are necrotizing and encircled by a red halo. Initially they have a dry, raised, white-yellowish center that becomes purple to black on turning necrotic. With appropriate treatment, the necrosed core sloughs off, disclosing a bright red, shiny bed of granulation tissue. The oral mucosal infections caused by the other gram-negative bacteria are clinically indistinguishable. They are identical in color, character, course, and distribution. Typical lesions are raised, creamy to yellow-white, moist, glistening, and non-purulent, with a smooth edged growth seated on painful, red, superficial mucosal ulcers and erosions. Any part of the oral cavity may be affected, but the dorsum and undersurface of the tongue, palatal and gingival mucosa, and lips are the most common sites. Oral staphylococcal and streptococcal infections, while not nearly as numerous as those of aerobic gram-negative bacilli, still constitute approximately 10% of all oral infections in patients receiving cancer chemotherapy. Because of drug-induced neutropenia, lesions produced by many of these normally pyogenic bacteria present as dry, raised patches, yellow-brown to black with little or no pus. Diagnosis of bacterial infections can be made by culturing samples of the lesions on selected media, determining the species by conventional methods.

Existing oral infections, such as those that accompany periodontal and pulpal disease, are often exacerbated during cancer chemotherapy. One study reported up to 22% of leukemic patients who practiced limited oral hygiene had such infections, down to a low of 5% of those who practiced good oral hygiene.

VIRAL INFECTIONS

Herpes simplex virus (HSV) is the most common viral pathogen associated with oral lesions in patients receiving myelosuppressive chemotherapy or bone marrow transplant. It is common to find patients that have had prior infection with HSV, since antibodies are found in the serum of 30%–100% of the general adult population in America. Once the host resistance is compromised by cytoreductive therapy in those who harbor the latent virus, reactivation of the virus occurs, leading to severe oral and potentially disseminated infection. Primary infections with HSV can occur in this population, but are extremely rare. Patients who harbor latent herpes simplex virus have antibody against the virus that may be detected in their sera, and are therefore seropositive. The patients are at risk for reactivation of the virus with immunosuppression. In contrast, patients without antibodies to the virus are seronegative and are unlikely to develop herpes simplex virus infection with immunosuppression. The incidence and severity of herpes simplex infection depend on the intensity of the immunosuppression experience by the patient. Bone marrow transplantation patients who receive intensive chemotherapy alone or with total body irradiation present the highest risk for reactivation of severe herpes simplex viral infections. Approximately 50%–90% of BMT patients who are seropositive for HSV will develop HSV infections, usually within the first 3 weeks after transplantation. Similarly, a large proportion of patients with acute leukemia or others receiving intensive chemotherapy will experience reactivation of HSV during periods of immunosuppression.

The clinical presentation consists of severely ulcerated and painful oral mucosa, often without the telltale fever blisters as a clue to its infectious cause. The most important systemic consequence of HSV infection is local barrier breakdown, facilitating entry of commensal oral microorganisms into the circulation, which can lead to sepsis by oral organisms such as alpha-hemolytic streptococci. In intensely treated leukemia and bone marrow transplant patients, HSV can also spread to other organs, resulting in esophagitis, tracheitis, pneumonitis, or widely disseminated disease. Before acylovir was available, 5%–10% of HSV infected patients undergoing bone marrow transplantation died. This infectious cause of oral mucositis is frequently indistinguishable from noninfectious (direct) mucositis caused by chemotherapy or radiotherapy.

Another significant yet much less common viral infection seen in immunosuppressed cancer patients is herpes zoster (varicella). Acute zoster infections of the oral cavity generally involve activation within the trigeminal, glossopharyngeal, or the vagal somatic sensory ganglia with a unilateral eruption in the distribution of one or more of the nerve branches. When it affects the mandibular division of the fifth cranial nerve, it generally produces painful vesicles on the tongue, palate, buccal gingival mucosa, and/or floor of the mouth. Coalescence of vesicles may occur, and healing may be delayed; as with herpetic stomatitis, breakdown of the oral mucosa may facilitate entry of commensal oral organisms into the circulation, which can lead to sepsis.

Other oral viral infections such as herpangina (coxsackie group a) occur very infrequently in immunosuppressed cancer patients.

DIAGNOSIS OF ORAL INFECTIONS

The complex interaction of infectious pathogens in the oral cavity and the host defense is still relatively poorly understood. We need to understand better the early steps in pathogenesis of infections at the mucosal barrier. Currently, the diagnosis of any of these oral infections is primarily based on the clinical findings and history, which take into account a thorough knowledge of underlying disease behavior, chemotherapeutic agents used and their toxicities, and antimicrobial agents administered and the organisms' sensitivities. We are just beginning to use the oral cavity as a window to detect or even possibly predict systemic infections. For high risk patients, routine monitoring of the oral cavity as well as posterior pharynx and nares should be performed routinely. In cases where there is a suspected infection, such as spiking fevers, cultures should be attained to help determine the identity of the causative organism(s). Serologic studies may be of limited value because of frequent blood transfusions and the often compromised immunologic response. Biopsy and histologic evaluation including special stains may be justified in certain cases. Diagnostic confirmation may be delayed for several days after empirical therapy has begun.

MANAGEMENT OF ORAL INFECTIONS

Empirical systemic antimicrobial therapy is generally started when infection is suspected; the choice of agents is discussed in a separate chapter (Chapter 59). Early administration of vigorous oral antifungal prophylaxis, and aggressive treatment of confirmed fungal infection, are essential. The topical prophylactic antifungal regimen is maintained to prevent further seeding of systemic pathogens via the breakdown in the oral mucosa barrier.

In some cases, debridement of necrotic tissues may increase the effectiveness of systemic and topical therapy. It should be performed with great care, since undue violation of normal underlying tissue may predispose to further spread of infection. Patients should be adequately anesthetized and even sedated, or have the procedure performed under general anesthesia in certain cases. In selected circumstances, surgical intervention may be essential to survival, as in the treatment of mucormycosis.

ORAL HEMORRHAGE

Hemorrhage is a common oral complication of cancer chemotherapy. The most important single contributing factor is the thrombocytopenia that results from the drug-induced myelosuppression. The lower the platelet count, the greater the possibility of oral bleeding. Oral bleeding is uncommon at platelet counts above 50,000/mm^3. The chances of such hemorrhage at levels below 30,000/mm^3 is greater than 50%. While thrombocytopenia is the identifiable cause in approximately 90% of patients receiving chemotherapy who manifest bleeding of the mouth, there are other notable causes and contributing factors such as disseminated intravascular coagulation, hypofibrinogenemia, and vitamin K deficiency. Almost half of chemotherapy patients who experience oral hemorrhage have such coagulation factor deficiencies.

Bleeding from oral tissues is generally quite distressing to both the patient and health care worker. Blood loss is difficult to assess due to patient salivation, emesis, or the patient swallowing. Oral hemorrhages can originate in any part of the mouth, with the lips, tongue, and gingiva the most common sites. Generally, the hemorrhages are caused by trauma. The hemorrhage is usually dark red, oozing, and may be intermittent and have a single or multiple bleeding sites. Soft, friable clots form, break away, and then reform. Most oral hemorrhage can be controlled locally, but in rare cases, it can become life-threatening. Hemorrhage into the tongue, or parapharyngeal, or paratracheal spaces, may rapidly induce respiratory distress. Rupture of a major vessel may lead to exsanguination or, in rare cases, hepatic coma may result from nitrogen overload secondary to swallowed blood in the hepatocompromised patient.

Local control is obtained by direct pressure, with gauze pads or rolled cotton directly applied to the bleeding points and maintained until hemostasis is achieved. This can be supplemented by applying a topical thrombin to gauze to act as a hemostatic agent. It is of utmost importance that good visualization of the isolated bleeding area be obtained prior to applying local pressure. Microfibrillar collagen powder can be applied to localized areas of gingival bleeding. If generalized or multifocal oral bleeding occurs, microfibrillar collagen powder can be placed in a custom-made acrylic oral carrier/mouth guard lined with vaseline impregnated gauze and sprinkled with the topical thrombin. The clear mouth guard allows observation of bleeding control. While the patient is wearing the mouth guard, it should be removed two to three times daily, cleaned, disinfected, and new liner placed. Because sensitization to foreign protein can occur, an additional hemostatic agent should be used only for fresh hemorrhage. Also, during the period of healing, vigorous mouth rinses should be avoided along with use of straws by the patient to avoid dislodging the friable clots. Once healing is adequate and re-epithelialization has begun, gentle oral hygiene procedures may be resumed. Also, during the period of bleeding the patient can eat soft or liquid diet and may require nutritional supplementation. For severe hemorrhages, or those not controlled well with local measures, the patient is best managed with transfusion of HLA-compatible fresh frozen platelets or cryoprecipitate until bone marrow recovery restores hemostatic control.

ORAL GRAFT-VERSUS-HOST DISEASE

Patients who undergo autologous as well as allogeneic bone marrow transplantation may develop acute or chronic graft-versus-host disease (GVHD). This may manifest as mucosal erythema, atrophy, and ulceration, or as vesicullobullus, or lichenoid lesions. GVHD may resemble other autoimmune diseases including lichenplanus, pemphigoid or, systemic sclerosis, lupus erythematous, or Sjrôegren's syndrome. Diagnosis may easily be confused with candidiasis or herpetic stomatitis, and definitive diagnosis may be obtained only by biopsy looking for specific microscopic features seen in minor and major salivary glands. Once a diagnosis of GVHD has been established, generally systemic therapy is initiated; in some cases topical steroids such as decadron elixir may provide additional relief.

PEDIATRIC CONSIDERATIONS

Short-term oral complications seen in children are similar to those seen in adults. However, children can acquire additional long-term sequelae. Acute manifestations of cancer therapy seen in both children and adults include mucositis and ulceration, fungal, viral, and bacterial infections, bleeding, and pain. However, because children are actively growing and developing, cancer treatment creates additional long-term problems unique to the pediatric patient. As modern therapy results in increasingly improved survival for a variety of pediatric cancers, long-term sequelae of treatment are beginning to emerge. Some more recent studies involving combined radiation and chemotherapy have shown oral complications can be up to three times more common in children than in adults. The increased mitotic index in children is thought to be responsible for their greater susceptibility to complications of cancer therapy. The nature and severity of these treatment sequelae depend upon a number of factors: the type and location of the tumor, the age of the patient, the dose of the radiation therapy, the aggressiveness of the chemotherapy, the status of oral and dental health, and the level of dental care before, during, and after therapy.

The long-term sequelae seen in children but not in the adult population include disturbances of oral and dental development. These chronic problems involve impaired growth and development of hard and soft tissues which may result in orofacial asymmetry, xerostomia, dental caries, trismus, and a wide variety of dental abnormalities. The latter include delayed tooth eruption, altered dental root development with shortening and thinning of the roots, enamel opacities, enamel grooves and pits, small teeth, small crowns, and failure of tooth development and eruption. In teeth with underdeveloped roots secondary to cancer therapy, even minimal periodontal disease will result in early loss of teeth. Long-term studies involving pediatric cancer patients indicate that chemotherapy mainly induces qualitative disturbances of dentin and enamel, whereas irradiation induces qualitative and quantitative changes.

Preventive oral protocols for the pediatric population are much the same as for the adult cancer patient. It is clear that all sources of oral infection, such as dental caries, abscessed teeth, and gingivitis, should be resolved prior to cancer therapy. During therapy, an oral care program for children is needed that includes oral hygiene methods appropriate for the child's medical status and for the age of the child, so that either the child can administer or have the family member or health care worker provide the preventive service. The oral care program for the child should include an antimicrobial agent for the prevention of secondary infection such as chlorhexidine gluconate (Peridex®), and a caries prevention regimen as well.

These children may have lifelong dental problems requiring periodic routine dental, orthodontic, prosthodontic, or orthagnathic procedures. It is imperative that supervised consistent oral care with meticulous oral hygiene and a regular dental recall schedule be implemented for these patients. This is key to maintenance of dental health care in children cured of their cancer. In addition, the emotional and psychological consequences of orofacial deformities and oral dysfunction in these children deserve more attention as increasing numbers of these patients survive.

The potential for development of secondary malignancies in these survivors is a serious delayed sequelae of a successful cancer therapy. Although a majority of secondary malignancies reported in children consist of leukemia or lymphomas, soft tissue and bone sarcomas can occur in an irradiated site. The possibilities of secondary malignancies arising in these children should heighten the clinician's awareness of this potential problem.

Providing education and information to the patient and family is essential for maximum treatment compliance. The direct involvement of the family results in improved adherence to treatment protocols and therefore enhances the patient's quality of life.

PREVENTION OF ORAL COMPLICATIONS

Oral Evaluation and Treatment Prior to Cancer Therapy

Patients who are about to undergo myelosuppressive therapy are at a major risk for sepsis, which in fact is the major cause of death in these individuals. In addition, the patient's reduced ability to fend off infection is coupled with the loss of oral epithelial integrity as a consequence of the direct stomatotoxic effects of chemo- and radiation therapy. Therefore, the objectives of a screening program for this group of patients include the identification of sites of asymptomatic oral infection, or potential oral infection and identification of sources and sites of chronic irritation. The components of a comprehensive pre-treatment assessment include history, consultation, clinical examination, and radiographic examination. The history should include both medical and dental histories. The patient should be asked specifically about the frequency and extent of past dental care, the age and condition of existing prostheses, oral soft tissue lesions, including traumatic lesions, candidiasis, and herpes simplex infections, and oral symptoms, including periodontal or tooth pain or sensitivity or gingival bleeding or swelling, pericoronitis, or impairments of salivary function. A consultation with the patient's former dentist may be helpful to confirm earlier treatments, and in some cases it may be helpful to obtain past dental radiographs for comparison. The clinical examination should include extra-oral soft tissue of the head and neck and intra-oral soft tissue examination. Periodontal screening should include tooth mobility, gingival inflammation, loss of gingival attachment and alveolar bone and subduration, and oral hygiene level. The hard tissue examination should include existing prostheses, orthodontic appliances, tooth vitality, where appropriate, and document defective restorations, caries, and fractured or broken teeth, and partially erupted teeth, especially third molars which are susceptible to pericoronitis. The radiographic examination should minimally be a panoramic for even the edentulous patient, and appropriate periapical and interproximal radiographs (bitewings) for the dentate patient. Supplemental films and imaging studies as needed, for example sinus films, magnetic resonance imaging, or computerized tomography, may be indicated in rare instances.

Pre-induction treatment planning for the oral cavity is designed to render the area clean and free from existing sources of irritation and infection. It should include: 1) for the dentate patient, thorough cleaning, removal of all calculus, prophylaxis, and fluoride treatment, 2) restoration of all carious lesions or defective restorations, 3) resolution of periodontal pathology, 4) resolution of periapical pathology with endodontic treatment, possibly including apicoectomy, 5) extraction of teeth that are not restorable or amenable to other treatments, including impacted teeth predisposed to pericoronitis, 6) for patients either partially dentate or edentulous wearing removable prosthetic devices, a comprehensive fitting and meticulous cleaning, and 7) a thorough review of possible oral complications and preventive measures to be instituted by the patient during and after the cancer therapy.

The obvious concern for the dentist in providing these services would be sequencing considerations. Hematologic status of the patient, granulocyte count, and platelet count should be at levels appropriate for the planned treatment. Also, indwelling catheters require prophylactic antibiotic coverage according to the regimen recommended by the American Heart Association for heart murmurs.

Oral Care During Chemotherapy

Proper oral hygiene must be stressed even before the onset of chemotherapy. The daily routine should include inspection of the oral cavity either by the health care professional or by the patient if treatment is rendered on an out-patient basis. Examination should be made for redness, blisters, ulcers, or coatings. The patients may be allowed to maintain flossing of teeth unless there are low platelet or low neutrophil counts. In addition to this daily routine, mouth cleansing should be performed after each meal and before bed time, or, if the patient is not eating, this should be done approximately once every 6 hours throughout the day. Mouth cleansing should be performed after emesis. This includes removal of partial or complete dentures, and for those who are dentate, brushing with an ultrasoft toothbrush and an American Dental Association approved, non-abrasive fluoride tooth paste. Toothettes should be used instead of a tooth brush if significant bleeding is experienced or platelets are low. The oral cavity may then be rinsed with a salt and soda solution. This is to be followed by an antifungal regimen of either nystatin (10–15 cc swish and swallow q.i.d. or nystatin popsicles sucked on and allowed to slowly dissolve q.i.d.) or Chlotrimazole troche (allowed to dissolve slowly in the mouth q.i.d.) for those with low neutrophil count. This is to be followed a half hour later by an antimicrobial mouthrinse, such as chlorhexidine gluconate, 0.012%, 15 cc swish for 30 seconds then expectorated.

If the patient develops mucositis, the patient needs to be cautioned to avoid citrus fruits, highly acidic foods, spicy foods, extremes in food temperature, and crusty or rough foods. They may also increase their salt and soda rinses to every 2 hours. Also, when patients become xerostomic and their lips are dry, they may add a lip lubricant, such as Blistex. If the discomfort from the mucositis is not managed by the other oral agents, another mild analgesic mouth rinse, such as viscous lidocaine, dyclonine, or diphenhydramine mixed with milk of magnesia can be used every 3–4 hours. Special concern for those patients who wear removable dentures is that as therapy progresses and weight loss ensues, dimensional changes may occur in the oral cavity and result in poorly fitting dentures. A resilient tissue conditioner may be used to provide increased comfort, retention, and adaptability. However, in cases of significant oral mucositis the patients may be more comfortable and at less risk for further tissue damage by leaving the prostheses out until healing occurs.

Post-Chemotherapy Oral Care

The patient may return to routine oral care if after at least two weeks from the last chemo or radiation treatment they no longer have signs or symptoms of mucositis, or their neutrophil count is greater than 1,000 and platelets greater than 40,000. This is the time of remission of the malignancy and recovery of the patient's normal function. This is also a time in which indicated dental treatment that could not be done earlier may be done, for example, dental prophylaxis, restorative, or periodontal, endodontic, or exodontic procedures.

Patients who have noted post-treatment oral sequelae such as xerostomia may continue the saline and bicarbonate rinses and/or begin using oral lubricants or artificial salivas such as Xero-lube or Oralube. Also because of these individuals' predisposition to rampant caries, additional instructions may include avoidance of sucrose or sweetened foods that bathe the teeth in sugar. The xerostomic patient with teeth may also be placed on supplemental topical fluorides as neutral *p*H 1% fluoride gel brushed on once or twice daily or acidulated 0.4% stannous fluoride gel either brushed on or applied inside a soft vinyl mouth guard for the upper and lower teeth for a 5-minute period per day. Patients receiving topical fluoride are also instructed not to rinse, eat, or drink for at least one half hour after application of the fluoride and preferably to use it at bed time so that the effect may be a continuation of reaction with enamel throughout the night.

RADIATION THERAPY PATIENTS

Patient Selection

All patients whose radiation therapy portal includes the oral cavity are at risk for significant oral complications, and therefore should have an assessment and any indicated dental treatment completed prior to the start of radiation. Patients at risk for oral complication include those with a primary malignancy of the head and neck whose field of radiation will include the pituitary or salivary glands or will have an exited portal that includes the oral cavity, and Hodgkin's lymphoma patients who receive mantle field radiation.

ORAL COMPLICATIONS IN HEAD AND NECK IRRADIATION

Radiation, like chemotherapy, can affect normal cells as well as tumor cells, and several types of oral tissues can display negative effects of radiation. Tissue damage from radiation can be either direct or indirect. Direct radiation injury destroys or damages susceptible cells, causing a loss or disruption of tissue function. The indirect effects result from decreased vascularity and subsequent tissue alterations. The direct and indirect radiation effects on the oral cavity are discussed in the following paragraphs.

Oral mucositis or stomatitis secondary to head and neck irradiation is the direct result of the radiation effect on the basal cell layer of the oral epithelium. The epithelium lost due to normal function is not replaced due to the slowing or the cessation of cell replication and maturation, causing eventual thinning of tissue and ulceration. This can manifest as early as the first week, but usually begins approximately 2 weeks after the initiation of radiation therapy and lasts approximately 2 to 3 weeks following the last radiation treatment. These patients also have a predisposition to the development of opportunistic oral infections, especially *Candida albicans,* and should be treated aggressively since it cannot exacerbate the underlying mucositis. Patients receiving head and neck radiation, unlike those on chemotherapy, do not appear to have an increased incidence of HSV reactivation. The management of radiation mucositis is much like that for chemotherapy mucositis with the exception of the use of chlorhexidine gluconate mouth rinses, which only show benefit in the first few weeks of radiation therapy and thereafter can have a negative effect. This is thought to be due to the xerostomia and lack of salivary mucins which are necessary in the binding of the chlorhexidine.

Xerostomia is a very common result in patients whose salivary glands lie within the port of head and neck irradiation. It usually begins within the first week of radiation therapy due to the edema and inflammatory infiltration of the salivary glands. Eventually, glandular fatty degeneration, necrosis, and small blood vessel fibrosis will occur. Radiation appears to have more of an effect on the serous portion of the salivary glands than on the mucous component. Therefore, saliva generally becomes thicker and more difficult for the patients to manage. The *p*H of the saliva will also decrease significantly and other salivary components decrease quantitatively. Irreversible salivary gland changes generally require dosages of between 4,000 to 6,000 cGy. Management of the xerostomia is generally palliative, through the use of oral alkaline rinses and artificial saliva preparations. Some patients will find these substitutes to be very effective, while others receive the same benefit from sipping frequently from a small bottle of water.

Recently, the FDA approved pilocarpine hydrochloride, Salagen, for head and neck cancer patients with radiation-induced dry mouth. This prescription product has been clinically proven to relieve radiation-induced xerostomia in some patients by stimulating saliva production from functioning salivary glands. The recommended starting dose is one 5 mg tablet tid.

Radiation caries, or, better termed, xerostomia-associated caries can affect all teeth, including those that were not in the radiation port. This decay, which is often rampant and difficult to control, is probably due to several factors. As mentioned earlier, there is a change in the quality and constituents of saliva. The reduced volume of saliva decreases the dilution of bacterial acids, reduced buffering capacity of the saliva increases oral acidity, and the reduction of salivary immunoglobulin A contributes to a proliferation and shift to the oral microbial flora. Also, with the decrease in ability of saliva to lubricate food, patients tend to shift to a diet that is high in refined carbohydrates that also in turn have a tendency to adhere to oral structures. The two most common surfaces involved in radiation caries are the cervical areas and the cusp tips of teeth. As decay progresses, it eventually results in amputation of the tooth crown.

The prevention of radiation caries is the hallmark of therapy. Meticulous oral hygiene measures must be implemented to reduce the load of oral bacteria that will induce dental decay. Patients must be taught careful oral hygiene techniques including tooth brushing and dental flossing as well as daily fluoride treatments to be continued for the rest of their lives. Patients should be followed for oral hygiene evaluation and therapy frequently, generally between every 3 to 6 months.

Once the carious process is clinically obvious often no treatment is possible other than full mouth extractions or full mouth endodontics (root canal therapy) and extensive prosthetic replacement.

Ageusia (loss of taste) or dysgeusia (alteration of taste) can occur during and persist after radiation therapy. The loss of taste may occur as early as the second week of therapy, with regeneration of cells occurring within 4 months after therapy has ended. Permanent taste changes may result, however, with bitter and acidic perception more affected than sweet and salty. This can be a major quality of life issue for many patients. The management of loss of taste involves avoidance of highly flavored or spiced foods and frequent rinses with a non-irritating oral rinse such as isotonic saline or saline bicarbonate.

Trismus, the limitation of movement of the mandible, may also occur if the temporomandibular joint or muscles of mastication have been irradiated. The initial inflammation of the muscles and joint during radiation may be followed by fibrous scarring of those muscles afterwards. There is little chance to recover opening once trismus occurs. All patients with radiation therapy portals that include the oral musculature should perform routine jaw opening exercises. These exercises should include maximal opening and closing or a stretching of the jaws by placing the thumb on the palate and using the fingers of the other hand pressing the lower jaw against the pressure of the lower hand under the chin. These exercises should be performed for 2 minutes each and should be repeated 4 times daily. Jaw-opening devices as molt mouth props or more simple devices like multiple tongue blades taped together may be used in jaw-opening exercises as well.

Osteoradionecrosis (ORN) is the most severe consequence of head and neck radiation. This can be defined as an open area of exposed bone within a field of previous radiation which is present for at least 3 months. This is a result of obliterative endarteritis, the reduction of blood flow to the area of bone secondary to head and neck radiation. More simply, the irradiated bone is rendered devitalized. Osteora-dionecrosis typically presents as an area of denuded bone after tooth extraction or soft tissue trauma and can lead to complete necrosis and loss of large sections of the jaw. ORN is more frequent in the mandible and has been associated with higher doses of radiation therapy and with poor oral hygiene and extensive oral disease in patients with poor dental repair. The most effective treatment for ORN is prevention. The elimination of any potential sources of oral infection prior to radiation therapy is critical. For those who develop ORN, treatment is usually conservative debridement of exposed bone, hyperbaric oxygen therapy, and possibly systemic antibiotics.

Dental Care and Radiation Therapy

Pre-irradiation management begins with the evaluation of the hard and soft oral tissues that should proceed concurrently with the tumor diagnostic work-up and treatment planning. The evaluation should include a complete oral examination and appropriate radiographs, generally, a panorex (even if the patient is edentulous), interproximal dental x-rays (bitewings), and appropriate periapical radiographs. As with the chemotherapy patient, all calculus and plaque should be removed and the patient taught proper oral hygiene to reduce stomatitis during radiation therapy and caries afterwards. Teeth that are nonrestorable, severely periodontally involved, or have periapical radiolucencies should be removed. Use an alveolectomy and primary closure of all mandibular extraction sites to facilitate healing by surgically eliminating poorly supported alveolar bone and reducing the site of extraction defects. Carefully remove mandibular tori, sharp mylohyoid ridges and exostoses to minimize post-surgical wound dehiscence and exposed bone. Extract partially impacted teeth and diseased or symptomatic impacted teeth. Be aware of the increased risk of prolonged healing of the bony defects created by extractions and delay radiation for as long as possible. The surgical sites should be well healed or at least covered with granulation tissue prior to the initiation of radiation therapy. The oncologic effect of this delay (generally 7 to 10 days) must be weighed against the increased possibility of osteoradionecrosis. All caries and defective restorations should be restored and any planned periodontal treatment or endodontic therapy should be completed prior to the initiation of radiation. Impressions of the teeth can also be made prior to radiation for fabrication of custom fluoride applicators. Patient education must also be accomplished at this time, including a review of the possible oral side effects of radiation and the importance of oral hygiene during and after irradiation, especially for the dentate patient. It is important to note that patients with indifferent oral hygiene attitudes, gingival inflammation, heavy calculus, and pocket depths less than 3 millimeters may be more at risk for dentoalveolar pathosis than a patient with greater periodontal pocket depths and fewer risk factors.

Routine dental care is generally contraindicated during radiation therapy because of the oral discomfort and the impairment of the ability of the oral tissues to heal during radiation therapy. Even the daily oral hygiene must be altered or stopped including the daily application of fluoride until mucositis subsides. Weekly dental follow-up visits should be scheduled during radiation therapy to assess the degree of reaction and to provide or prescribe palliative care and emotional support. Within 2 to 4 weeks after radiation therapy, the patient should have a dental follow-up to review oral hygiene and trismus preventive exercises as well as to detect trismus or soft tissue/bone necrosis in its early stages. Good dental care including the treatment of infection is necessary following radiation therapy. Root canal therapy is preferred over extractions. Occasionally, teeth must be extracted, in a previous field of radiation treatment. Ideally, hyperbaric oxygen therapy should be employed prior to the extraction or if hyperbaric oxygen is not available, minimally, adequate coverage with antibiotics is suggested. Currently, loading doses of penicillin VK, 2 grams followed by 500 mg 4 times daily for 7 to 10 days, or until the bone is covered with soft tissue, is recommended. For penicillin allergic patients, erythromycin is used, 1 gram followed by 250 mg four times daily. Post-operatively, monitoring for delayed healing of alveolar ridge wounds is imperative; consider initiating hyperbaric oxygen therapy when exposed bone persists for several months or with a diagnosis of ORN.

Because these patients remain at risk for many different oral complications for the remainder of their lives, especially the dentate patients should be closely followed by their dentist every 3 to 6 months.

REFERENCES

Barasch A, Safford MM. Management of oral pain in patients with malignant diseases. Compend Contin Educ Dent XIV(11):1376–1383, 1993

Bergman OJ. Oral infections and septicemia in immunocompromised patients with hematologic malignancies. J Clin Microbiol 26:2105–2109, 1988.

Consensus Development Conference on Oral Complications of Cancer Therapies: Diagnosis, Prevention, Treatment. NCI Monogr 9:1990

Dahllöf G, Rozell B, Forsberg, C Borgström B. Histologic changes in dental morphology induced by high dose chemotherapy and total body irradiation. Oral Surg Oral Med Oral Path 77(1):56–60, 1994

Dreizen S, McCredie KB, Bodey GP, et al. Quantitative analysis of the oral complications of antileukemia chemotherapy. Oral Surg, 68:650–653, 1986

Dreizen S, McCredie KB, Bodey GP, et al. Microbial mucocutaneous infections in acute adult leukemia: Results of an 18-year inpatient study. Postgrad Med 79:107–118, 1986

Ferretti GA, et al. Chlorhexidine for prophylaxis against oral infections and associated complications in patients receiving bone marrow transplants. J Am Dent Assoc, 114:461, 1987

Greenberg MS, Cohen SG, McKitrick JC et al. The oral flora as a source of septicemia in patients with acute leukemia. Oral Surg 53(1):32–36, 1982

Jaffe N, Toth BB, Hoar RE et al. Dental and maxillofacial abnormalities in long-term survivors of childhood cancer: Effects of treatment with chemotherapy and radiation to the head and neck. Pediatrics, 73(6):816–823, 1984

Lockhart PB, Clark J. Pretherapy dental status of patients with malignant conditions of the head and neck. Oral Surg, Oral Med, Oral Path, 77(3):236–241, 1994

Marciani RD, Ownby HE. Osteoradionecrosis of the jaws. J Oral Maxillofac Surg, 44:218–223, 1986

Marciani RD, Ownby HE. Treating patients before and after irradiation. JADA, 123:108–112, 1992

Marx RE, Johnson RP, Kline SN. Prevention of osteoradionecrosis: A randomized prospective clinical trial of hyperbaric oxygen versus penicillin. J Am Dent Assoc, 111:49–54, 1985

Peterson DE: Bacterial infections: periodontal and dental disease. In Peterson DE, Sonis ST (eds): Oral Complications of Cancer Chemotherapy, pp. 79–91. The Hague, Martinus Nijhoff, 1983

Peterson DE, Sonis ST (eds): Oral Complications of Cancer Chemotherapy. Boston, Martinus Nijhoff, 1983

Peterson DE, Elias EG, Sonis, ST (eds): Head and Neck Management of the Cancer Patient. Boston: Martinus Nijhoff Publishers, 1986

Redding SW, Montgomery M (eds). Dentistry in Systemic Disease. 1st ed. Portland, Oregon: JBK Publishing, 1990

Rosenberg SW, Lepley JB. Mucormycosis in leukemia. Oral Surg 54(1):26–32, 1982

Rosenberg SW: Oral complications of cancer chemotherapy—A review of 398 patients. J Oral Med 41(2):93–97, 1986

Rosenberg SW, Kolodney H, Wong GY, et al. Altered dental root development in long-term survivors of pediatric acute lymphoblastic leukemia: A review of 17 cases. Cancer 59:1640–1648, 1987

Schubert MM, Sullivan KM, Morton TH, et al. Oral manifestations of chronic graft-vs-host disease. Arch Intern Med 144:1591–1595, 1984

Shannon IL, Trodahl JN, Starcke EN: Remineralization of enamel by a saliva substitute designed for use by irradiated patients. Cancer 41(5):1746–1750, 1978

Simon AR, Roberts MW. Management of oral complications associated with cancer therapy in pediatric patients. J Dent Child 58:384-389, Sept/Oct 1991

Sonis ST, Kunz A. Impact of improved dental services on the frequency of oral complications of cancer therapy. Oral Surg 65:19–22, 1988

Wright WE, Haller JM, Harlow SA et al. An oral disease prevention program for patients receiving radiation and chemotherapy. J Am Dent Assoc 11:43–47, 1985

John S. Macdonald, Daniel G. Haller, Robert J. Mayer, Eds. *Manual of Oncologic Therapeutics*, Third Edition.

66. ALOPECIA

Claudia A. Seipp

Alopecia is a common and distressing side effect of a variety of antineoplastic agents and scalp irradiation. Drugs and conditions that interfere with cell division are responsible for alterations in the phases of hair growth. Since no safe and effective method exists to prevent this loss, most patients choose to cover their heads with wigs, scarves, turbans, or hats during this time. Although drug-induced alopecia is almost always reversible, this hair loss can cause a negative body image, alter interpersonal relationships, and arouse enough anxiety to cause some patients to reject potentially curative treatment.

Frank discussion of alopecia by physicians and nurses acknowledging the patient's anxiety is helpful in allowing the patient to begin to prepare for the impact of hair loss. Although the use of wigs is not entirely satisfactory for all patients, caregivers can offer support with some practical explanations as to when hair loss can be anticipated while emphasizing the expected time of regrowth. Often the presence of a spouse, family member, or friend during this discussion with the patient is helpful in placing the problem in perspective.

Scalp irradiation does not cause uniform hair loss. Epilation may begin at doses of 500 cGy; the prospects for hair regrowth diminish with increasing doses. Skin doses greater than 4000 cGy may produce total and permanent alopecia. Radiation ports of extremities that have received 5000 cGy to 6000 cGy have been noted to be hairless 10 years after treatment. At lower total doses, regrowth of hair may begin 8 to 9 weeks after cessation of therapy. Frequently the new hair is different in character from the pretreatment hair.

The rate and extent of hair loss in any chemotherapy program depends on the drugs used, their doses, the frequency of the cycle repetition, and the excretion of the drug. Obviously, different effects can be anticipated when drugs are administered by bolus infusion compared to continuous infusion. Often hair loss is caused by more than one drug used in combination therapy.

Although chemotherapeutic agents differ in the extent to which they can cause alopecia, a wide range of single agents and combinations may have this effect (Table 66–1). Doxorubicin and cyclophosphamide are common cytologic agents known to cause epilation after only two cycles at doses above 50 mg/m^2 and 500 mg/m^2 respectively. Alopecia can be expected with other single agents such as those listed in Table 66–1 or their combinations. Long-term therapy may result in loss of pubic, axillary, and facial hair as well as scalp hair.

Hair regeneration may begin 1–2 months after therapy is discontinued. Alteration in color and texture of hair may occur; hair may be a lighter or darker shade and may be curlier as it regrows.

When hair loss occurs, nurses and clinicians can suggest wigs or head covering with stylish scarves, turbans, or hats. Wigs should be selected before hair loss begins so that the patient is prepared when alopecia occurs and so that hair color and style can be matched. Hairpieces are tax-deductible medical expenses and are covered by some medical insurance policies. Several small private businesses have been developed by former patients who distribute or sell head coverings of various designs. A national American Cancer Society rehabilitation program called "Look Good, Feel Better" has been developed specifically to assist women to compensate for hair loss and skin changes during cancer treatment. Volunteer beauticians and cosmetologists help patients look and feel more comfortable with changes in their appearance such as dry, discolored, or blotching skin, discolored nails, and alopecia. Information is available to patients through an ACS central hotline 1-800-395-LOOK which gives directions for contacting local resources.

Over the past 25 years, interventions have been proposed to attempt to prevent scalp hair loss from chemotherapy. The rationale for these procedures is to prevent drug circulation to the hair follicles by causing temporary vasoconstriction with either an occlusive scalp tourniquet or localized hypothermia. The pharmacokinetics of the drugs to be used must be understood, with occlusion of the superficial scalp veins beginning before the drugs are given and, to be effective, extending beyond the time of the peak plasma drug levels.

Various types of scalp icing devices have been manufactured by several different American companies. Although the Food and Drug Administration had initially approved the marketing of cooling caps intended to cause localized scalp hypothermia, early in 1990 the FDA reviewed these applications and became concerned that the safety and efficacy of these devices had not been substantiated by adequate clinical data. The regulatory agency addressed the following concerns: the potential for scalp metastasis posed by the use of these devices, the potential for reducing drug circulation to other anatomic sites beyond the scalp such as the skull and possibly the brain, the effectiveness of preventing hair loss, and how specific cytologic doses and other variables affected the results achieved. Therefore, the FDA halted the commercial distribution of these devices and, 3 years after their withdrawal, no company has come forward with supporting clinical evidence of reasonable safety and effectiveness.

Therefore, limitations of safety and inconclusive and conflicting reports of the results of the usefulness of scalp hypothermia should be factors discussed with patients seeking information about these devices and hair preservation techniques.

Previous studies have found that providing individual at-

TABLE 66–1. SINGLE AGENTS WITH POTENTIAL TO INDUCE REVERSIBLE ALOPECIA

Amsacrine	5-Fluorouracil
Bleomycin	Hydroxyurea
Cyclophosphamide	Ifosfamide
Dactinomycin	Methotrexate
Daunorubicin	Mitomycin
Doxorubicin	Melphalan
Epirubicin	Taxol
Etoposide	Vinblastine
Vincristine	

The degree of onset of alopecia is dependent upon dose, schedule of sequences, rate of delivery, route of delivery, and various combinations of agents

tention, continuity of care from physicians and nurses, support from other patients, and information given in advance about the occurrence of alopecia, all facilitated better adaptation during this period of stress. Knowledge that hair would regrow at the end of therapy helped patients plan strategies to minimize the anxiety of hair loss.

BIBLIOGRAPHY

Camp-Sorrell D. Scalp hypothermia devices: current status. ONS News 7(8):1, Sept. 1991

Keller JF, Blausey LA. Nursing issues and management in chemotherapy-induced alopecia. Onc Nurs Forum 15(5):603–607, 1988

"Look Good, Feel Better", ACS, telephone 1-800-395-LOOK

Wagner L, Bye MG. Body image and patients experiencing alopecia as a result of cancer chemotherapy. Cancer Nurs 2(5):365–369, 1979

John S. Macdonald, Daniel G. Haller, Robert J. Mayer, Eds. *Manual of Oncologic Therapeutics*, Third Edition.

67. REHABILITATION FOR MUSCULOSKELETAL IMPAIRMENTS AND THEIR DISABILITY IN CANCER PATIENTS

Lynn H. Gerber
Charles L. McGarvey

INTRODUCTION

Musculoskeletal dysfunction in patients with cancer may occur as a result of direct tumor invasion, metastatic spread, or the indirect effects of antineoplastic management (*i.e.*, surgery, chemotherapy, radiation or immunotherapy). Tumors most likely to affect the musculoskeletal system are presented in Table 67–1. While medical management has proven effective in the improvement of life expectancy of patients with cancer, many of the treatment modalities currently utilized contribute to pain, muscle weakness, limitation of joint motion or stability, and decreased endurance. These musculoskeletal impairments often result in functional limitations which delay or inhibit the patient's ability to return to previous life activities. A review of the effects of cancer treatments on the musculoskeletal system is presented in Table 67–2. In addition, Table 67–3 summarizes rehabilitation programs with treatment goals and interventions for deficits typically seen in these patients.

PATIENT EVALUATION

Rehabilitation professionals such as physiatrists and physical, occupational, and speech therapists, are responsible for assisting patients in achieving maximum function. Treatment planning depends on an initial evaluation which begins with a thorough examination of all musculoskeletal and neurological systems in order to determine the presence of any functional deficits. A comprehensive history includes questions regarding the patient's work environment, activities of daily living (*i.e.*, grooming, dressing, eating, bathing, mobility, communication, toileting habits, and avocational pursuits.) A number of instruments have been designed and published over the past few years in an attempt to reliably measure many of these functional and quality of life domains.[1] Scientific and economic issues related to the need for better measures of functional outcome and appropriate reimbursement for rehabilitation services have facilitated the regular use of these standard measurement tools by rehabilitation professionals as a integral part of clinical evaluation. Scores from such instruments as the Sickness Impact Profile (SIP), Functional Independence Measure (FIM), Assessment of Motor and Process Skills (AMPS), and Symptom-Limited Graded Exercise Test (SLGXT) are being included in documentation and will eventually form the basis for assessing functional impairment and attainment of functional goals. (See References).

SPECIFIC PROBLEMS

Six problems frequently encountered by cancer patients are worthy of special note:

1. Deconditioning Effects of Immobility

Bedridden patients suffer significant complications as a result of immobility. These include decubiti, osteoporosis, joint contractures, and disuse atrophy. *Early referral* of these patients to rehabilitation would promote prevention of such complications and subsequent earlier return to function. Treatment modalities include use of foam pads, mattresses, and splints to prevent decubiti. Use of a Stryker frame is beneficial in preventing pressure sores and use of a tilt-table can assist in reducing the incidence of autonomic hypotension. Active and active assisted range of motion exercises performed daily prevent the formation of muscle tightness and joint contracture. Progressive ambulation incorporates both cardiopulmonary and skeletal muscle systems to promote the patient's maximum efficiency in returning to routines of daily life (ADL), facilitating earlier release from the hospital. Recent investigations of the beneficial physiological effects of aerobic exercise administered to patients with cancer have focused on $V0_2<$ max body weight and composition. Data are now available to help guide clinicians in the appropriate prescription and administration of this form of exercise based on sound cardiopulmonary principles.[2,3]

2. Mobility and Self Care Deficits

Acute and long-term effects of surgery, radiation, and chemotherapy employed as single agents or in combination often have traumatic or toxic impact on motor and sensory systems. Problems with balance, coordination, proprioception, and gross and fine motor skills occur routinely in these patients. Common problems include: difficulty walking independently, eating and communicating effectively, and in

TABLE 67–1. TUMORS AFFECTING THE MUSCULOSKELETAL SYSTEM

SYSTEM INVOLVED	CLINICAL SIGNS AND SYMPTOMS
Bone and Soft Tissue (osteogenic, Ewing's soft-tissue sarcoma, rhabdomyosarcoma)	Extremity pain or swelling or fracture
Central Nervous System (glioma, astrocytoma, neuroblastoma)	Hemiplegia, hemiparesis, coordination deficit
Cord Lesions (ependymoma, astrocytoma)	Motor or sensory loss, paraplegia, or quadraplegia
Metastases to Bone (carcinoma—breast, lung, prostate)	Back and rib cage pain or fracture, hip, and shoulder pain or fracture, limps, inability to bear weight
Remote Effects of Tumor	
Carcinoma (breast, pelvic organs, gastrointestinal tract)	Proximal muscle weakness with a dermatopolymyositis picture
Small cell carcinoma	Eaton-Lambert syndrome—weakness improving with exercise
Lymphoma	Motor loss
Lung tumors	Sensory or motor loss

completing such basic functions as dressing, grooming, and toileting, which are necessary for the patient's safe discharge to home.

Speech and swallowing should be evaluated using an oral motor exam and modified barium swallow and ultrasound. Dietary modification or tube feeding and the use of alternative communication aides may be needed.

Early referral to rehabilitation would allow for assessment of these deficits and facilitate the provision of exercise programs, assistive devices, gait aides, and communication sys-

TABLE 67–2. EFFECTS OF CANCER TREATMENT ON THE MUSCULOSKELETAL SYSTEM

	INTERVENTION					
		CHEMOTHERAPY		RADIATION		
MUSCULOSKELETAL DEFICIT	SURGERY	EARLY	LATE	EARLY	LATE	IMMUNOTHERAPY
Atrophy/weakness	x					x
Contracture/fibrosis	x				x[1]	
Wound problems/ decubitis ulcer	x			x		x
Edema	x	x			x	x
Gait abnormalities (motor/ sensory)	x	x[2]			x	
Joint instability	x					
Neuropathy (motor/ sensory)	x	x[2]	x[2]		x	
Decreased endurance (cardiotoxicity)			x[3]	x		x
Central nervous system involvement (balance UMN, LMN)[6]	x	x[4,5]	x[4,5]	x	x	

[1]Especially when more than 6000 cGy are administered

[2]Vincristine and cisplatin

[3]Doxorubicin

[4]Intrathecal methotrexate

[5]Cytarabine

[6]*UMN*, upper motor neuron lesion; *LMN*, lower motor neuron lesion

TABLE 67–3. MUSCULOSKELETAL DEFICITS AND REHABILITATION INTERVENTION

STAGE	POTENTIAL PROBLEM	COURSE OF ACTION		GOAL
		TREATMENT	FREQUENCY OF TREATMENT	
PREOPERATIVE	Delayed referral to rehabilitation medicine	Initiate referral requesting: rehabilitation evaluation and treatment	One to two visits	Maintenance
		Identify risk factors of primary treatment		
	Delay in rehabilitation intervention	Educate in preliminary exercise program		
POSTOPERATIVE				
ACUTE STAGE Bedrest Postoperative days 1 to 4	Atrophy	Isometrics, active range of motion	Once daily	Prevention, restoration
	Range of motion	Passive range of motion		
	Contracture	Static bracing, stretching		
	Pain	Electroanalgesia		
	Weakness	Isometrics		
	Decubiti	Functional bracing, body positioning		
	Neuropathy	Functional bracing		
INTERMEDIATE STAGE Limited activity Postoperative day 4 to discharge	Weakness	Isokinetics, electrostimulation	Twice daily	Restoration
	Decreased stamina	Aerobic exercise		
	Range of motion	Active and active-assisted range of motion, mobilization		
	Pain	Heat, cold, electroanalgesia		
	Gait deficits	Progressive ambulation and assistive devices		
	Joint instability	Temporary bracing with thermoplastic appliance		
	ADL* limitations	Assess ADL needs and provision of equipment		
POSTDISCHARGE STAGE Unrestricted activity	Range of motion	Active and active-assisted range of motion	Depends on musculoskeletal deficits and strategy of treatment (*i.e.*, chemotherapy and/or irradiation)	Maintenance, restoration
	Decreased stamina	Aerobic exercise		
	Weakness	Isotonic exercise		
	Pain	Heat, cold, electroanalgesia		
	Edema	Pneumatic compression and pressure gradient sleeves		
	Neuropathy	Permanent bracing, electrostimulation		
	Gait deficits	Permanent prosthesis/orthesis		
	Role adjustment	Evaluation and referral to appropriate counseling service		

*ADL, activities of daily living

tems. Should there not be ample time or resources available to address these needs before hospital discharge, then a referral to a home health agency would be appropriate for obtaining rehabilitation services.

3. Pain Management

Acute and severe pain in patients with cancer is best managed by the medical team utilizing the appropriate pharmacological agents (see Chapter 56, Pain). However, patients with low level pain syndromes (*i.e.*, myalgia, arthralgia, hyperesthesia) who do not require pharmacological intervention often respond to non-invasive physical agents such as local heat, cold, electrical stimulation, and exercise. The Agency for Health Care Policy and Research (AHCPR) published a set of guidelines in March, 1994, recommending the safest and most effective methods to manage pain in patients with cancer.[4] Included in these recommendations is a section on nonpharmacological management.

4. Metastasis

Metastasis of the primary tumors may be to such vital organs as the brain or the spine, both of which may result in musculoskeletal and neurological deficients. Metastasis to the brain often presents with neurological signs similar to those seen in patients who have been diagnosed with a cerebral vascular accident (CVA) or head trauma, and require appropriate neurodevelopmental re-training of their central nervous system.

Metastasis to the spine may result in vertebral fracture or spinal cord compression. Instability of the spine with resultant extradural spinal cord compression occurs in approximately 5% of patients with cancer, for whom the primary treatment is radiation therapy.[5] Orthopedic stabilization is sometimes attempted with decompression laminectomy followed by fixation with Harrington, Luque, or more recently, Contrel-Dubousset instrumentation. External bracing with a lumbosacral (L-S) corset, thoracolumbosacral orthosis (TLSO), or spinal jacket is rarely beneficial or biomechanically effective in controlling translational or rotational forces affecting the spine during normal movements.

5. Immunosuppression

The most common effect of chemotherapy and total body irradiation is myelosuppression. Patients so treated exhibit signs and symptoms of decreased stamina and generalized weakness. This is especially true for patients being prepared for bone marrow transplantation (BMT). Rehabilitation programs emphasizing incremental exercise and activity post bone marrow transplantation have been developed[6] and have proven very effective in reducing the effects of immobility and immunosuppression. Therapists assist patients in activities such as range of motion, strengthening, and aerobic conditioning as tolerated, in accordance with acceptable hematological levels.[7]

Long-term complications of BMT include graft-versus-host disease (GVHD) and chronic pulmonary infection and respiratory failure. While no controlled trials have demonstrated long-term benefits from ROM or aerobic conditioning, there is some published clinical evidence indicating that these activities may indeed be beneficial.[8]

6. Neuropathy, Instability and Amputation

New approaches in the medical management of patients with osteosarcoma and advanced or recurrent melanoma have been reported which have improved local tumor control and in some cases have increased the number of patients in remission.

Historically, patients with osteosarcoma of the extremity received amputation as a definitive treatment for local tumor control. However, evolving surgical and chemotherapeutic strategies have promoted limb salvage/sparing techniques which employ the use of endoprosthetic devices and the concomitant administration of multi-agent chemotherapy.[9] Complications involving functional deficits due to the failure of endoprosthetic devices or the necessary excision of major peripheral nerves have required quick and aggressive intervention by rehabilitation. The provision of orthotic devices to improve joint stability and decrease abnormal pressures over insensitive areas often prevents further morbidity and preserves the patient's ability to function independently.

In advanced or recurrent melanoma, oncologists have reported the efficacy of isolated limb perfusion (ILP) with various chemotherapeutic agents (*i.e.*, melphalan) and biological response modifiers (*i.e.*, tumor necrosis factor, TNF, and interferon) where mild to moderate limb toxicity has been reported.[10] Complications resulting from these procedures include transient peripheral neuropathy, edema, skin breakdown and vascular compromise with tissue necrosis. As a result of these complications, rehabilitation of these patients is often protracted and requires careful daily monitoring of the skin for areas of pressure combined with an active program of exercises and progressive ambulation. Amputation of the extremity is sometimes an inevitable complication which then requires a significant intervention in preparing and implementing a prosthetic program for the patient.

SUMMARY

Acute and long-term morbidity of patients with cancer may be due to invasion of the primary tumor, metastatic spread, or the side effects of antineoplastic treatment. Many of the musculoskeletal and neurological deficits occurring may be prevented or effectively managed through early referral of these patients to the rehabilitation department for assessment and treatment of these conditions. Individuals interested in more detailed information regarding the principles and practice of rehabilitation of cancer patients should consider reviewing the articles and books listed in the References and Bibliography sections below.

REFERENCES

1. McGarvey C. Quality of life assessment of cancer patients: A review of the literature. Rehabilitation in Oncology 7(1)10–12, 1989
2. MacVicar MG, Winningham ML, Nickel JL. Effects of aerobic interval training in cancer patients' functional capacity. Nursing Research 38:348–51, 1989
3. Guidelines for Exercise Testing and Prescription, 4th ed. American College of Sports Medicine. Philadelphia: Lea & Febiger, 1991:178–80
4. Management of Cancer Pain Guideline Panel: management of cancer pain. Clinical Practice Guideline No. 9. U.S. Department of Health and Human Services, Public Health Service, Agency for Health Care Policy and Research. AHCPR Publication No. 94–0592. March 1994:75–88
5. Harper GR. Recognition and treatment of extradural spinal cord compression. Clinical Cancer Briefs 3–13, 1984
6. Hicks JE. Exercise for cancer patients. In Basmajian JV,

Wolf SL, (eds): Therapeutic Exercise, 5th ed. Baltimore: Williams & Wilkins, 1990:351–69

7. James MC. Physical therapy for patients after bone marrow transplant. Physical Therapy 67:946–52, 1987
8. Turner-McGlade J, Decker W, Fehir K. Cardiopulmonary changes in bone marrow transplant patients: effects of an exercise program. J Cardiopul Rehabil 120:405, 1988
9. Meyer WH, Malawer MM. Osteosarcoma. Clinical features and evolving surgical and chemotherapeutic strategies. Pediatric Clinics in North America 38(2):317–48, 1991
10. Thompson JF, Gianoutsos MP. Isolated limb perfusion for melanoma: effectiveness and toxicity of cisplatin compared with that of melphalan and other drugs. World Journal of Surgery 16(2):227–33, 1992

BIBLIOGRAPHY

Fisher A. Assessment of motor and process skills. Research Edition 7.0. Ft. Collins, CO, Colorado State University, 1994

Funtional Independence Measure (FIM) Copyright 1986, Uniform Data System for Medical Rehabilitation

Gerber LH, Levinson S, Hicks JE et al. Evaluation and management of disability: rehabilitation aspects of cancer. In Devita VT, Hellman S, Rosenberg SA (eds): Cancer: Principles & Practice of Oncology, 4th ed. Philadelphia, JB Lippincott, 1993:2538–69

Levinson SF. Rehabilitation of the patient with cancer or human immunodeficiency virus. In DeLisa JA, Gans BM (eds): Rehabilitation Medicine: Principles and Practice, 2nd ed. Philadelphia, JB Lippincott, 1993:916–33

MacVicar MG, Winningham ML, Nickel J. Effects of aerobic interval training on cancer patients' functional capacity. Nursing Research 38(5):348–51, 1989

McGarvey CL (ed). Physical Therapy for the Cancer Patient. New York, Churchill Livingstone, 1990

Sickness Impact Profile (SIP) Bergner M, Bobbitt RA, Kressel S et al. The sickness impact profile: development and final revision of a health status measure. Intl J Health Serv 6:393–415, 1976

John S. Macdonald, Daniel G. Haller, Robert J. Mayer, Eds. *Manual of Oncologic Therapeutics*, Third Edition.

68. HEMATOPOIETIC GROWTH FACTORS: APPROPRIATE UTILIZATION IN CANCER THERAPY

George D. Demetri

Current cytotoxic therapies for malignant diseases are distressingly nonspecific, with an unfavorable therapeutic index due to associated toxicities. In addition to damaging and killing neoplastic cells, cytotoxic chemotherapeutic agents also damage and kill normal cells, and rapidly dividing cells are, in general, especially sensitive to such damage. These nonspecific toxicities may be physiologically innocuous (although damaging to the cancer patient's quality of life, as with the alopecia resulting from damage to the hair follicles) or they may be medically critical, limiting the oncologist's ability to treat the patient successfully. In the latter category falls the insult to blood cell production caused by myelotoxic chemotherapy. Myelosuppression is a well-known toxicity associated with most anticancer chemotherapeutic drugs. The avoidance of severe, life-threatening myelosuppressive toxicities has always been an important consideration in testing novel chemotherapeutic agents and in designing new combination chemotherapy regimens. From the earliest days of cytotoxic agents in the treatment of cancer, myelosuppression was simply a toxicity to be avoided, with no ability of the oncologist to improve the underlying ability of the patient to resist the undesirable toxicities of the therapy. With the introduction of hematopoietic growth factors into the routine clinical practice of oncology in 1991, oncologists suddenly found themselves in possession of potent tools with which to manipulate host hematopoiesis to minimize the myelosuppressive toxicities of chemotherapy. This, in turn, promises to improve the therapeutic index of anticancer chemotherapy. This chapter reviews the data supporting the clinical effectiveness of hematopoietic growth factors, as well as the limitations of these data. The overall challenge now in medical oncology will be to use these agents in a manner that optimizes clinical outcomes for patients while recognizing the potential for inappropriate use.

BACKGROUND: CLINICAL RELEVANCE OF MYELOSUPPRESSION

The clinical impact of myelosuppressive toxicities was noted early in the development of cytotoxic agents as therapy for acute leukemia. Bodey and coworkers reported the inverse relationship between the clinical risk of severe infectious complications and both the depth and duration of severe neutropenia.[1] Similar observations relating the duration of severe thrombocytopenia to hemorrhagic complications in acute leukemia patients were also reported from this same era.[2] These complications of myelosuppression were truly life-threatening and decreased the overall beneficial impact of aggressive therapy for leukemia.[3] Over the ensuing decades, the field of oncology has extrapolated from these data in leukemics to the cytotoxic chemotherapy of common solid tumors. It is important to note that the therapy of leukemia is generally quite different from chemotherapy for solid tumors (Table 68-1). Thus, the risks noted in the more intensive therapy of leukemia might be an exaggeration of the risks seen with standard cytotoxic therapies of solid tumors. On the other hand, the risks of standard solid tumor chemotherapy may be low simply because the regimens were developed specifically to avoid toxicities, not to optimize antitumor responses or overall clinical outcomes. This simple fact underlines a crucial point upon which clinical usefulness of the hematopoietic growth factors is based: there may be a clinically relevant dose–response relationship between chemotherapy and anticancer effectiveness. The importance of chemotherapy dose remains far more a point of speculation and theoretical extrapolation from preclinical modeling than a clinical fact documented in numerous rigorous, prospective, controlled randomized trials. Nevertheless, several lines of retrospective analyses have converged on the theory that chemotherapy dose may be a crucial determinant of the clinical effectiveness of chemotherapy.[4–7] It is clear that chemotherapy dose is a direct determinant of chemotherapy-associated toxicities for most drugs: for example, 7000 mg/m^2 of cyclophosphamide is reproducibly associated with severely low neutrophil nadir counts and occasional severe thrombocytopenia, whereas the more standard cyclophosphamide dose of 600 mg/m^2 is only mildly myelosuppressive, with a fair amount of interpatient variability in the depth and duration of neutropenia and generally without clinically important thrombocytopenia. To make rational decisions about chemotherapy dose, practicing oncologists require research that rigorously demonstrates increased efficacy with higher-dose, more toxic regimens to justify the increased levels of adverse effects. It has been difficult to study chemotherapy dose–response over a broad dose range because of the unacceptable risk of infectious complications, bleeding, and death with very-high-dose regimens. However, with the hematopoietic growth factors, it is clear that increased dose ranges may be made somewhat more tolerable and safe, so that rigorous proof or refutation of the

TABLE 68–1. DISTINCTIONS BETWEEN STANDARDS FOR ANTILEUKEMIA THERAPY AND SOLID TUMOR CHEMOTHERAPY

LEUKEMIA CHEMOTHERAPY	STANDARD SOLID TUMOR CHEMOTHERAPY
Induction (heavily myelotoxic) followed by consolidation and maintenance months later	Repetitive cycles, mild–moderate myelosuppression
Aplasia therapeutically desirable and unavoidable	Hypoplasia avoided as dose-limiting, aplasia totally unacceptable
Thrombocytopenia accepted and common	Thrombocytopenia unacceptable
Inpatient treatment, prolonged period acceptable	Generally outpatient treatment, short periods of hospitalization
High degree of risk acceptable	Low risk acceptable
Curative intent	Generally palliative intent with uncommon exceptions

chemotherapy dose-response may finally be obtained in the next few years of cancer clinical trials.

BIOLOGY OF HEMATOPOIESIS

To optimize the clinical use of hematopoietic growth factors, it is necessary to recognize the physiologic roles played by these molecules in the complex process of hematopoiesis. Hematopoiesis is an intricately orchestrated interaction of stem/progenitor cells, soluble and cell-bound "factors" (*i.e.*, proteins and glycoproteins that regulate cell growth, differentiation, and function), non-hematopoietic "stromal" cells (such as vascular endothelium and bone marrow fibroblasts), and physical issues such as cell-to-cell contact. Although still far from completely understood, the physiological mechanisms by which humans control the production of blood cells of different lineages have been identified in detail since the 1960s. The hierarchical arrangement of blood cells, ranging from the most immature stem cell to the mature, fully-differentiated, functional elements of the peripheral blood, is schematized in Figure 68–1. Hematopoietic "growth" factors may act at any level of the hierarchy, based on their individual biology and the expression of specific receptors on the surface of responsive target cells. Hematopoietic "cytokines" may, in fact, be a preferable term to describe these molecules, since they are multifunctional. In addition to inducing "growth," most of these molecules affect differentiation and activate effector cell functions in the target cell populations (Table 68–2). There is a functional overlap between several of the molecules that regulate the process of blood cell growth and differentiation.[8,9] The true physiologic rationale for this overlap remains somewhat speculative, but it certainly has practical implications. Oncologists should understand the general level of the hierarchy at which a given hematopoietic growth factor acts *in vitro*. This may well predict the activity *in vivo* and may allow a more rational match between the desired therapeutic effect and the physiologic activity of the native molecule.

CLINICAL STUDIES OF HEMATOPOIETIC GROWTH FACTORS

The preclinical studies, in both *in vitro* and non-human *in vivo* testing, of hematopoietic growth factors suggested that these molecules might possess clinical activity which would be useful. It is important to broadly separate the hematopoietic growth factors into those active on different lineages (*e.g.*, leukocytes, red blood cells, and platelets). The most comprehensive clinical trial data exist for hematopoietic growth factors with leukocyte-lineage activity, while somewhat less exists for erythroid-active factors. The least amount of data exist for hematopoietic growth factors active either on the megakaryocyte/platelet lineage or on very primitive, multipotent stem/progenitor cells.

Another issue complicating the interpretation of data in this field is that there are several hematopoietic growth factors with somewhat overlapping activity profiles, such as GM-CSF and G-CSF. Beyond that, there are often studies that use different recombinant versions of the same native molecule.[10] For example, the clinical research literature regarding GM-CSF is based on studies of (1) **glycosylated** recombinant human GM-CSF (produced by genetically-engineered yeast and known generically as Sargramostim [the generic names of these biological agents are capitalized for some obscure reason] and (2) **non-glycosylated** recombinant human GM-CSF (produced by genetically-engineered *E. coli* bacteria and known generically as Molgramostim). Similarly, the clinical research literature regarding G-CSF is based on studies of (1) a **non-glycosylated** recombinant human G-CSF (produced by genetically-engineered *E. coli* bacteria and known generically as Filgrastim) and (2) a **glycosylated** recombinant human G-CSF (produced by genetically-engineered mammalian cells and known generically as Lenograstim). Patent disputes run rampant in this field and have dictated the boundaries of availability of these agents. The G-CSF of North America is Filgrastim, where commercial distribution of "Lenograstim" was forbidden by patent

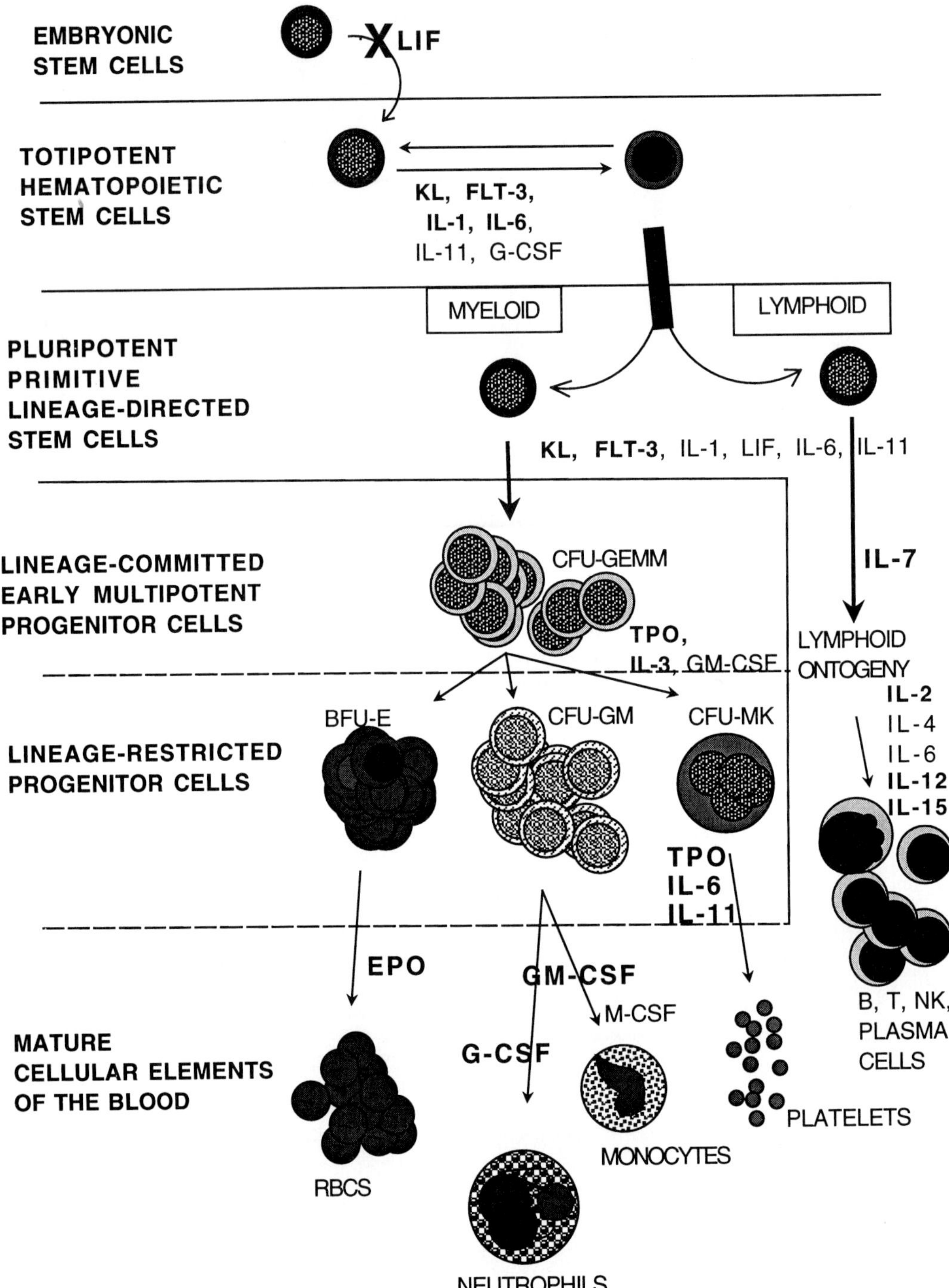

Figure 68–1. The hierarchy of blood cells.

TABLE 68–2. SELECTED HEMATOPOIETIC CYTOKINES: OVERVIEW OF BIOLOGICAL ACTIVITIES

NAME	PRIMARY STIMULATORY ACTIVITY
COLONY-STIMULATING FACTORS	
Granulocyte colony-stimulating factor (G-CSF)	Proliferation of mature progenitor cells Neutrophil-specific differentiation Neutrophil effector cell function (phagocytosis, killing)
Granulocyte-macrophage colony-stimulating factor (GM-CSF)	Proliferation of multipotent mature progenitor cells Multispecific differentiation (neutrophils, monocyte/macrophage, eosinophil Neutrophil, monocyte, eosinophil effector cell function (phagocytosis, killing)
Macrophage colony-stimulating factor (M-CSF, also known as CSF-1)	Proliferation of mature progenitors Monocyte/macrophage differentiation Monocyte/macrophage effector function
Multi-CSF (now known as interleukin-3, IL-3)	Proliferation of more immature progenitors Multipotent differentiation Monocyte, eosinophil effector function
INTERLEUKINS	
IL-1	Very immature cells Megakaryocytic differentiation Wide spectrum of nonhematopoietic cells
IL-2, IL-12, IL-15	T-lymphocytes, NK cells Proliferation and functional activation
IL-6, IL-11	Very immature cells Megakaryocytic differentiation Acute phase response
IL-7	Primitive lymphoid cells
OTHERS	
Erythropoietin	Erythroid-specific differentiation
c-*kit* ligand (also known as stem cell factor, *Steel* factor, and mast cell growth factor)	Primitive multipotent cells (?true stem cells) Mast cell growth and differentiation Mast cell activation/degranulation Synergism with other factors
c-*mpl* ligand (also known as thrombopoietin)	Megakaryocyte/erythroid proliferation and differentiation
FLT3/FLK2 ligand	Primitive multipotent cells (?true stem cells) Synergism with other factors

agreement (both versions of G-CSF are available in Europe, Japan, and Australia). The only GM-CSF commercially available in North America as of 1995 is Sargramostim, while in Europe both versions are available due to the manner in which registration by the European analog of the Food and Drug Administration was sought and approved. If there are differences between these versions of the same native human molecule (either in associated side effects or in specific activity and efficacy), the research literature from Europe may not apply to the American practice of medicine with different recombinant human growth factors. Although this may seem like a trivial or obvious point, it needs to be kept in mind for any rational interpretation of the research literature and the extrapolation to clinical practice.

EARLY CLINICAL TRIALS OF G-CSF AND GM-CSF: TOXICITIES AND STIMULATION OF LEUKOCYTE PRODUCTION

The earliest clinical trials of hematopoietic growth factors with activity on leukocytes (e.g., GM-CSF and G-CSF) confirmed that these molecules could stimulate human leukocyte production in a dose- and schedule-dependent manner.[11–14] Additionally, certain early studies in patients with marrow failure states suggested that these agents might stimulate leukocyte production even in the setting of impaired host hematopoiesis.[15–17]

Besides the obvious clinical activity in stimulating host hematopoiesis *in vivo*, the toxicity profiles associated with these agents was remarkably benign, particularly in comparison with high-dose infusional IL-2 (another recombinant human hematopoietic growth factor that was entering clinical development at around the same time as GM-CSF and G-CSF). The most common adverse effect noted with both GM-CSF and G-CSF is a mild to moderate ache in bones, particularly the lower back and pelvis. The etiology of this "medullary pain" remains poorly understood, although it is routinely attributed to the rapid proliferation of marrow elements. The pain is clearly dose-related, with more severe pain noted at very high doses of G-CSF. The kinetics of this pain indicate that the onset is immediately prior to full hematologic recovery in the peripheral blood, when the myeloid elements of the marrow are most active. Additionally, in the setting of autologous bone marrow transplantation, this pain is usually not noted, suggesting that if there is a "clearing-out" of the bulk of the marrow cellularity, this pain does not arise. Whether the pain is truly due to physical pressure from rapid expansion of marrow cellularity or whether other mediators, such as prostaglandins or other inflammatory mediators, might be released locally by large numbers of marrow elements, remains poorly understood. If it occurs, the bony pain associated with either G-CSF or GM-CSF usually is easily managed by acetaminophen administration, without the need for more potent nonsteroidal anti-inflammatory agents or narcotic analgesics.

Occasional transient skin rash has been an associated clinical toxicity with either G-CSF or GM-CSF. The toxicity profile in the literature suggests that other side effects from G-CSF are exceedingly rare (including rare fevers). No dose-limiting toxicities (other than bony pain) have been reported for G-CSF (Filgrastim) at any dose (highest clinical doses tested have been in the range of 115 μg/kg per day.[18,19] On the other hand, the toxicity profile with GM-CSF seems more complex and common.[20] Certainly, there is a higher incidence of GM-CSF–related toxicities with higher doses of GM-CSF. The phase I testing of any new drug or biologic routinely tests for the maximal tolerated dose of that agent, which may not necessarily be the optimal dose of that agent for clinical use. This seems particularly true for GM-CSF. The phase I toxicity studies of the Molgramostim version of GM-CSF showed biologic effects at the lowest doses tested (< 5 μg/kg per day) with higher doses of GM-CSF (>30 μg/kg per day) clearly inducing dose-limiting toxicities such as pleuropericarditis, thrombotic complications, and third-spacing of fluid.[12] Although they are biologically intriguing, these severe GM-CSF-related toxicities may have nothing whatsoever to do with routine clinical practice, if the molecule is clinically efficaceous at lower doses. Thus, the toxicity literature must be interpreted cautiously. Appropriate utilization of the hematopoietic growth factors will be based on a thorough understanding of the clinical dose-response for these agents.

The relative safety of G-CSF and GM-CSF was impressive in phase I toxicity trials, but more impressive was the evident activity on leukocyte production. Clearly, these molecules were able to stimulate host hematopoiesis and increase numbers of leukocytes. The mechanisms by which these agents stimulate peripheral leukocytosis differ somewhat. G-CSF stimulates more rapid differentiation of immature progenitor cells into mature neutrophils,[21] whereas GM-CSF diminishes the time required for cells to traverse the cell cycle and allows faster proliferation of committed progenitor cells.[22] The clinical activity of either molecule is apparent within 1 to 2 days of dosing. The kinetic response of neutrophilia to G-CSF may be somewhat more rapid than GM-CSF because of its action on the most mature lineage-restricted progenitor cell pool. GM-CSF induces a leukocytosis over days in the absence of a myelosuppressive stimulus, and this response may be somewhat more sustained following discontinuation of GM-CSF dosing than would be seen with G-CSF because of the stimulation and expansion of a more immature multilineage pool of progenitor cells. The clinical activities of both G-CSF and GM-CSF in this regard are thus relatively predictable based on their *in vitro* spectrum of activity.

Definitive Randomized Studies of Hematopoietic Growth Factors: Background to Trial Designs

Having demonstrated clinical activity in phase I studies, investigators were faced with the task of proving that stimulation of leukocyte production in humans would be clinically useful and beneficial. After all, the increased numbers of circulating leukocytes induced by G-CSF or GM-CSF represent only a laboratory finding: a "surrogate endpoint" for other, more meaningful clinical endpoints such as lower rates of infection or fewer toxic deaths from aggressive therapy. It was theoretically possible that the high circulating leukocyte levels might have no clinical activity, and trials were necessary to determine whether these leukocytes were truly functional effector cells. This was suggested by laboratory studies of G-CSF or GM-CSF-exposed leukocytes in which increased phagocytosis and oxidative killing of microbial targets were reported.[23,24] However, other early trials had reported abnormalities in the motility of leukocytes produced under the stimulation of GM-CSF, suggesting that GM-CSF might not induce the production of optimal effector cells.[25] G-CSF and GM-CSF also were noted to have different effects on the expression of certain neutrophil adhesion molecules such as L-selectin, which might affect the ability of neutrophils to traffic to sites of inflammation or infection.[26,27] It was clear that the level of circulating leukocytes might be a misleading indicator of clinical activity for these hematopoietic growth factors. The challenge was to design and interpret clinical trials to prove that the CSF-stimulated leukocyte production had clinically relevant beneficial impacts on endpoints other than a laboratory value.

Based on the activity seen in the phase I trials of G-CSF and GM-CSF, pivotal randomized phase III trials were designed. Relatively few phase II studies were performed with these molecules to define the optimal doses for effect, the optimal schedule of administration, or the variety of clinical effects noted with differing myelotoxic drugs. This fact has continued to plague the field, with relatively little definitive data on these important aspects concerning the use of GM-CSF and G-CSF. Nevertheless, both molecules have a rather broad therapeutic index (although the therapeutic index for G-CSF is more broad than for GM-CSF due to the increased incidence of side effects with higher doses of GM-CSF), and it was possible to reasonably estimate a dose of both molecules that would most probably confer clinical benefit to patients undergoing myelosuppressive therapy for cancer.

The most successful trials that studied either GM-CSF or G-CSF shared one basic tenet: to show that stimulation of leukocyte production is associated with improved clinical outcomes of any sort, the myelosuppression under study must be relatively severe. Simply put, the myelotoxicity of therapy must be reproducibly present and clinically problematic without CSF use to show a difference from its amelioration. While the clinical scenarios used in the research studies were reasonable models and assumptions to study the *in vivo* activity of GM-CSF and G-CSF, these clinical trial scenarios of severe myelosuppression may not necessarily be relevant to the vast majority of anticancer regimens for common solid tumors (See Table 68–1). This may prove an important problem in extrapolating from the available research data to formulate a strategy for optimal utilization of these agents in practice.

To interpret the available data as the justification for rational use of G-CSF or GM-CSF, it is important to define some terms. Most of the original clinical research studies were aimed at testing the ability of either G-CSF or GM-CSF to prevent infectious complications of myelosuppressive therapy **before** any complications had ever occurred. This strategy for use of hematopoietic growth factors is known as "primary prophylaxis" of infectious complications, and represents the preemptive use of these agents to prevent potential adverse clinical events (such as fever with neutropenia). Other potential strategies for the use of G-CSF or GM-CSF include the following:

> Secondary prophylaxis is the attempt to prevent **subsequent** recurrences of an infectious complication after one such episode has already occurred. For example, if a patient had experienced an episode of fever with neutropenia during her second cycle of chemotherapy given without an adjunctive CSF, the use of CSF during the subsequent third cycle of chemotherapy to prevent a recurrence of an infectious complication would typify the use of CSF as secondary prohylaxis.
>
> Therapeutic use of G-CSF or GM-CSF is defined as the use of these agents to actively treat a clinical problem. For example, if a patient to whom adjunctive G-CSF or GM-CSF had *not* been prescribed experiences an episode of bacterial sepsis with neutropenia, beginning dosing of CSF concurrent with initiation of parenteral broad-spectrum antibiotics would represent the use of CSF with "therapeutic" intent. Other examples of CSF use with "therapeutic" intent would be the use of these agents to treat clinical disorders other than the myelosuppression of cancer chemotherapy, such as marrow failure states or congenital neutropenias.

The vast majority of clinical trials have evaluated the ability of these agents to improve clinical outcomes when used in the strategy of primary prophylaxis. It is critical to note this point as one interprets the research literature and attempts to draw conclusions for non–research-based clinical practice.

Randomized Studies of G-CSF as Primary Prophylaxis

The pivotal study of G-CSF was a multicenter, randomized, prospective, double-blinded, placebo-controlled clinical trial. This study used a fairly aggressive dosing regimen of CAE chemotherapy (cyclophosphamide, doxorubicin, etoposide) in patients with previously untreated small cell lung cancer. These patients were randomized to receive CAE either with placebo or with active G-CSF as primary prophylaxis. The study was conducted in the United States,[28] and a replicate study was performed in Europe.[29] The United States study was designed so that any episode of infectious complication (such as fever with neutropenia) would trigger the patient to "cross-over" to receive unblinded active G-CSF. The European study kept patients on the treatment arm to which they were originally randomized (G-CSF or placebo) for the entire duration of protocol therapy with no cross-over. Despite these differences in study design, the data from these two randomized studies are quite consistent. Both studies showed that patients receiving these cytotoxic drugs at the doses employed experienced a median of 6 days of severe neutropenia if the chemotherapy was given with placebo; this was reduced to only 3 days of similarly severe neutropenia in the patients receiving adjunctive G-CSF. It is important to look beyond the simple surrogate laboratory endpoint of neutrophil counts to clinical outcome endpoints. The patients who received this very myelosuppressive regimen without G-CSF in both studies suffered exceptionally high rates of infectious complications, such as fever with neutropenia prompting admission to the hospital (57% of placebo-treated patients receiving these doses of CAE in the first cycle); the addition of G-CSF as an adjunct to the supportive care of these patients decreased the incidence of infectious complications by 50% (*i.e.*, a 28% incidence of fever with neutropenia in the group receiving G-CSF). Correlating with these diminished rates of fever with neutropenia is a decreased incidence of hospitalization for management of infectious complications. This is a tautology, however, since the operational rules of the clinical trial required that patients with fever and neutropenia be admitted to hospital (as would have been standard practice in most institutions in 1988). Additionally, there were certain clinical indicators that suggested that the duration of hospitalization and duration of parenteral antibiotic administration were also decreased in the group receiving G-CSF. Interpretation of data relevant to hematologic recovery from chemotherapy beyond the first cycle in both studies is complicated by differences in the chemotherapy dose reductions between treatment arms. Nevertheless, it is clear that G-CSF can be shown to diminish certain clinically relevant toxicities of aggressive myelotoxic chemotherapy. This is taken as proof that the increased levels of circulating neutrophils produced in response to pharmacologic dosing of G-CSF are indeed fully functional effector cells. On the basis of these randomized data and prior pilot studies, the Filgrastim recombinant version of G-CSF was approved for commercial distribution by the United States Food and Drug Administration (FDA) in February 1991. The FDA approval was remarkably broad in scope, allowing the use of G-CSF as an adjunct to myelosuppressive chemotherapies of all types in the treatment plan for all types of non-myeloid malignancies.

Pivotal Randomized Trial of GM-CSF: "Primary Prophylaxis" with ABMT

The strategy to test the impact of GM-CSF in oncology took a somewhat different route. Most of the pivotal data for GM-CSF were generated in the setting of extremely high-dose chemotherapy or chemoradiotherapy with autologous bone marrow transplantation (ABMT). Pilot studies of GM-CSF had suggested an acceleration of leukocyte recovery following ABMT compared to historic control.[29–31] The definitive study of the Sargramostim (yeast-produced, glycosylated) version of GM-CSF was a randomized, prospective, double-blinded, placebo-controlled clinical trial performed at three academic transplant centers using patients with a variety of lymphoid malignancies who were undergoing ABMT.[32] In a sense, this was a test of GM-CSF as primary prophylaxis, since it was administered before any infectious complications occurred. In this trial, the group receiving GM-CSF exhibited significantly more rapid leukocyte recovery following ABMT than the group receiving placebo. This translated into a more rapid discharge from hospital (on the order of 1 week earlier than the placebo group) and a lower requirement for parenteral antibiotics in the group receiving adjunctive GM-CSF. Despite GM-CSF, fever during the pancytopenic nadir remained a universal finding in all patients, but this was expected based on the severity of myelosuppression associated with the high-dose cytotoxic therapy employed. Fewer documented infections and fewer fungal infections were noted in the group receiving adjunctive GM-CSF. This study, in addition to much pilot data, led to FDA approval of the Sargramostim version of GM-CSF in February 1991. However, based on the pivotal trial that had been conducted in the setting of ABMT, the approval was far more limited than that granted for G-CSF; FDA approval for GM-CSF covered the use of this molecule only as an adjunct to patients with non-myeloid malignancies undergoing ABMT.

Limitations of Data from Pivotal Studies of G-CSF and GM-CSF: Implications for Practice

While the development of G-CSF and GM-CSF are impressive tales of technology assessment and commercialization, these molecules present enigmatic problems for the practice of oncology, which will be detailed in the following sections.

RELEVANCE OF CLINICAL TRIAL DATA TO ROUTINE PRACTICE

In the vast majority of cases of cancer treated with cytotoxic therapy, the incidence of infectious complications does not approach the 60% to 100% incidence noted in the pivotal trials of G-CSF or GM-CSF. This indicates that the data may be directly applicable only to the small subset of patients treated with exceptionally myelotoxic regimens and with ABMT high-dose approaches. The routine application of CSFs as primary prophylaxis may be a somewhat excessive extrapolation of the data to less myelosuppressive clinical scenarios.

WHICH PATIENTS SHOULD RECEIVE ADJUNCTIVE CSF SUPPORT?

The optimal strategy for CSF use remains open to discussion. Certainly, one might reasonably question the routine use of CSFs as primary prophylaxis in all patients with non-myeloid malignancies treated with any myelosuppressive chemotherapy. Although this broad definition would technically be covered under the FDA-approved indication for G-CSF, no one (not even the commercial vendor of G-CSF) would think this represents the most appropriate use of the CSFs. The vast majority of patients are not receiving myelosuppressive chemotherapy at doses sufficiently potent to induce high rates of clinical problems. For example, the vast majority of patients receiving adjuvant CMF (cyclophosphamide, methotrexate, 5-fluorouracil) or 5-FU/levamisole chemotherapy for breast or colon cancer, respectively, do not experience clinically relevant infectious complications. In these patients, the routine application of CSF support would likely be overtreatment. On the other hand, in selected high-risk patients, the judicious use of CSF support might truly be appropriate and clinically beneficial. The efficacy of CSF support in high-risk populations (*e.g.*, the very elderly or patients with severe co-morbid disease) requires further study.

PRIMARY OR SECONDARY PROPHYLAXIS?

As noted earlier, most of the clinical trial data have studied the use of CSFs as primary prophylaxis. In one randomized study of G-CSF, placebo-treated patients who experienced an infectious toxicity with a prior cycle of chemotherapy were crossed over to receive G-CSF in the subsequent cycle.[28] This is the clinical test of G-CSF when used as secondary prophylaxis. G-CSF as secondary prophylaxis was able to stimulate accelerated neutrophil recovery and diminish the incidence of infectious complications. Thus, limited prior chemotherapy does not abrogate the ability of G-CSF to stimulate hematopoiesis. Secondary prophylaxis may be very reasonable for optimizing CSF use, since the patient population would be selected on the basis of clinical parameters (*i.e.*, prior poor tolerance of chemotherapy) and would represent a more restricted subset than in a "primary prophylaxis" strategy. On the other hand, if a patient is at very high risk for toxicity or if any toxicity might be excessively morbid, a strategy of primary prophylaxis might still be more reasonable for that individual. This will likely remain an area of active debate, since medical judgement is fundamental to this and excessively strict rules governing the prescribing behavior of physicians may not recognize the complexity of medical decision-making.

CLINICAL DIFFERENCES BETWEEN G-CSF AND GM-CSF

There are no trials in which G-CSF has been concurrently tested in a randomized fashion against GM-CSF. GM-CSF has been tested in clinical settings less myelotoxic than ABMT with somewhat mixed results. One randomized prospective study of GM-CSF versus placebo as support of myelosuppressive chemotherapy for lymphoma patients indicated certain improvements in clinical outcomes in a subset of patients.[33] However, the incidence of clinical intolerance to GM-CSF made the beneficial findings not applicable to the entire study population, and no comparison to G-CSF was attempted in that trial. Similar findings have been noted in other randomized studies of GM-CSF with myelosuppressive chemotherapy for small cell lung cancer[34] or germ cell tumors.[35] In summary, the 20% incidence of fevers associated with GM-CSF administration reported in the literature might confound the ability of investigators to show a beneficial impact of GM-CSF support on rates of fever with neutropenia. On the other hand, that may not be the only (or even the most important) clinical indicator of activity. If the desired therapeutic endpoint is "full hematologic recovery adequate to allow repetitive administration of chemotherapy according to a certain schedule," it is possible that GM-CSF and G-CSF might have clinically similar effects. It is also critical to note that the different recombinant versions of GM-CSF (glycosylated versus non-glycosylated, Sargramsostim versus Molgramostim) have never been compared to each other in a rigorous randomized manner. Thus, while certain investigators have suggested that a particular molecular version of recombinant GM-CSF might be less toxic and equally efficacious than another, this remains unproven. In contrast to GM-CSF, G-CSF has never proven its clinical efficacy in a rigorous, randomized, placebo-controlled clinical trial in the setting of ABMT. Nonetheless, given the strength and consistency of large numbers of studies using G-CSF to support high-dose chemotherapy with bone marrow transplantation, the FDA has recently approved the use of G-CSF for ABMT as well. As with GM-CSF, the different recombinant molecular versions of G-CSF (glycosylated versus non-glycosylated, Lenograstim versus Filgrastim) have never been rigorously compared in a randomized clinical trial. Differences in areas such as specific activity, bioavailability, pharmacodynamics, and toxicities have seemed to remain more in the province of biopharmaceutical marketing than in the domain of clinical investigation, unfortunately. Far more work needs to be done to understand the clinical differences between these agents and how they should be used optimally for clinical oncology and hematology.

RELEVANCE OF OUTCOMES STUDIED TO CURRENT PRACTICE

The clinical endpoints most beneficially affected by the adjunctive use of GM-CSF or G-CSF were hospitalization and the incidence of infectious complications, respectively. The management of infectious complications of chemotherapy is evolving. Certain low-risk subsets of patients presenting with fever and neutropenia syndromes have been identified, and such patients may enjoy perfectly acceptable clinical outcomes if managed by appropriate outpatient strategies rather than by inpatient hospitalization. Additionally, the criteria for discharge of patients undergoing ABMT have evolved similarly over the past several years, with an increased sense of safety regarding earlier discharges as the field has matured. With ABMT, it is impossible to assess how much of the increase in earlier discharges may be due to CSF utilization, since these agents have been universally used in that setting after 1991. Nevertheless, for routine non-transplant chemotherapy, the changing spectrum of management of fever with neutropenia may diminish somewhat the clinical benefits of CSF support to chemotherapy.

SIGNIFICANCE OF CHEMOTHERAPY DOSE INTENSITY

Dose intensity is often used as a justification for CSF support. Nearly all clinical trials have demonstrated an increased ability of patients to tolerate higher dose intensities of chemotherapy with equivalent toxicities if adjunctive CSF support has been given. This leads to the obvious question: how clinically significant are such increases in dose intensity? The controversy surrounding dose intensity continues to generate more heat than light, although randomized clinical trial data are finally beginning to appear. Although beyond the scope of this review, most data support the hypothesis that a certain threshold of chemotherapy dose must be attained to achieve optimal clinical anticancer efficacy. This is supported, for example, by the large randomized study performed by the Cancer and Leukemia Group B in patients with early breast cancer.[36] Additionally, prospective studies testing the importance of higher-than-standard doses of chemotherapy are in progress. The results of these studies will be absolutely critical to the rational use of CSFs in clinical practice. If non-myelosuppressive chemotherapy were to be shown to have efficacy equal to myelosuppressive chemotherapy, the clinical utility of the CSFs to ameliorate myelosuppressive toxicities would clearly be much less important in practice.

COSTS OF PROVIDING ADJUNCTIVE CSF SUPPORT

This is a major issue in the current climate of cost-control in health care. The prospective research studies of G-CSF and GM-CSF did not specifically address the costs of these agents. For novel chemotherapy agents with primary antineoplastic activity, cost may be somewhat less of an issue. However, for supportive care agents such as G-CSF or GM-CSF that have not been shown to increase survival in standard chemotherapy or ABMT for solid tumors, a great deal of scrutiny has been applied to the sizeable costs of these agents.[37] Certain analyses have suggested that the adjunctive use of CSFs would be cost-saving.[38,39] These analyses are based on the potential savings that accrue from keeping patients out of the hospital for management of toxicities. The ability to keep patients out of the hospital with G-CSF or GM-CSF is based on the assumption that patients need to be in the hospital to begin with. If the rates of hospitalization are low, it is difficult to show any savings with CSF use, since the primary "big ticket" determinant of cost is the hospitalization incidence and duration. Thus, changes in practice patterns that will affect the incidence of hospitalization (*e.g.*, in the routine management of fever and neutropenia) will have important effects on the cost analyses of CSF use. In the setting of ABMT, though, with the attendant prolonged hospitalizations of 3 to 4 weeks, most analyses support the fact that the routine application of CSF support is objectively cost-saving. This seems clear and helpful to justify CSF use with ABMT. It is difficult to determine how cost analyses should be used to guide the use of CSFs in less myelosuppressive settings. All agents used to treat cancer patients cost money, and valid analyses of "cost-effectiveness" have been performed for very few drugs or procedures used in clinical oncology. Thus, the "value" of CSF support to ameliorate myelosuppressive toxicities must be studied and not simply measured by an arbitrary standard of "cost savings." We do not require that ondansetron or other novel supportive care agents provide cost savings for them to be very useful clinically. On the other hand, most patients would be very willing to pay dearly for the symptomatic relief offered by ondansetron, and thus the clinical value of that agent based on the quality-of-life impact is clear. The quality-of-life impact of the CSFs has not been as rigorously assessed in practice. Such data might help guide the appropriate use of CSFs in non-ABMT settings. If CSFs were very inexpensive, this would not be an issue at all. However, the CSFs as commercially available are not inexpensive, and the challenge for oncologists is to determine where the clinical value of these agents equals or exceeds the costs. Certainly, injudicious use of CSFs can induce important "financial toxicities." Additionally, different strategies of CSF use can be important determinants of the cost.[40]

DOSE AND SCHEDULE OF CSFS

The CSFs, like many biologic agents, present interesting problems that diverge from the traditional path of oncology drug development. For example, these agents are highly active over a wide dose range. There may not be significantly increased clinical efficacy at higher doses, and the optimal bioactive dose may not be synonymous with the maximal tolerated dose. The doses of GM-CSF (250 μg/m^2/day) and G-CSF (5 μg/kg/day) that have become widely accepted and FDA-approved may not be the truly optimal doses. Current research in progress is attempting to define more specifically the CSF dose–response curve and the relevance of CSF schedule of administration to clinical outcome. Early phase II clinical trials that evaluated differences between CSF doses or schedules were based on very small patient numbers.[41–43] Certainly, with GM-CSF it is clear that too high a dose is excessively toxic and can interfere with clinical activity and tolerance.[34] However, lower doses of GM-CSF may be equivalently effective with better tolerance and thus may have a more favorable therapeutic index. Clinically important questions relevant to CSF schedule (such as whether the initiation of CSF dosing can be delayed a few days in a chemotherapy cycle or whether the CSF can be stopped earlier in the cycle), although seemingly mundane, may have an enormous impact on the use of CSF in routine practice and will be relevant to issues of cost-effectiveness. There may also be important issues of toxicities of CSFs relevant to schedule of administration. For example, the administration of CSF concurrently with certain chemotherapy drugs has been noted to paradoxically **increase** the myelotoxicity of chemotherapy.[44] This may be due to the increased cell cycling of progenitor cells induced by the CSF at the same time high concentrations of cytotoxic drug are present. A similar mechanism has been postulated to account for the increased myelotoxicity of large-field radiation therapy when administered concurrently with GM-CSF.[45] On the basis of these observations, a reasonable schedule of CSF administration outside of a clinical trial would be to avoid the concurrent dosing of CSF with chemotherapy or large-field radiation therapy.

THERAPEUTIC USE OF CSFS

As defined earlier, the "therapeutic" use of hematopoietic growth factors is defined as the administration of these agents to treat an acute (or chronic) problem, not to prevent problems. In the setting of chemotherapy-induced myelosuppression, "therapeutic" use of GM-CSF or G-CSF is widely used in the routine practice of oncology with a paucity of objective research data to justify the use in that setting. There has been one multicenter, prospective, randomized, placebo-controlled clinical trial to evaluate the worth of G-CSF versus placebo as an adjunct to empiric antibiotics and hospitalization for patients admitted with fever and neutropenia.[46] This trial is far from definitive, due largely to the fact that patients with fever and neutropenia represent an extremely heterogeneous group of patients with highly variable clinical outcomes. In the modern era of routine, broad-spectrum antibiosis, mortality from infectious complications of even the most myelosuppressive chemotherapy regimens is vanishingly rare (although still occurring at a finite low rate). This study showed that the therapeutic use of G-CSF was able to diminish time to recovery from severe neutropenia by approximately 1 day; this "surrogate endpoint" of a beneficial impact of G-CSF on neutrophil recovery was statistically significant. The improvement in hematologic recovery did not lead to a significant decrease in the lengths of hospital stays in this patient population, however. The clinical relevance of the accelerated neutrophil recovery may have been somewhat masked by the operational rules of the study design: patients were required to remain as hospitalized inpatients until their neutrophil counts had recovered **and** they had remained absolutely afebrile for several days post-recovery. This stringent standard may have been the standard of care when the study was designed in the late 1980s, but the current practice of oncology is based on more flexible guidelines for discharge from the hospital tied more closely to neutrophil recovery and clinical stability than the temperature curve *per se*. Thus, this study may have underestimated some impact of G-CSF to diminish hospital stays to some degree. Alternatively, it is possible that for the vast majority of patients, starting a CSF during the period of nadir neutropenia may be too late to significantly affect the time to hematologic recovery. In this study, there were trends which suggested that the group of patients receiving G-CSF may have had a more consistent time to neutrophil recovery; in other words, the G-CSF may diminish the risk of "outliers" who might otherwise experience excessively prolonged recovery from myelosuppressive chemotherapy. Further research will be required to decide whether the costs of "therapeutic" CSF administration as adjuncts to standard antibiotics in the setting of acute infectious complications from chemotherapy justify this application. Additionally, very little research has rigorously evaluated the use of GM-CSF in this setting, although GM-CSF might activate a more broad spectrum of immunologic effector cells.

OTHER INDICATIONS FOR CSFS BEYOND SUPPORTIVE CARE WITH CHEMOTHERAPY

The "therapeutic" use of G-CSF and GM-CSF may extend far beyond simple supportive care of myelosuppressive chemotherapy. Perhaps the most clear indication of therapeutic benefit in this regard has been in the setting of patients with congenital or acquired disorders of neutrophil production. A large randomized trial has been conducted in patients with severe chronic neutropenia in which G-CSF dosing has been shown to impact favorably on the clinical course, with decreased incidence and severity of infections and a higher quality of life for the patients.[47] Limited data suggest that GM-CSF may not be as consistently active as G-CSF in stimulating clinically useful levels of leukocytes in patients with certain congenital marrow failure states.[48,49] Hematopoietic growth factors have also been used in several pilot research studies to stimulate hematopoiesis in patients with myelodysplasia (MDS) and other marrow failure states.[15-17,50-52] One randomized study of G-CSF versus observation in patients with high-grade MDS (specifically refractory anemia with excess of blasts [RAEB] and RAEB in transformation) has now failed to show a survival benefit to the use of G-CSF.[53] The use of hematopoietic growth factors in MDS must be considered investigational, and the optimal treatment for such patients, in general, remains participation in relevant clinical research trials. The clinical comparisons of G-CSF with GM-CSF in the treatment of marrow failure states remain anecdotal, and more certainly needs to be learned about the activities and toxicities of these agents in this "therapeutic" setting before their use should be widely employed. New research avenues are also being explored using hematopoietic growth factors in the "therapeutic" setting, but these remain highly investigational and of unproven benefit at this time. For example, studies are evaluating the worth of CSFs as adjuncts to antibiotics in the therapy of patients with high-risk pneumonias or refractory infections. It is likely that stimulation of cellular immunity may also be of potential utility in diseases such as drug-resistant tuberculosis, but these trials are only now in the earliest stages of conception.

IS THE PHYSICIAN LIABLE FOR NON-USE OF CSF SUPPORT?

The medicolegal aspects of hematopoietic growth factors have been of some concern to many practicing physicians. Specifically, if a CSF is **not** used in prophylaxis and the patient subsequently suffers an infectious complication of therapy, would the physician be liable for the medical decision? While beyond the scope of this review to examine this issue in adequate depth, it seems important to note that in no study of CSF use as supportive care of solid tumor chemotherapy has there been any survival advantage noted in the group of patients receiving the CSF compared to placebo. Thus, fears of liability should not guide medical practice in this regard so much as the physician's medical assessment of the patient's risk of infection and the patient's ability to handle an infection if one were to occur.

SHOULD CSFS BE USED TO SUPPORT THE CYTOTOXIC THERAPY OF PATIENTS WITH LEUKEMIA?

Much concern has been raised about the potentially dangerous ability of CSFs to stimulate the proliferation of leukemia cells, particularly cells of myeloid leukemias. Clonogenic leukemia cells, in general, retain sensitivity to the stimulatory effects of hematopoietic growth factors *in vitro*. The clinical significance of this laboratory finding, though, remains unclear, since the hematopoietic growth factors also may enhance cellular differentiation. The balance *in vivo* of CSF action might be tilted in favor of differentiation of the leukemic clone; alternatively, the balance might be shifted toward stimulation of the normal stem/progenitor cell pools. In essence, the only way to answer this question of safety and efficacy is with a randomized clinical trial. At least three prospective randomized trials have now been reported, with somewhat overlapping results.[54–56] In all three studies, there has been no obvious clinical danger from the use of adjunctive G-CSF or GM-CSF to support the initial cytotoxic induction therapy of patients with acute myelocytic leukemias. No rapid regrowth of leukemias has been noted in this setting, as was feared from the *in vitro* studies on leukemia cells. Two of these three studies have documented a clinical benefit to the use of CSF in the treatment of leukemia patients.[54,55] One of the studies, presented in abstract form, has observed an actual survival benefit in the group receiving GM-CSF compared to placebo.[55] Another randomized study of GM-CSF in AML patients has noted no clinically relevant differences between GM-CSF support or placebo.[56] In general, the use of CSF support for patients with myeloid malignancies remains investigational pending further data reporting, but consistently data now suggest that CSF use may be quite safe in this setting of severe myelotoxicity.

DOES CSF SUPPORT IMPROVE OUTCOMES FOR PATIENTS WITH AIDS?

The first clinical trial of GM-CSF was undertaken in patients with AIDS-related leukopenia.[11] Several trials have since valuated the use of hematopoietic growth factors in this clinical setting.[57,58] Overall, the literature suggests that the infectious complications of AIDS may not be successfully overcome simply by stimulation of neutrophils. On the other hand, the ability of G-CSF or GM-CSF to overcome some of the myelosuppressive aspects of antiretroviral agents such as AZT may allow the more effective administration of those agents.[59,60] At this point, many investigators are attempting to define an appropriate role for CSFs in the management of patients with AIDS, but this too remains poorly defined and somewhat investigational.

WHAT WILL DETERMINE PHYSICIAN PRESCRIBING BEHAVIOR OF HEMATOPOIETIC GROWTH FACTORS AS ADJUNCTS TO MYELOSUPPRESSIVE CHEMOTHERAPY?

Many factors will drive this issue. The primary issue should be the medical risk to the patient of the myelosuppressive regimen. Obviously, host factors such as patient age, co-morbid diseases, and performance status will be important considerations. Most importantly, too, the American Society of Clinical Oncology has begun a data-driven Practice Guidelines Development process to steer oncologists toward the most rational use of these agents. Finally, more complete data will be critical to the most optimal use of these agents in a variety of clinical scenarios. Future studies, to affect clinical practice patterns, will need to take into account issues of cost, as well as quality of life, patient preferences, effectiveness in practice settings outside traditional academic centers, and other non-traditional parameters.

HEMATOPOIETIC GROWTH FACTORS ACTIVE ON OTHER LINEAGES BESIDES LEUKOCYTES

This is an area of intensive investigation. Currently, the only other FDA-approved hematopoietic growth factor is recombinant human erythropoietin (EPO). EPO has been shown to decrease the incidence of red blood cell transfusion requirements in a heterogeneous population of anemic cancer patients in large multicenter prospective placebo-controlled trials.[61] However, the most appropriate use of EPO remains a subject of much controversy. Again, issues of appropriate patient selection and cost-effectiveness are paramount in considering the optimal clinical use of EPO. Nevertheless, with better data, one can be hopeful that EPO may yet be a useful addition to the supportive care regimens of patients with cancer. Several thrombopoietic agents are under active clinical investigation, including IL-1,[62] IL-3,[63] the GM-CSF/IL-3 fusion molecule known as PIXY321,[64,65] IL-6,[66] and IL-11.[67] Much enthusiasm has greeted the recent report of the cloning and characterization of the ligand for c-*mpl*, which may be the true physiologic thrombopoietin.[68–70] However, this molecule has not yet undergone the test of even the earliest phase I toxicity testing in humans, and it is premature to predict its clinical efficacy. Nevertheless, it seems not excessively hopeful to posit that clinicians will soon have tools to stimulate platelet production just as they currently have tools that stimulate the production of leukocytes and erythrocytes.

COMBINATIONS OF HEMATOPOIETIC GROWTH FACTORS

In vitro, combinations of hematopoietic growth factors are most often synergistic rather than additive. Whether the same would hold true to any clinically relevant degree *in vivo* remains to be seen. At this time, there are no data to indicate that combinations of hematopoietic growth factors are in any way deleterious compared to single agents. There are no indications of premature marrow failure or "lineage-steal" in studies where combinations of hematopoietic growth factors were given to support chemotherapy (such as G-CSF + EPO[71] or G-CSF + IL-6[72]). Hematopoietic growth factors active on primitive progenitor cells and true stem cells are being identified.[9, 73–75] The clinical utilities of these early-acting molecules remain to be tested, but they may prove useful in increasing the quality of autologous cellular products (such as peripheral blood stem/progenitor cells). Additionally, such molecules are critical to most laboratory research protocols for gene transduction and gene therapy initiatives. If "gene therapy" ever becomes clinically more disseminated, these hematopoietic growth factors will certainly prove indispensable to the process.

FUTURE DIRECTIONS AND CURRENT RECOMMENDATIONS FOR PRACTICE

The most appropriate use of the hematopoietic growth factors remains a subject of intense discussion, controversy, and investigation. Much of the utility of the leukocyte-active agents (G-CSF and GM-CSF) is tied to the delivery of heavily myelosuppressive chemotherapy. If a patient is at high risk from a severely myelosuppressive regimen, these agents certainly have a proven track record of diminishing the risks and accelerating the expected hematologic recovery as primary prophylaxis. However, this will come at a certain cost. For extremely myelosuppressive treatments such as ABMT, all would agree that the hematopoietic stimulation offered by G-CSF or GM-CSF is not only effective but also cost-effective. For less myelotoxic applications, however, it may be most prudent to hold CSF support for the more selected subset of patients in whom hematologic tolerance is suboptimal or who have already exhibited a clinical complication of therapy. This strategy may well decrease the costs of CSF use in general while maximizing the benefits to selected and appropriate patients. The area of hematopoietic supportive care is evolving rapidly, and clinicians should stay current with the research literature. This will drive a rational, data-based decision-making process that takes into account medical appropriateness, the effectiveness of these agents, as well as the complexity and variety of situations encountered by medical oncologists and hematologists in clinical practice.

REFERENCES

1. Bodey GP, Buckley M, Sathe YS, Freireich EJ: Quantitative relationship between circulating leukocytes and infections in patients with acute leukemia. Ann Intern Med 64:328–340, 1966
2. Gaydos LA, Freireich EJ, Mantel N, et al. The quantitative relation between platelet count and hemorrhage in patients with acute leukemia. N Engl J Med 266:905, 1962
3. Hersh EM, Bodey GP, Niles BA, Freireich EJ: Causes of death in acute leukemia—a ten-year study of 414 patients from 1954–1963. JAMA 193:99, 1965
4. Frei E III, Canellos GP: Dose: a critical factor in cancer chemotherapy. Am J Medicine 69:585–594, 1980
5. Henderson I, Hayes DF H, Gelman R: Dose-response in the treatment of breast cancer: a critical review. J Clin Oncol 6:1501–1515, 1988
6. Hryniuk W, Bush H: The importance of dose intensity in chemotherapy of metastatic breast cancer. J Clin Oncol 2:1281–1288, 1984
7. Demetri GD, Griffin JD: Hematopoietic growth factors and high-dose chemotherapy: will grams succeed where milligrams fail? [comment]. J Clin Oncol 8:761–764, 1990
8. Metcalf D: Hematopoietic regulators: redundancy or subtlety? Blood 82:3515–3523, 1993
9. Moore MAS: Clinical implications of positive and negative hematopoietic stem cell regulators. Blood 78:1–19, 1991
10. Zoon KC, Cohen RB, Gerrard T: Regulatory issues involved in hematopoietic growth factor approval. Seminars in Oncology 19:432–440, 1992
11. Groopman JE, Mitsuyasu RT, DeLeo MJ, et al: Effect of recombinant human granulocyte-macrophage colony-stimulating factor on myelopoiesis in the acquired immunodeficiency syndrome. N Engl J Med 317:593–598, 1987
12. Antman K, Griffin J, Elias A, et al: Effect of recombinant human granulocyte-macrophage colony-stimulating factor on chemotherapy-induced myelosuppression. N Engl J Med 319:593–598, 1988
13. Gabrilove JL, Jakubowski A, Fain K, et al: Phase I study of granulocyte colony-stimulating factor in patients with transitional cell carcinoma of the urothelium. J Clin Invest 82:1454–1461, 1988
14. Morstyn G, Campbell L, Souza LM, et al: Effect of granulocyte colony stimulating factor on neutropenia induced by cytotoxic chemotherapy. Lancet 1:667–672, 1988
15. Vadhan-Raj S, Keating M, LeMaistre A, et al: Effects of recombinant human granulocyte-macrophage colony-stimulating factor in patients with myelodysplastic syndromes. N Engl J Med 317:1545–1552, 1987
16. Vadhan-Raj S, Buescher S, Broxmeyer HE, et al: Stimulation of myelopoiesis in patients with aplastic anemia by recombinant human granulocyte-macrophage colony-stimulating factor. N Engl J Med 319:1628–1634, 1988
17. Negrin RS, Haeuber DH, Nagler A, et al: Treatment of myelodysplastic syndromes with recombinant human granulocyte colony-stimulating factor. A phase I-II trial. Ann Intern Med 110:976–984, 1989
18. Demetri GD, Griffin JD: Granulocyte colony-stimulating factor and its receptor. Blood 78:2791–2808, 1991
19. Lieschke GJ, Burgess AW: Granulocyte colony-stimulating factor and granulocyte-macrophage colony-stimulating factor (parts I and II). New Engl J Med 327:28–35, 99–106, 1992
20. Demetri GD, Antman KHS: GM-CSF: preclinical and clinical investigations. Semin Oncol 19:362–385, 1992
21. Lord BI, Bronchud MH, Owens S, et al: The kinetics of human granulopoiesis following treatment with granulocyte

colony-stimulating factor in vivo. Proc Natl Acad Sci USA 86:9499–9503, 1989

22. Aglietta M, Piacibello W, Sanavio F, et al: Kinetics of human hemopoietic cells after in vivo administration of granulocyte-macrophage colony-stimulating factor. J Clin Invest 83:551–557, 1989
23. Rose RM: The role of colony-stimulating factors in infectious disease: current status, future challenges. Semin Oncol 19:415–421, 1992
24. Sullivan R, Griffin JD, Simons ER, et al: Effects of recombinant human granulocyte and macrophage colony-stimulating factors on signal transduction pathways in human granulocytes. J Immunol 139:3422–3430, 1987
25. Peters WP, Stuart A, Affronti ML, et al: Neutrophil migration is defective during recombinant human granulocyte-macrophage colony-stimulating factor infusion after autologous bone marrow transplantation in humans. Blood 72:1310–1315, 1988
26. Griffin J, Spertini O, Ernst T, et al: Granulocyte-macrophage colony-stimulating factor and other cytokines regulate surface expression of the leukocyte adhesion molecule-1 on human neutrophils, monocytes, and their precursors. J Immunol 145:576–584, 1990
27. Demetri GD, Spertini O, Pratt ES, et al: GM-CSF and G-CSF have different effects on expression of the neutrophil adhesion receptors LAM-1 and CD11b. Blood 76 (suppl1): 178a (abstract 704), 1990
28. Crawford J, Ozer H, Stoller R, et al: Reduction by granulocyte colony-stimulating factor of fever and neutropenia induced by chemotherapy in patients with small-cell lung cancer. N Engl J Med 325:164–170, 1991
29. Trillet-Lenoir V, Green J, Manegold C, et al: Recombinant granulocyte colony stimulating factor reduces the infectious complications of cytotoxic chemotherapy. Eur J Cancer 29A:319–324, 1993
30. Brandt SJ, Peters WP, Atwater SK, et al: Effect of recombinant human granulocyte-macrophage colony-stimulating factor on hematopoietic reconstitution after high-dose chemotherapy and autologous bone marrow transplantation. N Engl J Med 318:869–876, 1988
31. Nemunaitis J, Singer JW, Buckner CD, et al: Use of recombinant human granulocyte-macrophage colony-stimulating factor in autologous marrow transplantation for lymphoid malignancies. Blood 72:834–836, 1988
32. Nemunaitis J, Rabinowe SN, Singer JW, et al: Recombinant granulocyte-macrophage colony-stimulating factor after autologous bone marrow transplantation for lymphopid cancer. N Engl J Med 324:1773–1778, 1991
33. Gerhartz HH, Engelhard M, Meusers P, et al: Randomized, double-blind, placebo-controlled, phase III study of recombinant human granulocyte-macrophage colony-stimulating factor (rhGM-CSF) as adjunct to induction treatment of high-grade malignant non-Hodgkin's lymphomas. Blood 82:2329–2339, 1993
34. Hamm JT, Schiller J, Oken MM, et al: Dose ranging study of recombinant human granulocyte-macrophage colony stimulating factor in small cell lung cancer. Proc Am Soc Clin Oncol 12:335 (abstract 1118), 1993
35. Bajorin DF, Schmoll H-J, Kantoff PW, et al: Recombinant human granulocyte-macrophage colony-stimulating factor as an adjunct to conventional-dose ifosfamide-based chemotherapy for patients with advanced germ-cell tumors: a randomized trial. J Clin Oncol 13:79–86, 1995
36. Budman DR, Wood W, Henderson IC, et al: Initial findings of CALGB 8541: a dose and dose intensity trial of cyclophosphamide (C), doxorubicin (A), and 5-Fluorouracil (F) as adjuvant treatment of stage II, Node+, female breast cancer. Proc Am Soc Clin Oncol 11:51 (abstract #29), 1992
37. Lyman GH, Lyman CG, Sanderson RA, Balducci L: Decision analysis of hematopoietic growth factor use in patients receiving cancer chemotherapy. J Natl Cancer Inst USA 85:488–493, 1993
38. Glaspy J, Bleecker G, Crawford J, et al: The impact of therapy with recombinant granulocyte colony stimulating factor (GCSF) on the health care costs associated with cancer chemotherapy. Blood 78 (supp 1): 7a, 1991
39. Gulati SC, Bennett CL: Granulocyte-macrophage colony-stimulating factor (GM-CSF) as adjunct therapy in relapsed Hodgkin Disease. Ann Intern Med 116:177–182, 1992
40. Nichols CR, Fox EP, Roth BJ, et al: Incidence of neutropenic fever in patients treated with standard-dose combination chemotherapy for small-cell lung cancer and the cost impact of treatment with granulocyte colony-stimulating factor. J Clin Oncol 12:1245–1250, 1994
41. Morstyn G, Campbell L, Lieschke G, et al: Treatment of chemotherapy-induced neutropenia by subcutaneously administered granulocyte colony-stimulating factor with optimization of dose and duration of therapy. J Clin Oncol 7:1554–1562, 1989
42. Gianni A, Bregni M, Siena S, et al: Recombinant human granulocyte-macrophage colony-stimulating factor reduces hematologic toxicity and widens clinical applicability of high-dose cyclophosphamide treatment in breast cancer and non-Hodgkin's lymphoma. J Clin Oncol 8:768–778, 1990
43. Neidhart JA, Mangalik A, Stidley CA, et al: Dosing regimen of granulocyte-macrophage colony-stimulating factor to support dose-intensive chemotherapy. J Clin Oncol 10:1460–1469, 1992
44. Meropol NJ, Miller LL, Korn EL, et al: Severe myelosuppression resulting from concurrent administration of granulocyte colony-stimulating factor and cytotoxic chemotherapy. J Natl Cancer Inst (USA) 84:1201–1203, 1992
45. Bunn JPA, Crowley J, Hazuka M, et al: The role of GM-CSF in limited stage SCLC: a randomized phase III study of the Southwest Oncology Group (SWOG). Proc Am Soc Clin Oncol 11:292 (abstract 974), 1992
46. Maher D, Green M, Bishop J, et al: Randomized, placebo-controlled trial of Filgrastim (r-metHuG-CSF) in patients with febrile neutropenia (FN) following chemotherapy. Proc Am Soc Clin Oncol 12:434 (abstract 1498), 1993
47. Dale DC, Bonilla MA, Davis MW, et al: A randomized controlled phase III trial of recombinant human granulocyte colony-stimulating factor (Filgrastim) for treatment of severe chronic neutropenia. Blood 81:2496–2502, 1993
48. Freund MR, Luft S, Schober C, et al: Differential effect of GM-CSF and G-CSF in cyclic neutropenia [letter]. Lancet 336:1990
49. Welte K, Zeidler C, Reiter A, et al: Differential effects of granulocyte-macrophage colony-stimulating factor and granulocyte colony-stimulating factor in children with severe congenital neutropenia. Blood 75:1056–1063, 1990
50. Vadhan-Raj S, Buescher S, LeMaistre A, et al: Stimulation

of hematopoiesis in patients with bone marrow failure and in patients with malignancy by recombinant human granulocyte-macrophage colony-stimulating factor. Blood 72:134–141, 1988

51. Schuster MW, Thompson JA, Larson R, et al: Randomized trial of subcutaneous granulocyte-macrophage colony-stimulating factor (GM-CSF) versus observation in patients (PTS) with myelodysplastic syndrome (MDS) or aplastic anemia (AA). Proc Am Soc Clin Oncol 9:205 (Abstract 793), 1990
52. Negrin RS, Haeuber DH, Nagler A, et al: Maintenance treatment of patients with myelodysplastic syndromes using recombinant human granulocyte colony-stimulating factor. Blood 76:36–43, 1990
53. Greenberg P, Taylor K, Larson R, et al: Phase III randomized multicenter trial of G-CSF vs. observation for myelodysplastic syndromes (MDS). Blood 82 (suppl 1): 196a (abstract 768), 1993
54. Ohno R, Tomonaga M, Kobayashi T, et al: Effect of granulocyte colony-stimulating factor after intensive induction therapy in relapsed or refractory acute leukemia. N Engl J Med 323:871–877, 1990
55. Rowe JM, Andersen J, Mazza JJ, et al: Phase III randomized placebo-controlled study of granulocyte-macrophage colony stimulating factor (GM-CSF) in adult patients (55–70 years) with acute myelogenous leukemia (AML). A study of the Eastern Cooperative Oncology Group (ECOG). Blood 82:329a (Abstract #1299), 1993
56. Stone R, George S, Berg D, et al: GM-CSF v. placebo during remission induction for patients >60 years old with de novo acute myeloid leukemia: CALGB study #8923. Proc Am Soc Clin Oncol 13:304 (abstract #992), 1994
57. Groopman JE: Status of colony-stimulating factors in cancer and AIDS. Semin Oncol 17:31–41, 1990
58. Groopman JE, Feder D: Hematopoietic growth factors in AIDS. Semin Oncol 19:408–414, 1992
59. Levine JD, Allan JD, Tessitore JH, et al: Recombinant human granulocyte-macrophage colony-stimulating factor ameliorates zidovudine-induces neutropenia in patients with acquired immunodeficiency syndrome (AIDS). Blood 78:3148–3154, 1991
60. Miles SA, Mitsuyasu R, Moreno J, et al: Combined therapy with recombinant granulocyte colony-stimulating factor and erythropoietin decreases hematologic toxicity from zidovudine. Blood 77:2109–2117, 1991
61. Abels RI: Use of recombinant human erythropoietin in the treatment of anemia in patients who have cancer. Semin Oncol 19 (suppl 8): 29–35, 1992
62. Smith II JA, Longo DL, Alvord WG, et al: The effects of treatment with interleukin-1 alpha on platelet recovery after high-dose carboplatin. N Engl J Med 328:756–761, 1993
63. D'Hondt V, Weynants P, Humblet Y, et al: Dose-dependent interleukin-3 stimulating of thrombopoiesis and neutropoiesis in patients with small-cell lung carcinoma before and following chemotherapy: A placebo-controlled randomized Phase Ib study. J Clin Oncol 11:2063, 1993
64. Vadhan-Raj S, Papadoupoulos N, Burgess M, et al: Optimization of dose and schedule of PIXY321 (GM-CSF/IL-3 fusion protein) to attenuate chemotherapy (CT)-induced multilineage myelosuppression in patients with sarcoma. Proc Am Soc Clin Oncol 12:470 (abstract 1640), 1993
65. Vose JM, Anderson J, Bierman PJ, et al: Initial trial of PIXY321 (GM-CSF/IL-3 fusion protein) following high-dose chemotherapy and autologous bone marrow transplantation (ABMT) for lymphoid malignancy. Proc Am Soc Clin Oncol 12:366 (abstract 1237), 1993
66. Demetri GD, Bukowski RM, Samuels B, et al: Stimulation of thrombopoiesis by recombinant human interleukin-6 (IL-6) pre- and post-chemotherapy in previously untreated sarcoma patients with normal hematopoiesis. Blood 82 (suppl 1) 367a, 1993
67. Gordon MS, Hoffman R, Battiato L, et al: Recombinant human interleukin eleven (Neumega rhIL-11 growth factor; rhIL-11) prevents severe thrombocytopenia in breast cancer patients receiving multiple cycles of cyclophosphamide (C) and doxorubicin (A) chemotherapy. Am Soc Clin Oncol 13:133 (abstract 326), 1994
68. Kaushansky K, Lok S, Holly RD, et al: Promotion of megakaryocyte progenitor expansion and differentiation by the c-Mpl ligand thrombopoietin. Nature 369:568–571, 1994
69. Wendling F, Maraskovsky E, Debili N, et al: c-Mpl ligand is a humoral regulator of megakaryocytopoiesis. Nature 369: 571–574, 1994
70. Metcalf D: Thrombopoietin — at last (editorial). Nature 369:519–520, 1994
71. Demetri GD, Renaud R, Blumsack R, et al: Combination cytokine support of dose-intensified cyclophosphamide/doxorubicin (CD) chemotherapy with concomitant G-CSF (G) plus erythropoietin (EPO). Proc Am Soc Clin Oncol 13:434, 1994
72. Hamm J, Crawford J, Figlin R, et al: A phase I/II study of the simultaneous administration of recombinant human Interleukin-6 (rhIL-6; *E. coli*) and Neupogen® (rhG-CSF, *E. coli*) following ICE chemotherapy in patients with advanced non-small cell lung carcinoma. Proc Am Soc Clin Oncol 13:332 (abstract 1100), 1994
73. Spangrude GJ, Smith L, Uchida N, et al: Mouse hematopoietic stem cells. Blood 78:1395–1402, 1991
74. Witte ON: Steel locus defines a new multipotent growth factor. Cell 63:5, 1990
75. Lyman S, James L, VandenBos T, et al: Molecular cloning of a ligand for the FLT3/FLK2 tyrosine kinase receptor — A proliferative factor for primitive hematopoietic cells. Blood 82:87a (abstract 335), 1993

John S. Macdonald, Daniel G. Haller, Robert J. Mayer, Eds. *Manual of Oncologic Therapeutics*, Third Edition.

VIII. BONE MARROW TRANSPLANTATION

69. ALLOGENEIC BONE MARROW TRANSPLANTATION FOR TREATMENT OF MALIGNANCY

Frederick R. Appelbaum

In this chapter, the indications for allogeneic marrow transplantation in the treatment of malignant diseases are reviewed, and the general technique and associated complications are discussed.

INDICATIONS

Acute Myelogenous Leukemia (AML)

Allogeneic marrow transplantation is the only form of therapy that can cure patients who fail to achieve an initial remission, with cure rates of 15%–20% reported in this setting. Therefore, all patients less than age 55 with newly diagnosed AML should be human leukocyte antigen (HLA)-typed along with family members soon after diagnosis to allow those who fail initial induction to be transplanted without delay. Allogeneic transplantation can cure 25%–30% of patients with AML in second remission and 35% of patients in first relapse, results which are better than those achieved with conventional chemotherapy; thus these settings are clear indications for allogeneic marrow transplantation. The best results with transplantation have been obtained when carried out in first remission, with cure rates of 50%–65% reported from large series. In prospective controlled trials, marrow transplantation in first remission cures 40% to 64% of patients, whereas chemotherapy cures 19% to 24%. However, since the conduct of these trials, there have been important advances both in chemotherapy and transplantation, casting some doubt about their current relevance. Further, whether transplantation in first remission is superior to the combination of initial chemotherapy plus transplantation as salvage therapy if patients relapse is unknown. Autologous marrow transplantation for acute myelogenous leukemia in first and second remission in several pilot studies has yielded results not very dissimilar from those obtained with syngeneic or allogeneic marrow. In general, relapse rates after autologous transplantation are substantially higher than after allogeneic transplantation, while deaths from transplant-related complications are somewhat less. In the few studies where allogeneic and autologous transplantation have been compared head-to-head, a small survival advantage has been found with allogeneic transplantation.

Acute Lymphocytic Leukemia

As for acute myelogenous leukemia, allogeneic transplantation for acute lymphocytic leukemia in relapse or second remission almost certainly provides a higher likelihood of long-term survival than continued chemotherapy, and thus is an indication for transplantation. Survival rates of 15%–25% have been reported for patients transplanted for chemotherapy resistant disease and 30%–40% for patients in second remission. Transplantation in first remission has resulted in 30% to 65% survival in selected studies, but prospective studies comparing transplantation to chemotherapy have not been completed. Autologous transplantation of acute lymphocytic leukemia in second remission has resulted in 10% to 25% disease-free survival rates at 2 years in several pilot studies. No large prospective randomized comparison of autologous transplantation with conventional chemotherapy has been completed.

Chronic Myelogenous Leukemia

Allogeneic (or syngeneic) marrow transplantation is the only known curative therapy for chronic myelogenous leukemia, with 5-year disease-free survival rates of 15% to 20% for patients in blast crisis, 20% to 30% for accelerated-phase patients, and 60% to 70% for patients transplanted during chronic phase. For chronic-phase patients, time from diagnosis to transplant appears to influence outcome of transplantation, with the best results obtained in patients transplanted within 1 year of diagnosis and progressively worse results with longer delays. Thus, at present transplantation soon after diagnosis (*i.e.*, within the first year) is indicated. There is, at present, no established role for autologous marrow transplantation for chronic myelogenous leukemia.

Malignant Lymphoma

Allogeneic marrow transplantation can cure 10% to 20% of patients with recurrent malignant lymphoma resistant to conventional therapy, and preliminary results suggest cure rates of 40% for patients transplanted in first relapse or second remission. Although no formal comparative trials have been completed, these results appear superior to those achieved with salvage chemotherapy. The outcome of allogeneic transplantation during first remission has not been determined. Disease histology (Hodgkin's disease, high-grade non-Hodgkin's lymphoma, or intermediate-grade non-Hodgkin's lymphoma) has not been shown to affect results dramatically. Retrospective and prospective studies comparing allogeneic and autologous transplantation for malignant lymphoma show a higher relapse rate with autologous transplantation, but less transplant-related mortality, resulting in equivalent survival.

Myelodysplasia

Allogeneic marrow transplantation is the only form of therapy with curative potential for myelodysplasia. Results appear better in patients with refractory anemia without excess blasts, where cure rates of 60% to 70% have been reported, and are somewhat worse in patients with refractory anemia with excess blasts, with cure rates of 25% to 40%. Given the variable course of myelodysplasia, transplantation is generally reserved for patients with a poor prognosis, including those with life-threatening cytopenias or an increase in marrow blasts above 5%.

Multiple Myeloma

Allogeneic marrow transplantation is being increasingly used for therapy of multiple myeloma. Overall survival rates among patients who have failed first-line chemotherapy have averaged 30% to 35% at 5 years after transplant and, importantly, studies demonstrate a plateau in disease-free survival, suggesting these patients are cured. Autologous transplantation has also been studied as treatment for myeloma and while responses are common, there is as yet little evidence that this approach is curative.

Other Hematologic Malignancies

Long-term survival has been documented following transplantation for chronic lymphocytic leukemia, hairy cell leukemia, and various myeloproliferative syndromes, but the number of patients reported in any of these disease categories is, as yet, small.

Solid Tumors

There are few indications for allogeneic transplantation in solid tumors. The only clear indication is in the treatment of neuroblastoma, where high-dose therapy followed by marrow transplantation can cure 15% of relapsed patients and up to 40% of Stage IV patients transplanted in remission. In breast cancer, testicular cancer, and other tumors generally considered to be responsive to conventional dose chemotherapy, high-dose therapy with autologous marrow transplantation has been studied, and long-term survival has been reported in some patients. There is no evidence that allogeneic transplantation represents an advantage over autologous transplantation in these settings.

The indications for allogeneic marrow transplantation are also influenced by a number of factors in addition to the specific disease, such as donor source, patient age, performance status, and life goals. Syngeneic (twin) transplantation is relatively well-tolerated, and therefore the availability of an identical twin donor broadens the indications for transplantation. Among non-twin transplant recipients, younger patients and those with a good performance status do better, again widening the indications. Conversely, the indications are more limited for older patients, those with poor performance status, and those with only a partially matched or unrelated donor.

DONOR SELECTION

Identical twins, when available, are the best possible donors. Although relapse rates may be less following allogeneic transplantation, the relative lack of complications with syngeneic marrow favors its use. Syngenicity is established by human leukocyte antigen (HLA) typing, mixed leukocyte culture tests, erythrocyte antigen typing, erythrocyte enzyme electrophoretic determinations if the patient has not been recently transfused, and, when available, by pathologic reports of the placenta. Physical identity from birth is usually, although not absolutely, reliable.

Allogeneic transplants are most commonly performed between siblings genotypically identical for HLA. The genes encoding HLA are located on chromosome 6 and are co-dominantly expressed. Thus, the probability of HLA identity between any two siblings is 25%, and given the average family size in the United States, the chance of a patient having an HLA-matched sibling is approximately 35%. HLA genotypic identity is determined by demonstrating identity for HLA class I and class II determinants. HLA class I antigens (usually referred to as HLA-A and HLA-B) are defined primarily through the use of alloantisera in microcytotoxicity assays. Using this method, 20 different HLA-A antigens and 40 HLA-B antigens have been defined. HLA class II antigens are encoded by genes located within the HLA-D region and are termed DP, DQ and DR. DR and DQ antigens can be identified by alloantisera. Identification of DP requires cellular techniques, such as mixed lymphocyte culture (MLC) reactions or homozygous typing cells (HTC), or more recently developed molecular techniques, such as the use of sequence-specific oligonucleotide probe (SSOP) hybridization. SSOP is performed by using the polymerase chain reaction to amplify the gene sequence encoding HLA-D and then using oligonucleotide probes which hybridize with unique proteins of the different class II genes. SSOP has largely replaced the use of MLC or HTC in most large laboratories.

While the best results have generally been obtained with the use of HLA-genotypically matched sibling donors, most data suggest that use of family donors identical with the patient for one haplotype but mismatched for a single locus on the other (A, B or D) results in a higher incidence of graft-versus-host disease (GVHD), but survival similar to use of matched sibling donors. The use of donors mismatched for two or more loci results in more graft rejection, more graft-versus-host disease, and poorer survival. The formation of the National Marrow Donor Program has led to a dramatic increase in the use of matched unrelated donors. Currently more than 1,000,000 normal individuals have volunteered to serve as marrow donors in the United States, making the chance of finding an A, B and D matched unrelated donor approximately 50%. From the time a search is initiated, on average 4 to 5 months elapse before the transplant can be performed. Analysis of the first several hundred patients undergoing transplant from a matched unrelated donor suggests that GVHD will be more common than with a matched family member, and long-term cure rates will be slightly lower. Marrow transplantation can be carried out despite major ABO blood group incompatibility. However, to avoid hemolysis, incompatible red cells must be removed from the marrow inoculum by centrifugation or sedimentation, or, alternatively, isoagglutinins must be removed from the patient's blood by immunoadsorption or plasma exchange.

The use of autologous marrow or peripheral blood stem cells is discussed in Chapter 70.

PREPARATIVE REGIMENS

The preparative regimens used prior to marrow transplantation must be capable of eradicating the malignancy and must be sufficiently immunosuppressive to prevent the patient from rejecting the marrow graft. One commonly used regimen combines cyclophosphamide, 60 mg/kg/daily for 2 days, with 12 Gy to 15.75 Gy total body irradiation (TBI) delivered as daily 2– or 2.25–Gy fractions. Variations of this theme have substituted etoposide, cytarabine, or melphalan for the cyclophosphamide, have added various agents to the cyclophosphamide, and have delivered the total body irradiation either as a single fraction or hyperfractionated over several days. Several regimens rely on chemotherapy only. One commonly used regimen employs busulfan, 4 mg/kg/daily for 4 days, and cyclophosphamide 60 mg/kg/daily for 2 days. Relatively few prospective randomized studies comparing preparative regimens have been performed. A study comparing cyclophosphamide plus 12 Gy TBI with cyclophosphamide plus busulfan as treatment for patients with AML in first remission found the TBI containing regimen to be superior. A second trial compared the same 2 regimens as treatment for patients with CML in chronic phase and found the 2 regimens to be equivalent. The choice of preparative regimens is influenced by the particular clinical situation. Patients with more resistant malignancies require regimens of greater intensity, while older patients and those with co-morbid diseases may only be able to tolerate less aggressive regimens.

MARROW ASPIRATION AND INFUSION

Marrow is usually obtained from the donor's anterior and posterior iliac crests with the donor under spinal or general anesthesia. A marrow volume equivalent to 10 ml to 15 ml/kg donor body weight is obtained, with each aspirate site limited to 3 ml to 5 ml to avoid excessive dilution with peripheral blood. The marrow is placed in heparinized tissue culture media and filtered through 0.3-mm and 0.2-mm screens to remove bone spicules and fat. Subsequent processing of the marrow may involve T-cell depletion to avoid GVHD, or red cell depletion in the ABO-incompatible setting. If no processing is necessary (as in the case of a straightforward ABO-matched allograft), the marrow is directly infused into the patient. Marrow infusion usually is without complication, although patients occasionally may develop fever and a cough with mild shortness of breath. Slowing the infusion is usually successful in alleviating these symptoms. The risk of marrow donation is small but definable; in Seattle there were 6 serious but nonfatal complications among 1220 consecutive donations.

ENGRAFTMENT

Peripheral blood counts usually begin to increase within 1 to 2 weeks of transplant. The granulocyte count reaches $100/mm^3$ by day 16 and $1000/mm^3$ by about day 26. Platelets recover with or slightly after granulocytes. Engraftment can be documented using several cytogenetic techniques, including identification of sex chromosomes if donor and recipient are not sex-matched, the use of unique chromosomal polymorphisms identified by banding, or restriction fragment-length polymorphism analysis. If the patient has not received recent red cell transfusions, polymorphic red cell enzymes can be used to monitor engraftment as well. Prospective randomized trials suggest that hematopoietic growth factors (GM-CSF or G-CSF) can accelerate engraftment if given post-transplant.

COMPLICATIONS OF MARROW TRANSPLANTATION

Chemoradiotherapy Toxicities

The immediate toxicities seen following the standard cyclophosphamide-TBI preparative regimen are nausea, vomiting, fever, parotitis, and mild skin erythema. Occasionally, patients develop hemorrhagic cystitis despite bladder irrigation and, rarely, acute hemorrhagic carditis. Oral mucositis develops at about 5 to 7 days post-transplant. By 10 days most patients have developed complete alopecia and are profoundly pancytopenic.

Within 1 to 4 weeks of transplant, approximately 10% of patients present with a syndrome of ascites, tender hepatomegaly, and jaundice, which represents veno-occlusive disease of the liver. There is no proven effective therapy for veno-occlusive disease beyond aggressive supportive care. Recent preliminary studies suggest that therapy with alprostadil (prostaglandin E1) or tissue plasminogen activator may reverse some of the manifestations of veno-occlusive disease, but the potential toxicities of these approaches are considerable. Patients with pretransplant hepatitis of whatever cause appear to have a higher incidence of veno-occlusive disease.

Idiopathic interstitial pneumonia, which is thought to be a direct chemoradiotoxicity, is seen in 5% to 10% of patients between 30 and 90 days from transplant. The disease has a case fatality rate of approximately 50% and no clearly effective therapy.

Late complications of the preparative regimen include decreased growth velocity in children and delayed development of secondary sex characteristics. Most men become azoospermic, and most postpubertal women develop ovarian failure, which should be treated. Thyroid dysfunction, usually well compensated, has been reported. Cataracts develop in 10% to 20% of patients. The toxicities listed above are those associated with a cyclophosphamide-total body irradiation regimen. Other preparative regimens are associated with different and sometimes unexpected arrays of toxicities.

Graft Failure

Occasionally following transplantation, marrow function either does not return, or after a period of recovery, marrow function is lost. Graft failure is seen more commonly in patients with extensive marrow fibrosis pretransplant, in recipients of HLA-mismatched or T-cell-depleted marrow, and in patients prepared with regimens that do not include total body irradiation. Occasionally, graft failure may result from exposure to myelosuppressive agents post-transplant (trimethoprim-sulfamethoxazole, methotrexate, or cimetidine) or may presage disease recurrence. The obvious first step in patients with graft failure is to remove all potentially myelosuppressive agents. A reasonable next step is to attempt a trial of granulocyte-macrophage colony stimulating factor (GM-CSF); published studies suggest that 40% to 50% of patients will respond favorably to such a trial. If patients do not respond, further therapy depends, in part, on whether persistent host lymphocytes in peripheral blood or marrow can be detected either by cytogenetic analysis, leukocyte enzyme analysis, or in the mismatched setting, by HLA typing. If no residual host cells are detected, simple marrow reinfusion is sometimes followed by recovery of hematopoiesis. If persistent host cells are found, the patient should receive further immunosuppression before a second transplant is performed. A commonly used second preparative regimen combines cyclophosphamide, 50 mg/kg/daily for 4 days, with antithymocyte globulin. No evidence exists to suggest whether the initial marrow donor or an alternative is preferable.

Graft-Versus-Host Disease

GVHD is thought to be the result of allogeneic T-cells transfused with the graft or developing from it, which react with targets of the genetically different host. Significant acute GVHD developing during the first 3 months has rarely been reported following syngeneic or autologous transplantation, and following allogeneic transplantation is found in 30%, 50% and 70% of HLA-identical, one-antigen and two-antigen mismatched donor-recipient pairs given post-transplant methotrexate and cyclosporine. Acute GVHD is characterized by an erythematous maculopapular skin rash that favors the palms and soles, followed by diarrhea, often with abdominal pain and ileus, and liver disease characterized by rises in bilirubin, transaminases, and alkaline phosphatase. Skin, liver and endoscopic intestinal biopsies along with upper gastrointestinal and small bowel follow-through are all useful in diagnosis. Acute GVHD is more commonly seen in older patients. The very high incidence of GVHD seen when no post-transplant immunosuppression is used suggests that some form of prophylaxis is necessary. Methotrexate and cyclosporine are about equally effective. The use of a combination of cyclosporine and methotrexate compared with either agent alone has been shown to result in a lower incidence of GVHD in all age groups and an overall improved survival. T-cell depletion of marrow by most methods, while effective in diminishing GVHD, has been associated with an increased incidence of marrow graft rejection and an increased incidence of leukemic relapse. Accordingly, studies are underway testing the use of partial T-cell depletion, adding back a fixed number of T-cells post-transplant, or the use of interleukin-2 (IL-2) after engraftment. Treatment of established GVHD involves the use of steroids, antithymocyte globulin, and monoclonal antibodies against T-cells.

Approximately 20% to 40% of patients surviving more than 6 months after allogeneic marrow transplantation will develop chronic GVHD. This disorder looks like a collagen-vascular disease with malar erythema, sclerodermatous changes, sicca syndrome, arthritis, obliterative bronchiolitis, and in some cases bile duct degeneration and cholestasis. Chronic GVHD is seen more often in patients who had acute GVHD and is also age related. Single-agent prednisone is, at present, standard treatment of chronic GVHD and is effective in 50% to 70% of cases. Cyclosporine, azathioprine, and thalidomide are useful in some cases. Because patients with chronic GVHD are susceptible to bacterial infections they should receive prophylactic trimethoprim-sulfamethoxazole and/or penicillin, especially if immunosuppressive agents are still being given.

Infectious Complications

Nearly all patients develop granulocytopenia and fever during the first 2 or 3 weeks post-transplant, and in about one third of patients positive blood cultures are found. Gram-positive organisms predominate (about 20% of cases) but gram-negative organisms (10%) and fungi (2%–5%) are also seen. Accordingly, it is standard practice to treat febrile granulocytopenic patients with broad spectrum antibiotics, and in many centers, broad spectrum antibiotics are initiated once patients become granulocytopenic, even if afebrile, to prevent septicemia. The addition of fluconazole prophylaxis reduces the incidence of *Candida* infections. Treatment of granulocytopenic patients who remain febrile despite antibiotic and antifungal prophylaxis is a difficult issue and depends, in part, on the individual patient's condition as well as the infection experience at the particular treatment center. Amphotericin B is frequently added to the treatment of patients who remain febrile and granulocytopenic for 3 to 4 days despite broad spectrum antibiotic treatment. Prophylactic granulocyte transfusions can prevent early infections, but have not been shown to affect survival. Similarly, laminar airflow isolation prevents infection, but has been shown to improve survival only in patients transplanted for aplastic anemia, not leukemia. With current methods of supportive care, the risk of death due to infection during the early granulocytopenic period is low, roughly 5%.

The most important infections occurring in the interval between successful engraftment and day 100 are viral or protozoan. Approximately 75% of patients with detectable antibody to cytomegalovirus (CMV) pretransplant have some evidence of CMV activation post-transplant. Often, activation is asymptomatic, and manifests only by a rise in antibody titer or viral excretion in the urine. However, approximately 50% of patients who excrete virus post-transplant have, in the past, gone on to develop symptomatic infection. CMV may cause hepatitis, fever with marrow suppression, or a gastrointestinal syndrome associated with nausea, vomiting, and abdominal pain. The most serious result of CMV activation is CMV pneumonia, which in the past occurred in roughly 15% of patients and had a case fatality rate of about 85%. Primary CMV infection can be prevented in CMV seronegative patients by the sole use of CMV seronegative blood products. More recently it has been shown that treatment of CMV seropositive patients who excrete CMV post-transplant with ganciclovir can prevent the development of symptomatic infection. Similarly, ganciclovir has been used from the time of engraftment to prevent CMV disease. While effective, ganciclovir suppresses marrow function in at least 15% of patients.

Herpes simplex infection can contribute to the severity of early oral mucositis and, in some cases, results in esophagitis, bronchopneumonia, and (rarely) encephalitis. Systemic acyclovir, 250 mg/m^2 every 8 hours intravenously, is effective in the treatment of established herpes simplex infection after marrow transplant and, if used as prophylaxis starting one week before transplant and continuing for 4 weeks after transplant, can prevent herpes simplex reactivation in over 90% of seropositive patients.

Pneumonia due to *Pneumocystis carinii*, although previously a problem in 5% to 10% of transplant recipients, can be prevented by treating the patient with oral trimethoprim-sulfamethoxazole at a dose of 75 mg/m^2 twice daily for 1 week pretransplant, and then resuming treatment 2 days per week once the granulocyte count exceeds 500/mm.^{3}

Late infections (more than 3 months post-transplant) usually are due to varicella-zoster virus or, in patients with chronic GVHD, recurrent bacterial infections. Varicella-zoster infections most often present as localized zoster, but about one third of untreated patients disseminate and 15% to 20% of varicella-zoster infections present as varicella. The case-fatality rate of disseminated varicella-zoster occurring during the first 9 months post-transplant, if untreated, is 35%. Thus, all such patients should be treated with either acyclovir (500 mg/m^2 every 8 hours) or vidarabine (10 mg/kg/day). As noted earlier, we recommend continuing trimethoprim-sulfamethoxazole and/or penicillin, in hopes of reducing late bacterial infections in patients with chronic GVHD.

Post-Transplant Relapse

Patients who relapse post-transplant can sometimes achieve a worthwhile clinical remission with standard chemotherapy, especially if the duration from transplant to relapse is long. Some patients have been successfully retransplanted, but attempts at second transplants within the first year of transplant are rarely, if ever, successful. Patients with CML who relapse after an allogeneic transplant often respond to interferon-α. Recently, infusion of donor buffy coat to patients who have relapsed after allogeneic transplant has been reported to result in a surprisingly high incidence of complete remission, especially in patients with CML.

Referral of Patients for Marrow Transplantation

Physicians with patients who may be candidates for marrow transplantation should contact a marrow transplant center as soon as possible. The center can provide information about the relative risks and benefits of transplantation, the method of donor identification, and the process of transferring a patient for transplant. Transplantation is usually, but not invariably, covered by most comprehensive health insurance policies.

REFERENCES

Anderson JE, Appelbaum FR, Fisher LD et al. Allogeneic bone marrow transplantation for 93 patients with myelodysplastic syndrome. Blood 82:677–681, 1993

Biggs JC, Horowitz MM, Gale RP et al. Bone marrow transplants may cure patients with acute leukemia never achieving remission with chemotherapy. Blood 80:1090–1093, 1992

Blaise D, Maraninchi D, Archimbaud E et al. Allogeneic bone marrow transplantation for acute myeloid leukemia in first remission: A randomized trial of a busulfan-cytoxan versus cytoxan-total body irradiation as preparative regimen: A report from the Groupe d'Etudes de la Greffe de Moelle Osseuse. Blood 79:2578–2582, 1992

Chao NJ, Forman SJ, Schmidt GM et al. Allogeneic bone marrow transplantation for high-risk acute lymphoblastic leukemia during first complete remission. Blood 78:1923–1927, 1991

Chopra R, Goldstone AH, Pearce R et al. Autologous versus allogeneic bone marrow transplantation for non-Hodgkin's lymphoma: A case-controlled analysis of the European bone marrow transplant group registry data. J Clin Oncol 10:1690–1695, 1992

Clift RA, Appelbaum FR, Thomas ED. Editorial: Treatment of chronic myeloid leukemia by marrow transplantation. Blood 82:1954–1956, 1993

Hansen JA, Mickelson EM, Choo SY et al. Clinical bone marrow transplantation: Donor selection and recipient monitoring. In: Rose NR, De Macario EC, Fahey JL et al. (eds): Manual of Clinical Laboratory Immunology. Washington, D.C., American Society for Microbiology, 1992:850–866

Horowitz MM, Gale RP, Sondel PM et al. Graft-versus-leukemia reactions after bone marrow transplantation. Blood 75:555–562, 1990

Kernan NA, Bartsch G, Ash RC et al. Analysis of 462 transplantations from unrelated donors facilitated by The National Marrow Donor Program. N Engl J Med 328:593–602, 1993

Vogelsang GB, Hess AD, Santos GW. Acute graft-versus-host disease: Clinical characteristics in the cyclosporine era. Medicine 67:163–174, 1988

John S. Macdonald, Daniel G. Haller, Robert J. Mayer, Eds. *Manual of Oncologic Therapeutics*, Third Edition.

70. AUTOLOGOUS BONE MARROW TRANSPLANTATION

Philip J. Bierman
James O. Armitage

Interest in autologous bone marrow transplantation (ABMT) resulted from the observation that splenic shielding could protect mice from lethal doses of radiation. The first attempts at using ABMT to treat radiation-induced myelosuppression were reported more than 40 years ago. Later attempts at using this technique to treat malignancies were hampered by inadequate chemotherapy and deficiencies in supportive care. The first series of patients treated with ABMT were reported in the late 1970s, and use of this technique has rapidly increased. Data from the International Autologous Bone Marrow Transplant Registry indicate that more than 6000 autologous marrow transplants are performed annually, and the number is increasing at a rate of 20% each year.

RATIONALE

The use of ABMT is based on the fact that certain chemotherapeutic agents exhibit steep dose-response curves against some tumors. Relatively small increases in the dose of a drug may thereby result in large increases in tumor cell kill. If the dose-limiting toxicity of a drug is due to myelosuppression rather than extramedullary toxicity, patients can be "rescued" from the effects of high-dose therapy with stored autologous bone marrow. Therefore, ABMT should be thought of as supportive care that allows the use of higher doses of therapy than would otherwise be possible.

Certain agents may display steep dose-response curves, yet be poor choices for dose escalation if their limiting toxicity is due to damage to organs such as lungs or liver, rather than myelosuppression. Drugs most widely used for dose escalation in transplant preparative regimens include alkylating agents such as cyclophosphamide, melphalan, thiotepa, and busulfan. Other commonly used agents include etoposide, carmustine, carboplatin, and cytarabine. Many regimens also include total-body irradiation (TBI). ABMT allows the doses of these agents to be escalated several-fold.

ABMT is now being used more frequently than allogeneic bone marrow transplantation (BMT). A major advantage of ABMT is the lack of need for a donor. In addition, morbidity and mortality rates from ABMT are lower than those rates from allogeneic BMT because of the absence of graft-versus-host disease and the lack of need for prolonged immunosuppression. Autologous bone marrow transplantation can safely be performed on patients in their seventh decade. A disadvantage of ABMT is the risk of reinfusing malignant cells into the recipient, although the clinical importance of this risk is unclear. A second disadvantage of ABMT relates to the loss of the immunologic antitumor effect mediated by donor cells in an allogeneic transplant. Patients who receive allogeneic transplants for leukemia have lower relapse rates than those who receive transplants from an identical twin (syngeneic). This "graft-versus-leukemia effect" does not occur after ABMT.

DESCRIPTION OF PROCEDURE

Bone marrow is withdrawn from the posterior iliac crests in the same manner as an allogeneic marrow harvest. Approximately 500 to 1000 cc of bone marrow, representing 2 to 4 × 10^8 nucleated cells/kg are collected in media containing anticoagulant. After filtration and depletion of erythrocytes, the marrow is preserved in glycerol or dimethylsulfoxide (DMSO), or a mixture of hydroxyethyl starch and DMSO. These agents act as cryoprotectants to prevent the formation of ice crystals. The marrow is then placed in a −80°C freezer or frozen at a controlled rate and stored in liquid nitrogen at −196°C. Autologous marrow has been successfully transplanted after more than 9 years of storage.

Transplantation requires a dedicated team of physicians, nurses, and support from ancillary services. Most institutions have a separate "transplant unit" with some form of air filtration. After receiving high-dose therapy, the stored marrow is thawed in a water bath and immediately infused into a central vein. Hematopoietic recovery begins approximately 10 to 14 days after transplantation. Randomized trials have shown that hematopoietic growth factors, such as granulocyte-macrophage colony-stimulating factor and granulocyte colony-stimulating factor, shorten the period of neutropenia after ABMT by approximately 1 week. In addition, use of growth factors after transplantation results in fewer infections and shortened hospital stays, although improvements in overall survival have not been demonstrated.

PERIPHERAL STEM CELL TRANSPLANTATION

More than 20 years ago it was recognized that hematopoietic progenitor cells can be found in the circulating blood and in bone marrow of humans. These cells can be collected and used to re-establish hematopoietic function following high-dose therapy in exactly the same manner as autologous bone marrow. Peripheral blood stem cells can be collected by processing 7 to 10 liters of blood through an apheresis machine. Usually, several collections of 3 to 4 hours each are required to obtain sufficient cells, but sometimes only one collection is required. The number of circulating progenitor cells is increased several-fold on recovery from chemotherapy-induced myelosuppression or after receiving hematopoietic growth factors. These "mobilization" techniques allow peripheral stem cells to be collected more rapidly and result in shorter periods of hematopoietic recovery after transplantation. The peripheral stem cells are cryopreserved and reinfused after high-dose therapy in the same manner as autologous bone marrow.

Autologous peripheral stem cells have several advantages over autologous bone marrow. Peripheral stem cells may be collected without the need for general anesthesia required for an autologous bone marrow harvest. Several studies have shown that hematopoietic recovery may be more rapid following peripheral stem cell transplantation (PSCT), compared with ABMT. In addition, it has been reported that there may be less malignant contamination with peripheral stem cells, although the clinical significance of this observation is unknown. The ability to collect peripheral stem cells has the greatest advantage for patients who might be candidates for ABMT but whose marrow is unsuitable. These patients include those with marrow metastasis and those with hypocellular marrow. The use of PSCT is increasing rapidly, and some investigators have advocated replacing ABMT with this technique. Both ABMT and PSCT are supportive care that allows the use of high-dose therapy, and clinical results are similar with either technique. In this discussion, the term ABMT applies to both types of transplantation unless otherwise specified.

PURGING

The use of ABMT carries the risk of reinfusing malignant cells, which might cause relapse. Although malignant cells are undoubtedly present in many harvests, it is not known whether such cells are clonogenic, whether the cells survive cryopreservation and thawing, or whether the number of reinfused cells is sufficient to cause a relapse. Because relapse after ABMT most commonly occurs at sites of prior disease, it is believed that most relapses are due to failure of the conditioning regimen rather than reinfusion of contaminated marrow. However, recent retroviral studies have demonstrated that at least some relapses following ABMT for acute myelogenous leukemia, chronic myelogenous leukemia, and neuroblastoma may result from the infused autologous marrow.

Several pharmacologic and physical methods may be used to "purge" malignant cells from bone marrow. Pharmacologic methods use agents such as 4-hydroperoxycyclophosphamide and mafosfamide, which are incubated with the marrow before cryopreservation. The main physical purging methods use monoclonal antibodies directed against antigens on the surface of malignant cells. The monoclonal antibodies may be conjugated to potent toxins, such as ricin. Alternatively, malignant cells may be lysed with complement. A third method of purging with monoclonal antibodies uses magnetic microspheres coated with anti-antibodies. These spheres bind to the antibody-coated tumor cells, which can be separated by passing the marrow through a magnetic field. Positive selection techniques can also be used to separate cells expressing the CD34 antigen, which is present on pluripotent progenitors, but not on most malignant cells. These techniques can deplete the marrow of 4 or 5 logs of tumor cells, although the clinical benefits of purging remain controversial in most circumstances.

TRANSPLANT REGIMENS

Preparative regimens used for ABMT are similar to those used for allogeneic BMT. These regimens can be conveniently divided into those that contain total-body irradiation (TBI), and non–TBI-containing regimens. Regimens that contain TBI have been associated with a higher rate of pulmonary complications, but there is little evidence that any regimen is superior in a given clinical situation.

CLINICAL RESULTS

Leukemia

ACUTE MYELOGENOUS LEUKEMIA

High-dose therapy followed by ABMT has extensively been used as consolidation therapy for AML patients in first complete remission. Leukemia-free survival rates of 30% to 60% have been noted in a number of studies. Relapse rates are similar to those seen following syngeneic BMT, which indicates that residual disease, rather than reinfusion of malignant cells, is responsible for a major portion of the relapses.

Comparisons of autologous and allogeneic BMT for AML have generally shown higher relapse rates following ABMT. This graft-versus-leukemia effect is offset by the higher transplant-related mortality associated with allogeneic transplantation. Some reports have noted longer survival following allogeneic BMT for patients in first complete remission. Data from the North American Autologous Bone Marrow Transplant Registry and preliminary results from randomized trials show no difference in leukemia-free survival between recipients of allogeneic and recipients of autologous transplants for acute myelogenous leukemia in their first complete remission. Some evidence supports the use of purging for ABMT for acute myelogenous leukemia in first remission. Leukemia-free survival for patients receiving ABMT for acute myelogenous leukemia in early first relapse or second complete remission is approximately 30%.

ACUTE LYMPHOBLASTIC LEUKEMIA

Most autografts for acute lymphoblastic leukemia have used purged marrow. Leukemia-free survival rates are 40% to 50% for acute lymphoblastic leukemia patients who underwent transplantation in first remission. It is unclear whether these results are better than those of standard chemotherapy. Leukemia-free survival is approximately 30% for patients who underwent transplantation in second remission. Comparative trials of allogeneic transplantation and ABMT for acute lymphoblastic leukemia have shown lower relapse rates, but similar survival after allogeneic BMT. Trials comparing ABMT with standard consolidation therapy in first remission are under way.

CHRONIC MYELOGENOUS LEUKEMIA

ABMT for chronic myelogenous leukemia has usually been performed using cells stored from patients in the chronic phase. Transplants performed in such patients when their disease progresses may establish some degree of Philadelphia chromosome–negative hematopoiesis in as many as 50% of patients. Leukemia-free survival is less than 10% at 2 years, and it is unclear whether overall survival is prolonged. There is now increasing interest in performing ABMT for patients in the first chronic phase. In some series, more than 50% of patients have become partly or completely Philadelphia chromosome–negative. Although leukemia-free survival is less than 10% at 3 years, some patients have remained Philadelphia chromosome–negative for more than 4 years. No randomized studies have been performed, although one retrospective report noted improved 5-year survival in a group of chronic myelogenous leukemia patients autografted during the chronic phase, compared with historical controls.

Multiple Myeloma

Among patients with advanced or relapsed myeloma, relatively high complete remission rates of 25% to 30% are noted after ABMT. Transplant-related mortality is under 5% at experienced centers. Outcome is better in patients who have sensitive disease at the time of transplantation. Other factors associated with better prognosis include low beta$_2$-microglobulin levels, interval from diagnosis to BMT of less than 1 year, and non–immunoglobulin A subtype. Despite high response rates, ABMT in these patients does not appear to have curative potential, and it is unknown whether survival is prolonged, compared with standard therapy.

Autologous transplantation has also been used as part of an intensive initial treatment strategy. This approach is associated with high complete response rates, and 3-year disease-free survival rates of 75% to 80% have been reported. Some institutions have reported improved overall survival in patients treated with this form of aggressive initial therapy, compared with patients receiving conventional chemotherapy.

Non-Hodgkin's Lymphoma

Fewer than 10% of patients with relapsed non-Hodgkin's lymphoma can be cured with conventional salvage chemotherapy. This has led to the wide use of ABMT for relapsed and refractory non-Hodgkin's lymphoma, which accounts for approximately 25% of transplants reported to the North American Autologous Bone Marrow Transplant Registry. Most transplants have been performed for intermediate- and high-grade histologic subtypes. Retrospective analyses comparing ABMT with standard salvage chemotherapy have shown a survival advantage in favor of transplantation for non-Hodgkin's lymphoma patients who have had a relapse. Prospective comparisons are under way.

It is common practice to administer a brief course of conventional salvage chemotherapy to non-Hodgkin's lymphoma patients who have had a relapse before giving them high-dose therapy and ABMT. Failure-free survival rates of 40% to 50% are seen for patients who are sensitive to conventional salvage therapy before ABMT (sensitive relapse), and 10% to 15% for patients who are resistant to salvage chemotherapy (resistant relapse). Patients who are refractory to primary therapy are rarely cured with ABMT. Other variables associated with improved outcome include normal LDH, absence of bulky disease, and less extensive therapy before transplantation. Non-Hodgkin's lymphoma patients who achieve only partial remission with initial chemotherapy may achieve prolonged disease-free survival rates of 50% following ABMT.

Mortality rates from ABMT are below 5% at many institutions. This has led to trials of ABMT as consolidation therapy for poor-prognosis patients in first complete remission. Such patients can be identified by the presence of such factors as increased LDH, poor performance status, and advanced stage. Several trials have shown that ABMT in this situation can be performed with little or no mortality. Survival rates appear better than those for historical controls. A prospective randomized European trial showed a trend in favor of improved disease-free survival for high-risk patients who underwent transplantation in first remission.

There is no convincing evidence in favor of purging for intermediate-grade non-Hodgkin's lymphoma. Like AML, allogeneic BMT for non-Hodgkin's lymphoma is associated with a lower relapse rate than ABMT. This effect is offset by the higher transplant-related mortality of allogeneic BMT, and overall results are similar. Allogeneic BMT may be preferred for patients with lymphoblastic lymphoma.

Relatively few transplants have been performed for low-grade non-Hodgkin's lymphoma. Most marrows have been purged with monoclonal antibodies directed against B cells. Failure-free survival rates of 30% to 40% have been reported. These rates appear to be better than those for historical controls, although it is unclear whether overall survival is improved. Results of PSCT and purged ABMT for low-grade non-Hodgkin's lymphoma are similar. The use of ABMT as part of initial therapy for patients with low-grade non-Hodgkin's lymphoma is being examined. Prolonged follow-up will be required to evaluate these results.

Hodgkin's Disease

Prolonged failure-free survival following ABMT has been reported in 25% to 50% of patients with relapsed Hodgkin's disease. Factors associated with improved outcome include good performance status, fewer prior chemotherapy regimens, initial remission longer than 1 year, and absence of B symptoms at relapse. A recent randomized European study showed improved event-free survival for patients with relapsed and refractory Hodgkin's disease undergoing ABMT, compared with those who received conventional doses of salvage chemotherapy. Patients who fail to enter complete remission or have a relapse within 1 year of initial remission have a poor outcome with standard salvage chemotherapy. Results of ABMT in these patients appear to be better than those in patients who have undergone conventional salvage chemotherapy. Failure-free survival rates of 50% to 85% have been reported for patients who had transplants after initial remissions that exceed 1 year. Mortality rates after ABMT may be less than 5%, and it may be appropriate to recommend ABMT to any Hodgkin's disease patient who has had a relapse from chemotherapy.

Like for non-Hodgkin's lymphoma patients, there is evidence that the survival for high-risk Hodgkin's disease patients may be prolonged if ABMT is performed in first complete remission. Prospective randomized studies to test this hypothesis are under way.

Solid Tumors

BREAST CANCER

Breast cancer is now the most common indication for ABMT in North America. Patients with metastatic disease have a poor prognosis, with a median survival of under 2 years. Other poor prognostic groups include women with Stage II disease and more than 10 positive lymph nodes and patients with locally advanced disease or inflammatory carcinoma. Preclinical and clinical evaluations of conventional chemotherapy administered in the adjuvant setting and for metastatic disease show a dose-response effect. This provides a strong rationale for the use of dose escalation in breast cancer.

Several trials of high-dose chemotherapy with ABMT for patients with metastatic disease show complete response rates of 35% to 40%. These results are higher than those seen with conventional doses of chemotherapy for metastatic disease, although no comparative trials have been performed. Long-term disease-free survival rates of 15% have been observed for patients with metastatic disease. Patients with sensitive disease and those with non bulky disease seem to respond best. Hormone-receptor negativity, liver metastases, and use of prior adjuvant chemotherapy are adverse prognostic factors. Randomized trials are under way to compare ABMT with standard maintenance chemotherapy for patients with metastatic breast cancer.

The clinical evidence supporting the concept of dose intensity for adjuvant breast cancer has led to trials of high-dose therapy followed by ABMT as adjuvant therapy for high-risk patients. Trials of adjuvant BMT in high-risk patients (those with six to ten, or more than ten involved nodes or those with locally advanced disease) have yielded prolonged remissions in more than 70% of patients. These results are superior to those of historical controls. Several cooperative trials are under way to test the value of adjuvant high-dose therapy with ABMT for patients with Stage II breast cancer with more than ten involved lymph nodes. Other trials are examining similar strategies for women with Stage III or inflammatory breast cancer.

NEUROBLASTOMA

High-dose therapy followed by ABMT results in 2-year disease-free survival of approximately 15% for children with relapsed or refractory neuroblastoma. Most patients have received purged marrow, although the value of purging is unclear. Intensive conventional induction chemotherapy followed by high-dose chemotherapy, and ABMT is generally recommended as initial therapy for patients with Stage IV and high-risk Stage III disease. Disease-free survival at 2 years is 20% to 40% for these patients.

GERM CELL NEOPLASMS

Phase II trials have shown high response rates for patients who have refractory germ cell neoplasms or those who have failed conventional salvage chemotherapy. Long-term disease-free survival has been noted in 15% to 20% of such patients. Trials are under way to test this approach for consolidation therapy of certain high-risk patients in first complete remission.

OTHER SOLID TUMORS

High-dose therapy with ABMT has been used less frequently for a number of other solid tumors, including glioblastoma, ovarian carcinoma, malignant melanoma, soft-tissue sarcoma, and small cell lung carcinoma. Results have generally been disappointing, although high response rates for ovarian cancer, brain tumors, and sarcomas have been noted in some situations. It is hoped that ongoing trials will clarify the role of ABMT in these malignancies.

SUMMARY

High-dose therapy followed by ABMT or PSCT is being used with increasing frequency. Improvements in supportive care, such as hematopoietic growth factors, as well as better patient selection and increased experience have made this form of therapy easier, safer, and less expensive. The morbidity and expense associated with ABMT are similar to those associated with prolonged courses of conventional chemotherapy in many situations. Transplants are now being performed on an outpatient basis. Follow-up studies show that the majority of patients who remain in remission after ABMT return to normal functional status.

Transplantation is still a relatively new technique, however. Patients require prolonged follow-up to assess the ultimate results of therapy. Late relapses have been observed, and other complications, such as myelodysplastic syndromes, are being described. Few randomized controlled trials have been performed, and the results of ABMT may be due to selection bias. Results from such trials will need to be reported before the ultimate role of ABMT in various malignancies can be defined. Patients should be entered in these trials whenever possible.

BIBLIOGRAPHY

Attal M, Huguet F, Schlaifer D et al. Intensive combined therapy for previously untreated aggressive myeloma. Blood 79:1130, 1992

Bierman PJ, Bagin RG, Jagannath S et al. High dose chemotherapy followed by autologous hematopoietic rescue in Hodgkin's disease: Long term follow-up in 128 patients. Ann Oncol 4:767, 1993

Coiffier B, Philip T, Burnett AK et al. Consensus conference on intensive chemotherapy plus hematopoietic stem-cell transplantation in malignancies: Lyon, France, June 4–6, 1993. J Clin Oncol 12:226, 1994

Goldman JM. Autografting for chronic myeloid leukaemia—palliation, cure or nothing? Leuk Lymph 7(suppl):51, 1992

Gorin NC, Aegerter P, Auvert B et al. Autologous bone marrow transplantation for acute myelocytic leukemia in first remission: A European survey of the role of marrow purging. Blood 8:1606, 1990

Jagannath S, Vesole DH, Glenn L et al. Low-risk intensive therapy for multiple myeloma with combined autologous bone marrow and blood stem cell support. Blood 80:1666, 1992

Kessinger A. Utilization of peripheral blood stem cells in autotransplantation. Hematol Oncol Clin North Am 7:535, 1993

Linker CA, Ries CA, Damon LE et al. Autologous bone marrow transplantation for acute myeloid leukemia using busulfan plus etoposide as a preparative regimen. Blood 81:311, 1993

Nemunaitis J, Rabinowe SN, Singer JW et al. Recombinant granulocyte-macrophage colony-stimulating factor after autologous bone marrow transplantation for lymphoid cancer. N Engl J Med 324:1773, 1991

O'Shaughnessy JA, Cowan KH. Dose-intensive therapy for breast cancer. JAMA 270:2089, 1993

Peters WP, Ross M, Vredenburgh JJ, et al. High-dose chemotherapy and autologous bone marrow support as consolidation after standard-dose adjuvant therapy for high-risk primary breast cancer. J Clin Oncol 11:1132, 1993

Philip T, Armitage JO, Spitzer G et al. High-dose therapy and autologous bone marrow transplantation after failure of conventional chemotherapy in adults with intermediate-grade or high-grade non-Hodgkin's lymphoma. N Engl J Med 316:1493, 1987

Reece DE, Connors JM, Spinelli JJ et al. Intensive therapy with cyclophosphamide, carmustine, etoposide ± cisplatin, and autologous bone marrow transplantation for Hodgkin's disease in first relapse after combination chemotherapy. Blood 83:1193, 1994

Shpall EJ, Stemmer SM, Bearman SI et al. Role of autotransplantation in treatment of other solid tumors. Hematol Oncol Clinics North Am 7:663, 1993

Vose J, Anderson JR, Kessinger A, et al. High-dose chemotherapy and autologous hematopoietic stem-cell transplantation for aggressive non-Hodgkin's lymphoma. J Clin Oncol 11:1846, 1993

John S. Macdonald, Daniel G. Haller, Robert J. Mayer, Eds. *Manual of Oncologic Therapeutics*, Third Edition.

IX. PARANEOPLASTIC SYNDROMES

71. ENDOCRINE EFFECTS

Donna Glover

Of all of the paraneoplastic processes, those related to ectopic polypeptide hormone production are the most frequent and best understood. Most of the patients described in the literature fail to fulfill all of the criteria necessary to prove ectopic hormone production by the malignant cells. These criteria include the following:

1. Increased hormone levels.
2. Decrease in the hormone level after removal or treatment of the tumor.
3. Persistent hormone elevation after removal of the normal gland that secretes the substance.
4. An arteriovenous gradient of hormone levels across the tumor vascular bed.
5. Demonstration that the tumor cells *in vitro* both synthesize and secrete the hormone.

Recently, with more sensitive radioimmunoassay techniques, investigators have found that ectopic hormone production is more common than previously reported. Many patients may have elevated hormone levels without clinical symptoms.[1,2] This may be due to the fact that many of these hormones are high-molecular-weight precursors, fragments, or submits which are biologically inactive. Some hormones may be elevated for years before patients develop signs of excess hormone production (*e.g.*, increased growth hormone levels leading to acromegaly). Occasionally, physiologic feedback mechanisms will inhibit hormone secretion from the normal gland, resulting in decreased hormone levels. Many tumors that produce ectopic hormones will secrete more than one substance that may be biologically active. Rarely, these multiple hormones may counterbalance clinical signs that would have developed otherwise.[1]

GROWTH HORMONES

Elevated growth hormone levels have been detected in patients with lung and gastric carcinoma. Several investigators have proposed that elevated growth hormone levels may lead to hypertrophic pulmonary osteoarthropathy. However, prospective studies have not consistently shown significantly higher growth hormone levels in patients with hypertrophic pulmonary osteoarthropathy compared with patients who do have this syndrome. Although patients may have elevated growth hormone levels, cancer patients rarely live long enough to develop acromegaly.[3] Acromegaly may occur in association with slow-growing carcinoids. Five acromegalic patients with growth hormone excess were cured after removal of their bronchial carcinoids.[4]

Ectopic production of growth hormone-releasing factor has also been detected in human lung tumors and carcinoids. Twelve cases of acromegaly with pituitary enlargement have been described in association with carcinoid. These patients had elevated growth hormone-releasing factor levels. Skull radiographs showed symmetrical enlargement of the sella. In this setting, acromegaly developed over a short time period (generally 2 to 6 years). Based on these studies, several endocrinologists have proposed that Type I multiple endocrine neoplasia may be secondary to a slow-growing functional adenoma that produces multiple hormones and releasing factors.[5]

ECTOPIC ADRENOCORTICOTROPHIC HORMONE SECRETION

Ectopic adrenocorticotrophic hormone (ACTH) secretion was the first paraneoplastic endocrine syndrome described in the early 1900s. ACTH is elevated from a large prohormone into its active form. The promolecule can circulate with no clinical side effects, because it is biologically inactive and unable to bind to tissue receptors. The prohormone is divided into other active hormonal segments, melanocyte-stimulating hormone and three hormones that have opiate-like activity (beta-lipotropic hormone (LPH), beta-endorphin, and meta-enkephalin.)[1]

The majority of patients with clinical signs from ectopic ACTH production present with hypokalemic metabolic alkalosis. Since most patients have advanced malignancy, they do not live long enough to develop a Cushingoid habitus. However, with extremely high cortisol levels, patients may develop diabetes, hypertension, edema, muscle wasting, central obesity, moon faces, buffalo humps, and striae.[3] Rarely, patients will experience alterations in mental status, fatigue, or anorexia from the effects of the opiate-like peptide fragments.[7,8]

The most common tumor associated with ectopic ACTH production is small cell lung cancer, which accounts for 50% of patients with the clinical syndrome. High cortisol levels have also been described in both adenocarcinoma and large cell carcinoma of the lung.[2,9,10] However, less than 5% of patients with lung cancer will develop Cushing's syndrome.[11-13] Other tumors associated with this paraneoplastic process include carcinoids, thymoma, neural crest tumors (such as pheochromocytomas, neuroblastomas, paragangliomas, islet cell tumors, medullary carcinoma of the thyroid), and rarely bronchial adenomas.[6, 14,15] All other tumors arising in other locations had small cell anaplastic or carcinoid histology on review.[(1,15-17,18]

Using a radioimmunoassay technique for ACTH, a high proportion of patients without Cushing's syndrome have high ACTH levels in their blood and tumor extracts.[1] Many patients may have increased fasting cortisol levels with or without dexamethasone suppression, but only a small proportion of patients will have the full-blown clinical syndrome.[1]

Fifteen percent of patients with Cushing's disease have ectopic ACTH production.[1] The diagnosis should be excluded in patients with small cell anaplastic carcinomas and neuroendocrine tumors in the presence of hypokalemic alkalosis or a Cushingoid habitus. A plasma ACTH level over 200 pg/ml is suggestive of the diagnosis. The plasma cortisol should be over 40 μg/dl at 8 A.M. to 6 P.M. without diurnal variation. A dexamethasone suppression test should be performed. Patients should receive 2 mg of dexamethasone every 6 hours for eight doses followed by an 8 A.M. cortisol and ACTH blood level. In 95% of cases with ectopic ACTH production, the ATH and cortisol were not suppressed with dexamethasone (<40% below baseline).[1]

The treatment for ectopic ACTH secretion is effective antitumor therapy. Potassium stores should be repleted. Unless there is a significant antitumor response, the patient will deteriorate from corticosteroid excess and tumor progression.[1]

GONADOTROPHINS

The gonadotrophin hormones include follicle-stimulating hormone (FSH), luteinizing hormone (LH), and human chorionic gonadotrophin (HCG).[9,10,19] Normally, FSH and LH are produced by the pituitary; HCG is produced by the placenta in pregnant women.[1] Increased production of gonadotrophins can lead to gynecomastia in the male, oligomenorrhea in premenopausal women, and precocious puberty in children. Hyperthyroidism has also been reported in association with elevated HCG levels, which cause thyroid stimulation. Elevated gonadotrophin levels have been reported in association with pituitary tumors, choriocarcinoma, nonseminomatous germ cell tumors, hepatoblastomas, and non-small cell lung cancer.[9,10,19-21]

Precocious puberty has been described in children with hepatoblastomas that secrete ectopic gonadotrophins. Gynecomastia rarely occurs in patients with elevated HCG levels, except those with carcinoma of the testicle or lung.[10,22]

Increased FSH and LH levels have not been described in association with malignancy, except in association with pituitary tumors. Elevated alpha and beta subunits of HCG frequently occur in patients with nonseminomatous germ cell tumors of the testicle and with gestational trophoblastic disease. In these diseases, HCG serves as a tumor marker that is followed to determine the efficacy of chemotherapy. Low levels of HCG have been detected in patients with carcinoma of the lung, colon, breast, pancreas, stomach, and islet cell carcinomas.[9,10]

HYPERTHYROIDISM

Isolated cases of ectopic thyroid-stimulating hormone secretion have been reported in association with malignancy. However, these patients do not have clinical signs or laboratory studies to suggest a hyperthyroid state.[23] HCG has thyroid-stimulating capabilities. Hyperthyroidism has been reported in less than 8% of patients with HCG elevation secondary to nonseminomatous testicular cancer, choriocarcinoma, and hydatidiform mole.[10,24] In these cases, the hyperthyroid state resolves as the HCG levels decline with effective antineoplastic therapy.[1,25]

ECTOPIC PROLACTIN SECRETION

Elevated prolactin levels have been described in three patients with undifferentiated lung cancer, small cell lung cancer, and adenocarcinoma of the kidney. Only one patient had signs of galactorrhea. Following tumor resection or regression after radiotherapy, prolactin levels fell to normal range.[9,10]

REFERENCES

1. Bunn PA, Minna JD. Paraneoplastic syndromes. In DeVita VT, Hellman S, Rosenberg SA (eds): Cancer: Principles & Practice of Oncology, pp 1797–1842. Philadelphia, JB Lippincott, 1985
2. Jeffcoate WJ, Rees LH. Adrenocorticotropin and related peptides in nonendocrine tumors. Curr Top Exp Endocrinol 3:57–74, 1978
3. Ennis CG, Cameron DP, Berger HG. On the etiology of hypertrophic pulmonary osteoarthropathy in bronchogenic carcinoma: Lack of relationship of elevated growth hormone levels. Aust N Z J Med 3:157–161, 1973
4. Sonksen PH, Ayres AB, Braimbridge M et al. Acromegaly caused by pulmonary carcinoid tumors. Clin Endocrinol 5:505–513, 1976
5. Scheihauer BW, Carpenter PC, Bloch B, Brazeau P. Ectopic secretion of a growth hormone-releasing factor. Report of a case of bronchial carcinoma tumor. Am J Med 76:605–606, 1984
6. Odell WD. Endocrine complications of cancer. In Calabresi P, Schein PS, Rosenberg SA (eds). Medical Oncology, pp 240–243, New York, Macmillan, 1985
7. Guillemin R. Endorphins, brain peptides that act like opiates. N Engl J Med 296:226–228, 1977
8. Hughes J. Opioid peptides and their relatives. Nature 278:394–395, 1979
9. Blackman MR, Rosen SW, Weintraub BD. Ectopic hormones. Adv Intern Med 23:85–113, 1978
10. Lees LH. The biosynthesis of hormones by nonendocrine tumors — a review. J Endocrinol 67:14–175, 1975
11. Eagan RT, Maurer LH, Forcier RJ, Tulloh M. Small cell carcinoma of the lung: Staging, paraneoplastic syndromes, treatment, and survival. Cancer 33:527–532, 1974
12. Lokich JJ. The frequency and clinical biology of the ectopic hormone syndromes of small cell carcinoma. Cancer 50:2111–2114, 1982
13. Singer W, Kovacs K, Ryan N, Horvath E. Ectopic ACTH syndrome: Clinicopathological correlations. J Clin Pathol 31:591–598, 1978
14. Azzopardi JG, Williams ED. Pathology of "nonendocrine" tumors associated with Cushing's syndrome. Cancer 22:274–286, 1968
15. Skrabanek P, Powell D. Unifying concept of non-pituitary ACTH secreting tumors: Evidence of common origin of neural-crest tumors, carcinoids, and oat-cell carcinomas. Cancer 42:1263–1269, 1978
16. Ghali VS, Garcia RL. Prostatic adenocarcinoma with carcinoidal features producing adrenocorticotrophic syndrome. Immunohistochemical study and review of the literature. Cancer 54:1043–1048, 1984
17. Lojek MA, Fer MF, Kasselberg AC et al. Cushing's syndrome with small cell carcinoma of the uterine cervix. Am J Med 69:140–144, 1980
18. Werner S, Jacobsson B, Bostrom L et al. Cushing's syndrome due to an ACTH-producing neuroendocrine tumor in the nasal roof. Acta Med Scan 217:235–240, 1985
19. Odell WD, Wolfsen AR. Humoral substances associated with cancer. Ann Rev Med 29:379–406, 1978
20. Faiman C, Colwell JA, Ryan RJ et al. Gonadotropin secretion from a bronchogenic carcinoma. N Engl J Med 277:1395–1399, 1967
21. Vaitukaitis JL, Ross GT, Braunstein GD, Rayford PL. Gonadotropins and their subunits: Basic and clinical studies. Recent Prog Horm Res 32:289–321, 1976
22. Skrabanek P, Kirrane J, Powell D. A unifying concept of chorionic gonadotropin production in malignancy. Invest Cell Pathol 2:75–85, 1979
23. Hennen G. Characterization of a thyroid stimulating factor in human cancer tissue. J Clin Endocrin Metab 27:610–614, 1967
24. Odell WD, Bates RW, Rivlin RS et al. Increased thryoid function without clinical hyperthyroidism in patients with choriocarcinoma. J Clin Endocrinol Med 23:658–668, 1963
25. Cave WT Jr, Dunn JT. Choriocarcinoma with hyperthyroidism: Probable identity of the thyrotropin with human chorionic gonadotropin. Ann Int Med 85:60–63, 1976

John S. Macdonald, Daniel G. Haller, Robert J. Mayer, Eds. *Manual of Oncologic Therapeutics*, Third Edition.

72. HEMATOLOGIC EFFECTS

Edward J. Lee
Charles A. Schiffer

Hematologic paraneoplastic syndromes may affect either the cellular elements of blood or the coagulation system, or may involve abnormal circulating immunoglobulins. Anemia, thrombocytopenia, and granulocytopenia are typical consequences of both cancer and its treatment. The recognition of a hematologic abnormality as a paraneoplastic manifestation requires the clinician to be alert to the setting in which these syndromes appear and to be able to distinguish such manifestations from the more common direct effects of cancer and its treatment.

PARANEOPLASTIC SYNDROMES AFFECTING THE CELLULAR ELEMENTS OF BLOOD

Erythrocytosis

Increased red blood cell production occurs in as many as 10% to 20% of patients with cerebellar hemangioblastomas, 1% to 5% of patients with renal tumors, and less frequently in patients with hepatomas, adrenal tumors, and various other malignancies. Many such tumors are nonmalignant, including uterine fibroids, adrenal adenomas, and renal cysts. Increased levels of erythropoietin have been found in tumor extracts from some patients with cerebellar hemangiomas and hypernephromas, but in only half of all patients with erythrocytosis can elevated erythropoietin levels be found to account for the erythrocytosis. Malignant or benign renal tumors may compress the renal artery, with a resultant decrease in renal blood flow leading to increased erythropoietin secretion and erythrocytosis. Regardless of definable cause, if the underlying tumor is successfully treated, the erythrocytosis usually resolves as well. Recurrence of the erythrocytosis may herald recurrence of the neoplastic process.

The erythrocytosis associated with tumors rarely produces the clinical signs or symptoms associated with erythrocytosis of other etiologies. Not uncommonly, the elevated hematocrit is found incidentally when evaluating a patient with a known tumor. When severe (*i.e.*, hematocrit > 55%), it is necessary to distinguish tumor-related erythrocytosis from other causes such as polycythemia vera (PV), hemoglobinopathy, smoking, pulmonary disease with hypoxia, right-to-left cardiac shunts, hypoventilation, or intravascular volume contraction ("stress" polycythemia). Physical examination, arterial blood gas, P50 measurement, hemoglobin electrophoresis, and radio-isotopic red cell mass/ blood volume studies may be helpful in excluding other causes of secondary erythrocytosis. Occasionally, the distinction between tumor-associated erythrocytosis and PV may be difficult. Both are associated with elevated red cell mass, and obvious splenomegaly does not occur in all patients with PV. The erythrocytosis of PV will not resolve with treatment of an underlying malignancy and is usually associated with elevations of white cell or platelet counts. Serum erythropoietin determinations may be helpful, since elevated levels are virtually never found in unphlebotomized patients with PV.

Management consists of treatment of the underlying condition. The presence of erythrocytosis is not necessarily indicative of metastatic disease, and does not preclude an attempt at curative resection in the absence of evidence of metastatic disease. Phlebotomy is not indicated on a chronic basis for asymptomatic patients, although such treatment might be considered in patients with a history of thromboembolic disease. Individuals with marked elevations of red cell mass in whom surgery is planned should undergo phlebotomy prior to general anesthesia to minimize the chance of complications due to thrombosis or low-flow states.

Anemia

Anemia is a very common complication of cancer and its treatment. Direct involvement of bone marrow by malignancy, radiation, and chemotherapy all may have substantial impact on red cell production. Red cell survival may be affected by blood loss or splenomegaly. The etiology of anemia may be difficult to define. Nonetheless, certain clear-cut paraneoplastic syndromes have distinguishing clinical characteristics.

PURE RED CELL APLASIA

Isolated severe anemia due to absent red cell production without associated thrombocytopenia or leukopenia is rare. Approximately 50% of all patients with acquired pure red cell aplasia (PRCA) have thymomas. A variety of immunologic or autoimmune phenomena such as hypogammaglobulinemia, paraproteinemia, antinuclear antibodies, or autoimmune hemolytic anemia have been described in patients with PRCA. Patients with thymomas tend to be female (3–5:1), and 15% may have associated myasthenia gravis. Little is known about the pathogenesis, which may involve suppressor T-cells. The clinical manifestations are severe reticulocytopenic anemia with an absence of red cell precursors in the bone marrow. In some patients with thymomas, other hematologic abnormalities may occur, such as leukopenia or thrombocytopenia. Patients with lymphoproliferative malignancies, particularly chronic lymphocytic leukemia, may have PRCA either related to infection with human parvovirus B19 (HPV) or to expansion of large granular lymphocytes. Treatment with intravenous gammaglobulin may be effective if infection with HPV has been documented.

Folic acid deficiency or chemo/radiation therapy effect must be excluded if leukopenia or thrombocytopenia are also present. Treatment of thymoma with surgery or radiation is not uniformly successful in reversing the anemia, with only 25% of patients with PRCA recovering adequate red cell production. Corticosteroids, splenectomy, or immunosuppressive therapy may be useful.

A small number of patients has been reported in whom PRCA was followed by the development of carcinoma in 6 weeks to 5 years. There is little information regarding treatment of patients with cancer and PRCA.

AUTOIMMUNE HEMOLYTIC ANEMIA

Autoimmune hemolytic anemia (AIHA) may occur in patients with lymphoid malignancies or, less commonly, in patients with solid tumors such as ovarian carcinoma. Approximately 10% of patients with chronic lymphocytic leukemia and a lesser number of patients with lymphomas (usually of B-cell origin) will have AIHA at some time during their course. Patients may present initially with symptoms of anemia with incidental identification of the underlying disease, or the hemolytic process may be well compensated with only a mild decrease in hemoglobin and hematocrit. Except in patients recently treated with radiation or chemotherapy, the reticulocyte count is usually elevated. The anemia may be severe and may be associated with a palpable spleen, pallor, and jaundice. Peripheral blood smears show spherocyte formation, and laboratory investigation may demonstrate markedly decreased or absent haptoglobin and elevated indirect bilirubin and lactate dehydrogenase. If hemolysis is due to a "warm" reactive antibody, the direct Coombs' test is usually positive with immunoglobulin G (IgG) and complement on the red cell surface. If hemolysis is due to a "cold" reactive antibody, usually immunoglobulin M (IgM), the diagnosis may be suspected by examining a tube of anticoagulated blood for spontaneous red cell agglutination. In cold agglutinin disease, red cell indices may be spuriously and markedly elevated, and other red blood cell parameters may be abnormal due to agglutination of red cells in the chambers of automated cell counters. Warming the blood to 37° C eliminates most of the abnormalities and the visible agglutination. The Coombs' test is positive but will show only complement when cells are tested at 37°C.

Treatment of AIHA due to a warm reactive antibody usually consists of corticosteroids (*e.g.*, prednisone, 1–1.5 mg/kg per day) to control the hemolytic process, followed by treatment of the underlying disease when hemolysis has been controlled. It is recommended that chemotherapy or radiation to large ports be delayed whenever possible, until stabilization of hemolysis has occurred, because antineoplastic therapy can impair the ability of the bone marrow to maintain red blood cell production. Thus, when compensated hemolysis is present, chemotherapy given prior to obtaining adequate control of hemolysis with steroids can result in severe anemia complicated by difficulties cross-matching blood because of the autoantibodies. Nonetheless, treatment of the underlying disease is necessary following steroids in order to sustain the steroid-induced remission.

After a response in the underlying disease is obtained, steroid therapy should be tapered slowly over 2 to 3 months, and the patient followed periodically by hematocrit, reticulocyte count, and direct Coombs' testing. Recurrence of disease is often heralded by recurrent hemolysis, and with a resistant neoplasm, hemolysis may be difficult to control with corticosteroids. Splenectomy is sometimes helpful in the management of selected patients.

Management of cold agglutinin-induced hemolysis is more difficult because corticosteroids and splenectomy are ineffective. Treatments of the underlying disease with chemotherapy, radiation therapy, and transfusion with red blood cells are the major therapeutic interventions.

MICROANGIOPATHIC HEMOLYTIC ANEMIA

Severe microangiopathic hemolytic anemia (MAHA) is an unusual complication of cancer, but may go unrecognized when present in a mild form due to the frequency with which anemia occurs in the setting of cancer and its treatment. Microangiopathic changes are often seen in the setting of disseminated intravascular coagulation (DIC), but MAHA is distinctly unusual as a sequela of DIC alone. MAHA caused by underlying solid tumors is often associated with clinical and laboratory evidence of DIC, including hemorrhagic and thromboembolic events. MAHA must also be distinguished from AIHA in which the direct Coombs' test is positive. MAHA is virtually always associated with a negative direct Coombs' test. MAHA can be found with the mucin-producing adenocarcinomas, with gastric carcinoma being the most commonly associated malignancy. The pathogenesis in these diseases has not been defined, although damage to red cells may be due to intravascular fibrin deposits, pulmonary vascular tumor emboli, or pulmonary vascular intimal hyperplasia. MAHA may also develop in patients with hemangiomas, probably on the basis of mechanical trauma to red blood cells passing through abnormal tumor vessels (Kasbach-Merrit Syndrome).

The clinical manifestations depend on the severity of the anemia. Patients may present with marked anemia with reticulocytosis. The hallmark of MAHA is the presence of schistocytes in the peripheral blood smear. Elevated bilirubin, hemoglobinemia, hemoglobinuria, and hemosiderinuria all may occur, and thrombocytopenia is common if DIC is also present.

Treatment for MAHA other than therapy for the underlying tumor is not generally effective. Heparin is not effective in reducing red blood cell transfusion requirements, although it could be considered if there is evidence of DIC. Occasionally, relapse of disease may occur with MAHA, and evidence of malignancy should be looked for in appropriate patients for whom no other obvious explanation of anemia exists.

The hemolytic-uremic syndrome (HUS) (MAHA, thrombocytopenia, and renal dysfunction) may occur in patients without malignancy or other precipitating cause. In such situations, dialysis (when necessary) and plasma infusion or exchange are the mainstays of treatment, and are variably successful. HUS may also occur following marrow ablative chemotherapy and bone marrow transplantation (BMT), the use of cyclosporine-A, mitomycin-C, or platinum-based regimens. Discontinuing cyclosporine-A is often successful in reversing renal dysfunction with subsequent clearing of schistocytes from the smear, and resolution of MAHA, but HUS following mitomycin-C, platinum-based chemotherapy, or BMT is less responsive to treatment. A variety of approaches including aggressive plasma exchange, intravenous infusions of high doses of gammaglobulin, and the use of staph protein A columns have not convincingly altered the poor prognosis of HUS in these settings.

Hyperleukocytosis and Leukemia

Patients with leukemia may present with marked elevation of the white blood count. Such patients may represent true emergencies if the underlying disease is acute myeloid leukemia or chronic myelogenous leukemia in blast crisis. If the circulating white blood cell count and differential indicate that more than 100,000 blasts/μl are present, then immediate treatment is necessary. The blast cells in patients with myeloid leukemias are relatively large and much less deformable than red cells, lymphocytes, lymphoblasts, or mature granulocytes. In the capillary circulation, sludging of cells with impairment of blood flow and subsequent disruption of vascular endothelium may occur. Should this occur in the central nervous system, then catastrophic hemorrhage may follow, particularly with concomitant thrombocytopenia or coagulation abnormalities. Circulatory impairment may also occur without hemorrhage. Patients may present with lethargy or confusion without focal neurologic findings. Patients may also be hypoxic, sometimes with pulmonary infiltrates related to sludging in the pulmonary microcirculation. Caution and clinical correlation are recommended in interpreting the results of laboratory tests in patients with marked elevation of blast counts. "Pseudohypoxia" and "pseudohypoglycemia" can develop because of *in vitro* metabolic activity of the leukocytes, while "pseudohyperkalemia" can be a consequence of disruption and release of potassium from blast cells after blood drawing and clotting.

Patients with hyperleukocytosis should not routinely receive red blood cell transfusions, because whole-blood viscosity may increase markedly with subsequent slowing of blood flow in the microcirculation. If necessary, red cells should be given slowly, with caution, preferably in conjunction with measures described below to lower the white blood cell count. Single units of red blood cells may be split into aliquots that can be given over a prolonged interval.

Treatment consists of rapid lowering of the white blood cell count. If the diagnosis and plan for chemotherapy are known, then definitive treatment should be instituted immediately, preceded only by allopurinol administration. Patients should be well hydrated with crystalloid and monitored for the occurrence of a tumor lysis syndrome manifested by hyperphosphatemia, hyperkalemia, hypocalcemia, and renal insufficiency. If definitive therapy has not yet been decided because the results of special studies (*e.g.*, cytochemical stains) are not yet available, then hydroxyurea, 3 g/m^2 can be administered orally, again following allopurinol. This dose, if effective, can be repeated when the white count rises.

Leukopheresis using cell-separator machines can be a useful temporizing measure in addition to chemotherapy by mechanically removing large quantities of circulating blasts within 2 to 3 hours. Such treatment should be considered in symptomatic patients in whom chemotherapy cannot be initiated immediately because of hyperuricemia, renal dysfunction, or other medical problems.

The role of radiation therapy in such emergencies is controversial. Theoretically, single-dose cranial irradiation (400 cGy), which has virtually no toxicity, results in effective cytotoxicity in areas where circulating antineoplastic agents may not penetrate due to circulatory impairment. There are no clinical data about the efficacy of this maneuver and it is variably used in different centers. There are insufficient data to justify prophylactic use of this modality, although it may be appropriate for patients who are symptomatic from hyperleukocytosis.

If hyperleukocytosis occurs in patients with acute or chronic lymphocytic leukemia, circulatory problems usually do not occur because of the relatively smaller cell size; urgent treatment is therefore not generally necessary. Similarly, patients with high numbers of circulating mature granulocytes do not require emergent intervention.

Granulocytosis

Leukemoid reactions of substantial proportions may be seen in cancer patients without bone marrow involvement by tumor. Differential white blood cell counts show primarily an increased number of mature granulocytes. Leukocytosis of lesser proportions occurs in many patients. Other causes such as inflammation or infection should be excluded, but in some patients no obvious cause other than cancer can be identified. Gastric, bronchogenic, pancreatic carcinoma, melanoma, central nervous system tumors, Hodgkin's disease, and large cell lymphomas may all be associated with leukocytosis. The pathogenesis is unknown. Chronic myelogenous leukemia can usually be distinguished by the presence of more immature elements and/or basophils in the peripheral blood, leukocyte alkaline phosphatase, splenomegaly, or, if necessary, by cytogenetic or molecular analysis for the presence of a Philadelphia chromosome.

Granulocytosis requires no treatment, and the syndrome has no known complications.

Eosinophilia

Eosinophilia, defined as an increase in the eosinophil count to more than 700/μl, may occur in cancer patients as a consequence either of radiation therapy or splenectomy performed as part of a staging or diagnostic evaluation. In addition, patients with myeloproliferative syndromes such as polycythemia vera and chronic myelogenous leukemia, solid tumors such as lung cancer, and as many as 20% of the patients with Hodgkin's disease may have mild eosinophilia. Marked elevation of the eosinophil count can occur in Hodgkin's disease, but relatively infrequently.

Other causes of eosinophilia should also be considered, such as allergic reactions or, rarely in North America, invasive parasitic infections. Eosinophilia is not useful as a marker of tumor activity, although on occasion recurrence of eosinophilia may be associated with recurrence of disease in a patient with Hodgkin's disease. There are no complications of eosinophilia associated with malignant disease, and specific therapy is not necessary.

Granulocytopenia

Granulocytopenia occurs commonly in patients who have been treated with radiation or chemotherapy, but very rarely as a direct complication of malignant disease. Patients with thymoma can have suppression of all or any hematopoietic cell line as an isolated finding. The mechanism is unclear (see Pure Red Cell Aplasia). Treatment consists of treatment of the underlying disease. Disorders of large granular lymphocytes (natural killer or NK cells) are often associated with a decrease in circulating granulocytes and the presence of an increased number of lymphocytes bearing CD16, 56 or 57. Initial treatment, following a careful diagnostic evaluation, usually consists of corticosteroids.

Thrombocytosis

As many as one third of all cancer patients may have an elevated platelet count (>400,000/μl). The underlying disease may be a solid tumor, Hodgkin's disease, or non-Hodgkin's lymphoma. Inflammatory processes, bleeding, iron deficiency, and post splenectomy syndrome must also be considered as diagnostic possibilities. Rarely, a myeloproliferative syndrome with thrombocytosis may coexist with a nonhematologic malignancy. Concomitant granulocytosis or erythrocytosis may suggest this possibility.

Complications of thrombocytosis, such as bleeding or thrombosis, occur primarily when other factors compromise blood flow, as may occur in patients with both elevated red blood cell mass and thrombocytosis, or with atherosclerosis. The isolated thrombocytosis associated with malignancy is rarely associated with any complications and therefore does not require specific therapy. Should surgery be required, the majority of patients do not need to have the platelet count lowered. However, in the rare patient with extreme reactive thrombocytosis (>2,000,000/μl), it may be advisable to lower the platelet count prior to surgery with either plateletpheresis or hydroxyurea and to consider postoperative anticoagulation if ambulation is delayed.

Thrombocytopenia

Thrombocytopenia occurs in patients with various forms of cancer, most frequently as a result of chemotherapy or radiation therapy. Thrombocytopenia also is seen in those patients with MAHA and DIC, in whom platelets may be consumed intravascularly (these disorders are considered earlier in this chapter). A syndrome resembling autoimmune thrombocytopenia (AITP) has been associated with Hodgkin's disease (HD, incidence approximately 2%), and less commonly with non-Hodgkin's lymphoma (NHL), chronic lymphocytic leukemia, acute lymphocytic leukemia, solid tumors, or bone marrow transplantation. Care must be taken to exclude nonimmune causes of thrombocytopenia, such as thiazide diuretics, DIC, and sepsis as well as immune thrombocytopenia related to drugs such as quinidine, cephalosporins, and trimethoprim-sulfamethoxazole. The diagnosis may be suspected in patients receiving treatment for HD, NHL, or other disease if thrombocytopenia occurs out of proportion to granulocytopenia. In patients with HD, the occurrence of AITP does not necessarily imply relapse or progression of disease, whereas in NHL progressive disease is usually apparent.

A bone marrow examination in AITP will show an abundance of megakaryocytes. Initial treatment consists of corticosteroid therapy (the equivalent of 1 mg/kg/day of prednisone). As with all patients with AITP, response to this treatment is often less than optimal. As many as 60% to 70% of patients may fail to achieve a sustained complete response. In most patients, however, the platelet count will improve. Splenectomy may be associated with a complete response in as many as 50% of patients. Intravenous gammaglobulin administration is often associated with a transient increase in platelet count, but rarely with sustained response. Early splenectomy is therefore recommended if patients are steroid dependent or refractory. However, AITP may occur in patients with HD who have undergone splenectomy as part of the evaluation of extent of disease. Immunosuppressive drugs may be useful in these patients. Little data exist on other therapeutic options such as danazol or Rh immune globulin. Platelet transfusions should be reserved for patients with significant hemorrhagic complications and should not be given routinely.

PARANEOPLASTIC SYNDROMES OF THE COAGULATION SYSTEM

A broad spectrum of abnormalities of the coagulation system frequently can lead to clinically evident thromboembolic disease; the reader is referred to a comprehensive review by Seifter and Bell cited at the end of the chapter.

Acute DIC or chronic DIC with associated complications of thrombophlebitis, arterial emboli and nonbacterial thrombotic endocarditis, circulating inhibitors of coagulation factors, and abnormal circulating proteins that may lead to hemorrhagic diatheses have all been described in cancer patients. Any malignant disease may be complicated by DIC. In nonhematologic malignancies, a prospective study of 108 patients with cancer disclosed laboratory evidence of abnormal coagulation studies in 68% of patients. The tumors most commonly associated with DIC are mucin-producing adenocarcinomas such as pancreatic, gastric, lung, prostate, or colon. Clinical disease may be seen as a consequence of these abnormalities in as many as 10% of all patients with cancer. DIC can also occur with any type of acute leukemia, but acute promyelocytic leukemia (APL; French-American-British classification M3) is virtually always associated with an acute DIC, probably on the basis of the release of a procoagulant contained in the abnormal granules of the leukemic promyelocyte.

Acute Disseminated Intravascular Coagulation

The principles of management of acute DIC have been developed in APL and may be applied to the rare patient with a solid tumor in whom this complication occurs and treatment is indicated.

Formerly, the hemorrhagic complications of APL heralded a difficult clinical course, with poorer survival of patients when compared with that of other types of acute leukemia. Currently, because of improved management of acute DIC, the short-term prognosis for patients presenting with APL has improved, and the long-term prognosis may be better. DIC also occurs in the variant of APL known as "microgranular" APL, which cannot be identified as APL except with the use of electron microscopy, cytogenetics, or, more recently, molecular techniques. Unfortunately, these procedures frequently require more than 1 week to complete, and the earliest indication of this variant APL may be the appearance of significant DIC. Thus, the physician must be sensitive to the earliest sign of coagulopathy in all patients with acute leukemia.

Patients may present with profound anemia and bleeding from multiple sites including mucus membranes, venipuncture, and bone marrow sites. Occasionally, patients may present with only laboratory evidence of DIC. Prolongation of the prothrombin time (PT) is one of the earliest routinely detectable abnormalities, along with the development of fibrin degradation products (FDP). These are usually followed by decreasing levels of fibrinogen and increase in the partial thromboplastin time (PTT) as the DIC accelerates either with increasing tumor burden or cytotoxic chemotherapy. In some patients the manifestations of DIC may not occur until cell lysis accelerates following chemotherapy, and in most patients, the DIC is most active shortly after initiation of chemotherapy.

The cornerstone of management of acute DIC is aggressive transfusion support in patients receiving chemotherapy to treat the underlying cause. Patients with active bleeding or those with significant laboratory evidence of DIC, such as marked elevations of the PT or marked decreases in the fibrinogen concentration, should be aggressively transfused with platelets to maintain the platelet count above 35,000 to 40,000/μl until bleeding or DIC subsides. Frequent transfusions may be required initially. Intravenous vitamin K, clotting factor replacement with fresh frozen plasma, or cryoprecipitate if the fibrinogen level is less than 75 mg/dl are mainstays of therapy. Each platelet transfusion generally contains approximately 500 mls of plasma. Thus, the platelet transfusion itself may be sufficient to replace depleted coagulation factors and fibrinogen.

The role of heparin is controversial. Heparin can decrease the acute DIC, and the administration of moderate doses (200 units/kg/24 hours) by continuous infusion often results in disappearance of clinical hemorrhage and improvement in laboratory parameters such as fibrinogen level, PT, and PTT. A reasonable approach to the management of acute DIC in patients with APL is to treat all patients with platelets and optimize their coagulation system while reserving heparin therapy for patients with hemorrhagic complications. Treatment with heparin can generally be discontinued within 5 to 7 days when coagulation parameters begin to improve. Surgical interventions, such as the placement of Hickman catheters, should be delayed whenever possible to allow the DIC to subside. Intramuscular and subcutaneous injections should be avoided. Antifibrinolytic agents have also been used in patients with APL to control coagulopathy with equivalent success rates compared to the use of heparin or aggressive transfusion therapy. Familiarity with one of these approaches is necessary for optimal care of such patients.

Recently, high remission rates using all-trans retinoid acid (ATRA) in patients with APL have been reported. This agent may become the standard treatment depending on the results of currently ongoing randomized trials. The use of ATRA is usually associated with rapid normalization of the fibrinogen level, and prothrombin time with concurrent resolution of the hemorrhagic diathesis. Thus it may be possible to provide less aggressive transfusion therapy once such improvements are noted.

When acute DIC complicates the course of patients with solid tumors, the etiology is most commonly sepsis, and heparin is not indicated.

Chronic Disseminated Intravascular Coagulation

Chronic DIC, with complications of venous thrombosis, embolic disease, nonbacterial thrombotic endocarditis, and less frequently hemorrhage, is one of the most frequent and challenging problems faced by the cancer physician. In general, fluctuating abnormalities of screening blood tests occur in these patients, punctuated by episodes of thromboembolic disease or hemorrhage. Thus, the earliest sign of DIC may be prolongation of the PT, high fibrinogen levels, or the presence of FDP. Patients may present with thrombophlebitis, pulmonary or arterial emboli, or hemorrhage. Other patients may be discovered to have DIC only through screening and blood tests. In a review of 182 patients with chronic DIC, Sack and colleagues found that 68% of patients had at least one episode of thrombophlebitis, and 53% had more than one episode. Fewer patients had hemorrhagic manifestations (42%) or arterial thrombi (25%). Nonbacterial thrombotic endocarditis (NBTE) was found in 23% of patients at autopsy. There was a high correlation between the presence of arterial emboli and NBTE, in that 79% of those with emboli who underwent autopsy had NBTE. In these patients the aortic and mitral valves were affected equally. Involvement of the right-sided heart valves was rare and always in conjunction with left-sided valvular involvement. Commonly associated tumors were pancreatic, lung, prostate, and gastric carcinomas. In this series, 27% of patients received antineoplastic therapy of some sort. In approximately half of those treated, some control of the manifestations of chronic DIC was obtained for a period of time.

Anticoagulant therapy was given to 30% of the patients reviewed. This group overlaps the group that received antineoplastic therapy in that 27 patients received both antitumor and anticoagulant therapy. Although the efficacy of anticoagulation was unclear, no patient responded to warfarin therapy after failing to respond to heparin, and recurrence of symptoms often occurred following discontinuation of anticoagulation. Patients who did not experience recurrent symptoms received either effective antineoplastic therapy or long-term anticoagulation therapy with either heparin or warfarin. Thus, after initial presentation with an episode of thrombophlebitis, patients should receive anticoagulation therapy with heparin and may benefit from long-term anticoagulation. Data from this large series suggest that oral anticoagulation may be less effective than heparin. Anticoagulation should be continued until either a response to antineoplastic therapy occurs or hemorrhagic complications occur.

The use of thrombolytic therapy should also be considered in patients presenting with deep venous thrombosis. In addition to all of the usual contraindications to the use of streptokinase or urokinase, including hemorrhage, recent surgery, central nervous system abnormalities, and severe hypertension, occult metastasis in the central nervous system should also be excluded, because treatment with thrombolytic therapy might result in central nervous system hemorrhage. If no contraindications to thrombolytic therapy are present, streptokinase or urokinase therapy may be the optimal treatment with preservation of venous valvular architecture, thereby avoiding a second episode in the same anatomical distribution. Thrombolytic therapy should then be followed by heparin treatment, as in the treatment of thrombophlebitis not associated with malignancy. The use of thrombolytic therapy should be weighed against the potential for response to chemotherapy in patients with widespread metastatic disease. The risk of bleeding is prohibitive in patients whose coagulation parameters are already markedly abnormal.

In view of the strong association between arterial emboli and NBTE, and the danger of exacerbating hemorrhage in embolic areas, thrombolytic therapy should not be given to patients with cancer presenting with arterial emboli and should be reserved for ambulatory patients with good performance status who have thrombophlebitis or pulmonary emboli. Heparin is indicated in patients with arterial emboli and NBTE, but such patients have an extremely poor prognosis because the underlying neoplasm is usually advanced and refractory to treatment.

PARANEOPLASTIC SYNDROMES ASSOCIATED WITH PARAPROTEINS

Coagulopathy

Patients with multiple myeloma or Waldenstrom's macroglobulinemia may have abnormal hemostasis and coagulation related to the effects of the paraprotein on what might otherwise be normal clotting factors and platelets. Prolonged bleeding times suggesting abnormal platelet function have been described in some patients. Coating of platelets with paraprotein and subsequent decrease in platelet function in response to agonists may be responsible. Paraproteins can inhibit fibrin monomer aggregation, act as inhibitors of factor VIII, act as nonspecific inhibitors or, rarely, bind factor X (amyloidosis). Patients may present with either hemorrhagic diatheses or thrombotic complications. When stable, chemotherapy for the underlying malignancy is the treatment of choice. Patients with intractable bleeding may benefit from plasmapheresis because the abnormalities in clotting function may be related to the level of the paraprotein. When plasmapheresis is performed, initiation of chemotherapy is also indicated, as ongoing paraprotein synthesis should also be reduced. Since most IgM and IgA is distributed in the intravascular space, one apheresis procedure is often adequate to stabilize clinical problems and to allow time for chemotherapy to decrease production of the paraprotein. Only 40% to 50% of IgG is intravascular. Because equilibration between intravascular and extravascular spaces occurs over 1 to 2 days after apheresis with redistribution of IgG to the intravascular space, further apheresis procedures may be necessary with IgG paraproteins. However, deficiencies of clotting factors may also occur in patients with plasma cell dyscrasias. Plasmapheresis of patients with specific factor deficiencies may exacerbate bleeding tendencies. Thus, careful evaluation of patients prior to plasmapheresis is necessary.

Hyperviscosity

Hyperviscosity occurs in multiple myeloma and Waldenstrom's macroglobulinemia because of either increased quantity of an IgM paraprotein in the blood or the polymerization of IgA or IgG paraproteins resulting in increased whole blood viscosity. Patients present with signs and symptoms related to decreased blood flow, such as headaches, dizziness, epistaxis, seizures, hearing loss, and the slow onset of alterations in mental status. Physical findings may include sausage-shaped retinal vein engorgement, retinal hemorrhage, signs of congestive heart failure, and hemorrhage. Coagulation abnormalities and anemia may be present, but a decreased hematocrit may also reflect an expanded plasma volume with a nearly normal red cell mass. Blood or serum viscosity may be measured by a variety of techniques and is expressed as a ratio to the viscosity of water. Normal serum viscosity is 1.4 to 1.8 relative to water. Symptoms secondary to hyperviscosity can occur at serum viscosities greater than 4 and are common with serum viscosities greater than 6.

Treatment of hyperviscosity by plasma exchange is effective in reversing both signs and symptoms. Treatment of the underlying disease is also appropriate in order to interrupt further production of the paraprotein.

Patients with hyperviscosity and anemia must be approached with caution. Transfusion with red blood cells may rapidly increase whole blood viscosity and precipitate cerebrovascular accidents, retinal hemorrhage, myocardial infarctions, or pulmonary edema. If transfusion is needed, each unit should be given extremely slowly.

BIBLIOGRAPHY

Antman KH, Skarin AT, Mayer RJ et al. Microangiopathic hemolytic anemia and cancer: A review. Medicine 58:277–384, 1979

Berchtold P, McMillan R. Therapy of chronic idiopathic thrombocytopenic purpura in adults. Blood 74:2309–2317, 1989

Loughran TP. Clonal diseases of large granular lymphocytes. Blood 82:1–14, 1993

Petz LD, Garratty G. Acquired Immune Hemolytic Anemias. New York, Churchill Livingstone, 1980

Pruzanski W, Shumak KH. Biologic activity of cold-reacting autoantibodies. N Engl J Med 297:538–542, 297:583–589, 1977

Rodeghiero F, Avvisati G, Castaman G et al. Early deaths and anti-hemorrhagic treatments in acute promyelocytic leukemia. A GIMEMA retrospective study in 268 consecutive patients. Blood 75:2112–2117, 1990

Sack GH, Levin J, Bell WR. Trousseau's syndrome and other manifestations of chronic disseminated coagulopathy in patients with neoplasms: Clinical, pathophysiologic, and therapeutic features. Medicine 56:1–37, 1977

Seifter EJ, Bell WR. Coagulation abnormalities in patients with cancer. In Schiffer CA (ed): Clinics in Oncology, Vol 2. Philadelphia, WB Saunders 1983:657–704

John S. Macdonald, Daniel G. Haller, Robert J. Mayer, Eds. *Manual of Oncologic Therapeutics*, Third Edition.

73. REMOTE EFFECTS OF CANCER ON THE NERVOUS SYSTEM

Joan E. Mollman

The phrase "remote effects of cancer on the nervous system" is sometimes used to describe all of the non-metastatic neurologic complications that occur in patients with cancer, including opportunistic infections, metabolic disturbances, vascular complications, treatment neurotoxicity, and the paraneoplastic syndromes. The focus here will be limited to the paraneoplastic syndromes, a group of disorders many of which now appear to be immunologically linked to the presence of cancer in the body. The paraneoplastic syndromes can be categorized based on their specificity for an association with cancer or on the type of tumor with which they are usually associated. Some are most commonly associated with solid tumors, while others are associated with hematologic malignancies.

Some syndromes are so specific for suggesting the presence of an occult neoplasm that once the diagnosis of the syndrome is made, an aggressive search for tumor should be undertaken. These include Lambert-Eaton myasthenic syndrome (LEMS), paraneoplastic cerebellar degeneration (PCD), paraneoplastic encephalomyelitis (PEM), and opsoclonus-myoclonus (OM). They are most commonly associated with solid tumors, especially small cell lung cancer (SCLC), breast cancer, ovarian cancer, other female genital tract tumors, and neuroblastoma (Table 73–1). The onset of neurologic symptoms is generally subacute occurring over weeks to a few months. Symptoms may present prior to the discovery of tumor by 2 or more years. If no tumor is found at the time of the initial diagnosis, the patient should be followed closely and re-evaluated aggressively for two years. The tumors are often quite small when found, suggesting that something about the presence of the paraneoplastic syndrome contributes to limiting the growth of the tumor. While there are isolated reports of improvement of the clinical paraneoplastic syndrome with treatment of the tumor alone, this is the exception rather than the rule. The majority of patients who have a treatable syndrome require specific therapy for the paraneoplastic symptoms.

The most significant recent advance in these disorders is the discovery of antibodies in the serum of many of the patients. Different distinct antibodies with different target antigens have been identified in LEMS, PCD, PEM, and OM. While the etiologic significance has not been determined in all of the disorders, RNA transcripts for the target antigen in LEMS, the voltage-gated calcium channel, have been identified in SCLC. It is postulated that the presence of antigen in the tumor leads to an autoimmune response in the patient. Regardless of their role in the pathophysiology of these disorders, the presence of antibody provides a positive test so that paraneoplastic syndrome no longer has to be a diagnosis of exclusion. The absence of an antibody in the serum of a patient with a typical clinical presentation does not exclude the diagnosis; however, the presence of an antibody can reassure the physician that it is cost effective to carry out an exhaustive search for certain tumors.

A few paraneoplastic syndromes are more often seen in the setting of hematologic malignancies. Subacute motor neuronopathy is a paraneoplastic syndrome most commonly associated with lymphomas, particularly Hodgkin's lymphoma. The POEMS syndrome (polyneuropathy, organomegaly, endocrinopathy, monoclonal protein, and skin changes) is often the harbinger of an osteosclerotic myeloma. All of these specific paraneoplastic syndromes will be described in more detail below.

There are other neurologic disorders that appear to occur with increased frequency in patients with cancer but occur with sufficient frequency in the general population that diagnosing the disease does not warrant the same diligent search for an underlying malignancy. These include sensorimotor axonal polyneuropathy, dementia, chronic inflammatory demyelinating polyneuropathy, and Guillain-Barré syndrome. Still it is important to appreciate that the presence of a tumor may be the only associated risk factor for these disorders in a particular patient. A search for a thymoma but not other tumors should be undertaken in patients who are newly diagnosed with myasthenia gravis. There probably is a slightly increased incidence of malignancy in patients over 40 who have dermatomyositis or polymyositis and do not have an underlying collagen vascular disorder. However, the increase in incidence compared to a control group was not statistically significant in one study, and the types of associated tumors are quite varied. In addition, in one retrospective study no unsuspected malignancies were found in patients who underwent exhaustive diagnostic studies. Therefore, it is not cost effective to carry out an extensive search for a malignancy in patients with dermatomyositis or polymyositis who do not have other suggestive symptoms or signs. Since breast and lung are the two most commonly associated tumors, it is reasonable to perform mammography and do a chest X-ray. It has been suggested that amyotrophic lateral sclerosis is sometimes caused by an underlying malignancy, but a review of the literature revealed only two patients in whom the presence of malignancy and motor neuron disease seemed to be more than a chance occurrence of

TABLE 73–1. PARANEOPLASTIC SYNDROMES

SYNDROME	USUAL TUMOR	ANTIBODY	ANTIGEN	TREATMENT
LEMS	SCLC	Anti-VGCC	VGCC Synaptotagmin	Plasmapheresis or IVIG
PCD	Breast, ovary, other female genital tract, Hodgkin's lymphoma	Anti-Yo	Purkinje cell	None
PEM	SCLC	Anti-Hu	DNA-binding Protein	None
OM	Neuroblastoma (children) Breast, SCLC (adults)	Unknown Anti-Ri	 Unknown	ACTH corticosteroids
Subacute motor Neuronopathy	Hodgkin's lymphoma, other lymphomas	None known		Supportive measures
POEMS	Osteosclerotic myeloma	None Known		Treat myeloma

See text for abbreviations.

two common disorders in an aging population. Patients who do not fit the usual age profile, who have a predominance of lower motor neuron findings, and who have sensory complaints deserve a chest X-ray and mammogram.

LAMBERT-EATON MYASTHENIC SYNDROME (LEMS)

Lambert-Eaton myasthenic syndrome is the most common of the paraneoplastic syndromes, occurring in nearly 3% of 150 SCLC patients studied prospectively. It is a disorder of neuromuscular transmission characterized clinically by proximal muscle weakness, reduced or absent deep tendon reflexes, a general feeling of fatigue, and frequently autonomic symptoms such as dry mouth, impotence, or constipation. The weakness often improves, and deep tendon reflexes may return with exercise. The electrophysiologic correlate of this phenomenon is a small initial compound muscle action potential that increases in amplitude with repetitive stimulation or after a brief period of maximal contraction of the muscle. The weakness is due to a decrease in the presynaptic quantal release of acetylcholine secondary to a decrease in calcium influx in the presynaptic nerve terminal. With repetitive stimulation or maximal voluntary contraction, acetylcholine accumulates in the synaptic cleft, allowing for a more normal post-synaptic response. The autonomic symptoms are due to involvement of the nicotinic cholinergic neurons. Only about 60% of patients with LEMS will have an associated tumor even after years of follow-up. Of those, 90% will have SCLC.

Lambert-Eaton myasthenic syndrome is the first of the paraneoplastic syndromes to have its pathophysiology defined. More than 10 years ago it was demonstrated that IgG from the plasma of patients with LEMS reproduced the syndrome when injected into mice. Within five years the target antigens had been identified as the voltage-gated calcium channel (VGCC) and a closely associated protein, synaptotagmin. More recently it has been demonstrated that small cell lung cancer cells express at least two classes of VGCC, including one that is bound by serum IgG from patients with LEMS.

Treatment for LEMS includes treating the underlying tumor coupled with plasma exchange or intravenous immunoglobulin (IVIG) therapy. More immediate relief of weakness may be achieved with 3,4-diaminopyridine, which prolongs the activation of the VGCC, thus enhancing release of acetylcholine from the presynaptic nerve terminals.

PARANEOPLASTIC CEREBELLAR DEGENERATION (PCD)

The clinical features of paraneoplastic cerebellar degeneration are those of a disorder of both mid-line and hemispheric cerebellar dysfunction. Within a few weeks patients may go from being normal to profoundly disabled by severe dysarthria, limb and truncal ataxia, and head titubation. Abnormal eye findings are prominent, including nystagmus, disruption of smooth pursuit, ocular dysmetria, and opsoclonus. While lethargy, mental decline, or weakness may signify a more generalized encephalitis, cerebellar dysfunction is the dominant clinical picture. Autopsy specimens consistently reveal a diffuse loss of Purkinje cells throughout the cerebellar cortex.

This paraneoplastic syndrome is most commonly associated with breast, ovarian, and female genital tract tumors, but is also seen in patients with Hodgkin's disease and small cell lung cancer. An anti-Purkinje cell antibody, originally designated anti-Yo, can be identified in the serum of many of the patients who have breast, ovarian, or genital tract carcinomas but not in the serum of patients with Hodgkin's disease or other solid tumors. The antibody typically stains cytoplasm and proximal dendrites of Purkinje cells. It appears that the antigen is a protein that binds DNA and may regulate transcription.

Unlike LEMS patients, those with paraneoplastic cerebellar degeneration generally do not respond to treatment of their tumor, plasmapheresis, or other immune suppression, and end up severely debilitated. While there are isolated reports of improvement with removal or treatment of the underlying tumor, this occurs only rarely.

PARANEOPLASTIC ENCEPHALOMYELITIS (PEM)

Paraneoplastic encephalomyelitis encompasses a group of clinically distinct syndromes, including subacute sensory neuronopathy and limbic encephalitis, that share a common pathology. These disorders are most commonly associated with small cell lung cancer. Though the pathologic picture generally reveals patchy loss of neurons in many areas including cerebral cortex, cerebellum, brainstem, spinal cord, dorsal root ganglia, and autonomic ganglia, the clinical presentation is usually dominated by evidence of involvement in a particular area of the nervous system. Subacute sensory neuronopathy (SSN) is the most common of these disorders, occurring in 1–2% of patients with SCLC. The clinical picture is one of subacute onset of numbness, paresthesias, and loss of deep tendon reflexes. Painful burning paresthesias are not uncommon. Neurologic examination reveals loss of vibratory and joint position sensation out of proportion to loss of pin-prick sensation and temperature. Strength is preserved, but many patients are severely disabled by the loss of proprioception. As with PCD the course of SSN is rarely altered by treating the underlying tumor or various immunosuppressive measures. The painful paresthesias may respond to Tegretol, Dilantin, or tricyclic antidepressants. Patients should be referred for occupational and physical therapy to help them adjust to their disabilities.

Limbic encephalitis is a less common presentation of paraneoplastic encephalomyelitis. The clinical presentation is one of subacute deterioration of memory, particularly short-term memory. The first case described was of a London bus driver who could recount every detail of his bus route but could not remember what he had had for breakfast nor why he was in the hospital. Even more uncommon presentations of PEM include a cerebellar syndrome clinically indistinguishable from PCD; brainstem encephalitis manifested by vertigo, ataxia, nausea, vomiting, nystagmus, or bulbar palsies; myelopathy; and autonomic neuropathy.

OPSOCLONUS-MYOCLONUS (OM)

Paraneoplastic opsoclonus-myoclonus is characterized by nearly continuous involuntary saccadic eye movements in any direction, often associated with involuntary blinking and myoclonus of the limbs, trunk, pharyngeal muscles, and diaphragm. The opsoclonus usually persists when the eyes are closed and during sleep and may be aggravated by voluntary change in gaze or visual pursuit. Ataxia of the limbs and trunk is also commonly present, as may be irritability or change in cognitive function. The onset is usually abrupt.

The syndrome occurs more commonly in children than adults. Approximately half of the childhood cases are associated with an underlying neoplasm, usually neuroblastoma. The incidence in children with neuroblastoma is approximately 2% to 3%. The majority of adult cases of OM are associated with breast carcinoma or SCLC. Opsoclonus in adults may also be present as part of the picture of SCD or PEM, but when opsoclonus and myoclonus are the predominant features of the neurologic syndrome, prognosis for neurologic recovery is improved. There is no uniform pathologic pattern in OM patients, and the brainstem and cerebellum may even be normal at autopsy.

No antibody has been identified in children with OM and neuroblastoma, but circumstantial evidence suggests an immune mechanism. Neuroblastomas resected from children with OM show a high incidence of infiltration by mononuclear cells, and the presence of OM in children with neuroblastomas is an indicator for a good prognosis independent of other prognostic variables. In adults with breast cancer an anti-neuronal nuclear antibody called anti-Ri or ANNA Type 2 has been identified. Though the staining pattern in the CNS is indistinguishable from the anti-Hu antibody, the target antigens appear to be different. This antibody has not been detected in children with neuroblastoma or adults with SCLC and has not been detected in children with nonparaneoplastic OM.

Both children and adults with OM often respond to ACTH or corticosteroids. In addition, permanent remission of symptoms has been brought about in the majority of children with neuroblastoma by removal of the underlying tumor. Nevertheless, as many as half of children with OM will be left with residual impairment of cognition or cerebellar function despite an initial good response to steroids. Some adult patients have relentlessly progressed to death in spite of steroids and successful treatment of the underlying tumor.

SUBACUTE MOTOR NEURONOPATHY

Subacute motor neuronopathy is a disorder that has been described almost exclusively in malignant lymphoma, particularly Hodgkin's disease. The clinical picture consists of the subacute onset of progressive lower motor neuron weakness that may be asymmetric. Unlike Guillain-Barré syndrome, sensory complaints are rare, and bulbar musculature is generally spared. The weakness usually stabilizes and begins to improve after weeks to months, independent of the course of the underlying neoplasm. Nerve conduction studies are usually normal or only mildly decreased, but denervation is prevalent on electromyography. Protein may be mildly elevated in the cerebrospinal fluid.

This disorder has been reported almost exclusively in the setting of a known tumor, and no antibodies have been identified. The most prominent pathologic features include loss of anterior horn cells and demyelination of anterior nerve roots. A viral etiology has been hypothesized because the pathologic features are similar to those of old poliomyelitis, and viral particles were reported in the anterior horn cells of one patient. In addition, a similar neurologic syndrome has been produced in mice by infection with murine leukemia virus. No virus has yet been isolated from humans with this disorder.

Treatment should consist of supportive care with physical and occupational therapy while the disorder runs its course.

POEMS

There is a particular association between paraproteinemias and peripheral neuropathies. All patients with a peripheral neuropathy of unknown cause should have a serum protein electrophoresis and immunoelectrophoresis. Paraproteinemia will be present in approximately 10% of these patients, and they should be evaluated for a plasma cell dyscrasia. In addition to these predominantly motor or sensorimotor peripheral neuropathies, a distinct syndrome of hepatosplenomegaly, lymphadenopathy, endocrinopathy, hyperpigmentation, thickening of the skin, anasarca, hirsutism, hyperhidrosis, and peripheral neuropathy has been reported in patients with osteosclerotic myeloma. This has been designated the POEMS syndrome, for polyneuropathy, organomegaly, endocrinopathy, monoclonal protein, and skin changes. The skin changes are particularly distinct in their very tough, leather-like quality. The syndrome is seen predominately in men, and dramatic resolution of symptoms may be brought about by treatment of the underlying myeloma with radiation or surgical excision. One study suggests that the abnormalities in multiple organ systems are secondary to immunoglobulin binding of the pituitary gland.

BIBLIOGRAPHY

Bohan A, Peter JB, Bowman RL, Pearson CM. A computer-assisted analysis of 153 patients with polymyositis and dermatomyositis. Medicine 56:255–286, 1977

Erlington GM, Murray NMF, Spiro SG, Newsom-Davis J. Neurological paraneoplastic syndromes in patients with small cell lung cancer. A prospective survey of 150 patients. J Neurol Neurosurg Psychiatry 54:764–767, 1991

Kelly JJ, Kyle RA, Miles JM, O'Brien PC, Dyck PJ. The spectrum of peripheral neuropathy in myeloma. Neurology 31:24–31, 1981

Lakhanpal S, Bunch TW, Ilstrup DM, Melton LJ. Polymyositis-dermatomyositis and malignant lesions: Does an association exist? Mayo Clin Proc 61:645–653, 1986

Oguro-Okano M, Griesmann GE, Wieben ED et al. Molecular diversity of neuronal-type calcium channels identified in small cell lung carcinoma. Mayo Clin Proc 67:1150–1159, 1992

Posner JB. Paraneoplastic syndromes. Neurologic Clinics 9:919–936, 1991

Reulecke M, Dumas M, Meier C. Specific antibody activity against neuroendocrine tissue in a case of POEMS syndrome with IgG gammopathy. Neurology 38:614–616, 1988

Rosenfeld MR, Posner JB. Paraneoplastic motor neuron disease. Adv Neurol 56:445–459, 1991

Schold SC, Cho E-S, Somasundaram M, Posner JB. Subacute motor neuronopathy: A remote effect of lymphoma. Ann Neurol 5:271–287, 1979

Vincent A, Lang B, Newsom-Davis J. Autoimmunity to the voltage-gated calcium channel underlies the Lambert-Eaton myasthenia syndrome, a paraneoplastic disorder. TINS 12:496–502, 1989

John S. Macdonald, Daniel G. Haller, Robert J. Mayer, Eds. *Manual of Oncologic Therapeutics*, Third Edition.

74. CUTANEOUS SIGNS OF INTERNAL MALIGNANCY

Daniel B. Dubin
Richard Allen Johnson

A working knowledge of the cutaneous markers for malignancy can aid in the timely diagnosis and treatment of neoplastic disorders. The dermatologic manifestations of internal cancer fall into three categories: direct cutaneous involvement, genodermatoses, and acquired paraneoplastic conditions. The acquired paraneoplastic disorders can be further subclassified into those tightly, possibly, and weakly associated with internal malignancy. Skin findings associated with only cutaneous neoplasia are not included in the ensuing discussion.

The internal cancers that have been reported to invade the skin by either vascular dissemination or direct extension are listed in Table 74–1. Cutaneous metastasis often forebodes advanced disease and a poor prognosis, regardless of the primary malignancy.[1] Metastases to the skin can be the presenting sign of malignancy, particularly in patients with carcinoma of the breast or upper respiratory tract. Typical carcinomatous metastases tend to be asymmetrically distributed, firm nodules of either skin-color, red, purple, or blue hue. Often, these metastatic lesions involve areas of skin near the site of the primary tumor.

Distant cutaneous metastasis is also possible, and the scalp is a particularly common site for such lesions. Scalp metastasis may appear as an area of hair loss referred to as alopecia neoplastica. Periumbilical lymph node metastasis, also known as Sister Mary Joseph nodule, has been classically associated with gastric carcinoma, although colon, ovarian, and pancreatic carcinoma can also produce umbilical metastasis.

Overall, carcinoma of the breast is the most common source of cutaneous carcinomatosis. The clinician should be aware of three pathologically distinct patterns of cutaneous invasion. Inflammatory breast carcinoma presents as an asymmetric red, warm, indurated mammary plaque that mimics erysipelas. Histopathology of these lesions reveals extensive tumor involvement of dermal and subcutaneous lymphatics. Carcinoma en cuirasse is marked by a firm, infiltrated mammary plaque that on microscopic examination shows relatively few tumor cells scattered throughout a markedly fibrotic dermis.

Paget's disease of the breast appears as a red, edematous, eczematous mammary plaque whose histopathology is typified by tumor cells percolating through the epidermis. Extramammary Paget's disease, whose pathogenesis is similar to that of its mammary counterpart, frequently involves the perineal structures and has been associated with gastrointestinal or genitourinary tumors (12–25%), underlying eccrine or apocrine carcinoma (25%), and local neoplastic changes in the intraepidermal portion of the sweat duct.

Leukemia or lymphoma cutis often resembles carcinomatous cutaneous metastases, presenting as firm nodules or plaques. The distribution of the skin lesions may have some diagnostic significance, as truncal involvement is characteristic of acute leukemia and chronic lymphocytic leukemia, whereas facial lesions are more suggestive of chronic myelogenous leukemia.[2] Gingival infiltrates are particularly common in monocytic leukemia. Although these hematologic malignancies rarely present initially with cutaneous infiltrates, such lesions can provide easily accessible tissue for preliminary pathologic diagnosis.

The skin represents the most common presenting site for Kaposi's sarcoma.[3] In the 1990s, the appearance of this vascular tumor should raise a strong suspicion for human immunodeficiency virus (HIV) infection because approximately 15% of cases initially manifest with epidemic or HIV-associated Kaposi's sarcoma. Autopsy series have demonstrated that 90% of HIV-infected individuals with cutaneous Kaposi's sarcoma also have internal organ involvement. Aside from epidemic Kaposi's sarcoma, three additional clinical variants have been described. African (endemic) Kaposi's sarcoma tends to afflict young, black, adult males in the sub-Saharan region of Africa. Excluding cases of HIV-associated African Kaposi's sarcoma, immunosuppression is not a feature of the endemic variant. Classic Kaposi's sarcoma develops in male patients of Mediterranean or Eastern European ancestry and can be associated with an underlying hematologic malignancy. The fourth variant of Kaposi's sarcoma is linked to iatrogenic immunosuppression, most commonly seen in solid organ transplant recipients. When disfiguring or painful, cutaneous Kaposi's sarcoma can often be locally controlled by radiotherapy, cryotherapy, or intralesional vinblastine injection.

Stewart-Treves syndrome connotes the development of angiosarcoma in an area of lymphedema.[4] Although originally described as arising in the edematous arm of a patient who underwent radical mastectomy, angiosarcoma can develop in a chronically edematous extremity without precedent tumor. The cutaneous nodules tend to have a bluish color and frequently ulcerate. The Stewart-Treves variant of angiosarcoma metastasizes early and carries a poor prognosis.

Because the cutaneous manifestations of the genodermatoses (Table 74–2) often predate the expression of internal malignancy, it is important to identify affected individuals early so that they can be enrolled in appropriate cancer screening protocols. Molecular dissection of the paraneoplastic genodermatoses, such as neurofibromatosis 1, basal

TABLE 74–1. DIRECT CUTANEOUS INVOLVEMENT BY INTERNAL MALIGNANCY

Metastatic carcinoma or melanoma (ocular, meningeal)
Kaposi's sarcoma
Lymphoma/leukemia cutis
Paget's disease: mammary and extramammary
Stewart-Treves syndrome (angiosarcoma)
Malignant histiocytosis

cell nevus syndrome, von Hippel-Lindau syndrome, and tuberous sclerosis, has revealed putative tumor-suppressor genes, which may be operant in the development of sporadic neoplasia.[5–7]

Table 74–3 presents a list of relatively common dermatoses most often associated with benign disease, which, in the appropriate context, may spur an investigation for internal malignancy. For example, clubbing is most frequently a mundane finding in patients with chronic pulmonary, gastrointestinal, or cardiovascular disease. However, its significance as a marker for lung cancer is enhanced by a clinical scenario of recent 50-pound weight loss, hemoptysis, and a smoking history of 150 packs per year.

Strict criteria have been proposed for determining whether or not a true link exists between an acquired dermatosis and a particular internal malignancy: (1) uncommon dermatosis, (2) strong temporal linkage, and (3) strong association with specific internal cancer(s).[8] However, the most stringent test for a putative paraneoplastic disorder remains establishing a direct pathophysiologic connection between the cutaneous disorder and a pre-existing internal malignancy. The cutaneous manifestations elaborated in Table 74–4 are relatively uncommon acquired dermatoses that best satisfy the aforementioned criteria and thus prompt a thorough search for internal malignancy.

TABLE 74–2. GENODERMATOSES

DISORDER	SKIN FINDINGS	ASSOCIATED TUMOR(S)
Basal cell nevus syndrome	Basal cell nevi, palmar and plantar pits	Medulloblastoma, astrocytoma, ameloblastoma, ovarian carcinoma
Dyskeratosis congenita	Reticular hyperpigmentation, nail dystrophy, leukokeratosis, palmar hyperkeratosis	Oropharyngeal and manual squamous cell carcinoma (SCC)
Fanconi's anemia	Reticular hyperpigmentation	Leukemia, mucosal SCC, breast carcinoma
Hemochromatosis	Hyperpigmentation	Hepatocellular carcinoma
Howel-Evans syndrome	Diffuse thickening of palms and soles	Esophageal carcinoma
Cowden's disease	Facial trichilemmomas, oral papillomas, acral keratoses	Breast, uterine, and thyroid carcinoma
Neurofibromatosis 1	Café-au-lait macules (CALM), neurofibromas	Neurofibrosarcoma, malignant schwannoma, pheochromocytoma, carcinoid, astrocytoma
Multiple endocrine neoplasia Type IIb	Mucosal neuromas	Pheochromocytoma, thyroid carcinoma
Maffucci's syndrome	Multiple hemangiomas	Chondrosarcoma
Peutz-Jeghers syndrome	Pigmented macules of lips, buccal mucosa, digits	Gonadal tumors and lung, breast, and gastrointestinal (GI) carcinomas
Gardner's syndrome	Epidermoid cysts	GI carcinoma
Tuberous sclerosis	Ash leaf spots, facial angiofibromas, shagreen patches, CALM	Gliomas, ependymomas
Muir-Torre syndrome	Multiple sebaceous neoplasms	GI and genitourinary carcinoma
von Hippel-Lindau syndrome	Facial vascular angiomas	Pheochromocytoma, renal cell carcinoma, cerebellar hemangioblastomas
Ataxia-telangiectasia	Conjunctival telangiectasia, progeric hair and skin changes, CALM, hypopigmented macules	Leukemia, lymphoma
Chédiak-Higashi syndrome	Hypopigmentation of hair and eyes	Lymphoma
Turcot's syndrome	Pigmented nevi, CALM	Gliomas
Werner's syndrome	Subcutaneous tissue atrophy, scleroderma-like changes, alopecia	Sarcomas
Wiskott-Aldrich syndrome Bruton's agammaglobulinemia	Eczema	Lymphoma, leukemia

TABLE 74–3. POTENTIAL CLUES TO MALIGNANCY

SIGN/SYMPTOM	ASSOCIATED MALIGNANCY
Erythroderma	Hodgkin's disease, cutaneous T-cell lymphoma (CTCL)
Hyperpigmentation	Oat cell carcinoma of the lung
Leukoderma (depigmentation)	Ocular melanoma
Jaundice	Hepatocellular carcinoma, pancreatic carcinoma, cholangiocarcinoma, metastatic involvement of liver
Pallor	Myelophthesic malignancy
Palmar erythema	Primary or secondary hepatic malignancy
Pyoderma gangrenosum	Leukemia, myeloma, polycythemia vera
Urticaria	Leukemia, lymphoma, polycythemia vera
Urticaria pigmentosa	Leukemia, lymphoma, systemic mastocytosis
Clubbing	Intrathoracic malignancies
Fat necrosis	Pancreatic carcinoma
Pruritus	CTCL, lymphoma
Xanthoma (planar variety only)	Leukemia, lymphoma, myeloma
Coagulopathy (disseminated intravascular coagulation, marantic endocarditis)	Nonspecific
Cachexia	Nonspecific
Herpes zoster	Nonspecific

Basex syndrome, erythema gyratum repens, and hypertrichosis lanuginosa acquisita are exceedingly rare dermatoses whose appearance virtually clinches a diagnosis of internal malignancy. However, for some of the "paraneoplastic" dermatoses, it is essential to rule out benign etiologies before rashly pursuing an extensive evaluation for internal malignancy. For example, recently acquired acanthosis nigricans can be highly suggestive of adenocarcinoma of the gastrointestinal tract, given the absence of a family history (*i.e.*, inherited form of acanthosis nigricans), endocrinopathy, or intake of medications such as nicotinic acid, niacinamide, diethylstilbestrol, glucocorticoids, or oral contraceptives. Likewise, it is important to exclude cholesterol-lowering drugs, granulomatous disease, endocrinopathy, and nutritional deficiency before definitively linking acquired ichthyosis to internal malignancy.

A few of the paraneoplastic disorders listed in Table 74–4 have direct pathophysiologic links to the primary malignancy. The characteristic skin findings (see Table 74–4) of both cryoglobulinemia and primary amyloidosis are due to the extravascular deposition of immune cell paraproteinemias. The flushing, gastrointestinal distress, asthma, and cardiovascular symptoms characteristic of carcinoid syndrome are secondary to tumor-elaborated vasoactive amines and/or peptides. Akin to Eaton-Lambert syndrome, paraneoplastic pemphigus is thought to be an autoimmune disorder wherein distinct autoantibodies against keratinocyte and basement membrane antigens trigger blistering of the skin.[9] Superficial migratory thrombophlebitis is most likely related to the tumor elaboration of procoagulant factors.[10] The papillomatous epidermal hyperplasia in acanthosis nigricans may be due to tumor production of epidermal growth factors.[11]

Once zinc deficiency is excluded, the presence of necrolytic migratory erythema is strongly suggestive of glucagonoma. However, the pathophysiologic mechanism by which elevated glucagon levels cause the characteristic skin changes has not been elucidated. Although malignancy has been found in only 15% of patients with Sweet's syndrome, its predilection to coincide with hematologic malignancies suggests a significant link.[12] Pyoderma gangrenosum, a neutrophilic dermatosis akin to Sweet's syndrome, has also been linked to hematologic neoplasms[13]; however, this condition is more frequently associated with inflammatory bowel disease. Multicentric reticulohistiocytosis is a rare disorder that has a 25% association with cancer.

Dermatomyositis just misses the list of strongly linked disorders for three reasons: a distinct pathophysiologic mechanism has not been established, no specific tumor type has been linked to this paraneoplastic disorder, and case-control retrospective studies have not unequivocally identified a significant association.[14] Thus, no more than routine cancer screening guided by age, history, and physical examination is currently recommended for patients with dermatomyositis. Signs such as multiple acrochordons, multiple seborrheic keratoses (Leser-Trelat),[15] pemphigus/pemphigoid, and palmoplantar keratoses are so highly prevalent as background "noise" in the adult population that specific associations with malignancy are difficult to prove. Some reports have shown a significant association between cancer and deep venous thrombosis of the leg. However, it is not clear whether this association is due to an increased incidence of occult cancer or an increased prevalence of pre-existing malignancy and its attendant morbidity.

TABLE 74–4. STRONGLY LINKED TO INTERNAL MALIGNANCY

PARANEOPLASTIC DISORDER	SKIN FINDINGS	ASSOCIATED TUMOR(S)
Acanthosis nigricans	Velvety hyperpigmented flexural patches	Gastrointestinal carcinoma (GI)
Acquired ichthyosis	Fish scale–like eruption	Lymphoma, Hodgkin's disease
Basex syndrome	Red-purple scaling plaques over ears, digits, nose	Aerodigestive squamous cell carcinoma
Carcinoid syndrome	Deep red facial flushing	Neuroendocrine tumors
Cronkhite-Canada syndrome	Alopecia, nail changes, pigmented macules	Colon carcinoma
Cryoglobulinemia	Acral cyanosis, purpura	Myeloma, Waldenström's macroglobulinemia, lymphoma, leukemia
Erythema gyratum repens	Urticarial, polycyclic plaques	Lung, GI, genitourinary (GU) carcinoma
Hypertrichosis lanuginosa acquisita	Fine generalized hypertrichosis	Lung, colon carcinoma
Multicentric reticulohistiocytosis	Translucent yellow to red papules	GI, lung, liver, ovarian carcinoma, sarcoma
Necrolytic migratory erythema	Red, scaling, eroded plaques over periorificial areas and extremities	Glucagonoma
Paraneoplastic pemphigus	Bullous eruption with distinct immunopathology	Lymphoma, leukemia, sarcoma
Primary amyloidosis	Pinch purpua, waxy papules, macroglossia	Myeloma
Superficial migratory thrombophlebitis	Tender red nodules along course of superficial vein	Pancreas, GI, GU, lung carcinoma
Sweet's syndrome	Red-purple nodules, plaques	Acute myelogenous leukemia (AML), myelodysplastic syndrome, adenocarcinoma

REFERENCES

1. Lookingbill DP, et al. Cutaneous metastases in patients with metastatic carcinoma. J Am Acad Dermatol 29:228–236, 1993
2. Bluefarb EM (ed). Leukemia cutis. Springfield, IL, Charles C Thomas, 1960
3. Martin RW et al. Kaposi sarcoma. Medicine 72:245–261, 1993
4. Stewart FW, Treves N. Lymphangiosarcoma in postmastectomy lymphedema. Cancer 1:64–81, 1948
5. Epstein EH. The morbid cutaneous anatomy of the human genome. Arch Dermatol 129:1409–1423, 1993
6. Nellist et al. Identification and characterization of the tuberous sclerosis gene on chromosome 16. Cell 75:1305–1315, 1993
7. Latif F et al. Identification of the von Hippel-Lindau disease tumor suppressor gene. Science 260:1370–1420, 1993
8. Curth HO. Skin lesions and internal carcinoma. In Andrade R, Gumport SL, Popkin GL (eds). Cancer of the skin. Philadelphia, WB Sanders 1308–1341, 1976
9. Anhalt GJ et al. Paraneoplastic pemphigus. N Engl J Med 323:1729–1735, 1990
10. Lesher JL. Thrombophlebitis and thromboembolic problems in malignancy. Clin Dermatol 11:159–163, 1993
11. Ellis DL et al. Melanoma, growth factors, acanthosis nigricans, the sign of Leser-Trelat, and multiple acrochordons. N Engl J Med 317:1582–1587, 1987
12. Cohen PR, Kurzrock R. Sweet's syndrome and malignancy. Am J Med 82:1220–1226, 1987
13. Duguid CM, Powell FC. Pyoderma gangrenosum. Clin Dermatol 11:129–133, 1993
14. Bernard P, Bonnetblanc J. Dermatomyositis and malignancy. J Invest Dermatol 100:128s–132s, 1993
15. Ramper FHJ, Schwengle LEM. The sign of Leser-Trelat: does it exist? J Am Acad Dermatol 21:50–55, 1989

BIBLIOGRAPHY

Lynch HT, Frichot BC. Skin cancer, and heredity. Semin Oncol 5:67–84, 1978

McLean DI, Haynes HA. Cutaneous manifestations of internal malignancy. In Fitzpatrick TB, Eisen AZ, Wolff K et al (eds). Dermatology in general medicine. 4th ed. New York, McGraw-Hill, 2229–2248, 1993

Poole S, Fenske NA. Cutaneous markers of internal malignancy, parts I and II. J Am Acad Dermatol 28:1–13, 147–164, 1993

Thiers BH. Dermatologic manifestations of internal cancer. CA Cancer J Clin 36:130–148, 1986

Worret WI. Skin signs and internal malignancies. Int J Dermatol 32:15, 1993

John S. Macdonald, Daniel G. Haller, Robert J. Mayer, Eds. *Manual of Oncologolic Therapeutics*, Third Edition.

APPENDICES

APPENDIX A. GRADING OF TOXICITY

Over the years investigators have devised various schemes for the quantitative or semiquantitative grading of chemotherapy toxicity. Such schemes are necessary to ensure some level of standardization in the reporting of toxicity and to provide an objective basis for dose modification in the course of treatment. Until recently, the lack of a commonly accepted set of criteria has prevented the reporting of toxicity in a standardized format. In early 1988 the clinical cooperative groups in the United States finally agreed upon a set of common toxicity criteria for clinical trials of systemic therapy (see Table A–1). With a few exceptions, the definitions of the various grades of each toxicity are an amalgam of the individual definitions that have been in use for years in the various cooperative groups. As experience with this system accumulates, some modification and supplementation will no doubt be necessary.

Readers should consult Table A–1 for definitions of the grades (1 through 4) of the various toxicities referred to throughout this manual.

TABLE A–1. COMMON TOXICITY CRITERIA FOR CANCER CLINICAL TRIALS

TOXICITY	GRADE 0	GRADE 1
BLOOD/BONE MARROW		
White blood cell count	≥4.0	3.0–3.9
Platelets	WNL (within normal limits)	75.0–normal
Hemoglobin	WNL	10.0–normal
Granulocytes/bands	≥2.0	1.5–1.9
Lymphocytes	≥2.0	1.5–1.9
HEMORRHAGE (CLINICAL)	None	Mild, no transfusion
INFECTION	None	Mild
GASTROINTESTINAL		
Nausea	None	Able to eat reasonable intake
Vomiting	None	One episode in 24 hours
Diarrhea	None	Increase of 2–3 stools/day over pretherapy baseline
Stomatitis	None	Painless ulcers, erythema, or mild soreness
LIVER		
Bilirubin	WNL	—
Transaminase (serum glutamic-oxaloacetic transaminase, serum glutamate pyruvate transaminase)	WNL	≤2.5 × N
Alkaline phosphatase or 5′ nucleotidase	WNL	≤2.5 × N
Liver—clinical	No change from baseline	—
KIDNEY AND BLADDER		
Creatinine	WNL	<1.5 × N
Proteinuria	No change	1+ *or* <0.3 g/dl *or* <3 g/liter
Hematuria	Negative	Micro only
ALOPECIA	No loss	Mild hair loss
PULMONARY	None or no change	Asymptomatic, with abnormality in pulmonary function tests (PFTs)
HEART		
Cardiac dysrhythmias	None	Asymptomatic, transient, requiring no therapy
Cardiac function	None	Asymptomatic, decline of resting ejection fraction by less than 20% of baseline value
Cardiac—ischemia	None	Nonspecific T wave flattening
Cardiac—pericardial	None	Asymptomatic effusion; no intervention required
BLOOD PRESSURE		
Hypertension	None or no change	Asymptomatic, transient increase by greater than 20 mmHg (D) or to >150/100 mm Hg if previously WNL. No treatment required

TABLE A–1. COMMON TOXICITY CRITERIA FOR CANCER CLINICAL TRIALS (*Continued*)

GRADE		
2	3	4
2.0–2.9	1.0–1.9	<1.0
50.0–74.9	25.0–49.9	<25.0
8.0–10.0	6.5–7.9	<6.5
1.0–1.4	0.5–0.9	<0.5
1.0–1.4	0.5–0.9	<0.5
Gross, 1 to 2 units transfusion per episode	Gross, 3 to 4 units transfusion per episode	Massive, >4 units transfusion per episode
Moderate	Severe	Life threatening
Intake significantly decreased but can eat	No significant intake	—
Two to five episodes in 24 hours	Six to ten episodes in 24 hours	More than 10 episodes in 24 hours, or requiring parenteral support
Increase of 4 to 6 stools/day, or noctunal stools, or moderate cramping	Increase of 7 to 9 stools/day, or incontinence, or severe cramping	Increase of ≥10 stools/day or grossly bloody diarrhea, or need for parenteral support
Painful erythema, edema, or ulcers, but can eat	Painful erythema, edema, or ulcers, and cannot eat	Requires parenteral or enteral support
<1.5 × N	1.5–3.0 × N	>3.0 × N
2.6–5.0 × N	5.1–20.0 × N	>20.0 × N
2.6–5.0 × N	5.1–20.0 × N	>20.0 × N
—	Precoma	Hepatic coma
1.5–3.0 × N	3.1–6.0 × N	>6.0 × N
2–3+ *or* 0.3–1.0 g/dl *or* 3–10 g/liter	4+ *or* >1.0 g/dl *or* >10 g/liter	Nephrotic syndrome
Gross, no clots	Gross + clots	Requires transfusion
Pronounced or total hair loss	—	—
Dyspnea on significant exertion	Dyspnea at normal level of activity	Dyspnea at rest
Recurrent or persistent; no therapy required	Requires treatment	Requires monitoring, or hypotension, or ventricular tachycardia, or fibrillation
Asymptomatic, decline of resting ejection fraction by more than 20% of baseline value	Mild congestive heart failure, responsive to therapy	Severe or refractory congestive heart failure
Asymptomatic, ST and T wave changes suggesting ischemia	Angina without evidence for infarction	Acute myocardial infarction
Pericarditis (rub, chest pain, ECG changes)	Symptomatic effusion; drainage required	Tamponade; drainage urgently required
Recurrent or persistent increase by greater than 20 mm Hg (D) or to >150/100 mm Hg if previously WNL. No treatment required	Requires therapy	Hypertensive crisis

(continued)

TABLE A–1. COMMON TOXICITY CRITERIA FOR CANCER CLINICAL TRIALS *(Continued)*

	GRADE	
TOXICITY	0	1
Hypotension	None or no change	Changes requiring no therapy (including transient orthostatic hypotension)
NEUROLOGIC		
Sensory	None or no change	Mild paresthesias, loss of deep tendon reflexes
Motor	None or no change	Subjective weakness; no objective findings
Cortical	None	Mild somnolence or agitation
Cerebellar	None	Slight incoordination, dysdiadochokinesia
Mood	No change	Mild anxiety or depression
Headache	None	Mild
Constipation	None or no change	Mild
Hearing	None or no change	Asymptomatic, hearing loss on audiometry only
Vision	None or no change	—
SKIN	None or no change	Scattered macular or papular eruption or erythema that is asymptomatic
ALLERGY	None	Transient rash, drug fever ≥ 38°C (100.4° F)
FEVER IN ABSENCE OF INFECTION	None	37.1°–38.0° C (98.7°–100.4° F)
LOCAL SKIN/SOFT TISSUE	None	Pain
WEIGHT GAIN/LOSS	<5.0%	5.0%–9.9%
METABOLIC		
Hyperglycemia	<116	116–160
Hypoglycemia	>64	55–64
Amylase	WNL	<1.5 × N
Hypercalcemia	<10.6	10.6–11.5
Hypocalcemia	>8.4	8.4–7.8
Hypomagnesemia	>1.4	1.4–1.2
COAGULATION		
Fibrinogen	WNL	0.99–0.75 × N
Prothrombin time	WNL	1.01–1.25 × N
Partial thromboplastin time	WNL	1.01–1.66 × N

TABLE A–1. COMMON TOXICITY CRITERIA FOR CANCER CLINICAL TRIALS (*Continued*)

GRADE		
2	3	4
Requires fluid replacement or other therapy but not hospitalization	Requires therapy and hospitalization; resolves within 48 hours of stopping the agent	Requires therapy and hospitalization for >48 hours after stopping the agent
Mild or moderate objective sensory loss; moderate paresthesias	Severe objective sensory loss or paresthesias that interfere with function	—
Mild objective weakness without significant impairment of function	Objective weakness with impairment of function	Paralysis
Moderate somnolence or agitation	Severe somnolence, agitation, confusion, disorientation, or hallucinations	Coma, seizures, toxic psychosis
Intention tremor, dysmetria, slurred speech, nystagmus	Locomotor ataxia	Cerebellar necrosis
Moderate anxiety or depression	Severe anxiety or depression	Suicidal ideation
Moderate or severe but transient	Unrelenting and severe	—
Moderate	Severe	Ileus > 96 hours
Tinnitus	Hearing loss interfering with function but correctable with hearing aid	Deafness not correctable
—	Symptomatic subtotal loss of vision	Blindness
Scattered macular or papular eruption or erythema with pruritus or other associated symptoms	Generalized symptomatic macular, papular, or vesicular eruption	Exfoliative dermatitis or ulcerating dermatitis
Urticaria, drug fever ≥ 38° C (100.4° F), mild bronchospasm	Serum sickness, bronchospasm requires parenteral medication	Anaphylaxis
38.1°–40.0° C (100.5°–104.0° F)	>40.0° C (104.0° F) for less than 24 hours	>40.0° C (104.0° F) for more than 24 hours or fever accompanied by hypotension
Pain and swelling, with inflammation or phlebitis	Ulceration	Plastic surgery indicated
10.0%–19.9%	≥20.0%	—
161–250	251–500	>500 or ketoacidosis
40–54	30–39	<30
1.5–2.0 × N	2.1–5.0 × N	>5.1 × N
11.6–12.5	12.6–13.5	≥13.5
7.7–7.0	6.9–6.1	≤6.0
1.1–0.9	0.8–0.6	≤0.5
0.74–0.50 × N	0.49–0.25 × N	≤0.24 × N
1.26–1.50 × N	1.51–2.00 × N	>2.00 × N
1.67–2.33 × N	2.34–3.00 × N	>3.00 × N

John S. Macdonald, Daniel G. Haller, Robert J. Mayer, Eds. *Manual of Oncologic Therapeutics*, Third Edition.

APPENDIX B. PERFORMANCE STATUS AND QUALITY OF LIFE

Early in the evolution of cancer treatment, it became clear that the functional status of the patient at diagnosis or at the start of treatment is a major determinant of outcome. This finding has been confirmed repeatedly across a broad spectrum of tumor types. The underlying basis for the dependence of outcome on functional status is probably that a patient's ability to function in the activities of daily living is often related to tumor burden or, in some cases, to the location of tumor in particularly critical sites, such as the central nervous system.

Table B–1 shows the two scales that are most commonly used to measure the performance status (PS) of individual patients. The Karnofsky scale extends from 100 (asymptomatic, fully functional) to 0 (dead) in steps of 10; integers not divisible by 10 are undefined and should not be used. The Zubrod or Eastern Cooperative Oncology Group (ECOG) scale is a five-point system that effectively telescopes the Karnofsky categories into a somewhat simpler scheme (Table B–2).

Although these scoring systems have been criticized for their lack of precision and interobserver reproducibility, their use in clinical trials has established PS as a major prognostic factor for most cancers. The clinician should, therefore, become familiar with both scoring systems, since they are referred to widely in the literature and since PS is the basis for much clinical decision making. In addition to the value of PS as a prognostic indicator, longitudinal estimates of PS as

TABLE B–1. KARNOFSKY PERFORMANCE STATUS SCALE

DEFINITION	%	CRITERIA
Able to carry on normal activity and to work. No special care needed.	100	Normal; no complaints; no evidence of disease.
	90	Able to carry on normal activity; minor signs or symptoms of disease.
	80	Normal activity with effort; some signs or symptoms of disease.
Unable to work. Able to live at home and care for most personal needs. Varying amount of assistance needed.	70	Cares for self. Unable to carry on normal activity or to do active work.
	60	Requires occasional assistance but is able to care for most needs.
	50	Requires considerable assistance and frequent medical care.
Unable to care for self. Requires equivalent of institutional or hospital care. Disease may be progressing rapidly.	40	Disabled; requires special care and assistance.
	30	Severely disabled; hospitalization is indicated, although death not imminent.
	20	Very sick; hospitalization necessary; active supportive treatment necessary.
	10	Moribund; fatal processes progressing rapidly.
	0	Dead.

(Karnofsky, DA, Abelmann WH, Craver LF, Burchenal JH: The use of the nitrogen mustards in the palliative treatment of carcinoma. Cancer 1:634–656, 1948)

TABLE B–2. ECOG PERFORMANCE STATUS SCALE

SCORE	DEFINITION	KARNOFSKY EQUIVALENT
0	Asymptomatic	100
1	Symptomatic, fully ambulatory	80–90
2	Symptomatic, in bed less than 50% of day	60–70
3	Symptomatic, in bed more than 50% of day but not bedridden	40–50
4	Bedridden	20–30

(Zubrod CG, Schneiderman M, Frei E et al: Appraisal of methods for the study of chemotherapy in man: Comparative therapeutic trial of nitrogen mustard and triethylene thiophosphoramide. J Chron Dis 11:7–33, 1960)

therapy progresses are valuable indicators of the net effect of the disease and its treatment on the patient.

As a measure of functional status, PS should not be confused with "quality of life," a more complex construct of which functional status is but one aspect. Improved quality of life is an important goal of cancer treatment, and investigators with a psychosocial orientation are currently striving to develop instruments that furnish valid measures of the quality-of-life construct. It seems clear that no simple measure will serve this purpose and that the various measures of quality of life may have to be tailored to the requirements of the various cancers individually. (See Aaronson NK, Beckmann J [eds]: *The Quality of Life in Cancer Patients*. New York, Raven Press, 1987.)

John S. Macdonald, Daniel G. Haller, Robert J. Mayer, Eds. *Manual of Oncologic Therapeutics*, Third Edition.

APPENDIX C. MEASURES OF THERAPEUTIC EFFECT

Throughout this manual, reference is made to many different kinds of measures of therapeutic effect. These fall into four general categories: (1) extent of tumor shrinkage; (2) duration of tumor control; (3) duration of survival; (4) improvement in symptom control, functional status, and quality of life. The first three categories are discussed here; functional status and quality of life are the subject of Appendix B.

MEASURES OF TUMOR SHRINKAGE

For solid tumors presenting as bidimensionally measurable masses, the most commonly used response criteria depend on estimates of the extent of tumor burden reduction with treatment. There are no universally accepted definitions for the several categories of response, but the sample definitions that follow are fairly typical:

1. Complete response (CR): Disappearance of all evidence of disease for at least 4 weeks
2. Partial response (PR): A decrease of at least 50% in the sum of the products of two diameters of all (or a selected subset of) measurable lesions for at least 4 weeks, without progression of any lesion or the appearance of new lesions
3. Minor response (MR): Objective shrinkage of tumor of magnitude not meeting the criteria of PR
4. Stable disease (SD): No significant change in the size of measurable lesions
5. Progression (Prog): Increase of more than 25% (or 50%) in the sum of the products of two diameters of measurable lesions as described in item 2 in this list.

Because the definitions of these response categories are not standardized, the reader wishing to compare the results of different clinical trials reports should make very certain that the response criteria are comparable; apparently minor differences in definition (for example, defining PR as 50% shrinkage of "the measured lesion," "measured lesions" selected retrospectively, or "the sum of the products of all measurable lesions") may make major differences in the reported response rate.

In cases in which bidimensionally measurable disease is not present by either clinical examination or radiologic imaging, other kinds of criteria must be used. Such presentations as lymphangitic lung disease, lytic bone metastases, or ill-defined areas of contrast enhancement on computed tomography of the brain require individualized criteria. Although a striking therapeutic response is usually discernible in each of these three examples, quantifying response is generally not possible, and the distinction between PR and MR loses meaning.

For tumor types in which circulating markers regularly reflect tumor burden, changes in marker levels may be added as additional criteria of response. Finally, the criteria suitable for solid tumors are clearly inappropriate for disorders that do not present as discrete masses, and diseases such as the leukemias and myeloma require a set of response criteria that are appropriate to the clinical behavior of these tumors.

DURATION OF TUMOR CONTROL

Many different terms are in common use to describe the duration of beneficial effect (Table C–1), and the reader should be alert to the sometimes subtle differences in their definitions. These definitions are not completely standard either; for example, some investigators measure duration of response from the start of therapy, rather than from the time that the existence of a response has been ascertained.

TABLE C–1. DURATION OF TUMOR CONTROL

TERM	APPLIES TO	MEASURED FROM	MEASURED TO
Duration of response	All responders	Date response ascertained	Date progression ascertained
Progression-free interval (time to progression)	All patients on treatment	Date therapy started (or date randomized)	Date progression ascertained
Disease-free interval (disease-free survival, relapse-free survival)	Complete responders (to any therapeutic modality)	Date rendered disease free	Date of relapse

SURVIVAL

The least ambiguous measure of therapeutic effect, survival measures the duration from some starting point (*e.g.*, diagnosis, start of therapy, and time of randomization) to death. Survival data are generally uninterpretable without reference to a control group treated in some other way. In considering analyses of survival, the reader must know whether all deaths are being treated as events or whether noncancer deaths are treated as censored observations. This distinction between all-cause mortality and cancer-related mortality may be crucial in interpreting results from the literature.

John S. Macdonald, Daniel G. Haller, Robert J. Mayer, Eds. *Manual of Oncologic Therapeutics*, Third Edition.

APPENDIX D. PDQ: LINKING HEALTH CARE PROFESSIONALS, PATIENTS, AND POLICY-MAKERS WITH CANCER RESEARCH RESULTS

Susan Molloy Hubbard
Anne Lewis Thurn

One of the major challenges that health care professionals face is how to keep up with what is important in the medical literature. Results from a 1989 survey on information management of 520 primary care practitioners and opinion leaders demonstrated that two thirds of the physicians surveyed considered the volume of medical literature to be unmanageable.[1] Seventy-eight percent of physicians surveyed reported difficulty in screening out irrelevant data when reviewing the medical literature. Health care professionals are not alone in their need for current medical information. Patients and their families are faced with the arduous task of interpreting the information they are given or have sought out themselves to make well-informed decisions about their own care. Lastly, those who bear the responsibility of making policy decisions on health care issues must have access to state-of-the-art medical information.

A high priority objective of the International Cancer Information Center (ICIC) of the National Cancer Institute (NCI) is to improve access to medical knowledge by developing computerized systems to accelerate the transfer of useful information from clinical research into clinical practice. PDQ (Physician Data Query), the NCI's comprehensive cancer information database, was developed to assist in this effort.

PDQ first became available to health professionals in 1984. Since then, the scope of the information it contains has expanded, not only for health care professionals and policy-makers but also for patients and their families. It is composed of three main types of information:

1. Full-text statements based on the published literature that reflect the current state-of-the-art information on the treatment, supportive care, prevention, and screening of cancer, as well as information about selected anti-cancer drugs still under clinical evaluation
2. Summaries of research protocols under evaluation in clinical trials
3. Directories of physicians and organizations that provide cancer care.

PDQ has been described as a knowledge base as distinguished from a data base because instead of simply presenting basic information and leaving its interpretation to the user, it incorporates expert opinion into its selection of literature by synthesizing it into concise summaries and recommendations. By assisting the user in making the transition from data published in the current literature to readily usable information, PDQ provides a practical way for health care professionals, patients, and policy-makers to keep up with advances in the medical literature. For those who are interested in studying the results of current research more closely, PDQ includes full citations and abstracts for each reference cited. Another feature that helps make the information in PDQ available to a broad audience is the fact that in most implementations it is completely menu-driven and does not require the knowledge of a specialized searching language.

TREATMENT INFORMATION

PDQ contains prognostic and treatment information on the major types of cancer in children and adults, including information on AIDS-related malignancies. For each major type of cancer, there is a detailed statement on prognosis, staging, and treatment directed to the information needs of health care professionals. Key citations to the literature are referenced and abstracts of these citations are available for review by the user. A limited number of brief statements on less common cancers are also included. PDQ also provides treatment statements for patients and their families which contain similar information but are written in non-technical language.

SUPPORTIVE CARE INFORMATION

PDQ contains supportive care statements describing the pathophysiology and treatment of common complications of cancer and its treatment, such as pain, hypercalcemia, and nausea or vomiting. Each statement generally contains an overview, information on etiology, assessment and management, and references to the current literature.

SCREENING AND PREVENTION INFORMATION

The screening information in PDQ includes statements on screening for nine cancers, including breast, cervical, oropharynx, skin, colorectal, prostate, testicular, ovarian and gastric. Each statement contains a summary of the available data concerning screening for that particular disease site, the levels of evidence for that summary (Table D–1) and information on the significance and evidence of benefit for the summary statement. The statements also include references to the current literature that support the information in the statement.

In early 1994, information on cancer prevention was added to PDQ. The first statements to be included in PDQ were on prevention of aerodigestive cancers, colorectal cancer, and skin cancer. Similar in format to the PDQ information on screening, these statements also contain a summary of data concerning prevention for that particular disease site, levels of evidence for that summary (Table D–2), and information on the significance and evidence of benefit for the summary statement.

DRUG INFORMATION

PDQ contains information on 11 anticancer agents currently under clinical evaluation. The information provided includes a description of each drug, its mechanism of action, indications and contraindications, interactions, dose schedules and modifications, and pharmaceutical information.

TABLE D–1. PDQ SCREENING STATEMENT LEVELS OF EVIDENCE

1. Evidence obtained from at least one randomized controlled trial
2. Evidence obtained from controlled trials without randomization
3. Evidence obtained from cohort or case-control analytic studies, preferably from more than one center or research group
4. Evidence obtained from multiple-time series with or without intervention
5. Opinions of respected authorities based on clinical experience, reports of expert committees

The criteria listed above are used by members of the PDQ Screening and Prevention Editorial Board to evaluate available data on screening. Available information is summarized and is assigned appropriate level(s) of evidence to assist the user in making decisions regarding screening.

TABLE D–2. PDQ PREVENTION STATEMENT LEVELS OF EVIDENCE

1. Evidence obtained from at least one randomized controlled trial with:
   a. A cancer mortality endpoint
   b. A cancer incidence endpoint
   c. An accepted validated intermediate endpoint (*e.g.*, large adenomatous polyps for colorectal prevention)
2. Evidence obtained from controlled trials without randomization with:
   a. A cancer mortality endpoint
   b. A cancer incidence endpoint
   c. An accepted validated intermediate endpoint (*e.g.*, large adenomatous polyps for colorectal prevention)
3. Evidence obtained from cohort or case-control analytic studies, preferably from more than one center or research group with:
   a. A cancer mortality endpoint
   b. A cancer incidence endpoint
   c. An accepted validated intermediate endpoint (*e.g.*, large adenomatous polyps for colorectal prevention)
4. Evidenced obtained from multiple-time series with or without intervention with:
   a. A cancer mortality endpoint
   b. A cancer incidence endpoint
   c. An accepted validated intermediate endpoint (*e.g.*, large adenomatous polyps for colorectal prevention)
5. Ecologic studies (descriptive) (*e.g.*, international patterns studies, migration studies) with:
   a. A cancer mortality endpoint
   b. A cancer incidence endpoint
   c. An accepted validated intermediate endpoint (*e.g.*, large adenomatous polyps for colorectal prevention)
6. Opinions of respected authorities based on clinical experience or reports of expert committees (*e.g.*, any of the above study designs using non-validated surrogate endpoints)

The criteria listed above are used by members of the PDQ Screening and Prevention Editorial Board to evaluate available data on cancer prevention. Available information is summarized and is assigned appropriate level(s) of evidence to assist the user in making decisions regarding prevention.

THE REVIEW PROCESS

A major rationale for developing the system as an on-line database was the desire to use computer technology to maintain its currency because a database can be updated much more quickly than a textbook. The information in PDQ is peer-reviewed by five core Editorial Boards, one for each type of information covered by the cancer information statements: adult treatment, pediatric treatment, supportive care, screening and prevention, and drugs undergoing clinical evaluation. Board members have the task of translating information culled from the medical literature into medical knowledge that can be effectively used by health professionals.

The core Boards are comprised of 65 cancer specialists, the majority of whom are not government employees. Each core Editorial Board is supplemented by an Advisory Board that reviews the statements at least once each year. The Advisory Boards are comprised of over 100 physicians and other health care professionals with special expertise in the prevention, screening, treatment, and supportive care of cancer. Members of the core and Advisory Boards oversee the development and maintenance of the cancer information in PDQ. The core Boards meet regularly to discuss recent literature, and to develop new state-of-the-art statements or to revise existing statements. Recommendations on the scientific literature are based on the clinical expertise of the core and Advisory Editorial Board members.

To assist Board members in reviewing the medical literature effectively and promptly, a process has been developed to provide them with appropriate information (Fig. D–1). Each month, professionals review the tables of contents of more than 70 biomedical journals to identify articles of potential relevance. After reviewing these articles, NCI staff forward the articles of highest potential relevance and scientific validity to appropriate Board members.

The Board members suggest and the Editor-in-Chief chooses topics that should be discussed at the next Board meeting. Important changes to the state-of-the-art statements, such as the deletion or addition of a treatment option to the list of standard treatment options, are discussed by the Board during meetings. In cases in which there is disagreement about the interpretation of data, PDQ statements address the controversial nature of the topic.

CLINICAL TRIALS

PDQ contains more than 1500 summaries of clinical trials that are open or approved for patient accrual, including protocols for cancer treatment, supportive care, and screening and prevention. For each trial, detailed summaries are prepared from the original protocol document, ensuring the uniformity and accuracy of the content. PDQ protocols can be retrieved by diagnosis, treatment modality, phase, locality, and drug name, or a combination of these parameters. All protocols supported by the NCI are listed in PDQ. Board members review protocols submitted by investigators who are not directly supported by the NCI prior to inclusion of their protocol in PDQ. The criteria for evaluating voluntary protocol submissions are shown in Table D–3. Foreign protocols and clinical trials that are not supported by the NCI are included after review and approval using a process sanctioned by the PDQ Editorial Board. In addition, there are more than 7000 summaries of protocols that have been completed or are no longer accepting patients. PDQ provides a source of information on previous and ongoing clinical cancer research whether the results are positive or negative. For physicians and policy-makers, the ability to easily retrieve this data is essential to the responsible planning of cancer treatment resources.

DIRECTORIES

Physician Directory

The PDQ Physician Directory contains more than 20,000 names, addresses, and telephone numbers, of physicians who devote a major portion of their clinical practice to the treatment of cancer patients. Also included is information on medical specialties, oncologic subspecialty board certification, and organizational affiliations of the physicians listed.

Physicians listed in the membership directories of major oncologic societies or organizations (Tables D–4 and D–5), and clinical investigators who have protocols in PDQ and/or are members of NCI sponsored Clinical Trials groups are also listed in this directory.

Organization Directory

The PDQ Organization Directory contains information on over 2500 health-care institutions that provide care for cancer patients and over 4000 facilities accredited by the American College of Radiology for mammography screening. Information on organizations is retrievable by name and/or city, state, country, and/or zip code.

ACCESS

A wide range of mechanisms for gaining access to PDQ exists. Some have been developed by the NCI and others by private vendors. These mechanisms fall into two general categories: on-line time-sharing systems with dial-up or Internet access, and "local" implementations that reside on a single computer or a local area network for use by individuals or groups of individuals. Local access to PDQ is currently available as a licensed product from the NCI for installation on a personal computer or local area netwrok. PDQ is also offered as a local system on CD-ROM by two commercial sources. Subscriptions to the CD-ROM products are sold on an annual basis and are updated monthly. They can be pur-

TABLE D–3. PDQ VOLUNTARY PROTOCOL REVIEW CRITERIA

1. Is the study reasonable in design?
2. Is it based on rational scientific information?
3. Is it likely to yield some useful information?
4. Is it unduly risky to patients?
5. Are the entry criteria clear and complete?
6. Is the statistical section complete?

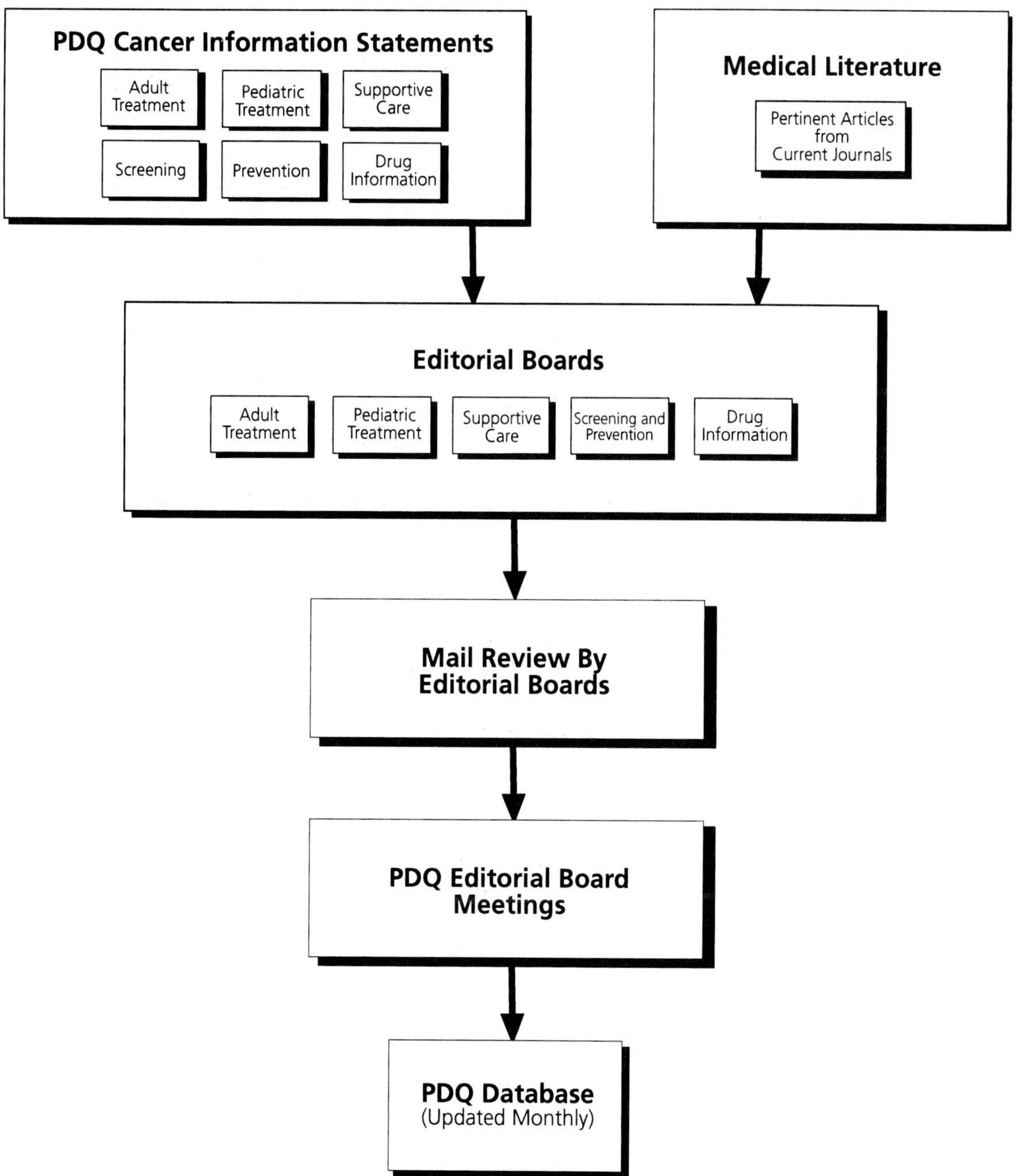

Figure D–1. The Editorial Board review process used to maintain and update the PDQ database is shown schematically here. Board members are provided with copies of the current cancer information statements and with pertinent articles from the current literature. Controversial topics or areas of special interest are discussed at regularly scheduled Board meetings. When PDQ is updated each month, changes suggested by the Editorial Boards are incorporated.

TABLE D–4. MEDICAL SOCIETIES LISTING THEIR PHYSICIAN MEMBERS IN PDQ

American Academy of Dermatologists
American College of Mohs Micrographic Surgery and Cutaneous Oncology
American College of Radiation Oncology
American College of Surgeons (Fellows)
American Society of Clinical Oncology
American Society of Colon and Rectal Surgeons
American Society for Head and Neck Surgery
American Society of Hematology
American Society of Pediatric Hematology/Oncology
American Radium Society
American Society of Therapeutic Radiology + Oncology
American Urologic Association
Society of Head and Neck Surgeons
Society of Gynecologic Oncologists
Society of Pelvic Surgeons
Society of Surgical Oncology
Society of Urologic Oncology

chased to run on a DOS-based personal computer or a local area network. A number of non-local mechanisms for using PDQ are also available. In 1994, more than 60,000 domestic and 7,000 foreign centers have access to the cancer information databases on the MEDLARS system of the National Library of Medicine. this includes 8000 student access accounts. There are currently 15 principal foreign MEDLARS centers that offer access to PDQ for foreign medical institutions and physicians. An on-line service operated by the European Organization for Research and Treatment of Cancer (EORTC) makes PDQ available to its participating organizations in Europe. PDQ is also licensed to commercial vendors and academic and non-profit health care organizations with computerized medical information systems.

TABLE D–5. ORGANIZATIONS LISTING THEIR INSTITUTIONAL MEMBERS IN THE PDQ DATABASE

American Association of Cancer Institutes
Association of Community Cancer Centers
Clinical and Comprehensive Cancer Centers funded by the NCI
Clinical Cooperative Groups funded by the NCI and their affiliates
Community Clinical Oncology Program (CCOP) grantees
European Organization on Research and Treatment of Cancer (EORTC)
Hospitals with organized cancer programs certified by the ACS Commission on Cancer
Mammography screening facilities approved by the American College of Radiology

Advances in technology have allowed facsimile (fax) boards to be placed inside personal computers so that the computer can act as a fax machines, sending and receiving documents simultaneously. When coupled with digital voice technology and software that interprets user selections from a touch-tone telephone, information from a database like PDQ can be delivered to a caller without human intervention. In 1991, NCI staff began distributing the cancer information statements from PDQ using fax on-demand technology. The CancerFax service allows users to dial into one of the NCI's computers from a fax machine and retrieve a facsimile image of any of PDQ's cancer information statements (including treatment for health care professionals or patients, supportive care, drug or screening and prevention). Additional information and important news items, such as reanalyses of NSABP trial results, are also available through CancerFax. Much of the information is available in both English and Spanish. The service is in operation 24 hours each day and there is no cost to the user other than the cost of the telephone call to 1-301-402-5874 in Bethesda, Maryland. Over 50,000 CancerFax requests were fulfilled in 1993, and CancerFax currently fulfills over 5000 requests each month.

In July of 1992, the NCI introduced CancerNet, an electronic service that enables computer users to obtain free access to selected PDQ and other cancer-related information 7 days a week via Internet electronic mail. Access to CancerNet data was expanded in 1993 by implementing it on Internet Gopher Servers in the United States, Japan, and Singapore. CancerNet is also available on FedWorld, an electronic bulletin board system (BBS) produced by the National Technical Information Service that provides information from federal agencies as well as a gateway to over one hundred federal agency BBS's. Current use of CancerNet via E-mail is approximately 5000 requests each month, and 30% of these requests come from outside the United States. Internet Gopher Servers fulfill 20,000 requests each month, 40% of which come from outside the United States.

In addition to PDQ information, CancerFax and CancerNet contain fact sheets on various cancer-related topics produced by the NCI's Office of Cancer Communications (OCC), selected news items, information about ordering patient information and publications from the NCI, citations and abstracts from CANCERLIT for selected types of cancer, and PDQ availability information.

THE NCI'S INFORMATION ASSOCIATES PROGRAM

The Information Associates Program (IAP) is a membership program open to health professionals and organizations worldwide. The program was started in 1994 to establish a better link between the ICIC and the health care professionals it serves. The program provides members with direct access to the scientific information services of the ICIC, including the *Journal of the National Cancer Institute*, *Journal Monographs*, the PDQ database, patient education materials from the Office of Cancer Communications, and bulletins from the NCI. Members can access this information through many electronic information vehicles: toll-free fax (CancerFax), a dial-up BBS, and the Internet. Trained representatives are available via a toll-free customer service line to assist members (1-800-624-7890 in the United States or 301-816-2083 outside the United States). The BBS contains the PDQ database; information on ICIC products and services; late-breaking news from the NCI; the table of contents and abstracts from issues of the *Journal of the National Cancer Institute*; Fact Sheets from the Office of Cancer Communications; selected abstracts from CANCERLIT on a variety of clinical topics; E-mail capability, and an electronic conferencing capability. The annual membership fee is $100 for domestic members and $150 for international members.

CANCER INFORMATION SERVICE

Another means of retrieving information from PDQ is through the Cancer Information Service (CIS). The CIS, a nationwide network of 19 regional offices supported by the NCI, uses PDQ extensively to fulfill its objective of providing information on cancer to patients and their families, health professionals, and the general public. CIS offices can be reached anywhere in the country by dialing 1-800-4-CANCER (1-800-422-6237).

In 1995, the NCI will begin operation of a toll-free PDQ database search service designed to respond to the needs of physicians and other health professionals.

REFERENCE

1. Williamson JW, German PA, Weiss R, Skinner EA, and Bowes F: Health science information management and continuing education of physicians. A survey of 110:151–160, 1989.

John S. Macdonald, Daniel G. Haller, Robert J. Mayer, Eds. *Manual of Oncologic Therapeutics*, Third Edition.

INDEX

Page numbers followed by an f indicate a figure; numbers followed by a t indicate a table.